Veterinary Anaesthesia

Veterinary Anaesthesia

Principles to Practice

Second Edition

Alexandra H. A. Dugdale *MA, VetMB, PhD, PGCert(LTHE), DVA, Dip.ECVAA, FHEA, MRCVS*
ChesterGates Veterinary Specialists CVS (UK), Ltd.
Cheshire, UK

Georgina Beaumont *BVSc(Hons.), MANZCVS (Veterinary Anaesthesia,*
Emergency and Critical Care), Dip.ECVAA, MRCVS
Christopher Beaumont Consulting Ltd.
Manchester Veterinary Specialists
Manchester, UK

Carl Bradbrook *BVSc, CertVA, Dip.ECVAA, MRCVS*
Anderson Moores Veterinary Specialists
Winchester, UK

Matthew Gurney *BVSc, CertVA, PgCertVBM, Dip.ECVAA, MRCVS*
Anderson Moores Veterinary Specialists
Winchester, UK

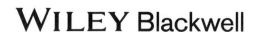

This edition first published 2020
© 2020 John Wiley & Sons Ltd

Edition History
John Wiley & Sons (1e, 2016)

The right of Alexandra H. A. Dugdale, Georgina Beaumont, Carl Bradbrook, and Matthew Gurney to be identified as the authors of this work has been asserted in accordance with law.

Registered Offices
John Wiley & Sons, Inc., 111 River Street, Hoboken, NJ 07030, USA
John Wiley & Sons Ltd, The Atrium, Southern Gate, Chichester, West Sussex, PO19 8SQ, UK

Editorial Office
9600 Garsington Road, Oxford, OX4 2DQ, UK

For details of our global editorial offices, customer services, and more information about Wiley products visit us at www.wiley.com.

Wiley also publishes its books in a variety of electronic formats and by print-on-demand. Some content that appears in standard print versions of this book may not be available in other formats.

Library of Congress Cataloging-in-Publication Data

Names: Dugdale, Alex, 1966– author. | Beaumont, Georgina, author. |
    Bradbrook, Carl, author. | Gurney, Matthew, author.
Title: Veterinary anaesthesia : principles to practice / Alexandra H. A.
    Dugdale, Georgina Beaumont, Carl Bradbrook, Matthew Gurney.
Description: Second edition. | Hoboken, NJ : Wiley-Blackwell, 2020. |
    Includes bibliographical references and index.
Identifiers: LCCN 2020013288 (print) | LCCN 2020013289 (ebook) | ISBN
    9781119246770 (paperback) | ISBN 9781119246756 (adobe pdf) | ISBN
    9781119246787 (epub)
Subjects: MESH: Anesthesia–veterinary | Handbook
Classification: LCC SF914 (print) | LCC SF914 (ebook) | NLM SF 914 | DDC
    636.089/796–dc23
LC record available at https://lccn.loc.gov/2020013288
LC ebook record available at https://lccn.loc.gov/2020013289

Cover Design: Wiley
Cover Images: © Alexandra H. A. Dugdale

Set in 9.5/12.5pt STIXTwoText by SPi Global, Pondicherry, India
Printed and bound by CPI Group (UK) Ltd, Croydon, CR0 4YY

C9781119246770_240124

Contents

Preface

Welcome to the second edition of *Veterinary Anaesthesia: Principles to Practice*, which only really came to fruition thanks to all the encouraging messages received in response to the first edition.

The updating and expansion took a little while longer than originally intended, but I and my co-authors hope that this edition remains a 'go-to' source of information for veterinary nurses, veterinary practitioners, veterinary students, and particularly, post-graduate students studying for professional veterinary anaesthesia qualifications.

We also hope to share our fascination, passion, and sheer enjoyment of the subject and wish you all 'Happy Reading!'

Acknowledgements

My very grateful thanks are extended to my co-authors: Georgina Beaumont, Carl Bradbrook, Fran Downing, Nicki Grint, and Matt Gurney, and also to Kate Brooks for her amazing artwork.

In addition, I would like to thank all my work colleagues and students, past and present, for their unending encouragement and support.

And finally, my heartfelt thanks to Jayadivya Saiprasad at Wiley-Blackwell for having more patience than anyone I know!

About the Companion Website

This book is accompanied by a companion website:

www.wiley.com/go/dugdale/veterinary-anaesthesia

Scan this QR code to visit the companion website
The website contains downloadable figures, appendices, self assessment questions and answers from the book.

1

Concepts and Mechanisms of General Anaesthesia

LEARNING OBJECTIVES

- To be able to define general anaesthesia.
- To be able to discuss general anaesthesia in terms of its component parts, i.e. the triad of general anaesthesia.
- To be able to define balanced anaesthesia.

1.1 Definitions

Anaesthesia literally means 'lack of sensation/feeling' (from *an* meaning 'without' and *aesthesia* pertaining to 'feeling'). Therefore, general anaesthesia means global/total lack of sensations, whereas local anaesthesia relates to lack of sensation in a localised part of the body.

General anaesthesia can be defined as a state of unconsciousness produced by a process of controlled, reversible, intoxication of the central nervous system (CNS), whereby the patient neither perceives nor recalls noxious (or other) stimuli.

General anaesthesia is, however, often referred to as the state of the patient when the three criteria in the triad of general anaesthesia have been met.

1.1.1 The Triad of General Anaesthesia

1) **Unconsciousness**: no perception or memory (therefore including **amnesia**), of any sensory, or indeed motor, event.
2) **Analgesia** (or, more correctly in an unconscious patient, **antinociception**): can also be thought of as suppressed responses/reflexes to nociceptive sensory inputs.
3) **Suppressed reflexes**: autonomic (e.g. haemodynamic, respiratory and thermoregulatory) and somatic (e.g. proprioceptive reflexes such as the righting reflex).
   - Suppression of somatic reflexes can be useful, e.g. it can provide a degree of **muscular weakness/relaxation**.

- Suppression of autonomic reflexes can be a nuisance (see Chapter 18 on Monitoring), but **autonomic stability** can be a desirable component of anaesthesia and is often listed as a fourth component.

All these components could potentially be achieved in a patient following administration of a single 'anaesthetic' drug but, e.g. if that drug did not have very good analgesic properties, then large doses would be required to produce sufficiently 'deep' unconsciousness to reduce the response to noxious stimuli. Such deep anaesthesia is often associated with extreme depression of the CNS and homeostatic reflexes (Table 1.1).

An alternative approach, therefore, would be to produce each component (of the 'triad') separately by administering several drugs, each of which targets one component more specifically. This latter approach is theoretically advantageous because, by 'titrating to specific effect', relatively smaller doses of each individual drug tend to be sufficient, thereby minimising both each individual drug's, and the overall, side effects. This 'polypharmacy' approach is often referred to as **balanced anaesthesia**.

1.1.2 Balanced Anaesthesia

The administration of a number of different drugs, each with different actions, given during the immediate perioperative period, to produce an overall state of general anaesthesia, which fulfils the criteria of unconsciousness, analgesia, and muscle relaxation.

Veterinary Anaesthesia: Principles to Practice, Second Edition. Alexandra H. A. Dugdale, Georgina Beaumont, Carl Bradbrook, and Matthew Gurney.
© 2020 John Wiley & Sons Ltd. Published 2020 by John Wiley & Sons Ltd.
Companion website: www.wiley.com/go/dugdale/veterinary-anaesthesia

Table 1.1 Summary of effects of general anaesthesia.

Central Nervous System Depression
- Loss of consciousness
- Damping of reflexes
  - Cardiovascular → Hypotension
  - Respiratory → Hypoventilation
  - Thermoregulatory → Hypothermia
  - Postural → Reduced muscle tone
- Central modulation of nociception (hopefully providing analgesia/antinociception)

Cardiovascular System Depression (→ Hypotension)
- Reflex (e.g. baroreflex) suppression (centrally and peripherally)
- Changes in autonomic balance
- Changes in vasomotor tone (drug effects, centrally and peripherally)
- Myocardial depression
  - Direct (drugs)
  - Indirect (e.g. hypoxaemia, hypercapnia [acidosis])

Respiratory Depression (→ Hypoventilation; resulting in hypercapnia/hypoxaemia)
- Reflex suppression (↓ventilatory response to ↑PCO_2 [↓pH], and ↓PO_2)
- Reduced respiratory muscle activity (↓ sighing and yawning)
- Alveolar collapse/small airway closure (atelectasis)
- Reduced functional residual capacity
- Ventilation/perfusion mismatch

1.1.2.1 Components of the Peri-operative Period

- **Pre-operative assessment**: patient stabilisation; provision of (pre-emptive) analgesia.
- **Premedication**: anxiolysis/sedation and initiation/continuation of analgesia provision if not already provided.
- **Induction** of anaesthesia.
- **Maintenance** of anaesthesia; provision of muscle relaxation; continuation of analgesia/antinociception provision.
- **Recovery** from anaesthesia (sometimes referred to as 'reanimation'): aftercare; continuation of ('preventive') analgesia provision.

1.2 The Depth of General Anaesthesia

Some texts refer to various stages and planes of anaesthesia that try to mark the progression of the continuum between consciousness and death. When ether was used as the sole anaesthetic agent, five 'degrees' of progression through ever 'deeper' stages of anaesthesia in people, from consciousness to deep coma, were described by John Snow; Overton did similar for chloroform. Guedel developed Snow's ideas further and, in 1937, produced a chart outlining the patient's responses at each of four successive stages of diethyl ether anaesthesia. This was developed still

further by Artusio in 1954, who divided Guedel's stage 1 into three planes.

Table 1.2, included purely for historical interest, describes the features of diethyl ether anaesthesia in the dog, after Guedel. The features of these stages and planes, however, do not necessarily apply similarly to other inhalant agents, and apply even less to injectable agents, to say nothing of the combination of inhalational and injectable agents that can be administered when balanced anaesthesia is practised. Furthermore, the chart is not necessarily transferrable to other species.

So, when we do not want to use ether, when we need to consider species other than dogs, when we prefer to practise 'polypharmacy' to achieve the desired state/depth of general anaesthesia, and when we add surgical stimulation to the anaesthetised patient (because depth of anaesthesia is not only related to the 'dose' of drug/s administered, but is also dependent upon the degree of stimulation [usually surgery] at the time), we should still monitor the patient's physiological responses to, and status during, anaesthesia, which are considered in more detail in Chapter 18.

Although Table 1.2 is included purely for interest, it is important to note that during induction of anaesthesia, stage II (involuntary excitement/movement) may be witnessed; and during recovery from anaesthesia, all the stages are traversed in the reverse order, such that emergence excitement/delirium (stage II) may be observed.

1.3 Mechanisms of Action of General Anaesthetic Drugs

Compounds that exert general anaesthetic effects exhibit a wide diversity of chemical structure and can be administered by injection (usually intravenously), or by inhalation. Although a unifying target for their action has been sought, the diversity in their structure makes a single target site unlikely.

Nevertheless, Meyer (1899) and Overton (1901), independently, reported that anaesthetic potency was strongly correlated with lipid solubility which sparked interest in lipid membranes as the site of action. It was variously hypothesised that anaesthetic agents may exert a non-selective physical perturbation of a lipid site within the membrane or possibly perturb the volume or fluidity of the membrane itself. That physical dissolution of lipid-soluble agents within plasma membranes caused their expansion, sparked the 'critical volume' and 'membrane expansion' hypotheses, with some demonstration of pressure-reversal. The **lipid theory**, however, had several problems, including the fact that some isomers with identical lipid solubilities had different anaesthetic potencies, not all anaesthetic

Table 1.2 Stages of ether anaesthesia in the dog, after Guedel.

Stage of anaesthesia	Depression of CNS	MM colour	Pupil size	Eyeball activity	Breathing
Stage I: stage of voluntary movement/excitement	?Sensory cortex	N / flushed	Small	Voluntary	Rapid/irregular
Stage II: stage of involuntary movement/excitement 'delirium'	Motor cortex Decerebrate rigidity	Flushed	Dilated	Increased	Irregular
Stage III (light surgical): plane 1	Midbrain	Flushed / N	Smaller	Increased	Slow/regular
Stage III (moderate surgical): plane 2	Spinal cord	N	Miotic	Fixed, ventral rotation	Slow/regular
Stage III (deep surgical): plane 3	Spinal cord	N / pale	Miotic	Ventral rotation	Large abdominal component
Stage III (excessive surgical): plane 4	Spinal cord	Pale	Bigger	Central	Abdominal/shallow
Stage IV: paralysis (death follows respiratory and subsequent cardiac arrest)	Medulla	Pale/cyanotic	Mydriatic	Central	None/agonal gasps

Stage	Pulse rate & BP	Palpebral reflex	Corneal reflex	Swallowing	Cough	Pedal withdrawal	Comments
I	Rapid/high	+	+	+	+	+	Analgesia?
II	Rapid/high	+	+	+	+	+	Unconscious
III (plane 1)	N/N	Poss slight	+	-	+	+	Some lacrimation persists
III (plane 2)	N/N	-	Slight	-	-	-	
III (plane 3)	Rapid/low	-	-	-	-	-	
III (plane 4)	Rapid (or slow)/low	-	-	-	-	-	Anal reflex poor
IV	'Shocky'	-	-	-	-	-	Anal/bladder sphincters relax

N = normal.

Changes tabled above refer specifically to those observed during ether anaesthesia in the dog.

Surgical stimulation may alter haemodynamic and respiratory variables via autonomic reflexes which persist into stage III, planes 2–3.

effects were reversible with applied pressure, and small temperature changes could also change membrane volume but without anaesthetic effects.

Although microtubule and even bubble theories have also been proposed, the biggest step forwards came with the discovery, by Franks and Lieb (1984) that anaesthetic agent potency correlated with inhibition of firefly luciferase, a large globular protein. This **protein theory** was a turning point for research and focused attention on proteins as potential targets for anaesthetic agents, in particular membrane receptors and ion channels that control ionic permeabilities.

Accepting that anaesthesia results from reversible CNS depression, it is plausible that either enhancement of inhibitory neurotransmission and/or inhibition of excitatory neurotransmission could produce a state of unconsciousness. Anaesthetics have therefore been proposed to act by modulation of such neurotransmission.

The main inhibitory neurotransmitter in the brain is gamma-aminobutyric acid (GABA), and the main excitatory neurotransmitter is **glutamate**. Between them, these neurotransmitters act at several key synaptic, ligand-gated ion channels: GABA at $GABA_A$ receptors; and glutamate at N-methyl-D-aspartate (NMDA), alpha-amino-3-hydroxy-5-methyl-4-isoxazolepropionic acid (AMPA) and kainate receptors. (Although primarily ligand-gated, the NMDA receptor also displays a voltage-dependent magnesium block.) The majority of anaesthetic agents have been shown to interact with at least one of these targets.

Barbiturates, benzodiazepines, neuroactive steroids, propofol and, to a lesser extent, the volatile agents, have been shown to be **positive allosteric modulators of the $GABA_A$ receptor**; that is, they produce little direct effect alone (except barbiturates and alfaxalone at higher doses), but enhance GABA-mediated chloride currents in post-synaptic membranes. This produces membrane hyperpolarisation with consequent reduction in neuronal activity, resulting in depressant effects. The different anaesthetic agents, however, appear to have different preferred sites of allosteric modulation within the receptor complex. Furthermore, variations in both receptor structure (many different isoforms exist), and distribution (not only throughout the CNS but also between pre-, extra-, and post-synaptic sites), increases the possibilities for differential effects.

Ketamine, nitrous oxide and xenon are **NMDA receptor antagonists,** again having different sites of action within the receptor complex. These anaesthetic agents reduce the activation/permeability of NMDA receptors to calcium and sodium, thus reducing excitation of the neurone, resulting in overall depression. NMDA receptors are also involved in the development of nociceptive- and memory-processing, hence NMDA receptor antagonists produce analgesic, anti-hyperalgesic, anti-allodynic, and other effects.

More recently, the volatile anaesthetic agents have also been shown to interact with a family of so-called tandem-pore-domain or **two-pore-domain potassium (K_{2P}) channels**, which are widely expressed in the brain and have roles in regulation of sleep and membrane excitability generally. Local anaesthetic agents also have actions at these channels.

Finally, many anaesthetics have also been shown to affect other, unrelated, receptors, resulting in a multitude of possible side effects: these are often undesirable but may, on occasion, be beneficial. Some of these **other sites of action** include: glycine receptors, other glutamate receptors, cholinergic receptors, potassium channels (e.g. voltage-gated, ATP-sensitive, etc.), voltage-gated calcium channels, voltage-gated sodium channels, and others (e.g. hyperpolarisation-activated cyclic nucleotide-gated non-selective cation channels such as neuronal HCN1).

From this multiplicity of sites of action, we can begin to see how 'balanced' anaesthesia developed; that is, the administration of several different anaesthetic agents, each with a slightly different site/mode of action (or spectrum of activities), to produce an overall state of what we refer to as 'general anaesthesia', with, hopefully, fewer overall side effects because usually a lower dose of each agent suffices.

No matter which drug/s we use to produce general anaesthesia, our main objective is to maintain tissue perfusion, with delivery of oxygen and removal of waste products. If this fails, we can expect increased patient morbidity and mortality. There are no safe anaesthetics; there are only safe anaesthetists.

References

Franks, N.P. and Lieb, W.R. (1984). Do general anaesthetics act by competitive binding to specific receptors? *Nature* 310: 599–601.

Meyer, H.H. (1899). Zur Theorie der Alkoholnarkose. *Archiv für Experimentelle Pathologie und Pharmakologie* 42 (2–4): 109–118. https://doi.org/10.1007/BF01834479.

Overton, C.E. (1901). Studien über die Narkose zugleich ein Beitrag zur allgemeinen Pharmakologie. Jena, Switzerland: Gustav Fischer.

Further Reading

Campagna, J.A., Miller, K.W., and Forman, S.A. (2003). Mechanisms of actions of inhaled anesthetics. *The New England Journal of Medicine* 348: 2110–2124.

Foster, P. (2003). How deep is the sleep? Looking into anaesthesia depths. *Southern African Journal of Anaesthesia and Analgesia* 91: 6–8.

Jones, R.S. (2002). A history of veterinary anaesthesia. *Annales de Veterinaria de Murcia* 18: 7–15.

Kaul, H.L. and Bharti, M. (2002). Monitoring depth of anaesthesia. *Indian Journal of Anaesthesia* 46: 323–332.

Lambert, D.G. (2010). Mechanisms of action of general anaesthetic drugs. *Anaesthesia and Intensive Care Medicine* 12: 1410143.

Laws, D., Verdon, B., Coyne, L., and Lees, G. (2001). Fatty acid amides are putative endogenous ligands for anaesthetic recognition sites in mammalian CNS. *British Journal of Anaesthesia* 87: 380–384.

Lugli, K.A., Yost, C.S., and Kindler, C.H. (2009). Anaesthetic mechanisms: Update on the challenge of unravelling the mystery of anaesthesia. *European Journal of Anaesthesiology* 26: 807–820.

Mashour, G.A., Forman, S.A., and Campagna, J.A. (2005). Mechanisms of general anesthesia: From molecules to mind. *Best Practice and Research Clinical Anaesthesiology* 19: 349–364.

Matta, J.A., Cornett, P.M., Miyares, R.L. et al. (2008). General anesthetics activate a nociceptive ion channel to enhance pain and inflammation. *Proceedings of the National Academy of Science, USA* 105: 8784–8789.

Pascoe, P.J. and Steffey, E.P. (2013). Introduction to drugs acting on the central nervous system and principles of anesthesiology. In: Veterinary Pharmacology and Therapeutics, 9e (eds. J.E. Riviere and M.G. Papich), 183–210. Ames, Iowa, USA: Wiley-Blackwell.

Schupp, M. and Hanning, C. (2003). Physiology of sleep. *British Journal of Anaesthesia: CEPD Reviews* 3: 69–74. *(Distinguishes sleep from general anaesthesia; useful information on effects of sleep deprivation for the anaesthetist).*

Tranquilli, W.J. and Grimm, K.A. (2015). Introduction: use, definitions, history, concepts, classification and considerations for general anesthesia. In: Veterinary Anesthesia and Analgesia: The Fifth Edition of Lumb and Jones (eds. K.A. Grimm, L.A. Lamont, W.J. Tranquilli, et al.), 3–10. Ames, Iowa, USA: Wiley Blackwell.

Urban, B.W. and Bleckwenn, M. (2002). Concepts and correlations relevant to general anaesthesia. *British Journal of Anaesthesia* 89: 3–16.

Weir, C. (2006). The molecular mechanisms of general anaesthesia: dissecting the GABA$_A$ receptor. *Continuing Education in Anaesthesia, Critical Care and Pain.* 6: 49–53.

Whelan, G. and Flecknell, P.A. (1992). The assessment of depth of anaesthesia in animals and man. *Laboratory Animals* 26: 153–162.

Self-test Section

1 Induction excitement occurs during which classical 'stage' of anaesthesia?
  A Stage I
  B Stage II
  C Stage III
  D Stage IV

2 The main inhibitory and excitatory neurotransmitters in the brain are, respectively:
  A GABA and glycine
  B Glutamate and GABA
  C Glycine and glutamate
  D GABA and glutamate

2

Patient Safety

LEARNING OBJECTIVES

- Provide an overview of risk in veterinary anaesthesia.
- Provide an overview of medical error and how risk can be reduced.

2.1 Introduction

In 1999, the U.S. Institute of Medicine released its report 'To Err Is Human', highlighting the enormity of the problem of medical error and harm, and catapulting human patient safety firmly into both the public and health sector psyches worldwide. Human patient safety research subsequently rose by almost twofold in the first 5 years alone and the focus shifted from malpractice (fault/blame of the individual/team) to organisational culture (fault/blame of the organisation/procedures). As a result of the research in human patient safety, six main target areas have been identified:

- Hospital acquired infection
- Surgical complications
- Medication errors
- Device complications
- Identification errors
- Death

The World Health Organisation (WHO) has already targeted the first 3 of these with its 2005 'Clean Care is Safer Care', 2008 'Safe Surgery Saves Lives' and 2017 'Medication Without Harm' Global Patient Safety Challenges. The implementation of hand-washing protocols (Clean Care) and peri-surgery checklists (Safe Surgery) has had a significant, positive impact on patient safety with improved outcomes demonstrated in many countries (high, low, and middle income) and it is hoped that the Medication Without Harm campaign will yield similar results by reducing medication errors.

Over the past 30 years, advancements in veterinary anaesthesia have led to improved anaesthetic risk for cats, dogs, and horses, particularly in ill patients (Table 2.1). However, veterinary patient safety has only recently emerged as a subject in its own right, over the last 10 years, with increases in patient safety publications and a shift in focus from primarily mortality risk reporting, to reporting on broader aspects of safety culture.

2.2 Anaesthetic Risk

Anaesthesia, and veterinary medicine in general, carries the risk of inadvertent medical error and/or harm. An understanding of the patient, human and system factors that contribute to anaesthetic error and risk, and those that may mitigate it, is of key importance to anaesthetists. Of all Veterinary Defence Society claims made against veterinary practices in the UK, only 2% related to anaesthesia (2013–2014). However, as in human medicine, focus group work indicates that the rate of actual significant events occurring is likely to be higher. The worst outcome of error and harm is death (usually of a patient, rarely the death of a member of staff or the public) and in the UK National Health Service there are approximately 7000 significant events or near misses for every catastrophic significant event. Similar data for veterinary medicine is currently unavailable.

Veterinary Anaesthesia: Principles to Practice, Second Edition. Alexandra H. A. Dugdale, Georgina Beaumont, Carl Bradbrook, and Matthew Gurney.
© 2020 John Wiley & Sons Ltd. Published 2020 by John Wiley & Sons Ltd.
Companion website: www.wiley.com/go/dugdale/veterinary-anaesthesia

Table 2.1 Peri-anaesthetic risk of mortality (%) reported for various species. Human mortality figures are shown as rate and percentage. Rates vary according to study year, country, and methodology. Healthy = ASA 1–2; ill = ASA ⩾3.

Species	Overall risk (%)	Risk healthy (%)	Risk ill (%)	Country	Year
Cats	0.29	0.18	3.33	UK	1990
	0.24	0.11	1.4	UK	2008
Cats and dogs (pooled)	1.35	0.12	4.77	France	2012
Dogs	0.23	0.11	3.12	UK	1990
	0.17	0.05	1.33	UK	2008
	1.29	0.33	4.06	Spain	2013
	0.65	0.28	1.74	Japan	2017
Equine	1.9	0.9	7.8	International	2002
	1.6	0.9	—	International	2004
	1.1	0.9	1.6	UK	2016
Great apes	0.88	—	—	USA	1986
	1.35	—	—	UK	2007
Rabbits	1.39	0.73	7.37	UK	2008
	4.8	—	—	UK	2018
Guinea pigs	3.8	—	—	UK	2008
Ferrets	0.33	—	—	UK	2008
Hamsters	3.66	—	—	UK	2008
Chinchillas	3.29	—	—	UK	2008
Rats	2.01	—	—	UK	2008
Other small mammals	1.72	—	—	UK	2008
Budgerigars	16.33	—	—	UK	2008
Parrots	3.94	—	—	UK	2008
Other birds	1.76	—	—	UK	2008
Reptiles	1.49	—	—	UK	2008
Human					
Adult	8.8:100 000 (0.0088%)	—	—	Netherlands	2001
	4.7:100 000 (0.0047%)	0.4:10 000 (0.0004%)	—	France	2006
	1:57 023 (0.0018%)	7% of deaths	93% of deaths	Australia and New Zealand	2017
Child	1–7:10 000 (0.01–0.07%)	—	—	International	2011
Neonate	19–24:10 000 (0.19–0.24%)	—	—	International	2011

- **Significant events** are deviations from the usual medical care that are considered undesirable or that pose a risk of unnecessary harm to the patient, whether or not actual injury occurs as a result (also called safety incidents, critical incidents, or critical events)

- **Catastrophic significant events** are those that result in major harm or death of the patient
  - Major harm: sickness or injury leading to long-term incapacity/disability and/or increased duration of hospitalisation by more than 15 days and/or subject to statutory reporting

– Catastrophic harm: irreversible health effects and/or multiple permanent injuries or death
- A **near miss** is a significant event that specifically did not result in harm (on this occasion)

For the risk of mortality for selected species, see Table 2.1. The majority of veterinary peri-anaesthetic mortality occurs during maintenance of, or recovery from, anaesthesia. Systemically healthy animals (American Society of Anesthesiologists [ASA] physical status classification 1 and 2) are, unsurprisingly, at a lower risk of death than unhealthy (≥ASA 3) animals. See below for more information on ASA classification. Veterinary peri-anaesthetic mortality is generally reported as a percentage, whilst human mortality is reported as a rate.

2.2.1 Factors Affecting Anaesthetic Risk

The factors affecting anaesthetic risk are listed below; not all are patient-related. The duration of anaesthesia and surgery are particularly related to risk.

- Patient's health
- Urgency: elective or emergency procedure
- Surgery: surgeon's experience, duration of surgery, type of surgery, gravity of surgery, surgery that involves the airway/lungs and interferes with the anaesthetist's 'space'
- Facilities available (surgical and anaesthetic): equipment, drugs, referral hospital, general practice or field
- Help available and experience of available personnel
- Anaesthetist: experience, duration of surgery (tiredness/vigilance/boredom), type of surgery
- Duration of anaesthesia and surgery

2.2.1.1 Patient Factors
Poor oxygen delivery to the tissues means trouble. Tissues susceptible to hypoperfusion/hypoxia are:

- Central nervous system (visual cortex)
- Myocardium
- Kidneys
- Liver

To reduce peri-operative morbidity and mortality, we must consider the effects of anaesthesia on any disease processes already present and the problems that those disease processes pose for anaesthesia.

We can improve the overall safety of anaesthesia with adequate pre-operative assessment, medical treatment and stabilisation of the patient where possible, and anticipation of the possible complications.

Familiarity with an anaesthetic technique is often a more important safety factor than the theoretical pharmacological advantage of an unfamiliar drug/technique.

A **careful history and thorough clinical examination** will reveal any problem areas. If there is time, further work-up may be warranted, such as laboratory tests, imaging or electrodiagnostics. The whole peri-anaesthetic period (including the pre-operative and post-operative periods) can then be tailored to suit each individual animal (see Chapter 18 on monitoring).

2.2.1.1.1 Body Mass
Is the animal overweight or too skinny, even debilitated? Is there a recent history of weight gain or loss? For obese animals, try to assess what their lean mass ought to be (See Chapter 40 on Obesity).

2.2.1.1.2 Age
Very young (neonatal) and very old (geriatric) animals may require dose adjustments (see Chapter 37 on neonates and Chapter 38 on geriatrics). Some chronologically old animals act as if they are still very young and some very young animals act as if they are very old, so be aware that the animal's chronological (true) age may not match its physiological/behavioural age. An animal's response to anaesthesia often matches its physiological age more than its chronological age.

2.2.1.1.3 Pre-existing Conditions
Hypovolaemia, cardiac disease, or respiratory disease may compromise the patient's ability to maintain adequate tissue perfusion/oxygen delivery, even before the physiological insult of anaesthesia.

Exercise tolerance is the **best indication of how compromised an animal is by its cardiac and/or respiratory disease**. Resting heart and breathing rates are also useful, especially in dogs.

Renal, hepatic, endocrine, neurologic, allergic, neoplastic, and musculoskeletal pathology/disease/dysfunction can all influence anaesthetic risk through derangements, or alterations, in:

- Homeostasis (glucose and electrolytes, acid–base, coagulation, thermoregulation, paraneoplastic syndromes, etc.)
- Drug pharmacokinetics and pharmacodynamics
- Drug interactions by pre-existing medicines or nutraceuticals (that may or may not be given under veterinary direction)
- Pain

2.2.1.1.4 ASA Physical Status Classification
Having completed the history and clinical examination, the animal is assigned to one of the ASA physical status classes (basic class descriptors are given below but, in line with the original medical classification system, a recent veterinary version has been devised with exemplars for

each class, see further reading), as this can help to decide whether anaesthesia can proceed, or whether further investigations or patient stabilisation are warranted first.

1) Normal healthy animal; no detectable underlying disease (cannot be an emergency)
2) Mild systemic disease, but causing no obvious clinical signs or incapacity (animal compensating well)
3) Severe systemic disease, causing clinical signs (animal not compensating fully, substantial functional limitations)
4) Severe systemic disease that is a constant threat to life
5) Moribund and not expected to survive without the procedure
E) Add 'E' to any class to denote an emergency (where a delay in treatment significantly increases the threat to life or limb)

2.2.1.1.5 Stabilisation

Pre-operative support/stabilisation should be considered, which could involve:

- Anxiolysis/sedation
- Analgesia
- Pre-oxygenation/oxygen supplementation
- Fluid therapy/diuresis
- Attention to thermoregulatory requirements
- Medical support (e.g. for diabetes or cardiac arrhythmias)
- Surgical procedures (e.g. tracheostomy, chest, or pericardial drainage)

Appropriate monitoring should be considered and may be instigated in the pre-operative phase. Take extra care with very young, old or thin animals, and those with endocrinopathies or liver disease. Hypothermia will delay recovery. Remember that hypoglycaemia may be a confounding factor in very young animals, those with insulinomas, or poorly controlled diabetes mellitus.

2.2.1.1.6 Pre-anaesthetic Fasting

Feeding has traditionally been suspended for varying durations (averaging 6–12 hours), before premedication/anaesthesia because of the risk of vomiting or regurgitation, and subsequent aspiration. Whilst some agents can stimulate vomiting (e.g. morphine, α2 agonists), this usually occurs during the 'onset' of sedation or premedication. Occult (undetected) gastro-oesophageal reflux (GOR), however, appears to be more common than regurgitation (where material refluxing from the stomach through the cardia becomes visible in the pharynx); but both can result in oesophagitis and even oesophageal stricture, and both pose the additional risk of aspiration

pneumonitis. GOR has been reported to occur in around 25+% of dogs and around 12% of cats; regurgitation in around 1% of patients, and aspiration/chemical pneumonitis (Mendelson's syndrome) in <1%. Material of adverse pH reaching the nasopharynx undetected can also result in choanal stricture.

The barrier pressure across the cardia (i.e. the difference between lower oesophageal sphincter pressure [LOSP] and intragastric pressure [IGP]) is important in determining whether GOR/regurgitation may occur. (Species differences exist in the muscular composition of the lower oesophagus: striated muscle is present in dogs and ruminants, whereas only smooth muscle is present in horses and cats.)

Lowered barrier pressure (increased risk of GOR/regurgitation), occurs with either decreased LOSP and/or increased IGP. Opioids, sedatives, anaesthetic, and ancillary drugs can reduce LOSP (and many of these also delay gastric emptying); and a recent large meal or drink can increase IGP, but so can factors increasing intra-abdominal pressure in general. Increased gastric acidity can also reduce LOSP, whereas reducing the acidity of gastric contents (with food or antacids) can help to increase LOSP.

Suggested **predisposing factors for GOR/regurgitation appear to include: opioid administration** (butorphanol > morphine >> pethidine), **age** (very young and very old), **increased intra-abdominal pressure** (e.g. obesity, pregnancy, abdominal surgery), **history of gastrointestinal disease** (including brachycephalics), **deep-chested conformation**, and **multiple changes in patient position** (common in orthopaedic patients undergoing pre- and post-operative imaging). Use of laryngeal mask airways has been reported to increase the risk of occult GOR in kittens.

As for aspiration pneumonitis, this most commonly appears to follow occult GOR. Whilst predisposing factors facilitating aspiration might include use of supra-glottic airway devices compared with suitably-inflated cuffed endotracheal tubes, the severity of the pneumonitis depends not only upon the volume, physical composition and pH of aspirated material but also on other factors, including the patient's ASA physical status.

A single optimum duration for denying access to food before anaesthesia/surgery is unlikely to exist because it will depend upon: the species (dogs appear more prone than cats), the individual patient, its health status (including pre-existing pathologies which may predispose to GOR, regurgitation or delayed gastric emptying), what meal size/s and intervals are usually adhered to, and what type of food is usually fed (wet or dry; caloric content and composition in terms of fat/carbohydrate [including fibre types]/protein).

At the spring 2019 meeting of the Association of Veterinary Anaesthetists (AVA), lively debate was held regarding opinions for food and water withhold before anaesthesia. This was sparked by recent changes to human guidelines following recognition that prolonged fasting is associated with dehydration, thirst, hunger, irritability (patients are often referred to as being 'hangry' = hungry and angry), and adverse metabolic consequences including the promotion of insulin resistance. Although no veterinary consensus was reached due to the many factors involved, one suggestion was:

- For dogs and cats, a light meal (supplying up to around half of the daily energy requirements), of 'wet' (canned) food, of low fat and low fibre composition (so as not to increase gastric emptying time), may be offered (4-)6 hours before premedication. (If dry, fatty, or high protein content food is given, then 10+ hours should be allowed before premedication.) (For puppies and kittens, see Chapter 37.)
- Water should be freely available: up to the time of premedication (or, if a restriction time is felt necessary, then access to water should be allowed up to one to two hours before 'anaesthesia' [which could be interpreted as premedication or induction]).

Should regurgitation be observed, then suction, with or without oesophageal warm-water lavage (this may be preferred for acidic material), may be indicated (taking care to protect the airway). This author also flushes the nasal passages with warm water in a retrograde fashion, ensuring the nasopharynx is cleared of material, to reduce the risk of choanal mucosal damage and subsequent stricture.

Delayed gastric emptying (due to stress, anaesthesia, and surgery), might also increase nausea and possibly delay resumption of feeding post-operatively. The subject of when to re-introduce feeding post-operatively, and with food of what quantity, frequency, and composition, remains to be discussed.

See Chapters 30, 33, and 35 for horses and farm species.

2.3 Error

Medical error is the failure to correctly complete an intended action, or the implementation of a wrong plan to achieve the goal. Errors may be **latent**, due to the system (e.g. poorly designed systems/procedures/buildings), or **active**, due to the people (e.g. dose/technical error).

High-reliability organisations (e.g. nuclear power, aviation, rail networks) recognise that people will always be fallible, particularly in high risk/stressful/emotional situations, and so they focus on constructing systems with as few latent risk factors as possible so that people are less likely to find themselves in a situation where they can err. Safe industries also assume that errors will, at some point, occur and so they build in vigilance and damage-control to these systems. This protects employees, clients, and the public from error by:

- Minimising the risk of an error occurring in the first place
- Vigilantly looking for errors
  - Errors are detected quickly and reliably, allowing rapid correction/management
  - Errors are reported and reviewed to enable system improvements, staff training (or re-training) and further research/learning
- Actively managing errors to reduce their impact

It is interesting to note that medical professionals perceive themselves as less fallible than aviation pilots do. This denial of normal, human fallibility reflects a problematic discrepancy in safety culture and attitude towards risk between medicine and high-reliability organisations. It also sets medical professionals up for failure and the emotional and psychological distress that accompanies it. Veterinary professionals have similar levels of perfectionism, workplace complexity, moral conflict and expectations of professional infallibility (for themselves and each other) as our medical counterparts, and these unrealistic professional expectations contribute to poor mental health and career dissatisfaction. Recent safety culture studies have revealed significant overlap and commonality between veterinary and medical errors.

2.3.1 Latent (System) Error

Latent errors are often foreseeable and include:

- Communication
  - Within and between teams; written, oral and behavioural
  - Clinical handovers and transitions are particularly susceptible to communication error, especially when performed informally/without structure
  - Unwillingness or failure to ask for help
- Non-technical skills
  - Non-technical skills are cognitive, social, and personal resource skills that complement technical skills
  - The importance of non-technical skills in patient safety culture and efficient, edifying working relationships is well documented in high reliability organisations and human medicine
- Leadership (individuals or organisations)
  - Failure to take charge of situations or to clearly allocate/identify roles

- Failure to acknowledge strengths/contributions of team members
- Failure to acknowledge weaknesses (of team members and self) and provide appropriate support/supervision
- Weak industry regulation
- Product or equipment design flaws
  - Standards for veterinary products are not as robust or well developed as for human products, e.g. there is no requirement for veterinary anaesthetic machines to be fitted with hypoxic guards
  - Many drugs are similarly packed and look identical in an unlabelled syringe
    - If possible, similarly packaged or named products should be separated
- Productivity
  - Time and financial pressures
  - Inefficient and under-staffing
  - Over-time and shift structure
- Organisational failure
  - Lack of safety systems and protocols
  - Institution of policies or procedures that are not fit for purpose
- Owners
  - Poor compliance or refusal of recommended treatment
  - Loss to follow-up or further investigations
  - Conflicting owner: animal needs
    - Legally, animals are personal property; laws pertaining to property rights may conflict with laws safeguarding animal welfare, resulting in marked moral stress
- Veterinary specific
  - Animal behaviour, e.g. aggression or ability to out-run the veterinarian
  - Inability to control the surroundings, e.g. procedures performed in the field

2.3.2 Active Error

Active errors are often difficult to foresee and include:

- Cognitive limitations
  - Slips: the action is not carried out as planned, often due to distraction
  - Lapses: the action is missed out entirely, may be due to distraction but includes deliberate omissions where the individual believes it will not cause harm
  - Mistakes: the wrong action is carried out but the individual believes it to be the correct action
    - Rule-based: the incorrect application of previous learning

- Knowledge-based: the individual has never known the correct solution and has come to the wrong conclusion whilst attempting to work the problem out
  - Conformational bias: the individual sees what they expect to see instead of what is actually there
  - Memory failure
- Individual factors
  - Fatigue: 17 hours without sleep results in a reduction of psychomotor performance equivalent to a blood alcohol concentration of 50 mg/dl; and 24 hours of sleep deprivation reduces performance equivalent to a blood alcohol concentration of 100 mg/dl (the current UK legal driving limit is 80 mg/dl)
  - Illness, emotional distress, and stress all significantly impair decision-making
- Lack of technical ability
  - Failure of supervision and support, particularly of junior staff
  - Attempting a task beyond the training, capability or experience of the individual; this can be accompanied by emotional stress if the individual is aware of the deficiency but feels pressured into continuing with the course of action regardless
- Deliberate negligence/harm
  - Perpetrators of deliberate negligence/harm should be formally disciplined and criminal charges may be appropriate; thankfully this is an uncommon cause of error and harm

Most significant events are caused by multiple errors (the Swiss-cheese model), often arising from different levels within the organisation. Active (human) error, communication, and leadership are consistently the top three contributors to medical errors. Initial research indicates that this may also hold true for veterinary errors. An understanding of the types and patterns of error in veterinary medicine provides the opportunity to develop interventions to minimise risk and may highlight individuals that require additional (re)training, or systems that require review and overhaul.

2.3.3 Cost of Error

Error has medical, psychosocial, and financial costs. The medical cost of error is borne through patient morbidity and/or mortality, i.e. the harm. The psychosocial cost is the emotional and psychological impact of error on the patient, owner, and staff member(s). It is important to remember that staff may become the hidden (second) victim(s) of an error and can experience significant emotional and psychological distress requiring appropriate support and counselling. The financial cost lies in rectifying the error, which often requires additional treatment/hospitalisation, and the cost of litigation against the practice that erred.

Of the estimated 237 million medication errors occurring in the UK each year, most (72%) have little or no potential to cause harm and many are detected before reaching the patient (near misses). Despite this, it is estimated that medication errors alone cost the UK National Health Service £98.5 million per year, requiring an additional 181,626 hospital bed-days, directly causing the death of 712 people and contributing to the death of an additional 1,708 people.

As there is no mandatory reporting in veterinary medicine, accurate information on the true magnitude and cost of veterinary error is, at this time, lacking.

2.3.4 Responding to Error

When responding to an error, the following questions should be considered:

- Was the harm deliberate?
  - If so, disciplinary action is required
- Were staff physically or mentally impaired (e.g. fatigue, distress, substance abuse, injury)?
  - If so, the staff involved require support
    - Disciplinary action may or may not be required (and may be harmful in some instances)
- Were established policies, protocols, and procedures followed correctly?
  - If not, the staff involved require additional (re)training
    - Disciplinary action may or may not be required (and may be harmful in some instances)
- Would the same error have occurred if different, similarly skilled staff members had been exposed to the same circumstances?
  - If so, the system causes/allows error and accountability for the error is shared with the organisation's leadership
    - The system must be changed so that harm is avoided rather than encouraged
- Has the same, or a similar, harm occurred previously?
  - If so, the repetitive safety failing must be addressed whether by systems overhaul if the system is at fault or, if a particular staff member has repeatedly caused the harms, by performance review

2.4 Safety Culture

The safety culture of an organisation is the product of individual and group values, attitudes, perceptions, competencies, and patterns of behaviour that determine the commitment to, and the style and proficiency of, an organisation's health and safety management. Organisations with a positive safety culture are characterised by communications founded on mutual trust, by shared perceptions of the importance of safety and by confidence in the efficacy of preventive measures.

ACSNI Human Factors Study Group (1993)

Committed and engaged management, active employee participation and honest and blame-free communication are crucial for a healthy safety culture. Organisations with healthy safety cultures: monitor and review significant errors, proactively implement changes and training to reduce future risk, and cultivate a no blame environment. Checklists, significant event reporting, drills/training, and established, written procedures improve safety whilst also aiding in the development of a healthy safety culture. For example:

- Purposeful, regular team training (e.g. practical resuscitation training, handover training) improves teamwork, communication, and non-technical skills
- Checklists help to prevent errors due to cognitive limitations whilst also developing teamwork and non-technical skills

2.4.1 Checklists

Checklists help to prevent significant events by avoiding reliance on memory and vigilance, and by standardising common procedures. They promote teamwork, communication, and flat safety hierarchies. Checklists have been shown to improve outcomes in a variety of veterinary applications including:

- Small animal anaesthesia and surgery
- Equine anaesthesia
- Cardiology
- Clinical pathology laboratories
- Patient discharges to the owner

Checklists are used to ensure that the basic, common tasks that should always be completed *are* always completed (e.g. open the adjustable pressure limit valve before the animal is connected to the breathing system). A good checklist should be:

- Concise and focused on critical interventions/events, with no more than nine steps
- Brief, taking no more than 60 seconds to complete
- Actionable: every step is linked to a clear action
- A verbal exercise undertaken between multiple team members

- Modified only following collaboration with representatives of all of the team members who will be using it
- Tested before it is formally launched; feedback from testing feeds into additional improvements and facilitates collaboration
- Integrated into the existing framework; using the checklist should be the norm

Peri-operative checklists pertinent to anaesthesia have been developed by the WHO and the AVA, in conjunction with Jurox UK, and are freely accessible online. These documents comprise three separate checklists: one for before induction ('sign in'), one for before first incision ('time out') and one for surgery end, before everyone leaves theatre ('sign out'). The AVA has also produced a comprehensive anaesthetic workstation checklist for use daily and an abridged checklist for use between patients.

2.4.2 Significant Event Reporting

Significant event reporting is critical to the advancement of safety culture and development of strategies and tools that promote safety in veterinary practice. Significant event reporting acts as a sentinel, providing an early warning system for potential problems, before significant harm occurs. In human medicine, up to 20% of acute care patients experience at least one significant event during their hospitalisation. Of these significant events, ~65% result in minimal or no harm, providing an opportunity for corrective measures to be made before a patient is permanently disabled, or killed.

Many, larger veterinary practices and corporates have begun to implement significant event reporting systems. In the UK, the VetSafe voluntary reporting system was launched in 2019 to capture, report, and develop solutions for veterinary errors and harm. The VetSafe reporting system is operated by the Veterinary Defence Society Ltd (UK) and is available to their members. In addition to the anonymised collation and analysis of practice incidents, reports made via VetSafe form the first notification to the insurer (i.e. the Veterinary Defence Society) of an event that might result in a claim against the practice.

2.4.3 Drills/Training

Scenario training enhances teamwork, communication, situational awareness, and practical performance during high stress events, such as cardiopulmonary-cerebro resuscitation

(CPCR). Standardised drills/training also aim to improve adherence to protocols and guidelines

2.4.4 Established Protocols and Procedures

Organised, well-documented, written protocols and procedures aim to reduce the likelihood of cognitive limitation contributing to error by providing staff with evidence-based, safe and appropriate frameworks to work within. Familiarisation with the protocols and procedures and clear cognitive aids (algorithms, checklists, dosage charts, etc.) enable staff to provide a consistent standard of care across the team. Examples of written protocols and procedures include (non-exhaustive):

- RECOVER (REassessment Campaign On VEterinary Resuscitation) guidelines for CPCR (2012)
- Handover mnemonics, e.g. I-PASS (Illness severity, Patient summary, Action list, Situation awareness and contingency planning, Synthesis by receiver) or SBAR (Situation, Background, Assessment, Recommendation)
- Anaesthetic workstation checks
- Medication checks, e.g. double-checking doses and dispensed medication
- Controlled drug management (including disposal)
- Treatment pathways, e.g. management of hypotension, patient temperature, local anaesthetic toxicity, etc.
- Standard procedures for managing clinical scenarios, e.g. aggressive patients, intravenous catheter care, fire action plans, etc.

2.5 Where to Get Help

Humans make errors. Veterinarians make errors. When we do err, we may suffer emotional and psychological distress. This is called **second victim syndrome**. This includes feelings of isolation, shame, denial, and a sense of being unsupported. It is important that vets affected by these issues are able to talk about them in a safe way and receive the support they need.

In many countries, independent, confidential support is available 24 hours a day, 365 days a year, from organisations such as the Samaritans (UK, Republic of Ireland, Australia, New Zealand, Thailand, Singapore, Hong Kong) **and Lifeline** (Australia).

Reference

Health and Safety Commission (1993). ACSNI Study Group on Human Factors. 3rd Report: Organising for safety. Health and Safety Commission. London: HMSO.

Further Reading

ACT Academy (2018). Quality, service improvement and redesign tools: SBAR communication tool – situation, background, assessment, recommendation. https://improvement.nhs.uk/resources/sbar-communication-tool (accessed July 2019).

Alef, M., von Praun, F., and Oechtering, G. (2008). Is routine pre-anaesthetic haematological and biochemical screening justified in dogs? *Veterinary Anaesthesia and Analgesia* 35: 132–140.

Allegranzi, B., Storr, J., Dziekan, G. et al. (2007). The first global patient safety challenge "Clean Care is Safer Care": from launch to current progress and achievements. *Journal of Hospital Infection* 65: 115–123.

Arbous, M.S., Grobbee, D.E., van Kleef, J.W. et al. (2001). Mortality associated with anaesthesia: a qualitative analysis to identify risk factors. *Anaesthesia* 56: 1141–1153.

Armitage-Chan, E.A. (2014). Human factors, non-technical skills, professionalism and flight safety: their roles in improving patient outcome. *Veterinary Anaesthesia and Analgesia* 41: 221–223.

Armitage-Chan, E., Maddison, J., and May, S.A. (2016). What is the veterinary professional identity? Preliminary findings from web-based continuing professional development in veterinary professionalism. *Veterinary Record* 178: 318–323.

Australian and New Zealand College of Anaesthetists (2017). Safety of anaesthesia – A review of anaesthesia-related mortality reporting in Australia and New Zealand 2012–2014. Report of the Mortality Sub-Committee.

Baker, R.G., Norton, P.G., Flintoft, V. et al. (2004). The Canadian adverse events study: the incidence of adverse events among hospital patients in Canada. *Canadian Medical Association Journal* 170: 1678–1686.

Barach, P. and Small, S.D. (2000). Reporting and preventing medical mishaps: lessons from non-medical near miss reporting systems. *British Medical Journal* 320: 759–763.

Bille, C., Auvigne, V., Libermann, S. et al. (2012). Risk of anaesthetic mortality in dogs and cats: an observational cohort study of 3546 cases. *Veterinary Anaesthesia and Analgesia* 39: 59–68.

Boysen, I.I.P.G. (2013). Just culture: a foundation for balanced accountability and patient safety. *The Ochsner Journal* 13: 400–406.

Brodbelt, D.C., Blissitt, K.J., Hammond, R.A. et al. (2008). The risk of death: the confidential enquiry into perioperative small animal fatalities. *Veterinary Anaesthesia and Analgesia* 35: 365–373. *(CEPSAF.)*.

Burton, D., Nicholson, G., and Hall, G.M. (2004). Endocrine and metabolic response to surgery. *Continuing Education in Anaesthesia, Critical Care and Pain* 4: 144–147.

Catchpole, K.R., De Leval, M.R., McEwan, A. et al. (2007). Patient handover from surgery to intensive care: using formula 1 pit-stop and aviation models to improve safety and quality. *Pediatric Anesthesia* 17: 470–478.

Clarke, K.W. and Hall, L.W. (1990). A survey of anaesthesia in small animal practice: AVA/BSAVA report. *Veterinary Anaesthesia and Analgesia* 17: 4–10.

De Miguel-Garcia, C., Dugdale, A., Pinchbeck, G.L., and Senior, J.M. (2013). Retrospective study of the risk factors and prevalence of regurgitation in dogs undergoing anaesthesia. *The Open Veterinary Science Journal* 7: 6–11.

Dugdale, A.H.A. and Taylor, P.M. (2016). Equine anaesthesia-associated mortality: where are we now? *Veterinary Anaesthesia and Analgesia* 43: 242–255.

Dugdale, A.H.A., Obhrai, J., and Cripps, P.J. (2016). Twenty years later: a single-centre, repeat retrospective analysis of equine perioperative mortality and investigation of recovery quality. *Veterinary Anaesthesia and Analgesia* 43: 171–178.

Elliott, R.A., Camacho, E., Campbell, F., Jankovic, D., Martyn St James, M., Kaltenthaler, E., Wong, R., Sculpher, M.J., and Faria, R. (2018). Prevalence and economic burden of medication errors in the NHS in England: Rapid evidence synthesis and economic analysis of the prevalence and burden of medication error in the UK. Policy Research Unit in Economic Evaluation of Health & Care Interventions, Universities of Sheffield and York.

Fordyce, P.S. (2017). Welfare, law and ethics in the veterinary intensive care unit. *Veterinary Anaesthesia and Analgesia* 44: 203–211.

Gil, L. and Redondo, J.I. (2013). Canine anaesthetic death in Spain: a multicentre prospective cohort study of 2012 cases. *Veterinary Anaesthesia and Analgesia* 40: e57–e67.

Hartnack, S., Bettschart-Wolfensberger, R., Driessen, B. et al. (2013). Critical incidence reporting systems – an option in equine anaesthesia? Results from a panel meeting. *Veterinary Anaesthesia and Analgesia* 40: e3–e8.

Haynes, A.B., Weiser, T.G., Berry, W.R. et al. (2011). Changes in safety attitude and relationship to decreased postoperative morbidity and mortality following implementation of a checklist-based surgical safety intervention. *BMJ Quality & Safety* 20: 102–107.

Hofmeister, E.H., Quandt, J., Braun, C., and Shepard, M. (2014). Development, implementation and impact of simple patient safety interventions in a university teaching hospital. *Veterinary Anaesthesia and Analgesia* 41: 243–248.

Institute of Medicine (2000). *To Err Is Human: Building a Safer Health System*. Washington, DC: The National Academies Press https://doi.org/10.17226/9728.

Itami, T., Aida, H., Asakawa, M. et al. (2017). Association between preoperative characteristics and risk of anaesthesia-related death in dogs in small-animal referral hospitals in Japan. *Veterinary Anaesthesia and Analgesia* 44: 461–472.

Jothiraj, H., Howland-Harris, J., Evley, R., and Moppett, I.K. (2013). Distractions and the anaesthetist: a qualitative study of context and direction of distraction. *British Journal of Anaesthesia* 111: 477–482.

Johnston, G.M., Eastment, J.K., Wood, J.L.N., and Taylor, P.M. (2002). The confidential enquiry into perioperative equine fatalities (CEPEF): mortality results of Phases 1 and 2. *Veterinary Anaesthesia and Analgesia* 29: 159–170. *(CEPEF 1 & 2 summary.)*.

Johnston, G.M., Eastment, J.K., Taylor, P.M., and Wood, J.L.N. (2004). Is isoflurane safer than halothane in equine anaesthesia? Results from a prospective multicentre randomised controlled trial. *Equine Veterinary Journal* 36: 64–71. *(CEPEF 3.)*.

Kinnison, T., Guile, D., and May, S.A. (2015). Errors in veterinary practice: preliminary lessons for building better veterinary teams. *Veterinary Record* 177: 492–496.

Kinnison, T., Guile, D., and May, S.A. (2015). Veterinary team interactions, part 2: the personal effect. *Veterinary Record* 177: 541–546.

Lamata, C., Loughton, V., Jones, M. et al. (2012). The risk of passive regurgitation during general anaesthesia in a population of referred dogs in the UK. *Veterinary Anaesthesia and Analgesia* 39: 266–274.

The Lancet (2008). WHO's patient-safety checklist for surgery. *The Lancet* 372: 1).

Lee, H.W., Machin, H., and Adami, C. (2018). Peri-anaesthetic mortality and nonfatal gastrointestinal complications in pet rabbits: a retrospective study on 210 cases. *Veterinary Anaesthesia and Analgesia* 45: 520–528.

Lienhart, A., Auroy, Y., Péquignot, F. et al. (2006). Survey of anesthesia-related mortality in France. *Anesthesiology* 105: 1087–1097.

Masters, N.J., Burns, F.M., and Lewis, J.C.M. (2007). Peri-anaesthetic and anaesthetic-related mortality risks in great apes (Hominidae) in zoological collections in the UK and Ireland. *Veterinary Anaesthesia and Analgesia* 34: 431–442.

Mayhew, D., Mendonca, V., and Murthy, B.V.S. (2019). A review of ASA physical status – historical perspectives and modern developments. *Anaesthesia* 74: 373–379.

McMillan, M. (2014). Checklists in veterinary anaesthesia: why bother? *Veterinary Record* 175: 556–559.

McMillan, M. (2014). New frontiers for veterinary anaesthesia: the development of veterinary patient safety culture. *Veterinary Anaesthesia and Analgesia* 41: 224–226.

McMillan, M. and Darcy, H. (2016). Adverse event surveillance in small animal anaesthesia: an intervention- based,

voluntary reporting audit. *Veterinary Anaesthesia and Analgesia* 43: 128–135.

McMillan, M.W. and Lehnus, K.S. (2018). Systems analysis of voluntary reported anaesthetic safety incidents occurring in a university teaching hospital. *Veterinary Anaesthesia and Analgesia* 45: 3–12.

Mellanby, R. and Herrtage, M. (2004). Survey of mistakes made by recent veterinary graduates. *Veterinary Record* 155: 761–765.

Mellin-Olsen, J., Staender, S., Whitaker, D.K., and Smith, A.F. (2010). The Helsinki declaration on patient safety in anaesthesiology. *European Journal of Anaesthesiology* 27: 592–597.

Michou, J.N., Dugdale, A.H.A., and Cripwell, D. (2019). Achieving safer anaesthesia with ASA. www.alfaxan.co.uk/news/achieving-safer-anaesthesia-with-asa (accessed July 2019).

Oxtoby, C., Ferguson, E., White, K., and Mossop, L. (2015). We need to talk about error: causes and types of error in veterinary practice. *Veterinary Record* 177: 438–444.

Oxtoby, C., Mossop, L., White, K., and Ferguson, E. (2017). Safety culture: the Nottingham Veterinary Safety Culture Survey (NVSCS). *Veterinary Record* 180: 472–479.

Oxtoby, C. and Mossop, L. (2019). Blame and shame in the veterinary profession: barriers and facilitators to reporting significant events. *Veterinary Record* 184: 501–507.

Paterson, N. and Waterhouse, P. (2011). Risk in pediatric anesthesia. *Pediatric Anesthesia* 21: 848–857.

Perrin, H.C. (2017). Improving safety through changes to the practice culture. *Veterinary Record* 180: 470–471.

Reason, J. (2000). Human error: models and management. *British Medical Journal* 320: 768–770.

Reinersten, J.L. (2000). Let's talk about error. *British Medical Journal* 320: 730.

Schnittker, R. and Marshall, S.D. (2015). Safe anaesthetic care: further improvements require a focus on resilience. *British Journal of Anaesthesia* 115: 643–645.

Sexton, J.B., Thomas, E.J., and Helmreich, R.L. (2000). Error, stress, and teamwork in medicine and aviation: cross sectional surveys. *British Medical Journal* 320: 745–749.

Shaw, R., Drever, F., Hughes, H. et al. (2005). Adverse events and near miss reporting in the NHS. *BMJ Quality & Safety* 14: 279–283.

Sideri, A.I., Galatos, A.D., Kazakos, G.M., and Gouletsou, P.G. (2009). Gastro-oesophageal reflux during anaesthesia in the kitten: comparison between use of a laryngeal mask airway or an endotracheal tube. *Veterinary Anaesthesia and Analgesia* 36: 547–554.

Smith, A.F., Pope, C., Goodwin, D., and Mort, M. (2008). Interprofessional handover and patient safety in anaesthesia: observational study of handovers in the recovery room. *British Journal of Anaesthesia* 101: 332–337.

Starmer, A.J., Sectish, T.C., Simon, D.W. et al. (2013). Rates of medical errors and preventable adverse events among hospitalized children following implementation of a resident handoff bundle. *Journal of the American Medical Association* 310: 2262–2270.

Starmer, A.J., Spector, N.D., Srivastava, R. et al. (2012). I-PASS, a mnemonic to standardize verbal handoffs. *Pediatrics* 129: 201–204.

Starmer, A.J., Spector, N.D., Srivastava, R. et al. (2014). Changes in medical errors after implementation of a handoff program. *New England Journal Medicine* 371: 1803–1812.

Stelfox, H.T., Palmisani, S., Scurlock, C. et al. (2006). The "To Err is Human" report and the patient safety literature. *BMJ Quality & Safety* 15: 174–178.

Stones, J. and Yates, D. (2019). Clinical risk assessment tools in anaesthesia. *BJA Education* 19: 47–53.

Tivers, M. (2015). Reducing error and improving patient safety. *Veterinary Record* 177: 436–437.

Tivers, M. and Adamantos, S. (2019). Significant event reporting in veterinary practice. *Veterinary Record* 184: 498–499.

Turner, M. (2018). Patient safety first. *Veterinary Record* 182: 607.

van Beuzekom, M., Boer, F., Akerboom, A.S., and Dahan, A. (2013). Perception of patient safety differs by clinical area and discipline. *British Journal of Anaesthesia* 110: 107–114.

The Veterinary Record (2016). Reducing error and blame in practice. *Veterinary Record* 179: 559–560.

Waters, A. (2017). The importance of learning from errors. *Veterinary Record* 181: 521.

Weiss, M., Hansen, T.G., and Engelhardt, T. (2016). Ensuring safe anaesthesia for neonates, infants and young children: what really matters. *BMJ Archives of Disease in Childhood* 101: 650–652.

Whitaker, D.K., Brattebo, G., Smith, A.F., and Staender, S.A.E. (2011). The Helsinki declaration on patient safety in anaesthesiology: putting words into practice. *Best Practice & Research Clinical Anaesthesiology* 25: 277–290.

White, M.C., Randall, K., Capo-Chichi, N.F.E. et al. (2019). Implementation and evaluation of nationwide scale-up of the surgical safety checklist. *British Journal of Surgery* 106: e91–e102.

Self-test Section

1 What are non-technical skills?

2 It is important that checklists:
   A Are very detailed and descriptive
   B Take less than 60 seconds to complete
   C Contain as many steps as possible
   D Focus on unique or uncommon events

3 True or False? If an error would have happened irrespective of the staff member involved, latent, system factors are most likely the root cause and the system should be reviewed and amended accordingly.

3

Pain

LEARNING OBJECTIVES

- To be able to define pain (International Association for the Study of Pain [IASP] definition).
- To be able to outline the neurophysiological pain pathways and different sites for intervention.
- To be able to recognise the importance of pre-emptive analgesia and outline the concept of preventive analgesia.
- To be able to discuss the concept of multimodal analgesia.
- To be familiar with the different classes of analgesic drugs available, their proposed mechanisms of action, and their associated side effects.

3.1 Introduction

Two of the main challenges facing vets are to recognise when an animal is in pain and how to treat that pain adequately.

In 1979, the IASP published a definition of *pain* **as an unpleasant sensory and emotional experience associated with actual or potential tissue damage, or described in terms of such damage**. Since 1996, an accompanying note has been added to this definition, which states: **The inability to communicate in no way negates the possibility that an individual is experiencing pain and is in need of appropriate pain-relieving treatment.**

A 'working definition of animal pain', proposed by Molony and Kent (1997) following extensive work with farm species, was: 'an aversive sensory and emotional experience, representing awareness by the animal of damage to, or threat to the integrity of, its tissues ... producing changes in physiology and behaviour ... which help to reduce or avoid the damage, reduce the likelihood of recurrence and promote recovery'.

Although acute pain can be beneficial because it can help protect against injury and enable healing; chronic unrelenting pain is detrimental to health, physiologically (homeostatically), immunologically, and psychologically and it can result in suffering and distress. Such chronic pain is referred to as maladaptive pain.

3.2 Evolution of Pain

Even in the 'primordial soup' it seems reasonable to assume that organisms that had some way of detecting and reacting to noxious stimuli had an evolutionary advantage, indeed it has been shown that protozoa can respond to certain noxious stimuli. We find similarity between higher order organisms in the anatomy and physiology of their nervous systems, such that it may be reasonable to assume that the way in which they respond to pain is similar.

The expression of pain has probably evolved differently in different species. Social animals (e.g. dogs, monkeys) may cry out in pain to get help from others. Prey species tend to hide pain. Predators preferentially attack weak animals, so it is not in the interests of prey species (e.g. sheep, cattle, horses) to express pain or distress signals. In both groups, however, there are similar increases in glucocorticoid and β-endorphin release when 'painful' or stressful conditions exist.

Veterinary Anaesthesia: Principles to Practice, Second Edition. Alexandra H. A. Dugdale, Georgina Beaumont, Carl Bradbrook, and Matthew Gurney.
© 2020 John Wiley & Sons Ltd. Published 2020 by John Wiley & Sons Ltd.
Companion website: www.wiley.com/go/dugdale/veterinary-anaesthesia

3.3 The Different Types and Qualities of Pain

You may hear pain referred to as:

- Somatic *versus* visceral
- Superficial *versus* deep
- Fast (transmitted by Aδ fibres) *versus* slow (transmitted by C fibres)

3.3.1 The IASP Refers to Different Types of Pain

Nociceptive

- Pain that arises from actual or threatened damage to non-neural tissue and is due to the activation of nociceptors.

Neuropathic

- Pain caused by a lesion or disease of the somatosensory nervous system, either peripherally or centrally.

Nociplastic

- Pain that arises from altered nociception despite no clear evidence of actual or threatened tissue damage causing the activation of peripheral nociceptors or evidence for disease or lesion of the somatosensory system causing the pain.

3.3.2 Pain Components

- **Sensory/discriminative:** allows determination of the site of origin of the pain and the stimulus intensity, duration and quality.
- **Motivational/affective/behavioural:** results in cortical arousal, neuroendocrine responses, limbic system responses (fear/anxiety and behavioural responses), and activation of reflexes, such as the withdrawal reflex. Limbic system responses can feed back to the cortex to enhance the individual's perception of the input. It is important to realise that **fear and anxiety can enhance the perception of pain**.
- **Cognitive/evaluative:** the higher-level information processing that exists in humans and possibly animals.

3.3.3 Pain Signal Acquisition, Processing, and Recognition

Figure 3.1 outlines the following steps:

1) Signal **transduction**: A noxious stimulus (mechanical, thermal, or chemical), is converted into an electrical signal at a nociceptor. Aδ nociceptors are mechano-thermal and rapidly adapting, whereas C fibres are polymodal and slowly adapting. (Polymodal nociceptors respond to a variety of signals: heat, cold, mechanical pressure, chemical.)

Figure 3.1 Simplified pain pathway.

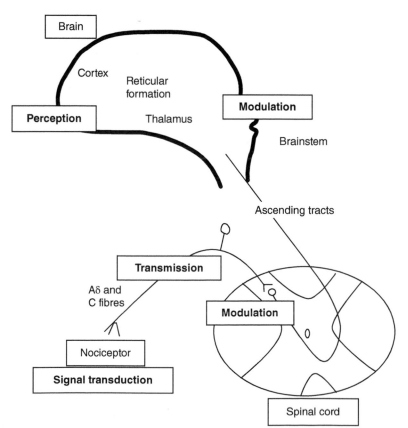

2) **Transmission** of the nerve impulse along the nerve fibre (Aδ or C fibre), to the dorsal horn of the spinal cord.

3) **Modulation** of incoming 'pain information' at various sites within the central nervous system (CNS) (e.g. dorsal horn of spinal cord, brainstem, and higher centres). Acutely, this may be in the form of hypoalgesia (reduced pain sensation), in order to allow an animal to escape from a predator; but more chronically, it can be responsible for 'sensitisation' to pain inputs, e.g. hyperalgesia and allodynia (see below).

4) **Projection:** although Figure 3.1 shows ascending pain information crossing the midline, in more primitive (sub-primate) species, the nociceptive tracts often ascend bilaterally and tend to be more diffuse.

5) Conscious **perception** of pain.

These five steps provide the main sites for drug intervention, as will be discussed below.

Nociception could be termed **physiological pain**. It tends to be **acute** and involves transduction, transmission, and modulation of signals arising from stimulation of nociceptors by noxious stimuli; and when carried to completion, results in the conscious perception of pain. For pain to be perceived, consciousness is required, some degree of brain analysis occurs, emotions may be displayed, and memory and learning occur. Animals under an adequate depth of general anaesthesia are incapable of perceiving painful stimuli, but the first three steps of nociception can still occur. It is, however, good practice to provide antinociception (with drugs that target the earlier stages of the pain pathway) to patients under general anaesthesia.

What has been called **pathological pain** tends to be **chronic** and occurs when excessively intense or prolonged stimuli induce tissue damage that results in extended discomfort and abnormal sensitivity. It can take several forms: including inflammatory, neuropathic, and nociplastic or sympathopathic (i.e. where the autonomic nervous system becomes involved), which are not mutually exclusive.

3.3.3.1   Features of Physiological Pain

- Much is due to Aδ fibre activity.
- The 'pain' is acute, transient, and localised.
- The 'pain' is stimulus-specific and rapidly adaptive (see below).
- One could argue that it has protective functions, in that it may prevent further tissue damage; and it may promote 'learned avoidance' responses.

3.3.3.2   Features of Pathological Pain

- Much is due to C fibre activity that produces a dull ache.
- The 'pain' is persistent/chronic (outlasts the stimulus duration) and diffuse.

- The 'pain' is not stimulus-specific and is slowly adaptive.
- Chronic/maladaptive pain is not generally protective (it offers no useful biological function or survival advantage), but is debilitating and increases patient morbidity.

3.3.3.3   Adaptation to Painful Stimuli

Unlike the situation for most other sensory neurons, the **adaptation that occurs in pain fibres (especially C fibres) tends to be a sensitisation** rather than a fatigue, especially in the situation of pathological pain. It is important to remember that **pain is a dynamic and multidimensional experience** and that neuronal plasticity is important in the 'progression' of pain.

3.4   The Pain Pathway

3.4.1   Afferent Fibres

- Aδ (myelinated) fibres relay 'fast pain' (e.g. mechanical pain, cuts, pin-pricks); sometimes called **epicritic pain**. The conduction velocity is 5–20 m/s.
- C (unmyelinated) fibres relay 'slow pain' (e.g. dull pain, burning pain, aches); sometimes called **protopathic pain**. The conduction velocity is 0.5–1 m/s. (Not all C fibres are nociceptive and a subgroup called pruritoceptors are responsible for itch transduction.)

Aδ and C fibres have peripheral sensory receptors (nociceptors), which respond to various noxious stimuli. These fibres transmit signals from the periphery to the **dorsal horn of the spinal cord** and have their cell bodies in the dorsal root ganglia or trigeminal ganglia. Both fibre types synapse with second-order neurons primarily in Rexed's laminae I (marginal cells) and II (the substantia gelatinosa) of the dorsal horn.

Three basic responses to such incoming signals occur in the dorsal horn:

- The signal may invoke a spinal/segmental reflex (e.g. withdrawal type response) because interneurons may synapse with motor fibres in the ventral roots to form reflex arcs.
- The signal may be projected to the brain via the spinocervicothalamic tract, which is ipsilateral (compared to the spinothalamic tract in primates which is contralateral), to the thalamus, reticular formation, and cortex.
- The signal may undergo some processing (modulation).

The main neurotransmitter between the primary nociceptive afferents and second-order neurons is glutamate, which produces an excitatory signal, but several other neurotransmitters may be co-released, including substance P, aspartate, calcitonin gene related peptide (CGRP), vasoactive intestinal polypeptide (VIP), and nitric oxide (NO).

If the original stimulus was intense enough, or caused enough tissue damage, then an inflammatory reaction will have been initiated. This involves the release of cytokines and inflammatory mediators (prostaglandins [PG], histamine, bradykinin) that result in the typical signs of inflammation: warmth ('calor'), swelling ('tumor'), erythema ('rubor') and pain ('dolor'). The pain occurs because these mediators are **algogens**. Some of them stimulate nociceptors directly to elicit pain (e.g. histamine), and others decrease the threshold of nociceptors at the site of inflammation (e.g. PG), and as time progresses, of nociceptors around the site too.

3.4.2 Hyperalgesia

Hyperalgesia is an increased sensitivity to a normally painful stimulus. It occurs at the site of injury (primary hyperalgesia) due to inflammatory mediators either activating or sensitising the nociceptors (**peripheral sensitisation**), lowering their thresholds for firing, and it spreads to the surrounding non-injured tissues (secondary hyperalgesia) due to events in the spinal cord (**central sensitisation**).

3.4.3 Allodynia

Allodynia is a painful response to a normally innocuous stimulus. *Allodynia* refers to previously 'silent' high threshold mechanoreceptors that become recruited to relay pain information, e.g. when tissue inflammation reduces their thresholds (part of the **peripheral sensitisation**). Besides this peripheral change, there is also a 'central' component to this altered interpretation of information/allodynia (part of the **central sensitisation**).

3.4.4 Gate Control Theory

The sensory nerve synapses in the dorsal horn of the grey matter are the first site where neurotransmitters and neuromodulators influence the further propagation of the signal. This is also where some modulation may occur. The so-called **gate control theory** (Melzack and Wall) (Figure 3.2) was put forward in an attempt to try to explain this. The signal may, or not, then travel up the spinal cord (possibly on the contralateral side, although species differences exist). Most of these ascending pathways are in the spinoreticular and spinothalamic tracts of the spinal cord, and there are probably several levels of 'gating' in these ascending pathways.

If the mechanoreceptor fibre (Aβ) is inactive, the gate is open for onward and upward C fibre transmission. However, activity in the Aβ fibre can close the gate, so that C fibre transmission is interrupted. In simple terms, the gate theory highlights that a painful nerve signal has to 'cross over or

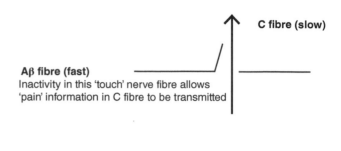

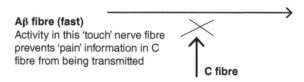

Figure 3.2 Gate control theory.

through' many 'gates' (other synapses) before that signal will be further transmitted. This is why, e.g. when you bang your elbow, it hurts; but if you rub it, it hurts less.

Descending pathways in the spinal cord, both **inhibitory** and **facilitatory**, also exist, and can influence the gating processes.

3.4.5 Neuroplasticity/Neuromodulation

This is how the perception of a painful stimulus changes over time. This is an important feature of the CNS response to pain. There are two main types of adaptation: desensitisation and central sensitisation.

3.4.5.1 Desensitisation
If there is a persistent painful stimulus, and if the animal continuously feels the same degree of pain, then that animal may not be able to behave and function normally. It is physiologically beneficial for the CNS to modify its response to these signals so that the level of pain is decreased, that is for **desensitisation** to occur. This is a more medium- to long-term response to a painful stimulus and **does not always occur**. The mechanisms by which it is mediated are poorly understood but the descending pathways (see below) are thought to be involved. Desensitisation is not widely recognised in the clinical setting.

3.4.5.2 Central Sensitisation
At the level of the dorsal horn, there is an activity-dependent plasticity in response to prolonged or intense noxious stimuli, known as **central sensitisation** (Figure 3.3). This results in augmentation of subsequent signals (to the higher centres) that are not related to the intensity or duration of

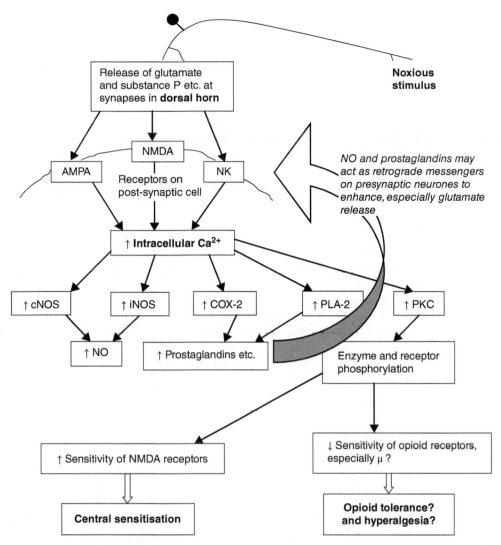

Figure 3.3 Pathway of central sensitisation. AMPA and NMDA receptors are glutamate receptors; NK1 (neurokinin 1) receptor is a substance P receptor; cNOS, constitutive nitric oxide synthase; iNOS, inducible nitric oxide synthase; COX-2, cyclooxygenase 2 (inducible); PLA2, phospholipase A2; PKC, protein kinase C; NO.

the initial stimulus. **Central sensitisation** has been documented in dogs with osteoarthritis (OA) from cruciate ligament disease and hip dysplasia and should be considered in all cases of chronic pain. (Although central sensitisation is initially thought to be an adaptive response to pain that encourages the animal to develop protective behaviour, it may become maladaptive in the long-term.) The mechanisms involved are complex, but we know that N-methyl D-aspartate (NMDA) receptors are key. The result is that any subsequent painful stimulus is likely to be perceived as being more painful. It is this central sensitisation that led to the practice of **pre-emptive analgesia** in which analgesics are given before the pain starts, so that they are working when the noxious stimulus occurs; and **preventive analgesia** whereby analgesics are administered for as long as the pain is expected to last. The result is that any subsequent

pain is easier to control than if analgesic treatment had been delayed until after the noxious stimulus had occurred. Central sensitisation can result in changes to the CNS that may last much longer than minutes or hours.

NMDA receptors control non-specific cation channels (allowing Na^+ and Ca^{2+} influx and K^+ efflux) in nerve fibres and are involved in memory and learning and synaptic plasticity in general. NMDA receptors are unusual because they are both voltage-gated and ligand-gated and both conditions must be satisfied for them to open. In order to open, the receptor requires initial membrane depolarisation (e.g. following opening of other ion channels), which displaces Mg^{2+} from the channel so that glutamate binding can then open it. Glutamate is an excitatory neurotransmitter. Glycine (usually thought of as an inhibitory neurotransmitter) is a co-agonist for the NMDA receptor: its binding promotes glutamate's binding and action. NMDA receptors/channels activate slowly and remain activated (open) for a relatively lengthy time (several hundred milliseconds) so they are well placed for their role in neuroplasticity. Prolonged ion fluxes, especially the influx of calcium (the channel's main permeability) can affect intracellular processes and signalling, including the activation of enzymes, altered gene expression and synthesis and activation of receptors. For the patient, this means increased transmission of signals to higher centres and increased pain perception.

Ketamine, pethidine, and one of methadone's isomers (d-methadone), can antagonise NMDA receptor activation by glutamate. This can prevent central sensitisation and can even reverse it once it has occurred. Ketamine, at subanaesthetic doses, is commonly used in the treatment of chronic pain states. Nitrous oxide and xenon also have some NMDA antagonistic actions, and even benzodiazepines may modulate NMDA receptor activity. In a chronic pain setting both amantadine and memantine are used for their NMDA antagonist effect.

You may hear the term *wind-up*, which many people use interchangeably with *central sensitisation*. However, in the strictest terms, *wind-up* is a laboratory phenomenon, whereby repetitive (low frequency) and prolonged C fibre input to the dorsal horn can result in reduced firing thresholds of dorsal horn neurons. Temporal and spatial summation of depolarisation increases the likelihood of NMDA receptor activation, which then results in enhanced and prolonged depolarisation of dorsal horn neurons, which finally increases the overall response. This wind-up is only seen during the period of actual repetitive stimulation. *Hyperalgesia* strictly refers to a patient's overall exaggerated response to a given painful stimulus; whereas *sensitisation/hypersensitivity* refers to an exaggerated response of an individual neuron to a noxious stimulus.

Non-neuronal cells such as **astrocytes** and **microglia** are also recognised as having a role in the transmission, propagation, and maintenance of pain.

3.4.5.3 Pain Pathways in the Brain

Projection neurons arise from the dorsal horn of the spinal cord and innervate various higher centres that together constitute the pain matrix, including the thalamus, midbrain peri-aqueductal grey (PAG), pontine locus coeruleus (LC), parabrachial area (PBA, at the junction of the midbrain and pons), nucleus of the solitary tract (nucleus tractus solitarius, NTS, in the dorsomedial medulla) and rostroventral medulla (RVM), which also contains the nucleus raphe magnus (NRM), which lies between the caudal pons and the rostral medulla. From the thalamus, billions of nerve fibres run to all parts of the brain including the cerebral cortex (where the signal is probably first perceived as pain), the reticular activating system (sleep/wake centre), and the limbic system (emotion). All these neuronal connections and communications result in what we experience as pain, but they also influence further transmission and interpretation of the signal. For example, the limbic system that deals with emotion has a huge influence over perception of pain.

3.4.5.4 Descending Control Pathways

There are a number of descending control pathways (Figure 3.4) through which the brain can exert a modulatory effect on nerve fibres involved in the transmission of pain. We usually talk of descending inhibitory pathways, but descending facilitatory pathways also exist.

The four tiers of descending modulation are considered to be:

- Cortex and thalamus.
- Peri-aqueductal grey (PAG) matter in the midbrain.
- PBA (at junction of midbrain and pons), LC (in the pons), NRM (located in the caudal pons and rostral medulla), nucleus tractus solitarius (NTS, in dorsomedial medulla), and the wider RVM (that contains important ON–OFF serotonergic cells).
- Caudal medulla oblongata and spinal cord (dorsal horns).

Descending control plays a role in acute and chronic pain and further understanding shows the interplay between cognitive functions and homeostatic mechanisms as well as incoming nociceptive signals. One important part of the brain that controls some of these pathways is the PAG matter in the middle of the brain, which has a high concentration of opioid receptors. The PAG receives input from the somatosensory and anterior cingulate cortices, the amygdala, thalamus, and hypothalamus as well as direct nociceptive input from ascending pathways. The RVM is the final relay point where ON cells facilitate nociception and OFF cells inhibit it. Although descending inhibition is thought to work on many levels of the CNS, it is thought to be most important at the spinal level. The power of this descending inhibition is great, allowing people to run away from a crashed car that is on fire, despite having suffered broken legs in the crash; this is called **stress-induced analgesia** and depends primarily upon endocannabinoids.

The descending pathways are poorly understood but we know that a wide range of neurotransmitters are involved, such as gamma-aminobutyric acid (GABA), serotonin, glutamate, noradrenaline (norepinephrine), dopamine, acetylcholine, adenosine, and endorphins. Noradrenaline plays a role in pain inhibition through activation of spinal

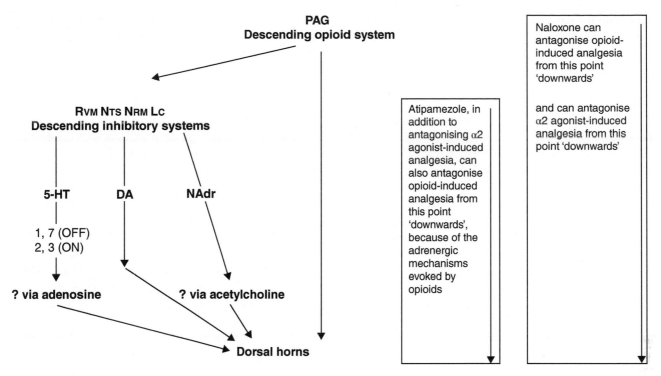

Figure 3.4 Some descending pathways.

α2 adrenoreceptors. Serotonergic neurons in the RVM influence nociceptive processing depending upon the serotonin receptor sub-type that is activated; however, this mostly favours facilitation. Activity in the RVM also influences spinal NMDA activity and may play a role in central sensitisation.

These neurotransmitters are an important focus for the development of novel pharmacological analgesic agents. The descending pathways have also helped us understand how current analgesics may work. We now know that, e.g. nitrous oxide stimulates the endogenous opioid system; which stimulates the descending spinal noradrenergic system (involving α2 receptors); which stimulates a cholinergic system, resulting in analgesia via modulation at the dorsal horns. You are probably familiar with how closely the effects of opioids and α2 agonists resemble each other; this is because the opioidergic and noradrenergic systems are closely linked (Figure 3.4). Figure 3.3 gives a more complex overview in which you can see why NMDA antagonists are so useful in preventing central sensitisation, and even reversing it, and they appear to prevent the development of tolerance to opioids and may even reverse it.

3.4.5.5 Opioid-Induced Hyperalgesia (OIH)

In both experimental and clinical settings, very high (and also clinical) doses of full μ agonist opioids (fentanyl, morphine, remifentanil) can increase NMDA receptor responsiveness and create hypersensitivity to pain (which is associated with a 'tolerance' to opioids). Giving more opioid in these circumstance does not produce analgesia, but hyperalgesia. The NMDA receptor is thought to play a role in the development of OIH because NMDA receptor antagonists (ketamine) have been shown to reduce the hyperalgesia. Does this mean that we should be careful of using opioids for pre-emptive analgesia? It probably means that we should be careful of using very high doses of opioids, and for long periods (especially if patients are not in that much pain), and perhaps be careful not to use very high doses of opioids in premedication before noxious stimulation occurs, unless we combine their use with an NMDA antagonist (e.g. low dose ketamine). We must practice balanced analgesia. We must also ask, however, whether persistent pain is simply the effect of inadequate analgesia or could it actually be OIH.

3.4.5.6 Visceral and Referred Pain

Visceral nociceptors differ from somatic nociceptors in not having differentiated special endings; which partly explains why visceral pain is usually diffuse and poorly localised. But many mechanoreceptors are also present in viscera with both low and high thresholds. Visceral nociceptors show a graded response to increasing stimulus intensity (e.g. distension, ischaemia, inflammation, chemical), i.e. **visceral stimuli are intensity-coded** ranging from physiological to noxious. The viscera have a low density of innervation (only 7% of spinal afferents project from viscera), and the nerves have huge and overlapping receptive fields. The innervation density of skin compared with viscera is around 100 : 1, with the ratio of Aδ : C fibres for skin being 1 : 2, compared with viscera, where the ratio is 1 : 8–10. C fibres are truly polymodal, they can transduce mechanical, chemical, and thermal information. Temporal and spatial summation of visceral 'nociceptor' activity is important.

Visceral organs may have two different extrinsic sensory afferent pathways, e.g. bladder and distal colon send signals in the pelvic and splanchnic nerves, via their respective ganglia, to the dorsal horn. In the spinal cord, visceral afferents arborise widely and converge on the same second order spinal neurons as other non-visceral (somatic) sensory nerves, which is referred to as **somato-visceral convergence** of information. Visceral afferents may be associated with autonomic fibres (and some use the same ganglia). In some disease states autonomic effects may accompany visceral nociception.

Somato-visceral convergence explains the concept of referred pain (synalgia). This visceral nociception is not perceived at the site of origin, rather at an adjacent or distant somatic site. The pain is usually referred to superficial somatic structures innervated by the same segmental spinal nerve that supplies the affected viscus (or up to one or two segments either side). For example, angina pectoris is the upper arm pain associated with the visceral (heart) pain.

3.4.6 Pre-emptive and Preventive Analgesia

It is recognised that if analgesia (true analgesia being better than hypoalgesia) can be provided before a noxious stimulus is applied, then any subsequent pain experienced is of lesser intensity and duration, and is more easily controllable with analgesic drugs because the initiation and establishment of peripheral and central sensitisation is prevented (or at least reduced). This is called **pre-emptive analgesia** and has been documented in dogs with both opioids and non-steroidal anti-inflammatory drugs (NSAIDs).

A one-off dose of analgesic/hypoalgesic given before surgery, however, may have only a limited duration of action and may not outlast the pain and inflammation that follows surgical intervention, and therefore will not continue to pre-empt all post-operative pain. It is for this reason that analgesia should be provided before surgery and should be continued into the post-operative period for as long as the pain is likely to be present. The concept of this **provision and continuation of pre-emptive analgesia** is what is called **preventive analgesia**. In this case, both the establishment and the maintenance of peripheral and central sensitisation are prevented or reduced. The aim here is to provide analgesia for as long as the pet is painful.

3.4.7 Other Aspects of Pain

The **placebo effect** occurs when a patient obtains pain relief after taking a pharmacologically inactive or inert compound. About 20% of patients respond to a placebo analgesic; demonstrating a strong psychological component to pain.

The **nocebo effect** can modulate the outcome of a given therapy in a negative way, as do placebo effects in a positive way. Underlying mechanisms are both psychological and possibly neurobiological, and can actually be triggered by a clinician explaining the effects of a drug to a patient.

Psychological pain is the pain experienced by a patient when there is no apparent pathology, although it usually follows a previous painful incident (now look back at the definition of *pain*).

Phantom pain occurs when an individual perceives pain from a part of the body that has been removed (e.g. limb, kidney, tooth). There have been a few case reports of the phantom complex/phenomenon in animals (see Chapters 12–14 on local anaesthetics and Chapter 43 on orthopaedic concerns).

3.5 Analgesia

- *Analgesia* is defined as a lack of pain sensation.
- *Hypoalgesia* is defined as a reduction of pain sensation to a more tolerable level.
- *Antihyperalgesia* is defined as the prevention, and/or reversal of, sensitisation to pain.

By definition then, analgesia is the absence of all pain, but most of the methods we use to try to achieve analgesia are only partially successful, so we only really effect hypoalgesia. The term *analgesia* is often used loosely to mean both true analgesia and also hypoalgesia. We probably should be using the terms: *hypoalgesics* (e.g. for opioids, which raise the threshold to pain AND alter its perception); *antihyperalgesics* (for drugs that help to reset increased central sensitisation such as NSAIDs and NMDA antagonists); and *true analgesics* (e.g. for local anaesthetics). For patients under general anaesthesia, and therefore unable to consciously perceive pain, the term *antinociception* is preferred to analgesia or hypoalgesia.

We can achieve analgesia/ hypoalgesia/antinociception by:

- **Pharmacological agents**
- **Surgical intervention (e.g. neurectomy)**
- **Nerve stimulation (e.g.** transcutaneous electrical nerve stimulation [TENS], **acupuncture)**

3.5.1 Pharmacological Agents

These can be aimed at different points along the pain pathway as outlined below.

3.5.1.1 Interrupt the Pain Pathway at the Site of Noxious Signal Transduction

Local anaesthetics will prevent nociceptor activation. Anti-inflammatories (e.g. **NSAIDs**) will also reduce nociceptor stimulation by reducing the amount of inflammatory mediators in the 'sensitising soup' produced at the site of tissue injury. We also know that α2 receptors and opioid receptors are expressed in inflamed tissues, so **opioids** and **α2 agonists** may have peripheral actions too. We are also learning that drugs like corticosteroids and NSAIDs have central actions in addition to their peripheral actions.

3.5.1.2 Interrupt the Pain Pathway at the Site/s of Signal Transmission

These sites are the peripheral and central neurons. **Local anaesthetics** prevent nerve conduction and can be used for, e.g. nerve blocks, ring blocks, and neuraxial anaesthesia.

3.5.1.3 Affect Modulation of the Signal

This reduces 'onward' transmission/projection to higher centres by affecting activity at receptors in the dorsal horns and higher centres, including opioid receptors, α2 adrenoreceptors, NMDA receptors and other ion channels. **Opioids, α2 agonists** and **NMDA receptor antagonists** can be administered systemically or neuraxially. **Tramadol, tapentadol, tricyclic antidepressants,** and **anticonvulsants** (e.g. **gabapentinoids**) can also be used.

3.5.1.4 Reduce Perception of Incoming Signals in the Higher Centres

This can be achieved by anxiolysis, sedation, or general anaesthesia, using **anxiolytics/sedatives** (phenothiazines, α2 agonists, benzodiazepines, trazodone, gabapentin), **opioids** (provide some sedation), and **injectable and inhalational general anaesthetic agents**.

This chapter focuses on the main groups of analgesic drugs that veterinarian anaesthetists are likely to come across.

3.5.2 Multimodal ('Balanced') Analgesia

This concept has two components:

1) The pain pathway can be interrupted at more than one site; and the more sites that can be targeted, the better will be the overall analgesia provision.
2) To maximise the analgesia provision using drugs from different classes with complementary analgesic activities, whilst simultaneously minimising the overall side effects for the patient.

3.5.3 Sequential Analgesia

Sequential analgesia was once commonly used, especially in small rodents. It refers to the administration of a potent μ agonist (e.g. morphine) pre-operatively, which was then (especially after 'mild' surgery), partially antagonised post-operatively (e.g. by buprenorphine or butorphanol), in the hope of minimising the side effects of the full μ agonist (drowsiness), whilst maintaining decent analgesia (by the partial agonist or agonist/antagonist). This is of interest academically however not commonly used in clinical practice.

3.6 Opioids

Throughout most of recorded history, the opium poppy (*Papaver somniferum*) has been used to provide pain relief. Morphine is still the mainstay of analgesic therapy for severe pain in human medicine, although with a more recent focus on opioid-sparing, given the adverse effects seen with these drugs in both the acute period and longer-term effects (see opioid-induced hyperalgesia in section 3.4.5.5.).

Terminology for this group of compounds includes:

- **Opiates** are drugs derived from the opium poppy (e.g. morphine, papaveretum, codeine).
- **Opioids** are drugs that work in a similar manner to morphine.
- **Narcotic analgesics** are basically any of the opioids as they provide analgesia, but can also induce a state similar to sedation or euphoria (a sense of well-being) called narcosis.

Opioids exert their effects by binding to opioid receptors. Originally it was thought that opioid receptors could only be found in the CNS. It is now known that they also occur in the periphery, such as in the gastrointestinal (GI) tract and in the joints (especially with inflammation). Opioid receptor distribution in the CNS (and probably elsewhere) differs among species (and probably to some extent among individuals of the same species), so that different species/individuals may respond differently to different opioids and/or may require different doses. For instance, μ receptor agonists in humans tend to cause narcosis, whereas in horses (and cats) they can cause increased locomotor activity and excitement (in large doses). Another example is that some birds and reptiles have more κ-receptors in their CNS and so respond better to κ-receptor agonist than μ-receptor agonist analgesics.

3.6.1 Opioid Receptors

The known receptor types are listed below (although listed by the chronological order in which they were cloned, the traditional classification [Greek letters: δ, κ, μ] is most popular, although the terms delta opioid [DOP]; kappa opioid [KOP]; and mu opioid [MOP] receptors are also acceptable):

- **OP-1 (δ, delta, DOP) receptor** (*δ1, δ2*).
- **OP-2 (κ, kappa, KOP) receptor** (*κ1, κ2*).
- **OP-3 (μ, mu, MOP) receptor** (*μ1, μ2, μ3*).
- **σ, sigma** is no longer classified as an opioid receptor. It is now thought to be closely associated with NMDA receptors, perhaps the phencyclidine (PCP) binding site.
- **ε, epsilon** is the theoretical receptor for the endogenous β-endorphins, but has only been found in rat vas deferens; its existence elsewhere has yet to be proven.
- **Nociceptin opioid (NOP) receptor/novel opioid receptor-like 1 (ORL-1) receptor/Orphanin FQ peptide receptor/OP4**: the role of this receptor is uncertain, but it may help set the thresholds to pain, and may be involved in neuronal plasticity and tolerance to opioids. (Note that the old *κ3* receptor is now thought to be NOP receptor.)

The receptors shown in italics are some of the subtypes of each receptor that have been identified, although their clinical relevance remains to be determined.

The different receptors mediate their effects mainly via G-protein interactions, resulting in, e.g. membrane ion permeability changes or intracellular enzyme activation or inhibition.

3.6.2 Endogenous Ligands

- Pro-opiomelanocortin → β endorphin → acts on MOP (μ) and DOP (δ) receptors.

- Pro-enkephalin → (Met)enkephalin, (Leu)enkephalin and metorphamide → act on DOP (δ), [KOP (κ) and MOP (μ)] receptors.
- Pro-dynorphin → dynorphin A, dynorphin B, α-neoendorphin, β-neoendorphin → act on KOP (κ), [(DOP (δ) and MOP (μ)] receptors.
- Unknown precursor → endomorphin 1 and endomorphin 2 → act on MOP (μ) receptor.
- Pre-pro N/O FQ → N/O FQ → acts on NOP receptor.

The location of the receptors in the CNS determines their effects. In the spinal cord (dorsal horn) opioid receptor activation inhibits the release of primary pain neurotransmitters (e.g. glutamate, substance P). There are a large number of opioid receptors in the PAG matter where their activation stimulates descending pain control systems, so opioids are very effective against pain, and especially C fibre second pain or dull pain. There are not so many opioid receptors in the reticular formation ('state of arousal' centre) and opioids are less effective against sharp pain (the reticular formation is an important reception site for sharp pain information). Opioid receptors are, however, found in the limbic system and are probably involved in the emotional aspect of pain. It seems that NOP receptors and N/O FQ are also involved in pain information processing.

3.6.3 Opioid Effects

In addition to analgesia, opioids produce a number of other effects, which differ between agents and species: some of these are outlined in Table 3.1. All opioids tend to produce analgesia at lower doses than those required for sedation. Animals in pain tend to suffer fewer/less severe side effects than non-painful animals.

Table 3.1 Comparison of opioid receptor effects.

	MOP (μ) receptor	KOP (κ) receptor	DOP (δ) receptor
Analgesia			
• Supraspinal	+++	–	–
• Spinal	++	+	++
• Peripheral	++	++	–
Respiratory depression	+++	–? Antitussive	++? Antitussive
Pupil	Miosis (dog); mydriasis (cat, horse)	Miosis	Mydriasis
Gastrointestinal motility	↓↓	↓?	↓↓
Euphoria	+++	–	–
Dysphoria	–	+++	–
Sedation	++	++	–
Dependence	+++	+	–

3.6.3.1 Respiratory Depression

Opioids reduce the sensitivity of the respiratory centre to changes in blood carbon dioxide tension and can cause respiratory depression. This effect does not seem to be as great a problem in the common veterinary species as it is for humans, unless the potent MOP (μ) receptor agonists, such as fentanyl, alfentanil, and remifentanil are administered in high doses intravenously.

Potent MOP (μ) receptor agonists, such as fentanyl, can occasionally cause chest-wall rigidity ('wooden chest'), a sort of splinting of the respiratory (and sometimes also the abdominal) muscles, which can compromise ventilation. Artificial ventilation may be necessary, but may also be difficult to provide effectively unless naloxone and/or a neuromuscular blocker is administered. This is documented in humans, but studies in dogs have been unable to replicate this effect, even at high doses, although anecdotal reports have suggested that it may, sporadically, occur.

3.6.3.2 Cardiovascular Effects

Cardiovascular effects are wide ranging and depend upon the agent and species, the most common being bradycardia which is dose- and opioid-dependent. Some opioids (particularly morphine and pethidine), can cause histamine release that may lead to hypotension (which may result in compensatory reflex tachycardia). Morphine can cause a centrally mediated (vagomimetic) hypotension and bradycardia. Etorphine and carfentanil can cause massive hypertension.

3.6.3.3 Gastrointestinal Effects

In animals that can vomit, many opioids act on the chemoreceptor trigger zone (CTZ; not protected by the blood–brain barrier) in the medulla (CNS) to initiate vomiting. However, most opioids also act on the vomiting centre itself (inside the blood–brain barrier) to produce anti-emetic effects. The more fat-soluble the opioid (e.g. methadone compared with morphine) the more likely it is to rapidly cross the blood–brain barrier, so its emetic activity (action in the CTZ) is offset by its anti-emetic activity (action in the vomiting centre), so no vomiting occurs.

In general, with the exception of pethidine (see below), opioids increase the smooth muscle tone of the GI tract, resulting in an overall reduction in propulsive peristaltic activity and a risk of post-operative ileus. Sphincter tone is also increased. Sometimes evacuation (defecation) occurs before sphincter tone increases. Pethidine is spasmolytic due to its anticholinergic (parasympatholytic) effects. It is also spasmolytic on the biliary and pancreatic duct sphincters. (Dogs probably do not have a true sphincter of Oddi, whereas cats do.)

3.6.3.4 Urinary Effects

Opioids, particularly MOP (μ) receptor agonists, tend to cause urinary retention, whether administered systemically or neuraxially. Although the mechanisms are incompletely understood, it appears that a decrease in detrusor muscle tone is at least partly responsible.

3.6.3.5 Temperature

There have been reports of increased body temperatures after opioid administration, especially in cats, horses, and cattle. The mechanisms are not fully understood but alongside opioid effects on the thermoregulatory centre, species, individual patient, and environmental factors likely also play a role.

3.6.3.6 Metabolism

Metabolism is hepatic, with biliary and urinary excretion of the metabolites, so with any active metabolites there is the potential for entero-hepatic recycling.

3.6.3.7 Pruritus

Although generally uncommon following systemic opioid administration, pruritus can occur as a complication of neuraxial opioid administration. Following systemic administration, it appears that direct activation of peripheral mast cell/basophil degranulation may be caused by opioids, a response which can be reduced by administration of anti-histamines (H_1 blockers); although true anaphylaxis may also occasionally occur, which may be life-threatening. Pruritus following neuraxial opioid administration, however, appears to be caused by a central MOP (μ) receptor-mediated effect, as naloxone is effective in its treatment.

3.6.3.8 Ocular

Opioids reduce the blink rate in several species and corneal lubrication is advised.

3.6.4 Classification of Opioids

Opioids can be classified according to their chemical structure. The phenanthrene family includes morphine, hydromorphone, oxymorphone, diamorphine (heroin), codeine, buprenorphine, and butorphanol. The benzomorphans include pentazocine. The phenylheptylamines include methadone. The phenylpiperidines include pethidine, fentanyl, alfentanil, remifentanil, and sufentanil. The phenylpropylamines include tramadol and tapentadol.

Opioids may also be classified according to whether they are naturally occurring, semi-synthetic, or synthetic. Naturally occurring opioids include morphine, codeine, thebaine, and papaverine. Semi-synthetic opioids include diamorphine and buprenorphine. Synthetic compounds include pethidine, methadone, fentanyl, alfentanil, remifentanil, tramadol, and tapentadol.

Opioids are, however, classified for clinical use depending upon the receptors they mainly act upon and their effects on those receptors. However, many opioids have effects on more than one receptor type as shown in Table 3.2.

The terms *receptor affinity* and *potency* can be confusing when applied to the opioids. Affinity for receptor types is shown in Table 3.2, but an opioid's affinity for a receptor does not give any information about its efficacy. For example, naloxone (an antagonist) has the same (and probably slightly greater) affinity for the MOP (μ) receptor as morphine (an agonist); but they have opposite effects.

When discussing potency, the context should be clarified. Potency can be described in terms of affinity for a receptor or in terms of clinical efficacy (dose required for a certain effect, e.g. ED_{50}), as in Table 3.3. The more potent an opioid is, the lower the dose required for a given effect.

Alfentanil has a more rapid onset and shorter duration of action than fentanyl. The more rapid onset is because its pKa is lower. The shorter duration is because its volume of distribution is less (it is more protein bound and less lipid soluble), which allows more rapid clearance; and it is not taken up by the lungs. It also has no active metabolites, whereas fentanyl has a partially active metabolite norfentanyl. Fentanyl has the greater lipid solubility and can accumulate in fatty tissues.

3.6.4.1 Full MOP (μ) Receptor Agonists
3.6.4.1.1 Morphine
Dose: 0.1–1.0 mg/kg (lower end of range for cats and horses) IM, IV, SC

Morphine is the 'gold standard' analgesic to which others are compared. It can cause histamine release if administered IV. The dose interval is two to four hours (dogs, horses); four to six hours (cats) after IM or IV administration. Morphine has poor bioavailability if administered orally. It can cause vomiting. It can also be administered neuraxially and intra-articularly. Cats have poor glucuronyl transferase activity, so there is slow glucuronidation of morphine; and they tend to produce less morphine-6-glucuronide than morphine-3-glucuronide. Morphine-6-glucuronide is an even more potent analgesic than the parent morphine. Morphine-3-glucuronide is inactive (or may have some antagonistic properties).

Table 3.2 Relative receptor affinities of some opioids.

	MOP (μ) receptor	KOP (κ) receptor	DOP (δ) receptor
Pethidine	++	+/−	−
Morphine	+++	+/−	+/−
Methadone	+++	−	−
Fentanyl	+++	−	−(+)
Alfentanil	+++	−	−
Etorphine	+++	++	++
Buprenorphine	+++ (partial agonist)	++ (antagonist)	+/−
Butorphanol	++ (agonist/antagonist)	++ (agonist)	−
Naloxone	+++ (antagonist)	++ (antagonist)	+ (antagonist)

Table 3.3 Relative analgesic efficacies (partly explained in terms of access to central opioid receptors).

Analgesic efficacy	% protein binding	Drug	pKa	Lipid solubility
1	30	Morphine	7.9	Low
1/10	70	Pethidine	8.5	Medium
100	80	Fentanyl	8.4	Very high
10–25	90	Alfentanil	6.5	High
1000	90	Sufentanil	8	Very high
50	70–90	Remifentanil	7.1	Medium

3.6.4.1.2 Pethidine (meperidine)

Dose: 3.5–10 mg/kg IM, SC (not IV because of potential histamine release)

Pethidine is less potent than morphine (about 1/10th). Duration of effect 45–60+ minutes in dogs (at about 5 mg/kg), probably nearer 120 minutes in cats (at about 10 mg/kg) (the dose interval is often quoted as 1–2 hours), and duration probably nearer to 30 minutes in horses and cattle. It has anticholinergic spasmolytic effects. Pethidine is said to be vagolytic (whereas other opioids tend to be vagomimetic), and is supposed, therefore, not to lower the heart rate; although this supposed vagolytic effect may be partly due to histamine release and the reflex tachycardic response to a fall in arterial blood pressure. There are, however, conflicting reports of the effects of pethidine on heart rate. A reduction in heart rate, reported with high (10 mg/kg) doses, may be due to pethidine's agonistic action on α2B receptors, which results in peripheral vasoconstriction with subsequent increase in arterial blood pressure followed by reflex bradycardia. Pethidine also has some direct negative inotropic effect (via calcium channel blockade) at doses >3.5 mg/kg, but this may have little clinical relevance. One of its metabolites, norpethidine, has some analgesic activity and can cause seizures at high doses, but this is highly unlikely to be a problem with clinical usage. Pethidine also has local anaesthetic-like activity; and is antagonistic at NMDA receptors.

3.6.4.1.3 Methadone

Dose: 0.1–0.4+ mg/kg IM, IV, SC (0.1–0.5 mg/kg for cats)

Methadone is clinically very similar to morphine, except it does not tend to initiate vomiting because of its greater lipid solubility, so it crosses the blood–brain barrier to produce anti-emetic effects in the vomiting centre at the same time that it reaches the CTZ (outside the blood–brain barrier) where it has emetic effects. (Morphine reaches the CTZ much earlier than the vomiting centre, so emesis occurs initially.) This also means that the peak activity is quicker after methadone (about 5 minutes after IV administration) than after morphine (about 10–20 minutes after IV administration). Methadone may have a longer duration of action than morphine and it is slightly cumulative, despite having no active metabolites, due to its high lipid solubility and ability to cause some hepatic enzyme inhibition. Its NMDA antagonistic effects (d-isomer [S-methadone] only) may be useful; but the majority of analgesia comes from the l-isomer (R-methadone), which has agonist activity at MOP (μ) receptors. Measurable plasma concentrations have been demonstrated following the SC route of administration, but have not been correlated with analgesia to date, probably because plasma concentrations do not necessarily reflect the effect-site concentrations.

3.6.4.1.4 Papaveretum

Dose: 0.2–1.0 mg/kg IM (0.1–0.3 mg/kg for cats)

This is a mixture of morphine and other opiate alkaloids. Its effects are very similar to morphine. Papaveretum can cause histamine release if given IV. It appears to provide a very effective neuroleptanalgesic combination along with acepromazine for aggressive animals.

3.6.4.1.5 Fentanyl

Dose: 0.001–0.005 mg/kg IV

Fentanyl is a very potent analgesic and is useful for controlling intra-operative pain. It has a fast onset of action (within 1–2 minutes), and a short effective half-life of about 10 minutes making it suitable for repeated boluses or infusions, at least in the short- to medium-term. It is, however, a potent respiratory depressant, so that mechanical ventilation is often required in anaesthetised patients. It also tends to cause bradycardia which may require treatment with anticholinergics. Fentanyl has a very large volume of distribution and long elimination half-life due to its high fat solubility, such that too many repeated doses or too prolonged an infusion, may result in accumulation of the drug.

Fentanyl is combined with fluanisone (a butyrophenone) in the product **Hypnorm**™ (marketed as a neuroleptic anaesthetic/analgesic for rabbits, rats, mice, and guinea pigs).

Transdermal fentanyl patches that slowly release fentanyl at a constant rate are available; the fentanyl then being readily absorbed across the skin. The 'dose rate' required is 2–5 μg/kg/h; and patches are available with release rates of 12.5, 25, 50, 75, and 100 μg/h (corresponding to patches with fentanyl contents of 1.25, 5, 7.5, and 10 mg). For patch application, the hair should be shaved off to ensure that the patch actually contacts the skin; the dorsum of the neck is a good place; and the edges of the patch can be secured with tissue glue before a light bandage is applied. Heavy bandaging may result in local vasodilation secondary to a thermal insulating effect, which may result in too rapid drug absorption. After patch application in dogs, peak plasma concentrations take about 20 hours to be achieved and last for 72 hours; in cats, plasma concentrations take 12 hours to peak, and patches last for 5 days. Beware local skin lesions and the effects of, e.g. heat pads, which cause local vasodilation and increase absorption. For horses, one 10 mg patch per 150 kg body mass is suggested; onset time is about 1–3 hours and duration about 32–48 hours.

Alfentanil, sufentanil, and remifentanil are synthetic analogues of fentanyl with even shorter half-lives and can be administered as boluses and infusions intraoperatively for analgesia. Remifentanil is metabolised by non-specific plasma and red blood cell cholinesterases, and its elimination is therefore independent of hepatic function, which is very useful in cases with hepatic disease. However, its duration of action is so short that when an infusion is terminated, other analgesics must be 'on board' to ensure continuation of analgesia.

3.6.4.1.6 Etorphine

This is an extremely potent MOP (μ) receptor agonist reputedly having 10000 times the analgesic potency of morphine. It is a highly dangerous drug in the case of accidental self-administration, and its use should not be contemplated unless antagonists are available. In the UK, etorphine gained notoriety as part of the cocktail that made up 'Large Animal Immobilon'. Immobilon™ is only available in packs that also contain its antagonist, Revivon™ (diprenorphine).

3.6.4.2 Partial MOP (μ) Receptor Agonists
3.6.4.2.1 Buprenorphine

Dose: 0.005–0.02 mg/kg IM, IV, SC, or oral (buccal) transmucosal (OTM)

Buprenorphine has a very high affinity for MOP (μ) receptors, but is generally considered to have only partial agonist activity at these receptors. In 2008, however, a consensus group concluded that, at clinical doses, buprenorphine behaves as a full MOP (μ) receptor agonist as regards analgesia, whereas it behaves as a partial agonist (displaying a ceiling effect) for respiratory depression, which usefully limits this particular opioid side effect. Interestingly, work in dogs has demonstrated no additional analgesia with 0.04 mg/kg buprenorphine versus 0.02 mg/kg, perhaps defining a change from full to partial agonist activity, and the existence of a ceiling effect, between these doses. Buprenorphine has also been reported to have a bell-shaped dose–response curve, where very high (higher than likely to be used clinically) doses produce lesser analgesic effects than lower doses, possibly because partial agonist activity begins to offset full agonist activity at these huge doses. Finally, some sources report an antagonistic action at KOP (κ) receptors.

Buprenorphine is licenced for use in dogs, cats, and horses. It has a slow onset time (about 30 minutes), but a correspondingly long duration of action of about 6–8 hours. It has shorter durations of action in some pain models and some other species (about two hours in sheep). The drug has poor oral bioavailability (if swallowed) because of first-pass metabolism, but is well absorbed in cats following OTM administration of the solution intended for injection at 0.02 mg/kg. Analgesia was poorer when 0.01 mg/kg was used. Unfortunately, similarly good OTM absorption does not occur in dogs because of their different salivary

pH, although there are reports of buprenorphine being delivered OTM at 0.12 mg/kg providing analgesia similar to IV 0.02 mg/kg in dogs. Two recent formulations of buprenorphine have been released in the UK for sublingual administration: 0.2 mg/ml (10 ml); and 0.8 mg/ml (30 ml). Horses have similar salivary pH to cats (~9), and OTM administration offers a useful alternative route for administration in needle-shy animals. Buprenorphine patches (70 µg/h) have also been evaluated in dogs for transdermal delivery and have been shown to provide comparable analgesia to SC 0.02 mg/kg buprenorphine with both groups documenting analgesia compared to no treatment.

3.6.4.3 Agonist–Antagonists
3.6.4.3.1 Butorphanol

Dose: 0.2–0.5 mg/kg IM, IV, SC, dogs and cats; (0.05–0.2 mg/kg horses)

This drug is the source of much confusion in anaesthesia and pharmacology textbooks. It is generally considered to be an agonist–antagonist with affinity for both MOP (μ) and KOP (κ) receptors. It has weak partial agonist effects (and therefore, in the presence of full μ agonists, can demonstrate antagonistic effects) on MOP (μ) receptors and mainly agonist effects on KOP (κ) receptors. In the majority of studies, it also has a short duration of action of about 45 minutes (but may be longer, up to 1–2 hours, even up to 5 hours, depending upon dose, species, and circumstance). Butorphanol is also a potent antitussive and it was first licenced for this use.

Butorphanol is now commonly used in the UK in various combinations with α2 agonists (i.e. medetomidine/ketamine/butorphanol combinations in small animals, especially cats; and α2-agonist/butorphanol combinations in horses). Butorphanol has been associated with excitement and dysphoria in horses, dogs, and cats. Whereas dysphoria is more likely following butorphanol; euphoria is more likely after buprenorphine. Nevertheless, and especially in combination with acepromazine, α2 agonists, or benzodiazepines, butorphanol appears to have synergistic sedative effects.

Although in theory butorphanol and buprenorphine are more potent analgesics than morphine (two to five times), pharmacological studies have shown that the agonist-antagonists tend to have a ceiling effect for analgesia, beyond which higher doses do not provide greater analgesia. Full MOP (μ) agonists should therefore be chosen for patients in severe pain.

3.6.4.4 MOP (μ) Receptor Antagonists
3.6.4.4.1 Naloxone

Dose: 0.04–1.0 mg/kg

Naloxone is a pure antagonist with affinity for all three opioid receptors. It is used mainly to antagonise the effects of full or partial MOP (μ) receptor agonists. **It has a short duration of action of less than an hour so repeated doses may be required**.

3.6.4.4.2 Others

Peripherally-acting mu-opioid receptors antagonists (PAMORAs), such as methyl-naltrexone and alvimopan, have been administered in the hope of reducing the peripheral (principally, GI), side effects of opioids, without being able to cross the blood–brain barrier to reduce their analgesic effects.

3.6.5 Clinical Use of Opioids

There are a number of applications where opioids may be used in veterinary medicine:

- Treatment of pain
- Neuroleptanalgesia (see Chapter 4 on premedication)
- As part of a **balanced analgesia** regimen (**multimodal pain therapy**)
- As part of a **balanced anaesthesia** regimen
- As neuraxial analgesics (see Chapters 12, 14 & 16 on local/regional anaesthetic/analgesic techniques)
- As antitussives
- As spasmolytics (pethidine)
- To decrease gut motility (antidiarrhoeals, e.g. codeine)

There are two main considerations before using opioids. The first (apart from choosing the right drug at the right dose), is to make sure there are no contra-indications for use such as respiratory depression, increased intra-cranial pressure, oesophageal, or biliary/pancreatic duct obstruction. The second involves the legal implications, as many opioids are controlled drugs. Several opioids have NMDA antagonist effects when tested at supraclinical doses, meaning this effect is likely not achieved at the clinical doses quoted above, however, may be achieved with neuraxial use.

3.7 Corticosteroids

Corticosteroids are extremely effective anti-inflammatory drugs and as such, can be thought of as having analgesic properties. It is controversial as to whether corticosteroids have any direct analgesic action. They are included in this chapter because clinically they can be a potent tool in some circumstances.

The effects of corticosteroids include:

- Altered carbohydrate, lipid, and protein metabolism
- Altered fluid and electrolyte balance
- Immunosuppression
- Anti-inflammatory action (inhibit PLA2)
- Inhibit catechol-O-methyl transferase, and up-regulate β adrenergic receptor expression to facilitate the effects of catecholamines

3.7.1 Anti-Inflammatory Actions

Glucocorticoids enter the cell and bind to cytoplasmic receptors. The steroid–receptor complex then enters the cell nucleus where it affects expression of various genes.

Depending upon the cell, steroids can have a multitude of anti-inflammatory effects:

- Corticosteroids enhance the synthesis of lipocortin 1, which **inhibits PLA2**, therefore there will be a **reduction of PLA2 products**, i.e. a decrease in arachidonic acid and platelet activating factor (PAF) production. (PAF is a vasodilator, increases vascular permeability and is a potent chemotaxin.) Arachidonic acid is a 20-carbon fatty acid that contains four double bonds. Its chemical name is e**icosa**-(20) **tetra** (four double bonds)-e**noic** acid (or ETE for short) (Figure 3.5).
- **Increased amount/activity of IκBα**, which normally inhibits nuclear transcription factor kappa B (NFκB is a transcription factor that promotes cytokine production).
- **Secondary to reduced NFκB activity, a reduction in generation of COX-2 products**, i.e. decrease in arachidonic acid metabolites, so decreased PG/thromboxane (TX)/leukotriene (LT) production.
- **Secondary to reduced NFκB activity, a reduction in generation of iNOS products**, i.e. decreased NO. (NO is a potent vasodilator.)
- **Membrane stabilising effects**, so reduction of mast cell degranulation (histamine release); and decreased lysosomal enzyme release.

3.7.2 Potency and Routes of Administration

The glucocorticoids have variable mineralocorticoid effects (Table 3.4).

Glucocorticoids can be administered by a wide variety of routes depending upon the product formulation:

- Intravenous
- Intramuscular
- Oral
- Inhalation (e.g. beclomethasone)
- Intra-articular
- Extradural
- Topical

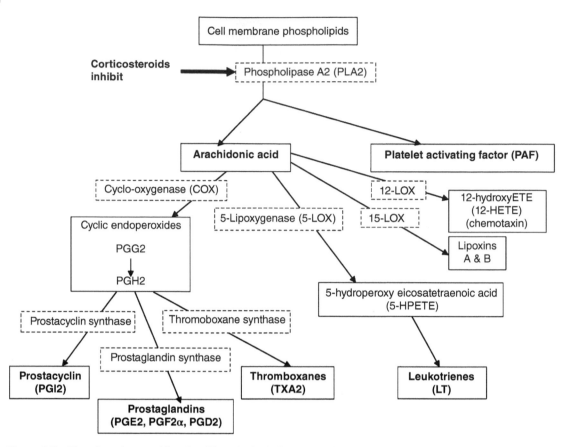

Figure 3.5 Site of corticosteroid action. The principal eicosanoids (arachidonic acid metabolites) are the PGs, TXs, and LTs. Others include the lipoxins. The term *prostanoids* is often reserved for just the PGs and TXs.

Table 3.4 Relative effects of common corticosteroids at 'equivalent' doses.

Drug	Anti-inflammatory action	Relative Glucocorticoid action	Relative Mineralocorticoid action	Duration (hours)
Cortisol	1	1	1	8–12
Hydrocortisone	1	1	1	8–12
Methylprednisolone	5	5	0.5	12–36
Betamethasone	25	30	0	36–72
Dexamathasone	25	30	0	36–72

3.7.3 Side Effects

Side effects are numerous and include:

- Immunosuppression
- Hypothalamo-pituitary axis suppression
- Abortion, so care is required in pregnant animals
- May result in GI and renal compromise secondary to reduction in prostaglandin production; beware combination with NSAIDs
- Laminitis in susceptible animals (although likely to be rare)
- Delayed wound healing; beware with corneal ulceration

3.8 Non-steroidal Anti-inflammatory Drugs (NSAIDs)

NSAIDs include any drug with anti-inflammatory properties that is not a steroid. NSAIDs specifically are drugs that inhibit formation of PGs and TXs from arachidonic acid. NSAIDs classically have **anti-inflammatory, analgesic,** and **antipyretic** effects. The two main groups are enolic acids and carboxylic acids.

The enolic acids include:

- Pyrazolones (e.g. dipyrone, tepoxalin)
- Pyrazolidines (e.g. phenylbutazone)
- Oxicams (e.g. piroxicam, meloxicam)

The carboxylic acids include:

- Salicylic acids (e.g. aspirin)
- Acetic acids (e.g. phenylacetic acids such as diclofenac and eltenac)
- Propionic acids (e.g. ketoprofen, carprofen, ibuprofen, vedaprofen)
- Fenamic acids (e.g. meclofenamic acid, tolfenamic acid)
- Nicotinic acids (e.g. flunixin)

The specific COX-2 inhibitors (the coxibs such as firocoxib, robenacoxib) are pyrazoles (see later). Despite their theoretically better safety profile, their use has been associated with procoagulant and adverse cardiovascular effects (stroke and myocardial infarction; due to vasoconstriction, and hypercoagulation, possibly due to more inhibition of PGI_2 production than of TXA_2 production) in humans, and rofecoxib was withdrawn from the market. Such effects have not yet been reported in veterinary species.

3.8.1 Effects of NSAIDs

Although the different drugs may be structurally and pharmacokinetically dissimilar, their main mechanisms of action (and side effects) tend to be shared. These mechanisms include:

- **Peripheral actions:** anti-inflammatory, analgesic, anti-endotoxic, antithrombotic, antispasmodic.
- **Central actions:** primarily analgesic and antipyretic effects. The analgesic effects may include antihyperalgesic effects (neuromodulation).

More specifically, NSAIDs have the following effects:

- **Anti-inflammatory** via cyclo-oxygenase (COX) inhibition.
- **Antipyretic** via COX inhibition.
- **Analgesic** by several possible mechanisms.
- **Antihyperalgesic** by preventing sensitisation to pain via COX inhibition effects (i.e. they decrease PG synthesis), and NMDA receptor effects (see below under analgesia and antihyperalgesia).
- **Reversal of central plasticity** documented in human OA patients with etoricoxib.
- **Anti-endotoxic effects** via COX inhibition and reduction of NFκB activity, which is normally important in amplifying the various inflammatory, complement, and coagulation cascades.

- **Antithrombotic effects** via platelet COX inhibition, reduction of TXA_2 production, and thus reduction of platelet aggregation.
- **Weak antispasmodic effects** via inhibitory action on GI tract smooth muscle.
- **Chondroprotection (versus chondrodestruction)**, is often debated for NSAIDs, but is difficult to demonstrate in the face of their anti-inflammatory effects.
- **Potential interference with bone healing**, is postulated between days 3 and 14 after fracture, when COX expression would normally increase. Other factors, however, are also involved in fracture repair and further work is necessary to determine the magnitude of NSAID effect.

3.8.1.1 COX Inhibition

NSAIDs inhibit COX enzymes (Figure 3.6). COX enzymes act on arachidonic acid (a product of cell membrane phospholipid breakdown, especially in damaged cells); inhibition of COX enzymes therefore reduces PG and TX synthesis. (Cyclo-oxygenase used to be called prostaglandin G/H synthase. Conversion of arachidonic acid to prostanoids requires an initial two-step process; firstly, PGG_2 is produced from arachidonic acid by the COX active site of the enzyme, but is unstable, and is quickly converted to PGH_2 by the POX [peroxidase] active site of the enzyme, or by other POXs, e.g. glutathione peroxidase.)

Certain NSAIDs (tepoxalin and ketoprofen) also inhibit 5-LOX and thus reduce LT production, which results in anti-inflammatory and anti-bronchospasm effects, LTs being important inflammatory mediators. Classic NSAIDs are contra-indicated in asthmatic patients because inhibition of COX results in the shunting of more arachidonic acid down the 5-LOX pathway, with more LT production, which can worsen asthma attacks (NERD [NSAID Exacerbated Respiratory Disease/distress] syndrome).

3.8.2 COX Isoforms

- There are two main isoforms of COX: **COX-1** and **COX-2**.
- COX-3 may be a splice variant of COX-1 and seems to be expressed in the CNS (see later).
- Many NSAIDs are non-selective inhibitors of both forms of COX.
- COX-1 is the constitutively expressed enzyme in many tissues, and its inhibition results in reduction of the production of many housekeeping 'good' PGs. Most adverse side effects of NSAIDs are associated with inhibition of COX-1.
- COX-2 is inducible in many tissues. The gene for COX-2 is activated by both inflammatory and proliferative

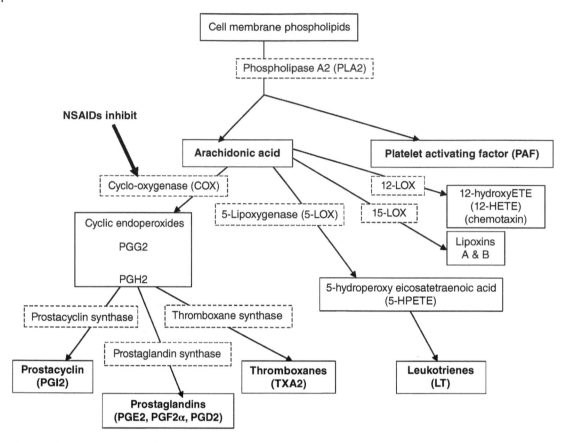

Figure 3.6 Site of NSAID action.

stimuli (e.g. inflammatory cells) and products include the inflammatory PGs (some of which enhance pain transmission or even act as direct algogens).

It used to be thought that inhibition of COX-1 had detrimental effects by interfering with the housekeeping PGs, especially in the kidneys and GI tract. Such housekeeper PGs are involved in the autoregulation of renal blood flow, renin secretion and tubular transport; and in the regulation of gastric mucosal blood flow, production of the protective mucus/bicarbonate layer in the stomach, modulation of gastric acid and enzyme secretion, epithelial cell restitution and gut motility. Inhibition of housekeeper PG production may therefore result in the well-known renal and GI side effects, hence the drive for NSAIDs which preferentially inhibited COX-2.

However, COX-2 is involved in the angiogenesis of wound healing and is constitutively expressed in the kidneys. Both COX-1 and COX-2 are constitutively expressed in the CNS, and COX-1 products may also contribute to the inflammatory response. So, instead of wanting to inhibit only COX-2, a little COX-1 inhibition might actually be OK, and perhaps care should be exercised in how much COX-2 inhibition is produced.

In humans the selective COX-2 inhibitor rofecoxib was withdrawn from the market following an increased incidence of acute myocardial infarction in older people. This selective inhibition reduces inflammation- or shear-stress-induced vascular endothelial prostacyclin production (by COX-2), which is responsible for vasodilation and reduced platelet aggregation. With no concurrent reduction in COX-1, platelet TXA_2 production continues unchecked (enhancing platelet aggregation and vasoconstriction), with resultant adverse effects. It is clear that a balance between COX-1 and COX-2 inhibition is required.

There is often much debate about the **COX ratio** for the NSAIDs (usually the ratio of IC_{50} for inhibition of COX-1 versus the IC_{50} for inhibition of COX-2, but sometimes reported the other way round). It is this that leads to the classification of NSAIDs being COX-2 preferential, selective, or specific. These are usually derived from *in vitro* studies, and are highly dependent upon the type of assay used and the cell line. They may be difficult to translate to the *in vivo* situation and must never be extrapolated between species. Of key importance is that such assays are conducted at therapeutic plasma concentrations. The whole blood assay is said to be the gold standard.

3.8.2.1 Anti-inflammatory Actions

COX inhibition, and therefore reduced production of prostaglandin E_2 (PGE2; especially in polymorphonuclear leucocytes), and PGI_2 and PGD_2 (especially in mast cells) prevents vasodilation, histamine release, and bradykinin production. Thus, NSAIDs reduce erythema, oedema, and exudation. Migration of leucocytes towards the inflammatory focus is also reduced and the potential for self-perpetuating chronic inflammation is decreased.

Leukotrienes are generally pro-inflammatory, by being chemotactic to inflammatory cells, and by increasing vascular permeability. They are also potent bronchoconstrictors, although their effects on vascular tone vary (some cause vasoconstriction, others may cause vasodilation). 5-LOX inhibition should therefore contribute to the anti-inflammatory effect of NSAIDs which also inhibit COX.

Some NSAIDs also inhibit activation of NFκB (which is normally responsible for the production of inflammatory mediators). NSAIDs may also inhibit free radical generation, may inhibit metalloproteinases and possibly also inhibit lysosomal enzyme release.

3.8.2.2 Analgesia and Antihyperalgesia

PGs released during inflammation are involved in causing hyperalgesia, both peripherally, by sensitising (reducing the firing threshold of) nociceptors, and centrally in the dorsal horns of the spinal cord (and possibly higher centres) via their actions at prostanoid receptors. Some COX-2 products (PGs) may act as direct algogens in the periphery too.

Whilst NSAIDs produce their anti-inflammatory/antinociceptive/analgesic effects through inhibition of PG production (and therefore PG action), peripherally and possibly centrally too, there is growing evidence for centrally-mediated prostaglandin-independent antinociceptive effects. These may include an increase in CNS kynurenate (kynurenic acid), a naturally occurring metabolite of tryptophan, which is an endogenous antagonist at the glycine binding site of the NMDA receptor for glutamate. Thus, NSAIDs may be able to reduce the activation of NMDA receptors by glutamate. **NSAIDs are much more effective if given before inflammation/pain occurs, because their early administration combats the development of peripheral and central sensitisation.**

3.8.2.3 Antipyretic Effects

Endogenous pyrogens (e.g. IL-1), are released by inflammatory cells and increase PGE-type prostaglandin production in the hypothalamus, which elevates the set point for temperature regulation, resulting in fever. NSAIDs inhibit PGE production, which results in the restoration of normal body temperature.

3.8.2.4 Effects on Cartilage

Some NSAIDs appear to have chondroprotective effects *in vitro*, e.g. carprofen at low doses, although a systematic review of RCTs in humans was unable to support this clinically.

3.8.2.5 GI Effects

PGI_2 and PGE_2 (COX-1 products) are GI protective as they decrease gastric acid production whilst increasing mucous and bicarbonate production. Thus, their inhibition can increase the risk of gastric ulceration; but COX-2 has an important role in ulcer healing. In human medicine, gastro-protectant strategies are often used alongside NSAID treatment. One novel drug combination is the tagging of NO (a vasodilator) onto the NSAID, producing a so-called NO-NSAID, to provide some GI protection.

Gastro-protectants include PGE analogues (misoprostol), proton pump inhibitors (e.g. omeprazole), anti-H_2 histamines (e.g. cimetidine, ranitidine, famotidine), sucralfate, and the antacids (e.g. aluminium or magnesium hydroxide).

Aspirin can also cause direct toxicity to the gastric mucosa through the topical irritant effects of salicylate, but aspirin and other NSAIDs are also proposed to cause mitochondrial oxidative injury (through uncoupling of oxidative phosphorylation) in gastric (and possibly other intestinal) mucosal epithelial cells into which they are absorbed. (NSAIDs are weakly acidic, so in the acidic environment of the stomach, they become less ionised and so are more lipophilic, aiding cellular uptake, but they can then become ion-trapped in the cells as they re-ionise at the less acidic intracellular pH.) Oral phenylbutazone (as used in horses) can bind to feed components and is suggested to later be released in the large intestine resulting in the production of ulcerative lesions, particularly in the right dorsal colon where conditions are also acidic due to production of volatile fatty acids, perhaps through a similar oxidative injury mechanism. Flunixin and meloxicam have also been implicated in similar pathology. Several potential mechanisms and predisposing factors have been suggested, including the enterohepatic recycling of NSAIDs, resulting in delivery of relatively high concentrations of NSAIDs (in bile) into the duodenum, which is a common site of ulceration (see Further Reading). One interesting feature is the change in balance between 5-LOX and 15-LOX activities, with an increase in 5-LOX products (LTs, pro-inflammatory), and a decrease in 15-LOX products (lipoxins, which are anti-inflammatory). Therefore, it seems that GI ulceration may be due to at least three mechanisms: reduced mucosal (especially gastric) protection, direct cell damage (possibly through oxidative mechanisms), and increased LT production that promotes inflammation.

The question of whether NSAIDs should be given with or without food, and if with food, then with what type of food, remain to be fully evaluated. In rats, when NSAIDs were taken after fasting, gastric mucosal damage occurred; whereas when NSAIDs were taken with food, there were more intestinal lesions. Although it is generally thought that taking NSAIDs with food delays their onset of action but does not reduce their overall bioavailability, it is suggested to give robenacoxib on an empty stomach (for dogs), so as not to reduce its efficacy as it may bind to food components (which, perhaps does reduce its bioavailability). NSAID treatment, particularly by the oral route, is often withheld from animals that are anorexic, but further work is required to fully understand the potential GI toxicities of NSAIDs, administered by different routes, under these circumstances.

3.8.2.6 Renal Effects

PGE_1 and PGE_2 are renal vasodilators, especially during hypotension and hypovolaemia. (Remember that under general anaesthesia, it is not unusual for a slight reduction in arterial blood pressure to occur.) NSAIDs inhibit the production of these protective PGs, resulting in renal hypoperfusion, especially in patients in whom hypotension or hypovolaemia may be a problem (i.e. anaesthetised patients). The renal medulla is most susceptible to ischaemic damage.

Renin production is partly controlled by PGs in the kidney, so NSAIDs can reduce renin production. This could lead to hypoaldosteronism, which results in reduced sodium and water retention and increased potassium retention, but hyperkalaemia is quite a rare consequence of NSAID administration. More commonly, slight fluid (sodium, chloride, and water) retention occurs with NSAID administration because of inhibition of a variety of renal effects of PGs. That is, PGs can alter regional renal blood flow and increase glomerular filtration rate (GFR), so they tend to promote sodium, chloride, and water excretion (partly via increasing GFR, and partly by inhibition of Na^+, Cl^-, and water reabsorption in the loop of Henle), and they antagonise the effect of anti-diuretic hormone (although they increase renin production); these effects being offset by NSAIDs. PGs, however, are not primary regulators of basal renal function in normal individuals, so the side effects of NSAID treatment on fluid and electrolyte imbalances are more likely to be seen in patients with a degree of pre-existing renal dysfunction.

3.8.2.7 Platelet Effects

Platelet aggregation is reliant on the balance of platelet-produced TXA_2 and vascular endothelium-produced PGI_2. TXA_2 promotes platelet aggregation (and vasoconstriction), whereas PGI_2 has anti-aggregation (and vasodilation)

effects. Some NSAIDs, especially aspirin and ketoprofen, limit platelet TXA_2 production, whilst allowing vascular endothelium PGI_2 production (i.e. vascular endothelial cells can generate new COX whereas platelets cannot); hence producing an antithrombotic effect. Aspirin's effect on platelet COX (TXA_2 production) is irreversible, because of covalent binding to the enzyme and an inability of platelets to synthesis new COX enzyme. There have been several reports of 'excessive bleeding' during surgery in otherwise healthy animals following ketoprofen administration. The COX-2 selective drugs (coxibs such as rofecoxib) appear to preferentially inhibit vascular endothelial COX-2 driven PGI_2 production, thus potentially resulting in adverse procoagulant effects.

3.8.2.8 Hepatotoxicity

The precise metabolism and excretion of NSAIDs varies between species. This is why phenylbutazone is so dangerous to humans (hence its European Union ban in food animals). Generally, both phase I and phase II hepatic metabolic pathways are important. Therefore, care should be taken with NSAIDs in animals with impaired liver function. (NSAIDs are all highly protein bound too, so caution is advised in patients with hepatic disease, where plasma proteins [albumin] may be low.) NSAIDs themselves may cause some liver damage, e.g. long-term use of phenylbutazone in old horses has been associated with hepatotoxicity. Excretion of metabolites is mainly via urine, although some are also excreted via bile, which provides the potential for some enterohepatic recirculation, especially if there are active metabolites (e.g. phenylbutazone is metabolised to oxyphenbutazone). There have been occasional reports of acute hepatic dysfunction in Labradors after treatment with carprofen, but no explanation has been put forward.

3.8.3 Side Effects

The side effects of NSAIDs include:

- GI ulceration: protein losing enteropathy; haemorrhage.
- Renal medullary/papillary ischaemia/necrosis: acute renal failure (especially if the patient is also hypovolaemic/hypotensive).
- Hepatotoxicity (how reversible?).
- Possible embryotoxicity/teratogenicity, especially in the first trimester, especially aspirin.
- Bone marrow toxicity and blood dyscrasias (sometimes irreversible).
- Haemorrhagic diatheses (especially the older COX-1 inhibitors such as aspirin); beware patients with pre-existing coagulopathies.
- Delayed parturition (beware use near parturition).

- Premature closure of ductus arteriosus (beware administration to pregnant animals).
- Worsening of bronchoconstriction in asthmatics, possibly by diverting more arachidonic acid down the 5-lipoxygenase pathway. Leukotrienes are known to enhance bronchial reactivity, they are chemo-attractants for inflammatory cells, and can induce changes in vascular permeability.
- Chondrodestruction: especially articular cartilage (e.g. phenylbutazone).

3.8.4 Available Drugs

3.8.4.1 General Notes
3.8.4.1.1 Absorption of NSAIDs
Mainly administered via oral or parenteral (IV or SC) routes. NSAIDs are well absorbed from the GI tract, but food may interfere with absorption. NSAIDs are weak acids, therefore they are relatively unionised in the acidic environment of the stomach and as such, are more lipophilic and cross the gastric mucosa more easily.

3.8.4.1.2 Distribution of NSAIDs
Highly plasma protein bound, about 95–99%, except aspirin (50–80%). (Phenylbutazone is thought to bind irreversibly to plasma proteins.) NSAIDs should be used with care in cases of hypoproteinaemia or where other highly protein-bound drugs are used concurrently (e.g. angiotensin converting enzyme [ACE] inhibitors).

Leakage of plasma proteins at sites of inflammation and the acid pH of inflamed tissue leads to intracellular ion-trapping of NSAIDs at the site where they are really needed. This may explain why you can detect a clinical effect from a NSAID, even though its plasma concentration may not be in the therapeutic range.

3.8.4.1.3 Metabolism and Excretion of NSAIDs
Hepatic metabolism is important. Renal excretion is determined by the degree of plasma protein binding (and therefore concentration of free drug), and urine pH. As stated above, the metabolism varies between species. **NSAIDs of the propionic acid group are chiral compounds**, and exist as two different enantiomers; the S(+) and R(−) forms; the available solutions are usually racemic (50 : 50) mixtures of these. The S(+) form is usually the most potent enantiomer where COX inhibition is concerned. The different enantiomers may have different pharmacokinetics and pharmacodynamics because of differing stereochemistry; and stereoselective processes are often species-related. *In vivo,* chiral inversion usually occurs, so that the R(−) form is converted into the S(+) form. This **unidirectional chiral inversion** occurs to differing extents with different drugs in different species, but interestingly, carprofen does not appear to undergo chiral inversion in the horse, calf, dog, cat, or human. The non-chiral NSAIDs may also have differing pharmacokinetics between species.

Different patients with different types of pain may respond differently to different NSAIDs; so if one NSAID does not appear to work, try another, but ideally allow a minimum 'washout' period between different NSAIDs based on 5× the half-life of the drug being discontinued (which often means a minimum of about five days). Individual patients may also differ in their tolerance to different NSAIDs. No one NSAID currently marketed is safer or more efficacious than any other.

None of the currently licenced NSAIDs has been safety tested in neonates and all summaries of product characteristics (SPCs) carry warnings to avoid their use in animals generally <6 weeks old.

3.8.4.2 Acetylsalicylic Acid/Aspirin/Sodium Salicylate
Not generally used for pain management but for its antithrombotic effect in patients with clotting disorders such as cats with aortic thromboemboli. Doses not well established; aspirin has a long half-life in dogs (8–12 hours) and even longer in cats (20–40 hours). Beware GI side effects. The reader is referred to specialist texts for further dosage information.

Cats: ¼ of 75 mg junior aspirin PO, every two to three days
Dogs: 10 mg/kg PO, q12 hours
Cattle: see Chapter 33
Pigs: see Chapter 35

3.8.4.3 Carprofen
For horses, cattle, dogs, and cats. Available in injectable and orally administered forms, but not licenced for oral administration in cats. In horses and cats, carprofen has a long half-life of about 24 hours. Its exact actions may be different in different species, but carprofen is reported to be a weak COX (COX-2 > COX-1) inhibitor, although this may not entirely account for its actions.

- Licenced for pre-operative administration in dogs (may be continued 24 hours later)
- Licenced for pre-operative administration in cats (single perioperative dose only)

3.8.4.4 Cimicoxib
For treatment of pain and inflammation associated with OA and management of peri-operative pain due to orthopaedic or soft tissue surgery in dogs. Oral tablet. Licence claims that pharmacokinetics are not altered in renal disease although this does not indicate that cimicoxib is safer than another NSAIDs in renal disease.

3.8.4.5 Deracoxib

The first licenced coxib in the USA for pain associated with OA and dental disease in dogs. COX-1 sparing and COX-2 selective.

3.8.4.6 Firocoxib

For dogs only. To date, only an oral preparation is available. A highly selective (preferring/specific?) COX-2 inhibitor, with possibly few GI and renal side effects, but reportedly has a low safety margin (three and five times the licenced dose produces adverse effects).

3.8.4.7 Flunixin Meglumine

For horses, cattle, and pigs. Flunixin is available in injectable and orally administered forms. It is a potent analgesic for equine colic and can mask pain and the cardiovascular effects of endotoxaemia-related Systemic Inflammatory Response Syndrome (SIRS). Therefore, care should be exercised over its administration to horses with colic. Flunixin is commonly combined with an antibiotic in preparations designed for farm animal practice, e.g. treatment of calf pneumonia. See Chapters 33 and 35.

3.8.4.8 Ketoprofen

For horses, cattle, pigs, dogs, and cats. Ketoprofen is reportedly as potent as flunixin in masking the signs of colic. It is only licenced for post-operative use as it has been reported to cause clotting problems. See Chapters 33 and 35.

3.8.4.9 Mavacoxib

A long-acting oral COX-2 inhibitor for the treatment of OA where therapy is required long-term. A monthly treatment for dogs (initial dose given, then repeated 14 days later, then monthly thereafter). At a dose of 2 mg/kg half-life is 44 days in most dogs although longer in some individuals.

3.8.4.10 Meclofenamic Acid

For horses only. Oral preparation only.

3.8.4.11 Meloxicam

For horses, cattle, pigs, dogs, and cats. COX-2 selective. The analgesic dose is often less than the anti-inflammatory dose (as for other NSAIDs), so higher doses are commonly administered peri-operatively. Studies document that dose reduction may be effective for long-term administration in dogs, but not to reduce below 60% labelled dose as below this dose, efficacy is reduced. See Chapters 33 and 35.

- The only NSAID formulated as a palatable syrup, chewable tablets, and in two concentrations, for easy administration.
- Licenced for pre-operative use in dogs and cats.

- Licenced for long-term use in dogs and cats.

3.8.4.12 Metamizole (Dipyrone)

In the UK, marketed as Buscopan compositum™, which also contains hyoscine butylbromide. For horses, cattle, pigs, and dogs. Causes localised tissue reaction if administered extravascularly. Because hyoscine is a parasympatholytic, an increase in heart rate commonly occurs after administration. Dipyrone is an interesting NSAID. It is a good anti-pyretic, a good anti-spasmodic, and a good anti-thrombotic (potentially useful in horses with endotoxaemia and in the early stages of disseminated intravascular coagulopathy [DIC]), but is a relatively poor anti-inflammatory. See also Chapters 33 and 35.

3.8.4.13 Phenylbutazone

For horses and dogs, phenylbutazone comes in a wide variety of preparations: injectable (IV only; very irritant to tissues if accidental extravascular administration occurs), granules, paste. Only available as tablets (not an injectable) for dogs, although currently no licenced oral product available in UK. Metabolised to oxyphenbutazone. Danilon Equidos™ contains the prodrug suxibuzone: this is metabolised to two active metabolites: phenylbutazone and oxyphenbutazone; and gamma hydroxyphenylbutazone, which is inactive.

3.8.4.14 Robenacoxib

For dogs and cats for acute surgical pain and osteoarthritic pain. Absorption is improved with an empty stomach. Robenacoxib was compared to meloxicam in a small number of dogs: at normal clinical doses, there was no evidence that robenacoxib provided superior patient comfort. Although studies in cats reported a beneficial effect of robenacoxib versus meloxicam, there was variation in surgical procedures between groups, making the comparison less robust.

3.8.4.15 Tolfenamic Acid

For cattle, pigs, dogs, and cats. Injectable and oral formulations. Some debate about whether preferential COX-2 inhibition. See Chapters 33 and 35.

3.8.4.16 Tepoxalin (No Longer Available)

For dogs. Was originally marketed as a drug of choice for OA flare-ups. A non-selective COX inhibitor (therefore strong COX-1 inhibition), and a 5-LOX inhibitor (although this action may be relatively short-lived *in vivo*). It was reported to selectively avoid gastric COX inhibition, which coupled with its 5-LOX inhibition, was supposed to provide an improved GI safety profile. It was claimed to have a 'renal sparing' effect because only 1% was renally excreted. It was available as 'fast melt' 'tablets' that stuck to the buccal mucosa and dissolved rapidly. The tablets consisted of a lyophilisate preparation, essentially micronised drug interspersed between the pores of a lyophilised gelatine–sugar matrix.

3.8.4.17 Vedaprofen

For horses and dogs. As with most oral NSAIDs, should be given with food (although some foods may interfere with absorption). Do not give to animals with oral lesions. Not licenced for horses <6 months old.

- Licenced for pre-operative dosing in horses.

3.9 Paracetamol (Acetaminophen)

Paracetamol is a non-acidic compound, and it is a para-aminophenol derivative. It is a good antipyretic, but usually referred to as a weak analgesic and weak anti-inflammatory. It appears to have mainly central actions (see below). **Cats** cannot glucuronidate phenols very well, so tend to develop methaemoglobinaemia and hepatic toxicity much more readily after paracetamol exposure than other species.

Not a classic COX-1 inhibitor, but may act on central (CNS) COX-3 (which may be a COX-1 splice variant). There is some debate about whether it is also a COX-2 inhibitor, and also some suggestions that it has more inhibitory activity at the POX active site of prostaglandin G/H synthase than at the truly COX-specific site. It used to be said that it had central actions through interference with the actions of arachidonic acid derivatives (with possible antihyperalgesic actions), but it has recently been discovered that paracetamol also acts as a prodrug; the active product being an endogenous cannabinoid, which produces analgesia. Paracetamol is first de-acetylated to para-aminophenol (PAP); this is then conjugated with arachidonic acid to form N-arachidonoylphenolamine (i.e. N-arachidonoylaminophenol, AM404), which is an endogenous cannabinoid. AM404 itself has weak actions on the CB1 receptor, but inhibits re-uptake of another endogenous cannabinoid, anandamide, which prolongs anandamide's actions on CB1 receptors in the CNS (with analgesic results), and N-arachidonoylphenolamine also appears to have agonist actions at one of the vanilloid receptors, so-called transient receptor potential non-selective cation channel, subfamily V, member 1 (TRPV1), which is important in the transmission and modulation of pain both centrally and peripherally. Furthermore, studies document an activating effect on the descending serotonergic pathways,

suggesting another mode of analgesia provision via descending inhibitory actions. Paracetamol also has anti-arrhythmic properties in dogs at higher doses.

- Dogs: 10 (−25) mg/kg PO, B-TID. Toxic dose c. 100mg/kg.
- **Cats: narrow therapeutic index, so contra-indicated.**
- Pigs: See Chapter 35.
- Licenced for dogs in UK as Pardale-V™ in combination with codeine (400 mg paracetamol; 9 mg codeine phosphate). Dose suggested as 33.3 mg/kg TID for up to five days only.
- Available as an IV preparation (off licence). Commonly used at 15 mg/kg IV TID.

Two separate studies investigated the use of either IV paracetamol or oral Pardale-V in dogs undergoing orthopaedic surgery and each suggested an analgesic benefit, although further work is required to confirm this in a prospective manner.

The mechanism of toxicity of paracetamol is related to the drug's metabolism. In dogs, paracetamol is normally metabolised in the liver, primarily by conjugation (glucuronidation more than sulphation pathway), and to a small extent, oxidation. If large doses are given, however, the glucuronidation and sulphation pathways become overwhelmed, so that the oxidation pathway becomes more active. The product of oxidative metabolism is N-acetyl-p-benzoquinoneimine (NAPQI or NABQI), which is a highly reactive oxidising (and alkylating) species. Normally, hepatic and red cell glutathione can deactivate this compound, but if large doses of paracetamol have been ingested, the glutathione is rapidly depleted, and glutathione synthesis may also be inhibited, allowing NAPQI to damage proteins, cell membranes (red cells and hepatocytes), cause methaemoglobin production and eventually lead to red cell lysis and hepatic necrosis. It has been suggested that PAP, rather than NAPQI, may be a major contributor to the formation of methaemoglobin, and that deficient arylamine N-acetyl transferase (NAT) in dogs and cats contributes to the methaemoglobinaemia seen in these species with paracetamol toxicity.

In cats, because their glucuronidation and sulphation pathways are less active, even small doses of paracetamol are metabolised via the oxidation pathway with the production of NAPQI. Cats also seem to have relatively low levels of glutathione. Hence, the narrow therapeutic index in this species.

Treatment is aimed at providing antioxidant (reductant) capacity. N-acetylcysteine is the preferred antidote as it is a precursor of glutathione and is also oxidised in the liver to form sulphate which helps the sulphation pathway for paracetamol metabolism. Ascorbic acid may also be used as an antioxidant; it is suggested that it may help convert methaemoglobin back to haemoglobin.

If treatment is to be continued for longer than the suggested five days, it would appear reasonable to monitor liver enzymes and function at regular intervals.

3.10 Piprants

Grapiprant (Galliprant®) is a non-cyclooxygenase inhibiting, PGE_2 EP4 receptor antagonist from the piprant class.

One of the prostanoids produced by degradation of arachidonic acid, PGE_2, binds to four receptors to mediate homeostatic functions and is involved in pain and inflammation via the EP4 receptor. Grapiprant works at the level of this receptor which is a specific target for pain. It has demonstrated efficacy for treatment of pain in dogs with OA when compared to a placebo. No evidence of gastric ulceration was found in dogs after a nine-month study even when doses of up to 15× the recommended dose were given. Some vomiting did occur in dogs, but this was not associated with GI pathology and if grapiprant was continued the vomiting resolved. Although safety of oral daily dosing of grapiprant has been demonstrated in cats at three different doses, no studies have been published demonstrating efficacy for treatment of OA in cats to date.

3.11 Local Anaesthetics

Not only can local anaesthetic agents be used to perform nerve blocks, but their systemic administration (lidocaine has been most commonly used) also provides analgesia (see Chapters 12–16 on local anaesthetics and techniques).

The systemic analgesic effects are thought to be due to several mechanisms including:

- Anti-inflammatory effects
- Effects on glycine signalling, which may result in inhibition of NMDA receptor activity
- Activation of TRPV1 channels
- Effects on other ion channels
- Inhibition of substance P binding to its receptors

3.12 α2-Adrenoceptor Agonists

Xylazine, romifidine, detomidine, medetomidine, and dexmedetomidine are the α2 agonists used in veterinary practice in the UK. They have a wide range of effects on the body and the CNS (see Chapters 4 on premedication and 28 on equine sedation). Like opioid receptors, α2 receptors are G-protein linked transmembrane receptors, which can be coupled to several types of effector mechanisms (e.g. voltage gated ion channels, adenyl cyclase). In the CNS, α2 receptor activation tends to have an inhibitory effect. Many α2 receptors are found in similar locations to opioid receptors in areas of the CNS involved with pain, and there is much interaction between the opioidergic and adrenergic systems, both of which may explain some of the synergistic effects seen when the two classes of drugs are administered together. However, because of the other effects of these drugs such as sedation, cardiovascular, and respiratory effects, the α2 agonists are seldom used as primary analgesics. Nevertheless, they are commonly used alongside other agents (e.g. opioids, ketamine) to produce combinations of sedation, anaesthesia, and analgesia. There are exceptions to this, however, e.g. xylazine can be useful to relieve the pain associated with equine colic as it is a potent spasmolytic as well as sedating and calming the horse, yet its effects are short lived and will not mask any signs of deterioration in colic cases; and α2 agonists may also be administered extradurally to provide analgesia.

3.13 Other Analgesic Drugs

3.13.1 Tramadol

Sometimes called an atypical opioid, tramadol is a synthetic 4-phenylpiperidine analogue of codeine with roughly 1/10th the potency of morphine. A racemic mixture of two enantiomers (+ and −), it is a centrally acting analgesic with both opioid and non-opioid effects, but with fewer side effects than true opioids. The major active metabolite in humans is O-desmethyltramadol (M1), via the hepatic cytochrome P450 system, which has six times the analgesic potency of tramadol itself. Production of the various metabolites is species-dependent (and possibly also individual-dependent). Metabolism involves demethylation and glucuronidation or sulphation; cats struggle with both the demethylation and the glucuronidation pathways.

Actions of tramadol include:

- Weak MOP (μ) receptor agonist (parent compound: very low affinity; M1 metabolite: 200 times greater affinity than parent compound).
- Weak direct α2 agonist action (M1 metabolite).
- Inhibition of re-uptake of noradrenaline (the − enantiomer); therefore, enhanced descending noradrenergic inhibitory activity in spinal cord.

- Inhibition of serotonin re-uptake, and enhancement of serotonin release (the + enantiomer); therefore, enhanced descending serotonergic inhibitory activity in spinal cord.
- May reduce the release of substance P.
- A possible NMDA receptor antagonism has also been suggested.

Efficacy in dogs is questionable, although tramadol has been shown to improve activity in cats with OA. These differences are likely to be due to species variation in metabolism.
   Dose:

- Dogs: 5 mg/kg TID failed to provide improvement in dogs with OA.
- Cats 3 mg/kg twice a day proved most effective in cats with OA.

Tramadol can also be administered systemically and neuraxially. Side effects include vomiting and drowsiness. Although tramadol can be administered alongside NSAIDs and gabapentin without any dose adjustments, it should be used with caution if tricyclic antidepressants, monoamine oxidase inhibitors, or serotonin re-uptake inhibitors are being taken because of the risk of **serotonin syndrome**. The serotonin syndrome (due primarily to increased serotonin activity in the CNS) can manifest as agitation or confusion, convulsions, increased muscle activity/rigidity/rhabdomyolysis (beware secondary renal failure), diarrhoea, autonomic instability (sometimes cardiovascular collapse), and fever; occasionally it can result in death.

3.13.2　Tapentadol

Tapentadol is another synthetic compound, also sometimes called an atypical opioid, with a dual mode of action, but, unlike tramadol, is not a pro-drug. It has agonist activity at the MOP (μ) receptor but has 50× less affinity at these receptors than morphine. It also inhibits noradrenaline re-uptake, which is likely its major mechanism for producing analgesia. It only weakly inhibits serotonin re-uptake which may not be sufficient to enhance its analgesic actions. Its activation of descending inhibitory pathways (both opioidergic and monoaminergic) explain its analgesic effects, which may differ in models of acute pain (where opioidergic effects are more relevant) and neuropathic pain (where monoamine re-uptake inhibition is more important). So far, only preliminary experimental work has been performed, although with promising results.

3.13.3　Ketamine

Although used as an anaesthetic induction agent, ketamine is also used to provide analgesia at sub-anaesthetic doses. Ketamine is a PCP congener. As discussed earlier, glutamate is an important excitatory neurotransmitter in the CNS and is involved in pain processing whereby pain responses are altered (i.e. neuroplasticity/modulation). Glutamate binds with four types of receptors, but the NMDA receptor has a key role in the processing and modulation of neural activity and in the development of memory. The NMDA receptor has binding sites for both glycine and glutamate, but its ligand-gated activity is also dependent upon membrane depolarisation (voltage-gating), whereby Mg^{2+} inhibition (Mg^{2+} possibly sits in the channel) is 'relieved'.

$$\text{Glycine + glutamate} \xrightarrow[\text{Membrane depolarisation}]{\text{NMDA receptor}} Ca^{2+} \text{ enters cell}$$

Ketamine is a non-competitive NMDA antagonist. It does not compete with glutamate for glutamate's binding site, but instead ketamine binds to the PCP-binding site (some sources suggest that this might also be the old sigma [σ] opioid receptor), which is probably located within the channel of the NMDA receptor. This 'channel blockade' is time-, concentration-, and stimulation-frequency (i.e. use)-dependent; it depends upon initial channel activation and opening, but once ketamine gains access to the channel, further Ca^{2+}, entry into the cell is inhibited.

Ketamine possibly has some opioid actions that may add to its analgesic effects. It has antagonistic actions at MOP (μ) receptors, but agonistic ones at KOP (κ) and DOP (δ) receptors.

Ketamine has sympathomimetic effects in that it produces a non-uniform stimulation of the sympathetic nervous system, inhibition of the parasympathetic nervous system, and also inhibits the re-uptake of noradrenaline (monoamine uptake 1 and 2), and so increases vascular tone, heart rate, and myocardial oxygen demand.

Ketamine has direct myocardial depressant effects in vitro (negative inotropy, possibly via voltage-gated calcium channel blockade), but this effect is usually masked by its sympathetic stimulatory effects and unlikely to be a concern if used at analgesic doses. However, shocky animals with depleted catecholamine stores may be more susceptible to overall cardiovascular depression.

Ketamine is a racemic mixture of two isomers:

- R(−) ketamine is a poor analgesic and is associated with excitatory/psychomimetic effects.
- S(+) ketamine is a potent analgesic with little excitatory/psychomimetic effects.

Unfortunately, with the standard racemic mixture, both effects are seen, and so ketamine is usually administered with some other agent/s to counter the excitatory effects.

The **analgesic properties of ketamine**, however, are such that it can be administered either in very small (sub-anaesthetic) doses (<1/10th induction dose, e.g. 0.1–0.5 mg/kg), or by infusion during anaesthesia (e.g. 10–20 μg/kg/min), and also in the post-operative period (e.g. 2–5 μg/kg/min) to provide excellent analgesia.

Ketamine is a basic compound and is available commercially as the hydrochloride salt (ketamine-HCl), therefore the solution is acidic (pH 3.5–5.5). Ketamine's pKa is 7.5; so at pH 4, most is present as the ionised (NH^+) form. At body pH (7.4), the equilibrium shifts so that almost equal quantities of the ionised and unionised forms are present; thus conferring both good water solubility and good lipid solubility. Combined with its low protein binding, the shift towards more of the unionised form (in the body) helps to enhance its passage across the blood–brain barrier. This property is also utilised in the neuraxial administration of ketamine.

Preparations that contain only the S(+) isomer have fewer undesirable side effects, but none are licenced for veterinary species, at least in the UK, and they tend to be expensive.

Because of ketamine's antagonistic actions at NMDA receptors, which are involved in the adaptation of the CNS to pain stimuli, it may have some promise as a treatment for chronic pain conditions such as phantom limb pain and hyperalgesia. In the meanwhile, other NMDA antagonists are available for use in the treatment of chronic pain states, such as **amantadine** (originally developed as an antiviral compound), which is available for oral administration. Amantadine works by increasing the rate of channel closure following activation of the NMDA complex. In conjunction with meloxicam in dogs with OA, amantadine was documented to improve activity and reduce lameness compared to meloxicam alone. This effect was noted after three to six weeks of treatment. Other reports in dogs and cats are anecdotal. Adverse effects are rare, but high doses may cause some agitation. **Memantine** is also an NMDA antagonist documented to improve compulsive disorders in dogs in combination with fluoxetine, but without documented efficacy as an analgesic despite anecdotal use.

There has been much speculation over whether exogenous **magnesium** can help to provide analgesia (via increased blockade of NMDA receptors). The results so far have been equivocal.

3.13.4 Nitrous Oxide (N_2O) and Xenon

N_2O has minimal cardiovascular and respiratory depressant effects, it is not metabolised and has very low blood solubility. For it to act as a general anaesthetic, it would have to be administered at a concentration of at least 90% of the inspired gases in humans; in animals it is even less potent. So, at normal atmospheric pressure, it could never be used as an anaesthetic agent (as we would not be able to deliver enough oxygen). It can, however, be used at sub-anaesthetic doses (normally 50–66% of the inspired gases) where it still provides analgesia.

N_2O has **NMDA receptor antagonist activities** and also **stimulates endogenous opioid production** (see earlier). N_2O is therefore a useful analgesic adjunct to anaesthesia (as part of balanced anaesthesia), where it not only has minimal adverse effects on the animal's physiology and homeostasis, but also reduces the requirements for other anaesthetic agents (and therefore their side effects). In addition, its low blood and tissue solubilities mean that it is rapidly eliminated (so long as ventilation is maintained; beware diffusion hypoxia), so it can be used perioperatively without risk of prolonging recovery from anaesthesia.

The major drawbacks with N_2O are the worry of prolonged exposure (by hospital staff) with the slight risk of neurological problems, teratogenic effects, and anaemia; and the environmental impact (nitrous oxide is a greenhouse gas and facilitates atmospheric ozone depletion).

Xenon has many of the properties of an ideal anaesthetic agent and can be used as such at normal atmospheric pressures (its MAC is about 70% in people). It also provides analgesia by mechanisms similar to nitrous oxide, yet pollution and toxicity are not problems because xenon is inert. Although its administration requires inhalation, which could limit its application to in-patients, the major drawbacks at the moment are its rarity and the expense of its production.

3.13.5 Other Drugs

- Antidepressants and anxiolytics (e.g. tricyclics, MAO inhibitors, selective serotonin re-uptake inhibitors)
- Anticonvulsants (e.g. gabapentin, pregabalin, topiramate, phenobarbital)
- Nerve growth factor (NGF) antagonists
- Cannabinoids
- Cholecystokinin (CCK) antagonists
- NK-1 receptor antagonists
- Ion channel blockers
- Bisphosphonates
- Soluble epoxide hydrolase (sEH) inhibitors

Antidepressants and anticonvulsants may modulate central pain processing pathways to alter pain perception. They may be useful in some chronic pain states, especially those associated with cancer and neuropathic pain. The tricyclic antidepressants, e.g. carbamazepine and amitriptyline have been used in the treatment of neuropathic pain states such as trigeminal neuralgia, and so are sometimes given to head-shaker horses where increased trigeminal nerve sensitivity is thought to exist. These drugs tend to inhibit the re-uptake of monoaminergic neurotransmitters (noradrenaline and serotonin), and thus are able to enhance activity in the descending monoaminergic inhibitory pathways and therefore aid in providing analgesia. Beware concurrent use with tramadol because of the risk of serotonin syndrome. Duloxetine, a selective noradrenaline re-uptake inhibitor, has analgesic effects in neuropathic and osteoarthritic pain in humans.

Gabapentinoids: gabapentin and **pregabalin** are GABA analogues, but seem not to produce their main effects (anticonvulsant, anxiolytic, analgesic) at GABA receptors. Instead, they **modulate and inhibit the actions of voltage-gated calcium channels** (such as can be up-regulated in chronic pain states), and so have been found useful in the treatment of chronic, especially neuropathic, pain states. Gabapentin reduces the activity of presynaptic voltage-gated calcium channels to reduce glutamate (an excitatory neurotransmitter) release. It may also modulate the activity of the post-synaptic glutamate receptors, both NMDA and non-NMDA types. Pregabalin also interacts with **voltage-sensitive potassium channels**. The $\alpha2\delta$ subunit of L-type voltage-gated calcium channels is highly expressed in C nociceptors, particularly after nerve injury, and is an analgesic target of gabapentinoids. Their analgesic effects in some pain states may, however, require previous activation of descending serotonergic pathways. Beware of gabapentin syrups produced for people as these often contain xylitol (an artificial sweetener), which is a potent inducer of insulin secretion and can cause profound hypoglycaemia, hypokalaemia, and even death in dogs.

Topiramate, another anticonvulsant, has been trialled in dogs with syringomyelia. It blocks voltage-gated sodium and calcium channels and inhibits excitatory glutamate actions (at AMPA and kainate receptors, but with no NMDA receptor effect); and enhances the inhibitory effects of GABA. It is also a carbonic anhydrase inhibitor so can reduce cerebrospinal fluid production.

Nerve growth factor (NGF) is important for sympathetic and sensory neurons during their development. It is released during inflammation and acts via the tyrosine kinase (TrkA) receptor expressed on nociceptors to produce hyperalgesia. Dogs with OA have been found to have increased NGF in synovial fluid compared with dogs with normal joints. **Monoclonal antibody antagonists** have been produced for dogs (**ranevetmab**) and cats (**frunevetmab**) with clinical studies currently assessing the potential benefits in arthritic patients.

NK-1 receptor antagonists such as maropitant citrate, which is marketed for its anti-emetic activity, may also have some visceral analgesic effects. NK-1 receptors are found in multiple locations throughout the body, including the CNS, and are activated by substance P to produce a variety of effects including nausea, vomiting, and pain. Substance P co-release with other neurotransmitters, such as glutamate, can occur from C fibres and Aδ fibres (about 50% of C fibres and about 20% of Aδ fibres in rats), but, importantly, such co-release correlates with the intensity of the noxious stimulus and appears important in the generation of chronic pain states. Small animal studies have shown reduced inhalation agent requirement when maropitant has been included in the anaesthetic protocols for neutering procedures, although the optimum dose of maropitant to provide clinically relevant analgesia, especially when opioid and NSAID analgesics are also administered, has not been determined.

Sensory nerves express different types of **sodium channels**. Those that are important for transmission of non-noxious stimuli are expressed in Aβ fibres and are called tetrodotoxin sensitive (TTXs) sodium channels. However, pain fibres (Aδ and C fibres) express both TTXs and tetrodotoxin resistant sodium channels (TTXr), the latter being important for the transmission of noxious stimuli. These may be up-regulated in chronic pain states, such that **TTXr antagonists** may be useful.

Neurons also express a range of voltage sensitive calcium channels, some of which can be inhibited by **cannabinoids** as well as the anticonvulsants (e.g. gabapentin). **Conotoxins** (from venomous snails such as *Conus magus*) are N-type calcium channel antagonists and have analgesic actions. One such is ziconotide, which has been administered intrathecally.

CCK, which acts as an endogenous opioid antagonist, is known to be up-regulated where there has been peripheral nerve injury. **CCK antagonists** may improve the analgesia afforded by opioids.

Resiniferatoxin (RTX) is a relative of **capsaicin** (the compound that makes chilli peppers 'hot'), and, like capsaicin, it has been shown to bind to vanilloid receptors, allowing excessive calcium influx into cells, which can result in their death. Only cells expressing the receptors are vulnerable, including pain fibres (C type especially). For some chronic pain states, chemical neuronal knock-out like this has been considered.

Sarapin is a distillate of alkaloids from the pitcher plant and has been used as a therapy or an adjunct in the treatment of many chronic and neuropathic pain states. It does not seem to have local anaesthetic type activity, despite often being used to perform 'regional analgesia'. Its mechanism of action is unknown.

Bisphosphonates (e.g. tiludronate disodium), although usually used for the treatment of hypercalcaemia, also appear to provide analgesia for patients with bone cancer and perhaps with inflammatory bone disorders (e.g. navicular disease in horses). Their mechanisms of action are incompletely understood, but in addition to inhibiting osteoclast activity (and stimulating osteoblast activity), they may have NMDA antagonistic actions.

sEH inhibitors prevent epoxy-fatty acid (EpFA) degradation. EpFAs are alternative metabolic products of arachidonic acid and tend to have anti-nociceptive effects. One inhibitor, t-TUCB (trans-4-{4-[3-(4-trifluoromethoxy-phenyl)-ureido]-cyclohexyloxy}-benzoic acid) has shown potential in an equine model of synovitis.

Note: Angiotensin-converting enzyme inhibitors (ACEi) are widely used in small animal medicine, yet they prevent the degradation of substance P and bradykinin and can upregulate the B2 bradykinin receptor. It has recently been suggested that ACEi therapy may have the undesirable side effect of promoting hyperalgesia.

3.14 Pharmacogenetics

Pharmacogenetics is the study of genetic variations that cause individual differences in response to therapeutic agents. It is well known that individual animals can have a unique response or non-response to a particular drug, and studies are beginning to unravel some of the underlying genetic differences.

Genetic mutations/polymorphisms in the cytochrome P450 system can have a huge influence on the individual's pharmacokinetics for a drug. More is also being learned about the Multi-Drug Resistance 1 (MDR1) gene (sometimes referred to as the ABCB1 gene). It encodes a transporter protein called P-glycoprotein ('permeability'-glycoprotein or P-gp), which is expressed by various tissues, including intestinal and renal tubular cells and brain capillary endothelial cells. This ATP-dependent transporter protein appears to be able to transport a number of structurally and functionally unrelated drugs to limit their oral absorption and CNS entry. Mutations in the MDR1 gene may result in poor function of the P-gp, which may increase susceptibility to the toxicity of several drugs. The most well-known example is the mutation present in Collies that results in their susceptibility to ivermectin toxicity because of an absence or functional deficiency of P-gp. It is also suggested that such mutations may increase the risk of toxicity to sedative and anaesthetic agents by allowing an increased concentration within the CNS.

The MC1R gene has also received attention. This encodes the melanocortin-1 receptor. Sex differences in pain and analgesic sensitivity have already been documented, especially in rodents; and in women, red hair is a useful phenotypic expression of MC1R mutations. Red-haired women have recently been shown to be more sensitive to thermal pain, more resistant to lidocaine, more sensitive to κ agonist opioids, and less sensitive to desflurane anaesthesia. This is likely to be an exciting area of research in the future.

3.15 Adjuncts to Analgesia

Notwithstanding the ability to provide analgesia with drugs, there are several other ways to improve patient comfort:

- **Support** such as fracture stabilisation (splints/bandages) and wound dressings.
- **Cardiovascular and respiratory support** such as resuscitation (IV fluids, supplemental O_2).
- **Nutritional support** aids wound healing.
- **Gentle surgery** and, e.g. the use of muscle relaxants.
- **Muscle relaxation,** e.g. diazepam to reduce the muscle spasms associated with neck and back pain with intervertebral disc disease.
- **Allay fear and anxiety** with judicious use of sedatives and tranquillisers as necessary (apprehensiveness increases perception of pain).
- **Provide a comfortable environment,** e.g. provide a quiet kennel at an appropriate temperature, a comfy bed, ensure food and water are available, provide light and dark (i.e. wake and sleep) times, assist grooming, provide tender loving care and quality time. Animals that are 'expressive' (e.g. dogs) when they feel pain seem to respond when they are petted or nursed by another animal (human or otherwise). This is not thought to be just a behavioural response. But the oxytocin and endorphins released in the brain appear to decrease the amount of pain being felt.
- **Ensure empty bladder and rectum** and prevent skin scalding.

- **Gentle physiotherapy** such as massage and passive range of motion exercises. Other types of physiotherapy that may be helpful in controlling pain are hot/cold compresses, laser treatment, ultrasound, magnetic field therapy, and gentle electrical stimulation like TENS.
- **Stimulation induced analgesia and acupuncture** attempt to utilise the body's own mechanisms for controlling pain by stimulating endogenous endorphin release or by stimulating certain afferent nerve fibres which activate inhibitory neurotransmission in the spinal cord (non-painful paraesthesia). The best-known example of this method is acupuncture, which uses segmental and extra-segmental stimulation (i.e. the stimulation is not localised to the part of the body from where the pain arises). Proponents of acupuncture say this method not only releases widespread endorphins but treats the 'whole body' response to pain.
- **TENS** is commonly employed by physiotherapists and doctors, and is used locally, near to the painful site (i.e. segmentally). It is mostly used to treat chronic back pain, and so its application may be limited in animals as such conditions may be difficult to diagnose. Percutaneous electrical nerve stimulation, similar to TENS but with skin penetration by the electrodes (and with some similarities to electroacupuncture), has gained recent attention for the treatment of head-shaking in horses.
- **Surgery** may seem obvious, but removing the cause of the painful stimulus is often the best way to provide relief from pain. This can involve immobilising a fractured bone, removing a foreign body, removing a tumour, removing a section of ischaemic intestine, or performing a neurectomy.

3.16 Euthanasia

Uniquely, as vets, we have the ability and the means to relieve unrelenting or uncontrollable pain and suffering in animals by euthanasia. This should always be done as humanely as possible with consideration to the animal, and, if applicable, the owner. In many circumstances, it may be helpful to view euthanasia as a positive action and the most humane treatment option.

3.17 Assessment of Pain

3.17.1 Pain Scoring

Pain assessment methods in animals tend to employ different scoring systems (numerical rating, visual analogue, or simple descriptive), which are used to attribute the presence and severity of various signs associated with pain. The recurrent problem is that these assessments are subjective and individual scorers differ widely in their interpretation of signs. They are used mainly to aid research into pain and are not always easily applicable to busy practice. However, the types of score whereby the observer interacts with the animal, and several aspects of its behaviour or physiology are assessed (so-called composite or multi-dimensional scales) seem to be superior.

The Glasgow Composite Measure Pain Scales are multidimensional pain scales validated for acute pain in dogs and cats. In their shortened forms (Figures 3.7 and 3.8), these pain questionnaires are also relatively easy to apply in a practice situation. The short form composite measure pain score (CMPS-SF) can be applied quickly and reliably in a clinical setting and has been designed as a clinical decision-making tool which was developed for dogs in acute pain. It includes 30 descriptor options within 6 behavioural categories, including mobility. Within each category, the descriptors are ranked numerically according to their associated pain severity and the person carrying out the assessment chooses the descriptor within each category which best fits the dog's behaviour/condition. It is important to carry out the assessment procedure as described on the questionnaire, following the protocol closely. The pain score is the sum of the rank scores. The maximum score for the 6 categories is 24, or 20 if mobility is impossible to assess. The total CMPS-SF score has been shown to be a useful indicator of analgesic requirement and the recommended analgesic intervention level is 6/24, or 5/20 (for non-ambulatory patients). The CMPS-Feline can be applied quickly and reliably in a clinical setting and has been designed as a clinical decision-making tool for use in cats in acute pain. It includes 28 descriptor options within 7 behavioural categories. Within each category, the descriptors are ranked numerically according to their condition. It is important to carry out the assessment procedure as described on the questionnaire, following the protocol closely. The pain score is the sum of the rank scores. The maximum score for the 7 categories is 20. The total CMPS-Feline score has been shown to be a useful indicator of analgesic requirement and the recommended analgesic intervention level is 5/20.

Our ability to assess chronic pain in dogs with OA has improved with validated tools (LOAD Liverpool Osteoarthritis in Dogs, COAST Canine Osteoarthritis Staging Tool, Canine Brief Pain Inventory, Helsinki Chronic Pain Index). For chronic pain states, Vetmetrica™ has also developed tools for dogs and cats. These assessments take into account the impact of pain and immobility on the animal's quality of life.

SHORT FORM OF THE GLASGOW COMPOSITE MEASURE PAIN SCALE

Dog's name _____   Date   /   /   Time

Hospital Number _____

Procedure or Condition _____

_____

In the sections below please circle the appropriate score in each list sum these to give the total score

A. Look at dog in Kennel
Is the dog

(i)		(ii)	
Quiet	0	Ignoring any wound or painful area	0
Crying or whimpering	1	Looking at wound or painful area	1
Groaning	2	Licking wound or painful area	2
Screaming	3	Rubbing wound or painful area	3
		Chewing wound or painful area.	4

In the case of spinal, pelvic or multiple limb fractures, or where assistance is required to

aid locomotion do not carry out section B and proceed to C

Please tick if this is the case ☐ then proceed to C

B. Put lead on dog and lead out of the kennel

When the dog rises/walks is it?

(iii)	
Normal	0
Lame	1
Slow or reluctant	2
Stiff	3
It refuses to move	4

C. If it has a wound or painful area including abdomen, apply gentle pressure 2 inches round the site

Does it?

(iv)	
Do nothing	0
Look round	1
Flinch	2
Growl or guard area	3
Snap	4
Cry	5

D. Overall

Is the dog?

(v)	
Happy and content or happy and bouncy	0
Quiet	1
Indifferent or non-responsive to surroundings	2
Nervous or anxious or fearful	3
Depressed or non-responsive to stimulation	4

Is the dog?

(vi)	
Comfortable	0
Unsettled	1
Restless	2
Hunched or tense	3
Rigid	4

Total Score (i+ii+iii+iv+v+vi) = _____

Figure 3.7 Short form of the Glasgow composite measure pain scale for dogs. *Source:* Reproduced from University of Glasgow (2008) with permission from NewMetrica Ltd.

Glasgow Feline Composite Measure Pain Scale: CMPS – Feline

Choose the most appropriate expression from each section and total the scores to calculate the pain score for the cat. If more than one expression applies choose the higher score

LOOK AT THE CAT IN ITS CAGE:

Is it?
Question 1
Silent / purring / meowing	0
Crying/growling / groaning	1

Question 2
Relaxed	0
Licking lips	1
Restless/cowering at back of cage	2
Tense/crouched	3
Rigid/hunched	4

Question 3
Ignoring any wound or painful area	0
Attention to wound	1

Question 4
a) Look at the following caricatures. Circle the drawing which best depicts the cat's ear position?

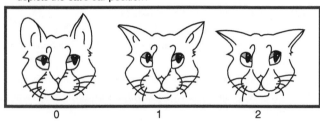

b) Look at the shape of the muzzle in the following caricatures. Circle the drawing which appears most like that of the cat?

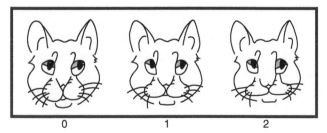

APPROACH THE CAGE, CALL THE CAT BY NAME & STROKE ALONG ITS BACK FROM HEAD TO TAIL

Question 5
Does it?
Respond to stroking	0

Is it?
Unresponsive	1
Aggressive	2

IF IT HAS A WOUND OR PAINFUL AREA, APPLY GENTLE PRESSURE 5 CM AROUND THE SITE. IN THE ABSENCE OF ANY PAINFUL AREA APPLY SIMILAR PRESSURE AROUND THE HIND LEG ABOVE THE KNEE

Question 6
Does it?
Do nothing	0
Swish tail/flatten ears	1
Cry/hiss	2
Growl	3
Bite/lash out	4

Question 7
General impression Is the cat?
Happy and content	0
Disinterested/quiet	1
Anxious/fearful	2
Dull	3
Depressed/grumpy	4

Pain Score ... /20

Figure 3.8 The Glasgow Composite Measure Pain Scale (CMPS)-Feline. *Source:* Reproduced from Universities of Glasgow and Edinburgh Napier (2015) with permission from NewMetrica Ltd.

Further Reading

Abbo, L.A., Ko, J.C., Maxwell, L.K. et al. (2008). Pharmacokinetics of buprenorphine following intravenous and oral transmucosal administration in dogs. *Veterinary Therapeutics* 9: 83–93.

Adelson, D., Lao, L., Zhang, G. et al. (2009). Substance P release and neurokinin 1 receptor activation in the rat spinal cord increases with the firing frequency of C-fibers. *Neuroscience* 161: 538–553.

Adrian, D., Papich, M., Baynes, R. et al. (2017). Chronic maladaptive pain in cats: a review of current and future drug treatment options. *The Veterinary Journal* 230: 52–61.

Andrews, F. and McConnico, R. (2009). Cause for concern: evidence that therapeutic dosing of nonselective NSAIDs contributes to gastrointestinal injury. *Equine Veterinary Education* 21: 663–664.

Angst, M.S. and Clark, J.D. (2006). Opioid-induced hyperalgesia. A qualitative systematic review. *Anesthesiology* 104: 570–587.

Ashley, F.H., Waterman-Pearson, A.E., and Whay, H.R. (2005). Behavioural assessment of pain in horses and donkeys: application to clinical practice and future studies. *Equine Veterinary Journal* 37: 565–575.

Azzam, A.A.H., McDonald, J., and Lambert, D.G. (2019). Hot topics in opioid pharmacology: mixed and biased opioids. *British Journal of Anaesthesia* 122: e136–e145.

Ballantyne, J.C., Loach, A.B., and Carr, D.B. (1988). Itching after epidural and spinal opiates. *Pain* 33: 149–160.

Barbarossa, A., Rambaldi, J., Giunti, M. et al. (2017). Pharmacokinetics of buprenorphine following constant rate infusion for postoperative analgesia in dogs undergoing ovariectomy. *Veterinary Anaesthesia and Analgesia* 44: 435–443.

Bardell, D. (2017). Managing orthopaedic pain in horses. *In Practice* 39: 420–427.

Belda, B., Enomoto, M., Case, B.C., and Lascelles, B.D.X. (2018). Initial evaluation of PetPace activity monitor. *The Veterinary Journal* 237: 63–68.

Bell, A. (2018). The neurobiology of acute pain. *The Veterinary Journal* 237: 55–62.

Bendinger, T. and Plunkett, N. (2016). Measurement in pain medicine. *BJA Education* 16: 310–315.

Blobaum, A.L. and Marnett, L.J. (2007). Structural and functional basis of cyclooxygenase inhibition. *Journal of Medicinal Chemistry* 50: 1425–1441.

Borland, K. and Rioja Garcia, E. (2019). Case report: possible opioid-induced hyperalgesia in a cat. *Companion Animal* 24: 246–248.

Bradbrook, C.A. and Clark, L. (2018). State of the art analgesia: recent developments in pharmacological approaches to acute pain management in dogs and cats: part 1. *The Veterinary Journal* 238: 76–82.

Bradbrook, C.A. and Clark, L. (2018). State of the art analgesia: recent developments in pharmacological approaches to acute pain management in dogs and cats: part 2. *The Veterinary Journal* 236: 62–67.

Bragg, D., El-Sharkawy, A.M., Psaltis, E. et al. (2015). Post-operative ileus: recent developments in pathophysiology and management. *Clinical Nutrition* 34: 367–376.

Carlino, E. and Benedetti, F. (2016). Different contexts, different pains, different experiences. *Neuroscience* 338: 19–26.

Carregaro, A.B., Freitas, G.C., Ribeiro, M.H. et al. (2014). Physiological and analgesic effects of continuous-rate infusion of morphine, butorphanol, tramadol or methadone in horses with lipopolysaccharide (LPS)-induced carpal synovitis. *BMC Veterinary Research* 21 (10): 966. https://doi.org/10.1186/s12917-014-0299-z.

Chabot-Dore, A.-J., Schuster, D.J., Stone, L.S., and Wilcox, G.L. (2015). Analgesic synergy between opioid and α2-adrenoceptors. *British Journal of Pharmacology* 172: 388–402.

Chapman, C.R. (2008). Progress in pain assessment: the cognitively compromised patient. *Current Opinion in Anaesthesiology* 21: 610–615.

Cohen, N.D. (2002). Right dorsal colitis. *Equine Veterinary Education* 14: 212–219.

Cook, V.L. and Blikslager, A.T. (2015). The use of nonsteroidal anti-inflammatory drugs in critically ill horses. *Journal of Veterinary Emergency and Critical Care* 25: 76–88.

Davis, J.L. (2017). Nonsteroidal anti-inflammatory drug associated right dorsal colitis in the horse. *Equine Veterinary Education* 29: 104–113.

De Boer, H.D., Detriche, O., and Forget, P. (2017). Opioid-related side effects: postoperative ileus, urinary retention, nausea and vomiting, and shivering. A review of the literature. *Best Practice and Research Clinical Anaesthesiology* 31: 499–504.

De, C., Williams, A.C., and Craig, K.D. (2016). Updating the definition of pain. *Pain* 157: 2420–2423.

Dietis, N., Rowbotham, D.J., and Lambert, D.G. (2011). Opioid receptor subtypes: fact or artifact? *British Journal of Anaesthesia* 107: 8–18.

Driessen, B. and Zarucco, L. (2007). Pain: from diagnosis to effective treatment. *Clinical Techniques in Equine Practice* 6: 126–134.

Dubin, A.E. and Patapoutian, A. (2010). Nociceptors: the sensors of the pain pathway. *The Journal of Clinical Investigation* 120: 3760–3772.

Eberspacher, E., Stanley, S.D., Rezende, M., and Steffey, E.P. (2008). Pharmacokinetics and tolerance of transdermal fentanyl administration in foals. *Veterinary Anaesthesia and Analgesia* 35: 249–255.

Ebert, E. (2012). Gastrointestinal involvement in spinal cord injury: a clinical perspective. *Journal of Gastrointestinal and Liver Disease* 21: 75–82.

Enomoto, M., Mantyh, P.W., Murrell, J. et al. (2019). Anti-nerve growth factor monoclonal antibodies for the control of pain in dogs and cats. *Veterinary Record* 184: 23.

Flecknell, P. (2018). Rodent analgesia: assessment and therapeutics. *The Veterinary Journal* 232: 70–77.

Fries, S. and Grosser, T. (2005). The cardiovascular pharmacology of COX-2 inhibition. *Hematology*: 445–451.

Ganesh, A. and Maxwell, L.G. (2007). Pathophysiology and management of opioid-induced pruritus. *Drugs* 67: 2323–2333.

Gleerup, K.B. (2018). Assessing pain in horses. *In Practice* 40: 457–463.

Gleerup, K. and Lindegaard, C. (2016). Recognition and quantification of pain in horses: a tutorial review. *Equine Veterinary Education* 28: 47–57.

Goldstein, J.L. and Cryer, B. (2015). Gastrointestinal injury associated with NSAID use: a case study and review of risk factors and preventative strategies. *Drug, Healthcare and Patient Safety* 7: 31–41.

Grint, N. (2017). Managing acute pain in dogs. *In Practice* 39: 346–354.

Guedes, A.G.P., Aristizabal, F., Sole, A. et al. (2018). Pharmacokinetics and antinociceptive effects of the soluble epoxide hydrolase inhibitor t-TUCB in horses with experimentally induced radiocarpal synovitis. *Journal of Veterinary Pharmacology and Therapeutics* 41: 230–238.

Hofmeister, E.H., Barletta, M., Shepard, M. et al. (2018). Agreement among anesthesiologists regarding postoperative pain assessment in dogs. *Veterinary Anaesthesia and Analgesia* 45: 695–702.

Hopster, K. and van Eps, A.W. (2019). Pain management for laminitis in the horse (review). *Equine Veterinary Education* 31: 384–392.

Howard, J., Aarnes, T.K., Dyce, J. et al. (2018). Pharmacokinetics and pharmacodynamics after oral administration of tapentadol hydrochloride in dogs. *American Journal of Veterinary Research* 79: 367–375.

Kissin, I. (2000). Preemptive analgesia. *Anesthesiology* 93: 1138–1143. ***(Should be read alongside Wolf CJ and Chong M–S 1993)***.

Lascelles, B.D.X., Court, M.H., Hardie, E.M., and Roberston, S.A. (2007). Nonsteroidal anti-inflammatory drugs in cats: a review. *Veterinary Anaesthesia and Analgesia* 34: 228–250.

Lascelles, B.D.X., Gaynor, J.S., Smith, E.S. et al. (2008). Amantadine in a multimodal analgesic regimen for alleviation of refractory osteoarthritis pain in dogs. *Journal of Veterinary Internal Medicine* 22: 53–59.

Lawson, A. (2019). Monitoring side effects of long-term NSAID use in dogs with chronic osteoarthritis. *In Practice* 41: 148–154.

Lee, M., Silverman, S., Hansen, H. et al. (2011). A comprehensive review of opioid-induced hyperalgesia. *Pain Physician* 14: 135–161.

Lisowski, Z.M., Pirie, R.S., Blikslager, A.T. et al. (2018). An update on equine post-operative ileus: definitions, pathophysiology and management. *Equine Veterinary Journal* 50: 292–303.

Liu, D., Ahmet, A., Ward, L. et al. (2013). A practical guide to the monitoring and management of the complications of systemic corticosteroid administration. *Allergy, Asthma and Clinical Immunology* 9: 30. http://www.aacijournal.com/cotent/9/1/30.

Madden, M., Gurney, M., and Bright, S. (2014). Amantadine, an N-methyl-d-aspartate antagonist, for treatment of chronic neuropathic pain in a dog. *Veterinary Anaesthesia and Analgesia* 41: 440–441.

Marchionatti, E., Larde, H., and Steagall, P.V.M. (2014). Opioid-induced adverse effects in a Holstein calf. *Veterinary Anaesthesia and Analgesia* 42: 229–230.

Marks, S.L., Kook, P.H., Papich, M.G. et al. (2018). ACVIM consensus statement: Support fot rational admnistratoin ofgastrointestinal protectants to dogs and cats. *Journal of Veterinary Internal Medicine* 32: 1823–1840.

Matsui, H., Shimokawa, O., Kaneko, T. et al. (2011). The pathophysiology of non-steroidal anti-inflammatory drug (NSAID)–induced mucosal injuries in stomach and small intestine. *Journal of Clinical Biochemistry and Nutrition* 48: 107–111.

McConkey, S.E., Grant, D.M., and Cribb, A.E. (2009). The role of Para-aminophenol in acetaminophen-induced methemoglobinemia in dogs and cats. *Journal of Veterinary Pharmacology and Therapeutics* 32: 585–595.

McDonald, J. and Lambert, D.G. (2015). Opioid receptors. *BJA Education* 15: 219–224.

McEntire, D.M., Kirkpatrick, D.R., Dueck, N.P. et al. (2016). Pain transduction: a pharmacologic perspective. *Expert Review of Clinical Pharmacology* 9: 1069–1080.

McFadzean, W.J.M. and Love, E.J. (2019). Perioperative pain management in horses (review). *Equine Veterinary Education* 31: 374–383.

Moll, X., Fresno, L., Garcia, F. et al. (2011). Comparison of subcutaneous and transdermal administration of buprenorphine for pre-emptive analgesia in dogs undergoing elective ovariohysterectomy. *The Veterinary Journal* 187: 124–128.

Molony, V. and Kent, J.E. (1997). Assessment of acute pain in farm animals using behavioural and physiological measurements. *Journal of Animal Science* 75: 266–272.

Monteiro, B.P. and Steagall, P.V. (2019). Chronic pain in cats, recent advances in clinical assessment. *Journal of Feline Medicine and Surgery* 21: 601–614.

Morton, C.M., Reid, J., Scott, E.M. et al. (2005). Application of a scaling model to establish and validate an interval level pain scale for assessment of acute pain in dogs. *American Journal of Veterinary Research* 66: 2154–2166.

Murrell, J. (2018). Perioperative use of non-steroidal anti-inflammatory drugs in cats and dogs. *In Practice* 40: 314–325.

Ossipov, M.H., Suarez, L.J., and Spaulding, T.C. (1989). Antinociceptive interaction between alpha 2 adrenergic and opiate agonists at the spinal level in rodents. *Anesthesia and Analgesia* 68: 194–200.

Ossipov, M.H., Dussor, G.O., and Porreca, F. (2010). Central modulation of pain. *The Journal of Clinical Investigation* 120: 3779–3787.

Ossipov, M.H., Morimura, K., and Porreca, F. (2014). Descending pain modulation and chronification of pain.

Current Opinions in Supportive and Palliative Care 8: 143–151.

Packiasabapthy, S. and Sadhasivam, S. (2018). Gender, genetics and analgesia: understanding the differences in response to pain relief. *Journal of Pain Research* 11: 2729–2739.

Patel, R. and Dickenson, H. (2016). Mechanisms of the gabapentinoids and α2δ-1 calcium channel subunit in neuropathic pain. *Pharmacology Research and Perspectives* 4: e00205. https://doi.org/10.1002/prp2.205.

Pathan, H. and Williams, J. (2012). Basic opioid pharmacology: an update. *British Journal of Pain* 6: 11–16.

Porreca, F., Ossipov, M., and Gebhart, G. (2002). Chronic pain and medullary descending facilitation. *Trends in Neurosciences* 25: 319–325.

Posner, L.P., Gleed, R.D., Erb, H.E., and Ludders, J.W. (2007). Post-anesthetic hyperthermia in cats. *Veterinary Anaesthesia and Analgesia* 34: 40–47.

Posner, L.P., Pavuk, A.A., Rokshar, J.L. et al. (2010). Effects of opioids and anesthetic drugs on body temperature in cats. *Veterinary Anaesthesia and Analgesia* 37: 3–43.

Rainsford, K.D. and Bjarnason, I. (2017). NSAIDs: take with food or after fasting? *Journal of Pharmacy and Pharmacology* 64: 465–469.

Rausch-Derra, L., Huebner, M., Wofford, J., and Rhodes, L. (2016). A prospective, randomized, masked, placebo-controlled multisite clinical study of grapiprant, an EP4 prostaglandin receptor antagonist (PRA), in dogs with osteoarthritis. *Journal of Veterinary Internal Medicine* 30: 756–763.

Rausch-Derra, L.C. and Rhodes, L. (2016). Safety and toxicokinetic profiles associated with daily oral administration of grapiprant, a selective antagonist of the prostaglandin E_2 EP4 receptor, to cats. *American Journal of Veterinary Research* 77: 688–692.

Reich, A. and Szepietowski, J.C. (2009). Opioid-induced pruritus: an update. *Clinical and Experimental Dermatology* 35: 2–6.

Reid, J., Nolan, A.M., Hughes, J.M.L. et al. (2007). Development of the short–form Glasgow Composite Measure Pain Scale (CMPS–SF) and derivation of an analgesic intervention score. *Animal Welfare* 16 (S): 97–104.

Reid, J., Nolan, A.M., and Scott, E.M. (2018). Measuring pain in dogs and cats using structured behavioural observation. *The Veterinary Journal* 236: 72–79.

Reid, J., Scott, E.M., Calvo, G., and Nolan, A.M. (2017). Definitive Glasgow acute pain scale for cats: validation and intervention level. *Veterinary Record* https://doi.org/10.1136/vr.104208.

Robertson, S.A. and Sanchez, L.C. (2010). Treatment of visceral pain in horses. *Veterinary Clinics of North America: Equine Practice* 26: 603–617.

Robinson, D.R. and Gebhart, G.F. (2008). Inside information: the unique features of visceral sensation. *Molecular Interventions* 8: 242–253.

Sawynok, J. (2016). Adenosine receptor targets for pain. *Neuroscience* 338: 1–18.

Schmid, V.B., Spreng, D.E., Seewald, W. et al. (2010). Analgesic and anti-inflammatory actions of robenacoxib in acute joint inflammation in dog. *Journal of Veterinary Pharmacology and Therapeutics* 33: 118–131.

Sharma, C.V. and Mehta, V. (2014). Paracetamol mechanisms and updates. *Continuing Education in Anaesthesia, Critical Care and Pain* 14: 153–158.

Sladky, K.K., Kinney, M.E., and Johnson, S.M. (2008). Analgesic efficacy of butorphanol and morphine in bearded dragons and corn snakes. *Journal of the American Veterinary Medical Association* 233: 267–273.

Slingsby, L., Taylor, P.M., and Murrell, J.C. (2011). A study to evaluate buprenorphine at 40 μg/kg compared to 20 μg/kg as a post-operative analgesic in the dog. *Veterinary Anaesthesia and Analgesia* 38: 584–593.

Smith, W.L., Urade, Y., and Jakobsson, P.-J. (2011). Enzymes of the cyclooxygenase pathways of prostanoid synthesis. *Chemical Reviews* 111: 5821–5865.

Soares, J.H.N., Henao-Guerrero, N., Pavlisko, N.D. et al. (2019). The effect of two doses of fentanyl on chest wall rigidity at equipotent doses of isoflurane in dogs. *Veterinary Anaesthesia and Analgesia* 46: 360–364.

Sostres, C., Gargallo, C.J., and Lanas, A. (2013). Nonsteroidal anti-inflammatory drugs and upper and lower gastrointestinal damage. *Arthritis Research and Therapy* 15 (Suppl 3): S3. http://arthritis-research.com/content/15/S3/S3.

Sparkes, A.H., Heiene, R., Lascelles, B.D.X. et al. (2010). ISFM and AAEP consensus guidelines: long-term use of NSAIDs in cats. *Journal of Feline Medicine and Surgery* 12: 521–538.

Steen, K.H., Steen, A.E., and Reeh, P.W. (1995). A dominant role of acid pH in inflammatory excitation and sensitization of nociceptors in rat skin, in vitro. *The Journal of Neuroscience* 15: 3982–3989.

Sun, Y., Gan, T.J., Dubose, J.W., and Habib, A.S. (2008). Acupuncture and related techniques for post-operative pain: a systematic review of randomised controlled trials. *British Journal of Anaesthesia* 101: 151–160.

Swallow, A., Rioja, E., Elmer, T., and Dugdale, A. (2017). The effect of maropitant on intraoperative isoflurane requirements and postoperative nausea and vomiting in dogs: a randomized clinical trial. *Veterinary Anaesthesia and Analgesia* 44: 785–793.

Szarvas, S., Harmon, D., and Murphy, D. (2003). Neuraxial opioid-induced pruritus: a review. *Journal of Clinical Anesthesia* 15: 234–239.

Treede, R.-D. (2018). The International Association for the Study of Pain definition of pain: as valid in 2018 as in 1979, but in need of regularly updated footnotes. *Pain Reports* 3: e643. https://doi.org/10.1097/RP9.0000000000000643.

Vanegas, H., Vazquez, E., and Tortorici, V. (2010). NSAIDs, opioids, cannabinoids and the control of pain by the central nervous system. *Pharmaceuticals* 3: 1335–1347.

Vineula-Fernandez, I., Jones, E., Welsh, E.P., and Fleetwood-Walker, S.M. (2007). Pain mechanisms and their implication for the management of pain in farm and companion animals. *The Veterinary Journal* 174: 227–239.

White, D.M., Mair, A.R., and Martinez-Tabaoda, F. (2017). Opioid-free anaesthesia in three dogs. *Open Veterinary Journal* 7: 104–110.

White, K., Targett, M., and Harris, J. (2018). Gainfully employing descending controls in acute and chronic pain management. *The Veterinary Journal* 237: 16–25.

Wiseman-Orr, M.L., Nolan, A.M., Reid, J., and Scott, E.M. (2004). Development of a questionnaire to measure the effects of chronic pain on health–related quality of life in dogs. *American Journal of Veterinary Research* 65: 1077–1084.

Woolf, C.J. and Chong, M.-S. (1993). Preemptive analgesia – treating post-operative pain by preventing the establishment of central sensitisation. *Anesthesia and Analgesia* 77: 362–379. ***(Best read in conjunction with Kissin [2000].).***

Yakamura, T., Sakimura, K., and Shimoji, K. (1999). Direct inhibition of the N-methyl-d-aspartate receptor channel by high concentrations of opioids. *Anesthesiology* 10: 1053–1063.

Yam, M.F., Loh, Y.C., Tan, C.S. et al. (2018). General pathways of pain sensation and the major neurotransmitters involved in pain regulation. *International Journal of Molecular Sciences* 19: 2164. https://doi.org/10.3390/ijms19082164.

Yeates, J. and Main, D. (2009). Assessment of companion animal quality of life in veterinary practice and research. *Journal of Small Animal Practice* 50: 274–281.

Zhang, B., Li, Q., Shi, C., and Zhang, X. (2018). Drug-induced pseudoallergy: a review of the causes and mechanisms. *Pharmacology* 101: 104–110.

Zubrzycka, M. and Janecka, A. (2000). Substance P: transmitter of nociception (minireview). *Endocrine Regulations* 34: 195–201.

Useful Textbook Resources

Clark, L. (2014). Pre-emptive or preventive analgesia – lessons from the human literature? *Veterinary Anaesthesia and Analgesia* 41: 109–112.

Duke-Novakovski, T., de Vries, M., and Seymour, C. (eds.) (2016). *BSAVA Manual of Canine and Feline Anaesthesia and Analgesia*, 3e. Gloucester, UK: BSAVA Publications.

Egger, C.M., Love, L., and Doherty, T. (eds.) (2014). *Pain Management in Veterinary Practice*. Iowa, USA: Wiley-Blackwell.

Flecknell, P. and Waterman-Pearson, A. (eds.) (2000). *Pain Management in Small Animals*. London, UK: WB Saunders.

Fox, S.M. (ed.) (2010). *Chronic Pain in Small Animal Medicine*. London, UK: Manson Publishing Ltd.

Fox, S.M. (ed.) (2014). *Pain Management in Small Animal Medicine*. Florida, USA: CRC Press (Taylor Francis Group).

Fox, S.M. (ed.) (2017). Multimodal management of canine osteoarthritis. In: 2e. Florida, USA: CRC Press (Taylor and Francis Group).

Gaynor, J.S. and Muir, W.W. (eds.) (2002). *Veterinary Pain Management*. Missouri, USA: Mosby Inc. (Elsevier Science).

Grant, D. (2006). *Pain Management in Small Animals: A Manual for Veterinary Nurses and Technicians*. Philadelphia, USA: Butterworth-Heinemann (Elsevier Science).

Lindley, S. and Watson, P. (eds.) (2010). *BSAVA Manual of Canine and Feline Rehabilitation, Supportive and Palliative Care*. Gloucester, UK: BSAVA Publications.

Mathews, K.A. (2008). Update on management of pain. *Veterinary Clinics of North America: Small Animal Practice* 38 (6): 1173–1490.

Self, I. (ed.) (2019). *BSAVA Guide to Pain Management in Small Animal Practice*. Gloucester, UK: BSAVA Publications.

Steagall, P., Robertson, S., and Taylor, P.M. (eds.) (2018). *Feline Anesthesia and Pain Management*. New Jersey, USA: Wiley-Blackwell.

Self-test Section

1 Define *pain*.

2 What do you understand by the term *preventive analgesia*?

3 In which clinical conditions has central sensitisation been documented?

4

Sedation and Premedication

Small Animals

LEARNING OBJECTIVES

- To be able to list the aims of premedication.
- To be able to discuss the properties of an ideal premedicant.
- To be familiar with the main groups of drugs, their effects, and their side effects.
- To be able to discuss the factors affecting the choice of these agents, to provide either sedation or premedication.

4.1 Premedication and Sedation

4.1.1 Why Use Premedication?

- To relieve anxiety in the patient, facilitating its handling for induction of anaesthesia. A co-operative patient also reduces the anxiety of the anaesthetist, which helps promote calm patient handling.
- To smooth the induction of anaesthesia (i.e. a gentle, more controlled, transition to a state of general anaesthesia is possible after premedication than if none is provided).
- Premedication can also reduce catecholamine release, which thereby reduces the risks of catecholamine-induced cardiac arrhythmias (especially during induction and early maintenance of anaesthesia).
- To smooth the maintenance phase of anaesthesia (should the premedication drugs have a sufficiently long duration of action).
- To smooth the recovery from anaesthesia (should the premedication drugs have a sufficiently long duration of action).
- To reduce the required doses of induction and maintenance anaesthetic agents and thus reduce their side effects.
- To provide analgesia (pre-emptively).
- To reduce muscle tone (to facilitate interventions/surgery).

- To reduce unwanted autonomic reflexes (e.g. anticholinergics may be considered where vagal reflexes are possible, e.g. ocular surgery).

The last four points show how premedication forms a valuable part of balanced anaesthesia.

4.1.2 Properties of an Ideal Premedicant or Sedative

An ideal sedative/premedication should:

- Allay fear and anxiety
- Be safe (have a high therapeutic index) and be effective in all species
- Be predictable (dose-dependent) and reliable
- Have a reasonably quick onset of action, and reasonable duration of action
- Be easily administered, perhaps by several different routes
- Its administration should be in a practical volume and its injection should not be irritant to tissues or unpleasant/painful for the animal
- Produce minimal cardiovascular, respiratory, and other side effects (e.g. diuresis, sweating)
- Possibly provide some analgesia and muscle relaxation
- Possibly provide amnesia

Veterinary Anaesthesia: Principles to Practice, Second Edition. Alexandra H. A. Dugdale, Georgina Beaumont, Carl Bradbrook, and Matthew Gurney.
© 2020 John Wiley & Sons Ltd. Published 2020 by John Wiley & Sons Ltd.
Companion website: www.wiley.com/go/dugdale/veterinary-anaesthesia

- Be miscible with other agents
- Be antagonisable (reversible)

No single drug fulfils all these criteria, but the drugs available are detailed below.

4.1.2.1 A Few Definitions

These terms may be difficult to distinguish in animals.

An **anxiolytic** is a drug that is said to produce a mental calming effect, characterised by a reduction in locomotor activity, reduced anxiety, and a lack of concern for, or interest in, the environment. Animals still maintain the ability to be aroused by stimuli, especially painful ones, but tend to be a little less jumpy and quieter to handle. The terms *anxiolytic*, *tranquilliser*, *ataractic*, and *neuroleptic* tend to overlap.

A **sedative** is a drug that produces a mental calming effect, characterised by sleepiness as well as disinterest in the environment, and generally a poorer responsiveness to stimuli than produced by an anxiolytic. However, animals may still be aroused. Sedatives are sometimes called hypnotics. Some drugs afford analgesia as well as sedation and are called sedative-analgesics.

Narcosis is the term coined to describe the sedation produced by opioid analgesics, hence 'narcotic analgesics'.

4.1.3 Phenothiazines

Acepromazine (acetylpromazine). Injectable 2 mg/ml for small animals; injectable 5 and 10 mg/ml for horses; 10 mg tablets for small animals; 35 mg/ml oral gel for horses.

Phenothiazines contain two benzene rings that are linked by a sulphur and a nitrogen atom. Chlorpromazine is taken as the prototype drug in this class because much work was done with it, but other phenothiazines are very similar. Different substitutions can alter the activity of the resulting compound, one interesting example being methotrimeprazine, which has some analgesic properties that are absent in other drugs of this group.

4.1.3.1 Actions

- Anti-adrenergic ($\alpha 1$ adrenoceptor blockade)
- Anti-dopaminergic (D1-like and D2-like receptor blockade)
- Anticholinergic (muscarinic receptor blockade)
- Antihistaminic (H_1 receptor blockade)
- Anti-serotonergic (5-HT receptor blockade)
- Local anaesthetic effects (ion channel blockade)
- 'Membrane' effects (sits in phospholipid bilayers)
- Anti-arrhythmic actions (possibly due to local anaesthetic effects, membrane stabilising effects, sedative effects

[through decreasing circulating catecholamines], or direct effects on myocardial receptors [$\alpha 1$ or $\alpha 2$])
- No analgesia (except methotrimeprazine)
- Smooth muscle spasmolytic effects (e.g. GI tract) due to anticholinergic effects
- Anti-thrombotic actions
- Possible anti-oxidant properties?
- Possible anti-inflammatory effects?

4.1.3.2 Effects

- Sedation
- Hypotension (due to vasodilation and reduced sympathetic tone)
- Hypothermia (due to vasodilation)
- Anti-emetic
- Anti-arrhythmic
- Antihistaminic

4.1.3.3 Pharmacology

Phenothiazines are highly protein bound (>90%). They are lipophilic (so cross the blood–brain barrier and placenta), and hydrophilic. They undergo hepatic metabolism; the metabolites being excreted in urine and faeces (via bile). Some metabolites have some activity. Metabolism follows the usual phase I and II biotransformation reactions. Hydroxylation with subsequent glucuronidation represents the principal metabolic pathway, but sulphation and demethylation also occur.

Phenothiazines have a wide variety of actions, mostly associated with depression of parts of the central nervous system (CNS) that assist in the control of homeostasis, these include vasomotor control, thermoregulation, hormonal balance, acid–base balance, and emesis.

4.1.3.4 Results of Administration

4.1.3.4.1 Mental Calming Effect

The primary reason for veterinary use. Mediated by anti-dopaminergic actions in the CNS (especially in the reticular activating system), including post-synaptic dopamine receptor blockade and inhibition of dopamine release, yet an increase in the rate of dopamine and norepinephrine turnover. Antihistaminic and anti-serotonergic actions may also contribute to the sedative effects. The result of all these actions is an overall decrease in motor activity, and an increase in the threshold for responding to external stimuli.

Centrally, dopamine receptors are found in the basal ganglia, the medulla (vasomotor and respiratory centres and the chemoreceptor trigger zone [CTZ]), and the hypothalamus. Peripherally, dopamine receptors are found, e.g. in the cardiovascular system and the kidneys. At least five types of G-protein coupled dopamine receptors have been described but they are grouped into two main families according to whether their activation results in an increase in intracellular cyclic adenosine monophosphate (cAMP) production (the D1-like receptor family, which includes D1 and D5 receptors) or whether their activation results in a decrease in intracellular cAMP production (the D2-like receptor family, which includes D2, D3, and D4 receptors).

On blood vessels, post-synaptic dopamine receptors are of the D1-like family and their activation promotes vasodilation; and pre-synaptic dopamine receptors are of the D2-like family and their activation results in reduced neurotransmitter (norepinephrine) release from the pre-synaptic terminal, which also promotes vasodilation. The peripheral anti-dopaminergic actions of phenothiazines would thus seem to favour vasoconstriction, but this effect is relatively mild compared to the alpha 1 receptor antagonism, hence overall, vasodilation prevails.

It is often said that low doses of acepromazine produce **tranquillisation/anxiolysis**, whereas higher doses produce **sedation**. The dose–response curve, however, rapidly reaches a plateau, after which increasing the dose only increases the duration of effect, not necessarily the degree of sedation. **Onset of action** depends upon the route of administration, but even after IV administration, it is suggested to wait 20–40 minutes, whilst leaving the patient undisturbed, for the full effect to occur. Sedation after acepromazine begins to wane after three to four hours, but can last up to six to eight hours, and can be prolonged by debility. However, acepromazine is unpredictable, and different responses can be seen in the same animal under different circumstances. The effects can also be overcome (temporarily) by an adequate stimulus, hence acepromazine is rarely used as the sole sedative agent. *See below for discussion about phenothiazines and benzodiazepines for noise-related sensitivities.*

Phenothiazines synergise with the CNS depressant effects of other sedative and anaesthetic agents, therefore the doses of these other agents can be reduced. Doxapram (an analeptic [CNS stimulant]) is suggested as an antagonist to excessive CNS depression caused by phenothiazines. (Amphetamines may also be useful.)

There may be species, breed, and individual sensitivities, and larger animals tend to be 'more sensitive' possibly because of allometric scaling. (Perhaps we should dose according to body surface area rather than to body weight; see later under dexmedetomidine.) Brachycephalics also tend to be 'more sensitive' to the effects of acepromazine (see below).

Occasionally, contradictory symptoms occur, such as generalised CNS stimulation and aggressiveness. At high doses, **extrapyramidal effects** can be seen, such as akathisia (increased locomotor activity and uncontrollable restlessness).

Neuroleptic Malignant Syndrome This may follow the use of phenothiazines and butyrophenones and its occurrence is possibly facilitated by dehydration, exhaustion, or CNS disease. The syndrome appears to be related to the anti-dopaminergic activity of the drugs. Clinical signs develop over one to three days and include:

- Hyperthermia
- Altered consciousness (excitement, restlessness, seizures, recumbency)
- Muscle rigidity (and damage leading to raised values of creatine kinase) due to extrapyramidal dysfunction (tremor/dystonia)
- Autonomic instability (tachycardia, labile blood pressure, sweating, salivation, urinary incontinence)

The differential diagnosis should include malignant hyperthermia, rhabdomyolysis, tetanus, serotonin syndrome and central anticholinergic syndrome (see below). Treatment is supportive and includes oxygen supplementation, fluid therapy, cooling, and possibly dantrolene. Occasional mortality occurs from acute renal failure, arrhythmias, pulmonary emboli, or aspiration pneumonia.

Central Anticholinergic Syndrome This occasionally occurs after administration of compounds with anticholinergic activity (atropine, pethidine, phenothiazines). Clinical signs are related to a decrease in the inhibitory actions of acetylcholine and include vacillation between hyperexcitability and depression, muscular incoordination, restlessness, anxiety, hallucinations, convulsions, coma, and signs of peripheral anticholinergic activity, such as tachycardia, dry mouth, dry skin, urinary retention. Diagnosis is confirmed by reversal of symptoms following physostigmine administration.

4.1.3.4.2 Cardiovascular Effects

Hypotension Due mainly to peripheral (systemic > pulmonary), α1 receptor blockade and the resulting vasodilation, but also, suppression of the sympathetic nervous system both centrally and peripherally, resulting in a slight change in autonomic balance towards an increased parasympathetic tone. Occasionally, the slight fall in blood pressure elicits a reflex tachycardia, but bradycardia has also been described. A slight negative inotropy occurs, probably due to the decrease in sympathetic tone. Beware in excited animals or those with pre-existing hypovolaemia.

Hypovolaemic animals try to maintain their blood pressure by increasing their sympathetic tone and vasoconstricting their periphery in order to centralise their remaining blood volume to supply vital organs. Acepromazine-induced peripheral vasodilation may overcome this compensatory response and result in a profound hypotension for which the animal can no longer compensate: syncope ('fainting') may result as cerebral perfusion is compromised (see below).

Syncope Cardiovascular collapse due to hypotension, usually accompanied by severe bradycardia, can lead to fainting. Dogs are quite susceptible to this, especially the brachycephalic breeds with their inherently high resting vagal tone, where acepromazine can further reduce their sympathetic tone, resulting in marked vagal dominance. Doses above 0.1 mg/kg have been reported to cause this in dogs whilst other authors report no such effect after 0.3 mg/kg. Acepromazine also increases the risk of respiratory obstruction in brachycephalics, because of the sedation and 'muscle relaxation' (including the pharyngeal muscles) produced. Lower doses (0.005–0.01 mg/kg) are recommended in brachycephalics with clinical airway obstruction.

Adrenaline Reversal (Dale's Vasomotor Reversal) Excited and apprehensive animals have high levels of circulating catecholamines. Catecholamines include epinephrine (adrenaline) and norepinephrine (noradrenaline). Norepinephrine is a vasoconstrictor (α agonist), but this action is antagonised by acepromazine. Epinephrine can act as a vasoconstrictor at high concentrations ($\alpha1$ [and $\alpha2$] effects), so can also be antagonised by acepromazine, but epinephrine preferentially produces vasodilation, especially at lower concentrations ($\beta2$ effects). When norepinephrine's and epinephrine's $\alpha1$ vasoconstrictive activity is blocked by acepromazine, then epinephrine's $\beta2$ vasodilative activity can prevail. Therefore, epinephrine's $\beta2$-induced vasodilation can enhance the $\alpha1$ blocking (i.e. vasodilatory) effects of acepromazine, and worsen the overall vasodilation and hypotension, resulting in **fainting**.

If hypotension becomes a problem, **treatment** is with **$\alpha1$ agonists** (e.g. phenylephrine), or ino-constrictors (e.g. ephedrine), and **intravenous fluids**.

The cardiovascular depressant effects of other anaesthetic agents can exacerbate the effects of phenothiazines.

Anti-Arrhythmic Effects Phenothiazines are said to reduce the incidence of catecholamine-induced cardiac arrhythmias in dogs under barbiturate and halothane anaesthesia (which increase the sensitivity of the myocardium to such arrhythmias). Suggested mechanisms include:

- Reduction of overall activity of the sympathetic nervous system (i.e. reduction of circulating catecholamines), and change of autonomic nervous system (ANS) balance to a more parasympathetic dominance.
- Local anaesthetic-like activity/membrane stabilising effects (acepromazine has been shown to decrease the

conduction velocity in cardiomyocytes, with a concomitant increase in the refractory period, a quinidine-like effect).
- Blockade of 'cardiac α(1 or 2?) arrhythmic receptors', combined with only a weak anticholinergic effect on the heart.

4.1.3.4.3 Respiratory Effects

The literature is confusing. Phenothiazines reduce the sensitivity of the respiratory centre to carbon dioxide and usually a slight reduction in respiratory rate is observed. There is normally little change (or a slight decrease) in tidal volume. Overall, minute ventilation is minimally reduced and blood gases remain almost unchanged.

The respiratory depressant effects of other sedative and anaesthetic agents can be enhanced by phenothiazines.

4.1.3.4.4 Anti-Emetic Effect

Phenothiazines inhibit dopamine (and histamine, serotonin (5-HT), and acetylcholine [ACH]), activity in the central CTZ. Their anti-emetic effect is especially good against the emetic effects of opioids (and possibly $\alpha2$ agonists).

Phenothiazines are less effective for the treatment of motion sickness (nausea and vomiting of vestibular origin), but may help to prevent it (perhaps due to anxiolysis). Sedation is an unwanted side effect when phenothiazines are used for their anti-emetic activity.

4.1.3.4.5 Antihistaminic Effects

Due to H_1 receptor blockade. Different phenothiazines have different antihistaminic potencies, but acepromazine should not be used prior to intradermal skin testing.

4.1.3.4.6 Pro- or Anticonvulsant Properties?

At one time, acepromazine was suggested to lower the seizure threshold in animals with epilepsy and so caution was advised regarding its use in animals with a history of seizures. This information was, however, related to chlorpromazine, not acepromazine. Two retrospective studies have confirmed that acepromazine does not increase the incidence of seizures in epileptic dogs.

At one time it was thought that acepromazine premedication in cases undergoing myelography could facilitate any seizure activity triggered by irritant radiographic contrast media. One study, however, reported no increase in seizure frequency when acepromazine was administered for premedication.

4.1.3.4.7 Anticholinergic Effects

Weak anti-muscarinic effects, mainly noted as anti-spasmodic effects in the GI tract, with slight reduction in GI tract secretions. Although acepromazine has been shown to be **spasmolytic**, its use has not been associated with any increased risk of ileus, possibly because of its sympatholytic properties. It does, however, cause relaxation of the cardiac sphincter, and may increase the risk of reflux and regurgitation.

Peripheral anti-dopaminergic effects on the GI tract add to the decreased gut motility, but tend to increase GI tract secretions.

4.1.3.4.8 Hypothermia

Due to depression of activity in the hypothalamic thermoregulatory centre, and to increased heat loss from the vasodilated periphery. Especially of concern in young or small-sized animals and with cold ambient temperatures.

4.1.3.4.9 Analgesia

Acepromazine is not analgesic. Methotrimeprazine appears to exert analgesic actions in its own right; however, other phenothiazines merely enhance the analgesia afforded by opioids and α2 agonists. Mechanisms may include dopaminergic, adrenergic, and local anaesthetic effects.

4.1.3.4.10 Local Anaesthetic Behaviour

Chlorpromazine may be the most potent in this respect. It can block sodium (and possibly other cation) channels.

4.1.3.4.11 Muscle Relaxation

Phenothiazines do not cause muscle relaxation as such, but do reduce general locomotor/muscle activity because of their anxiolytic effects; and they do decrease the muscle spasticity associated with ketamine. (Remember that side effects can include muscle tremors, rigidity, and akathisia).

4.1.3.4.12 Hepatic Effects

Acepromazine has no direct hepatotoxic actions, although may cause an increase in bile viscosity. Repeated dosing may result in hepatic enzyme induction.

4.1.3.4.13 Renal Effects

No direct toxic effects, but beware prolonged and severe hypotension. Phenothiazines may have mild diuretic effects via suppression of antidiuretic hormone (ADH) secretion, and/or via direct action on renal tubular dopamine receptors (especially D1) to decrease water and electrolyte reabsorption.

4.1.3.4.14 Hormonal Effects

Reduction in ADH, growth hormone and adrenocorticotropic hormone (ACTH, and therefore cortisol) secretion. Cortisol has permissive effects on the actions of catecholamines, and ADH has vasoconstrictor properties. Alongside the reduced catecholamine release (with anxiolysis/sedation), reduced cortisol and ADH can promote vasodilation and hypotension. The inhibition of ADH secretion may promote a mild diuresis.

Prolactin levels increase because of reduced secretion of prolactin-release-inhibiting hormone, and anti-dopaminergic activity in the pituitary. Increased prolactin levels can lead to gynaecomastia and galactorrhoea with long-term treatment (more a problem in humans). High doses may reduce follicular stimulating hormone (FSH) and luteinising hormone (LH) secretion and oestrus cycles may be suppressed. Data sheets caution against the administration of acepromazine to pregnant animals, although no specific studies have been performed to assess its safety during pregnancy.

4.1.3.4.15 Haematological Effects

A dose-dependent decrease in packed cell volume, platelet count, and total protein is seen within 30 minutes of administration in dogs, cows, and horses, thought to be due to splenic sequestration, and possibly to changes in the Starling forces across capillary beds. A slight reduction in white blood cell (WBC) count may be due to margination of cells.

Antithrombotic Effect Phenothiazines interact with the phospholipid bilayer membrane of platelets to inhibit aggregation via increasing membrane fluidity. Acepromazine's ability to decrease platelet count (splenic sequestration) and platelet function (decreased aggregation) is only transient and has never been reported to cause any increased risk associated with poor haemostasis in previously normal patients. Caution should, however, be exercised in animals with pre-existing coagulopathy, and, in particular, those with decreased platelet function (including von Willebrand's disease).

Blood Dyscrasias Leukopaenia and agranulocytosis have only been rarely associated with long-term administration of phenothiazines in humans.

Metabolic Effects Chlorpromazine causes a significant increase in plasma cholesterol in humans.

Other Effects No work has been done to establish the safety, or otherwise, of acepromazine in pregnant animals.

Phenothiazines **can exacerbate the effects of organophosphate compounds**, via reversible inhibition of acetylcholinesterase and pseudocholinesterase; (despite exhibiting atropine-like effects), so beware recent ectoparasite treatments.

Long-term treatment can sometimes result in **photosensitisation**, although this is mostly reported as a problem of chronic chlorpromazine administration in people.

4.1.3.5   Uses of Acepromazine in Small Animals
(For horses, see Chapter 28)

- Available as 2 mg/ml yellow solution (not to be confused with the equine 5 mg/ml or 10 mg/ml solutions); and as pale yellow 10 mg tablets.
- For sedation/premedication.
- As a tranquilliser/sedative during treatment of tetanus.
- Was once fashionable as a vasodilator in the treatment of arterial thromboembolic disorders in cats, but less commonly used now.
- As an aid to urethral relaxation in 'blocked cats' (but beware their intravascular volume status).
- Behavioural challenges. More effective options exist than oral acepromazine tablets (see below).

The dose is very variable and depends upon the size and nature of the animal, and on which other drug/s may be combined with it. Injectable acepromazine can be administered IM or IV, although, at least in cats, absorption after SC injection may also be adequate. Allow 20–40 minutes after injection (any route), and at least 40 minutes after oral administration, for it to take effect, and leave the animal undisturbed in quiet surroundings for this time for the best results.

The effects of phenothiazines are exacerbated by:

- Age – very old and very young
- Debility
- Renal disease
- Hepatic disease
- Hypovolaemia
- Congestive heart disease
- Beware in brachycephalics

4.1.3.5.1   *Dogs*
The injectable dose is 0.01–0.05 (reported even up to 0.1) mg/kg IM, or lower doses IV (0.005 mg/kg). Doses as low as 0.01 mg/kg IM can still cause syncope in hypovolaemic dogs. Use the lower doses in bigger dogs (applying allometric scaling, i.e. metabolic rate is more related to surface area than body mass); and extremely low doses in brachycephalics and sick dogs. The oral dose is generally 1 mg/kg but can vary from 0.25–3 mg/kg.

The **effect** tends to be **more predictable if combined with an opioid**, and lower acepromazine doses can often then be used too. Opioids have sedative properties which are enhanced by combination with other sedatives/tranquillisers. Increasing the dose of opioid tends to prolong the duration of sedation rather than increase the sedative effect. Such combinations provide **neuroleptanalgesia** (the combination of a neuroleptic/tranquilliser, and an analgesic), and include:

- acepromazine 0.01–0.03 mg/kg + methadone (0.1–0.5 mg/kg) IM
- acepromazine 0.01–0.03 mg/kg + morphine (0.1–0.5 mg/kg) IM
- acepromazine 0.01–0.03 mg/kg + pethidine (3.5–5 mg/kg) IM; never IV
- acepromazine 0.01–0.03 mg/kg + butorphanol (0.1–0.5 mg/kg) IM
- acepromazine 0.01–0.03 mg/kg + buprenorphine (0.02 mg/kg) IM

Sedation of aggressive dogs can be attempted with the combination of acepromazine and an opioid, with papaveretum (a mixture of opium alkaloids) being suggested as the best opioid. The papaveretum dose suggested is c. 0.2+ mg/kg. However, **never** trust any 'sedated-looking' dog, as some will be able to be aroused, even if only transiently, and bite. See below for more effective options.

4.1.3.5.2   *Cats*
The injectable dose is 0.05–0.1 mg/kg IM (or SC), and lower (e.g. half the dose) for IV administration. Again, very unpredictable, and possibly even more so than in dogs. Use lower doses (or avoid) in sick cats. Oral doses are the same as for dogs (i.e. c. 1 mg/kg PO), but rarely indicated.

More predictable sedation is obtained if acepromazine is combined with an opioid:

- Acepromazine c. 0.05 mg/kg + methadone (0.1–0.5 mg/kg) IM
- Acepromazine c. 0.05 mg/kg + morphine (0.1–0.2 mg/kg) IM
- Acepromazine c. 0.05 mg/kg + pethidine (5 mg/kg) IM or SC; never IV
- Acepromazine c. 0.05 mg/kg + butorphanol (0.1–0.5 mg/kg) IM
- Acepromazine c. 0.05 mg/kg + buprenorphine (0.02 mg/kg) IM

Allow 20–40 minutes for sedation to develop; it usually wanes in 3–4 hours, but can persist for about 7 hours. As well as these neuroleptanalgesic combinations, acepromazine has been used with ketamine in cats, to provide a state approaching full dissociative anaesthesia. Acepromazine offsets the muscle hypertonus associated with ketamine and can smooth induction and recovery from 'anaesthesia'. Doses recommended are acepromazine (0.05–0.1 mg/kg) + ketamine (c. 5+ mg/kg) IM or even SC. Allow at least 20 minutes for the full effect to occur. Doses up to 0.4 mg/kg were at one time suggested for cases of arterial thromboembolism.

4.1.4 Butyrophenones

Butyrophenones are even less predictable than pheno-thiazines and tend to cause excitement before sedation finally occurs. They are, however, potent anti-emetics. Butyrophenones are said to cause less cardiorespiratory depression and interference with thermoregulation than phenothiazines. Sedation occurs due to a combination of anti-dopaminergic, anti-adrenergic, and GABA-mimetic activity in the reticular activating system. Only two are licenced for use in veterinary species: azaperone in pigs, and fluanisone in rabbits, guinea pigs, mice, and rats, mar-keted in combination with fentanyl as Hypnorm™ (see Chapter 35 on pigs and Chapter 36 on rabbits).

4.1.5 Thioxanthenes

These are phenothiazine relatives and are used as anti-psychotics in people, e.g. zuclopenthixol. They have anti-dopaminergic (and therefore sedative) and anti-adrenergic actions, and also depress the release of many hypothalamic and pituitary hormones. Zuclopenthixol is available as the relatively long-acting injectable esters ('salts'): zuclopenthixol decanoate (long-acting) and zuclopenthixol acetate (shorter-acting), which may be useful to provide relatively long duration mild sedation for wild or feral animals.

4.1.6 Benzodiazepines

The benzodiazepines used in small animals are **diazepam** (licenced) and **midazolam** (not licenced). Zolazepam, in com-bination with tiletamine, is licenced (Telazol™ or Zoletil™) in some countries for IM and IV administration in dogs and cats, for sedation and anaesthesia, and can be used for capture chemi-cal restraint in a wide variety of wild/exotic species.

Midazolam is roughly twice as potent as diazepam and shorter acting, but this difference is often hard to detect clinically. Both can be well absorbed across mucous mem-branes. Midazolam has been used by the intranasal/trans-mucosal route for seizure control in dogs, and diazepam is also available in preparations for rectal administration. (Oral administration with subsequent absorption via the stomach and hepatic portal vein, results in significant first-pass metabolism, so doses must be increased [perhaps dou-bled] to be effective by this route.) Diazepam is irritant intramuscularly and has lower bioavailability by this route, so midazolam is preferred for IM use.

4.1.6.1 Actions
- Anticonvulsant
- Anxiolytic and sedative
- Muscle relaxation (skeletal muscle)

- Amnesic (anterograde; also some retrograde)
- **Not analgesic**

4.1.6.2 Pharmacology

Benzodiazepines consist of a core structure of a benzene ring fused to a diazepine ring. Midazolam is unusual in that it contains an imidazole ring. In acidic solution, this ring opens and the compound becomes water soluble, but, at pH >4, the ring closes and it becomes highly lipophilic. This unusual feature enables water-soluble salts to be prepared (commercially available solutions have pH 3.5), which can be administered IV or IM. The formulation of diazepam solubilised in propylene glycol should be administered only intravenously. Intramuscular deposition of this formulation results in poor bioavailability and causes discomfort on injection (because of the propylene glycol). **Propylene glycol** has also been blamed for haemolysis, cardiac arrhythmias, and hypotension. An alternative formulation of diazepam is available as an emulsion in soybean oil/ egg phosphatide/glycerol (intralipid™). It should only be administered IV as its bioavailability after intramuscular administration is poor. Diazepam adheres to certain types of plastic, possibly including those of syringes and IV fluid giving sets (equivocal results), so that any injections should be prepared immediately before administration.

Both diazepam and midazolam are highly protein bound (>95%). Hepatic metabolism results in a variety of metabolites, which are excreted in urine and faeces (via bile). Many of diazepam's metabolites are active, e.g. nor-diazepam [desmethyldiazepam], oxazepam, and temaze-pam, and there is potential for entero-hepatic recycling and cumulative effects. Repeated doses are also cumula-tive. Midazolam's metabolites, however, have very little activity, so it is better suited to administration by infu-sion, if that is necessary (see later). Diazepam has a slightly slower onset of action than midazolam after IV administration and may produce drowsiness lasting for several (4 up to 12+) hours (compared with 1–4 hours for midazolam).

4.1.6.3 Mechanisms of Action

Benzodiazepines act on specific benzodiazepine binding sites, which are associated with $GABA_A$ receptors, to enhance the affinity for, and/or action of, gamma-amin-obutyric acid (GABA), which is an inhibitory neurotrans-mitter. These receptors are found primarily in the brain and spinal cord. Benzodiazepines and barbiturates also enhance each other's binding at $GABA_A$ receptors, hence they can potentiate each other's GABA-ergic effects. Benzodiazepines increase the frequency of the $GABA_A$ receptor's chloride channel opening, whereas barbiturates increase the duration of its opening.

Benzodiazepines depress activity in the reticular activating system, by enhancing GABA actions, to produce sleepiness on a scale from **anxiolysis to sedation** (dose-dependent). Central GABA-enhancing activity explains their **anticonvulsant** effect. They also act in the spinal cord, where they depress internuncial neurotransmission, resulting in **postural muscle weakness**, via enhancement of inhibitory GABA effects, and possibly by potentiation of the inhibitory effects of glycine. This muscle weakness is often referred to as 'central' muscle relaxation.

Some texts also claim an anti-arrhythmic effect, probably more related to a reduction in circulating catecholamines with 'sedation' than any direct myocardial effects. (Beware preparations of diazepam in propylene glycol, as the latter may cause arrhythmias.) Benzodiazepines may also modulate NMDA receptor activity.

4.1.6.4 Results of Administration

4.1.6.4.1 Anxiolysis/Sedation

Somewhat dose-dependent, however, **disinhibition** (excitement [paradoxical] often associated with a 'change of character') can also occur.

4.1.6.4.2 Cardiovascular Depression

This is minimal, especially at lower doses. Midazolam, at higher doses (0.2+ mg/kg), causes more cardiovascular depression (some negative inotropy and vasodilation, which result in hypotension), than diazepam (the effects of which are negligible at this dose). Following higher dose midazolam administration, a transient fall in blood pressure and slight increase in heart rate occur.

4.1.6.4.3 Respiratory Depression

This is minimal at doses up to 0.2 mg/kg, but can enhance the respiratory depression caused by other anaesthetic agents and adjuncts. Respiratory depression is due to a reduced ventilatory response to carbon dioxide, and a slight relaxation of intercostal muscles producing less effective ventilation. It is more readily apparent in the anaesthetised patient. When used for anaesthetic co-induction with alfaxalone, midazolam 0.4 mg/kg IV caused more post-induction apnoea than alfaxalone alone. Another study showed that 0.25 mg/kg midazolam IV caused more post-induction apnoea if given before the alfaxalone compared with after it, but this was most likely due to a higher dose of alfaxalone being necessary (see below regarding an auto-priming technique).

4.1.6.4.4 Other Effects

There may be endocrine effects because benzodiazepines reduce plasma ACTH and cortisol concentrations, but the significance of this is not clear.

Diazepam may increase cardiac sphincter tone.

Liver enzyme induction may occur. Hepatic disease may slow metabolism, but renal disease, despite having unpredictable effects on drug volume of distribution and clearance, appears to require little dose adjustment. Beware hepatic disease if hypoproteinaemia is present, as there may be an increase in the proportion of 'free' (unbound) drug, so that an exaggerated response (overdose) is observed. Animals with portosystemic shunts may be hypoproteinaemic, and many are prone to seizures/hepatic encephalopathy (due to production/absorption of 'false neurotransmitters' from the gut), despite the common finding of increased circulating 'endogenous benzodiazepines'. Some clinicians will not use benzodiazepines in animals with portosystemic shunts because of the problems associated with protein-binding, drug metabolism, and the potential for increased likelihood of seizures due to either 'disinhibition' (inhibition of inhibitory pathways, and therefore excitement), or rebound seizures (i.e. exogenous benzodiazepines may help initially, but seizures can recur as their effect wears off).

The oral administration of diazepam in cats has been associated with the development of 'fulminant hepatic failure'; and many internal medicine clinicians do not favour its use in cats with or without hepatic disease.

4.1.6.5 Uses and Doses

- Use alone for anxiolysis/sedation

  Benzodiazepines are often used as the sole anxiolytic/sedative agent for paediatric, geriatric, and debilitated patients. Their use alone in fit healthy adult animals may result in CNS excitement reactions and possibly altered temperament, e.g. a previously quiet animal may become aggressive (due to **disinhibition**, the relief of inhibitions). The dose for either diazepam or midazolam is 0.1–0.4 mg/kg IV. For debilitated animals, try the lower dose. Although midazolam is twice as potent as diazepam, it is shorter acting, and halving the dose is not commonly practised. **Midazolam can also be administered IM**. As oral anxiolytics, benzodiazepines can be administered at 0.2–0.4 mg/kg PO every eight hours for cats (but see above and below regarding liver problems); and 0.5–2 mg/kg PO for dogs as required.

- In combination with opioids

  Benzodiazepines can be used in combination with opioids (morphine, methadone, pethidine, butorphanol, buprenorphine), or other sedative agents (acepromazine or α2 agonists). Dose 0.1–0.25 mg/kg IV.

- As a co-induction agent

  Benzodiazepines can be used as co-induction agents alongside, e.g. alfaxalone or propofol, to reduce the dose requirements of the anaesthetic agent. (The dose requirement for ketamine is difficult to lower, because of its dissociative effects.) Dose 0.1–0.25 mg/kg IV.

  It is debatable whether co-induction with midazolam and alfaxalone is of cardiovascular benefit, as cardiovascular depression is minimal with alfaxalone alone and so any dose reduction produces minimal measurable effects. However, improved post-induction ventilation has been shown when midazolam was used in conjunction with alfaxalone during an auto-priming co-induction technique, which enabled significant alfaxalone dose reduction (see below).

For this auto-priming co-induction technique: first give a 'priming' dose of induction agent (approx. ¼ of the calculated dose); then give the benzodiazepine (e.g. midazolam 0.25 mg/kg IV); and finally, give enough induction agent to facilitate tracheal intubation.

- As an adjunct to ketamine

Benzodiazepines offset the increased muscle tone that occurs with ketamine. Dose 0.1–0.25 mg/kg IV, with ketamine dose of 2.5 mg/kg.

Midazolam (0.1–0.25 mg/kg), can be used in conjunction with ketamine (c. 2.5–5+ mg/kg) IM (or IV using the lower doses) in ill or debilitated cats, to produce a more tractable patient, e.g. for insertion of an IV catheter, blood sampling, or minimally-invasive imaging procedures. Endotracheal intubation is, however, usually not possible because of retained gag and pharyngeal and laryngeal reflexes.

- To provide muscle relaxation

Benzodiazepines can be used in the treatment of tetanus and for 'muscle relaxation' to improve analgesia when intervertebral discs have prolapsed. They may be useful for urethral relaxation in 'blocked cats'. Dose 0.5–1 mg/kg IV; 0.5–5 mg/kg PO (but up to 10 mg/kg if necessary).

- To ease post-operative restlessness

Benzodiazepines can be given to calm patients with post-operative restlessness/emergence delirium, although alpha-2-agonists give a more predictable effect. Dose 0.25–0.4 mg/kg (some cardiorespiratory depression may occur at these higher doses). Ensure that the animal is pain-free, not suffering from opioid excitement, and ensure it has an empty bladder and is as comfortable as possible.

- Anxiolysis and amnesia for noise-related fear/anxiety or phobia responses (e.g. to fireworks)

Benzodiazepines are more suitable anxiolytics than phenothiazines and also provide useful amnesic (both retrograde and anterograde) effects. The use of, e.g. acepromazine alone, in noise-sensitive anxious dogs is not appropriate. (Although phenothiazines may produce sedation, they also compromise motor function, which gives owners an impression of their pet being relaxed. Phenothiazines, however, do not affect sensory input and thus leave these dogs suffering from negative emotional responses to the fireworks, whilst reducing their escape [motor] responses, which can have long-lasting effects on behavioural responses and also on physiological stress.) Benzodiazepines can have a variable effect in individuals and can occasionally result in paradoxical agitation that negates their benefit. Trial dosing is therefore recommended. Benzodiazepine-induced disinhibition can also lead to an alteration in the dog's behavioural response to their negative emotion and therefore a behavioural history should be taken before medication is prescribed to identify whether inhibition is present. Use of medication without addressing environmental factors, both physical in terms of provision of suitable hideouts and social in terms of owner behaviour, is not recommended. When treating, rather than managing, firework-related fear/anxiety or phobia responses, it may be beneficial to prescribe a selective serotonin re-uptake inhibitor (SSRI, e.g. fluoxetine) and combine this with a benzodiazepine during periods of unavoidable exposure to fireworks. Alprazolam is commonly used for this purpose at 0.01–0.05 mg/kg PO as required. Oral transmucosal dexmedetomidine gel has recently been licenced in the UK to reduce noise-related anxiety in dogs.

- As anticonvulsants

Benzodiazepines can be given for the treatment of convulsions/status epilepticus and can be administered by infusion if necessary. Midazolam is possibly a better choice as it does not adhere to plastic and is less cumulative. There is also no propylene glycol to worry about. Dose: diazepam 0.5 mg/kg IV; midazolam 0.25 mg/kg IV. Repeat every 10 minutes, up to a total of three doses. If struggling to get IV access, the dose can be administered per rectum. Alternatively, midazolam 0.5 mg/kg intranasally (transmucosally) is effective using a mucosal atomisation device (e.g. the nozzle from a kennel cough vaccine). Midazolam infusion rates are around 0.3 mg/kg/h (5 µg/kg/min) IV and are useful to reduce propofol requirements for status epilepticus patients. Caution in cats because of their difficulty with hepatic glucuronidation of phenolic compounds (i.e. those containing benzene rings).

- As appetite stimulants

For cats, diazepam can be given 0.1–0.2 mg/kg IV once before offering food. (Other agents, e.g. mirtazepine and cyproheptadine can also be considered.)

4.1.6.6 Antagonism

Flumazenil is a benzodiazepine antagonist and **sarmazenil** acts as a partial inverse agonist. Either can be used to antagonise the effects of benzodiazepines. Flumazenil is the most available, although expensive. The dose required depends upon the dose of agonist given and the length of time since its administration, however, a starting dose would be of the order of 10 µg/kg IV. The duration of antagonism provided by flumazenil is relatively brief and repeat doses may be necessary.

4.1.7 α2 Adrenoceptor Agonists

α2 adrenoceptor agonists are sedative drugs with analgesic and muscle relaxant properties. The licenced drugs for small animal use are **medetomidine** (1 mg/ml), **dexmedetomidine** (0.5 mg/ml, and oral transmucosal gel 0.1 mg/ml) and **xylazine** (20 mg/ml). Licenced drugs for horses are xylazine (20 mg/ml and 100 mg/ml), detomidine (10 mg/ml), and romifidine (10 mg/ml). Licenced drugs for cattle are xylazine (20 mg/ml) and detomidine (10 mg/ml). For more details on horses and farm species, see Chapters 28, 33, and 35. **Whether sedative effects outlast analgesic effects is equivocal.** Effects become apparent within 5 minutes of IM administration, but maximal sedation may take up to 20 minutes to be achieved. Duration of sedation is dose-dependent, but is of the order of 30–60 minutes after xylazine, and 30–180 minutes after medetomidine or dexmedetomidine.

4.1.7.1 Actions and Effects

α2 agonists act both centrally (at the spinal and supraspinal [brain], levels) and peripherally on G-protein coupled α2 adrenoreceptors. These are widely distributed in the body, although the exact numbers of receptors, their sensitivity, and their distribution in the body may vary among species and possibly with certain disease states. α2 receptors can also be found pre-synaptically and post-synaptically, whereas α1 receptors are generally post-synaptic. The actions of α2 agonists depend upon:

- Interaction with α2 (and α1) receptors
- Interaction with imidazoline receptors (I1, I2, and I3)
- 'Local anaesthetic type' activity via actions on ion channels
- 'Membrane effects', independent of specific receptor/ion channel effects

α2 adrenoceptor agonists produce the following effects:

- Anxiolysis
- Sedation
- Neuroprotection/possibly anticonvulsant?
- Analgesia
- Muscle relaxation
- Bradycardia
- Arterial blood pressure changes
- Thermoregulatory suppression, but peripheral vasoconstriction
- Emesis
- Reduction in GI tract motility and perfusion
- Uterine activity increases (depending upon species, drug, and whether gravid or non-gravid uterus)
- May be pro- or anti-arrhythmic?
- Endocrine changes (hyperglycaemia, diuresis)
- Coagulation (platelet aggregation) possibly enhanced?
- Ocular changes

4.1.7.2 Pharmacology

These compounds contain benzene rings. Some also contain a thiazine ring (e.g. xylazine), whereas others contain an imidazole ring (e.g. medetomidine, dexmedetomidine, and detomidine), and romifidine, whilst being an imidazoline derivative, does not contain an imidazole ring.

Due to their relatively high lipophilicity, they cross membranes easily, e.g. the blood–brain barrier, placental barrier, gut wall, and mucous membranes. Xylazine, medetomidine, and dexmedetomidine are not 'pure' α2 agonists, but show selectivity for interaction with α2 receptors. In this respect, medetomidine, and dexmedetomidine are much more selective for α2 receptors than α1 receptors; whereas xylazine is less α2 selective and has some, not insignificant, α1 activity also (Table 4.1). Imidazoline derivatives also have more activity at imidazoline (I1, I2, and I3) receptors, than thiazine derivatives.

4.1.7.2.1 Receptors

Alpha (α) Subtypes α1 and α2, are further subdivided into α1A, α1B, α1C, and α2A, α2B, α2C, and α2D (the rodent homologue of human α2A).

Beta (β) Subtypes β1, β2 and β3

Imidazoline 'Receptors' Imidazoline derivatives also interact with non-adrenergic, imidazoline-preferring binding sites (I receptors, also subdivided into I1, I2, and I3 types, with I2 being subdivided further into I2A and I2B). I1 receptors are G-protein coupled and are found in the brain (medulla oblongata and reticular formation), and adrenal medulla, renal epithelium, pancreatic islets, prostate, and platelets. Their stimulation produces a centrally mediated hypotension. I2 receptors are non-G-protein coupled and are present in the outer mitochondrial membrane in the cells of many tissues. I3 receptors are found in pancreatic β cells.

Table 4.1 Receptor selectivity of the common α2 agonists.

Drug	α2: α1 selectivity ratio
Clonidine	220:1
Xylazine	160:1
Detomidine	260:1
Medetomidine (mainly due to the dextro isomer, dexmedetomidine)	1620:1
Romifidine	340:1

Significant interaction occurs between α2 and I receptors. Central and peripheral imidazoline receptors may be responsible for some of the observed effects of α2 agonist drugs. These receptors are thought to have different signal transduction mechanisms compared with α2 receptors, but their activation may influence the activity of nearby α2 receptors. I2 receptors appear to be, or be associated with, allosteric binding sites on enzymes, especially monoamine oxidase (both MAOA and B), and their stimulation results in enzyme inhibition. Cardiac and neural mitochondrial I2 receptors may be involved in protection against ischaemia (see below). Some I2 receptors appear to be involved in the regulation of body temperature, food intake, and gut motility, whereas others are involved in pain modulation, especially in chronic pain states. I3 receptors increase insulin secretion from pancreatic β cells. I3 receptors may be associated with ATP-sensitive potassium channels.

Receptor Distribution
- Peripheral and central (spinal/supraspinal)
- Pre-synaptic (autoreceptors), post-synaptic, and extrasynaptic

α2A receptors are most prevalent in the CNS, whereas α2B receptors are most prevalent peripherally. α2A, α2B, and α2C receptors are thought to be involved in the analgesic actions of α2 agonist drugs. Different species have different receptor subtypes, distributions, and receptor densities.

Metabolism occurs mainly in the liver (particularly oxidative and hydrolytic breakdown), and metabolites are excreted in the urine. A small amount of unchanged parent compound may also be excreted in the urine. Many metabolites are produced, but most have minimal activity. Repeated doses may result in some apparent tolerance, which may be due to hepatic enzyme induction or receptor down regulation/desensitisation or perhaps the functionally-antagonistic effects of central α1 receptor stimulation (which result in arousal). However, medetomidine has also been reported to inhibit the Cytochrome P450 enzyme system.

4.1.7.3 Results of Administration
4.1.7.3.1 Anxiolysis and Sedation
Anxiolysis and sedation are produced by actions at **different sites** within the CNS. Sedation follows α2A agonism in the locus coeruleus in the brainstem; whereas anxiolysis follows suppression of activity in the reticular activating system. α2 agonist action at pre-synaptic receptors reduces neurotransmitter release, whereas their action at post-synaptic receptors results in membrane hyperpolarisation (and therefore reduced sensitivity to neurotransmission); the overall result being reduced synaptic transmission in the CNS. The sedation produced by α2 agonists resembles that produced by opioids, because α2 and opioid receptors are found in similar locations throughout the body, and these receptors also share common signal transduction pathways (involving G proteins), and common effector mechanisms (e.g. changes in ion permeabilities). α2 agonists and opioids are therefore synergistic.

The anxiolytic and sedative effects of the α2 agonist dose also depends upon the basal level of excitement of the animal at the time of drug administration. The more excited/stressed the animal, the less will be the observed sedative effects. Note that sedated animals may be stimulated to arouse transiently and can bite accurately in that short time. Never trust a sedated animal, even after combination of an α2 agonist with an opioid, which normally improves the reliability of the sedation.

4.1.7.3.2 Anaesthetic Sparing Effect
The anxiolytic/sedative, analgesic, and myorelaxant effects also allow reduction in dose requirements of other anaesthetic drugs (injectable and inhalational), and to a greater extent than after acepromazine or a benzodiazepine. These greatly reduced doses should also be administered IV slowly to effect. The circulation time is slowed after α2 agonist administration because of the reduction in cardiac output, so be patient, and wait one to two minutes before considering top-ups.

Anticonvulsant/Pro-convulsant? Low doses result in CNS depression and possible anticonvulsant activity. Higher doses, especially of the less 'pure' xylazine (i.e. less α2 selective), may result in stimulation, especially of α1 receptors, 'central excitement' and a pro-convulsant effect. CNS α1 receptor stimulation results in increases in cyclic guanosine monophosphate (cGMP) and nitric oxide (NO) activities, both of which are indicative of excitatory effects.

Neuroprotection (Cerebroprotection) It is well known that brain injury due to hypoxia/ischaemia is characterised by a series of events that most importantly includes 'excitotoxicity': the increased release of excitatory neurotransmitters, notably glutamate, which tend to result in a subsequent uncontrolled increase in intracellular calcium, and cell death. Amongst the factors potentially influencing these events is the balance between α1 receptor (excitatory) and α2 receptor (inhibitory) activity. Central I2 receptor activity is also important (see above).

Alpha 2 agonist infusions are commonly administered during intracranial surgery. Where raised intracranial pressure is a concern, the vasoconstrictive effects of α2 agonists reduce total intracranial blood volume, and therefore intracranial pressure, although they may reduce perfusion.

Diseased tissue may, however, respond differently. The neuroprotection (ischaemic preconditioning) afforded by the α2 agonists may also be helpful.

4.1.7.3.3 Analgesia

It appears that α2A, α2B, and α2C receptor interactions are involved, both peripherally (i.e. α2 receptors are present on nociceptors) and centrally. Centrally, the antinociceptive effects of alpha 2 agonists are more spinal than supraspinal and include a reduction of substance P activity and hyperpolarisation of dorsal horn neurons. Analgesia is similar to that afforded by opioids, and synergistic with it. Analgesia is said to be mostly visceral, but some 'surface' analgesia is also produced. As with the opioids, analgesia appears to correlate with cerebrospinal fluid (CSF) concentration of the drug; and these agents can also be used for epidural and true spinal/intrathecal (into the CSF), administration. The supraspinal analgesic effects of opioids include the activation of descending monoaminergic systems (noradrenergic and serotonergic) with resultant spinal actions. The spinal analgesic effects of α2 agonists therefore augment the supraspinal analgesic effects of opioids. These descending pathways also stimulate spinal cholinergic and purinergic (adenosine), systems. Hence intrathecally applied α2 agonists, adenosine, or acetylcholine (local acetylcholine concentration is usually increased by way of acetylcholinesterase inhibitors, e.g. neostigmine) can enhance opioid analgesia. Nitrous oxide increases endogenous opioid production, and its analgesic effects have much in common with the supraspinal opioid analgesic effects, in that the descending monoaminergic pathways are involved. Naloxone should antagonise both the supraspinal and spinal (including endogenous α2 effects) components of opioid analgesia; whereas atipamezole should only antagonise the spinal α2 effects (of opioids, or of exogenous α2 agonists), whilst leaving the supraspinal opioid effects untouched.

All α2 agonists have local anaesthetic-like actions (see below), but xylazine is the most potent in this respect. This property has been suggested to be due to their chemical structure closely resembling that of the local anaesthetics:

- Local anaesthetics: Aromatic group – amide or ester link – amino group
- α2 agonists: Aromatic group – link – hydrophilic part

The local anaesthetic-like actions of α2 agonists may be due to their ability to 'block' the I_h repolarisation current (hyperpolarisation-activated cation current), in a concentration-dependent manner, and has been proposed as the mechanism behind the prolonged duration of peripheral nerve blocks performed with dexmedetomidine in combination with local anaesthetic agents. α2 agonists, as well as

directly 'blocking' the I_h current, reduce norepinephrine release from nerve terminals, and this reduced availability of norepinephrine (which otherwise activates the I_h current) enhances their ability to reduce the repolarisation current. Interestingly, systemic α2 agonist administration has a similar, but smaller, effect, and may underlie why veterinary clinical studies (where α2 agonist premedication is common) have not yet documented improvements in analgesia when dexmedetomidine is combined with local anaesthetics for regional anaesthesia.

4.1.7.3.4 Cardiovascular Effects

The actual events depend upon the drug administered, its actions at adrenergic and imidazoline receptors, the dose, the route of administration, the species to which it is administered, and the individual (e.g. its level of excitement, pain, and stress). Table 4.2 outlines the cardiovascular distribution of common adrenoceptors and the effects of their stimulation.

Cardiovascular effects following, especially, **intravenous** administration are classically described as follows.

An **initial arterial hypertension** occurs due to peripheral post-synaptic α2 (especially α2B) receptor activation; and possibly also some α1 receptor activation; resulting in **peripheral vasoconstriction.** (If the α2 agonist is administered IM, then the initial hypertension is much less dramatic.)

This is followed by **bradycardia,** partly as a vagally-mediated baroreflex to the hypertension, but mainly due to central pre-synaptic α2 receptor and indeed I1 receptor activation causing a central sympatholysis (and a relative increase in parasympathetic tone), and also partly due to peripheral pre-synaptic α2 receptor activation resulting in reduced norepinephrine release at peripheral sympathetic nerve terminals in the heart. Bradyarrhythmias, such as S-A or A-V blocks, may also become apparent.

Finally, arterial blood pressure returns to near normal due to the central effects described above, and peripheral pre-synaptic α2 receptor activation, which reduces norepinephrine release, helping to relieve part of the previously induced peripheral vasoconstriction (but usually a slight vasoconstriction remains). Blood pressure therefore returns towards more normal values due to a combination of this reduced vasoconstriction and the slowed heart rate and reduction in cardiac output. The eventual state of the peripheral vasculature (i.e. usually a slightly increased peripheral vascular tone remains) and blood pressure (i.e. usually fairly near the original blood pressure, slightly above or slightly below) depends upon the balance among central and peripheral effects, the drug chosen, the dose chosen, the route of administration, the species, and the individual animal (health state and degree of excitement).

Table 4.2 Location of adrenoceptors in the cardiovascular system and results of their stimulation.

Receptor	Situation	Location	Effect of stimulation
α1	Post-synaptic	Vascular smooth muscle Myocardium?	Vasoconstriction +ve inotropy
α2	Post-/extra-synaptic	Vascular smooth muscle Endothelium?	Vasoconstriction Vasoconstriction or vasodilation
α2	Pre-synaptic	Vascular smooth muscle	Alleviation of vasoconstriction
β1	Post-synaptic	Vascular smooth muscle Myocardium	Vasodilation +ve inotropy +ve chronotropy
β2	Post-synaptic	Vascular smooth muscle Myocardium?	Vasodilation +ve inotropy +ve chronotropy

The bradycardia observed may be of the order of half the previous resting heart rate. A compensatory increase in stroke volume may be limited because of peripheral vasoconstriction (increased afterload), so cardiac output is thus dramatically reduced. Because the circulation is slowed, IV administration of anaesthetic agents should be done slowly to effect.

Peripheral mucous membranes look pale because of the vasoconstriction, and they may even appear cyanotic because of reduced perfusion (due to vasoconstriction), allowing a slower passage of blood through the capillary beds, and therefore more time for oxygen extraction by the tissues. Pulse oximeters may not pick up a good signal so the SpO_2 value will be low because with poor signal-to-noise ratio, the saturation reading tends towards 85–87% (see Chapter 18 on monitoring). Although the cardiac output is reduced overall, because there are effectively fewer peripheral tissues to perfuse, the 'central' tissues (i.e. the vital organs) are said not to have their perfusion or oxygenation compromised.

Pro-arrhythmic effects are suggested because occasionally bradyarrhythmias (which may be associated with ventricular escape beats) may occur as well as the bradycardia. Xylazine and medetomidine are also suggested to have direct myocardial depressant effects in the dog (negative inotropy), and have been blamed for sensitisation of the myocardium to catecholamine-induced arrhythmias. Protection against catecholamine induced arrhythmias, however, is documented. This may stem from the shift in ANS balance towards a more vagal dominance (central α and I effects), and protection (**preconditioning**) against myocardial ischaemia (**cardioprotection**) is afforded by interaction with I2 receptors, located in cardiomyocyte mitochondrial membranes.

Beware of using anticholinergics (especially atropine but also glycopyrrolate) to treat the bradycardia. Try a small dose of atipamezole instead (partial reversal/antagonism) if the heart rate falls below 30 bpm or where slow heart rates compromise blood pressure. Occasionally **fatal arrhythmias** and cardiac arrest have occurred following atropine administration, possibly because massive hypertension and tachycardia are induced, but the high afterload (peripheral vasoconstriction) remains, adding to cardiac workload. Also immense tachycardias reduce diastolic filling time (and coronary perfusion), so cardiac output can be further reduced, and myocardial oxygen supply further compromised in the face of increased demand. All this is bad news for the heart, especially if any degree of compromise pre-existed.

Continuing research, however, with **vatinoxan** (MK467), a peripheral-acting α2 adrenoceptor antagonist (i.e. does not cross the blood–brain barrier, and therefore should only antagonise the peripheral effects [side effects] of α2 agonists) shows promise. Studies to date have co-administered vatinoxan with dexmedetomidine and demonstrate reduced cardiopulmonary changes with no impact on (may even intensify) sedation in a variety of species.

4.1.7.3.5 *Respiratory Effects*
Respiratory effects are variable and are dependent upon species, drug, and dose. Furthermore, any drug that acts on the CNS to relieve anxiety, produce sedation, or alleviate pain is necessarily associated with some reduction in alveolar ventilation, which may reflect a reduction in metabolic rate.

With α2 agonists, although the respiratory rate may be reduced, the tidal volume may increase so that overall minute ventilation is not affected. Blood gases remain virtually unchanged. These statements are true for the 'lower' doses. In some species, notably ruminants, α2 agonists cause bronchoconstriction and pulmonary hypertension (pulmonary vasoconstriction), leading to pulmonary oedema and impaired oxygenation of blood with resultant hypoxaemia, which can be fatal. Care must be taken with their use in ruminants, especially small ruminants: calves, sheep, and goats. Large doses of detomidine (c. 300–500 μg/kg) do the same in horses. Interestingly, α2 agonists may offset pre-existing bronchoconstriction due to other causes (e.g. mediated by acetylcholine).

4.1.7.3.6 Muscle Relaxation

Postural muscles and smooth muscles seem to be affected. Postural muscle relaxation manifests as ataxia or recumbency. Reduced vigilance, accompanying anxiolysis/sedation, central actions, perhaps at imidazoline, glycine, and GABA$_A$ receptors and possible local anaesthetic actions, have all been suggested to be responsible.

Beware α2 agonist use in brachycephalics and animals with laryngeal paralysis, as pharyngeal and laryngeal muscle relaxation may further impair their already compromised 'airway'.

Lower oesophageal sphincter pressure is reduced, thus potentially increasing the risk of gastro-oesophageal reflux/regurgitation.

Their use in 'blocked cats' has been suggested to aid urethral relaxation to facilitate passage of a urinary catheter; but be aware of electrolyte disturbances (high potassium may cause bradycardia and arrhythmias), and intravascular volume status; and remember that these drugs can induce a diuresis, so urinary drainage must be established.

4.1.7.3.7 Hormonal Effects

- Decreased ADH secretion and responsiveness (increased urine production)
- Decreased renin secretion (due to action on renal α2 receptors)
- Decreased insulin secretion (due to action on α2 [and possibly also α1] receptors on pancreatic islet β cells) and, at least in some species (but not cats and dogs), increased glucagon secretion (due to action on α2 receptors on pancreatic islet α cells), all of which tend to increase plasma glucose. Effects at I3 receptors, however, may increase insulin secretion and offset these effects.
- Decreased ACTH secretion (central action), and therefore decreased cortisol (reduced stress response); there is uncertainty whether this might be beneficial
- Decreased catecholamines (sympatholysis/parasympathomimesis)
- Increased growth hormone

Arterial blood pressure effects from α and I receptor activation (changes in vasomotor tone and in ANS balance) are compounded by reduction in ADH (also called vasopressin) secretion and receptor responsiveness, and by the reduction in cortisol that normally has a permissive effect on the actions of catecholamines, and without which the effects of catecholamines, especially on vasomotor tone, are reduced.

Diuresis Reduced pituitary ADH secretion (secondary to α2 agonist effects in the hypothalamus) and also reduced ADH responsiveness in the kidney favour diuresis (most important mechanism).

- Reduced insulin (and, in some species, increased glucagon) secretion causes increased hepatic glycogenolysis and gluconeogenesis, and reduced peripheral tissue (skeletal and cardiac muscle and brown and white adipose tissue) insulin-dependent glucose uptake, causing hyperglycaemia, but this rarely results in glycosuria/osmotic diuresis (except in cattle; and the author has also documented this in horses receiving medetomidine infusions).
- Reduced renin (due to stimulation of renal α2 receptors) results in reduced angiotensin II, which favours an increase in glomerular filtration rate, natriuresis, and diuresis. (The reduced cardiac output may itself result in some reduction in renal blood flow and GFR, so perhaps the reduced renin/angiotensin helps to offset this.)
- Reduced angiotensin II also results in reduced aldosterone production (and possibly increased release of atrial natriuretic factor), which promotes the diuresis (and natriuresis).
- Reduced angiotensin II further reduces ADH production.
- The renin-angiotensin-aldosterone system may also be affected indirectly by the sedative and cardiovascular effects of α2 agonists.

Although normal micturition reflexes are maintained, urethral sphincter tone decreases, and overflow urine spillage may occur. Urine specific gravity and osmolality are reduced in inverse relation to the increase in urine volume. Glycosuria is not a common feature in small animals.

4.1.7.3.8 Uterine Effects

May affect uterine tone and intra-uterine pressure; exact effects appear to depend upon species and drug and whether the animal is pregnant. These agents, however, may cause utero-placental vasoconstriction that may compromise foetal viability. α2 agonists cross the blood–placental barrier easily and there is insufficient data about their safety in pregnant animals during foetal organogenesis. Their use is not recommended during pregnancy, especially during the last third.

4.1.7.3.9   GI Tract Effects

Gut motility is reduced (acetylcholine release is reduced from the pre-synaptic terminals of post-ganglionic para-sympathetic fibres in the gut wall), secretions (including saliva) are reduced, and gut blood flow is reduced. Gut transit time is prolonged. Beware if trying to perform a barium series. (Although acepromazine also prolongs gut transit time, some people prefer its use for such studies, if indeed sedation is required. Opioids also delay gut transit.) Lower oesophageal sphincter tone is reduced, encouraging gastro-oesophageal reflux/regurgitation.

Emesis may occur, especially if the animal is not starved before drug administration: possibly more common after xylazine than after (dex)medetomidine. Emesis tends to occur before maximum sedation is apparent; and occurs before gut motility is reduced. Cats may also vomit on recovery from sedation. At one time it was thought to be due to the initial transient hypertension, but now it is believed to be more likely due to α2 receptor activation in the CTZ or vomiting centre. Emesis is more likely when α2 agonists are administered alone (rather than when combined with an opioid). The use of α2 agonists is contra-indicated in cases with oesophageal obstruction and, e.g. gastric dilation/volvulus cases.

4.1.7.3.10   Thermoregulation

Central suppression of thermoregulation occurs, but reduction in heat production may be countered slightly by reduction in heat loss due to a slight overall peripheral vasoconstriction. Nevertheless, it is important to monitor the patient's temperature and guard against hypothermia. Both alpha and imidazoline receptor effects may be involved.

4.1.7.3.11   Haematological Effects

Cell counts and total protein may decrease slightly. Hyperglycaemia is common. Platelet aggregation is theoretically enhanced (α2 agonism), but is not reported to cause clinical problems. Packed cell volume is said to decrease due to splenic sequestration. Total protein is said to decrease due to a shift of fluid into the intravascular space secondary to hyperglycaemia.

4.1.7.3.12   Ocular Effects

Mydriasis (α2 receptors in radial [not circular] muscles of the iris are stimulated to contract), and aqueous humour production is reduced (α2 receptor activation in ciliary body). Despite mydriasis, which usually slows aqueous outflow, the overall tendency is for a decrease in intraocular pressure (IOP). ADH, prolactin, and cortisol are also important in the regulation of IOP, and imidazoline receptor effects may also be involved. Head position (relative to the body) can also influence IOP.

4.1.7.4   Uses and Doses

Care: These compounds can be absorbed across mucous membranes and have impressive cardiovascular and respiratory depressant effects in people, so beware any splashes into your eyes/mouth, or indeed prolonged skin contact, especially if any broken skin. Seek medical attention if **accidental self-administration** occurs; do not attempt to drive yourself to hospital.

4.1.7.4.1   Medetomidine

It is recommended that animals are fasted (fasting times are currently controversial, but four to six hours may be the minimum for food, whereas access to water should not be denied) prior to administration of medetomidine and dexmedetomidine.

- For sedation. Dose: dogs, 1–20 μg/kg IM (or the lower doses IV); cats, 10–50 μg/kg IM (or the lower doses IV), or up to 150 μg/kg if necessary, IM (or SC). Allow 10–20 minutes for peak effect following IM, duration is dose-dependent, e.g. 30–180 minutes. Useful for intradermal skin testing.
- In combination with an opioid, e.g. butorphanol, for sedation or premedication. Dose: dogs, 5–10 μg/kg medetomidine +0.1–0.5 mg/kg butorphanol IM (IV); cats, 10–50 μg/kg medetomidine +0.1–0.5 mg/kg butorphanol IM or SC.
- In combination with (an opioid and) ketamine for anaesthesia. Dose: dogs, c. 10–20+ μg/kg medetomidine (+ opioid) and + (or followed 5 minutes later by) c. 2.5–5 mg/kg ketamine IM; cats, c. 25+ μg/ kg medetomidine (+ opioid) + 5 mg/kg (range 2.5–7.5 mg/kg) ketamine IM.

4.1.7.4.2   Dexmedetomidine

The dosage for dogs is suggested in terms of body surface area (the data sheets provide a conversion chart for ranges of body weights) equivalent to between 3 and 40 μg/kg. In cats, a dose of 40 μg/kg based upon body mass is suggested in all instances. As with medetomidine, however, smaller doses may well suffice. Early reports suggested half the dose of medetomidine would give equivalent sedation with dexmedetomidine, but this may not be quite so exactly true.

- For sedation and premedication. Dose: dogs, 1–10 μg/kg IV, 5–20 μg/kg IM; cats, 5–20 μg/kg IV, or 5–40 μg/kg IM. Allow 3–5 minutes for peak effect IV, and 10–15 minutes after IM. Duration is dose-dependent, e.g. 30–180 minutes.
- For noise-related fear/anxiety in dogs, oral transmucosal dexmedetomidine can be applied: dose 125 μg/m^2 (syringe calibrated according to body weight to enable correct dosing), either at onset of observed anxiety or 30–60 minutes before the onset of the noise stimulus. Re-dosing can be performed every two to three hours for a maximum of 5 doses per period of noise-related anxiety.

4.1.7.4.3 Xylazine

Superseded by medetomidine & dexmedetomidine for small animals, but still used in shelter medicine in some regions of the world. It is recommended to withhold food for (for at least four to six hours) to reduce the risk of emesis.

- For sedation or premedication. Dose (dogs and cats), 1–3 mg/kg IM. Onset 5–15 minutes; duration up to 60 minutes (dose-dependent).
- In combination with any opioid to improve the reliability of sedation/premedication. Use the lower doses of xylazine with, e.g. pethidine (3.5–5 mg/kg, but up to 10 mg/kg if necessary in cats), morphine (0.1–0.2 mg/kg, but up to 0.5 mg/kg if necessary in dogs), methadone (0.1–0.5 mg/kg), buprenorphine (0.01–0.02 mg/kg), or butorphanol (0.1–0.5 mg/kg).
- In combination with (an opioid and) ketamine for anaesthesia. Dose: dogs, xylazine 1 mg/kg (lower doses in larger animals) followed 10 minutes later by ketamine c.10+ mg/kg IM; cats, xylazine 1 mg/kg administered alongside ketamine c.10+ mg/kg IM.

4.1.7.4.4. Epidural Administration

α2 agonists can theoretically be administered by the epidural (extradural) route, alone, or in combination with opioids and/or local anaesthetics. However, they can be rapidly absorbed into the systemic circulation, and so prior sedation or premedication with α2 agonists should be practised with caution. Xylazine has the most local anaesthetic effects, so expect a degree of motor blockade after extradural administration. Use of α2 agonists for small animal epidural injection is rarely reported. None of the products is licenced for administration by this route; all include preservatives, so no more than a single dose is recommended.

4.1.7.5 Antagonism

One of the advantages of the use of α2 agonists is the potential for their specific antagonism ('reversal'). Before the availability of specific antagonists, agents such as 4-amino-pyridine and doxapram (non-specific CNS stimulants), were used. There are a number of α adrenoceptor antagonists available, with differing α2:α1 selectivity:

- α1 > α2 prazosin
- α1 = α2 tolazoline
- α2 > α1 idazoxan, yohimbine
- α2 > > α1 atipamezole

4.1.7.5.1 Atipamezole

Atipamezole (5 mg/ml) is the most selective α2 antagonist available, and as such makes an excellent choice for antagonism of medetomidine and its dextro isomer, dexmedetomidine (the most selective α2 agonist available). It can also be used to antagonise the effects of the less α2 selective agents, although the doses are less well verified.

Antagonism (often called 'reversal') is occasionally accompanied by over-alertness, muscle tremors, tachycardia, transient hypotension (blockade of post-synaptic α2 receptors), panting, defecation, and vomiting (which some suggest may be a type of excitement reaction). Antagonism of the α2 agonist not only antagonises the sedative effects, but will also antagonise the analgesia, so care must be taken to ensure adequate analgesia is provided by other drugs (and remember that atipamezole may also reduce the effectiveness of opioids at the spinal level). Although antagonism of sedation becomes obvious soon after administration of atipamezole, the cardiovascular effects may not be completely antagonised at the doses most commonly used:

- Dose for **cats** = 2.5× the μg/kg dose of medetomidine (or 5× the μg/kg dose of dexmedetomidine), IM (equivalent to half the volume of medetomidine or dexmedetomidine administered).
- Dose for **dogs** = 5× the μg/kg dose of medetomidine (or 10× the μg/kg dose of dexmedetomidine), IM (equivalent to the same volume of medetomidine or dexmedetomidine administered).

The dose of atipamezole may be adjusted according to the time delay following administration of (dex)medetomidine. Atipamezole competes with (dex)medetomidine for receptor occupancy so **administration too soon can result in no effect**. It is also recommended that when ketamine has been combined with (dex)medetomidine, the (dex)medetomidine should not be antagonised for at least 20 minutes (cats) to 40 minutes (dogs) to reduce the chance of unveiling the excitement effects of residual active ketamine. Indeed, antagonism of medetomidine after combination with ketamine is not recommended at all in dogs because the excitement effects of residual ketamine, including seizure-like activity, may be unmasked, which is very unpleasant for the patient. Although domestic cats may also suffer the excitement effects of ketamine, they are less likely to display seizure-like activity, and ketamine is licenced as a sole anaesthetic agent for domestic cats, although not recommended.

To antagonise the effects of xylazine, again the xylazine dose administered and the time since its administration are important. Atipamezole doses from 50 to 250 μg/kg IM are recommended, starting at the lower dose and waiting at least five minutes for effect before giving further doses.

4.1.7.5.2 Vatinoxan

Vatinoxan (MK467) is a peripheral-acting α2 adrenoceptor antagonist (i.e. does not cross the blood–brain barrier and therefore should only antagonise the peripheral effects [side effects] of α2 agonists). Currently undergoing investigations, vatinoxan shows promise (see above).

4.1.8 Adjuncts to Premedication

4.1.8.1 Trazodone and Gabapentin

At the time of writing, oral trazodone (2–10 mg/kg as required [up to TID]; with 3 mg/kg as a useful starting dose) has become fashionable as an anxiolytic/sedative for dogs, especially for anxious patients travelling to veterinary clinics, whilst oral gabapentin (~50 mg/cat or up to approx. 20–30 mg/kg) has been shown to be useful for sedation of anxious cats (and possibly dogs), prior to presentation at veterinary clinics.

Gabapentin is more widely known as an analgesic for chronic, particularly neuropathic, pain states (See Chapter 3 on pain). Whether there is a behavioural advantage to this intervention is currently debatable.

Trazodone is an atypical antidepressant with mixed serotonergic agonist and antagonist activities (it is widely referred to as a serotonin antagonist and re-uptake inhibitor, SARI). The relatively recent increase in popularity of this drug for short-term use in dogs may be due to the recent reduced availability of acepromazine tablets. It should be used with caution in patients with renal and hepatic disease, although is safer than tricyclic antidepressants (TCAs) in patients with cardiac disease. Glaucoma, seizures, urinary retention, and severe liver disease are the main contraindications to its use. Although low doses may be used alongside SSRIs, serotonin syndrome is a recognised complication.

Serotonin syndrome is the group of symptoms due to serotonin toxicity that include:

- Hyperthermia
- Agitation
- Muscle tremors (even rhabdomyolysis)
- Seizures
- Dilated pupils
- Diarrhoea
- Increased sweating is reported in people, but may be less obvious in animals

Differential diagnoses should include neuroleptic malignant syndrome, malignant hyperthermia, central anticholinergic syndrome/toxicity, and heat stroke. Suspicion should be roused when a patient is receiving at least two medications with serotonergic actions, e.g.

selective serotonin re-uptake inhibitors (SSRIs), serotonin and noradrenaline re-uptake inhibitors (SNRIs), monoamine oxidase inhibitors (MAOIs), TCAs, ondansetron, metoclopramide, tramadol, pethidine, St. John's wort.

Treatment is mainly supportive, e.g. stop treatment with pro-serotonergic drugs if possible, employ active cooling, provide IV fluid therapy as required, benzodiazepines may help, but cyproheptadine (a serotonin antagonist) may be required.

4.1.9 Opioids

There is more information about opioids in Chapter 3 on pain. Although opioids are more usually combined with 'sedatives' (i.e. neuroleptanalgesia), they can be used alone to provide some sedation and analgesia with minimal cardiorespiratory depression. Analgesia occurs at lower doses than those necessary for sedation. Opioids alone can provide good sedation, but high doses, especially in pain-free animals, may cause excitement (cats and horses appear to be more susceptible to this than dogs), which is typified by increased (loco-)motor activity. Animals that are not experiencing pain will show excitement reactions after lower doses of opioids than those animals that are experiencing immense pain.

Opioids have central (brain [supraspinal] and spinal cord) actions, and also can act in the periphery, e.g. we now know that opioid receptors are expressed in inflamed tissue.

4.1.9.1 Opioid Receptors

The main opioid receptors are:

- Mu (μ) opioid receptor (MOP, also called OP3)
- Kappa (κ) opioid receptor (KOP, also called OP2)
- Delta (δ) opioid receptor (DOP, also called OP1)
- Nociceptin opioid receptor (NOP, also called OP4)

Table 4.3 outlines the opioid receptor preferences of the commonly used opioids.

Mu agonists are drugs such as morphine, methadone, pethidine, and fentanyl. Buprenorphine is a partial mu agonist. Butorphanol is a kappa agonist and is also variously described as either a partial mu agonist or a mu antagonist. Fentanyl is combined with a butyrophenone called fluanisone, as 'Hypnorm™', which is used for **neuroleptanalgesia** in mice, rats, rabbits, and guinea pigs. Etorphine was combined with acepromazine in large animal Immobilon™, which was used to provide **neuroleptanaesthesia** (i.e. etorphine is such a potent opioid, that its effects resemble those of general anaesthesia).

Table 4.3 The relative activities of some of the different opioids available at the various opioid receptors.

Drug	Mu opioid receptor	Kappa opioid receptor	Delta opioid receptor
Morphine	+++	+/−	+/−
Methadone	+++	−	−
Pethidine (meperidine)	++	+/−	−
Fentanyl	+++	−	−(+)
Etorphine	+++	++	++
Buprenorphine	+ + + (partial agonist)	++ (antag?)	+/−
Butorphanol	+ + (ag/antag?)	++	−
Naloxone (antagonist)	+++	++	+

Results of μ receptor stimulation include:

- Analgesia
- Sedation/narcosis
- Euphoria/increased locomotor activity
- Nausea/vomiting followed by constipation (decreased gut motility)
- Respiratory depression (more in humans than in animals)/cough suppression
- Panting (dogs with methadone)
- Miosis in dog and pig (mydriasis in horse and cat)
- Dependence

Results of κ receptor stimulation include:

- Analgesia
- Sedation
- Dysphoria/increased locomotor activity
- Slightly reduced gut motility
- Possibly some respiratory depression/may be antitussive
- Diuresis
- Miosis

Results of δ receptor stimulation include:

- Analgesia (possibly by modulation of μ receptor effects)
- Possible dysphoria/increased locomotor activity
- Reduced gut motility
- Respiratory depression (some say stimulation)/antitussive?
- Mydriasis

4.1.9.2 Results of Administration
The effects of opioid administration depend upon the opioid, the dose, the species treated, and how much pain that animal is in. Some generalisations, based on morphine and dogs are given below.

4.1.9.2.1 Analgesia
Table 4.4 summarises the relative analgesic potencies of commonly used opioids. Potency is related to dose: the

Table 4.4 Relative analgesic potencies of common opioids.

Drug	'Potency' (clinical efficacy as analgesic)
Morphine	1
Methadone	1
Pethidine	1/10
Fentanyl	100
Alfentanil	10–25
Remifentanil	50
Sufentanil	1000
Etorphine	10 000

more potent a drug, the lower the dose requirement. The doses used in clinical practice are given below. Pain scoring is advised to ensure duration of action is applicable to the individual.

Methadone Dogs 0.1–0.5 mg/kg IM, IV q. 2–4–6 hours. Administration by the SC route results in variable absorption and prolonged elimination. Panting and hypersalivation are not, however, necessarily reduced following SC dosing. In another study, whining, not considered to be a pain response, was actually increased when methadone was administered by the SC route.
Cats 0.1–0.5 mg/kg IM, IV q.2–4–6 h.

Morphine Dogs 0.1–0.5 mg/kg IM q. 2–4–6 h.
Cats 0.1–0.2 mg/kg IM q. 4–6–8 h.

Papaveretum (Included for Interest, Not Recommended) Crude mixture of opium alkaloids, including morphine, codeine.

Dogs 0.2 mg/kg ++ IM.
Cats 0.1–0.3 mg/kg IM.

Pethidine   Dogs 3.5–5 mg/kg IM or SC q. 1–2 h.
Cats 3.5–5(–10) mg/kg IM or SC q. nearer 2 h.

Buprenorphine   Dogs 0.01–0.02 mg/kg IM, IV, or SC q. 6–8 h. Recent studies have shown that, despite a previously thought unfavourable canine salivary pH, OTM buprenorphine (0.02 mg/kg) provides analgesia of similar duration, but poorer quality, to 0.02 mg/kg IV, whereas OTM buprenorphine 0.12 mg/kg provided a prolonged period (up to 24 hours) of good analgesia (but involves large volumes for administration).

Cats 0.01–0.02 mg/kg IM, IV, or SC (or buccal oral-transmucosal; delivered into cheek at 0.02 mg/kg) q. 6–8 h. In the USA there is an extended release preparation of buprenorphine for use in cats which is presented as a 1.8 mg/ml solution and licenced for once daily administration at a dose of 0.24 mg/kg SC. Published data are limited at this moment in time. An OTM formulation is available in the UK as a special.

Butorphanol   Dogs: 0.1–0.5 mg/kg IM, IV, or SC q. 1–2 h. Cats: 0.1–0.5 mg/kg IM, IV, or SC q. 1–2 h.

4.1.9.2.2   Bradycardia
Bradycardia may occur with minimal decrease in blood pressure, due to **vagomimetic** effects. A more profound hypotension results if histamine release occurs, e.g. pethidine IV or morphine IV stimulate histamine release. **Pethidine (meperidine)** is said to be less likely to induce bradycardia because of its vagolytic actions. Pethidine is often suggested in situations where bradycardia should be avoided (e.g. neonates depend upon a high heart rate to maintain their cardiac output, as they cannot vary their stroke volume very much). The heart rate therefore should not decrease, but a slight increase in heart rate may be observed (which may partly be a reflex response following histamine release with subsequent slight hypotension). At doses above 3.5 mg/kg, pethidine can cause slight direct myocardial depression (negative inotropy). Some texts suggest that at low doses, morphine is sympathomimetic. In horses, at 'normal' doses, morphine certainly seems to have some positive inotropic effects.

4.1.9.2.3   Respiratory Depression
Slight (but dose-dependent), respiratory depression occurs due to a decrease in sensitivity of the respiratory centre to carbon dioxide. Respiratory depression is much more of a worry in humans. In animals it is not a common problem, especially in animals in pain and at clinically appropriate doses; although IV boluses of, especially μ receptor agonists, can cause transient apnoea in anaesthetised animals. Cough suppression can be useful, e.g. in the treatment of kennel cough, or following laryngeal or tracheal surgery. Codeine and butorphanol are often used as antitussives. Methadone does cause panting in some dogs, but it is not known whether this is a form of respiratory side effect or whether this is due to thermoregulatory effects. In humans, and potentially also in dogs (see Chapter 3), large doses of fentanyl have been associated with a phenomenon called 'wooden chest' or 'splinted chest', which is associated with increased truncal skeletal muscle tone and reduced ventilatory ability. The mechanism of the rigidity is unclear but may be associated with the co-administration of other drugs which have anti-dopaminergic effects in the CNS, such as phenothiazines. Treatment may require administration of neuromuscular blockers and/or opioid antagonism to facilitate the provision of controlled ventilation.

4.1.9.2.4   Temperature
Dogs may pant, resulting in a slight reduction of body temperature. This is thought to be due to a re-setting of the temperature set point in the thermoregulatory centre. Postanaesthetic hyperthermia, lasting about five hours, has been documented in cats following hydromorphone administration.

4.1.9.2.5   GI Tract: Salivation, Nausea, Vomiting, Defecation
Less emesis is seen when animals are in pain prior to receiving opioids. Morphine and papaveretum (a crude opium poppy extract, containing mostly morphine, but some other opioids too) are the worst for causing vomiting.

Increased resting tone of GI tract, but reduced propulsive peristalsis (follows initial vomiting and defecation), and reduced GI tract secretions may occur. Opioids tend to increase sphincter tone, including those of the biliary and pancreatic ducts, ureters and urethra. Lower oesophageal sphincter tone, however, is reduced, with increased risk of gastro-oesophageal reflux. Pethidine, however, is spasmolytic, therefore an excellent choice where there may be ureteral colic, pancreatitis, or cholangiohepatitis. See Chapter 3 on pain for a discussion about the sphincter of Oddi.

4.1.9.2.6   Urinary Tract
Urine production may be decreased secondary to an increase in ADH secretion. Urine retention may occur due to increased urethral sphincter tone, although bladder tone tends to be increased too. Some people think this increase in ADH secretion is part of the stress response and not a true reflection of opioid activity. Pethidine may be favoured where ureteral colic or where urethral obstruction exists (and urethral catheterisation is being attempted), as it is spasmolytic.

4.1.9.2.7 Other Effects

- Miosis (but mydriasis in cats and horses, which are more sensitive to the excitement side effects of high dose opioids).
- Decreased blink rate may predispose to corneal ulceration: ocular lubricant recommended.
- Sedation.

For more information about opioids, see Chapter 3.

4.1.10 Anticholinergics

When ether was used for anaesthesia, its pungent odour stimulated respiratory tract secretions and salivation. To reduce problems of potential respiratory obstruction due to excessive secretions (especially in cats because of their small diameter airways and relatively greater mucous production compared to dogs), anticholinergic premedication used to be given as standard. Nowadays, the use of anticholinergics is reserved for emergency situations (resuscitation), or where vagal reflexes are encountered, e.g. during certain types of surgery (head/neck), or after administration of vagomimetic drugs such as potent opioids (e.g. remifentanil).

Atropine (0.6 mg/ml in UK) and **glycopyrrolate** (200 µg/ml) are most commonly used. Neither drug is a pure muscarinic receptor antagonist, as small doses can produce bradycardia. At one time, this bradycardia was thought to be due to central (CNS) actions, as it is more profound after atropine, which easily crosses the blood–brain barrier, or perhaps due to differential effects on SA and AV nodes. However, it is now thought that both compounds can exert weak agonistic actions on peripheral muscarinic receptors. The drugs may also have indirect sympathomimetic effects (i.e. they may inhibit the normal negative feedback of endogenous catecholamine release).

See also Chapter 17 on muscle relaxants because these agents are used in the 'reversal' of neuromuscular blockade to prevent the unwanted muscarinic side effects of anticholinesterases.

Some people advocate the use of anticholinergics when α2 agonists have been used because they feel uncomfortable with the bradycardias observed. The tachycardia that results from such anticholinergic administration, however, massively increases the myocardial work, and despite the increase in heart rate, the cardiac output is minimally increased, because the high afterload and fast heart rate (which decreases diastolic filling time) limit any increase in stroke volume. Moreover, if anticholinergics are administered alongside α2 agonists, they prevent the physiological, reflex-driven bradycardia, which means that very high

arterial blood pressures are reached, which can potentially rupture blood vessels (particularly in the brain and retina). For these reasons, caution is advised in the use of anticholinergics (especially atropine) in animals that have been given α2 agonists. Usually a first line of treatment for α2 agonist-induced bradycardia is to antagonise or partially antagonise the α2 agonist with an α2 antagonist, usually atipamezole.

Atropine is a natural alkaloid and a tertiary amine. Atropine has some local anaesthetic-like activity. Its elimination is rapid in dogs, with some metabolism to tropine, but much is excreted unchanged in the urine. Cats, rats, and rabbits (and possibly ruminants) have high blood concentrations of atropine esterase, thus promoting rapid clearance. Glycopyrrolate was originally developed as an antihistamine (H_2). It is a synthetic quaternary ammonium compound, hence it is also known as glycopyrronium.

4.1.10.1 Results of Anticholinergic Administration

- Bronchodilation (can increase dead space and facilitate rebreathing)
- Decreased respiratory secretions (watery part) and decreased ciliary activity (so there is reduced clearance of a more viscid mucous)
- Decreased watery part of saliva (so saliva becomes more viscid)
- Increased heart rate, with some increase in blood pressure
- Increased myocardial oxygen demand/heart work
- Tachyarrhythmias are possible
- Occasionally paradoxical bradycardia occurs (see above)
- Mydriasis
- Reduced tear production
- Reduced gut motility and GI tract secretions
- Reduced lower oesophageal sphincter tone (so increased risk of gastro-oesophageal reflux/regurgitation)
- Very little sedative effect

Glycopyrrolate does not cross the blood–brain barrier or placenta as it is highly ionised. Because of this, there is reportedly less chance of seeing paradoxical bradycardia, although this can still occur (see above). Its onset of action is much slower than atropine, even after IV injection (e.g. one to three minutes), therefore it is less useful in emergency situations.

It supposedly has a longer duration of action than atropine (but depends upon the species); 2–4 hours for cardiovascular effects (vs. 40–90 minutes for atropine), and even longer anti-sialogogue (and other GI tract) effects (e.g. can last several [~7] hours). It also reduces gastric acid secretion more than atropine (H$_2$ blocking effect). Altogether, it produces less dramatic cardiovascular effects but more potent GI effects than atropine. Tachyarrhythmias are less likely.

The dose of atropine for resuscitation/treatment of vagal reflexes in dogs and cats is 0.01–0.04 mg/kg IV. However, occasionally very fast tachycardias and tachyarrhythmias can occur at these doses if used in non-anaesthetised patients, so the lower doses (0.005–0.01 mg/kg IV) are usually administered for bradycardias, with the higher doses being reserved for asystole. (Note that further bradycardia [paradoxical] may occur, before tachycardia finally ensues.) Glycopyrrolate is less useful in emergencies than atropine as it takes longer to work, even after IV injection. The dose is (5−) 10 µg/kg IV.

Further Reading

Ansah, O.B., Raekallio, M., and Vainio, O. (1998). Comparison of three doses of dexmedetomidine with medetomidine in cats following intramuscular administration. *Journal of Veterinary Pharmacology and Therapeutics* 21: 380–387.

Badino, P., Odore, R., and Re, G. (2005). Are so many adrenergic receptor subtypes really present in domestic animal tissues? A pharmacological perspective. *The Veterinary Journal* 170: 163–174.

Camarata, P.J. and Yaksh, T.L. (1985). Characterisation of the spinal adrenergic receptors mediating the spinal effects produced by the microinjection of morphine into the periaqueductal gray. *Brain Research* 336 (1): 133–142.

Congdon, J.M., Marquez, M., Niyom, S., and Boscan, P. (2011). Evaluation of the sedative and cardiovascular effects of intramuscular administration of dexmedetomidine with and without concurrent atropine administration in dogs. *Journal of the American Veterinary Medical Association* 239: 81–89.

Davies, M.F., Reid, K., Guo, T.-Z. et al. (2001). Sedative but not analgesic alpha2 agonist tolerance is blocked by NMDA receptor and nitric oxide synthase inhibitors. *Anesthesiology* 95: 184–191.

Drynan, E.A., Gray, P., and Raisis, A.L. (2012). Incidence of seizures associated with the use of acepromazine in dogs undergoing myelography. *Journal of Veterinary Emergency and Critical Care* 22: 262–266.

Fagerholm, V., Haaparanta, M., and Scheinin, M. (2011). Alpha 2 adrenoceptor regulation of blood glucose homeostasis. *Basic and Clinical Pharmacology and Toxicology* 108: 365–370.

Garcia-Villar, R., Toutain, P.L., Alvinerie, M., and Ruckebusch, Y. (1981). The pharmacokinetics of xylazine hydrochloride: an interspecific study. *Journal of Veterinary Pharmacology and Therapeutics* 4: 87–92.

Gellai, M. and Edwards, R.M. (1988). Mechanism of alpha2-adrenoceptor agonist-induced diuresis. *American Journal of Physiology* 255: F317–F323.

Grint, N.J., Burford, J., and Dugdale, A.H.A. (2009). Does pethidine affect the cardiovascular and sedative effects of dexmedetomidine in dogs? *Journal of Small Animal Practice* 50: 62–66.

Honkavaara, A., Pypendop, B., Turunen, H., and Ilkiw, J. (2017). The effect of MK-467, a peripheral α2 adrenoceptor antagonist, on dexmedetomidine-induced sedation and bradycardia after intravenous administration in conscious cats. *Veterinary Anaesthesia and Analgesia* 44: 42–51.

Johard, E., Tidholm, A., Ljungvall, I. et al. (2018). Effects of sedation with dexmedetomidine and buprenorphine on echocardiographic variables, blood pressure and heart rate in healthy cats. *Journal of Feline Medicine and Surgery* 20: 554–562.

Jones, D.J., Stehling, L.C., and Zauder, H.L. (1979). Cardiovascular responses to diazepam and midazolam maleate in the dog. *Anesthesiology* 51: 430–434.

Khan, Z.P., Ferguson, C.N., and Jones, R.M. (1999). Alpha 2 and imidazoline receptor agonists; their pharmacology and therapeutic role. *Anaesthesia* 54: 146–165.

Kuusela, E., Vainio, O., Kaistinen, A. et al. (2001). Sedative, analgesic and cardiovascular effects of levomedetomidine alone and in combination with dexmedetomidine in dogs. *American Journal of Veterinary Research* 62: 616–621.

Leppanen, M.K., McKusick, B.C., Granholm, M.M. et al. (2006). Clinical efficacy and safety of dexmedetomidine and buprenorphine, butorphanol or diazepam for canine hip radiography. *Journal of Small Animal Practice* 47: 663–669.

McConnell, J., Kirby, R., and Rudloff, E. (2007). Administration of acepromazine maleate to 31 dogs with a history of seizures. *Journal of Veterinary Emergency and Critical Care* 17: 262–267.

Micieli, F., Chiavaccini, L., Lamagna, B. et al. (2018). Comparison of intraocular pressure and pupil size after premedication with either acepromazine or dexmedetomidine in healthy dogs. *Veterinary Anaesthesia and Analgesia* 45: 667–672.

Monteiro, E.R., Junior, A.R., Assis, H.M.Q. et al. (2009). Comparative study on the sedative effects of morphine, methadone, butorphanol or tramadol, in combination with acepromazine, in dogs. *Veterinary Anaesthesia and Analgesia* 36: 25–33.

Murahata, Y. and Hikasa, Y. (2012). Comparison of the diuretic effects of medetomidine hydrochloride and xylazine hydrochloride in healthy cats. *American Journal of Veterinary Research* 73: 1871–1880.

Murrell, J.C. and Hellebrekers, L.J. (2004). Medetomidine and dexmedetomidine: a review of cardiovascular effects and antinociceptive properties in the dog. *Veterinary Anaesthesia and Analgesia* 32: 117–127.

Murrell, J.C. (2016). Premedication and sedation. In: *BSAVA Manual of Canine and Feline Anaesthesia and Analgesia*, 3e (eds. T. Duke-Novakovski, M. de Vries and C. Seymour), 170–190. Gloucester, UK: BSAVA Publications.

Ossipov, M.H., Suarez, L.J., and Spaulding, T.C. (1989). Antinociceptive interaction between alpha 2 adrenergic and opiate agonists at the spinal level in rodents. *Anesthesia and Analgesia* 68: 194–200.

Posner, L.E., Gleed, D.G., and Ludders, J.W. (2007). Post-anesthetic hyperthermia in cats. *Veterinary Anaesthesia and Analgesia* 34: 40–47.

Pypendop, B., Honkavaara, A., and Ilkiw, J. (2017). Cardiovascular effects of dexmedetomidine, with or without MK-467, following intravenous administration in cats. *Veterinary Anaesthesia and Analgesia* 44: 52–62.

Restitutti, F., Raekallio, M., Vainionpaa, M. et al. (2012). Plasma glucose, insulin, free fatty acids, lactate and cortisol concentrations in dexmedetomidine-sedated dogs with or without MK-467: a peripheral $\alpha2$ adrenoceptor antagonist. *The Veterinary Journal* 193: 481–485.

Robinson, R. and Borer-Weir, K. (2015). The effects of diazepam or midazolam on the dose of propofol required to induce anaesthesia in cats. *Veterinary Anaesthesia and Analgesia* 42: 493–501.

Sanders, R.D. (2008). G-protein coupled receptors. *Handbook of Experimental Pharmacology* 182: 93–117.

Self, I.A., Hughes, J.M.L., Kenny, D.A., and Clutton, R.E. (2009). Effect of muscle injection site on preanaesthetic sedation in dogs. *Veterinary Record* 164: 323–326.

Sinclair, M.D. (2003). A review of the physiological effects of $\alpha2$ agonists related to the clinical use of medetomidine in small animal practice. *Canadian Veterinary Journal* 44: 885–897.

Soares, J.H.N., Henao-Guerrero, N., Pavlisko, N.D. et al. (2019). The effect of two doses of fentanyl on chest wall rigidity at equipotent doses of isoflurane in dogs. *Veterinary Anaesthesia and Analgesia* 46: 360–364.

Stepien, R.L., Bonagura, J.D., Bednarski, R.M., and Muir, W.W. (1995). Cardiorespiratory effects of acepromazine maleate and buprenorphine hydrochloride in clinically normal dogs. *American Journal of Veterinary Research* 56: 78–84.

Tobias, K.M. and Marioni-Henry, K. (2006). A retrospective study on the use of acepromazine maleate in dogs with seizures. *Journal of the American Animal Hospital Association* 42: 283–289.

Torneke, K., Bergstrom, U., and Neil, A. (2003). Interactions of xylazine and detomidine with alpha 2 adrenoceptors in brain tissues from cattle, swine and rats. *Journal of Veterinary Pharmacology and Therapeutics* 26: 205–211.

Tranquilli, W.J., Lemke, K.A., Williams, L.L. et al. (1992). Flumazenil efficacy in reversing diazepam or midazolam overdose in dogs. *Journal of Veterinary Anaesthesia* 19: 65–68.

Van Haaften, K.A., Eichstadt Forsythe, L.R., Stelow, E.A., and Bain, M.J. (2018). Efficacy of a single pre-appointment dose of gabapentin on aggression, anxiety and stress-related behaviors during feline transportation and veterinary examination. *Journal of Feline Medicine and Surgery* 20: 59–60. (Abstract presented at AAFP conference 2017.).

Valverde, A., Cantwell, S., Hernandez, J., and Brotherson, C. (2004). Effects of acepromazine on the incidence of vomiting associated with opioid administration in dogs. *Veterinary Anaesthesia and Analgesia* 31: 40–45.

Waterman, A.E., Kalthum, W., and Pearson, H. (1992). The influence of premedication with acepromazine on the pharmacokinetics of pethidine in the dog. *Journal of Veterinary Anaesthesia* 19: 85–86.

Self-test Section

1 Which of the following statements concerning acepromazine is true?
   A It causes hypertension
   B It provides analgesia
   C Administration results in emesis
   D It has some anti-arrhythmic properties

2 Which of the following would you be most reluctant to administer to neonates (one to two weeks old)?
   A Pethidine
   B Benzodiazepines
   C Medetomidine
   D Isoflurane

3 Which is true regarding dexmedetomidine?
   A It has an $\alpha2{:}\alpha1$ selectivity ratio greater than that of xylazine
   B It is licenced for epidural administration
   C Initial blood pressure change (following IV administration) is hypotension
   D It antagonises opioid analgesia

5

Injectable Anaesthetic Agents

5.1 Overview

Neurons are hyperpolarised either by increased inhibition or decreased excitation. Many injectable anaesthetic drugs potentiate or facilitate the effects of the inhibitory neurotransmitter gamma aminobutyric acid (GABA) at $GABA_A$ receptors (chloride channels) in the central nervous system (CNS). These agents may also inhibit L-type calcium channels and other ion channels (e.g. neuronal hyperpolarisation-activated cyclic nucleotide-gated non-selective cation channel 1 [HCN1]). All general anaesthetics also appear to stabilise the desensitised conformational state of the neuronal nicotinic acetylcholine receptor. See Chapter 1 for an overview of the mechanisms of general anaesthesia.

Routes of injection may be intravenous, intramuscular, intraperitoneal, or intraosseous (intramedullary), but the intravenous route is preferred and most commonly used; some agents do not lend themselves to other routes because of tissue irritation or poor bioavailability.

Injectable agents can be administered for **induction** of anaesthesia, and some are also suitable for **maintenance** of anaesthesia, if administered by intermittent top-ups, or continuous infusion.

5.2 Properties of an Ideal Injectable Anaesthetic Agent

- Rapid onset of action (fat soluble, crosses blood–brain barrier quickly)
- Smooth induction of anaesthesia
- Smooth recovery from anaesthesia
- Non-irritant to tissues
- Good bioavailability by any route of administration
- Short duration of action (generally advantageous; useful for top-up doses or for continuous infusion)
- Non-cumulative (useful for top-up doses or for continuous infusion)
- Rapid metabolism (even independent of hepatic, pulmonary, or renal function)
- No toxic or active metabolites or preservatives
- 'Reversible'
- Does not cause histamine release
- Minimal cardiorespiratory side effects (depression or stimulation)
- Produces a degree of muscle relaxation
- Produces a degree of analgesia
- Stable in storage (not degraded by heat or light)
- Stable in solution (not degraded by heat or light)
- Miscible with other agents
- Inexpensive with long shelf-life
- High therapeutic index
- No environmental pollution during manufacture, preparation, or use

5.3 Advantages and Disadvantages of Injectable Drugs

5.3.1 Advantages

- Little equipment needed (syringes, needles, intravenous catheters).
- Usually easy to administer.

Veterinary Anaesthesia: Principles to Practice, Second Edition. Alexandra H. A. Dugdale, Georgina Beaumont, Carl Bradbrook, and Matthew Gurney.
© 2020 John Wiley & Sons Ltd. Published 2020 by John Wiley & Sons Ltd.
Companion website: www.wiley.com/go/dugdale/veterinary-anaesthesia

- Induction of anaesthesia can be rapid and smooth.
- Delirium (anaesthesia stage II) rapidly traversed or avoided entirely.
- No environmental pollution during use.
- ± Relatively cheap.

5.3.2 Disadvantages

- Once given, retrieval is impossible.
- The patient must be weighed accurately in order to calculate the dose (should lean weight be used in obese patients, and what about pregnant patients?).
- Clinical signs of depth of anaesthesia may differ from those seen during inhalant anaesthesia (learning curve).
- When used as the sole anaesthetic agent, high doses are often necessary to produce sufficient depression of the CNS to prevent response to surgical stimulation.
  - Such high doses often produce profound cardiovascular and respiratory system side effects (usually depression).
- Not well tolerated by debilitated, hypovolaemic or septic/SIRS (systematic inflammatory response syndrome)/endotoxaemic animals, or by those suffering renal or hepatic impairment; therefore, doses should be reduced and given slowly to effect (unless you require rapid induction in order to gain rapid control of the airway).
- Some drugs have the potential for human abuse.
- Required volume of some agents may be cumbersome in Equidae/cattle.
- Risks of inadvertent self-administration.
- Manufacture (particularly sterilisation) has an environmental cost.

5.4 Response to Administration

The pharmacokinetic response to administration depends upon the following:

- Dose, concentration and rate of injection (if intravenous).
- Absorption from injection site (if not intravenous), i.e. bioavailability.
- Cardiac output (influences absorption from intramuscular or intraperitoneal sites, and also rate of delivery of drug from intravenous injection site to brain).
  - Cardiac output is influenced by heart rate and stroke volume; and these depend upon a number of factors such as autonomic tone, presence of dysrhythmias, systemic vascular resistance (afterload), myocardial contractility, blood volume (preload), and the effects of other sedative/anaesthetic drugs. See Chapter 18 on monitoring.

- Cerebral blood flow.
- Lipid solubility and ease of passage across the blood–brain barrier.
- Degree of ionisation in tissue fluids (depends upon body pH and drug's pKa; pKa is the pH at which half the amount of drug present is in its ionised form).
- Degree of protein binding (bound drug is 'unavailable'; free/unbound drug is active).
- Rate of redistribution to other tissues (and the mass of other tissues and their perfusion).
- Rate of metabolism and excretion.
- Do the lungs sequester or metabolise the drug?
- Are there any active metabolites?

5.5 Pharmacokinetic Body Compartments

If the blood is thought of as the central compartment, and injection being made into that, or absorption from an intramuscular injection site occurring into blood, then wherever the blood flows next, that is where the drug is next delivered.

We often read about:

- Vessel-rich tissues (vital organs: heart, brain, lungs, liver, kidneys).
- Intermediate vascularity tissues (muscles [and skin]).
- Vessel-poor tissues (fat).

If, however, a drug is administered into a systemic vein, the first tissue it reaches is the heart, quickly followed by the lungs, so the lungs are sometimes considered as a separate compartment. Also, muscle, skin and fat are differently perfused, so could be represented by three different compartments. The body could therefore be represented by five compartments:

- Lungs.
- Vessel-rich tissues (vital organs, importantly the brain).
- Vessel-moderate tissues (muscles [some people include skin]).
- Vessel-poor tissues (skin, tendons, bones, cartilage).
- Fat.

Some people place bones, cartilage, and tendons into a sixth group, which is also vessel poor, but with even slower equilibration than fat.

Each of these compartments has its own **time constant**. This is a measure of the time needed for that particular compartment to approach equilibrium with the central compartment (blood), once any change has occurred in the central compartment. The time constant is directly proportional to the volume of the compartment, and inversely proportional to its perfusion:

$$\text{Time constant} \propto \frac{\text{Volume of compartment}}{\text{Perfusion of compartment}}$$

When relatively lipophilic anaesthetic drugs are administered intravenously, they traverse the lungs before reaching the vital organs, and of these vital organs, the brain contains a large amount of lipid (white matter), so lipid-soluble drugs begin to equilibrate with the brain first. This is useful as it allows a relatively fast induction of anaesthesia. Other tissues with longer time constants have to wait longer for their chance to equilibrate (which is aided by a high lipid content in the tissue), but eventually this occurs as drug is redistributed away from the brain to the other compartments.

Body fat can be a huge compartment, with a large capacity; it can act as a store for lipophilic anaesthetic drugs (although it is usually slow to equilibrate because of poor perfusion), but such drugs have no anaesthetic effect when in adipose tissue. Redistribution of anaesthetic drugs away from the brain to a peripheral 'inactive' fatty store provides a useful method of 'awakening' from anaesthesia as the brain concentration falls.

Recovery from anaesthesia (re/awakening) may be partly dependent upon such redistribution, whereas eventual drug elimination also depends upon metabolism and excretion. Prolonged elimination results in an anaesthetic 'hangover'. Once elimination (redistribution, metabolism, and excretion) of the drug is underway, the plasma concentration starts to fall and drug can now leach out of the fat (and other) stores to fuel further elimination, until eventually elimination is complete.

5.6 Total Intravenous Anaesthesia (TIVA)

TIVA is the use of injectable anaesthetic agents to both induce and maintain anaesthesia. Administration can be by intermittent bolus injection or continuous infusion, with continuous infusion preferred because a more stable plane of anaesthesia is achieved. Partial intravenous anaesthesia (PIVA) is the co-administration of both injectable and inhalational anaesthetic agents. Supplemental intravenous anaesthesia (SIVA) is administration of injectable agents to reduce inhalation agent requirement, so, in effect, is akin to PIVA.

A balanced anaesthetic (polypharmacy) technique is required to deliver adequate analgesia and muscle relaxation for surgery, although respiratory depression, necessitating ventilatory support, is common during TIVA.

5.6.1 Minimum Infusion Rate (MIR)

In the 1970s the concept of **median effective dose (ED$_{50}$) for IV agents was expanded to the MIR, which is the minimum infusion rate of an anaesthetic agent at which 50% of patients are unresponsive to a surgical incision**. The MIR is a necessary concept for the development of **TCI** (target-controlled infusions), i.e. where the plasma concentration (or better, the effect-site/brain concentration) can be determined and the infusion tailored to maintain the required target concentration.

5.6.2 Effect-Site Equilibration Time

There is a time lag between injection of anaesthetic agent into a peripheral vein and loss of consciousness, called the effect-site equilibration time or biophase delay. Figure 5.1 outlines the features that help determine this time lag.

The **effect-site equilibration time** (the time lag for the drug to get from the blood across the blood–brain barrier and to its site of action in the brain) is **slower for propofol than thiopental**. It is about **three minutes for propofol** compared with about **one minute for thiopental** (in sheep, and probably similar in other species). The higher protein-binding of propofol and its higher pulmonary uptake (sequestration plus or minus some metabolism) may also contribute to this slower onset of 'effect'. In addition, propofol reduces cerebral blood flow during the induction process and this can also 'delay' onset of unconsciousness (especially if also administered by relatively slow injection). The effect-site equilibration time has not yet been determined for all anaesthetic drugs, in all species, and after different premedications. It is important, however, because the effect-site equilibration is not instantaneous, so if an induction agent is injected too rapidly, by the time the desired clinical effect is reached (e.g. endotracheal intubation is possible), an overdose has already been given because anaesthesia will continue to deepen beyond this intended end point, until effect-site equilibration finally occurs. Such overdoses (effectively over-deep anaesthesia) also tend to be associated with more profound side effects.

Many injectable anaesthetics also have a **context-sensitive half-time** whereby the half-life varies according to the 'context' of drug administration; the 'context' being the duration of its infusion. The *context-sensitive half-time* is defined as the time for the blood/plasma concentration to decline by 50% after an infusion (designed to maintain a steady state) has been stopped.

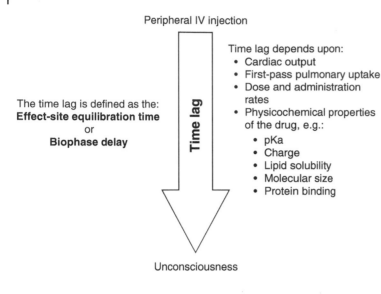

Peripheral IV injection

The time lag is defined as the:
Effect-site equilibration time
or
Biophase delay

Time lag depends upon:
- Cardiac output
- First-pass pulmonary uptake
- Dose and administration rates
- Physicochemical properties of the drug, e.g.:
  - pKa
  - Charge
  - Lipid solubility
  - Molecular size
  - Protein binding

Unconsciousness

Figure 5.1 The time lag between IV injection of an anaesthetic agent and the loss of consciousness, called the 'effect-site equilibration time' or 'biophase delay'.

5.6.2.1 Suggested Optimal Injection Times (to Avoid Overdosing)

- **Inject the chosen dose of thiopental over 10–30 seconds**; then wait a good 30 seconds (preferably 60 seconds) to assess the effect before deciding whether more is required.
- **Inject (infuse) the chosen dose of alfaxalone over about (30–)60 seconds**; then wait 45–60 seconds to assess the effect.
- **Inject (infuse) the chosen dose of propofol over about (one to)two minutes**; then wait one to two minutes to assess the effect.

Regardless of which drug is chosen, an intravenous catheter should be placed for its administration. A syringe-driver or infusion pump and premedicated, co-operative patient facilitate slow infusion rates and reduce the likelihood of overdoses.

5.7 Effects of Injectable Anaesthetic Drugs

Dose-dependent depression of the CNS resulting in a spectrum of effects ranging from **light sedation to deep anaesthesia** is a feature of most injectable anaesthetics. Few are analgesic. **Transient extrapyramidal dysfunction** (e.g. 'propofol twitches') may occur following administration of injectable anaesthetics. Extrapyramidal dysfunction is not thought to be representative of true seizures (i.e. EEG [electroencephalogram] recordings show sub-cortical activity, rather than cortical activity) but is likely due to inhibition of dopaminergic neurotransmission and excitation of sub-cortical pathways,

extended refractory periods within inhibitory pathways of the brainstem/spinal cord (see below) and/or glycine antagonism.

Cardiopulmonary effects are agent specific (see monographs below), but **generally dose-dependent**, and post-induction apnoea is a feature of many. **Post-induction apnoea** is more likely, and of longer duration, following rapid IV administration (and larger doses). Should assessment of laryngeal function be required, it should be performed during the induction of anaesthesia, prior to tracheal intubation.

Immunomodulatory, anti-inflammatory and anti-oxidative effects are agent-specific and have yet to be investigated for alfaxalone. Bacterial growth is supported by the unpreserved formulations of propofol > alfaxalone.

5.7.1 Extrapyramidal Dysfunction

Extrapyramidal symptoms (see Table 5.1) include dystonia (spasm of muscles or muscle groups) and dyskinesia (involuntary, uncontrolled movements).

The doses of anaesthetic required to cause extrapyramidal dysfunction are unknown and likely depend upon a number of factors, including individual patient and premedication. There are no definitive treatment guidelines for anaesthetic-induced extrapyramidal dysfunction. Benzodiazepine monotherapy rarely resolves clinical signs. In humans, dysfunction caused by antipsychotics or metoclopramide is treated with antimuscarinic medication, with or without a benzodiazepine. Antimuscarinic drugs resolve the symptoms of extrapyramidal dysfunction caused by drugs that either directly or indirectly inhibit dopaminergic neurotransmission. Commonly reported antimuscarinics used in humans include:

Table 5.1 Symptoms of extrapyramidal dysfunction.

Terminology	Description of abnormal movement
Akathisia	Motor restlessness manifesting as tension, nervousness and/or anxiety
Athetosis	Slow, involuntary, non-purposeful, writhing movements, affecting trunk and possibly proximal limb muscles
Ballismus	Appearance of flailing and ballistic, violent, undesired limb movements; usually rapid, non-purposeful and especially affecting proximal limb muscles
Bradykinesia	Slow movements
Chorea	Abrupt, involuntary, semi-purposeful or non-purposeful, often dance-like movements, especially affecting distal limb muscles
Choreoathetosis	Involuntary muscle contractions involving a combination of chorea and athetosis
Dyskinesia (often paroxysmal, i.e. episodic)	Involuntary, uncontrollable tremors and stiff jerking movements of face and body; may include oro-facial and oro-bucco-lingual dyskinesias, e.g. tongue thrusting, lip-smacking, excessive blinking
Dystonia	Intermittent or sustained involuntary spasms/contractions of muscles in the face, larynx, trunk, pelvis, and/or extremities
Oculogyric movement	Prolonged, upward deviation of the eyes
Opisthotonus	Spine and extremity hyperextension
Torticollus	Abnormal, asymmetrical head or neck position, typically twisted laterally with dorsiflexion

- Benzatropine (Cogentin™)
- Diphenhydramine (Benadryl™)
- Trihexyphenidyl (Artane™)

In dogs, there are now anecdotal reports of **successful treatment of extrapyramidal dysfunction with chlorphenamine** (a potent H_1 antagonist [actually an inverse agonist at H_1 receptors], with weak antimuscarinic activity), 0.1–0.3 mg/kg (maximum 10 mg/dog total) slowly IV.

5.8 Substituted Phenols

5.8.1 Propofol (2,6-di-Isopropyl Phenol)

- Most commonly marketed in the veterinary world as a 1% **macro-emulsion** (10 mg/ml), pH 7.8, in soybean oil, glycerol, and egg yolk lecithin (i.e. Intralipid™, one of the components used for intravenous nutrition); pKa 11.
  - The emulsion slowly settles, so it is recommended to shake the bottle before drug is withdrawn.
  - Both preserved (PropoFlo™ Plus, 28-day licence) and unpreserved (various brands, single-use) formulations are available.
  - Licenced for use in cats and dogs for anaesthetic induction and short-term maintenance (notably, >30 minutes is cautioned against in cats due to prolonged recoveries).
    - o Formulations containing preservative (benzyl alcohol) should not be used for anaesthetic maintenance,

as benzyl alcohol toxicity can occur after prolonged infusions in both dogs and cats.
  - **The unpreserved macro-emulsion formula** has been shown to support bacterial growth. The broached vial may be placed in a refrigerator (for further withdrawals that day), but any unused vial contents must be disposed of at the end of the day (within eight hours of) when the vial was first broached.
  - A modified, preservative-free, 1% propofol macro-emulsion (Propofol-Lipuro Vet™), in which the oil phase consists of **medium- and long-chain triglycerides** with soybean oil, egg lecithin, glycerol, and sodium oleate, is available for veterinary use; in humans, this formulation is associated with slightly less pain upon injection, possibly because of the reduced concentration of propofol present in the aqueous phase.
- A lipid-free (aqueous) **nano-droplet micro-emulsion** formulation of propofol was released for veterinary use (PropoClear™), but subsequently withdrawn due to an **unacceptable incidence of moderate–severe pain**, thrombophlebitis and injection site reactions (thought due to the rapid release of propofol from the tiny oil droplets and the subsequent high concentration of free propofol able to contact vascular endothelium).
- It is possible that propofol solubilised in cyclodextrins (aqueous solution), may become available in the future.
- 98% protein-bound, especially to albumin in blood.
- Highly lipid soluble.
- $GABA_A$ agonist.

- **Not (usually) irritant if extravascular deposition** occurs, but must be administered intravenously to be effective because absorption from, e.g. IM sites, is almost equalled by metabolism, so blood (and CNS) concentrations never reach those adequate for anaesthesia to occur.
- Occasionally, macro-emulsion causes **pain upon IV injection**.
  - Not reduced by warming/cooling, but overcome in man by injecting a little lidocaine first or by reducing the propofol concentration first reaching the endothelium, e.g. by dilution or slow injection.
- **Induction and recovery from anaesthesia are generally smooth and excitement-free**.
- **Recovery** after one injection is due to **redistribution and metabolism**, whereas after prolonged infusion, metabolism becomes more important as the tissues become saturated.
- **No hangover effect** because of rapid and 'complete' metabolism.
- **Very little accumulation** (**except cats, where its metabolism is slower**), so can be administered by continuous infusion for maintenance of anaesthesia.
  - **Extremely rapid metabolism in liver** and **also extrahepatic sites (possibly lungs, kidneys, and even GI tract)**.
    - Glucuronidation and hydroxylation are both important in the metabolism of this phenolic compound.
    - No active metabolites; metabolites undergo renal $\pm$ biliary, elimination.
    - Cats cannot metabolise drugs very well by glucuronidation, so propofol has the potential to be more cumulative in cats.
    - Metabolism in Greyhounds appears a little slower than in other dog breeds.
  - Some prolongation of recoveries may occur following longer (several hours) infusions in both dogs and cats (context-sensitive half-time).
  - If repeated doses or infusion are considered for cats, especially if multiple anaesthetics are required (e.g. for fractionated radiotherapy), beware phenol toxicity and the development of oxidative injury with Heinz body production (and the potential for haemolytic anaemia).
- **Urine often looks bright green/yellow** and stains easily, due to excretion of compounds akin to **azo-dyes**, called **quinols**.
- Occasional vomiting has been recorded upon recovery; sometimes appetite stimulation appears to occur.
- Cats may rub their faces on recovery.
- Dogs may develop extrapyramidal symptoms.
- **Not analgesic** or anti-analgesic.

- Slight direct myocardial depression (**negative inotropy**) and **venodilation**, so **blood pressure falls**.
  - The mechanism for venodilation appears to involve increased nitric oxide release from vascular endothelium (nitric oxide is a potent vasodilator), and reduced sympathetic tone.
  - **Baroreceptor sensitivity is reset** so that **reflex tachycardia (and sympathetically-mediated vasoconstriction) tend not to occur**; therefore the hypotension observed is actually more profound than that which occurs with other agents.
  - Causes mild arterial vasoconstriction at clinically relevant concentrations (higher doses cause arteriodilation), yet not sufficient to offset the fall in arterial blood pressure due to venodilation and negative inotropy.
- **Mild to moderate respiratory depression** occurs and **post-induction apnoea** can last for several minutes following rapid IV injection.
  - The duration of post-induction apnoea appears related to both the dose administered and the rate of injection.
  - Propofol is a **potent depressor of chemoreceptor function**, especially sensitivity to oxygen, and this may compound the post-induction apnoea seen, whereas thiopental and etomidate may stimulate chemoreceptor function slightly.
  - **Potentiates hypoxic pulmonary vasoconstriction** via inhibition of K_{ATP} channel-mediated vasodilation, but how this fits into the clinical picture remains to be determined.
- Mild bronchodilation may occur.
- Occasionally, especially if the patient is not pre-oxygenated, **cyanosis** may be detected after rapid IV injection. This may not be totally due to post-induction apnoea, but may be due to the opening up of intrapulmonary shunts (perhaps due to precapillary vasoconstriction or perhaps because pulmonary veins are more sensitive to the venodilation); it may also be due to transient effects on the binding of oxygen to haemoglobin.
- **Some muscle relaxation occurs**, but sometimes muscular spasms are observed (extrapyramidal signs).
- Over one third (36%) of cats will maintain a central eye when appropriately anaesthetised for orotracheal intubation (following acepromazine/morphine premedication).
- Laryngeal function can be assessed in lightly anaesthetised animals, but premedication is also important, with laryngeal function being well-preserved following premedication with acepromazine and butorphanol.
- **Cerebro-/neuro-protection:** propofol reduces cerebral metabolic rate, which results in autoregulatory cerebral

arterial vasoconstriction, thereby reducing cerebral blood flow, intracranial blood volume, and thence pressure; it maintains the coupling between cerebral metabolic rate and cerebral blood flow.

- Propofol infusions can be used to **aid the control of refractory status epilepticus**.
- **Reduces lower oesophageal sphincter tone** more in dogs than in cats; may promote gastro-oesophageal reflux.
- Propofol has been reported to cause **acute pancreatitis** in humans, even after one dose, perhaps due to the high lipid content of the propofol macro-emulsion.
  - Some vets are wary of its use in animals if pancreatitis has already been diagnosed or if they are at risk of developing it (e.g. pancreatic surgery).
- **Splenic engorgement** occurs (possibly secondary to venodilation), so caution is advised for splenectomies, gastric dilation/volvulus cases and some imaging procedures.
- **Variable effects on platelet aggregation** (low doses enhance it; high doses suppress it), but not reported to be a problem clinically.
- Conflicting evidence on the effect on intra-ocular pressure in dogs; premedication, head position, and gag-reflex stimulation during laryngoscopy/orotracheal intubation likely play a role.
- **Anti-oxidant effects** (possibly due to its structure resembling that of vitamin E, and it may enhance the cellular glutathione anti-oxidant system) may enhance neuro-/organo-protection.
- **Anti-inflammatory effects**, through suppressed PGE_2 production, reduced oxidation, and phagocytosis by neutrophils and macrophages, may be protective during acute lung injury, sepsis/SIRS/endotoxaemia and ischaemia-reperfusion injury syndromes.
- **Natural killer cell** function is preserved and so **no promotion of tumour metastasis**.
- Lipids (i.e. in the macro-emulsion formulation of propofol) may encourage lipid peroxidation, and under UV light, some lipid peroxidation occurs in the bottle.

  - When administered to cats every day for 6–7 consecutive days, malaise, anorexia, diarrhoea, and Heinz body formation were observed (but no haemolysis detected), suggesting some oxidative damage (all cats recovered within 24–48 hours).

5.8.1.1 Dose

- For induction of anaesthesia in unpremedicated dogs: 6.5 mg/kg.
- For induction of anaesthesia in unpremedicated cats: 8 mg/kg.

- After premedication, the induction dose is 1–4 mg/kg in dogs and 2–6 mg/kg in cats.
  - The actual dose required depends upon the premedicant and rate of propofol injection.
  - Dose reduction is more pronounced after slow injection or if an α2 agonist is included in the premedication.
- Slower IV injection, made 'to effect', instead of rapid IV bolus, enables lower doses to be used, with fewer consequent side effects (especially cardiovascular and respiratory).
- Propofol is minimally cumulative, so can be administered for maintenance of anaesthesia by 'top-ups' or continuous infusion (not recommended in cats; beware the formulation with benzyl alcohol preservative in cats and dogs).
- Infusion rate c. 0.1–0.4 mg/kg/min or less and often stepped-down with time.
  - Infusions are commonly administered alongside opioid (e.g. fentanyl or remifentanil) or α2 agonist (dexmedetomidine) infusions to reduce the propofol requirements and improve muscle relaxation.
  - Ventilatory support is likely to be required.

5.9 Neuro-active Steroids

5.9.1 Alfaxalone (3α-Hydroxy-5α-Pregnane-11,20-Dione)

- An aqueous solution of alfaxalone (10 mg/ml), solubilised in **2-hydroxypropyl beta cyclodextrin** (Alfaxan®); pH 6.5–7.0.
  - Licenced for use in dogs, cats, and rabbits for both induction and maintenance of anaesthesia.
  - Suitable for immersion anaesthesia of amphibians, reptiles, and fish.
  - Preserved (28-day licence) and unpreserved (single-use licence) formulations are available.
  - Has taken the place of Saffan™, which contained both alfaxalone and alfadolone, solubilised in cremophor EL (which caused problematic histamine release).
- **Plasma protein binding is low** (17.6–50%).
- Dual action at $GABA_A$ receptors: positive allosteric modulation of $GABA_A$ receptors at low doses, $GABA_A$ agonist at higher doses.
  - Also has some anti-muscarinic (M1 and M3) activity.
- Intravenous administration is recommended, but can be administered intramuscularly (off-licence).
  - Sedation-to-anaesthesia can be achieved (dose-dependent), but the volumes required may be limiting, especially for IM administration, in larger animals.
  - 2–5 mg/kg IM alfaxalone produces sedation in cats, dogs, pigs, Guinea pigs, rabbits, and rodents (lower

doses than these can be used but are generally combined with other sedative drugs).

- Volumes exceeding 0.5 ml/kg (= 5 mg/kg alfaxalone) per IM injection site are considered unacceptable.

- **No histamine release** with this formulation (unlike cremophor EL formulation).
- **No pain upon injection** and no tissue damage if accidental extravascular injection occurs.
- **Induction and recovery from anaesthesia are generally smooth and excitement-free.**
  - Some animals may exhibit delirium, trembling, paddling, and/or disorientation (these are possibly extrapyramidal signs), particularly early in the recovery period (more so than after propofol), but also possible at anaesthetic induction; premedication is advised.
- **Recovery** after one injection is due to **redistribution and metabolism** and there is **no hangover effect** because of rapid and 'complete' metabolism. Recovery after infusion depends more upon metabolism, which is rapid.
- Primarily **hepatic metabolism by oxidation (cytochrome P450), glucuronidation, and sulphation**, although renal, pulmonary, and cerebral sites of metabolism may also be involved.
- Primarily **renal elimination** of metabolites.
- Very rapidly **metabolised** and clinically non-cumulative, at clinically-recommended doses.
  - Cats exhibit non-linear pharmacokinetics: different doses exhibit different pharmacokinetic profiles.
  - Some prolongation of recoveries may occur following longer (several hours) infusions in both cats and dogs (context-sensitive half-time).
- **Not analgesic.**
- **Dose-dependent cardiovascular depression.**
  - Hypotension (due to a combination of direct myocardial depression and some peripheral vasodilation) is offset to some degree by a reflex tachycardia.
    - The baroreceptor reflex appears to be preserved.
  - Prolonged (15–30 minutes) tachycardia with normotension has been reported.
  - Higher doses cause more marked effects, and ventilatory support may be required if accidental overdose occurs.
- **Dose-dependent respiratory depression** after both IV and IM administration.
  - Transient hypoxaemia may accompany hypoventilation; oxygen supplementation is advised.
  - Animals may require ventilatory support during alfaxalone TIVA.
  - **Post-induction apnoea** is reported, with a slightly lower incidence than following propofol induction, and may be accompanied by hypoxaemia.
- **Reasonable muscle relaxation** but may be inadequate for some surgical procedures during TIVA; **premedication is recommended.**

- The majority of cats (~64%) maintain a central eye when appropriately anaesthetised for orotracheal intubation (following premedication with acepromazine and morphine).
- Laryngeal function can be assessed in lightly anaesthetised animals, but premedication is also important, with laryngeal function being well preserved following premedication with acepromazine and butorphanol.
- **Reduced cerebral metabolic rate** results in **proportional cerebral arterioconstriction** leading to **reduced cerebral blood flow and reduced intracranial pressure**; cerebral blood flow remains coupled to metabolic rate.
- Alfaxalone (and other 3α-hydroxy neurosteroids such as allopregnanolone and ganaxolone [3α-hydroxy-3β-methyl-5α-pregnan-20-one]) reduce EEG abnormalities associated with seizure activity and, in the ovine foetus and neonate, alfaxalone has been shown to exert a **neuroprotective** effect following hypoxic brain injury.
- **No effect on testosterone** concentration in male cats and cheetahs (despite being a progesterone analogue).
- **Reduced lower oesophageal sphincter pressure** in cats and dogs may predispose to gastro-oesophageal reflux.
- Stimulation of the **stress response**: plasma concentrations of both corticosterone and cortisol increased in rabbits after a single injection.

5.9.1.1 Dose

- For induction of anaesthesia in unpremedicated dogs: 2–4.5 mg/kg.
- For induction of anaesthesia in unpremedicated cats: 5 mg/kg.
- For induction of anaesthesia in unpremedicated rabbits: 3–10 mg/kg.
- After premedication, the induction dose is 0.5–2 mg/kg in dogs and cats, and 2–3 mg/kg in rabbits.
  - The actual dose required depends upon the premedicant.
  - Dose reduction is more pronounced after slow injection or if fentanyl or an α2 agonist is included in the premedication.
  - After very low induction doses, the animals may very suddenly awaken after 5–10 minutes because of rapid drug metabolism and possibly insufficient time for an adequate depth of volatile agent anaesthesia to be established.
- IV injection should be titrated, slowly, 'to effect'; doing this usually enables lower doses to be used, with fewer consequent side effects (especially cardiovascular and respiratory).
  - Should dilution be required to improve dosing-to-effect accuracy, it appears that normal saline is safe, at

least with the preservative-free formulation; and dilutions down to 2.5 and 1 mg/ml have been reported; but this constitutes off-licence use.

- Minimally cumulative, so can be administered for maintenance of anaesthesia by 'top-ups' or continuous infusion.
- Infusion rate c. 0.05–0.2 mg/kg/min and, ideally, stepped-down with time.

  - As for propofol, infusions are commonly administered alongside opioid (e.g. fentanyl or remifentanil) or α2 agonist (dexmedetomidine) infusions to reduce the alfaxalone requirements and improve muscle relaxation.
  - Ventilatory support is likely to be required.

5.10 Phencyclidine Derivatives/ Aryl-Cyclohexylamines

Three compounds, phencyclidine (PCP), tiletamine, and ketamine, have been used. PCP is the most potent and longest acting; tiletamine is intermediate; and ketamine is the shortest acting. Tiletamine is most often used in combination with the benzodiazepine zolazepam, in a mixture called Telazol™ (in the USA) or Zoletil™ (in Europe); for, especially, zoo or wild animal immobilisation/capture. Ketamine, although licenced for domestic animals (cats, dogs, horses, cattle, sheep, goats, and pigs), is also used widely in avian and exotic animal anaesthesia.

5.10.1 Ketamine Hydrochloride

- Aqueous solution, 10% (100 mg/ml), pH 3.5–5.5.
  - Around 50% protein-bound, and prefers α1-acid glycoprotein to albumin because it is a basic drug.
  - Prepared commercially as the hydrochloride salt, hence pH around 4, and is highly ionised in this aqueous solution; the drug is water- and lipid-soluble.
  - At body (blood) pH (7.4), it is roughly 50% ionised (because its pKa is 7.5), the unionised form is highly lipid-soluble and so, coupled with low protein binding, it **readily crosses the blood–brain barrier.**
  - **Racemic mixture**; S(+) isomer is 2–4× more potent than the R(−) isomer, and is less psychoactive (less emergence excitement).
- Can be administered IV or IM, and is **well absorbed across mucous membranes** (beware accidental self-administration).
- **Stings on IM injection** because of acidic pH.
- Ketamine is a **dissociative anaesthetic agent**; dissociative anaesthesia is characterised by:
  - Profound analgesia.

- Light sleep (there is much debate about whether this is true unconsciousness).
- Amnesia.
- Catatonia/catalepsy (trance-like immobility with a degree of muscle rigidity).
- Poor muscle relaxation; muscle rigidity/hypertonus/ spontaneous movements.
- Hypersensitivity to noise.
- Active cranial nerve reflexes: ocular (palpebral and corneal), and oral (gag/swallowing) reflexes persist, but do not guarantee a protected airway; salivation and lacrimation occur; nystagmus is commonly seen in horses.
- Transient convulsive-like activity is occasionally seen, especially in large felids and dogs and especially if premedication was poor.
- The thalamic and limbic systems seem to be stimulated, whereas higher centres/cortical activity are depressed/dissociated from any incoming signals.
  - Dissociative anaesthesia can be thought of as more of a **functional disorganisation of the CNS** rather than a generalised depression, such that the patient becomes 'disconnected' from its environment, both in terms of its interpretation of it, and its response to it. This results from a number of actions of ketamine in the CNS, including NMDA receptor antagonism and also possibly neuronal HCN1 cation channel inhibition.

- **Onset of action is relatively slow** (1–2+ minutes) because it produces dissociative effects, rather than conventional anaesthetic unconsciousness.
- Infusions are **cumulative**, as redistribution sites become 'saturated'.
  - Beware the effects of the **active metabolite** (norketamine) that, although providing some analgesia, can cause dysphoria.
- **Recovery** after one dose depends upon **redistribution** (ketamine itself is highly fat soluble) **and metabolism**, whereas after prolonged infusions, **metabolism and excretion** are more important.
- **Hepatic metabolism** (cytochrome P450 complex) occurs in most species, to some degree, with the production of an **active metabolite, norketamine**; this has about 20–30% of the activity of the parent compound in most species, but only 10% in cats.
  - The lungs, kidneys and intestines may also offer sites of metabolism.
  - Some texts suggest that ketamine can induce hepatic enzyme synthesis; others suggest it inhibits cytochrome P450 complex.
  - Metabolism is enantioselective (and R and S isomers may affect each other's metabolism).
  - Norketamine (the product of ketamine *N*-demethylation) can be excreted in the urine (and possibly also bile) or

be further metabolised/inactivated (by hydroxylation and subsequent conjugation, e.g. glucuronidation).

- Dogs and horses can metabolise norketamine (active) to its further metabolites, e.g. hydroxy-norketamine and dehydro-norketamine (inactive); ketamine and its metabolites undergo urinary or biliary excretion.
- Cats metabolise ketamine to norketamine only (no further metabolism to inactive compounds); both the ketamine and norketamine are excreted in the urine, so **beware cats with compromised renal function and with urine-voiding problems**.

- **Analgesia and anti-hyperalgesia**; appear to involve spinal, supraspinal, and even peripheral sites of action; ketamine can prevent, and also reverse, developed hypersensitivity to painful stimuli, even at sub-anaesthetic doses.
  - Ketamine may be a better anti-hyperalgesic (e.g. in chronic pain states) than analgesic (e.g. for surgical incisional type pain).
  - Ketamine may also have an important role in **preventing tolerance to opioid analgesics** and in preventing or treating the development of opioid-induced hyperalgesia.

- **Mild cardiovascular stimulation is seen in healthy animals**.
  - Ketamine is actually a direct myocardial depressant (i.e. a negative inotrope) and a direct vasodilator (these actions possibly partly via calcium channel blocking effects), but it also stimulates sympathetic nervous system activity (in a non-uniform fashion throughout the body), and so indirectly stimulates the cardiovascular system, with the overall effect of slightly increasing cardiac output, heart rate and blood pressure.
    - Cardiovascular stimulation is associated with increased circulating catecholamines (central sympathetic stimulation plus vagal withdrawal [leading to increased catecholamine release], and re-uptake 1 and 2 inhibition).
  - **Beware in shocky animals**, or those with sympathetic exhaustion or poor sympathetic reserves, because in these animals you will unmask ketamine's direct myocardial depressant effects and see some hypotension.
  - In hyperthyroid animals and those with adrenal tumours (i.e. phaeochromocytomas), ketamine may cause some arrhythmias, although it only minimally sensitises the myocardium to the arrhythmogenic effects of catecholamines.

- **Minimal respiratory depression**, perhaps a little **post-induction apnoea** after rapid IV bolus injection.
  - The ventilatory response to carbon dioxide is maintained, even enhanced, and hypoxic pulmonary vasoconstriction is also maintained.

- Occasionally **irregular or periodic breathing patterns** are observed and **apneustic breathing** may also occur (where there is an end-inspiratory pause, rather than an end-expiratory pause).

- Bronchodilation may occur, especially seen as a 'relief' of bronchospasm due to other causes.
- Active cranial nerve reflexes do not ensure a protected airway.
- **Increases intracranial pressure**: ketamine promotes cerebral blood flow but enhances blood flow over and above the demands of the cerebral circulation (so actually increases intracranial pressure).
- Ketamine may offer **cerebro-/neuro-protective** effects via calcium channel blockade, thereby reducing intracellular calcium accumulation; and also by blocking the effects of the potentially harmful excitotoxic neurotransmitter, glutamate at N-methyl-D-aspartate (NMDA) receptors.
  - However, it has also been reported to cause **neurotoxic** effects in rats and chronic seizure maintenance therapy with ketamine in humans has been linked to neurotoxicity (cerebellar and cerebral atrophy).
- Low-dose infusion may play a role in the **control of refractory seizures**.
- Intrathecal administration can cause lesions in the spinal cord, but the preservative chlorbutanol was probably to blame for these; hence preservative-free preparations are recommended for epidural and intrathecal administration (preservative-free solutions, especially of the more active S(+) isomer, are becoming available for epidural administration).
- **Does not appear to alter lower oesophageal sphincter tone**.
- Ketamine (+ benzodiazepine) can cause splenic engorgement.
- **Anti-inflammatory effects**, through suppression of natural killer cells, reduced oxidation and phagocytosis by neutrophils and macrophages, reduced NFκB activation, blunted TNF-α activity, and reduced pro-inflammatory cytokine production: may be protective during acute lung injury, SIRS/sepsis and ischaemia-reperfusion injury syndromes.
- **Impairment of natural killer cells promotes tumour metastasis**.
- Changes in intra-ocular pressure appear to be species-dependent, and increases may be associated with increased extra-ocular muscle tone.

5.10.1.1 Actions

The actions of ketamine include:
- Non-competitive NMDA antagonism (binds to PCP binding site of the NMDA receptor; at one time the PCP binding site of the NMDA receptor was proposed to be the σ opioid receptor).

- Antagonism at non-NMDA glutamate receptors.
- Actions at opioid receptors (μ antagonism, κ agonism, δ agonism).
- Actions at GABA$_A$ receptors (possibly anticonvulsant); this is controversial.
- Actions at nicotinic and muscarinic cholinergic receptors.
- Actions at monoaminergic receptors.
- Inhibition of re-uptake 1 and re-uptake 2 (i.e. monoamine uptake: noradrenaline (norepinephrine), serotonin (5-HT), and dopamine).
- Blockade of voltage-dependent calcium channels (L-type) and voltage-gated cation channels (e.g. HCN1).
- Has local anaesthetic-like activity (sodium channel blockade).
- Has anti-inflammatory/immuno-modulatory actions (as above and possibly via adenosine).
- May have anti-depressant effects in a subset of humans with major depressive disorder.

See Chapter 3 on pain for more information about NMDA, which binds to a subtype of glutamate receptors found in the CNS that are heavily involved in pain processing, especially the sensitisation to pain (resulting in hyperalgesia); and also memory processing and learning. Glutamate is an excitatory neurotransmitter. The analgesic and anti-hyperalgesic actions of ketamine may involve:

- NMDA antagonism.
- Descending monoaminergic pathway interactions.
- Opioid receptor interactions.
- Local anaesthetic type actions (may provide an extra benefit for epidural administration).
- Cholinergic effects (descending pathways).
- NOS inhibition.
- CNS dissociative effects.
- Reduction in pain memory formation.

5.10.1.2 Uses and Doses
5.10.1.2.1 Anaesthesia
Ketamine is used as an anaesthetic induction agent, usually following premedication, and often combined with a benzodiazepine or α2 agonist (to reduce the increased muscle tone produced by ketamine). It can be used in most species, but it is licenced (in the UK) for cats, dogs, horses, cattle, sheep, goats, pigs, and sub-human primates.

The dose varies, and depends upon premedication, but is commonly:

- 2.5 mg/kg for dogs.
- 2.5+ mg/kg for cats.
- 2.2 mg/kg for horses and farm animals.
- Higher doses are often required for birds and exotics.

- Routes of administration are IV, IM or even transmucosal.
  - Higher doses may be required IM in cats (40% bioavailable) compared to other species (e.g. 90–95% bioavailable in dogs and humans).

Ketamine can be administered for maintenance of anaesthesia either by top-up bolus doses or by infusion; commonly combined with other drugs (see Chapter 31 on field anaesthesia for horses), but is cumulative with prolonged infusions. For aggressive dogs, ketamine squirted into the mouth will be well absorbed across the oral mucosa to effect anaesthesia, but often the animals become quite hyperaesthetic (seizure-like activity may occur), if no sedative is administered first.

5.10.1.2.2 Analgesia
Ketamine can be administered in **sub-anaesthetic doses for analgesia** during surgery and/or post-operatively, or to treat other painful but non-surgical conditions. Doses are 0.1–0.5 mg/kg by any route (IV, IM, or SC); and further boluses may be administered, or a single bolus can be followed with an infusion at, e.g. 10–20 μg/kg/min intra-operatively, reducing to 2–5 μg/kg/min post-operatively in the conscious animal.

5.11 Barbiturates

Barbiturates are categorised according to their duration of action:

- Long acting: 8–12 hours
- Short acting: 45–90 minutes (e.g. pentobarbital)
- Ultrashort acting: 5–15 minutes for recovery to begin (e.g. thiopental, methohexital)

Duration of action also depends upon the dose administered. All barbiturates may induce hepatic enzymes. The barbiturates are no longer commercially available for the induction of anaesthesia in the United Kingdom, but pentobarbital is available as a euthanasia solution. See Chapters 30 and 33.

The pentobarbital euthanasia solution should not be used (diluted or not) for anaesthesia as the solution is not guaranteed to be sterile or free from pyrogens.

5.12 Carboxylated Imidazoles

5.12.1 Etomidate

Etomidate is the ester of a carboxylated imidazole. It is not licenced for veterinary use in the UK. Three preparations are available:

- Hypnomidate™: etomidate solubilised in aqueous solution (0.2%; 2 mg/ml), by 35% **propylene glycol**.
  - Propylene glycol can cause pain on injection, respiratory depression, hypotension, cardiac arrhythmias and direct myocardial depression (negative inotropy) all by itself, and can also be responsible for haemolysis, especially after large doses, e.g. prolonged infusions.
  - An increase in lactate is sometimes observed after propylene glycol administration because one product of its metabolism is lactate (see Chapter 22 on lactate).
- Etomidate-Lipuro™: etomidate presented in lipid emulsion (Lipofundin MCT/LCT™, which is similar to Intralipid™); 2 mg/ml.
- A drug matrix formulation for oral/transmucosal delivery in man; for sedation rather than anaesthesia.
  - Some of the preliminary work for this administration route was done in dogs.

5.12.2 Properties

- The propylene glycol solution has a pH of 6.9, and can cause **pain on injection**.
- **Extravascular injection can be mildly irritant** (due to the propylene glycol and/or the fact that the propylene glycol formulation is mildly hyperosmolar).
  - The lipid emulsion formulation does not cause pain on injection or venous/tissue irritation.
- The R(+) enantiomer (d isomer) is most active; hence the preparation contains only this enantiomer; the potency ratio of R : S enantiomers is said to be 5–10 : 1.
  - Etomidate is unique in that it shows **stereo-selectivity for GABA$_A$ receptors** and was one of the first drugs to be marketed as a single enantiomer rather than a racemic mixture.
- Moderate-to-high protein binding (75–76%), mainly to albumin in blood.
- Water soluble when highly ionised at acidic pH (the drug is weakly basic, pKa 4.2), but highly lipid soluble at body pH, when about 99% is unionised.
- GABA$_A$ agonist, weakly anti-nicotinic and anti-muscarinic.
- **No histamine release**.
- **Poor analgesia**.
- Induction and recovery quality is poor (mainly due to increased muscular activity), unless combined with other agents (e.g. benzodiazepines).
- After a single dose, **redistribution and metabolism** contribute to rapid recovery; after prolonged infusions, metabolism becomes more important (beware recent organophosphate treatment, as plasma esterases may be dysfunctional).
- **Very little accumulation; no active metabolites**.

- Useful for continuous infusions, but adrenal suppression may compromise the animal's post-operative 'recovery' and rehabilitation.
- **Rapid metabolism by liver *and* plasma esterases**, so not wholly dependent upon liver function.
  - A very small fraction of the parent drug may be excreted in the urine unchanged.
- Good cardiovascular stability; **minimal cardiovascular depression**; occasionally mild reduction in arterial blood pressure and possible slight increase in heart rate.
  - Slight negative inotropy.
  - No sensitisation of myocardium to catecholamine-induced arrhythmias.
- Occasionally causes **transient apnoea** after rapid IV injection.
  - **Transient mild respiratory depression** is proportional to the dose and speed of injection.
  - It does not inhibit hypoxic pulmonary vasoconstriction.
- Etomidate is an excellent hypnotic, but provides **poor muscle relaxation**.
  - Muscle hypertonus/myoclonus, especially during induction and recovery, are common with either IV formulation.
  - Muscle hypertonus is thought to be due to enhancement of monosynaptic spinal reflex activity.
  - Premedication is recommended (benzodiazepines provide useful muscle relaxation with minimal cardiovascular and respiratory effects).
- May be **cerebro-protective** as it decreases intracranial pressure through cerebral vasoconstriction and also reduces cerebral metabolic rate for oxygen and cerebral blood flow.
- **GI motility minimally affected**; occasionally vomiting is seen at induction or recovery, which is usually prevented by premedication and withholding food pre-operatively.
- May occasionally cause salivation.
- **Suppresses adrenocortical function** for 2–6 hours if healthy, and longer if unhealthy (6–48 hours, even after one dose), and therefore suppresses the stress response.
  - The mechanism of suppression of adrenocorticosteroid synthesis production is through inhibition of 11-β-hydroxylase and 17-α-hydroxylase.
  - There is still debate about whether this could be beneficial or detrimental, but this will also depend upon the individual patient's health status.
  - Beware its use in critically ill patients with poor adrenal function, as it may increase mortality.
  - Some people advocate supplementation with corticosteroids if a patient has known adrenocortical insufficiency and this drug is chosen.

– Newer (as yet, experimental) formulations (carbo-etomidate and methoxycarbonyl-etomidate [often called MOC-etomidate]) are less likely to suppress adrenal function; carbo-etomidate does so only during infusion, whilst MOC-etomidate has no N atom, which is required to inhibit 11-β-hydroxylase.

5.12.2.1 Dose

- About 1–3 mg/kg IV; premedication and/or co-induction is strongly recommended.

5.13 Injectable Volatile (Inhalational) Anaesthetic Drugs

Isoflurane and sevoflurane are volatile anaesthetic drugs, usually administered by inhalation, that can be emulsified in 30% lipid, or 15% lipid nano-emulsion, for intravenous administration. Intravenous administration of volatile anaesthetics may reduce the time taken to reach equilibration between the brain and tissues (compared to inhalational administration) as well as conferring a degree of organo-protection for the brain, heart, and kidneys through preconditioning; and the technique has been explored in dogs, pigs, mice, and rats. (See Chapter 8 on inhalational anaesthetics for more information.)

- Equivalent anaesthesia has been produced following both intravenous and inhalational administration.
- The **MAC (%) of isoflurane and sevoflurane is lower** for intravenous than inhalational administration.
  - **But** the total amount (g/h) required for an equivalent anaesthetic is the same, or greater, following intravenous administration.
  - The lipid carrier may increase the tissue solubility of the volatile anaesthetic, reducing the availability to equilibrate with alveoli.
    - Although there is **less respiratory excretion**, the patient's exhaled gases will still contain some volatile agents and therefore scavenging is still important.
- **Liver metabolism**, with subsequent renal excretion, may play a greater role in elimination following intravenous administration.
  - This may promote the development of toxic metabolites, such as trifluoroacetic acid (a strong acid) from isoflurane metabolism.
- Suspected **histamine release, causing facial oedema and moderate–severe hypotension**, has been observed with both formulations (lipid < nano-emulsion).
- **Respiratory acidosis**.
  - No difference between injectable or inhaled isoflurane.
  - Greater after intravenous sevoflurane than inhaled.

- Acute lung injury has been reported as a serious consequence, potentially due to the lipid carrier (lipoid pneumonitis).
- **Metabolic acidosis** is a feature and may be due to the lipid carrier; metabolic acidosis is particularly severe following intravenous isoflurane and may be exacerbated by the increased trifluoroacetic acid production.

5.14 Co-induction

Anaesthetic co-induction is the administration of a combination of drugs, for the induction of anaesthesia, whereby dose reductions of one or more of the drugs used should be possible, with a resultant decrease in the risk of cardiopulmonary and other adverse side effects. Usually veterinarians are aiming to reduce the dose of the injectable anaesthetic by combining it with a potent opioid or benzodiazepine. Co-induction may also be necessary to smooth the induction and provide adequate muscle relaxation for orotracheal intubation (e.g. ketamine and etomidate both cause increased muscle tone).

The order of administration is important:

- Potent opioids should be administered prior to the injectable anaesthetic.
- Benzodiazepines should be administered after deep sedation, or light anaesthesia, has already been achieved with the induction agent. This is called 'auto-priming', i.e. where a small proportion (c. ¼) of the estimated induction agent dose is given first, then the co-inductant and, finally, further induction agent is given, slowly, to effect. (See also Chapter 4 on sedatives).
  - Benzodiazepine administration prior to the injectable anaesthetic can be counter-productive as excitation may develop, then requiring a higher induction dose.
  - Midazolam, but not diazepam, enables propofol dose reduction.
  - Midazolam and diazepam enable alfaxalone dose reduction.
  - For best induction agent dose reduction, **benzodiazepine doses exceeding 0.3 mg/kg** are required, but at these doses, cardiorespiratory depression due to the benzodiazepine may be seen and may actually be counter-productive.
  - Anaesthetic sparing effects may (propofol) or may not (alfaxalone) extend into the maintenance period if following on with TIVA.
- In humans, lidocaine has been used to suppress the cough and cardiovascular responses to orotracheal intubation, thereby facilitating lower induction doses; however, **results have been somewhat equivocal in dogs**.

- In unpremeditated dogs, 1 mg/kg IV lidocaine prior to propofol anaesthetic induction neither attenuated the pressor response to orotracheal intubation nor reduced the occurrence of coughing.
- In dogs premedicated with methadone, 2 mg/kg IV lidocaine before propofol was found to attenuate the pressor response to endotracheal intubation (equivalent to 0.4 mg/kg topical laryngeal lidocaine), but the pressor response was thought to be already reduced due to the methadone premedication.

- o Cough suppression was also evident after IV lidocaine, but not after the smaller topical lidocaine dose.
- o No reduction in propofol dose requirement was found in this, or another, study using a lower lidocaine dose (1 mg/kg).
- **Lidocaine co-induction may, therefore, be useful for selected patients** in which avoidance of cough-induced increases in intracranial or intra-ocular pressures are warranted.

Further Reading

Akata, T., Izumi, K., and Nakashima, M. (2001). Mechanisms of direct inhibitory action of ketamine on vascular smooth muscle in mesenteric resistance arteries. *Anesthesiology* 95: 452–462.

Alkire, M.T., Hudetz, A.G., and Tononi, G. (2008). Consciousness and anesthesia. *Science* 322 (5903): 876–880.

Al-Rifai, Z. and Mulvey, D. (2016). Principles of total intravenous anaesthesia: basic pharmacokinetics and model descriptions. *BJA Education* 16: 92–97.

Amengual, M., Flaherty, D., Auckburally, A. et al. (2013). An evaluation of anaesthetic induction in healthy dogs using rapid intravenous injection of propofol or alfaxalone. *Veterinary Anaesthesia and Analgesia* 40: 115–123.

Anderson, S.L., Duke-Novakovski, T., and Singh, B. (2014). The immune response to anesthesia: part 2 sedatives, opioids and injectable anesthetic agents. *Veterinary Anaesthesia and Analgesia* 41: 553–566.

Baker, M.T. and Naguib, M. (2005). Propofol: the challenges of formulation. *Anesthesiology* 103: 860–876.

Barnes, T.R.E. and McPhillips, M.A. (1996). Antipsychotic-induced extrapyramidal symptoms: Role of anticholinergic drugs in treatment. *CNS Drugs* 6 (4): 315–330.

Bigby, S.E., Beths, T., Bauquier, S., and Carter, J.E. (2017). Effect of rate of administration of propofol or alfaxalone on induction dose requirements and occurrence of apnoea in dogs. *Veterinary Anaesthesia and Analgesia* 44: 1267–1275.

Borris, D.J., Bertram, E.H., and Kapur, J. (2000). Ketamine controls prolonged status epilepticus. *Epilepsy Research* 42: 117–122.

Braun, C., Hofmeister, E.H., Lockwood, A.A., and Parfitt, S.L. (2007). Effects of diazepam or lidocaine premedication on propofol induction and cardiovascular parameters in dogs. *Journal of the America Animal Hospital Association* 43: 8–12.

Cattai, A., Pilla, T., Cagnardi, P. et al. (2016). Evaluation and optimization of propofol pharmacokinetic parameters in cats for target-controlled infusion. *Veterinary Record* 178: 503. https://doi.org/10.1136/vr.103560.

Columb, M.O. and Hopkins, P.M. (2015). Programmes, guidelines and protocols- the antithesis of precision medicine? *British Journal of Anaesthesia* 115: 485–487.

Corrie, K. and Hardman, J.G. (2011). Mechanisms of drug interactions: pharmacodynamics and pharmacokinetics. *Anaesthesia and Intensive Care Medicine* 12: 156–159.

Covey-Crump, G.L. and Murison, P.J. (2008). Fentanyl or midazolam for co-induction of anaesthesia with propofol in dogs. *Veterinary Anaesthesia and Analgesia* 35: 463–472.

Deutsch, J., Jolliffe, C., Archer, E., and Leece, E.A. (2017). Intramuscular injection of alfaxalone in combination with butorphanol for sedation in cats. *Veterinary Anaesthesia and Analgesia* 44: 794–802.

d'Ovidio, D., Marino, F., Noviello, E. et al. (2018). Sedative effects of intramuscular alfaxalone in pet Guinea pigs (Cavia porcellus). *Veterinary Anaesthesia and Analgesia* 45: 183–189.

Dugdale, A.H.A., Pinchbeck, G.L., Jones, R.S., and Adams, W.A. (2005). Comparison of two thiopental infusion rates for the induction of anaesthesia in dogs. *Veterinary Anaesthesia and Analgesia* 32: 360–366.

Fawcett, W.J. and Jones, C.N. (2018). Bespoke intra-operative anaesthesia – the end of the formulaic approach? *Anaesthesia* 73: 1055–1066.

Flaherty, D. and Auckburally, A. (2017). Green discolouration of urine following propofol infusion in a dog. *Journal of Small Animal Practice* 58: 536–538.

Gambús, P.L. and Trocóniz, I.F. (2013). Pharmacokinetic-pharmacodynamic modelling in anaesthesia. *British Journal of Clinical Pharmacology* 79: 72–84.

Gaspard, N., Foreman, B., Judd, L.M. et al. (2013). Intravenous ketamine for the treatment of refractory status epilepticus: a retrospective multicenter study. *Epilepsia* 54: 1498–1503.

Gil, A.G., Silván, G., Villa, A., and Illera, J.C. (2012). Heart and respiratory rates and adrenal response to propofol or alfaxalone in rabbits. *Veterinary Record* 170: 444. https://doi.org/10.1136/vr.100573.

Grint, N.J., Smith, H.E., and Senior, J.M. (2008). Clinical evaluation of alfaxalone in cyclodextrin for the induction of anaesthesia in rabbits. *Veterinary Record* 163: 395–396.

Hanna, R.M., Borchard, R.E., and Schmidt, S.L. (1988). Pharmacokinetics of ketamine HCl and metabolite I in the cat: a comparison of i.v., i.m., and rectal administration. *Journal of Veterinary Pharmacology and Therapeutics* 11: 84–93.

Herbert, G.L., Bowlt, K.L., Ford-Fennah, V. et al. (2013). Alfaxalone for total intravenous anaesthesia in dogs undergoing ovariohysterectomy: a comparison of premedication with acepromazine or dexmedetomidine. *Veterinary Anaesthesia and Analgesia* 40: 124–133.

Herbert, G.L. and Murison, P.J. (2013). Eye position of cats anaesthetized with alfaxalone or propofol. *Veterinary Record* 172: 365–366.

Hill, A. (2004). Pharmacokinetics of drug infusions. *Continuing Education in Anaesthesia, Critical Care and Pain* 4: 76–80.

Hirst, J.J., Kelleher, M.A., Walker, D.W., and Palliser, H.K. (2014). Neuroactive steroids in pregnancy: key regulatory and protective roles in the foetal brain. *The Journal of Steroid Biochemistry and Molecular Biology* 139: 144–153.

Hopkins, A., Giuffrida, M., and Larenza, M.P. (2014). Midazolam, as a co-induction agent, has propofol sparing effects but also decreases systolic blood pressure in healthy dogs. *Veterinary Anaesthesia and Analgesia* 41: 64–72.

Hughes, J. and Bradbrook, C. (2016). Injectable anaesthetic induction agents. *Companion Animal* 21: 448–455.

Huynh, M., Poumeyrol, S., Pignon, C. et al. (2014). Intramuscular administration of alfaxalone for sedation in rabbits. *Veterinary Record* 176: 255. https://doi.org/10.1136/vr.102522.

Italiano, M. and Robinson, R. (2018). Effect of benzodiazepines on the dose of alfaxalone needed for endotracheal intubation in healthy dogs. *Veterinary Anaesthesia and Analgesia* 45: 720–728.

Jackson, A.M., Tobias, K., Long, C. et al. (2004). Effect of various anesthetic agents on laryngeal motion during laryngoscopy in normal dogs. *Veterinary Surgery* 33: 102–106.

Joliffe, C.T., Leece, E.A., Adams, V., and Marlin, D.J. (2007). Effect of intravenous lidocaine on heart rate, systolic arterial blood pressure and cough responses to endotracheal intubation in propofol-anaesthetized dogs. *Veterinary Anaesthesia and Analgesia* 34: 322–330.

Kästner, S.B.R. (2016). Intravenous anaesthetics. In: *BSAVA Manual of Canine and Feline Anaesthesia and Analgesia*, 3e (eds. T. Duke-Novakovski, M. de Vries and C. Seymour), 190–206. Gloucester, UK: BSAVA Publications.

Khan, K.S., Hayes, I., and Buggy, D.J. (2014). Pharmacology of anaesthetic agents 1: intravenous anaesthetic agents. *Continuing Education in Anaesthesia, Critical Care and Pain* 14: 100–105.

Kohrs, R. and Durieux, M.E. (1998). Ketamine: teaching an old drug new tricks. *Anesthesia and Analgesia* 87: 1186–1193.

Labuscagne, S., Zeiler, G.E., and Dzikiti, B.T. (2019). Effects of chemical and mechanical stimulation on laryngeal motion during alfaxalone, thiopentone or propofol anaesthesia in healthy dogs. *Veterinary Anaesthesia and Analgesia* 46: 435–442.

Liao, P.T., Sinclair, M., Valverde, A. et al. (2017). Induction dose and recovery quality of propofol and alfaxalone with or without midazolam coinduction followed by total intravenous anesthesia in dogs. *Veterinary Anaesthesia and Analgesia* 44: 1016–1026.

Maddern, K., Adams, V.J., Hill, N.A.T., and Leece, E.L. (2010). Alfaxalone induction dose following administration of medetomidine and butorphanol in the dog. *Veterinary Anaesthesia and Analgesia* 37: 7–13. (**Discusses dilution of alfaxalone**.).

Mellon, S.H. (2007). Neurosteroid regulation of central nervous system development. *Pharmacology & Therapeutics* 116: 107–124.

Michou, J.N., Leece, E.A., and Brearley, J.C. (2012). Comparison of pain on injection during induction of anaesthesia with alfaxalone and two formulations of propofol in dogs. *Veterinary Anaesthesia and Analgesia* 39: 275–281.

Minghella, E., Bensmansour, P., Iff, I. et al. (2010). Pain after injection of a new formulation of propofol in six dogs. *The Veterinary Record* 167: 866–867.

Mion, G. and Villevieille, T. (2013). Ketamine pharmacology: an update (pharmacodynamics and molecular aspects, recent findings). *CNS Neuroscience and Therapeutics* 19: 370–380.

Miroslav, P., Cherubini, G.B., and Palus, V. (2018). Neurogenic hyperkinetic movement disorders in dogs. *Companion Animal* 23: 230–235.

Mitek, A.E., Clark-Price, S.C., and Boesch, J.-M. (2013). Severe propofol-associated dystonia in a dog. *Canadian Veterinary Journal* 54: 471–474.

Musk, G.C., Pang, D.S.J., Beths, T., and Flaherty, D.A. (2005). Target-controlled infusion of propofol in dogs – evaluation of four targets for induction of anaesthesia. *The Veterinary Record* 157: 766–770.

Nakamura, K., Hatano, Y., Hirakata, H. et al. (1992). Direct vasoconstrictor and vasodilator effects of propofol in isolated dog arteries. *British Journal of Anaesthesia* 68: 193–197.

Natalini, C.C., Da Silva Serpa, P.B., Cavalcanti, R.L. et al. (2016). General anesthesia with an injectable 8% v/v sevoflurane lipid emulsion administered intravenously to dogs. *Veterinary Anaesthesia and Analgesia* 43: 271–280.

Natalini, C.C., Krahn, C.L., Serpa, P.B.S. et al. (2017). Intravenous 15% isoflurane lipid nanoemulsion for general anesthesia in dogs. *Veterinary Anaesthesia and Analgesia* 44: 219–227.

Norgate, D., Haar, G.T., Kulendra, N., and Veres-Nyeki, K.O. (2018). A comparison of the effect of propofol and alfaxalone on laryngeal motion in nonbrachycephalic and brachycephalic dogs. *Veterinary Anaesthesia and Analgesia* 45: 729–736.

Pai, A. and Heining, M. (2007). Ketamine. *Continuing Education in Anaesthesia, Critical Care and Pain* 7: 59–63.

Pascoe, P.J., Iliw, J.E., and Frischemeyer, K.J. (2006). The effect of the duration of propofol administration on recovery from anesthesia in cats. *Veterinary Anaesthesia and Analgesia* 33: 2–7.

Posporis, C., Wyatt, S., and Wessmann, A. (2018). Approach to canine paroxysmal dyskinesias. *Companion Animal* 23: 276–281.

Reddy, D.S. (2013). Role of hormones and neurosteroids in epileptogenesis. *Frontiers in Cellular Neuroscience* 7: 115. https://doi.org/10.3389/fncel.2013.0015.

Reeve, A.G. and Swenson, R.S. (2004). Chapter 26 Disorders of basal ganglia function. In: *Disorders of the Nervous System: A Primer*. Dartmouth Medical School https://www.dartmouth.edu/~dons/part_3/chapter_26.html.

Roberts, F. and Freshwater-Turner, D. (2007). Pharmacokinetics and anaesthesia. *Continuing Education in Anaesthesia, Critical Care & Pain* 7: 25–29.

Robinson, R. and Borer-Weir, K. (2013). A dose titration study into the effects of diazepam or midazolam on the propofol dose requirements for induction of general anaesthesia in client owned dogs, premedicated with methadone and acepromazine. *Veterinary Anaesthesia and Analgesia* 40: 455–463.

Rodríguez, J.M., Muñoz-Rascón, P., Navarrete-Calvo, R. et al. (2012). Comparison of the cardiopulmonary parameters after induction of anaesthesia with alphaxalone or etomidate in dogs. *Veterinary Anaesthesia and Analgesia* 39: 357–365.

Sánchez, A., Belda, E., Escobar, M. et al. (2013). Effects of altering the sequence of midazolam and propofol during co-induction of anaesthesia. *Veterinary Anaesthesia and Analgesia* 40: 359–366.

Sanders, R.D., Absalom, A., and Sleigh, J.W. (2014). 'For now we see through a glass, darkly': the anaesthesia syndrome. *British Journal of Anaesthesia* 112: 790–793.

Santos González, M., Torrent Bertrán de Lis, B., and Tendillo Cortijo, F.J. (2013). Effects of intramuscular alfaxalone alone or in combination with diazepam in swine. *Veterinary Anaesthesia and Analgesia* 40: 399–402.

Sear, J. (2010). Bonding, binding and isomerism. *Anaesthesia and Intensive Care* 12: 160–165.

Servin, F.S. and Billard, V. (2014). Surrogate measures, do they really describe anaesthetic state? *British Journal of Anaesthesia* 112: 787–790.

Schmitz, A., Portier, C.J., Thormann, W. et al. (2008). Stereoselective biotransformation of ketamine in equine liver and lung microsomes. *Journal of Veterinary Pharmacology and Therapeutics* 31: 446–455.

Schwarz, A., Kalchofner, K., Palm, J. et al. (2014). Minimum infusion rate of alfaxalone for total intravenous anaesthesia after sedation with acepromazine or medetomidine in cats undergoing ovariohysterectomy. *Veterinary Anaesthesia and Analgesia* 41: 480–490.

Sherer, J., Salazar, T., Schesing, K.B. et al. (2017). Diphenhydramine for acute extrapyramidal symptoms after propofol administration. *Pediatrics* 139: e20161135.

Sleigh, J., Harvey, M., Voss, L., and Denny, B. (2014). Ketamine – more mechanisms of action than just NMDA blockade. *Trends in Anaesthesia and Critical Care* 4: 76–81.

Smalle, T.M., Hartman, M.J., Bester, L. et al. (2017). Effects of thiopentone, propofol and alfaxalone on laryngeal motion during oral laryngoscopy in healthy dogs. *Veterinary Anaesthesia and Analgesia* 44: 427–434.

Strachan, F.A., Mansel, J.C., and Clutton, R.E. (2008). A comparison of microbial growth in alfaxalone, propofol and thiopental. *Journal of Small Animal Practice* 49: 186–190.

Suarez, M.A., Dzikiti, B.T., Stegmann, F.G., and Hartman, M. (2012). Comparison of alfaxalone and propofol administered as total intravenous anaesthesia for ovariohysterectomy in dogs. *Veterinary Anaesthesia and Analgesia* 39: 236–244.

Tamura, J., Ishizuka, T., Fukui, S. et al. (2015). The pharmacological effects of the anesthetic alfaxalone after intramuscular administration to dogs. *Journal of Veterinary Medical Science* 77: 289–296.

Thompson, K.R. and Rioja, E. (2016). Effects of intravenous and topical laryngeal lidocaine on heart rate, mean arterial pressure and cough response to endotracheal intubation in dogs. *Veterinary Anaesthesia and Analgesia* 43: 371–378.

Tuem, K.B. and Atey, T.M. (2017). Neuroactive steroids: receptors interactions and responses. *Frontiers in Neurology* 8: 422. https://doi.org/10.3389/fneur.2017.00442.

Tutunaru, A.C., Şonea, A., Drion, P. et al. (2013). Anaesthetic induction with alfaxalone may produce hypoxemia in rabbits premedicated with fentanyl/droperidol. *Veterinary Anaesthesia and Analgesia* 40: 647–659.

Ubogu, E.E., Sagar, S.M., Lerner, A.J. et al. (2003). Ketamine for refractory status epilepticus: a case of possible ketamine-induced neurotoxicity. *Epilepsy & Behavior* 4: 70–75.

Warne, L.N., Beths, T., Whittem, T. et al. (2015). A review of the pharmacology and clinical application of alfaxalone in cats. *The Veterinary Journal* 203: 141–148.

Waterman, A.E. (1983). Influence of premedication with xylazine on the distribution and metabolism of intramuscularly administered ketamine in cats. *Research in Veterinary Science* 35: 285–290.

Wilson, G.S. (2013). Ketamine: old dogs; new tricks. *South African Journal of Anaesthesia and Analgesia* 19: 24–26.

Yang, X.-L., Ma, H.-X., Yang, Z.-B. et al. (2006). Comparison of minimum alveolar concentration between intravenous isoflurane lipid emulsion and inhaled isoflurane in dogs. *Anesthesiology* 104: 482–487.

Yawno, T., Miller, S.L., Bennet, L. et al. (2017). Ganaxolone: a new treatment for neonatal seizures. *Frontiers in Cellular Neuroscience* 11: 246. https://doi.org/10.3389/fncel.2017.00246.

Yawno, T., Yan, E.B., Hirst, J.J., and Walker, D.W. (2011). Neuroactive steroids induce changes in fetal sheep behavior during normoxic and asphyxic states. *Stress* 14: 13–22.

Zanos, P., Moaddel, R., Morris, P.J. et al. (2018). Ketamine and ketamine metabolite pharmacology: insights into therapeutic mechanisms. *Pharmacological Reviews* 70: 621–660.

Zoff, A., Thompson, K., and Senior, M. (2016). Anaesthesia and drug interactions in dogs and cats. *In Practice* 38: 167–175.

Zonca, A., Ravasio, G., Gallo, M. et al. (2012). Pharmacokinetics of ketamine and propofol combination administered as ketofol via continuous infusion in cats. *Journal of Veterinary Pharmacology and Therapeutics* 35: 580–587.

Self-test Section

1 Which of the following reasons best explains ketamine's anti-hyperalgesic effects?
   A Its interaction with opioid receptors
   B Its antagonistic actions at NMDA receptors
   C Its interaction with $GABA_A$ receptors
   D Its ion channel blocking activities

2 Which statement is correct regarding co-induction with benzodiazepines?
   A Midazolam and diazepam are equally dose sparing for all injectable anaesthetic drugs.
   B The benzodiazepine must always be given before the injectable anaesthetic to ensure success.
   C Co-induction with alfaxalone will fail due to competitive inhibition at the $GABA_A$ binding site.
   D The benzodiazepine should be given after deep sedation/light anaesthesia has been achieved.

3 Which injectable anaesthetic is highly likely to promote the development of tumour metastasis?
   A Alfaxalone
   B Etomidate
   C Ketamine
   D Propofol

4 Regarding the use of benzyl alcohol preserved propofol formulations, which statement is incorrect?
   A It is not suitable for the prolonged maintenance of anaesthesia because the benzyl alcohol preservative will cause a potentially life-threatening toxicosis.
   B Only intravenous injection is effective; other parenteral (e.g. extravascular) injections are non-irritant (usually), but ineffective.
   C Causes hypotension by venodilation and slight negative inotropy, and blunts the baroreceptor reflex (no compensatory tachycardia).
   D The dose does not need to be reduced for hypoalbuminaemic patients, despite propofol being highly protein bound (98%), mostly to albumin.

6

Analgesic Infusions

6.1 Indications

- Provide multimodal analgesia in the peri-operative period
- Allow reduced volatile anaesthetic agent requirement
- Provide sedation
- Allow titration of analgesia according to patient requirement
- Chronic pain management

6.1.1 Advice

- Monitor autonomic indicators of nociception intra-operatively (heart rate, respiratory frequency, arterial blood pressure) to guide rate
- Evaluate the patient and adjust rate according to pain score post-operatively

6.2 Opioids

The opioid choices below are full μ opioid receptor agonists and their infusions can be used following premedication with other full μ receptor agonists, such as methadone. Controlled mechanical ventilation is required with alfentanil and remifentanil and higher doses (20 μg/kg/h) of fentanyl. Bradycardia is a potential side effect, which may require glycopyrrolate (5–20 μg/kg IV; start with 10 μg/kg). Doses given apply to cats and dogs unless otherwise stated.

6.2.1 Fentanyl

- Loading dose 1–5 μg/kg IV; intra-operative infusion 5–20 μg/kg/h; top-up bolus 2 μg/kg IV; post-operative infusion rate 1–5 μg/kg/h.
- IV bolus will cause transient apnoea.

6.2.2 Methadone

- Loading dose 0.3 mg/kg IV or IM; intra-operative infusion 0.1 mg/kg/h; top-up bolus 0.05 mg/kg; post-operative infusion rate 0.1 mg/kg/h.

- Effects of accumulation are seen as excessive sedation (dogs) and dysphoria (cats).
- Pharmacokinetics of fentanyl are better suited than methadone to administration by infusion.

6.2.3 Morphine

- Loading dose 0.1 + mg/kg IV (beware emesis), or IM; intra-operative infusion 0.1 mg/kg/h; top-up bolus 0.05 mg/kg; post-operative infusion rate 0.1 mg/kg/h.

6.2.4 Butorphanol

- Continuous infusions of butorphanol in horses have documented mixed results and the reader is directed to further reading for a wider discussion on this.

6.2.5 Alfentanil

- Loading dose 0.5–1.0 μg/kg IV; infusion c. 0.5–1.0 μg/kg/min; top-up bolus 0.5 μg/kg IV; post-operatively not recommended due to apnoeic potential.
- IV bolus will cause transient apnoea and beware profound bradycardia.

6.2.6 Remifentanil

- Loading dose not always required due to rapid onset, but 0.5–1.0 μg/kg IV can be used; infusion c. 0.5–1.0 μg/kg/min; post-operatively not recommended due to apnoeic potential.
- Remifentanil provides profound analgesia, but once the infusion is terminated (e.g. at the end of surgery), due to its rapid elimination, nociceptive input to the central nervous system is rapidly restored, causing increased pain intensity and requiring higher doses of analgesics.
- It is imperative that other forms of analgesia (e.g. methadone, NSAIDs, etc.) are provided before the infusion is terminated.

Veterinary Anaesthesia: Principles to Practice, Second Edition. Alexandra H. A. Dugdale, Georgina Beaumont, Carl Bradbrook, and Matthew Gurney.
© 2020 John Wiley & Sons Ltd. Published 2020 by John Wiley & Sons Ltd.
Companion website: www.wiley.com/go/dugdale/veterinary-anaesthesia

- Implicated in opioid-induced hyperalgesia (OIH).
- Both paracetamol and ketamine are documented to reduce OIH, so it may be advisable to use one or both concurrently with remifentanil.

If using alongside propofol for total intravenous anaesthesia (TIVA), start remifentanil at 0.1 μg/kg/min, three to four minutes before infusing propofol slowly to complete the induction. Continue propofol infusion at 0.1–0.2 mg/kg/min. If only a cardiovascular response occurs with surgical stimulation, then the remifentanil infusion rate should be increased; whereas if there is gross purposeful movement upon surgical stimulation, a small bolus (c. 1 mg/kg) of propofol should be administered and an increase in the propofol infusion rate should be considered. If neuromuscular blockers are administered, then there is unlikely to be gross purposeful movement (because the patient is paralysed) upon surgical stimulation. Therefore, autonomic responses should be monitored closely, but be aware of the vagomimetic response to remifentanil and also of the effects (and likely duration of action) of any administered anticholinergics.

6.2.7 Buprenorphine

Use of buprenorphine as a continuous infusion has been reported in dogs undergoing ovariohysterectomy. Dogs were premedicated with 15 μg/kg IV and then received an infusion of 2.5 μg/kg/h for 6 hours. Analgesia was supplemented with carprofen and local anaesthesia and no dogs required rescue analgesia. Norbuprenorphine (an active metabolite of buprenorphine, with agonist activities at kappa and nociceptin/orphanin FQ receptors) concentrations were negligible. Longer infusion times have not been studied.

6.3 Others

6.3.1 Ketamine

Ketamine can be administered at analgesic (sub-anaesthetic) doses. With intra-operative administration, the improved analgesia will reduce the requirement for maintenance anaesthetic agents (e.g. volatile or injectable agents). Alongside other analgesics, ketamine's NMDA antagonist actions provide synergistic multimodal analgesia.

- Loading dose 0.1–0.5 mg/kg IV; intra-operative infusion 10 μg/kg/min increasing to 20 μg/kg/min if responsive to surgery; post-operative analgesia 2–5 μg/kg/min. Salivation (perhaps indicative of nausea) sometimes seen and may necessitate reduction in rate of administration and/or treatment with an anti-emetic (e.g. maropitant).

- Transient bradypnoea seen with IV bolus: IM administration avoids this, but may require a higher dose (up to 1 mg/kg).
- Intramuscular ketamine, 0.5–1 mg/kg, is useful to control nociception during surgery where an infusion is not in use.
- Ketamine is an excellent option for post-operative pain where pain 'breaks through' despite opioid use. Infusion rate; 2–5 μg/kg/min (with or without initial loading dose of 0.2–0.5 mg/kg IV), but beware excitement in animals that are not under anaesthesia.

6.3.2 Lidocaine (Without Epinephrine or Preservative)

In humans, lidocaine is of particular benefit for acute hyperalgesia when opioids are not effective in treating pain.

Dogs: Loading dose 1–2 mg/kg; infusion 25–50 μg/kg/min. Debatable whether lidocaine causes nausea in dogs after c.24 hours, but salivation may be seen, especially at higher infusion rates, so consider the concurrent use of an anti-emetic, e.g. maropitant. Lidocaine infusion can be used to break the cycle of chronic pain at 25–50 μg/kg/min for 24 hours in dogs, often in combination with ketamine at 2–5 μg/kg/min.

Cats: Anaesthesia alters lidocaine pharmacokinetics in cats. Under anaesthesia, signs of intoxication (e.g. seizure activity) are difficult to determine; and furthermore, at lidocaine infusion rates sufficient for MAC reduction, cardiovascular depression (due to the lidocaine) in cats, has been demonstrated to be worse than that at an equivalent depth of volatile anaesthesia. Therefore, the use of lidocaine infusions is potentially restricted to conscious cats in the post-operative period. Published studies have only investigated short duration (maximum 6 hours) infusions and recommendations suggest rates of no greater than 50 μg/kg/min for a maximum of 2 hours before reducing the rate to 10–25 μg/kg/min for no more than a further 4 hours. If a loading dose is used, then 0.5 mg/kg is usually preferred over higher doses. Salivation can be seen at the higher infusion rates, especially if administered for prolonged durations. The author recommends ketamine infusions over lidocaine in cats.

Equine: Loading dose 1–2 mg/kg given IV **slowly** (over 5–10 minutes); infusion rate is usually 50 μg/kg/min but pharmacokinetics are affected by concurrent disease processes and anaesthesia so that lower or higher infusion rates may be more appropriate. A commercial 0.2% lidocaine solution (in 5% glucose) is available in 500 ml bags. Alternatively, 500 ml 2% lidocaine (without epinephrine) can be added to a 5 l bag of Hartmann's solution (ideally after first removing 500 ml of the Hartmann's solution), thus making a 0.2% solution (i.e. 2 mg/ml solution). This solution is suggested to be stable for 21 days.

6.3.3 Morphine–Lidocaine–Ketamine Infusion (MLK)

Morphine can be substituted with methadone at the same rates.

- Morphine loading dose 0.3–0.5 mg/kg IM; infusion 0.1 mg/kg/h.
- Lidocaine loading dose 0.5–1–2 mg/kg **slow** IV; infusion 25–50 μg/kg/min.
- Ketamine loading dose 0.1–0.5 mg/kg IV or IM; infusion 10–20 μg/kg/min.

Provides excellent analgesia: Be sure to reduce volatile agent. Continue infusion post-operatively at a lower rate. Although adding all three components to one infusion does not allow variation in administration rates of the individual components, it is simple to calculate.

The following recipe is a useful starting point.

After removing 46 ml from a 500 ml bag of normal saline or Hartmann's solution, add:

- 300 mg ketamine (= 3 ml of 100 mg/ml ketamine)
- 760 mg lidocaine (= 38 ml of 20 mg/ml [2%] lidocaine without epinephrine)
- 50 mg morphine or methadone (= 5 ml of 10 mg/ml morphine)

Infusion of this mixture intra-operatively can then be set at 1–2 ml/kg/h, which provides:

- 10–20 μg/kg/min ketamine
- 25–50 μg/kg/min lidocaine
- 1.7–3.3 μg/kg/min morphine

Post-operatively the infusion can be tapered down gradually whilst additional analgesia is provided by other means.

6.3.4 Dexmedetomidine

The α2 agonists provide sedation and analgesia with a MAC sparing (expect to deliver <1% isoflurane) effect. Analgesia in dogs is comparable to that with morphine infusion in clinical patients. Analgesia has been distinguished from sedation in neurophysiologic studies where >3 μg/kg/h was required for analgesia.

- Loading dose 2–5 μg/kg; intra-operative infusion rate 2.5–5 μg/kg/h; post-operative infusion rate 1–2.5 μg/kg/h.
- Expect bradycardia from dexmedetomidine.
- Decrease volatile agent.

See Chapter 28 for further details on α2 agonist and other infusions for sedation in horses. See also Chapter 3 for further details on pain and analgesics.

7

Intravascular Catheters/Cannulae

Some Considerations and Complications

LEARNING OBJECTIVES

- To be able to recognise the different types of intravascular catheters/cannulae.
- To be able to discuss the complications of intravascular (both venous and arterial) catheterisation/cannulation.
- To be able to devise a treatment plan for complications such as thrombophlebitis and venous air embolisation.

In human medicine, the word *catheter* refers to any tube longer than 12 cm that is inserted into a visceral or body 'cavity', and cannula to anything shorter, but usually denoting a tube inserted into a blood vessel; in veterinary medicine, *catheter* and *cannula* are used interchangeably.

Intravascular catheterisation is a common veterinary procedure and has been associated with reduced risk of peri-anaesthetic mortality in small animals. However, careful attention to technique and management are important to minimise the development of adverse events.

7.1 Veins for Catheterisation

- Cephalic vein (also accessory branches): dogs, cats, small ruminants, horses (Figure 7.1a)
- Saphenous vein: lateral saphenous vein (has cranial and caudal rami), commonly used in dogs as an alternative to cephalic vein (Figure 7.1b); medial saphenous vein preferred in cats and can be accessed in anaesthetised horses (Figure 7.2)
- Dorsal metatarsal (pedal) vein: dogs, cats, larger birds (Figure 7.3)
- Jugular vein: larger species, any species if 'central' venous catheterisation required (Figure 7.3)
- Femoral vein: medial saphenous vein drains into it, so that either the medial saphenous vein or the femoral vein can be catheterised using a long catheter to reach the caudal vena cava for 'central' venous access

- Auricular veins: marginal (lateral or medial), or intermediate branches; ease of catheterisation depends upon species, ear pinna size and shape (Figure 7.4)
- Lateral thoracic vein: larger species such as horses (Figure 7.5)
- 'Milk vein' (cranial superficial epigastric vein): cattle and pigs

7.2 Arteries for Catheterisation

Where possible, 'end arteries' should be avoided in order to prevent distal necrosis should occlusion of blood flow be caused during the 'life' of the catheter or as a complication of its placement. If in doubt, check for collateral supply by pulse palpation $\pm$ Doppler assessment.

Cannulatable arteries include:

- Caudal auricular artery (usually the intermediate/middle/central branch) on dorsal/caudal surface of pinna: camelids, dogs with large pinnae, horses, pigs, rabbits, large/small ruminants; beware associated veins (Figure 7.6)
- Transverse facial artery: horses (Figure 7.7); beware the close proximity of a vein and a branch of the facial nerve
- Mandibular artery: horses (Figure 7.8), small ruminants $\pm$ cattle; beware the close proximity of the parotid duct in horses
- Mandibular facial artery: horses, small ruminants $\pm$ cattle; this is a continuation of the mandibular artery where it courses up the cheek

Veterinary Anaesthesia: Principles to Practice, Second Edition. Alexandra H. A. Dugdale, Georgina Beaumont, Carl Bradbrook, and Matthew Gurney.
© 2020 John Wiley & Sons Ltd. Published 2020 by John Wiley & Sons Ltd.
Companion website: www.wiley.com/go/dugdale/veterinary-anaesthesia

(a)

(b)

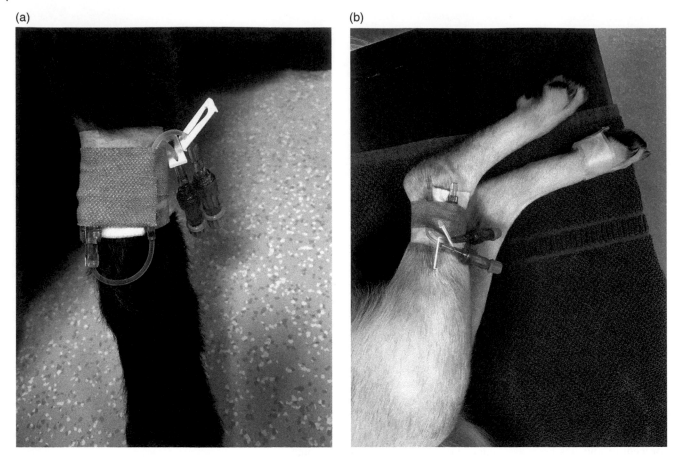

Figure 7.1 Catheterised cephalic vein in a conscious dog (a) and lateral saphenous vein in a sedated dog (b).

(a)

(b)

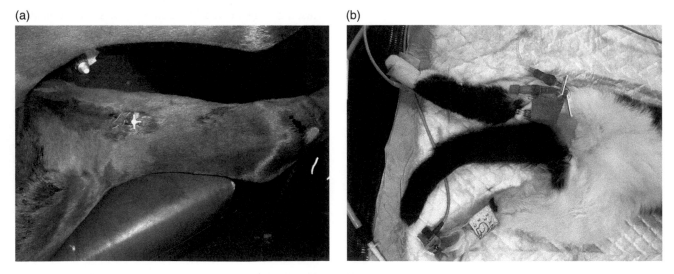

Figure 7.2 Catheterised medial saphenous vein in an anaesthetised horse (a) and cat (b).

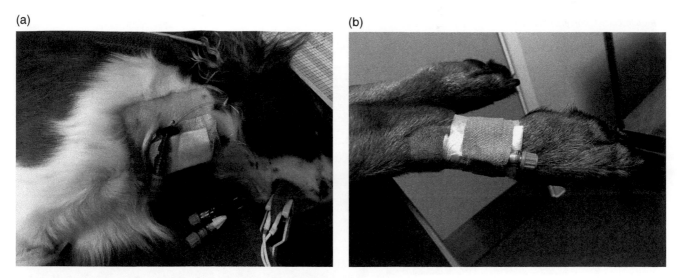

Figure 7.3 Catheterised jugular (a) and dorsal metatarsal (b) veins in sedated dogs.

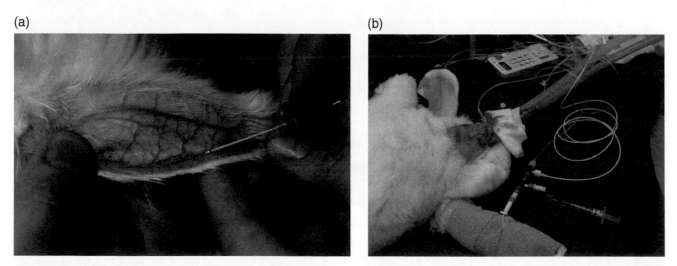

Figure 7.4 Catheterisation of a marginal ear vein in a rabbit (a); connection of a marginal ear vein catheter to infusions in a rabbit (b).

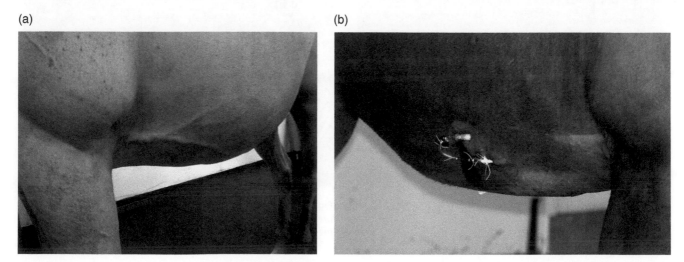

Figure 7.5 Equine left lateral thoracic vein and branches (a); right lateral thoracic venous catheter and short extension set in a horse (b). *Source:* Image courtesy Professor Derek Knottenbelt.

(a)

(b)

(c)

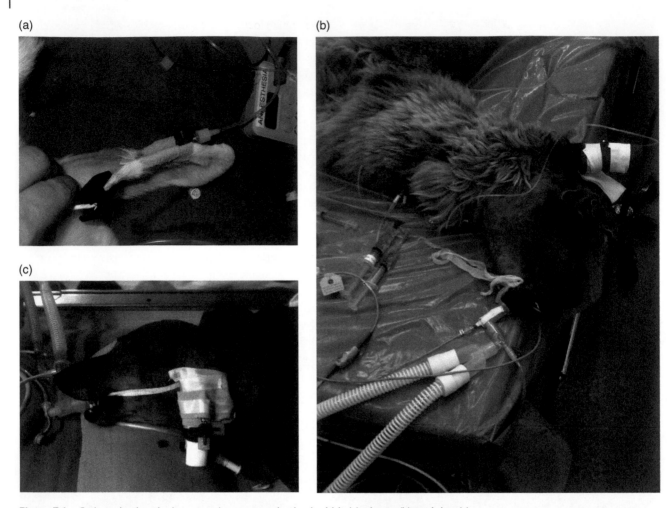

Figure 7.6 Catheterised auricular artery in an anaesthetised rabbit (a), alpaca (b), and dog (c).

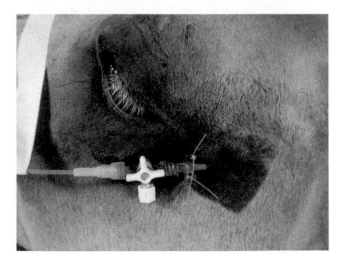

Figure 7.7 Catheterised transverse facial artery in an anaesthetised horse.

- Lingual artery: dogs
- Palmar carpal arch/metacarpal (median) arteries: dogs (Figure 7.9)

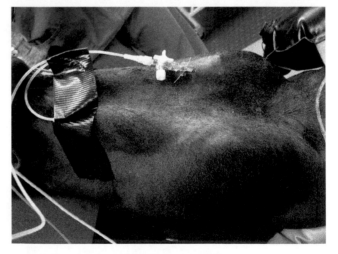

Figure 7.8 Catheterised mandibular artery connected to rigid pressure tubing via a three-way tap for arterial blood pressure measurement in an anaesthetised horse.

- Radial artery: pigs, occasionally other species
- Femoral artery: any species if access safe

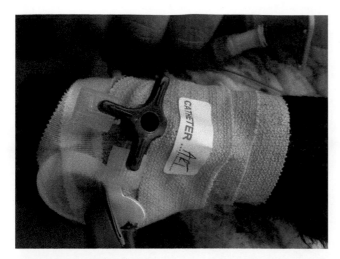

Figure 7.9 Catheterised palmar carpal arch artery in an anaesthetised dog.

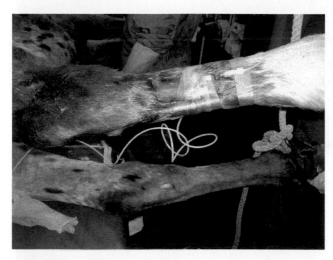

Figure 7.10 Catheterised dorsal/lateral metatarsal artery in an anaesthetised horse.

- Dorsal/lateral metatarsal artery: horses (Figure 7.10), ruminants; this artery is unusual in that there is no vein close by
- Cranial tibial artery (superficial branch): dogs, ±cats
- Dorsal metatarsal (pedal) artery: cats, dogs (Figure 7.11); beware associated vein (Figure 7.12)
- Plantar metatarsal artery (located medially): pigs
- Median (middle) caudal (coccygeal) artery: any tailed species (commonly cats and dogs)

7.3 Complications of Intravascular Catheterisation

There are marked discrepancies in outcomes, definitions, and design among studies investigating intravascular catheter complications. Most studies (human, but particularly

veterinary) focus on thrombophlebitis or catheter colonisation (see Table 7.1) rather than other, more common but less severe, complications. Overall vascular complication rates are reported at between 30 and 50% (cattle up to 100%) with catheter dysfunction rates of 15.8–35.6%. There are no apparent differences in bacterial colonisation rates of peripheral or central venous catheters in cats and dogs, though there may be in humans.

Arterial catheterisation is usually performed in order to allow continuous invasive blood pressure monitoring (see Chapter 18) but also allows the intermittent withdrawal of arterial blood for blood gas analysis (see Chapter 21). Complications are generally similar to those for venous catheters, but arterial catheters should remain in situ for shorter periods, certainly in non-intensive care patients. Generally septic complications are fewer than for venous catheters, but the sequelae may be limb-/appendage-threatening. The most frustrating complication is the misplacement into a vein, as many arteries are paralleled by veins (Figure 7.12).

Complications include:

- Local trauma (following difficult catheterisations, movement, or patient interference)
- Skin irritation/ulceration/erythema, particularly underneath connectors, and local (insertion site) inflammation
  - Cats: erythema 2.6–8.3%
  - Dogs: local inflammation 2.1–42%
  - Cats and dogs: skin irritation 14–22.2%, local inflammation 2.1%, erythema 1%
  - Humans: local erythema/irritation 1.9–2.3%
- Catheter-association pain
  - Humans: catheter-related pain 1.1–14%
- Extravasation of drugs/fluids ± associated periphlebitis/cellulitis/necrosis
  - Dogs: 1.8%
  - Humans: 10–28.1%
- Catheter dysfunction
  - Cats: bacterial colonisation 13–18.4% (any venous), 26% (central venous); mechanical obstruction 2.6–41.7%
  - Cats and dogs: bacterial colonisation 10.7–24.5% (any venous); mechanical obstruction 5.7–36%; malposition 3.7–14.8%
  - Dogs: bacterial colonisation 15.4–48.9% (risk increased by operator inexperience ~184–200%, and steroid administration 60%); mechanical obstruction 0.9–43.9%
  - Horses: bacterial colonisation 7.6–73%
  - Humans: bacterial colonisation 13.4–15.8% (venous) and 0.34–1% (arterial), catheter antimicrobial impregnation reduces risk by 9% (central lines); dislodgement 0.4–6%, (smaller catheter size increases risk);

(a) (b)

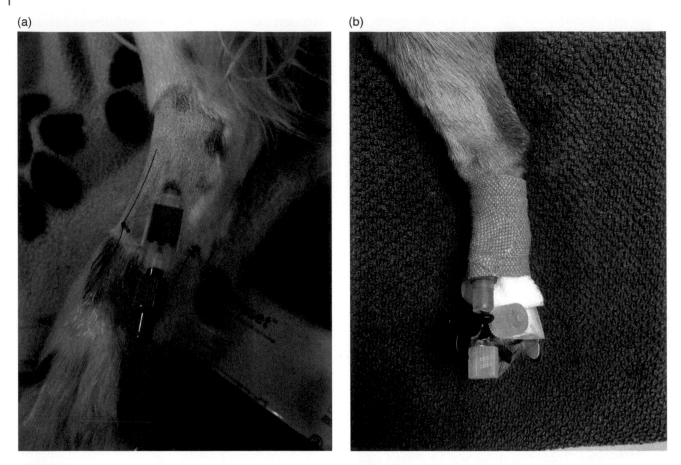

Figure 7.11 Catheterised dorsal metatarsal arteries in anaesthetised dogs using a 20 g arterial catheter with flow switch (a) secured with sutures, and a 22 g vascular catheter connected to a three-way tap (b) secured with tape.

(a) (b)

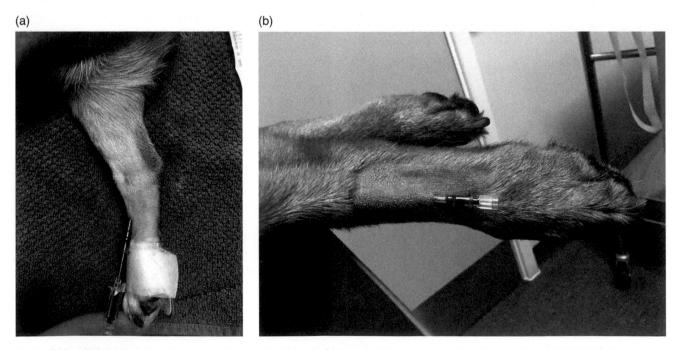

Figure 7.12 Catheterised dorsal metatarsal artery (a) and vein (b) in two different dogs noting the proximity of the artery to the vein. Care must be taken to avoid inadvertent puncture of the incorrect vessel.

Table 7.1 Pathogens associated with bacterial colonisation of catheters in a variety of domestic animal species.

Microbe	Species (proportion of positive cultures)
Acinetobacter species	Dogs (0–21.7%), horses (28.6%)
Achromobacter species	Dogs (1.8%)
Bacillus species	Dogs (2–7.2%)
Bacteroides species	Cats (12.5%)
Brochothrix species	Dogs (0.9%)
Burkholderia species	Dogs (16%)
Corynebacterium species	Dogs (0.9%)
Enterobacter species	Cats (37.5%), dogs (2–41.2%), horses (14.3%)
Enterococcus species	Cats (12.5–50%), dogs (1.8–14.3%), horses (14.3%)
Escherichia coli	Cats (25%), dogs (0–14.3%)
Kelbsiella species	Dogs (4–18%)
Lactobacillus species	Dogs (0.9%)
Micrococcus species	Dogs (5.4%), horses (14.3%)
Moraxella species	Dogs (2.7%)
Mucor species	Horses (14.3%)
Neisseria species	Dogs (0.9%)
Pasteurella species	Dogs (0.9%)
Proteus species	Dogs (2.9–5.4%)
Pseudomonas species	Dogs (2–57.1%), horses (14.3%)
Serratia species	Dogs (2–7.2%)
Staphylococcus species	Cattle, cats, dogs (10–11.8%), horses (14.3%)
Streptococcus species	Cats (12.5–50%), dogs (0.9–2.9%), horses

patient interference/removal 6%; extravasation/ obstruction 47%

- Haemorrhage/exsanguination (e.g. if cap becomes displaced, especially from a retrograde jugular venous catheter or an arterial catheter)
  - Humans: 0–8.7% (arterial)
- Haematoma formation
  - Cats and dogs: bruising 20.5%
  - Humans: haematoma 0–31% (arterial)
- Vessel cording and/or occlusion (thrombosis/embolism/ fibrosis/arterial spasm), may be temporary or permanent
  - Cattle (very limited evidence): thrombosis 20–100%, vessel cording ± pain 10–100%
  - Cats and dogs: arterial occlusion 18.8–22.3%
  - Humans: arterial occlusion 1.5–35% (temporary) and 0.09–0.2% (permanent)

- Phlebitis, thrombosis, and thrombophlebitis (if vein is catheterised) or thromboarteritis (if artery is catheterised)
  - Cats: phlebitis/thrombophlebitis 5.3%
  - Cats and dogs: thrombosis 2%
  - Dogs: phlebitis 10–46% (phlebitis may or may not increase the risk of catheter colonisation)
  - Horses: phlebitis 41%; thrombosis/thrombophlebitis 0.47–29% (lower in elective surgery, higher in colic)
  - Humans: phlebitis/thrombophlebitis 8.2–28.1% (larger catheter size increases risk); deep vein thrombosis 3.4–4.3%
- Infection: catheter-related blood stream infection (CRBSI), septic thrombophlebitis/arteritis or abscessation, local (insertion site) infection
  - Cats and Dogs: CRBSI 0.01–7.1%; local infection 4%; abscessation 1%
  - Dogs: CRBSI 0–10%
  - Humans: CRBSI 0.02–2%, catheter antimicrobial impregnation reduces risk by 2% (central lines); local infection 0–2.6%; arterial abscess 0–0.5%
- Fever
  - Cats: 21.1%
  - Dogs: 7.1%
  - Cats and dogs: 2%
- Embolisation of precipitate (incompatible fluid/drug combinations)
- Embolisation of catheter fragments (material failure [stress fracture], patient interference or poor placement/ removal technique where pieces are sheared off)
- Air embolisation (e.g. if catheterised vein is 'above' the heart; especially if cap becomes displaced from an anterograde jugular catheter with head held in normal position 'above' the heart)
  - Cattle: case reports only (arterial)
  - Cats, dogs, human infants, pigs: case reports only (venous)
  - Horses: 0–2.7% (venous)
  - Human adults: 0–0.2% (arterial)

The following notes focus on the problem of thrombophlebitis; its development, complications, prevention, and treatment options.

7.3.1 Thrombophlebitis

Thrombophlebitis can be associated with increased patient morbidity and mortality.

7.3.1.1 Potential Sequelae of Thrombophlebitis
- Vascular occlusion: limits IV access
- Bilateral jugular occlusion in horses results in congestion of nasal mucosa and, because horses are obligate

nose-breathers, respiratory distress, potentially necessitating emergency tracheostomy
- Endocarditis
- Distant organ thromboembolisation, with subsequent infarction, abscessation, and loss of function; emboli may lodge in pulmonary, coronary, cerebral, renal, mesenteric, or other vascular beds
- Bacteraemia/septicaemia if septic thrombophlebitis

7.3.1.2 Factors Involved in the Development of Aseptic Thrombophlebitis

- Mechanical irritation or trauma to the vessel wall, which triggers inflammatory (e.g. kinin) and coagulation cascades:
  - At the site of venepuncture.
  - At sites of 'contact' between the catheter and the intimal surface of the vessel (anywhere along the length of the catheter, but especially where it penetrates the vessel and at its tip).
  - Rapid infusions under pressure can cause endothelial or intimal injury at the site of impact (increased local turbulence, shearing forces and 'whipping' motion of catheter within vessel).
- Mechanical trauma to the valve leaflets (present in jugular veins) caused by the catheter and/or stylette will incite local inflammation and thrombus formation, as will multiple catheterisation attempts.
- Reaction to the 'foreign material' of the catheter results in the development of a 'fibrin sheath' (due to inherent thrombogenicity of catheter materials, surface properties and irregularities). Longer catheter dwelling times (>5 days) have been associated with an increased risk of thrombophlebitis in cats and dogs.
- Chemical irritation or trauma to the vascular endothelium or intima by the drugs and fluids administered can also cause thrombophlebitis, which is influenced by the characteristics of the drugs (pH, tonicity, temperature, and propensity to precipitate), and speed of delivery (i.e. turbulence of blood flow and potential for dilution).
- Patient factors:
  - Conditions favouring 'Virchow's triad', i.e. the three important factors for thrombus formation: slow blood flow, endothelial damage, and a hypercoagulable state.
    - Systemic inflammatory response syndrome (SIRS), sepsis (e.g. Salmonellosis), endotoxaemia, disseminated intravascular coagulopathy (DIC), hypoproteinaemia (e.g. protein-losing nephropathies and gastroenteropathies), and certain endocrinopathies (e.g. Cushing's disease) may all increase the risk of thrombophlebitis.

- Patients, e.g. certain colics or patients with neoplasia, can present in an early (perhaps covert) stage of DIC and have abnormal clotting profiles; in early DIC, antithrombin III is used up, so the tendency to clot outweighs the tendency to bleed, and catheters tend to clot with thrombophlebitis developing more readily in these patients (which are also the most likely to need prolonged vascular access).
  - Patient movement and interference with the catheter may reduce its 'in-dwelling' time considerably.
  - Small body size and extremes of age increase the likelihood for multiple attempts (risk factor for phlebitis) required for peripheral and central venous (jugular) catheterisation in cats and dogs.

7.3.1.3 Sources of Infection for Septic Thrombophlebitis

- Contamination of the catheter may occur during its insertion; careful aseptic technique is vital.
  - Microorganisms can gain access to the vessel via the breach made in the animal's integument.
  - The cleanliness of the animal's skin and its external environment are extremely important.
  - The cleanliness of the operator's hands is also vitally important.
- Haematogenous 'seeding' of microorganisms into sites of inflammation, thrombosis, or compromised tissue from distant infected foci.
  - Mild bacteraemias are common, but the liver and lungs normally do a good 'filtering' job, however, compromised/inflamed tissues favour bacterial colonisation.
- Contaminated fluids or drugs may be a source of infection, especially if 'home-made' where there is more chance of a breach in sterility during preparation.
  - Reconstituted preparations should be clearly labelled with discard dates/times.
- Patient factors that influence their susceptibility to septic thrombophlebitis include:
  - Malnutrition
  - Immuno-compromise (steroids and stress)
  - Existing infection
  - Coagulation abnormalities (e.g. DIC)

7.3.1.4 Aseptic Technique

The use of aseptic technique cannot be over-emphasised. Asepsis should be maintained during catheter insertion as well as maintenance. The hair should be clipped and a wide area of **skin cleansed, disinfected, and allowed to dry** prior to catheter insertion. Cleansing with a detergent is not advised prior to disinfection unless the skin is grossly contaminated with debris, e.g. mud, blood, saliva. Whilst there is some variation, studies in cattle, dogs, and humans indicate that 2% chlorhexidine in 70% isopropyl alcohol is a superior disinfectant to povidone iodine ± alcohol, or alcohol alone. In some instances, drapes may be necessary to reduce the potential for contamination from surrounding uncleansed skin/fur. Hands should be free of gross contamination, cleansed with an alcohol rub and preferably gloved. For long-stay catheter insertion, gloves should be worn. Where possible a 'no-touch aseptic technique' (Figure 7.13a) should be employed and special care should be taken to **avoid touching the catheter** during insertion.

Once the catheter is in situ, use of an extension set allows a 'stand-off' between the catheter's hub (important site for bacterial contamination, subsequent colonisation and access to subcutaneous tissues and the vessel) and the injection port. Using extension sets also reduces the potential for movement of the catheter within the vein (thus reducing intimal damage), and minimises disturbance at the skin entry site of the catheter, thus reducing further inflammation, bacterial colonisation and invasion. Initial human and horse studies indicate that the use of **70% isopropyl disinfectant catheter adaptor caps**, designed to be fitted over needle-free Luer ports when not in use, reduce the incidence of thrombophlebitis (Figure 7.13b). Further, larger studies are required to confirm these findings.

Some people advocate the use of antimicrobial ointments at the catheter insertion site. It is doubtful whether this helps, especially in the 'normal' horse or ruminant environment. The prophylactic use of systemic antibiotics only appears to enhance bacterial resistance, without precluding the development of infections, and is discouraged. Some people advocate bandaging the site of the catheter hub, using sterile dressings for the first layer. However, patient movement and recumbency still result in movement and displacement of the catheter and bandage, or contamination or wetting of the dressing which then 'wicks' microorganisms more quickly to the 'protected' site. It is, however, good practice to clean any blood away from the catheter insertion site after completion of its insertion, and to inspect the site regularly.

Hands should be cleansed and preferably gloved, before any medications are administered. If disinfectant caps are not used, injection ports should be swabbed with alcohol

(a)   (b)

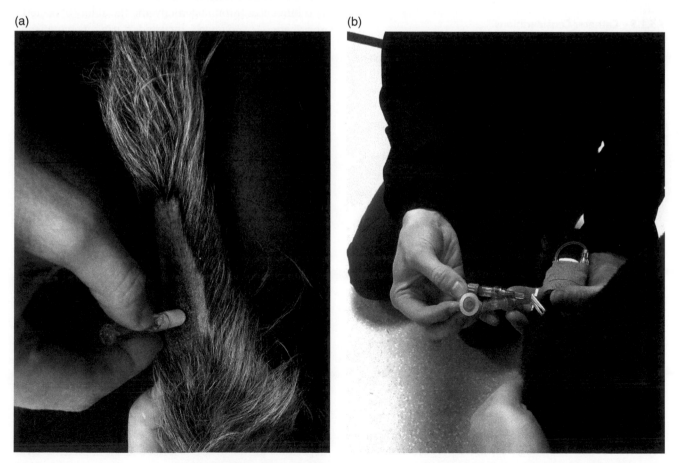

Figure 7.13 'No-touch' aseptic preparation of the skin using 2% chlorhexidine in 70% isopropyl alcohol (a); application of 70% isopropyl alcohol disinfectant catheter adaptor caps to the needle-free Y-extension set (b).

and allowed to dry before injections are made. The catheter and administration set should be treated as a 'closed' system wherever possible. Giving sets should be changed every 24–48 hours, depending upon the infusion, and connection sites swabbed before and after exchange. Disinfectant caps should be replaced once the alcohol impregnated swab dries out, or daily for total parenteral nutrition and lipid solutions.

All drugs and fluids administered should be sterile. (Be careful to maintain sterility if mixing solutions.) Bottle and container tops should be swabbed with alcohol and allowed to dry before withdrawing drugs or fluids.

The catheter insertion site and as much of the vein's superficial course as possible should be inspected daily, and preferably several times a day. At the first sign of catheter dysfunction or local heat/swelling or cording of the vein, the catheter should be withdrawn, taking cultures from the tip. The skin at the catheter entry site should be swabbed with alcohol and allowed to dry before removing the catheter, to reduce contamination of the tip before culture. Blood cultures can also be taken.

7.3.1.5 Catheter Considerations

- Anticipate duration of venous access required
- Catheter material: assess its thrombogenicity, surface properties, and security
- Safety, e.g. safety catheters and needle-free connectors to reduce sharps risks (see later, Figure 7.15a)
- Size (bore, length, and number of lumens) necessary to deliver anticipated medications
- Retrograde ('up', against blood flow) versus anterograde ('down', with blood flow) placement (for jugular veins)
- Placement technique: over-the-needle, through-the-needle, Seldinger (over a wire guide)
- Familiarity with placement technique (potential for venetrauma or contamination)
- Tonicity, pH, 'irritancy', quantity, rate of delivery, and temperature of drugs or fluids to be administered
- Continuous fluid administration or drug infusion versus intermittent dosing
- Presence of radiopaque markers (may dictate insertion site for imaging procedures)
- Antimicrobial impregnation (see below)
- Cost

Catheter impregnation with antiseptics or antibiotics reduced central line CRBSI in humans by 2% and colonisation by 9%. Impregnation had no effect on the risk of catheter related mortality, sepsis, insertion site infection, thrombophlebitis, thrombosis, bleeding, erythema, or pain.

7.3.1.5.1 Catheter Material Thrombogenicity

All catheter materials are thrombogenic, but some are less so than others. The materials are, in decreasing order of thrombogenicity:

- Polypropylene (most thrombogenic)
- Polyethylene
- Teflon (polytetrafluoroethylene)
- Siliconised rubber (silastic)
- Rubber
- Nylon
- Polyvinylchloride (PVC)
- Ethylene acrylic acid
- Polyurethane (least thrombogenic)

7.3.1.5.2 Catheter Softness

Temperature affects the softness of materials, especially plastics. Catheters of different materials, but with comparable softness at body temperature, can have similar thrombogenicities. Softness also affects the ability of the catheter to resist kinking, compression, and collapse.

7.3.1.5.3 Catheter Surface Texture

This influences thrombogenicity and the ability of bacteria to adhere. Any damage incurred during percutaneous placement, such as wrinkling of the tip, or kinking, can provide sites for thrombus formation and bacterial adherence. A small skin incision can be made prior to catheter insertion to reduce the potential for catheter damage, but the larger skin wound also increases the risk of bacterial ingress. Thick-skinned animals may well require a small skin incision and, occasionally, a cut-down may be required. Whether percutaneous insertion or insertion via cut-down is performed, the aim is to minimise tissue trauma and catheter damage.

7.3.1.5.4 Catheter Size

The shorter and narrower (relative to the vein) a catheter is, the less thrombophlebitis it will incite, however, the size chosen may be governed by the drugs and dose rates required to be given. Very short catheters are difficult to maintain within the vessel lumen because they are easily displaced by patient movement. The larger the catheter, relative to the size of the vessel, the greater the potential for vessel wall contact and the development of thrombophlebitis. Contact may occur anywhere along the catheter's length, but always occurs at the tip. Thrombophlebitis occurs locally at the venepuncture site and where the catheter tip touches the vessel wall. Between these sites, fibrin deposition 'grows' over the surface of the catheter to form the 'fibrin sleeve', this process is usually complete within 24 hours. This outer fibrin sheath presents an attractive site for bacterial colonisation. It becomes displaced and may embolise upon catheter removal.

7.3.1.5.5 Catheter Flushing

Fibrin deposition on the inner surface of the catheter is retarded by continual fluid administration, or frequent daily flushing with saline or heparinised saline (to provide a 'heparin lock').

Should heparinised saline be used? The use of heparinised saline for venous and arterial catheter care in humans has been called into question with several meta-analyses finding no benefit of heparinised (1–10 U/ml) saline over normal 0.9% saline in maintaining catheter patency. Similarly, in dogs no difference was found between flushing six-hourly with 10 U/ml heparinised saline or 0.9% saline. If heparinised saline is used, 2 U/ml is generally used for small animals and 5–10 U/ml for large animals.

How frequently should catheters be flushed? By convention, if continual fluid administration is not required, frequent catheter flushing every four to six hours has been advocated in both human and veterinary medicine. A recent, pilot study found that neither frequency of daily flushing (six-hourly versus once-a-day) or volume of 0.9% saline used (3 ml versus 10 ml) impacted catheter failure rates in hospitalised humans. In the absence of robust human or veterinary research, the current recommendation for either continual infusion or four to six hourly flushing remains.

7.3.1.5.6 Catheter Movement

To minimise catheter movement, placement of catheters over bony prominences, or where any part of the catheter is seated at a site of flexion, should be avoided. Once inserted, catheters must be firmly secured to reduce movement within the vein which incites inflammation and thrombosis and significantly contributes to catheter failure rates. The best site to ensure 'security' is at the catheter's hub. Careful security at this position helps to prevent the catheter moving laterally, backwards and forwards (into and out of the vein), 'reversing' out of the skin and vein entirely (especially a problem with short catheters inserted at sites of highly mobile skin), and 'whipping' around inside the vein. Sutures and superglue are invaluable (the stratum corneum is continually shedding, so glue needs to be re-applied every day) for large animals in particular, where circumferential taping is impractical. When securing a catheter with tape, care should be taken to **avoid kinking or bending of the catheter at the insertion site**, immediately below the hub. Tape should be applied to catheters in a neutral position with a preference for close conformity to the catheter hub rather than tight affixing to the limb/appendage. Extension sets reduce handling of the catheter

hub, minimising the potential for disturbance of the catheter seating.

There is no evidence that any one technique or material (or combination of materials) is superior to another for catheter fixation. Whichever technique for catheter fixation and maintenance is chosen, it should minimise catheter movement without impairing the daily evaluation of catheter function and vessel health (Figure 7.14).

7.3.1.5.7 Turbulent Blood Flow

Turbulence promotes catheter contact with the vessel wall and stimulates the formation of thrombophlebitis. Turbulence is greater with relatively large catheters, with rapid drug or fluid administration, and at sites of vessel branching (thus avoid siting the catheter tip at vascular branching sites).

7.3.1.5.8 'Up or Down' the Vein?

It is conceivable that catheters that are placed retrograde create more turbulence and have a greater tendency to 'whip' around inside the vessel, especially during drug or fluid administration. Thus, when intravascular access is required for more than a few hours, it is often advocated to place the catheter anterograde.

7.3.1.5.9 Techniques for Catheter Insertion

Most readers will probably be most familiar with **over-the-needle** catheters, which are sufficient for most situations. An over-the-needle catheter has a sharp stylette, trocar, or needle, which is necessary to penetrate the vein (Figure 7.15). The stylette is used as an introducer over which the catheter is then advanced into the vein. The stylette tip protrudes beyond the catheter tip. Upon insertion into a blood vessel, blood should 'flash back' into the hub of the stylette, but the whole assembly should be advanced a small distance further to ensure that the catheter's tip is also within the vessel; only then, when blood should still be flowing into the stylette hub, should the catheter be advanced from over the stylette into the vessel. Safety catheters have an additional sprung butterfly clip within the catheter hub that deploys over the tip of the stylette once it has been withdrawn from the catheter, reducing the risk of needle-stick injury (Figure 7.15a).

If, during advancement, the catheter does not run smoothly off the stylette into the vein, **never try to re-insert the stylette** into the catheter. Attempting this, risks shearing off the tip of the catheter, which may be carried in the blood stream and lodge in some distant organ such as the lungs, heart, or brain (Figure 7.16).

Through-the-needle catheters may be associated with a greater tendency for periphlebitis or cellulitis to develop, because the needle has a larger bore, and makes a larger hole

(a)

(b)

(d)

(c)

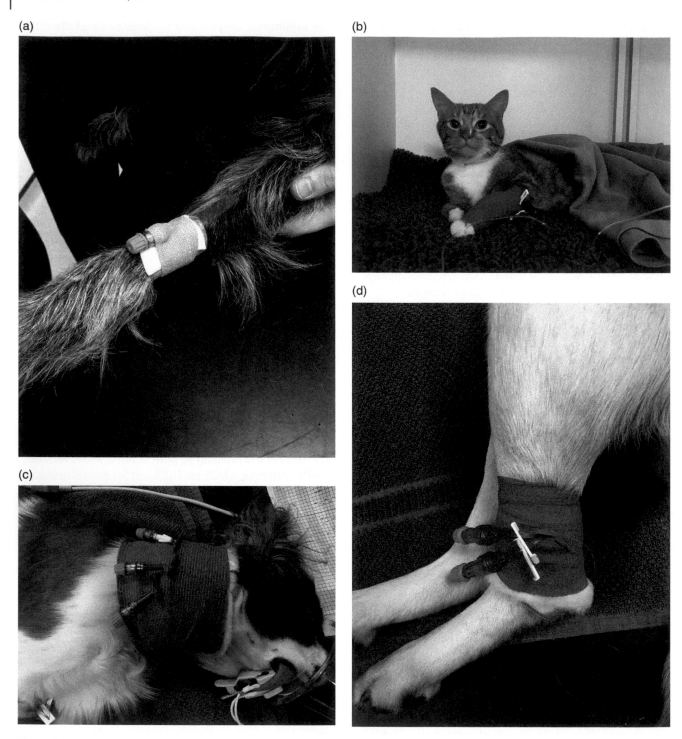

Figure 7.14 Catheter secured using tape with a small swab placed underneath the catheter hub to prevent pressure sores beneath the connection point (a); secured cephalic (b), jugular (c) and lateral saphenous (d) venous catheters wrapped with synthetic, soft bandaging, to prevent pressure sores beneath the connection points and line clamps, and covered with cohesive bandage. This hospital uses red cohesive bandage to indicate that an active intravascular line is below the bandage.

in the vein than the catheter itself, allowing extravascular leakage of blood and injectates. The needle must be retracted from the vessel, but cannot normally be removed from the catheter completely, so it is usually encased in a plastic shield to prevent it from causing damage to the patient or the catheter. A variation on this technique uses a large bore needle to introduce a peel-away sheath through which the catheter is inserted (Figure 7.17a). Finally, the toggles on the

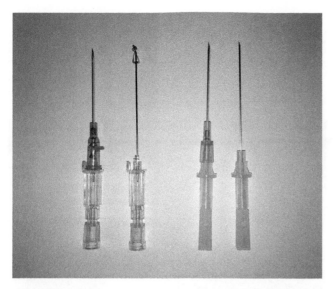

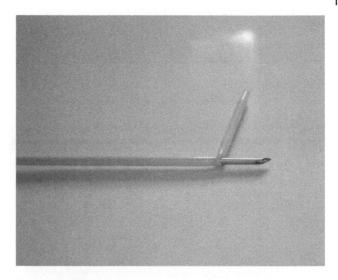

Figure 7.15 Over-the-needle safety catheter (a) and standard catheter (b).

Figure 7.16 Re-advancing the stylette may damage the catheter tip, which may subsequently shear off within the animal's blood vessel and embolise.

peel-away sheath are pulled to split the sheath so that it can be removed from the vessel (Figure 7.17b).

The **Seldinger technique** requires initial vascular access with a stout needle or temporary over-the-needle catheter, through which a flexible wire is then threaded (Figure 7.18 shows a Seldinger-type catheter kit). After completely withdrawing the needle (over the wire), a dilator is passed over the wire and twizzled to dilate the skin and vein entry sites to ensure easy passage of the soft, flexible catheter, so that it can pass through the skin and into the vein with minimal force or damage. After the dilator is withdrawn, the catheter is then introduced over the smaller diameter guidewire, before the wire is finally

removed and the catheter is secured in place. This technique can be very useful where small veins are difficult to access, or where central venous access is necessary (requiring long catheters). To avoid air entrainment, the vessel should be 'raised' (passive filling enabled by proximal occlusion) continuously until the catheter is correctly seated within the vessel. When using the Seldinger technique to place jugular catheters in small animals, the electrocardiogram (ECG) should be monitored to alert the operator to inadvertent contact of the myocardium with the introducer wire. Inadvertent myocardial contact with the metal wire generally produces ventricular premature complexes.

(a)

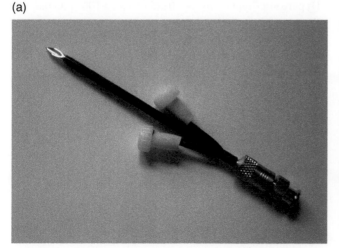

(b)

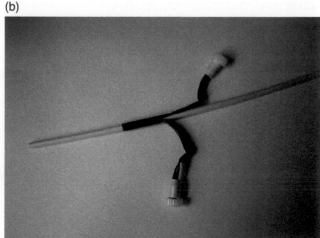

Figure 7.17 (a) Peel-away sheath over needle. The sheath is first inserted along with the needle, in the same way as an over-the-needle catheter is inserted. After the needle is withdrawn, the catheter is then inserted through the sheath which is finally peeled into two halves and removed from the vessel to leave only the catheter behind (b).

(a)

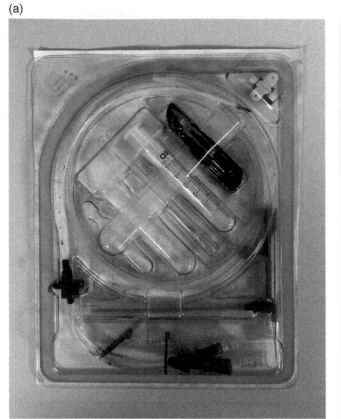

(b)

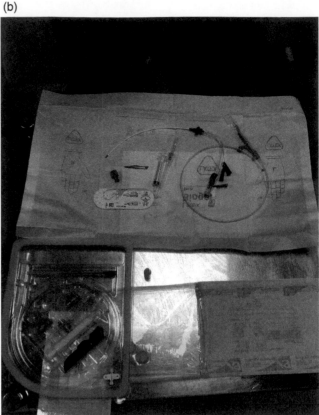

Figure 7.18 The components required for insertion of a catheter over a flexible guidewire: a scalpel blade, introducer needle (or over-the-needle catheter), the wire, a dilator, the catheter and short extension tube with injection caps which may be swapped for needle-free connectors. The wire is contained within a plastic casing to help control it and to prevent it from becoming contaminated during insertion. For catheters with a 'J' tip, the tip is retracted into the casing before the wire can be advanced through the needle. A 'J' tip prevents the wire from entering small vascular branches, however, it can sometimes cause problems during wire advancement such that this author may occasionally 'reverse' the wire direction so that a straight tip is advanced into the vein.

The reader is referred elsewhere for information regarding pulmonary arterial catheters, implantable vascular access ports and intra-osseous needles.

Familiarity with insertion technique and **operator experience** reduce the risk of infection in dogs and humans, probably due to a combination of better decision making for catheter siting and fewer catheterisation attempts with less vascular trauma. Attention to aseptic technique is of paramount importance.

7.3.1.5.10 Drug/Fluid Administration

Many drugs have acidic or alkaline pH (Table 7.2), are of unphysiological tonicity or osmolality, or may precipitate once in the blood. All of these factors may contribute to the 'irritation' caused to vascular endothelium. The speed of administration also affects local blood flow, may create turbulence and affects the dilution of the drug within the bloodstream.

Guaiphenesin (guaifenesin) is renowned for its ability to cause haemolysis, endothelial injury and thrombosis,

possibly following *in vivo* crystallisation. Sulpha drugs and tetracyclines are also well known for their tissue irritancy. Hypertonic/hyperosmotic fluids (e.g. >10% glucose and those used for parenteral nutrition), should always be administered by a large, preferably 'central', vein to minimise adverse effects by maximising the potential for dilution.

Table 7.2 Drug pH values.

Drug	pH
Normal (0.9%) saline	5–6.1
Hartmann's solution	6.4
Dextrose 5% solution	4.5
Phenylbutazone	8.8
Vitamin B complex	4
Ketamine	3.5–5.5
Thiopental	10.5

7.3.1.5.11 Aftercare

Prevention of complications requires consideration of all the above factors. Careful aseptic technique must be continued into the period of aftercare of the catheter. Aftercare must also include a heightened awareness of the potential for the development of thrombophlebitis, and thus the catheter site and vein must be carefully inspected at least daily (preferably at least four times daily), and the patient must be evaluated for signs of complications, such as pain, fever spikes, or depression.

Idle catheters (no use/flush for ≥24 hours) should be removed. Catheters that cause the patient pain when used/ flushed or inspected should also be removed.

7.3.1.6 Clinical Signs of Aseptic Thrombophlebitis

- Pain during administration of fluids/drugs through the catheter
- Swelling or induration along the vessel
- Abnormal filling or emptying of the vessel
- Thickening or 'cording' of the vein
- Stiff neck (if jugular vein)
- Swollen head if both jugular veins affected in horses (beware nasal oedema and respiratory obstruction in horses which are obligate nose-breathers)
- Typical ultrasonographic changes: irregular, hyperechoic, or mixed echogenic luminal mass

7.3.1.7 Clinical Signs of Septic Thrombophlebitis

Are the same as those for aseptic thrombophlebitis, but also include:

- Pain around the catheterisation site ± along the vessel
- Heat, swelling, erythema, oedema around the catheterisation site ± along the vessel
- Unexplained fever
- Depression

Note that septicaemia can develop in the absence of obvious signs of problems in the catheterised vein.

Ultrasonographic evaluation of affected veins may help to determine the extent of vessel obstruction or patency, and whether there is pocketing of infection. Ultrasound-guided aspiration is also possible if focal accumulations of non-flowing suppuration are observed. Such samples, collected aseptically, can then be submitted for laboratory evaluation.

7.3.1.8 Treatment Options

- Remove the catheter as soon as any problems are detected, and re-establish venous access in another, distant vein, if required. Avoid placing subsequent catheters in the same vessel as where the compromised catheter was. Remember to take swabs from the catheter tip, and preferably blood cultures from blood samples drawn aseptically from a distant site.
- Treat any underlying diseases.
- Topical hot packs and/or cold compresses.
- Topical anti-inflammatories such as dimethyl sulfoxide (DMSO), non-steroidal anti-inflammatory drugs (NSAIDs), possibly steroids.
- Topical antimicrobials.
- Topical nitroglycerine cream (vasodilator).
- Systemic anti-inflammatories (NSAIDs).
- Systemic antimicrobials.
- Excise any necrotic tissue and lance abscesses.
- Consider tetanus prophylaxis.

7.3.2 Air Emboli

Venous air emboli are more common, but **arterial** emboli can also occur (e.g. during flushing or laparoscopy). The lethal volume for air entrainment in rabbits was found to be 0.5–0.75 ml/kg versus 7.5–15 ml/kg in dogs. Horses can tolerate up to 0.25 ml/kg air being entrained before showing clinical signs, but the rate of entrainment is also important, with more than 0.5 ml/kg/min causing trouble. In dogs, up to 2–15 ml/kg gas (air, oxygen, or carbon dioxide) have been injected experimentally, and the clinical signs were volume-, rate-, and gas-dependent; rates over 0.69 ml/kg/min (air), were lethal, and over 0.75–1.5 ml/kg/min (oxygen), were problematic. Highlighting the impact of rate: 500 ml air injected rapidly caused clinical signs in horses whilst slow injection (over several hours) of 1400 ml in dogs was tolerated. Carbon dioxide is a very soluble gas, so causes the least trouble; nitrogen can be more problematic than oxygen.

7.3.2.1 Clinical Signs

If the patient is awake:

- Confusion, disorientation, agitation, or panic
- Muscle fasciculations
- 'Colicky' behaviour
- Blindness (may be delayed)
- Paresis
- Pruritus
- Dyspnoea
- Seizures (may be delayed)
- Sudden death

If the patient is anaesthetised:

- Decreased end-tidal carbon dioxide tension
- Decreased S_pO_2 (pulse oximetry: arterial haemoglobin oxygen saturation value)
- Decreased systemic arterial blood pressure
- Increased heart rate

- Possibly arrhythmias
- Possibly millwheel murmur
- Possibly pulmonary hypertension/oedema
- Possibly cardiopulmonary arrest

7.3.2.2 Treatment

Turn off any N_2O, as this will make any bubbles bigger. Stop intravascular injection/infusion whilst ascertaining the cause. Stop pneumatic drill use. If a venous 'hole' is the cause, reposition the patient so that the hole is below heart level, if possible; put pressure (a finger) on or occlude the site of the hole, or flood the site with sterile saline. Commence rapid intravenous fluids to increase the central venous pressure (CVP); and if the patient is under general anaesthesia, commence positive pressure ventilation ± positive end expiratory pressure if tolerated (these manoeuvres also increase CVP, which helps to put back-pressure on the 'open' vein to slow further entrainment of air). Chest compressions may be required to dislodge air from the right atrium if sufficient air was entrained to form an air-lock; or ultrasound-guided aspiration of air from cardiac chambers can be attempted. Following recovery from the acute episode, further symptomatic treatment may be required (e.g. corticosteroids, furosemide, and bronchodilators if pulmonary oedema develops; analgesia).

For further notes on central venous catheterisation, see Chapter 18 on monitoring.

Further Reading

Alexandrou, E., Ray-Barruel, G., Carr, P.J. et al. (2018). Use of short peripheral intravenous catheters: characteristics, management, and outcomes worldwide. *Journal of Hospital Medicine* https://doi.org/10.12788/jhm.3039.

Ashby, J. (2017). Peripheral intravenous catheter care in hospitalised cats and dogs. *Veterinary Nursing Journal* 32: 32–36.

Barr, E.D., Clegg, P.D., Senior, J.M., and Singer, E.R. (2005). Destructive lesions of the proximal sesamoid bones as a complication of dorsal metatarsal artery catheterization in three horses. *Veterinary Surgery* 34: 159–166.

Bradbury, L.A., Archer, D.C., Dugdale, A.H. et al. (2005). Suspected venous air embolism in a horse. *The Veterinary Record* 156: 109–111.

Calviño Günther, S., Sxhwebel, C., Hamidfar-Roy, R. et al. (2016). Complications of intravascular catheters in ICU: definitions, incidence and severity. A randomized controlled trial comparing usual transparent dressings versus new-generation dressings (the ADVANCED study). *Intensive Care Medicine* 42: 1753–1765.

Carr, P.J., Rippey, J.C.R., Cooke, M.L. et al. (2018). From insertion to removal: a multicenter survival analysis of an admitted cohort with peripheral intravenous catheters inserted in the emergency department. *Infection Control and Hospital Epidemiology* 39: 1216–1221.

Chanchaithong, P. and Ritthikulprasert, S. (2018). Prevalence of bacteremia in dogs admitted to an intensive care unit with intravenous catheterization. *Thai Journal of Veterinary Medicine* 48: 616–618.

Dolente, B.A., Beech, J., Lindborg, S., and Smith, G. (2005). Evaluation of risk factors for development of catheter-associated jugular thrombophlebitis in horses: 50 cases (1993–1998). *Journal of the American Veterinary Medical Association* 227: 1134–1141.

Dorey-Phillips, C.L. and Murison, P.J. (2008). Comparison of two techniques for intravenous catheter site preparation in dogs. *Veterinary Record* 162: 280–281.

Farrow, H.A., Rand, J.S., Burgess, D.M. et al. (2013). Jugular vascular access port implantation for frequent, long-term blood sampling in cats: methodology, assessment, and comparison with jugular catheters. *Research in Veterinary Science* 95: 681–686. (***For information on vascular access ports.***).

Fisk, N. (2018). A comparative study of disinfecting catheter caps and their effectiveness in the reduction of equine IV catheter related thrombophlebitis. *Veterinary Nursing Journal* 33: 74–78.

Geraghty, T.E., Love, S., Taylor, D.J. et al. (2009). Assessment of subclinical venous catheter-related diseases in horses and associated risk factors. *Veterinary Record* 164: 227–231.

Guzmán Ramos, P.J., Fernández Pérez, C., Ayllón Santiago, T. et al. (2018). Incidence of and associated factors for bacterial colonization of intravenous catheters removed from dogs in response to clinical complications. *Journal of Veterinary Internal Medicine* 32: 1084–1091.

Hay, C.W. (1992). Equine intravenous catheterization. *Equine Veterinary Education* 4: 319–323.

Jones, I.D., Case, A.M., Boag, S.A., and Rycroft, A.N. (2009). Factors contributing to the contamination of peripheral intravenous catheters in dogs and cats. *Veterinary Record* 164: 616–618.

Keogh, S., Flynn, J., Marsh, N. et al. (2016). Varied flushing frequency and volume to prevent peripheral intravenous catheter failure: a pilot, factorial randomized controlled trial in adult medical-surgical hospital patients. *Trials* 17: 348–357.

Lai, N.M., Chaiyakunapruk, N., Lai, N.A. et al. (2016). Catheter impregnation, coating or bonding for reducing central venous catheter-related infections in adults. *Cochrane Database of Systematic Reviews* (3): CD007878. https://doi.org/10.1002/14651858.CD007878.pub3.

Lankveld, D.P.K., Ensink, J.M., van Dijk, P., and Klein, W.R. (2001). Factors influencing the occurrence of thrombophlebitis after post–surgical long–term intravenous catheterization of colic horses: a study of 38 cases. *Journal of Veterinary Medicine A* 48: 545–552.

Levinson, A.T., Chapin, K.C., LeBlanc, L., and Mermel, L.A. (2018). Peripheral arterial catheter colonization in cardiac surgical patients. *Infection Control and Hospital Epidemiology* 39: 1008–1009.

Marsh, N., Webster, J., Mihala, G., and Rickard, C.M. (2015). Devices and dressings to secure peripheral venous catheters to prevent complications. *Cochrane Database of Systematic Reviews* 6: CD011070.

Marsh-Ng, M.L., Burney, D.P., and Garcia, J. (2007). Surveillance of infections associated with intravenous catheters in dogs and cats in an intensive care unit. *Journal of the American Animal Hospital Association* 43: 13–20.

Mooshian, S., Dietschel, S.L., Haggerty, J.M., and Guenther, C.L. (2019). Incidence of arterial catheter complications: a retrospective study of 35 cats (2010–2014). *Journal of Feline Medicine and Surgery* 21: 173–177.

Palkar, V., Patel, V., Jacob, C. et al. (2016). The impact of disinfectant cap implementation on central line-associated bloodstream infections. *Infec vtious Diseases* 48: 646–648.

Parkinson, N.J., McKenzie, H.C., Barton, M.H. et al. (2018). Catheter-associated venous air embolism in hospitalized horses: 32 cases. *Journal of Veterinary Internal Medicine* 32: 805–814.

Pusterla, N. and Braun, U. (1996). Prophylaxis of intravenous catheter-related thrombophlebitis in cattle. *Veterinary Record* 139: 287–289.

Rajaram, S.S., Desai, N.K., Kalra, A. et al. (2013). Pulmonary artery catheters for adult patients in intensive care. *Cochrane Database of Systematic Reviews* (2): CD003408. https://doi.org/10.1002/14651858.CD003408.pub3 *(For information on the risk:benefit of pulmonary artery catheters.)*.

Randolph, A.G., Cook, D.J., Gonzales, C.A., and Andrew, M. (1998). Benefit of heparin in peripheral venous and arterial catheters: systematic review and meta-analysis of randomized controlled trials. *British Medical Journal* 316: 9969–9975.

Reminga, C.L., Silverstein, D.C., and Drobatz, K.J. (2018). Evaluation of the placement and maintenance of central venous jugular catheters in critically ill dogs and cats. *Journal of Veterinary Emergency and Critical Care* 28: 232–243.

Scheer, B.V., Perel, A., and Pfeiffer, U.J. (2002). Clinical review: complications and risk factors of peripheral arterial catheters used for haemodynamic monitoring in anaesthesia and intensive care medicine. *Critical Care* 6: 198–204.

Seguela, J. and Pages, J.-P. (2011). Bacterial and fungal colonisation of peripheral intravenous catheters in dogs and cats. *Journal of Small Animal Practice* 52: 531–535.

Shah, P.S. and Shah, N. (2014). Heparin-bonded catheters for prolonging the patency of central venous catheters in children. *Cochrane Database of Systematic Reviews* (4): CD005983. https://doi.org/10.1002/14651858.CD005983.pub3.

Silver, H., Webster, K., Barlow, J., Sharman, M., and Alliso, A. (2017). Preliminary findings of an investigation into the efficacy of heparinised saline solution versus normal saline solution for maintaining patency of peripheral intravenous catheters in dogs. BSAVA Congress Proceedings, 519–520.

Spurlock, S.L. and Spurlock, G.H. (1990). Risk factors of catheter-related complications. Compendium on continuing education for the Practising. *The Veterinarian* 12: 241–248.

Tan, R.H.H., Dart, A.J., and Dowling, B.A. (2003). Catheters: a review of the selection, utilization and complications of catheters for peripheral venous access. *Australian Veterinary Journal* 81: 136–139.

Trim, C.M., Hofmeister, E.H., Quandt, J.E., and Shepard, M.K. (2017). A survey of the use of arterial catheters in anesthetized dogs and cats: 267 cases. *Journal of Veterinary Emergency and Critical Care* 27: 89–95.

Ueda, Y., Odunayo, A., and Mann, F.A. (2013). Comparison of heparinized saline and 0.9% sodium chloride for maintaining peripheral intravenous catheter patency in dogs. *Journal of Veterinary Emergency and Critical Care* 23: 517–522.

Unbeck, M., Förberg, U., Ygge, B.-M. et al. (2015). Peripheral venous catheter related complications are common among paediatric and neonatal patients. *Acta Paediatrica* 104: 566–574.

Webster, J., Osborne, S., Rickard, C.M., and Marsh, N. (2019). Clinically-indicated replacement versus routine replacement of peripheral venous catheters. *Cochrane Database of Systematic Reviews* (1): CD007798. https://doi.org/10.1002/1465185.CD007798.pub5.

White, R. (2002). Vascular access techniques in the dog and cat. *In Practice* 24: 174–192. (*Also includes notes on implantable vascular access ports and intraosseous needles.*).

Self-test Section

1 When considering the thrombogenicity of catheters, put the following catheter materials in order, from **most** thrombogenic **to least** thrombogenic:
   - Teflon
   - Polyurethane
   - Polyethylene
   - Nylon

2 What is the most important factor in minimising the risk of catheter related infection?

3 True or False? To reduce the risk of premature failure, catheters should **not** be placed in areas of flexion.

8

Inhalation Anaesthetic Agents

LEARNING OBJECTIVES

- To be able to discuss the basic pharmacology of the inhalation agents.
- To be able to list the properties of an ideal inhalation agent.
- To be able to define MAC.
- To be able to discuss the factors affecting agent choice.

8.1 Introduction

Inhalation agents, commonly volatile liquids or compressed gases (most are technically 'vapours'), can be administered by inhalation, for induction and/or maintenance of anaesthesia. Although all their actions remain to be determined, it appears that most enhance inhibitory activity at $GABA_A$ receptors (in the brain) and glycine receptors (in the spinal cord), whilst also possibly inhibiting excitatory effects at cholinergic (muscarinic and nicotinic) and glutamate receptors. The volatile agents also depress activity at various types of calcium channels; and may inhibit some types of sodium and potassium channel activities. See Chapter 1 for a brief overview of the mechanisms of anaesthesia.

8.2 Properties of an Ideal Inhalation Agent

- Easily vaporised at or near room temperature
- Non-flammable/non-explosive
- Stable on storage (not degraded by heat or light)
- Does not react with materials of anaesthetic breathing system or vaporiser
- Does not readily diffuse through materials of anaesthetic breathing system to pollute the operating environment
- Compatible with carbon dioxide absorbent
- Environmentally friendly; easily scavenged
- Non-irritant to mucous membranes; non-pungent, so that inhalation induction is not unpleasant
- Induction of anaesthesia and recovery from anaesthesia should be excitement-free
- Allows rapid control of anaesthetic depth (low blood solubility)
- Few cardiorespiratory side-effects
- Some analgesia would be an advantage
- Some muscle relaxation would be an advantage
- No renal, hepatic, lung, central nervous system (CNS), or other body tissue toxicity
- Minimally metabolised; any metabolites should be non-toxic and inactive
- Inexpensive
- Not requiring expensive vaporiser

Table 8.1 gives some physicochemical properties of inhalation agents for humans. For comparison, the blood/gas partition coefficient for nitrogen (N_2) is 0.0147. There are species differences, e.g. for the horse, the blood/gas

Table 8.1 Some properties of actual inhalation agents (based upon humans).

Agent	B·Pt °C	SVP(mmHg)	MWt	B/G	O/G	F/B	MAC (%)	Metab.
Desflurane	23.5	664	168	0.45	18.7	27	5.7 +	0.02%
Halothane	50.2	243	197	2.4	224	60	0.8	c. 20%
Isoflurane	48.5	238	184	1.4	98	45	1.3–1.6	0.2%
Nitrous oxide	−89	44 atm (cylinder pressure)	44	0.44–0.47	20	2.3	100–200	Inert
Sevoflurane	58.5	170	200	0.65	45	48	2.05 +	c. 2%
Methoxyflurane	104.7	23	165	13	825	495	0.16	20–80%
Xenon	−108.1	N/A	131	0.115	1.9	<10	60–71	Inert

Values may vary slightly, depending upon source.
B.Pt., boiling point at standard atmospheric pressure; SVP, saturated vapour pressure at 20 °C (except N_2O); MWt, molecular weight; B/G, blood/gas partition coefficient; O/G, oil/gas partition coefficient; F/B, fat/blood partition coefficient; Metab., metabolism; atm, atmospheres.

partition coefficients for halothane (no longer has UK marketing authorisation), isoflurane, and sevoflurane are 1.66, 0.92, and 0.46, respectively.

8.3 MAC

MAC (or *MAC-incision*) is defined as the minimum (originally, 'minimal') alveolar concentration of anaesthetic agent at which 50% of patients fail to respond, by gross purposeful movement (i.e. a motor response), to a standard supramaximal noxious stimulus (skin incision). It is defined in terms of percentage of 1 (standard) atmosphere pressure (be aware of altitude) and is analogous to a median effective dose 50% (ED_{50}) for immobility.

MAC values allow a comparison of inhalation agents by their potency, whereby potency is inversely proportional to the MAC value. Potency is directly proportional to the brain lipid solubility of the agents, which is reflected by the oil-gas partition coefficient. Table 8.2 shows MAC values for the commonly used inhalation agents in man and some of the domestic animal species.

As a basic rule of thumb, if a patient has an **end tidal anaesthetic agent concentration of 1.2–1.5 × MAC**, it is **highly unlikely to move at skin incision** (where that inhalation agent is the sole anaesthetic drug administered).

Several different MAC values are described for humans, such as MAC_{BAR} (where BAR means Blockade of Autonomic Response), which refers to the minimum alveolar concentration of inhalation agent at which the increase in heart rate and/or blood pressure provoked by skin incision is prevented in 50% of subjects. MAC_{BAR} is usually around 1–1.7 × $MAC_{incision}$. $MAC_{intubation}$ is the minimum alveolar concentration of inhalant that would inhibit movement and coughing during endotracheal intubation.

There is also MAC_{awake} (usually 0.3–0.5 × $MAC_{incision}$), which refers to the minimum alveolar concentration of agent at which 50% of subjects stop voluntarily responding to verbal commands (i.e. cessation of perceptive awareness) during induction of anaesthesia with that agent, or when 50% of subjects begin responding to verbal commands upon recovery from anaesthesia under that agent. For people, these various MAC values differ in the order: $MAC_{BAR} > MAC_{intubation} > MAC_{incision} > MAC_{awake}$.

Table 8.2 Some MAC values.

Species	Halothane	Isoflurane	Sevoflurane	Desflurane	Nitrous oxide
Human	0.76%	1.2%	1.93%	6.99%	105%
Dog	0.87%	1.3%	2.3%	7.2%	188–297%
Cat	1.1%	1.6%	2.6%	9.8%	255%
Horse	0.9%	1.3%	2.3%	7.6%	190–205%

Values may vary slightly, depending upon source.

For amphibious, laboratory, and other 'exotic' animals, the anaesthetic concentration required for loss of the righting reflex in 50% of the population has been advocated as a more appropriate end point for assessing clinically relevant anaesthetic potency, rather than MAC. This is particularly important in non-mammalian species (e.g. anurans) where the induction of anaesthesia may take many hours (compared to minutes, e.g. in dogs), despite a similar MAC. It is important to remember that the required concentration for loss of the righting reflex is probably more similar to MAC$_{awake}$ than MAC$_{incision}$, and is likely to be less than the concentration required for surgical procedures (i.e. noxious stimulation).

For birds, minimum *alveolar* concentration is re-defined as minimum *anaesthetic* concentration, as avian lungs contain air capillaries rather than alveoli.

8.3.1 MAC Is Not Affected by

- Duration of anaesthesia (unless patient becomes hypothermic, hypoxaemic, or hypercapnic)
- Gender
- Blood pH
- P_aCO_2 between 10 and 90 mmHg
- P_aO_2 between 40 and 500 mmHg
- Moderate anaemia
- Moderate hypotension (mean arterial pressure not below 50 mmHg)
- Hypertension

8.3.2 MAC Is Affected by

- Species (body size, i.e. MAC increases as the relative body surface area increases)
- Age: MAC is lower in the very young (neonates) and very old (geriatrics), but higher in young, growing, and fit animals
- $P_aO_2 < 40$ mmHg (profound arterial hypoxaemia), and $P_aCO_2 > 90$ mmHg (severe hypercapnia); both decrease MAC
- Hypotension (mean arterial pressure < 50 mmHg) decreases MAC
- Change in body temperature (for every 1 °C change in body temperature, MAC changes by 2–5% of its normothermic value; it decreases with hypothermia, and increases with hyperthermia; due to changes in basal metabolic rate and anaesthetic agent solubility)
- CNS depressant drugs (and some intracranial diseases) will reduce MAC
- CNS stimulant drugs will increase MAC

- Hyperthyroidism, and high levels of circulating catecholamines (excited or nervous animals; phaeochromocytoma) will increase MAC
- Pregnancy reduces MAC
- Hypernatraemia and hyperosmolality increase MAC
- Altitude: MAC increases with altitude (because it is expressed in terms of % of standard atmospheric pressure)

There is **controversy** about the MAC concept because the definition of *MAC* is highly dependent upon spinal reflex activity and spinal sites of action of anaesthetic agents. For this reason, claims that drugs have analgesic properties because they can cause MAC reduction, may not be valid.

8.4 Administration of Inhalation Agents

Inhalation agents may be administered for induction and/or maintenance of anaesthesia. Administration may be via:

- Face/nose mask
- Nasopharyngeal tube (insufflation)
- Nasotracheal tube
- Orotracheal tube (see Chapter 9 for potential problems associated with endotracheal tube use)
- Supra-glottic airway device
- Induction chambers: can be used for anaesthetic induction, but do not allow access to the patient
- (Intravenous injection of emulsified volatile anaesthetics [see Chapter 5])

8.4.1 Inhalation Induction

Inhalation induction may be accomplished by:

- Step-wise method, starting with just oxygen, and then slowly increasing the delivered inspired anaesthetic agent concentration, e.g. by a quarter to half a per cent every three or four breaths
- Delivering a high inspired concentration of anaesthetic agent from the outset (often called a 'crash induction')

Induction is said to be smoother if the first method is used; but induction is faster with the second. Most patients, especially if not premedicated, seem to traverse the 'involuntary movement/excitement stage' (Stage II) of anaesthesia as depth of anaesthesia increases towards a deeper, more surgical, plane, so be prepared for some 'struggling'. This period of struggling should be shorter when a high concentration is delivered from the outset. Inclusion of nitrous oxide may also speed the rate of induction through the second gas effect (see later).

8.5 Uptake and Elimination of Anaesthetic Agents

Inhalation agents produce anaesthesia via their effects in the CNS. **Depth of anaesthesia depends upon the concentration of the agent in the brain**. A better term than *concentration* would be *partial pressure* or *tension* because these agents are in the gas phase, and so their 'concentration' is usually measured in units of pressure.

When a patient breathes a mixture of oxygen and anaesthetic gas/vapour from a non-rebreathing system (so that each inhaled breath has the same composition), then the partial pressures of the agent in the alveoli, blood, and tissues (including brain) increase over time towards those of the inspired mixture.

Rate of induction (and recovery) **from inhalation anaesthesia is governed by the rate of change of anaesthetic agent partial pressure in the brain**. *Brain partial pressure of anaesthetic agent follows, with a slight delay, the change in its partial pressure in the alveoli.*

We cannot measure the 'brain concentration' of these agents, but we can measure the alveolar tension, or, at least the end tidal anaesthetic agent concentration, which is a surrogate measure for alveolar anaesthetic agent concentration (see Chapter 18 on monitoring).

Let us now consider the factors which affect the rate of change of the alveolar tension of anaesthetic agents, and therefore the uptake and elimination of these agents. **Kety curves** can be constructed, which are mathematical descriptions of anaesthetic uptake under defined conditions (Figure 8.1).

8.5.1 Factors Affecting Alveolar Anaesthetic Agent Uptake/Induction of Anaesthesia

- Inspired anaesthetic agent concentration
- Loss of agent (e.g. via diffusion through anaesthetic breathing system)
- Alveolar ventilation rate (and lung functional residual capacity, FRC)
- Uptake by blood and tissues

8.5.1.1 Inspired Anaesthetic Concentration

The deliverable inspired anaesthetic agent concentration depends upon the **volatility of the agent**, that is, its **boiling point** compared to room temperature. Its SVP at room or standard temperature will give you a clue about its volatility, e.g. at 20 °C, desflurane is very volatile (SVP = 700 mmHg, cf. standard atmospheric pressure of 760 mmHg), sevoflurane is much less volatile (SVP = 160 mmHg). The temperature at which the SVP equals atmospheric pressure is the agent's boiling point.

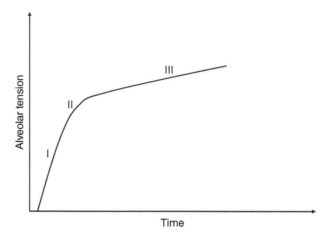

Figure 8.1 Kety curve. I is the initial rise: represents anaesthetic agent delivery to the lungs with alveolar ventilation. The gradient will be steeper with increased alveolar ventilation (for the same inspired concentration); II is the knee: represents initial equilibration between anaesthetic agent delivery to the alveoli by ventilation and removal of anaesthetic agent from the alveoli by pulmonary capillary blood flow; III is the slowly rising plateau: may also be represented by a series of knees and changing gradients, represents equilibration between other tissues, blood, and alveolar concentrations.

Increasing the **vaporiser setting** should increase anaesthetic agent delivery to the anaesthetic breathing system, and thereby to the alveoli, to hasten induction of anaesthesia. One utilisation of the **concentration effect** (see below), is called the **over-pressure technique**, when much more anaesthetic agent than is really required is initially delivered to the patient, to hasten anaesthetic induction. The vaporiser setting is then turned down as soon as the patient has achieved the desired level of anaesthesia to avoid an excessive depth of anaesthesia being reached.

The **design of the vaporiser** may also have some influence upon the achievable inspired anaesthetic agent concentration, e.g.:

- Temperature changes affect vaporisation, so temperature compensated (e.g. **Tec™**) vaporisers will give a more consistent output.
- Incorporation of wicks to increase the surface area for evaporation helps to increase the delivered anaesthetic agent concentration, as may increasing the operating temperature of the vaporiser. Thymol (a poorly volatile 'stabiliser' included with halothane) may affect vaporiser performance by clogging up wicks etc.
- Some vaporisers may be calibrated to deliver higher concentrations of agent than others. Most halothane and isoflurane vaporisers have a maximum calibrated output concentration of 5%, whereas others have a maximum output of 8%.

The inspired anaesthetic agent concentration cannot, however, be indefinitely increased because sufficient oxygen (usually a minimum of 33% is suggested for humans) must also be supplied to the patient.

If a circle (rebreathing) system is being used with the vaporiser out-of-circle (**VOC**), then, at the beginning of an anaesthetic, increasing the fresh gas flow into the circle will help to maintain the inspired anaesthetic agent concentration better (especially for agents which are highly soluble in the blood). It is common practice to denitrogenate both the circle and the patient (via its lung FRC) by using relatively high fresh gas flows for the first 10–20 minutes to hasten system equilibration. Using the smallest possible rebreathing bag (about 2× the patient's tidal volume), to minimise the circle's volume, will also help to maintain a higher anaesthetic agent concentration delivered to the patient by reducing the **time constant of the system** (see Chapter 9).

If using a vaporiser-in-circle (VIC), then increasing the fresh gas flow will tend to dilute the anaesthetic agent concentration in the circle. Higher flows through the vaporiser result in cooling and a reduction in evaporation; and higher flows do not become fully saturated during their passage through the vaporiser.

The **higher the blood solubility** of the agent, the **more pronounced** is the **effect of increasing the inspired anaesthetic agent concentration** on **hastening the speed of anaesthetic induction** (see below).

8.5.1.2 Loss of Anaesthetic Agent

This includes losses from the anaesthetic breathing system and/or the patient. Fresh soda lime can adsorb some of the anaesthetic agent from the anaesthetic breathing system. Different agents have different solubilities in the rubber or plastic hoses of the anaesthetic breathing systems, so this is another potential route for loss of agent from the breathing system. 'Loss' of anaesthetic agent from the patient's lungs into the blood and tissues is considered below, but loss from open body cavities or wounds, and to a small extent intact skin (especially anurans and other species that can respire via the skin), can also occur to the atmosphere.

8.5.1.3 Alveolar Ventilation

- Minute ventilation = respiratory frequency × tidal volume
- Tidal volume = alveolar volume + dead space volume
- Alveolar ventilation = respiratory frequency × alveolar volume
- Alveolar ventilation = respiratory frequency × (tidal volume – dead space volume)

The term *dead space volume* refers to the total, or physiological, dead space. This includes the anatomical dead space (the upper respiratory tract down to the respiratory bronchioles, i.e. where gaseous exchange does not normally occur), and the alveolar dead space (the relatively under-perfused or over-ventilated alveoli). Normally the physiological dead space is about one-third of the tidal volume, and therefore the alveolar volume is about two-thirds of the tidal volume. So, alveolar ventilation is about two-thirds of minute ventilation.

Alveolar ventilation therefore depends upon respiratory frequency and tidal volume (and also the dead space volume). Anything that increases minute ventilation and/or decreases dead space, results in increased alveolar ventilation and should facilitate an increase in the uptake of anaesthetic agent by enhancing the delivery of anaesthetic agent to the alveoli. Hyperventilation, either in an excited patient during inhalation induction, or by applying too rapid &/or too deep manual or mechanical ventilation, can hasten anaesthetic induction or depth change, especially for the agents with higher blood solubility.

Apparatus dead space should also be kept to a minimum because this acts like an extension of the patient's own dead space. Lower patient FRC also helps to hasten anaesthetic uptake, so in pregnant or bloated animals where the chest volume is reduced, slightly quicker anaesthetic agent uptake can be expected. Such patients also have smaller oxygen reserves due to their smaller FRC, so pre-oxygenation might be warranted.

The **higher the blood solubility** of the agent, the **more pronounced** is the **effect of increasing alveolar ventilation** on **hastening the speed of induction**.

8.5.1.4 Uptake by the Blood and Tissues

Blood uptake depends upon:

- **Solubility of agent in blood** (B/G partition coefficient)
- Pulmonary blood flow/perfusion (depends upon **cardiac output**)
- **Concentration gradient** between alveoli and blood
- **Diffusing capacity** of the lung (but this rarely causes problems unless there is severe lung disease)

Tissue uptake depends upon:

- **Solubility of agent in tissues**
- Tissue blood flow/perfusion (**cardiac output**)
- **Concentration gradient** between blood and tissue (equivalent to the arterio-venous concentration gradient)

The **more soluble the agent is in blood, the more is required to increase its partial pressure in the alveoli, and the slower the induction of anaesthesia** remembering that 'anaesthetic concentration in the brain follows, with a slight delay, that in the alveoli'. **The brain is in the vessel-rich tissue group, so has one of the first opportunities to receive anaesthetic agent delivered in the blood**. Brain contains a lot of lipid, and most of these agents have high lipid solubilities.

Compared with an agent of high blood (and tissue) solubility, an agent of low blood (and tissue) solubility is associated with a more rapid equilibration because only a small amount of anaesthetic agent need be dissolved in blood (and tissues) before equilibrium (with the delivered/alveolar concentration) is reached. **Low blood solubility is usually more desirable because induction and recovery are more rapid,** and **intra-operative anaesthetic depth changes can be achieved more rapidly**. Inhalant induction (and changes in anaesthetic depth) are therefore expected to be fastest with desflurane (desflurane > sevoflurane > isoflurane > halothane) due to its low blood and tissue solubilities. Methoxyflurane, on the other hand, is not only very soluble in blood and fat, but is also poorly volatile, so that inhalation induction is very slow, as is change of anaesthetic depth, but this does make it difficult to get patients too deep, too quickly. Therefore, despite its high potency (low MAC value), methoxyflurane's low volatility reduces the risks of overdose. Methoxyflurane is no longer available as an in-hospital anaesthetic agent in the UK but, because of its high solubility (hard to overdose) and analgesic properties, it has been favoured by first-responders/paramedics in Australia for some time and has recently been introduced into the UK for use in single-use inhalers (Penthrox™; affectionately known as the 'green whistle'). These are supplied with a 3 ml bottle of liquid methoxyflurane which is decanted into the inhaler when required; and also incorporate a chamber of activated charcoal on the expiratory side for scavenging. As these inhalers are much more lightweight and portable than Entonox cylinders (50 : 50, nitrous oxide: oxygen mixture, also analgesic), they are extremely useful when attending emergency trauma cases in remote/isolated areas.

The greater the alveolar concentration of anaesthetic agent that can be provided and the slower its removal or absorption from the alveoli, the more rapid is the rise in alveolar concentration of the agent (and therefore also of brain anaesthetic agent concentration), and, thereby the more rapid the anaesthetic induction. The alveolar anaesthetic agent tension may be increased by increasing the concentration of agent delivered (although there are usually limits to doing this, see above), which promotes its uptake: this is called the **concentration effect**; and the rate of rise of the alveolar anaesthetic agent tension is more rapid for agents of **low blood solubility**.

The alveolar anaesthetic agent tension may also be increased by the **second gas effect,** but it is only noticeable when the second gas is very much more insoluble and present at high concentration. For example, if nitrous oxide (the 'second gas') and a vapour (e.g. isoflurane) are both delivered to the patient in a stream of oxygen then because nitrous oxide is less soluble in blood (compared to isoflurane), and because it is administered at a much higher inspired concentration than the volatile agent (i.e. 50–66% compared to 1–3%), its uptake by blood and brain occurs, and is 'completed', more rapidly. Although nitrous oxide's solubility in blood is poor, some will dissolve; and at such high delivered concentrations, this small proportion of the large delivered concentration is still substantial enough to have an effect. The consequence, at this early stage of the induction, is that the initial rapid 'absorption' (removal) of nitrous oxide from the alveoli results in a relative increase in concentration of the gases left behind in the alveoli, i.e. isoflurane and oxygen. This in turn enhances the rate of rise of alveolar, and then brain, anaesthetic agent concentration, to hasten anaesthetic induction. The effect, however, is much less noticeable for volatile agents of lower blood solubility.

Anything that slows the rate of increase of alveolar anaesthetic agent tension will delay induction of anaesthesia. For example, if an **excited animal** is undergoing induction of inhalation anaesthesia, then its faster cardiac output (and pulmonary perfusion) will result in more rapid depletion of alveolar anaesthetic agent tension; and this delay in increase in alveolar anaesthetic agent tension can be thought of as reflected in a delay in increase in brain anaesthetic agent tension, and so induction of anaesthesia is also seen to be delayed. However, this is partly offset by a faster delivery of anaesthetic agent to the tissues (including brain) because of the greater cardiac output. In reality, the alveolar ventilation rate is also increased by excitement, and this also offsets the effects of increased cardiac output, so that induction may in fact be hastened.

In **shocky animals,** the lower cardiac output speeds induction of anaesthesia because alveolar anaesthetic agent concentration rises faster when alveolar perfusion is slow.

Changes in **cardiac output** and **alveolar ventilation** have **more effect** on the speed of induction with volatile anaesthetic agents of **higher blood (and tissue) solubilities** than those of lower blood solubilities.

Alveolar-to-blood and blood-to-tissue **concentration gradients** are greatest at the beginning of anaesthetic induction and reduce with time. Different body compartments equilibrate at different rates, according to their size and perfusion (see Chapter 5 on injectable agents where the concept of **different compartmental time constants** is discussed).

Equilibration among all body compartments takes time. The fat compartment can be huge and poorly perfused and therefore can take a long time to equilibrate, perhaps longer than the actual anaesthetic duration in clinical cases. Most agents are very soluble in fat, but interestingly, N_2O, and xenon are not. This equilibration time thus depends upon adipose tissue perfusion; how fat-soluble the agent is; how obese the patient is; and whether the agent is metabolised to any extent, which will delay this slow equilibration process further.

Various equations have been described to calculate uptake and elimination, or rather the rate of change of alveolar anaesthetic agent concentration. One is **Lowe's equation,** one version of which is:

$$\text{Rate of uptake of agent from alveoli}$$
$$= \lambda \mathbf{BG} \times \mathbf{CO} \times \left[\mathbf{P}(\mathbf{a} - \mathbf{v}) / \mathbf{P_{bar}} \right]$$

Where λBG is blood gas partition coefficient (measure of solubility), CO is cardiac output, and $P(a–v)/P_{bar}$ is the arterio-venous concentration (partial pressure) gradient, corrected for atmospheric pressure.

The rate of uptake of the anaesthetic agent from the alveoli is inversely related to the rate of induction/recovery or anaesthetic depth change.

The faster the anaesthetic agent is absorbed from the alveoli, the slower the alveolar concentration of the agent rises, the slower the brain concentration rises, and therefore the slower the anaesthetic induction.

Uptake and elimination curves can be represented as in Figures 8.2 and 8.3.

8.5.2 Factors Affecting Elimination of Inhalation Agents/Recovery From Anaesthesia

Such 'recovery' is sometimes referred to as 'eduction'. Just as recovery after cessation of an intravenous infusion of anaesthetic agent can be influenced by the duration of the drug infusion (the **context-sensitive half time,** see Chapter 5), a similar concept can be applied to inhaled anaesthetics: the **context-sensitive decrement time.** Again, the context refers to the duration of the anaesthetic, so context-sensitive decrement times vary according to the duration of anaesthesia, but are also affected by the solubility of the agent (especially in fat), the adiposity of the patient and whether the agent can be metabolised or is inert and eliminated exclusively by exhalation.

The context-sensitive decrement time for an inhaled anaesthetic agent is the time taken for the alveolar concentration or vital tissue (e.g. brain, heart, kidney, and liver, collectively called the vessel-rich group of tissues) concentration, to decrease by some fractional 'decrement' of the starting concentration; and depends upon the duration of anaesthesia (nominally at a constant alveolar concentration), which is considered to be the 'context'.

Following reduction of delivered (and therefore, alveolar) anaesthetic agent concentration, anaesthetic agent moves down the concentration gradients from the blood to the alveoli and from the tissues to the blood, and so its exhalation can continue (so long as alveolar ventilation continues).

Figure 8.2 'Wash-in' of anaesthetic agent (uptake). F_A/F_i, alveolar concentration of anaesthetic agent/ inspired concentration of anaesthetic agent.

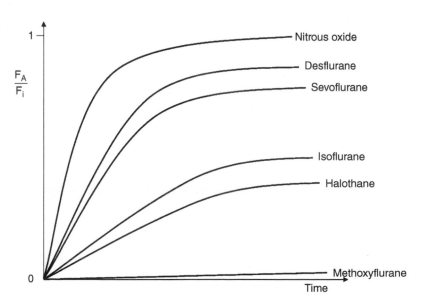

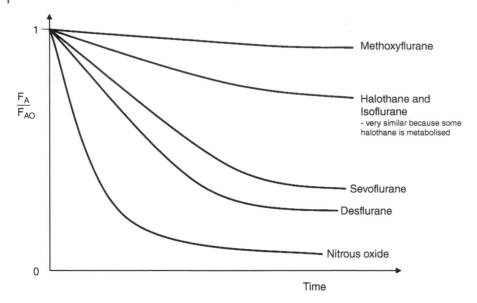

Figure 8.3 'Wash-out' of anaesthetic agent (elimination). F_A/F_{AO}, alveolar concentration of anaesthetic agent/alveolar concentration of anaesthetic agent just before vaporiser is turned off.

Recovery is therefore, influenced by:

- Inspired anaesthetic agent concentration
- Loss of agent from anaesthetic breathing system/patient (open wounds/body cavities)
- Alveolar ventilation
- Tissue/blood and blood/gas solubilities (and patient adiposity)
- Tissue perfusion
- Metabolism

The faster the inspired (and therefore alveolar) anaesthetic agent concentration can be reduced, the faster is re-awakening promoted, especially for agents of greater blood and tissue solubility. Switching off the vaporiser reduces the delivered anaesthetic agent concentration, and very rapidly if a non-rebreathing system is used. However, if a rebreathing system is used, the delivered anaesthetic agent concentration is slower to decrease, unless the fresh gas flow is increased and/or the rebreathing bag is emptied ('dumped') through the pop-off valve (into the scavenging system), several times (the system re-filled with oxygen after each dump), to hasten the rate of change of anaesthetic agent concentration circulating within the system. The inspired anaesthetic agent concentration cannot be reduced to below zero so there is only a limited amount you can do to reverse the concentration gradient between alveoli and blood/tissues/brain.

Alveolar ventilation is also important during recovery, although maintaining/increasing it has **most impact for the more blood/tissue soluble agents.**

Some anaesthetic agent will be **lost through** the **patient's wounds and any open body cavities,** and to a small extent, intact skin. Some agents may continue to be lost through the **anaesthetic breathing system tubing.**

The more tissue- and blood-soluble the agent, the slower its release back into the blood (and then the alveoli), and thus the slower the recovery. Tissue perfusion and cardiac output are again important. However, any **metabolism** of the agent is also important as it can accelerate the recovery.

Duration of anaesthesia potentially has a large influence, **especially for volatile agents with higher blood and tissue (especially fat), solubility:** the longer the anaesthetic duration, the more time these agents have to approach equilibrium with these tissues. The larger the body 'stores' that are built up (especially in the adipose tissues of obese patients), the longer it takes for the agent to be eliminated from those stores.

When using nitrous oxide, beware of the **Fink effect,** whereby **diffusion hypoxia** may occur. In this situation, the effect is **analogous to the second gas effect, but in reverse.** At the end of an anaesthetic, when the delivered concentrations of N$_2$O and, e.g. isoflurane, are reduced, N$_2$O, being least soluble, rapidly leaves the blood and floods into alveoli, thereby diluting the other gases present. Dilution of oxygen in the alveoli may reduce oxygen uptake, causing hypoxaemia and the so-called diffusion hypoxia, whereas dilution of isoflurane in the alveoli steepens the blood-alveolar concentration gradient, enhancing its elimination.

After short anaesthetics, recovery depends mainly upon exhalation, redistribution, and possibly some metabolism.

After long anaesthetics, recovery depends more upon the fat solubility of the agent, and how near saturation (equilibration), the tissues (especially fat), have become. Obese patients will have more prolonged recoveries after anaesthesia (especially if lengthy), with the more fat-soluble agents, isoflurane, or sevoflurane, than lean patients or following desflurane anaesthesia. Any **metabolism of the agent, however, helps hasten recovery**.

Elimination curves do not always exactly mirror uptake curves because of the context-sensitive decrement time (i.e. tissue solubilities, tissue accumulation and metabolism).

Halothane, though more blood- and fat-soluble than isoflurane, is also more metabolised and so recovery may not be much more prolonged following long anaesthetics with halothane cf. isoflurane. Sevoflurane is slightly more fat-soluble than isoflurane, so after long anaesthetics, even though sevoflurane has a lower blood solubility than isoflurane and is metabolised to a greater extent, the recovery times may not differ much because of sevoflurane's greater depot in fat. Desflurane is expected to result in more rapid recoveries than isoflurane in most instances, but may not always result in more rapid recoveries than sevoflurane due to sevoflurane's greater metabolism.

8.6 Halogenated Agents

These are the halogenated hydrocarbons (halothane) and the halogenated ethers (methoxyflurane, isoflurane, sevoflurane, and desflurane). Other halo-hydrocarbons of historical interest include chloroform, trichloroethylene, and cyclopropane. Other halo-ethers of historical interest include diethyl ether and methoxyflurane, although methoxyflurane is making somewhat of a comeback, as an analgesic, in human emergency/rescue situations.

As of August 2018, halothane no longer had marketing authorisation in the UK and is becoming less and less available/desired in the first world. Of the halo-ethers, isoflurane is most widely available, relatively cheaply, and is licenced for use in multiple species (dogs, cats, horses). Sevoflurane is currently only licenced for use in dogs and cats in UK.

All these agents, bar cyclopropane, were/are provided as volatile liquids (hence they are commonly known as the *volatile anaesthetic agents*), in either brown (to reduce degradation due to light) glass bottles: halothane, isoflurane, and desflurane (the bottle for desflurane is reinforced with a plastic jacket due to its great volatility near room temperature); or brown plastic or lacquer-coated aluminium bottles: sevoflurane. Cyclopropane was supplied in orange cylinders.

The **more fluorine** atoms in the molecule, the **more resistant to metabolism and degradation** it is; so there is a reduced requirement for stabilisers or preservatives to be included; there is a longer shelf-life; there is reduced flammability; there is less interaction with soda lime, but there is **less potency**, so **MAC increases**.

See Tables 8.1–8.4 for further details.

8.6.1 Effects of the Halogenated Agents

All agents cause **dose-dependent cardiovascular depression**, e.g. they reduce blood pressure (all agents produce similar mean arterial pressure reduction at equi-MAC doses); and they reduce cardiac output (halothane > isoflurane ≥ sevoflurane > desflurane).

The halogenated agents cause cardiovascular depression by a number of mechanisms, including:

- By direct myocardial depression (negative inotropy); (halothane >> isoflurane, sevoflurane > desflurane)

Table 8.3 The environmental impact of inhaled anaesthetic agents commonly used in veterinary anaesthesia.

	GWP$_{100yr}$	ODP	Atmospheric abundance (2014)*	Atmospheric lifetime (years)
Carbon dioxide	1.0	—	3.972×10^8	5–200
Desflurane	1525–2540	0	0.30	8.9–21
Halothane	50	1.56	0.0092	1.0–7.0
Isoflurane	328–571	0.03	0.097	3.2–5.9
Nitrous oxide	298–310	0.017	†	110–150
Sevoflurane	54–218	0	0.13	1.1–4.0

Values may vary slightly, depending upon source.
GWP$_{100yr}$, 100 year global warming potential compared to $CO_2 = 1$; ODP, ozone depletion potential compared to CFCs = 1; * global dry air mole fractions in parts per trillion (10^{-12}); † N_2O abundance was not determined as the contribution from anaesthesia could not be discriminated from other causes (e.g. industry and motorsports).

Table 8.4 A summary of various physicochemical and clinical characteristics of inhaled anaesthetic agents commonly used in veterinary anaesthesia. Values may vary slightly, depending upon source; cf. = compared with; cyt. P450 = cytochrome P450 microsomal enzyme system; des = desflurane; GWP_{100yr} = 100year global warming potential compared to CO_2 = 1; halo = halothane; HFIP = hexafluoroisopropanol; iso = isoflurane; NA = not applicable; ODP = ozone depletion potential compared to CFCs = 1; sevo = sevoflurane; TFA = trifluoroacetic acid; q4 = every 4 (from Latin *quaque*).

	Isoflurane	Sevoflurane	Desflurane	Halothane	Nitrous oxide	Xenon
Chemical formula	$C_3H_2OClF_5$	$C_4H_3OF_7$	$C_3H_2OF_6$	$C_2HBrClF_3$	N_2O	Xe
Chemical structure	(structural diagram)	(structural diagram)	(structural diagram)	(structural diagram)	(structural diagram) ^{54} Xe 131.3	
Chemical class	Ether Organic	Ether Organic	Ether Organic	Alkane Organic	Gas Inorganic	Noble gas Inorganic
First synthesised	1965	1968	1965	1951 (Suckling)	1772 (Priestly)	1898 (Ramsay and Travers)
First used clinically	1971	1990	1992	1956 (Johnstone)	1844 (limited, Wells, Hartford CT) 1863 (widespread, Colton, NYC)	1950s
Preservative?	No	Yes (water)	No	Yes (thymol)	No	No
Stable in soda lime?	Yes (unless desiccated & hot)	No (unless desiccated & hot)	Yes (unless desiccated & hot)	No	Yes	Yes
Stable in UV?	Yes	No	Yes	No	Yes	Yes
Toxic metabolites?	Minimal quantity of TFA	Fluoride ions HFIP	Negligible quantity of TFA	Hepatotoxicity by TFA Type 1 (enzyme derangement) Type 2 (autoimmune)	No	No

	Isoflurane	Sevoflurane	Desflurane	Halothane	Nitrous oxide	Xenon
Toxic breakdown products (in presence of CO₂ absorbents)?	CO (from O-CHF₂ moiety) **Iso** > Des	Compound A (C₄H₂OF₆)	CO Iso > **Des**	Possibly hydrofluoric acid (HF) and Compound BCDFE	No	No
Flammable/explosive?	No	No	No	No	Non-flammable Supports combustion of normally non-combustible substances	No
Warnings	GWP₁₀₀yr 328–571 ODP 0.03	GWP₁₀₀yr 54–218 Compound A nephrotoxicity in rodents (possibly due to metabolism within renal parenchyma) – not reported in other domestic species	GWP₁₀₀yr 1525–2540 Vaporiser requires uninterrupted power source	GWP₁₀₀yr 50 ODP 1.56 Avoid repeat GA within 3 months (autoimmune hepatotoxicity)	GWP₁₀₀yr 310 Denser than air Diffusion hypoxia risk Avoid >24 hours admin Avoid if Vit.B12/folate deficient Avoid use >q4 days.	3–6x denser than air. Appears to increase O₂ consumption [Little diffusion hypoxia observed] 1.4–1.5x increase in airway resistance compared to air or N₂O Care with cylinder filling ratio and storage
Analgesia?	No	No	No	No	Yes	Yes
Molecular weight (g/mol)	184	200	168	197	44	131
Liquid density (g/ml @ 20 °C)	1.85	1.52	1.47	1.86	1.42	NA
Boiling point (°C)	49	50	23.5	50	−89	−108
Saturated Vapour Pressure (mmHg at 20 °C)	240	160	700	243	NA [cylinder pressure: 4400 kPa; 0.75 filling ratio (0.67 if hot climate)]	NA [cylinder pressure: 3000 kPa]
(mmHg at 24 °C)	286	183	804	288		

(Continued)

Table 8.4 (Continued)

	Isoflurane	Sevoflurane	Desflurane	Halothane	Nitrous oxide	Xenon
ml vapour / ml liquid (20 °C)	195	182	211	227	NA	NA
Solubility coefficients:						
Water: gas/vapour (37 °C)					0.47	0.2
Olive oil: gas/vapour (37 °C)	91	47	18.7	224	1.4	1.9
Blood: gas/vapour (37 °C)	1.46	0.68	0.43	2.5	0.47 (cf. N_2 = 0.015)	0.12–0.14
Rubber: gas/vapour (20 °C)	60	29	19	190	1.2	Is soluble in rubber & silicone
PVC: gas/vapour (20 °C)	114	69	35	233	0	
Polyethylene: gas/vapour (20 °C)	58	31	16	128	0	
MAC (%)	1.3–2% (cat)	2.6–3.4% (cat)	9.8–10.2% (cat)	1–1.2% (cat)	255% (cat)	120% (dog)
	1.14% (cattle)	– (cattle)	– (cattle)	0.76% (calf)	223% (calf)	63–71% (human)
	1.2–1.5% (dog)	2.3–2.4% (dog)	7.2–10.3% (dog)	0.8–1% (dog)	188–297% (dog)	119% (pig)
	1.3–1.6% (horse)	2.3–2.8% (horse)	7–8% (horse)	0.9–1% (horse)	190–205% (horse)	85% (rabbit)
	1.15% (human)	1.6–2% (human)	6–7% (human)	0.7–0.8% (human)	105% (human)	161% (rat)
	1.45–1.8% (pig)	2–2.6% (pig)	10% (pig)	0.9–1.25% (pig)	162–195% (pig)	98% (rhesus monkey)
	2.05–2.12% (rabbit)	3.7% (rabbit)	8.9% (rabbit)	0.8–1.6% (rabbit)		
Metabolism (%)	0.2%	2–5%	0.02%	20–46%	0.004%	0%
Metabolism	Oxidation	Oxidation	Oxidation	Oxidation (cyt. P450: TFA) Anaerobic reduction: Br^- & F^-	Negligible. Elimination through lungs and skin	Negligible
Toxic effects	Fluoride liberation (Sevo > **Iso** > Des) – not clinically relevant	Fluoride liberation (**Sevo** > Iso > Des) – not clinically relevant HFIP production – not clinically relevant	Fluoride liberation (Sevo > Iso > **Des**) – not clinically relevant	Arrhythmias (sensitises to catecholamines) Hepatotoxicity: 1) Damage to microsomal enzymes and hepatocytes by TFA or other radicals 2) Immune response to TFA-induced novel haptens	Vit.B12 inactivation (normally a cofactor for methionine synthase) 1) Megaloblastic anaemia 2) Impaired DNA synthesis a) neurotoxicity b) agranulocytosis c) pancytopenia 3) Demyelination ± reduced fertility 4) Teratogen (folinic acid may be protective in rats)	Negligible

- By causing peripheral vasodilation; (isoflurane, sevoflurane, and desflurane >> halothane)
- By decreasing vascular reactivity and impairing tissue autoregulation so that tissue perfusion becomes more dependent upon the 'driving' arterial blood pressure; coronary autoregulation is suggested not to be affected
- Via CNS depression and reducing autonomic tone
  - These agents have sympatholytic and parasympatholytic properties, but sympathetic tone is generally reduced more than parasympathetic tone (halothane least parasympatholytic, desflurane most).

Some reflex tachycardia occurs with isoflurane, sevoflurane, and desflurane and this partly compensates for the reduction in blood pressure; however, this may not occur with halothane (due to a reduction in baroreflex activity/ relatively little vagolysis, although this is species-dependent), and thus there may be a slightly greater reduction in cardiac output seen with halothane compared with isoflurane, sevoflurane, and desflurane. In addition, the peripheral vasodilation caused by isoflurane, sevoflurane, and desflurane reduces the cardiac 'afterload', which may promote better cardiac output with these agents compared with halothane.

Greater respiratory depression (see below) tends to occur with isoflurane, sevoflurane, and desflurane, leading to the development of hypercapnia/respiratory acidosis (if ventilation is not supported). Hypercapnia itself, in certain circumstances, results in sympathetic stimulation which may help offset the decrease in cardiac output and arterial blood pressure. The institution of mechanical ventilation (to maintain normocapnia), may not only remove the cardiovascular supportive effects of hypercapnia/respiratory acidosis but, through the mechanical effects of increased intrathoracic pressure, may also impede venous return and further compromise cardiac output. Overall, there is greater cardiovascular depression induced by halothane (even though it causes slightly less respiratory depression) than the other agents at equipotent doses greater than 1.0 MAC.

Isoflurane and sevoflurane (and the other halo-ethers), do not sensitise the myocardium to the arrhythmogenic effects of catecholamines; whereas halothane (and the other halo-hydrocarbons) do. Paroxysmal atrioventricular (AV) dissociation may occur in cats. Ischaemic **pre- and post-conditioning of the myocardium, brain (and other organs including lungs, kidneys, liver, digestive tract, and skeletal muscles),** leading to reduced ischaemia-reperfusion injury and smaller infarct size in dog and rodent experimental models (and some small-scale human clinical trials) have been demonstrated with desflurane > sevoflurane > isoflurane. These effects, mediated by metabolic and mitochondrial mechanisms, are, however, attenuated by factors such as obesity and hyperglycaemia. The clinical relevance of pre- and post-conditioning remain to be fully investigated.

All agents cause some **dose-dependent respiratory depression** (isoflurane > halothane and sevoflurane). In some patients, however, sevoflurane appears to cause similar respiratory depression to isoflurane. Isoflurane has a more pungent smell and is more irritant to the respiratory mucosa. Desflurane is also very pungent (see below). Overall, it is said that minute ventilation decreases due to a reduction in tidal volume, with a slight, non-compensatory, increase in respiratory frequency; at higher 'doses', respiratory frequency then also tends to decrease (but the exact effects are species- and drug-dependent).

The halogenated agents cause respiratory depression by a number of mechanisms, including:

- By depressing the ventilatory response to CO_2
- By depressing hypoxic pulmonary vasoconstriction
- By almost abolishing the ventilatory response to hypoxia/ hypoxaemia
- By causing bronchodilation (which increases dead space); halothane & sevoflurane > all others

Hepatic and renal blood flow may be reduced because cardiac output and mean arterial blood pressure are reduced, and/or because splanchnic vasoconstriction occurs. Halothane hepatitis may occur in man (see below). The volatile agents undergo varying degrees of **hepatic metabolism**: halothane >> sevoflurane > isoflurane > desflurane. Halothane can be metabolised to trifluoroacetic acid (TFA) (see later under potential toxicities). Most volatile agents cause some hepatic **microsomal enzyme inhibition**. Halothane reduces blood flow in the hepatic portal vein and the hepatic artery; whereas isoflurane reduces flow in the hepatic portal vein but may slightly increase flow through the hepatic artery so that little overall change in hepatic perfusion occurs but an improvement in hepatic oxygenation may result.

All volatile inhalation agents appear to **inhibit insulin secretion**.

Cerebral blood flow is increased (due to vasodilation) (halothane > desflurane > isoflurane ≥ sevoflurane), but **cerebral metabolic rate is reduced** (which would normally result in some vasoconstriction due to autoregulation of cerebral blood flow, but this is blunted by volatile agents). Intracranial pressure tends to increase (dose-related) because of the overriding vasodilation. The effect on cerebral blood flow is much less pronounced (may be minimal) at 0.5 MAC and can be offset by hyperventilation, as hypocapnia promotes cerebral vasoconstriction (see Chapter 21). **Cerebral preconditioning** also occurs and appears to be partly via mechanisms involving nitric oxide, adenosine production, and activation of K_{ATP} channel activity, especially those in mitochondria. More chronic protective effects appear to be due to a reduction in cell apoptosis, the mechanism of which is unclear although it may include a reduction in intracellular calcium accumulation. Sevoflurane produces less cerebral vasodilation than the other agents at equi-MAC doses, and interferes less with cerebral autoregulation but may reduce the cerebral vasoconstrictive response to hypocapnia. Desflurane produces greater cerebral pre- and post-conditioning effects than the other agents, both acutely and more chronically.

All volatile agents may **trigger malignant hyperthermia** (reported in pigs, dogs, horses, cats, humans).

The volatile agents produce **poor analgesia** except for methoxyflurane (and the most pungent ones, isoflurane and desflurane, may even cause hyperalgesia).

All the volatile agents are **calcium channel (L, T, and possibly N type) blockers**, and their muscle relaxation effects (on cardiac, striated and vascular and other smooth muscle) may stem from reduced calcium entry into muscle cells and initial depletion of intracellular calcium stores, followed by reduced release from sarcoplasmic reticulum. The affinity of troponin C for calcium may also be affected.

Some **muscle relaxation** occurs, especially with the halo-ethers, but all the volatile agents potentiate the neuromuscular block produced by non-depolarising neuromuscular blocking agents (possibly due to calcium channel blocking effects).

All volatile agents **reduce lower oesophageal sphincter tone** and potentially increase the risk of gastro-oesophageal reflux/regurgitation, but there are species differences due to anatomical and physiological differences (i.e. smooth muscle/skeletal muscle components and muscle fibre configuration at the gastro-oesophageal junction).

All volatile agents cause a degree of **uterine relaxation** and uterine vasodilation, but halothane also appears to slow uterine involution.

In addition to the **$GABA_A$-mimetic effects** of the volatile agents, they are likely to have **other actions**, and, e.g. isoflurane has been shown to have NMDA receptor antagonist actions (so potentially provides some analgesia? See also Chapter 1).

Halothane requires inclusion of 0.01% poorly volatile **thymol** as a stabiliser/preservative. Methoxyflurane has **butylated hydroxytoluene** added as an antioxidant. Sevoflurane may degrade to acidic products in the presence of Lewis acids (usually metal oxides or halides, but thought to be primarily aluminium oxide impurities in glass) to form, e.g. hydrofluoric acid, which is a toxic volatile acid with a pungent smell even at sub-toxic doses. Hydrofluoric acid reacts with glass (silicon dioxide) to form silicon

fluorides (e.g. SiF_4 which is volatile, pungent, and highly toxic). Sevoflurane is now supplied in special plastic bottles or lacquer-coated aluminium bottles and **water** is added as its 'preservative' (a Lewis base [or Lewis acid inhibitor]) to prevent this degradation.

Desflurane has some special physical properties. Its SVP is high at room temperature, which alongside its low boiling point (23.5 °C), means that very high concentrations can be delivered to the patient. It requires a special temperature-controlled vaporiser (see Chapter 10 on vaporisers). Its low blood solubility means that induction, recovery, and anaesthetic depth change can be very rapid. Its low oil/gas solubility means that desflurane has a low potency, and therefore a high MAC. Desflurane is also very pungent, so is not suitable for inhalation inductions, at least in humans, where pulmonary (and other) 'pungent' receptors are stimulated by rapid increases in inspired desflurane concentrations and can result in 'sympathetic storms'. Desflurane may prove to be more suitable in veterinary species, but it is not yet licenced.

8.7 Nitrous Oxide

Nitrous oxide is produced by thermal decomposition of ammonium nitrate at 240 °C. It is supplied in white cylinders with French blue shoulders (completely blue cylinders may also be in circulation until 2025), as a **saturated vapour above liquid**. It is colourless and has a slightly sweet odour. It is non-flammable, but does support combustion.

A substance present in the gaseous phase is referred to as a **gas** when at a temperature above its critical temperature, and a **vapour** when at a temperature below its critical temperature.

The **critical temperature** is the temperature above which a 'gas' cannot be liquefied, no matter how much pressure is applied.

Cylinder pressure is 4400 kPa (~44 Atmospheres). The **critical temperature for nitrous oxide is 36.5 °C**. However, at room temperature (which is below this critical temperature), N_2O can be liquefied by compression, so that cylinders are filled with saturated vapour above a liquid. At constant temperature, the cylinder SVP (and therefore the **cylinder pressure gauge reading**), **does not decrease until all** the **liquid has evaporated**. Therefore, estimation of cylinder content is made by weighing the cylinder and comparing to empty weight. The empty weight (tare weight) of the cylinder should be stamped onto its neck. The density of N_2O is also stamped on the cylinder neck (0.001 872 6 kg/l). Density equals mass/volume; so volume remaining equals mass/density. (It is often easier to multiply the weight of the cylinder contents by 534; where

534 = 1/density.) Alternatively, because 1 mole of gas occupies 22.4 l at standard temperature and pressure (Avogadro's law), and as the molecular weight of nitrous oxide is 44, the cylinder content (in grammes) divided by the molecular weight, multiplied by 22.4, also gives an estimate of the number of litres remaining.

The **filling ratio** for N_2O cylinders in temperate climates like the UK is 0.75; whereas it is 0.67 in the tropics. The filling ratio is the ratio of the maximum weight of N_2O vapour and liquid that the cylinder should be filled with, compared to the weight of water the cylinder could hold, at around 16 °C. It is less in hotter climates because the relative under-filling reduces the potential for pressure build up (and cylinder rupture) with modest increases in environmental temperature.

If nitrous oxide is withdrawn rapidly from the cylinder, then adiabatic (rather than isothermal) cooling occurs as liquid agent evaporates (i.e. there is little time for heat energy to be transferred from the environment via the cylinder wall to the liquid agent within the cylinder). This can result in frosting of the cylinder (up to the level of remaining liquid within) and perhaps on the cylinder outlet too.

The **MAC of N_2O in man is 105%**, however, when administered at sub-anaesthetic doses, it affords useful analgesia. In man, inspired concentrations above 20% provide some analgesia, but animals generally need more than this. In animals, its MAC value is so high (**188% in dogs**, and **255% in cats**) that hyperbaric conditions are required in order to deliver it at sufficient dose to even contemplate any sort of anaesthesia without causing hypoxia. Instead N_2O is **administered to provide analgesia** at concentrations of 50–66%.

8.7.1 Mechanisms of Analgesic Effects

- N_2O activates the endogenous opioid system (in turn activating descending monoaminergic, cholinergic, and purinergic pathways)
- N_2O has NMDA receptor antagonist activity (and therefore can produce neurotoxic, as well as neuroprotective, effects)

8.7.2 Systemic Effects

Nitrous oxide causes **minimal overall cardiorespiratory depression**, and may even cause mild cardiovascular stimulation. Similar to ketamine, it causes direct negative inotropy that is balanced by sympathetic nervous system stimulation. The small rise in systemic peripheral vascular resistance often documented also occurs with increased inspired oxygen fractions (possibly reflecting increased tissue oxygen delivery and autoregulatory vasoconstriction).

Some references suggest pulmonary vascular resistance increases, whereas others suggest it decreases. High inspired oxygen concentrations tend to lower pulmonary vascular resistance (by offsetting hypoxic pulmonary vasoconstriction); but if apnoea occurs (due to oxygen oversufficiency), and hypercapnia follows, then hypercapnia can itself promote pulmonary vasoconstriction. Despite some texts suggesting caution with pre-existing pulmonary hypertension, if attention is paid to blood oxygenation, CO_2 tension, and FRC (lung volume can affect the pulmonary vascular resistance too), then the effects are minimal.

Nitrous oxide administration **reduces the MAC**, and therefore requirement, of other volatile anaesthetic agents, and so reduces side effects associated with larger doses of those agents too. N_2O appears to provide **very weak, or even no, ischaemic pre- and post-conditioning** effects. When administered alone, nitrous oxide increases cerebral metabolic rate, which increases cerebral blood flow and therefore also intracranial pressure.

In humans, its use may be associated with an increase in **postoperative nausea and vomiting** (PONV).

The blood/gas partition coefficient of N_2 is 0.0147; which is ~32× less soluble than N_2O (blood/gas partition coefficient of 0.47). **N_2O partitions into insoluble-gas-filled spaces**, and increases their volume or pressure, depending upon whether that compartment is distensible or not. That is, N_2O can enter such spaces faster than the already present, and even more insoluble gases, can leave. Such insoluble gases include nitrogen (beware air-filled spaces), hydrogen, and methane (beware rumens and large intestines in herbivorous creatures with fermentation occurring at various portions of their GI tracts). Problems can occur with, e.g. pneumothorax, gastric dilation/volvulus, and equine colics, if the distended viscus is not first decompressed, or if venous air emboli are likely, as N_2O can enhance their distension/size. The use of N_2O is equivocal in *healthy* horses, rabbits, and ruminants as, although one study documented an increase in the volume of the large intestine in healthy horses during anaesthesia which included N_2O, no untoward adverse clinical effects (e.g. post-operative colic) were documented. This author still suggests caution.

Nitrous oxide **can partition into air-filled endotracheal tube cuffs**, so their volume and pressure can increase if not initially inflated with a mixture of gases including nitrous oxide at their target concentrations. Some veterinarians prefer to inflate the tube cuff with sterile water or saline as a preventative measure against tracheal mucosal damage from this unplanned increase in cuff inflation.

Nitrous oxide can be used to encourage uptake of other inhalation agents at the beginning of an anaesthetic (by the second gas effect), either during inhalation induction or during the transition from intravenous induction to inhalation maintenance, but there is the potential for **diffusion hypoxia** at the end of the anaesthetic. Although the duration of this effect is probably only 2–5 minutes, most references advocate turning off the N_2O, and increasing O_2 flow about 10 minutes before turning off the volatile anaesthetic to prevent this.

The use of N_2O is often cautioned in anaemic patients because its use limits the inspired oxygen percentage that can be delivered. However, such patients lack haemoglobin as an oxygen carrier, so the additional amount of oxygen that can be dissolved in plasma by increasing the amount of oxygen the animal breathes, is actually very minimal.

Nitrous oxide may be a **very weak trigger of malignant hyperthermia**.

N_2O cannot be destroyed by scavenging (it is not adsorbed by activated charcoal), it can only be expelled into the atmosphere, where it is a **potent greenhouse gas** and adds to the destruction of the ozone layer and acid rain problems. It survives in the atmosphere for at least 150 years.

8.8 Xenon

Xenon is an inert, colourless, odourless gas. Its name means 'stranger'. It is very expensive to isolate from atmospheric gases (as a by-product of oxygen extraction by fractional distillation of liquefied air), because it is a trace element, present at no greater than 0.0875 ppm. It is supplied as a compressed gas in cylinders at pressures of ~30 Atmospheres although no standard size or international colour yet exists. Because it is a normal component of atmosphere and is inert, it is not a pollutant. It cannot be metabolised, is non-flammable and does not support combustion. It is only really affordable for use in closed system anaesthesia, to which it is suited because of its very low blood/gas partition coefficient. It diffuses easily through rubber and silicone, so plastic tubing is preferred. Xenon does not interact with soda lime.

Xenon causes minimal cardiovascular depression with mild sympathetic stimulation and is often described as being **cardiostable**. It causes some respiratory depression, and, unusually, causes a decrease in respiratory frequency and a slight increase in tidal volume, which almost compensates for the decrease in frequency. Xenon has higher density and viscosity than air (3.2× and 1.7×, respectively), so in high concentrations it may increase the resistance to breathing, and patients may require mechanical ventilation. It does not interfere with cerebral autoregulation; it **preserves cerebral blood flow: metabolism coupling,**

with little overall effect on cerebral blood flow. Its role in neuroanaesthesia seems promising. Xenon **provides ischaemic pre- and post-conditioning** effects, thereby being described as being organo- (e.g. cardio- and cerebro-/neuro-) protective. It **does not trigger malignant hyperthermia**.

Xenon's MAC of ~60–70% (in humans) allows a reasonable oxygen concentration to be delivered during xenon anaesthesia. Its MAC in dogs is nearer 120%, but it can be delivered at sub-anaesthetic doses to provide useful analgesia, through antagonistic effects at NMDA and AMPA receptors and also via stimulation of endogenous noradrenergic pathways. Xenon is said to be about 3× as analgesic as N_2O. Diffusion hypoxia and partitioning into 'insoluble gas'-/air-filled spaces should theoretically occur with Xe, but, despite its very low blood solubility (xenon is ~10× less soluble than nitrogen), because xenon is a big molecule, its 'diffusibility' is poor; thus, **partitioning is comparatively low**. Similar to N_2O, Xe can increase the risk of **PONV** above that associated with volatile agents.

8.9 Activated Charcoal

Activated charcoal is a very porous form of carbon, usually derived from wood or other organic materials after either heating to extreme temperatures (626–926 °C) in an inert gas, e.g. nitrogen, or argon (to prevent combustion) before exposure to oxygen to create the porous structure, or chemical treatment (with acid, alkali, or salt) before heating to create the porous structure.

The porous structure of activated charcoal gives it a huge surface area for the adsorption of organic molecules, which can form bonds with the myriad of exposed carbon atoms.

Activated charcoal is used as a detoxicant for inhaled or ingested toxins:

- Canisters of activated charcoal (e.g. Aldasorber™) can be used within waste anaesthetic agent scavenging systems for halogenated volatile anaesthetic agents only (but importantly NOT nitrous oxide).
- Activated charcoal filters can also be placed within a rebreathing anaesthetic breathing system (on both the inspiratory and expiratory limbs) as part of the treatment for unforeseen malignant hyperthermia, where they help to rapidly reduce the concentration of inhaled volatile anaesthetic agent.
- Activated charcoal filters can also be used to help ensure that modern anaesthesia workstations (with many internal and non-interchangeable, non-metal components which harbour vapour) can be made effectively

'vapour-free' (expected inhaled vapour <5 ppm), should patients prone to malignant hyperthermia be scheduled for general anaesthesia.

- The AnaConDa™ is a modified activated charcoal filter/reflector/HME device which adsorbs exhaled volatile agent yet desorbs most of the volatile agent during inhalation. Coupled with liquid agent injection (via a syringe-driver), agent evaporation within the device, and careful monitoring of inspired and exhaled anaesthetic agent concentrations, this device negates the requirement for a conventional vaporiser. The AnaConDa™ can be used with isoflurane and sevoflurane; whereas a similar device called the Mirus™ device, can be used with desflurane.

- Activated charcoal impregnated masks can be used by pregnant operating/recovery room personnel to reduce personal exposure.

- Slurries (or, less preferably, tablets/capsules) of activated charcoal can be given per-os or gavaged by stomach tube in order to help promote adsorption (and therefore reduce absorption and enterohepatic recirculation) of certain ingested toxins, to address residual gut lumen toxins following induction of emesis (where appropriate), or where inducing emesis is either contra-indicated or is too late to be effective after toxin ingestion. Most useful if it can be given within one to four hours after ingestion of non-polar toxins like salicylates and NSAIDs, barbiturates, and chocolate (theobromine and methylxanthines). May need to be given repeatedly to prevent enterohepatic recirculation. Does not work for substances like alcohol, ethylene glycol, xylitol, and metals.

8.10 Potential Toxicities

8.10.1 N$_2$O

N$_2$O can oxidise the cobalt within vitamin B12 (cobalamin), and therefore incapacitate this important co-factor for enzymes in intermediary metabolism, especially methionine synthase, which is important for (i) the folate cycle (important in purine and pyrimidine synthesis) and (ii) the S-adenosyl-methionine (SAM) cycle (which generates methyl donors); and hence, DNA and RNA synthesis, myelin synthesis, and homocysteine metabolism can all be affected by exposure to N$_2$O. Chronic exposure is therefore linked with anaemia (megaloblastic), leukopaenia, and neuropathies (demyelination types). Hyperhomocysteinaemia is implicated in cardiovascular disease, but the mechanisms are incompletely understood. Prolonged exposure has been anecdotally correlated with teratogenic effects, abortion, and infertility.

8.10.2 Reactive Radicals and Immunotoxicity

In humans, under normoxic conditions, a radical called trifluoroacetic acid (**TFA**) is produced during halothane metabolism, which binds to (acetylates) liver proteins to produce novel antigens ('haptens'), which can stimulate immune responses; the antibodies produced may also recognise normal host antigens. On subsequent halothane exposure, the immune response is greater, and can result in immune-mediated hepatic destruction, so called 'halothane hepatitis', with subsequent, fulminant hepatic failure. There is some suggestion (in humans) that prior exposure to halothane and subsequent exposure to isoflurane might also trigger hepatic failure.

Under hypoxic conditions, other active radicals can be produced (by a non-oxygen dependent pathway), which also result in hepatic damage, this time via lipid peroxidation. Fortunately, most veterinary species do not suffer the same problems as man, although there have been reports in rabbits, rats, and an alpaca cria.

Isoflurane and desflurane (but not sevoflurane), can be metabolised to produce tiny quantities of TFA and other similar compounds, usually insufficient to produce novel haptens for antibody production.

Sevoflurane is metabolised (c.2%) in the liver to produce hexafluoroisopropanol (**HFIP**) and free fluoride ions, but neither seem to cause significant hepatic or renal injury, probably because they are produced in such small quantities.

8.10.3 Free Fluoride Ions/Radicals

Large quantities of free fluoride ions are liberated, especially in the kidneys, during methoxyflurane degradation, and may be associated with the development of high output renal failure. (The exact mechanism/s of methoxyflurane-associated nephrotoxicity has/have not been determined, but may also involve dichloroacetic acid, another metabolite of methoxyflurane that is produced alongside the inorganic fluoride ions). In contrast, small quantities of free halide ions/radicals are produced by halothane > sevoflurane > isoflurane (and, very minimally, desflurane) degradation in liver and kidneys. Free fluoride ions can cause renal damage. Free fluoride ions compete with chloride ions at the chloride transporter in the ascending limb of the loop of Henle to result in 'high output renal failure'. Halothane halide radicals/ions (F, F$^-$, Cl, Cl$^-$, Br, and Br$^-$) may cause renal (and possibly hepatic) damage in Guinea pigs. (Bromide ions have also been reported to acetylate hepatic proteins, but the consequences of this are unclear.) Halothane and isoflurane may be degraded by ultraviolet light to produce free bromine and/or chlorine which can destroy ozone. Sevoflurane and desflurane do not contain chlorine or bromine atoms and are thought not to result in atmospheric ozone depletion.

8.10.4 Post-anaesthetic Cognitive Dysfunction

There is emerging evidence in rodents, non-human primates, and humans that general anaesthesia (inhalational but also injectable) in neonatal, paediatric, and geriatric sub-populations may cause lasting, adverse effects on neural morphology and cognitive function through neural apoptosis and altered synaptic connectivity. Mid-life adults do not appear to be affected; in fact, general anaesthesia may be neuroprotective during this life-stage.

8.11 Interaction of Inhalation Agents with CO_2 Absorbents

Degradation of all volatile agents by soda lime can occur and primarily decreases the amount of anaesthetic agent available to the patient. Fresh soda lime can also adsorb volatile agents, further reducing its availability to the patient. Degradation of volatile agents tends to be **more significant with desiccated and hot soda lime**. Absorbents in rebreathing systems desiccate if the fresh gas flow exceeds the minute ventilation or if oxygen (from a cylinder source and therefore 'dry') is inadvertently left flowing through the absorbent overnight or over a weekend.

The chemical interaction of volatile agents with absorbent can result in remarkable increases in temperature of the absorbent (57 °C with desflurane, 78 °C with isoflurane, 86 °C with halothane, 128 °C with sevoflurane), which again are more dramatic with desiccated absorbent (e.g. <100 °C with desflurane and 350–400 °C with sevoflurane). Spontaneous combustion has been reported in low flow anaesthesia systems with sevoflurane, dry soda lime, and high oxygen concentrations.

It has been suggested that **dry absorbent can be rehydrated** to ~13% water content by adding ~150 ml water (c. ½ a metric cup) per 1.2 kg desiccated absorbent, but this is a bad habit, so, preferably, the dry absorbent should be replaced with new fresh ('moist') absorbent.

8.11.1 Halothane

Reacts with soda lime (especially if hot and dry, and if a strong alkali is present as an activator) to produce **hydrofluoric acid** (HF), which is a potential **lung irritant**, and

Compound BCDFE (bromo-chloro-difluoro-ethylene), which can be **nephrotoxic** via the cysteine conjugate β lyase pathway (in rats). Addition of potassium permanganate to soda lime reduces production of BCDFE. Interestingly, hepatic metabolism of halothane can also produce small quantities of compound BCDFE.

8.11.2 Isoflurane

Very few problems, carbon monoxide (CO) production (see below) is a theoretical risk.

8.11.3 Sevoflurane

Dry soda lime can degrade sevoflurane to formaldehyde or formic acid. Hot and dry absorbents, especially if they contain activators (monovalent bases such as KOH and NaOH) lead to production of **Compound A** (which accumulates under conditions of low flow anaesthesia). Compounds B, C, D, and E have also been described. Compound A is fluoromethyl difluorotrifluoromethyl vinyl ether (an olefin). It undergoes hepatic glucuronidation, followed by renal metabolism (via the cysteine conjugate β lyase pathway, which is very active in rats) to yield a reactive **thiol** (and possibly free fluoride). The thiol can cause lung damage and the **free fluoride**, renal damage, although this has only been shown to be a clinical problem in rats. This may not be the full story though, so caution should be exercised with prolonged low flow anaesthesia especially with absorbents containing KOH or NaOH. Some sources state that CO_2 absorbents produce compound A with sevoflurane in the following order: baralyme > soda lime > KOH-free soda lime > activator-(KOH and NaOH)-free soda lime.

8.11.4 Compound A Production Is Increased if the Absorbent Is Dry and Hot and Contains Activators

Fresh baralyme contains less water than soda lime because its natural water of crystallisation is sufficient to get the normal CO_2 absorption reaction going (see Chapter 9). Being 'drier' than soda lime, it allows more degradation of volatile agents than soda lime, however, it is often marketed without activators, which are normally thought responsible for enhancing volatile agent degradation. Therefore, Compound A production may be less with activator-free baralyme than with soda lime, and even than with some KOH-free soda limes. Adding water to, and removing NaOH and KOH from, normally hydrated soda lime can reduce Compound A production dramatically. Several 'new generation' CO_2 absorbents are now available, tending to exclude caustic activators, and therefore less likely to result in significant Compound A production (e.g. LoFloSorb™ and Amsorb™).

8.11.5 Desflurane

Carbon monoxide production requires the presence of a di-fluoro-methoxy group (should not be possible with halothane and sevoflurane). Desflurane is initially degraded to trifluoromethane (also called 'fluoroform', CF_3H), a precursor of CO.

Again, CO production is **greatest with dry and hot absorbents and only with those which contain strong alkalis** (KOH, NaOH) as activators. Degradation to CO depends upon interaction with these strong alkalis. Production of CO with baralyme is said to be greater than with soda lime because baralyme is 'drier'. Interestingly, high carbon dioxide production by the patient may also influence the production of CO.

CO production is said to be in the order:

desflurane >> isoflurane >>>>>>> (sevoflurane ≡ halothane ≡ negligible)

8.12 Global Warming Potential

Halogenated organic compounds contribute directly to climate change through ozone depletion and by absorption of infrared radiation thereby impeding infrared escape through the atmosphere to space, and subsequently hindering the earth's cooling (global warming). Inhaled anaesthetics are halogenated organic compounds that are vented directly to the atmosphere after use and their global warming (GWP) and ozone depletion (ODP) potentials must be considered. As atmospheric lifetime impacts GWP, the 100-year average (GWP_{100yr}) is commonly used to compare molecules, using CO_2 as the comparator ($CO_2 \, GWP_{100yr} = 1$). The ODP depends upon how the molecule is halogenated, with greater ozone depletion caused by $Br^- >> Cl^-$ >>>>>>> ($F^- \equiv$ negligible); chlorofluorocarbons (CFCs) are the comparator (CFC ODP = 1). The impact on climate change of our inhaled anaesthetic agents is a function of atmospheric lifetime, atmospheric concentration, GWP, and ODP.

Environmental monitoring indicates that the atmospheric concentration of halothane has declined over the last decade, whilst concentrations of isoflurane, sevoflurane, and desflurane have increased, with the majority of anaesthetic gas emissions originating from the northern hemisphere. When developing an environmental strategy, it is important to remember that the total impact of inhaled anaesthetics on climate change also includes the environmental costs of production, packaging, and transport, which is not directly accounted for by GWP or ODP.

8.13 Chemical Formulae

8.13.1 Halo-ethers

Isoflurane

Sevoflurane

Desflurane

Methoxyflurane (not currently available for veterinary use in the UK)

8.13.2 Halo-Hydrocarbons

Halothane (no longer available for veterinary use in the UK)

Further Reading

Alkire, M.T., Hudetz, A.G., and Tononi, G. (2008). Consciousness and anesthesia. *Science* 322: 876–880. (***An excellent review of consciousness and anaesthesi.***).

Aranake, A., Mashour, G.A., and Avidan, M.S. (2013). Minimum alveolar concentration: ongoing relevance and clinical utility. *Anaesthesia* 68: 512–522.

Arch, A.M. and Harper, N.J.N. (2011). Xenon: an element of protection. *Trends in Anaesthesia and Critical Care* 1: 238–242.

Baker, M.T. (2007). Sevoflurane: are there differences in products? *Anesthesia and Analgesia* 104: 1447–1451.

Bates, N., Rawson-Harris, P., and Edwards, N. (2015). Common questions in veterinary toxicology. *Journal of Small Animal Practice* 56: 298–306.

Baumert, J.-H., Reyle-Hahn, M., Hecker, K. et al. (2002). Increased airway resistance during xenon anaesthesia in pigs is attributed to physical properties of the gas. *British Journal of Anaesthesia* 88: 540–545.

Baxter, P.J. and Kharasch, E.D. (1997). Rehydration of desiccated Baralyme prevents carbon monoxide formation from desflurane in an anesthesia machine. *Anesthesiology* 86: 1061–1065.

Baxter, P.J., Garton, K., and Kharasch, E.D. (1998). Mechanistic aspects of carbon monoxide formation from volatile anesthetics. *Anesthesiology* 89: 929–941.

Biber, B., Johannesson, G., Lennander, O. et al. (1984). Intravenous infusion of halothane dissolved in fat. Haemodynamic effects in dogs. *Acta Anaesthesiologica Scandinavica* 28: 385–389.

Bickmore, E.G. and Aziz, E. (2017). The use of activated charcoal filters in anaesthetic circuits in suspected malignant hyperthermia. *Anaesthesia* 72: 1415–1416.

Bilmen, J.G. and Hopkins, P.M. (2019). The use of charcoal filters in malignant hyperthermia: have they found their place? *Anaesthesia* 74: 13–16.

Birgenheier, M., Stoker, R., Westenskow, D., and Orr, J. (2011). Activated charcoal effectively removes inhaled anesthetics from modern anaesthesia machines. *Anesthesia and Analgesia* 112: 1363–1370.

Bovill, J.G. (2008). Inhalation anaesthesia: from diethyl ether to xenon. *Handbook of Experimental Pharmacology* 182: 121–142.

Bosenberg, M. (2011). Anaesthetic gases: environmental impact and alternatives. *South African Journal of Anaesthesia and Analgesia* 17: 345–348.

Brown, S.M. and Sneyd, J.R. (2016). Nitrous oxide in modern anaesthetic practice. *BJA Education* 16: 87–91. (***Reports on ENIGMA-I and ENIGMA-II.***).

Buhre, W., Disma, N., Hendrickz, J. et al. (2019). European Society of Anaesthesiology Task Force on Nitrous Oxide: a narrative review of its role in clinical practice. *British Journal of Anaesthesia* 122: 587–604.

Dai, T., Cheng, W., Yin, Q. et al. (2017). Minimum alveolar concentration: a reconsideration. *Translational Perioperative and Pain Medicine* 2: 13–16.

Eckenhoff, R.G. and Johansson, J.S. (1999). On the relevance of 'clinically relevant concentrations' of inhaled anaesthetics in *in vitro* experiments. *Anesthesiology* 91: 856–860.

Franks, N.P. (2008). General anaesthesia: from molecular targets to neuronal pathways of sleep and arousal. *Nature Reviews Neuroscience* 9: 370–386. (***A comprehensive review of the mechanisms of sleep, arousal and anaesthesia.***).

Gardner, A.J. and Menon, D.K. (2018). Moving to human trials for argon neuroprotection in neurological injury: a narrative review. *British Journal of Anaesthesia* 120: 453–468.

Guo, T.-Z., Davies, M.F., Kingery, W.S. et al. (1999). Nitrous oxide produces antinociceptive response via alpha$_{2B}$ and/or alpha$_{2C}$ adrenoceptor subtypes in mice. *Anesthesiology* 90: 470–476.

Ishizawa, Y. (2011). General anesthetic gases and the global environment. *Anesthesia and Analgesia* 112: 213–217.

Jones, R.S. (2016). Nitrous oxide: the nearly 'ideal' clinical sedative. *The Veterinary Journal* 212: 7–8.

Jones, R.S. and West, E. (2019). Environmental sustainability in veterinary anaesthesia. *Veterinary Anaesthesia and Analgesia* 46: 409–420. https://doi.org/10.1016/j.vaa.2018.12.008. (***An excellent review of veterinary anaesthesia and its environmental impact.***).

Kharash, E.D., Powers, K.M., and Artu, A.A. (2002). Comparison of Amsorb, sodalime and Baralyme degradation of volatile anesthetics and formation of carbon monoxide and compound A in swine *in vivo*. *Anesthesiology* 96: 173–182.

Kunst, G. and Klein, A.A. (2015). Peri-operative anaesthetic myocardial preconditioning and protection – cellular mechanisms and clinical relevance in cardiac anaesthesia. *Anaesthesia* 70: 467–482.

Lillehaug, S.L. and Tinker, J.H. (1991). Why do 'pure' vasodilators cause coronary steal when anaesthetics don't (or seldom do)? *Anesthesia and Analgesia* 73: 681–682.

Loveridge, R. and Schroeder, F. (2010). Anaesthetic preconditioning. *Continuing Education in Anaesthesia, Critical Care and Pain* 10: 38–42.

Lynch, C. (1999). Anesthetic preconditioning: not just for the heart? *Anesthesiology* 91: 606–608.

Moens, Y. and De Moor, A. (1981). Diffusion of nitrous oxide into the intestinal lumen of ponies during halothane-nitrous oxide anesthesia. *American Journal of Veterinary Research* 42: 1751–1753.

Mosing, M. and Senior, J.M. (2018). Maintenance of equine anaesthesia over the last 50 years: controlled inhalation of volatile anaesthetics and pulmonary ventilation. *Equine Veterinary Journal* 50: 282–291.

Mutoh, T., Nishimura, R., and Sasaki, N. (2001). Effects of nitrous oxide on mask induction of anesthesia with sevoflurane or isoflurane in dogs. *American Journal of Veterinary Research* 62: 1727–1733.

Neice, A.E. and Zornow, M.H. (2016). Xenon anaesthesia for all, or only a select few? *British Journal of Anaesthesia* 71: 1259–1272.

Olson, K.N., Klein, L.V., Nann, L.E., and Soma, L.R. (1993). Closed-circuit liquid isoflurane anesthesia in the horse. *Veterinary Surgery* 22: 73–78.

Pang, D.S.J. (2016). Inhalant anaesthetic agents. In: *BSAVA Manual of Canine and Feline Anaesthesia and Analgesia*, 3e (eds. T. Duke-Novakovski, M. de Vries and C. Seymour), 207–213. Gloucester, UK: BSAVA Publications.

Pasternak, J.J. and Lanier, W.L. (2010). Is nitrous oxide use appropriate in neurosurgical and neurologically at-risk patients? *Current Opinion in Anaesthesiology* 23: 544–550.

Porter, K.M., Dayan, A.D., Dickerson, S., and Middleton, P.M. (2018). The role of inhaled methoxyflurane in acute pain management. *Open Access Emergency Medicine* 10: 149–164.

Quasha, A.L., Eger (II), E.I., and Tinker, J.H. (1980). Determination and applications of MAC. *Anesthesiology* 53: 315–334.

Reed, R. and Doherty, T. (2018). Minimum alveolar concentration: key concepts and a review of its pharmacological reduction in dogs. Part 1. *Research in Veterinary Science* 117: 266–270.

Reed, R. and Doherty, T. (2018). Minimum alveolar concentration: key concepts and a review of its pharmacological reduction in dogs. Part 2. *Research in Veterinary Science* 118: 27–33.

Rodrigues Nunes, R., Duval Neto, G.F., Garcia De Alencar, J.C. et al. (2013). Anesthetics, cerebral protection and preconditioning. *Revista Brasileira de Anestesiologia* 63: 119–138.

Saleem Khan, K., Hayes, I., and Buggy, D.J. (2014). Pharmacology of anaesthetic agents II: inhalational anaesthetic agents. *Continuing Education in Anaesthesia, Critical Care and Pain* 14: 106–101.

Sanders, R.D., Franks, N.P., and Maze, M. (2003). Xenon: no stranger to anaesthesia. *British Journal of Anaesthesia* 91: 709–717.

Sanders, R.D. and Maze, M. (2005). Xenon: from stranger to guardian. *Current Opinion in Anaesthesiology* 18: 405–411.

Sanders, R.D., Weimann, J., and Maze, M. (2008). Biologic effects of nitrous oxide. *Anesthesiology* 109: 707–722.

Santangelo, B., Robin, A., Simpson, K. et al. (2017). The modification and performance of a large animal anesthesia machine (Tafonius®) in order to deliver xenon to a horse. *Frontiers in Veterinary Science* 4: 162.

Scarabelli, S. and Bradbrook, C. (2017). Inhalant anaesthetics. *Companion Animal* 22: 134–139.

Schallner, N. and Goebel, U. (2013). The perioperative use of nitrous oxide: renaissance of an old gas or funeral of an ancient relic? *Current Opinion in Anesthesiology* 26: 354–360.

Shan, J., Sun, L., Wang, D., and Li, X. (2015). Comparison of the neuroprotective effects and recovery profiles of isoflurane, sevoflurane and desflurane as neurosurgical pre-conditioning on ischemia/reperfusion cerebral injury. *International Journal of Clinical and Experimental Pathology* 8: 2001–2009.

Soares, J.H.N., Brosnan, R.J., Fukushima, F.B., and Hodges, J. (2012). Solubility of haloether anesthetics in human and animal blood. *Anesthesiology* 117: 48–55.

Sonner, J.M., Antognini, J.F., Dutton, R.C. et al. (2003). Inhaled anesthetics and immobility: mechanisms, mysteries and minimum alveolar anesthetic concentration. *Anesthesia and Analgesia* 97: 718–740.

Soro, M., Badenes, R., Garcia-Perez, M.L. et al. (2010). The accuracy of the anesthetic conserving device (Anaconda), as an alternative to the classical vaporizer in anaesthesia. *Anesthesia and Analgesia* 111: 1176–1179.

Stabernack, C.R., Brown, R., Laster, M.J. et al. (2000). Absorbents differ enormously in their capacity to produce compound A and carbon monoxide. *Anesthesia and Analgesia* 90: 1428–1435.

Strum, D.P. and Eger (II), E.I. (1994). The degradation, absorption and solubility of volatile anesthetics in soda lime depend on water content. *Anesthesia and Analgesia* 78: 340–348.

Sulbaek Andersen, M.P., Sander, S.P., Nielsen, O.J. et al. (2010). Inhalation anaesthetics and climate change. *British Journal of Anaesthesia* 105: 760–766.

Van Hese, L., Al tmimi, L., Devroe, S. et al. (2018). Neuroprotective properties of xenon in different types of CNS injury. *British Journal of Anaesthesia* 121: 1365–1368.

Vollmer, M.K., Rhee, T.S., Rigby, M. et al. (2015). Modern inhalation anesthetics: potent greenhouse gases in the global atmosphere. *Geophysical Research Letters* 42: 1606–1611.

Vutskits, L. and Xie, Z. (2016). Lasting impact of general anaesthesia on the brain: mechanisms and relevance. *Nature Reviews Neuroscience* 17: 705–717. (**An interesting review exploring post-anaesthetic cognitive dysfunction.**).

White, D. (2013). Uses of MAC. *British Journal of Anaesthesia* 91: 167–169.

Zhang, P., Ohara, A., Mashimo, T. et al. (1995). Pulmonary resistance in dogs: a comparison of xenon with nitrous oxide. *Canadian Journal of Anaesthesia* 42: 547–553.

Self-test Section

1   Define MAC$_{awake}$.

2   Rank desflurane, isoflurane, and sevoflurane in order of myocardial ischaemic preconditioning effect.

3   Which of the following statements about sevoflurane is true?

A   Sevoflurane sensitises the myocardium to the arrhythmogenic effects of catecholamines.

B   Sevoflurane causes very little sensitisation of the myocardium to the arrhythmogenic effects of catecholamines.

C   Sevoflurane causes cardiovascular depression/ hypotension mainly by direct myocardial depression.

D   Sevoflurane increases cardiac output through sympathetic nervous system stimulation

9

Anaesthetic Breathing Systems and Airway Devices

LEARNING OBJECTIVES

- To be able to recognise the most commonly used non-rebreathing and rebreathing systems.
- To be able to discuss the factors affecting choice of anaesthetic breathing system.
- To be able to determine the 'fresh gas flow' required to prevent rebreathing of carbon dioxide-rich exhaled gases for the commonly used non-rebreathing systems during spontaneous ventilation.
- To be able to determine appropriate 'fresh gas flows' for the safe use of rebreathing systems.
- To list the ways in which workplace pollution with anaesthetic gases can be reduced.
- To be familiar with the common problems associated with supraglottic airway and endotracheal tube (ETT) use.

9.1 Introduction

Anaesthetic breathing systems deliver oxygen and anaesthetic gases and vapours to the patient and allow elimination of carbon dioxide by means of one of three strategies:

1) Via one-way, non-rebreathing valves (valve-controlled systems), usually situated very close to the patient's mouth, as commonly used in resuscitation equipment
2) Through 'washout' (flow-controlled systems), i.e. the fresh gases continuously delivered to the breathing system effectively 'flush' the carbon dioxide-rich gases away from the patient's mouth and towards the scavenging system. Efficiencies of these systems depend upon the relationship between the fresh gas flow (FGF) and the patient's minute ventilation and the arrangement of components in the breathing system (see below)
3) By the inclusion of a chemical carbon dioxide absorbent

Anaesthetic breathing systems are broadly divided into:

- **Non-rebreathing systems**, which use strategy 2 above.
- **Rebreathing systems**, which use strategy 3 above.

9.2 Terminology

The term *rebreathing* can be quite confusing as the clinical definition of rebreathing (Nunn, 2008), states that: 'Rebreathing occurs when the inspired gas/es reaching the alveoli contain more carbon dioxide than can be accounted for by mere re-inhalation from/of the patient's dead space gas (which should contain negligible carbon dioxide)'. In the context of anaesthetic breathing systems, however, 'rebreathing' does NOT mean that it is permissible for carbon dioxide-rich exhaled gases to be re-inhaled.

FGF refers to those gases that emerge from the common gas outlet (CGO) of the anaesthetic machine, which is where the chosen anaesthetic breathing system attaches. The fresh gases usually consist of oxygen $\pm$ medical air $\pm$ nitrous oxide and may also pass through a vaporiser to 'pick up' volatile anaesthetic agent vapour.

Oxygen is administered at a higher percentage than present in atmospheric air, usually at a minimum of 33% of the inspired mixture. This has historical origins as, in anaesthetised humans, due to ventilation-perfusion mismatching, intrapulmonary shunts of up to 10–15% of cardiac output may develop, and, in order to overcome the

Veterinary Anaesthesia: Principles to Practice, Second Edition. Alexandra H. A. Dugdale, Georgina Beaumont, Carl Bradbrook, and Matthew Gurney.
© 2020 John Wiley & Sons Ltd. Published 2020 by John Wiley & Sons Ltd.
Companion website: www.wiley.com/go/dugdale/veterinary-anaesthesia

subsequent venous admixture (and therefore arterial oxygen desaturation), administration of c. 35% inspired oxygen was generally found sufficient. Note, in horses where intrapulmonary shunts of >20–30% of cardiac output may develop, even 100% inspired oxygen may be insufficient to overcome the ensuing systemic arterial desaturation.

With this figure of c. 33% inspired oxygen in mind, when using non-rebreathing systems, nitrous oxide can be delivered at c. 66%, making good use of its analgesic properties, at least in people (see Chapter 8). In contrast to the nitrous oxide : oxygen ratio of 2:1 used for non-rebreathing systems, there is more danger of supplying insufficient oxygen to the patient when using rebreathing systems, so nitrous oxide is either omitted (this is the safest strategy if you have minimal monitoring) or the nitrous oxide : oxygen ratio can be 1:1.

Minute ventilation (also known as minute respiratory volume) is usually estimated at around 200 ml/kg/min. Although often an over-estimate, using this figure should minimise the risk of carbon dioxide rebreathing when **calculating the FGFs required with non-rebreathing systems**.

Minute ventilation is the volume of air moved into (or out of) the lungs in one minute. This volume can be calculated as the product of tidal volume and respiratory frequency:

Minute ventilation =
Tidal volume × Respiratory frequency

The tidal volume is usually approximated to 10–20 ml/kg. The respiratory frequency will depend upon species and the presence of disease, but can be approximated to 10–20 breaths/min. The product of (10–20) and (10–20) is 100–400 ml/kg/min.

Most texts, however, quote **200 ml/kg/min** as the best mid-range approximation, but minute ventilation will be higher in panting animals.

The first part (about one-third) of an exhaled tidal breath consists of anatomical dead space gases (which are now warm and moist, but have not undergone any gaseous exchange), and the last part (about two-thirds) is from the alveoli, and therefore contains carbon dioxide; there is a little mixing of the two (Figure 9.1). Alveolar minute ventilation is therefore roughly two-thirds of the total minute ventilation.

9.3 Factors to Consider When Choosing a Breathing System

- Patient size (particularly lean body mass) and respiratory capability; consider the resistance offered by the system.
- Mode of ventilation: spontaneous or artificial (i.e. mechanical [or manual] ventilation, usually in the form of positive pressure ventilation).
- Requirement for economy of use of oxygen and anaesthetic gases and vapours.
- If you want to use a circle, do you want to use vaporiser out of circuit/circle (VOC) or vaporiser in circuit/circle (VIC); although the latter is not very commonly used?
- If you want to use low flow in a rebreathing system, are your flowmeters and vaporisers sufficiently accurate at these low flows?
- It is 'usual' to denitrogenate rebreathing systems at the start of the anaesthetic.
- Which inhalation agent/s do you want to use? N_2O, halothane, isoflurane, sevoflurane, desflurane (probably not yet xenon)?
- Be careful with the use of N_2O in rebreathing systems; ideally you should be able to measure the inspired oxygen concentration delivered to the patient.
- Expected length of procedure.
- Requirement for heat and moisture preservation (may partly depend upon length of procedure and size of patient).
- Necessity for sterilisation of equipment after procedure (you may wish to use a disposable breathing system).

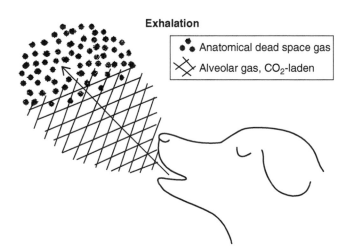

Exhalation

•• Anatomical dead space gas
⧓ Alveolar gas, CO_2-laden

Figure 9.1 Exhaled gases.

- 'Circuit drag' (location of surgery, e.g. head/mouth surgery) because anaesthetic breathing systems may affect surgical access too.
- Ease of scavenging (e.g. where is pop-off valve located?).

9.4 Non-rebreathing Systems

Non-rebreathing systems have been variously classified but Mapleson's classification is the best known and describes the different configurations in alphabetical order (A–F), according to their efficiency with respect to the FGF necessary to prevent rebreathing of CO_2 (Table 9.1). This text will, however, aim to use the actual names of the various breathing systems.

Common non-rebreathing systems:

- T-piece (Mapleson E [without bag]; Mapleson F [with bag])
- Bain (Mapleson D)
- Magill (Mapleson A)
- Lack (Mapleson A)

Table 9.2 illustrates the calculated FGFs for a 30 kg patient in different circumstances. Firstly, using a Bain system and with spontaneous breathing, FGF needs to be 2–4 × minute ventilation. Using oxygen alone, this requires 12–24 l/min. Some oxygen flowmeters are only calibrated up to 10, or even only 8 l/min, so cannot provide sufficient FGF for such a patient. One way round this is to use a combination of nitrous oxide (or medical air) and oxygen, but again, the flows required may be higher than the anaesthetic machine flowmeters are capable of delivering accurately (that is, nitrous oxide [and medical

Table 9.1 Fresh gas flows, in multiples of minute ventilation (MV), required to prevent rebreathing when using non-rebreathing systems during spontaneous and artificial ventilation.

Non-rebreathing system	FGF required to prevent CO_2 rebreathing during Spontaneous ventilation	FGF required to prevent CO_2 rebreathing during Artificial ventilation
T-piece	2 (−4) × MV	1 (−2) × MV
Bain	2 (−4) × MV	1 (−2) × MV
Magill	1 (−2) × MV	2 (−4) × MV*
Lack	1 (−2) × MV	2 (−4) × MV*

Note* that it is generally not recommended to use the Magill or Lack for prolonged provision of artificial ventilation as the actual FGFs required to prevent rebreathing cannot be easily predicted.

air] flowmeters are rarely calibrated beyond 15, or even 10 l/min). So, another option would be to provide artificial ventilation for this patient, thereby halving the FGF requirements with the Bain. A further option would, however, be choice of a more efficient breathing system if spontaneous ventilation is preferred, as represented here by the examples of FGFs required for a Lack system. It is also worth noting that at FGFs greater than around 15 l/min, vaporiser output may be less accurate. The ultimate option would, therefore, be choice of a rebreathing system (see Table 9.3).

From Table 9.3 it can be noted that these FGFs are much more achievable and produce much less wastage than those noted in Table 9.2. When using nitrous oxide in rebreathing systems, it is good practice to monitor the

Table 9.2 Examples of fresh gas flows (FGFs) required to prevent CO_2 rebreathing for a 30 kg patient, with estimated minute ventilation of 200 ml/kg/min (i.e. 6 L/min), during spontaneous ventilation and during the application of artificial ventilation with either a Bain or a Lack non re-breathing system and when using either oxygen alone of a combination of oxygen and nitrous oxide. Note that it is not usually advised to provide long-term artificial ventilation with a Lack.

Non-rebreathing system	FGFs required for Spontaneous ventilation		FGFs required for Artificial ventilation	
	O_2 (L/min)	$O_2 : N_2O$ (L/min : L/min)	O_2 (L/min)	$O_2 : N_2O$ (L/min : L/min)
Bain	12	4:8	6	2:4
	to	to	to	to
	24	8:16	12	4:8
Lack	6	2:4	12	4:8
	to	to	to	to
	12	4:8	24	8:16

Table 9.3 Illustration of fresh gas flows required for a 30 kg patient, with presumed oxygen requirement of 10 ml/kg/min (i.e. 300 ml/min), when using a circle rebreathing system with either oxygen alone or a combination of oxygen and nitrous oxide. No adjustments to FGF should be necessary to switch between spontaneous and artificial ventilation.

	FGFs required O_2 (l/min)	FGFs required $O_2 : N_2O$ (l/min : l/min)
Circle At start of anaesthetic, during denitrogenation and period of rapid uptake of anaesthetic agent by patient	2 to 4	1:1 to 2:2
Circle During maintenance phase, when anaesthetic depth is more stable	0.3	0.3:0.3

oxygen percentage delivered to the patient, or at least to measure oxygenation of the patient's arterial blood (pulse oximetry). It is important to check that the required gas flowmeters are calibrated to the small flows required. Some flowmeters are calibrated down to 100 ml/min whereas others may have their lowest calibration at 250 ml/min, which can limit the use of low flow anaesthesia in patients under 25 kg. Furthermore, when using flows of as little as around 250 ml/min, vaporiser output may not be accurate, thus anaesthetic agent monitoring is advised.

9.4.1 Magill and Lack (Mapleson A)

These function similarly; the Lack in its coaxial or parallel forms is basically like a coaxial or parallel Magill where the pop-off valve is placed at the anaesthetic machine end.

9.4.1.1 Magill

The Magill system is shown in Figure 9.2. The corrugated tube volume should be greater than the patient's (maximum) tidal volume to ensure no carbon dioxide rebreathing. The length of the tube in a standard Magill

system is around 1.1 m. The valve increases the system's resistance, therefore it is not generally used for animals <10 kg.

The characteristics of the Magill system are:

- **Generally used for animals >10 kg and up to around 70–80 kg (but see** Table 9.2 **and the explanation).**
- **FGF needs only to be 1 (−2)×minute ventilation during spontaneous breathing in order to prevent rebreathing of CO₂.** Animals that pant or have high breathing rates have a higher minute ventilation and may also require a relatively higher FGF to prevent rebreathing because of the shortened end-expiratory pause.
- **Quite an efficient system, conserving some of the anatomical dead space gases (warm and moist) for re-use.**
- **Modest apparatus dead space.**
- **Simple design, easy to use.**
- Easy to clean and sterilise.
- **Modest circuit drag** (heavy valve near animal's mouth).
- **Can be easily scavenged from, but scavenging tubing increases circuit drag.**
- **Cumbersome for head/dental surgery.**
- **Not ideal for prolonged artificial ventilation because rebreathing of carbon dioxide is encouraged,** *unless*: the FGF is doubled, adequate end-expiratory pauses are allowed, and nifty operation of the pop-off valve is carried out.

9.4.1.2 Lack

Figure 9.3 shows the coaxial Lack system and Figure 9.4 the parallel Lack system.

The characteristics of the Lack system are:

- **Very similar to the Magill, so FGF should be 1 (−2)×minute ventilation.** This system is **possibly slightly more efficient than the Magill for spontaneous breathing,** so **FGF need only be about 0.8 times minute ventilation, but** FGF requirements do seem to be inversely dependent upon the size of the animal, so that relatively larger animals cope better with relatively smaller FGF. Also animals which pant or have

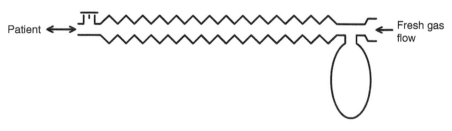

Figure 9.2 A Magill system.

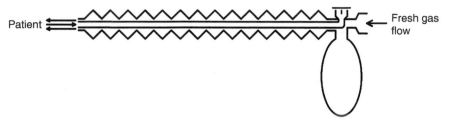

Figure 9.3 The coaxial Lack system.

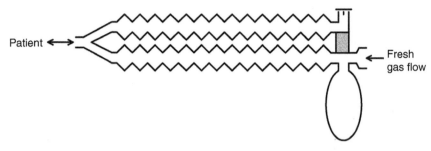

Figure 9.4 The parallel form of the Lack system.

high breathing rates may require higher FGF to prevent carbon dioxide rebreathing.

- **Generally used for animals >10 kg and up to around 70–80 kg (but see** Table 9.2 **and the explanation).**
- **Minimal apparatus dead space (especially the coaxial form).**
- **Resistance seems to be less (especially the parallel from) than that of the Magill,** perhaps because two-way gas flow down one tube does not occur to any great extent.
- **Slightly less circuit drag (valve away from animal's head), although there is a Y-piece in the parallel version, and a more bulky patient end in the coaxial form too** (inner tube is for exhalation, so must be relatively large diameter to reduce resistance; therefore outer tube is even bigger).
- **Beware prolonged artificial ventilation; must double FGF and allow long end-expiratory pauses to prevent carbon dioxide rebreathing. (It is best to use capnography to monitor inspired and expired CO_2 if artificial ventilation is necessary for more than the occasional breath.)**
- **To test the intactness of the inner tube in the coaxial Lack:** insert, as snugly as possible, the tip of an ETT into the patient end of the inner (expiratory) tube; close the pop-off valve (which is located at the 'far' end of this expiratory limb), and then attempt to blow down the ETT. If the inner tube is intact, there should be resistance to your exhalation, and the bag (on the inspiratory limb), should not move. If there is any bag movement, then there is probably a leak in the inner tube.

9.4.1.3 Mini Lack

A mini parallel Lack is available that can be used in patients down to about 2–3 kg. This system is supplied with an extremely low resistance valve and smooth bore tubing (to reduce resistance to breathing), and the tubing is also narrower (and may be shorter), with a special Y-piece with a small septum/shelf in it, to reduce apparatus dead space. The narrower tubing also reduces some of the inevitable mixing of gases, thus reducing the potential for rebreathing of CO_2-laden gases; and it reduces the consequent turbulence, inertia, and therefore resistance of the system.

9.4.1.4 Movement of Gases within the Magill System during Spontaneous Breathing

Figure 9.5 shows how rebreathing of carbon dioxide is avoided during spontaneous breathing. Figure 9.5a represents the situation during early inspiration when some anatomical dead space gases (no CO_2, but warm and moist) from the previous exhalation are inhaled. Figure 9.5b depicts the situation during late inspiration. Figure 9.5c shows the situation during early exhalation. Towards the end of exhalation and during the end-expiratory pause, most of the CO_2-laden exhaled gas is pushed out through the valve, i.e. the pop-off valve is 'popped open' when the pressure in the system builds up again as FGF continues to fill the bag and then the tubing (Figure 9.5d and e).

9.4.1.5 Movement of Gases within the Magill System during Artificial Ventilation

During prolonged artificial ventilation, be this manual or mechanical ventilation, there is a risk of causing the patient

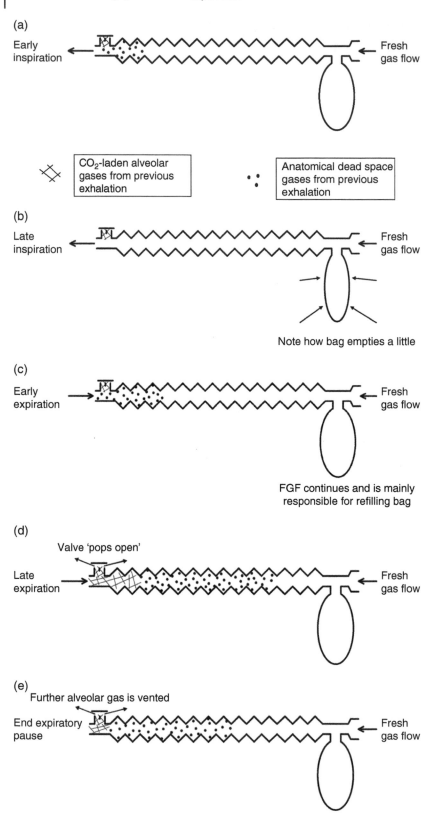

(a)

Early inspiration ← Fresh gas flow →

◇ CO₂-laden alveolar gases from previous exhalation

• Anatomical dead space gases from previous exhalation

(b)

Late inspiration ← Fresh gas flow →

Note how bag empties a little

(c)

Early expiration → Fresh gas flow →

FGF continues and is mainly responsible for refilling bag

(d)

Valve 'pops open'

Late expiration → Fresh gas flow →

(e)

Further alveolar gas is vented

End expiratory pause → Fresh gas flow →

Figure 9.5 Movement of gases within the Magill system during spontaneous breathing.

to rebreathe carbon dioxide. Imagine we are at the start of ventilating the patient's lungs, and the system is full of fresh gases from the anaesthetic machine. In order to get a reasonable chest inflation, we have to close the pop-off valve. Now we can squeeze the bag and we can appreciably empty the reservoir bag (Figure 9.6a). We now let the patient's chest deflate, i.e. let the patient exhale (we need to open the valve again too). The bag was so empty that both the exhaled gases from the patient and the fresh gases from the anaesthetic machine can enter the reservoir bag (Figure 9.6b).

After the first breath of artificial ventilation, during the end-expiratory pause, the FGF will purge much of the CO_2-laden gas from the tubing and out through the pop-off valve (if we remembered to open it again, and if we leave a long-ish end-expiratory pause). However, the

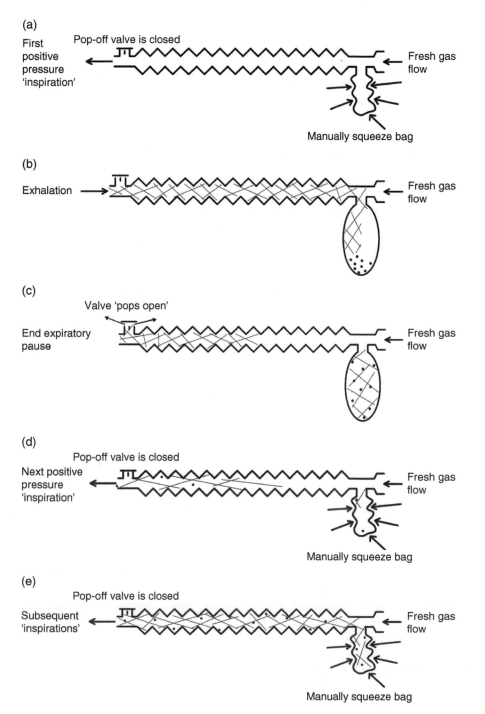

(a)

First positive pressure 'inspiration'

Pop-off valve is closed

Fresh gas flow

Manually squeeze bag

(b)

Exhalation

Fresh gas flow

(c)

Valve 'pops open'

End expiratory pause

Fresh gas flow

(d)

Pop-off valve is closed

Next positive pressure 'inspiration'

Fresh gas flow

Manually squeeze bag

(e)

Pop-off valve is closed

Subsequent 'inspirations'

Fresh gas flow

Manually squeeze bag

Figure 9.6 Movement of gases within the Magill system during artificial ventilation (manual or mechanical ventilation).

tubing tends not to be fully purged of CO_2-laden gas between breaths because it takes more FGF to refill the 'relatively empty' bag, so it takes longer to reach the breathing system pressure at which the valve 'pops open'. Some FGF, however, does enter the bag to dilute any CO_2 within it somewhat. The situation during the end-expiratory pause is shown in Figure 9.6c. Now imagine it is time for another inspiration. We need to close the pop-off valve again, and squeeze the bag again, but this time the tube and bag contain some CO_2 (Figure 9.6d). Imagine that we now give several more breaths. Breath by breath, as the patient's alveolar gas (CO_2-laden) continues to reach the reservoir bag, the concentration of CO_2 in the reservoir bag increases. Also, the tube is incompletely purged of CO_2-laden gas, especially if we allow only a relatively short end-expiratory pause. We can now see how the patient is forced to rebreathe much of its previously exhaled, CO_2-laden, gases. Therefore, the Magill and also the Lack (because it works in a similar fashion) are not very good for prolonged artificial ventilation (Figure 9.6e). However, if we:

- Increase the FGF (to c. $2\times$ minute ventilation (compared with $1\times$ minute ventilation for spontaneous breathing); and
- Remember to allow a long end-expiratory pause (i.e. do not ventilate too rapidly; we should not need to ventilate too rapidly anyway because we more than compensate for a slow rate by tending to give a larger tidal volume). This allows a long time for FGF to purge the tubing of CO_2 and further dilute what may be in the bag, then there is less potential for causing carbon dioxide rebreathing. So, it is possible to use the Magill and Lack for more prolonged artificial ventilation, but you must heed these rules. It also helps to use capnography as part of the patient's monitoring, as this will indicate increasing inspired and expired CO_2 values.

9.4.2 The T-piece

The original design (Ayre's T-piece) consisted of a T-shaped connector attached to a length of tube (the 'expiratory [reservoir] limb') and also to a fresh gas supply hose, which connects to the CGO on the anaesthetic machine (Figure 9.7).

The volume of the corrugated expiratory/reservoir limb should be greater than the patient's (maximum) tidal volume, or else outside air will be entrained during inspiration, which will dilute the O_2/N_2O and anaesthetic vapour being delivered to the patient. Normally the FGF, is at right angles to the direction of gas flowing into and out of the patient, but other configurations are possible (see below under T-piece modifications).

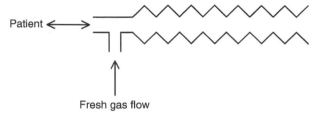

Figure 9.7 Ayre's T-piece (Mapleson E).

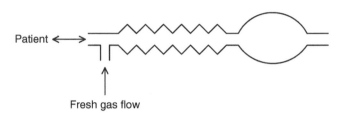

Figure 9.8 Jackson Rees modification of Ayre's T-piece (Mapleson F).

Using an original Ayre's T-piece, the patient's lungs can only be artificially ventilated by intermittent occlusion of the open end of the expiratory limb (e.g. using your thumb!), until the chest inflates, and then releasing the occlusion to allow exhalation, none of which allows for a very good pattern of ventilation (i.e. inflation tends to be too prolonged). The Jackson Rees modification of the Ayre's T-piece (Figure 9.8), in which an open-ended bag is placed at the end of the expiratory limb, allows much easier application of artificial ventilation because the open end of the bag can be occluded, and once the bag has filled sufficiently, it can be squeezed gently to create a much better (more rapid, more physiological) lung inflation. Squeezing the bag allows some assessment of the compliance of the lungs too. Bag movements can also be observed during spontaneous ventilation to allow some assessment of the patient's spontaneous breathing.

Characteristics of T-pieces:

- Used for **animals <10 kg.**
- **FGF needs to be 2–4$\times$ minute ventilation to ensure no carbon dioxide rebreathing**. If the animal is panting, there may be insufficient time for the FGF to purge the system of CO_2 between breaths, so you may need to increase the FGF further.
- **Minimal apparatus dead space:** *apparatus (or mechanical) dead space* is defined as an extension of the patient's own anatomical dead space. Anatomical dead space is the volume of the respiratory tree where no gas exchange occurs, i.e. the upper respiratory tract from the nares down to the respiratory bronchioles; but gases are still warmed and humidified. **Apparatus dead space** is recognised as the volume within the anaesthetic

breathing system between the incisor arcade and that part of the anaesthetic breathing system where the inspired and expired gas streams divide.

- **Low resistance**, especially in the Ayre's T-piece form. Once a bag is added, the resistance of the system may be increased slightly. To minimise this, a small 'cage' may be attached to the connector placed in the neck of the bag (referred to as a cage-mount connector), which ensures that the bag cannot flatten or deflate completely, because complete deflation increases the resistance to breathing.
- **Simple design, easy to use**.
- **Easy to clean** and sterilise.
- Cheap disposable versions available.
- **Modest circuit drag** because two (small) tubes are near the patient's mouth.
- **Can apply prolonged artificial ventilation (Jackson Rees modification best)**.
- **Not easy to scavenge from open-ended tube or bag** (and from the bag, without kinking the bag neck or outlet, thus risking cardiovascular compromise and/or lung damage).

9.4.2.1 How a T-piece Works
The movement of gases within a T-piece during spontaneous breathing is shown in Figure 9.9.

9.4.2.2 T-piece Modifications
9.4.2.2.1 The Y-piece
The Y-piece allows the fresh gas inlet to be angled towards the patient (Figure 9.10). This increases the resistance to exhalation (because exhalation is directly into the face of the oncoming FGF), and adds a slight positive pressure to inhalation, assisting inhalation. This continuous positive airway pressure (CPAP) is favoured in many human neonatal clinics because it reduces the tendency of the neonatal lungs to collapse. The Y-piece also reduces the functional apparatus dead space slightly by a flushing effect (during the end-expiratory pause) when fresh gases are still flowing (see below). Minimising the apparatus dead space minimises the risk of rebreathing.

9.4.2.2.2 The Cape Town Arrangement
This design brings the FGF entry point as close to the patient's mouth as possible, thus minimising apparatus dead space (which minimises the potential for rebreathing) and also provides CPAP (Figure 9.11).

9.4.2.2.3 Apparatus Dead Space and Functional Apparatus Dead Space
Functional apparatus dead space is greater with the original T-piece configuration (Figure 9.12a) than with the Y-piece configuration (Figure 9.12b).

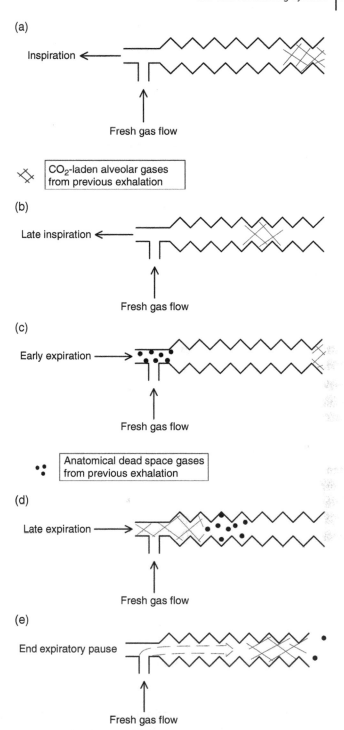

Figure 9.9 Movement of gases within a T-piece during spontaneous breathing. Note how during the end-expiratory pause the FGF helps purge carbon dioxide from the system.

9.4.2.2.4 Mapleson D System
One anaesthetic breathing system often sold as a T-piece is really a small Mapleson D system (Figure 9.13). It can be used in animals between about 3 and 10 kg because it has a low resistance valve and small bore corrugated tubing.

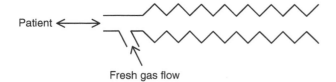

Figure 9.10 Modification at patient connector (Y-piece).

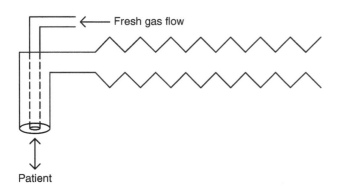

Figure 9.11 Cape Town arrangement.

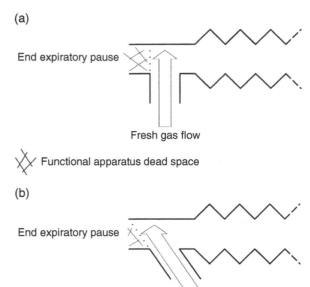

Figure 9.12 Functional apparatus dead space is greater with (a) the original T-piece configuration than (b) the Y-piece configuration.

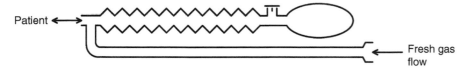

Figure 9.13 Mapleson D system.

9.4.3 Bain (Mapleson D) System

Bain modified the Mapleson D system by creating a coaxial tube arrangement. It functions similarly to the T-piece and has a broadly similar efficiency regarding rebreathing (Figure 9.14). The fresh gas **in**flow is through the **in**ner tube in a Ba**in**.

The **addition of valves usually adds resistance to a system,** which requires the animal to be able to generate higher pressures during breathing, which usually means more of a problem for smaller patients. The **coaxial arrangement** of tubes also **increases the resistance** compared with a parallel arrangement and increases the work of breathing for the patient.

The volume of the corrugated (expiratory/reservoir limb) tube and bag should be greater than the (maximum) tidal volume of the patient. Bain systems are usually available in three lengths: 1.8, 2.7 and 5.4 m. The longer the tube, the more the resistance to gas flows. However, animals >10 kg and up to about 80 kg can usually cope with these systems.

Very large dogs have high peak inspiratory flow requirements, and the relatively narrow tubing creates a higher resistance under these circumstances. Also the very high FGFs required for these large animals cause some of the CO_2-laden exhaled gases to be 'pulled' back towards the patient (the Venturi effect) to cause some rebreathing. Other possible problems for very large patients are that: some oxygen/medical air/nitrous oxide flowmeters do not provide high enough flows for larger animals, especially if using only oxygen and not, e.g. O_2/N_2O mixtures; and at very high FGF (e.g. >15 l/min), most vaporisers no longer deliver the concentration 'dialled up' (see Table 9.2).

The characteristics of the Bain system are:

- Used for **animals >10 kg and up to 70–80 kg (but see Table 9.2 and the explanation).**
- **FGF needs to be 2–4 × minute ventilation to prevent rebreathing during spontaneous breathing. Panting animals may require higher FGF.**
- **Inhaled fresh gases are thought to be warmed slightly by heat transfer from the warm exhaled gases in the surrounding tube (counter current system).**
- **Relatively low resistance (but greater than the T-piece).**

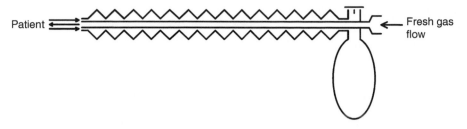

Figure 9.14 Bain system.

- **Minimal apparatus dead space**.
- Fairly simple design but **beware disconnection or leakage of inner tube** which facilitates rebreathing. **Test the intactness of the inner tube** by attaching the system to the CGO of the anaesthetic machine; then turn on say 2 l/min O_2 flow. Now occlude the patient end of the inner tube with a pen or pencil and watch the O_2 flowmeter indicator float (bobbin or ball); it should 'fall'. If it does not, the inner fresh gas delivery tube is broken or disconnected. An alternative test is the Pethick test. Connect the Bain system to the CGO and check the bag is not flat-empty. If it is, then use oxygen (either turn on the oxygen flow or use the oxygen flush facility) momentarily so as to ensure the bag has some contents (you may need to close the pop-off valve and occlude the patient end to do this). Then, with the patient end unoccluded, activate the oxygen flush valve. If the inner tube is intact, the fast oxygen flow through the inner tube should produce a Venturi effect at the patient end that draws gases from the outer tube and bag, so the bag should deflate and flatten. If the bag does not deflate, or even inflates, then the inner tube is not intact. Of both these tests, the inner tube occlusion test seems to be most sensitive and most preferred.
- **Minimal circuit drag**.
- **Easy to scavenge**.
- Disposable versions available.
- **Can be used for prolonged artificial ventilation.**
- **FGF can be reduced** to nearer 1×minute ventilation **for artificial ventilation, if** you either: (i) Aim to **hyper-ventilate slightly** (i.e. blow off a bit too much CO_2) because this hyperventilation is then 'offset' by the CO_2 rebreathing that follows the reduction in FGF. This is called **deliberate functional rebreathing**. **Alternatively**, (ii) you can aim to provide artificial ventilation with a **relatively large tidal volume and a relatively slow rate**, so the extra-long end-expiratory pause allows FGF to purge the system of CO_2-laden gases between breaths. However, it is **advisable to use capnography** to monitor for potential rebreathing during prolonged artificial ventilation (see Chapter 18).

9.5 Non-rebreathing Systems Compared with Rebreathing Systems

9.5.1 Advantages

- Simple construction, easy to use, generally easy to clean.
- No carbon dioxide absorbent necessary (possibly cheaper [but higher gas flows are required]; less resistance).
- Minimal apparatus dead space.
- Make the best use of precision vaporisers (i.e. the inspired vapour concentration delivered by the FGF should be that which is dialled up on the vaporiser).
- Lowish resistance (especially systems without valves; none have carbon dioxide absorbent).
- No need for denitrogenation of the system.
- Can use N_2O safely.
- Cheap disposable versions available.
- Can scavenge easily from most of the systems.

9.5.2 Disadvantages

- Poor economy because high FGF wastes lots of O_2 and medical air or N_2O; and high FGF also leads to high consumption of volatile inhalation agent, therefore much wastage.
- At FGFs much above 15 l/min, vaporiser output may be lower than the dialled up percentage.
- Must scavenge (lots of 'waste' gases to dispose of).
- Consider mode of ventilation (spontaneous versus artificial ventilation; remember problems associated with prolonged artificial ventilation with the Magill and Lack).
- The loss of rebreathable humidified and warmed gases with most systems promotes hypothermia and dehydration, especially in small patients; and results in reduced function of the respiratory mucociliary escalator, with increased potential for obstruction of the airways with drying secretions.
- High gas flows also increase the risk of cardiovascular embarrassment (through obstruction of venous return) and trauma to the lungs (potentially causing pneumothorax), should there be an obstruction to the anaesthetic breathing system outflow.

- For patients that develop malignant hyperthermia, it may not be possible to increase FGFs sufficiently to flush out the increased CO_2 produced by the patient, thus rebreathing systems (ideally 'new' and incorporating activated charcoal filters on the inspiratory and expiratory limbs) *may* be favoured, although the CO_2 absorbent can harbour halogenated agents.

9.6 Heat and Moisture Exchangers (HMEs)

HMEs, often with integral bacterial filters (HMEFs), are available that help conserve the warmth and humidity of exhaled gases. They consist of some form of membrane, usually impregnated with a hygroscopic chemical such as calcium chloride, and act as condensers ('artificial noses'). They are often used with non-rebreathing systems and in small patients undergoing long procedures. It may take up to 20 minutes of continued use for HMEs to reach their best performance. HMEs usually add little in the way of resistance, although they may add some apparatus dead space depending upon the size used, but they are available in several sizes to suit different patient sizes, and most have a gas sampling port to facilitate, e.g. sidestream capnography.

9.7 Pop-off or APL (Adjustable Pressure Limiting) Valves

A valve may be partly or fully open (Figure 9.15a). The valve leaflet/disc (which may be attached to a stem) rests on the valve's knife-edge seating; and depending how 'open' the valve is, variable tension is applied to a spring which acts on the valve disc. Now, when pressure within the system builds up and reaches the set pop-off pressure (determined by how tightly the spring holds the valve disc down onto the valve seating), then the valve leaflet lifts from the seating, and gases can escape, ideally into the scavenging system. When the valve is fully 'open', pressures as low as 1.5 cmH₂O within the breathing system are sufficient to lift the valve leaflet off its seating (it 'pops-off'), allowing excess gases to be vented through the valve and into the scavenging system. When the valve is fully 'closed' (Figure 9.15b), the valve leaflet is held tight against the valve seating by the spring. With old-fashioned valves, even very high pressures within the system could not open a 'closed' valve. However, modern valves now incorporate a safety relief mechanism that activates at higher pressures (usually c. 28–35 cmH₂O for human paediatric patients and 60 cmH₂O for human adults).

(a)

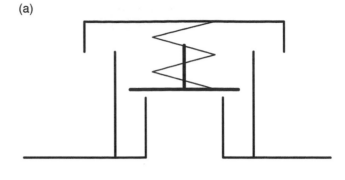

(b)

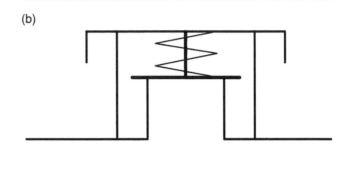

Figure 9.15 Adjustable pressure-limiting ('pop-off') valves in (a) the open and (b) the closed position.

9.8 Bag Terminology

The term *reservoir bag* is usually used for the bag in any breathing system where none of the patient's exhaled gases ever pass back into the bag. Strictly, this means only the bags in the Mapleson A systems (e.g. the Magill and Lack) where the bag is on the inspiratory limb, but beware when artificial ventilation is provided for more than a few breaths with these systems as exhaled gases will enter the bag. Some people also include the bags in the Jackson Rees modified Ayre's T-piece and Bain systems, saying that if none of the exhaled gases are actually rebreathed by the animal (i.e. they should all be flushed far enough downstream by the FGF) then the bags act only as reservoir bags.

The term *rebreathing bag* is used for the bag in any breathing system where the patient's exhaled gases can/do pass into the bag. Therefore, this is strictly the correct term for the bags in the Jackson Rees modified Ayre's T-piece, the Bain, and also the rebreathing systems like Waters' To and Fro and the circle.

The chosen bag should be of such a size that the capacity to which it may be easily distended must exceed the patient's tidal volume. Ideally, it should have a capacity of one to three times the patient's maximum tidal volume, which is roughly two to six times the patient's normal tidal volume. Although larger bags are safer (they more easily absorb volume/pressure increases, thus protecting the patient), they increase the time constant in rebreathing systems (i.e. they slow down the rate of change of anaesthetic agent concentration when the vaporiser setting is altered).

9.9 Hybrid Systems

9.9.1 The Humphrey ADE System and Circle

This is 'one' system that, by switching the position of a lever, or adding a carbon dioxide absorber canister with inspiratory and expiratory valves, can be converted between:

- A Magill/Lack type system (the Mapleson A) for best efficiency during spontaneous breathing.
- A Bain/T-piece type system (Mapleson D/E) for best efficiency during artificial ventilation.
- A circle with carbon dioxide absorbent, for best efficiency regardless of ventilation mode.

The system used to be available in coaxial and parallel forms, but now is marketed most commonly in the parallel form. The system requires regular maintenance and servicing but is very smartly engineered. It is supplied with narrow, smooth-bore hoses and a special low resistance pop-off valve (see below). It is marketed as being useful for patients between 30 g and 100 kg, by choosing the configuration most appropriate for the patient's size and needs. It is most commonly used in the A or D/E modes for patients <7–10 kg, whereas the circle configuration is usually preferred for patients >7–10 kg.

In the A configuration, it acts like a parallel Lack, whereas in the D/E configuration, it acts like a Bain/T-piece and is designed to allow artificial ventilation in this mode. It is therefore easy to switch between A (spontaneous breathing) and D/E configurations (artificial ventilation) without changing the FGF because the efficiency of the Mapleson A system for spontaneous breathing equals that of the Mapleson D system for artificial ventilation. In the 'A' mode, this system has been shown to be **even more efficient than a standard Magill or Lack** because the special design of the pop-off valve (a chimneyed, self-regulating, 4-phase exhaust valve) enables conservation of even more of the fresh gases and dead space gases during exhalation. Indeed, FGFs of around 100 ml/kg/min are sufficient to prevent rebreathing in many patients of <7–10 kg. The valve itself also provides around 1 cmH$_2$O positive end expiratory pressure, which may be advantageous.

A carbon dioxide absorber canister can be added, which also incorporates inspiratory and expiratory valves, enabling conversion of the system into a circle. The rebreathing bag becomes located on the inspiratory limb of the circle, which, alongside the special pop-off valve, helps to conserve fresh gases and improves the efficiency of the system.

9.10 Rebreathing Systems

These include a canister containing carbon dioxide absorbent to remove CO$_2$ from the gases in the system. They also tend to be used with FGF rates less than the patient's minute ventilation; but for the first 20 minutes or so of their use, the FGF is often higher. This allows the system, and indeed the patient's lung functional residual capacity (FRC), to be purged of 'air' (78% nitrogen), and allows a quicker increase in oxygen and anaesthetic vapour concentration to build up in the system. Using higher FGF for this 'nitrogen washout' or **denitrogenation** also reduces the chance of delivering an oxygen-poor gas mixture to the patient by discouraging nitrogen from building up in the system and diluting the gases delivered to the breathing system from the anaesthetic machine. After this initial denitrogenation phase, the FGF can be reduced so that the 'pop-off valve' (a safety release valve should the pressure of gases within the system exceed 'safe' levels) should not need to vent gases (and could even be closed) if the oxygen and anaesthetic inflows are reduced to become exactly equivalent to the patient's uptake; all exhaled carbon dioxide being absorbed. Such 'closed-system anaesthesia' is the perfect example of a 'low flow' technique (see below).

The patient's oxygen and anaesthetic demands can vary from minute to minute, depending upon factors such as patient size, metabolic rate, temperature, and depth of anaesthesia, making it is very difficult to perform true low flow (closed-system) anaesthesia (see below). Instead, we tend to supply a little extra oxygen and anaesthetic, allowing the excess 'gases' to vent through the pop-off valve, which is therefore left open.

Oxygen requirements are normally around 4–10 ml/ kg/min, but scale allometrically (disproportionately) with body mass, such that oxygen requirements vary according to metabolic body mass, which itself related to body surface area. As smaller animals tend to have relatively larger body surface areas, they also tend to have higher relative oxygen demands. For this reason, a safe minimum oxygen provision would be 10 ml/kg/min, especially for small animal patients.

Low flow has been variously defined, but one useful definition is that it is the situation when **O_2 flow rate equals the metabolic oxygen demand** (i.e. around 4–10 ml/kg/min).

Medium flow is the situation when the **FGF supplies more than the metabolic O_2 demand, but FGF is less than minute ventilation**.

High flow is the situation when **FGF exceeds minute ventilation**, e.g. most commonly used for non-rebreathing systems.

An example of how to use a circle system for a 30 kg Labrador:

- After induction of anaesthesia, a FGF of, say, 2 l/min could be used for the first 15–20 minutes. This could consist of only oxygen; or a 50:50 mixture of nitrous oxide and oxygen (i.e. 1 l/min nitrous oxide and 1 l/min oxygen); or a 50:50 mixture of medical air and oxygen (i.e. 1 l/min air and 1 l/min oxygen). Such a 'medium flow' facilitates stabilisation of the anaesthetic depth during a time of rapid uptake of volatile anaesthetic agent by the patient; and also, when the FGF does not include medical air (a source of nitrogen), facilitates denitrogenation of the circle and the patient's tissues
- The FGF could then be reduced to 1 l/min. Again, this could consist of only oxygen; or a 50:50 mixture of nitrous oxide and oxygen (i.e. 500 ml/min nitrous oxide and 500 ml/min oxygen); or a 50:50 mixture of air and oxygen (i.e. 500 ml/min air and 500 ml/min oxygen)
- After a further 15–20 minutes as above, if the anaesthetic depth is stable, the FGF could be reduced further to the estimated safe minimum oxygen requirement of 10 ml/kg/min. This would require an oxygen flow of 300 ml/min; or the oxygen requirement could be provided in a 50:50 mixture of 300 ml/min oxygen and 300 ml/min nitrous oxide (if the flowmeters are calibrated accurately at these low flows); or this could be provided as a mixture of 250 ml/min oxygen with 250 ml/min air (as the overall oxygen provision in this 500 ml/min mixture would be equivalent to 300 ml/min of 100% oxygen). Note that whatever the desired mixture of gases, the minimum oxygen requirement of 300 ml/min must be supplied
  - To enhance patient safety, it is recommended that the inspired oxygen percentage is monitored.
  - Monitoring end tidal anaesthetic agent concentration can help with anaesthetic depth management.
    - In order to change anaesthetic depth quickly, both the FGF and the vaporiser setting should be changed, even by relatively 'large' amounts.
    - Vaporisers tend to lose accuracy of their output at flows below about 250–500 ml/min.
  - If sidestream capnography (with sampling rates around 200 ml/min) is performed when low FGFs are

employed, it is important to return the sampled gases back to the breathing system after analysis, otherwise considerable 'loss' of gases occurs.

9.10.1 To and Fro

Figure 9.16 shows a To and Fro. Some of the first To and Fro systems were constructed using a Waters' canister to hold the carbon dioxide absorbent, hence these systems were known as Waters' To and Fro systems. The pop-off valve may be positioned as shown in Figure 9.16, or alternatively, be situated between the canister and the bag. The continually reversing gas flow creates **resistance due to inertia**. Extra resistance to breathing comes from the **carbon dioxide absorbent and valve**. A To and Fro system is usually used for **animals >10–15 kg**. The canister's capacity and rebreathing bag's capacity determine the maximum size of patient. **Rebreathing bags** should have a **capacity of 2–6 × the normal/resting tidal volume (i.e. 1–3 × the maximum tidal volume)**.

9.10.1.1 Problems with the Horizontal Canisters in a to and Fro System

No matter how well you fill the canister, the granules always 'settle' with time, so that a small channel, empty of granules, forms at the upper side of the canister (Figure 9.17a). Gases passing backwards and forwards, to and from the patient, will take the path of least resistance, and so will follow any channels because the path is unhindered by granules. Unfortunately, this **channelling** means that the gases do not contact so many of the granules, and so CO_2 absorption is very poor. The patient is then forced to breathe gases with a high carbon dioxide content.

Even if a canister is well-packed with granules, minimising channelling, the **absorbent becomes exhausted at the end of the canister nearest the patient first** because this is where the exhaled CO_2 first meets active granules (Figure 9.17b). As the granules become exhausted, the face of active absorbent moves further and further away from the patient, so more and more of the exhaled gases do not reach active absorbent. This **effectively increases the apparatus dead space of**

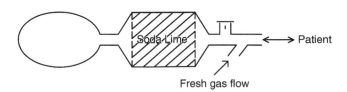

Figure 9.16 To and Fro.

Figure 9.17 Problems with horizontal canisters. (a) A small channel, empty of granules, may form at the upper side of the canister. (b) The soda lime becomes exhausted at the end of the canister nearest the patient first.

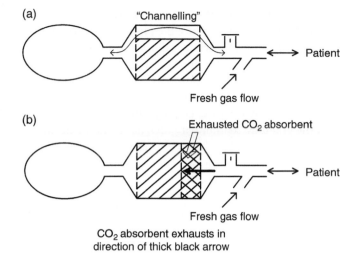

the system and can **lead to rebreathing of carbon dioxide**.

Because the patient's end tidal gases should reach/interact with active absorbent, the length of tubing between the patient and the canister should be kept as short as possible to keep the apparatus dead space, at least initially, as small as possible. This means that the canister must be close to the mouth, which is very **cumbersome, especially for dental or oral surgery**.

The other problem with this proximity of patient to canister is that because most absorbent granules are quite dusty, the **dust is easily inhaled by the patient** over this short distance. The dust is quite **irritant to the tracheobronchial tree** especially if the absorbent contains alkali, and can cause a chemical bronchitis. To reduce this prob-

lem, a piece of fine material, usually muslin, can be placed at the end of the canister nearest to the patient, to filter out some of the dust, but without excessively increasing the resistance of the system.

Although the absorber canister can be placed vertically, this is very difficult to achieve whilst maintaining the minimum tube length between patient and canister. Vertical canisters are much more easily employed in circle systems.

9.10.2   Circle Systems

The word 'circuit' strictly only applies to circle systems because of the circuitous flow of gases around the system (Figure 9.18).

Figure 9.18   Circle system.

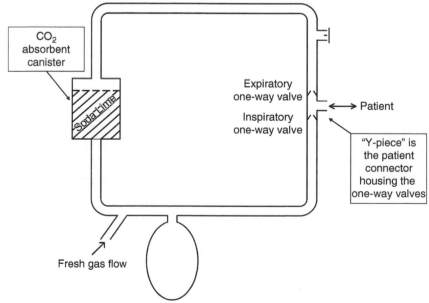

Carbon dioxide absorber canisters are usually supported in a vertical position to reduce the problems of channelling. The canister height : width ratio should ideally be 1:1. Usually canisters are not filled right to the top so that gases entering at the top of the canister can slow down. This helps to keep the circuit resistance to a minimum, whilst at the same time increasing the contact time between the gases and the granules, so improving CO_2 absorption efficiency.

Within the canister, the lowest resistance to gas flow is along the walls of the canister because one 'side' of the passage is the relatively smooth interior surface of the canister wall. This results in a sort of channelling of gas flow; so in order to minimise this, annular rings (baffles) are often placed within the canister to try to encourage (redirect) gases to flow more through the centre of the canister, where the gas flow comes into contact with granules on all sides.

The one-way inspiratory and expiratory valves may be housed in the Y-piece, or they can be moved further away from the patient. They are commonly located on the carbon dioxide absorber canister as 'turret' valves in some large animal circle systems. For maximum efficiency, however, they should be located within the Y-piece. For ease of construction, the pop-off valve is often placed nearer the bag and canister than shown in Figure 9.18, but this slightly reduces the efficiency of the system.

The **one-way valves** (inspiratory and expiratory) that help to **maintain the unidirectional/circular flow of gases around the circle** and the carbon dioxide absorbent granules do **add extra resistance** to breathing, and **so** circles are normally used for **animals >15 kg**. However, modern valves can be made of extremely lightweight materials, and the resistance they offer is much less than traditional valves, so that some makes of circles can be used on patients down to about 7 kg. These circles usually include appropriately scaled (small) absorber canisters, smaller rebreathing bags, and small-bore tubing which may even be smooth-bore too. These paediatric circles also tend to have special Y-pieces that have a septum in them, so that the mechanical/apparatus dead space is minimised, and therefore rebreathing of CO_2-laden gas is minimised.

There are many different designs for circles, but for best efficiency, a few rules should be followed:

- The rebreathing bag and the patient should be on opposite sides of the one-way (inspiratory and expiratory) valves. Rebreathing bags should have a capacity of two to six times the normal/resting tidal volume.
- The FGF entry point should not be between the patient and the expiratory valve.
- The pop-off valve should not be between the patient and the inspiratory valve.
- The rebreathing bag is best positioned between the FGF inlet and the inspiratory valve.

- The one-way valves are ideally positioned within the Y-piece as with this configuration, there is minimal mixing of dead space and alveolar gases. Furthermore, with this configuration, the pop-off valve may also be positioned within the Y-piece to allow more selective venting of alveolar (CO_2-laden) gas, which prolongs the 'life' of the absorbent. Circuit drag is, however, increased.

The 'normal' small animal (or adult human) circles can be used for patients up to about 135 kg (possibly up to 150 kg), with sufficiently large absorbent canister and rebreathing bag, but for animals larger than this, a large animal circle is required. Sometimes the size of the ETT determines which circle can be used, as the smaller tubes may not have connectors which are compatible with the Y-pieces of larger circles and vice versa.

The circle described above is used when the vaporiser for the inhalation agent of choice is situated out of the circle itself **(VOC)**. However, there are several designs of circles where a vaporiser can be incorporated into the circle **(VIC)**. These include the **Komesaroff machine** and the **Stephens circle**. (See Chapter 10 for information on vaporisers.) In-circle vaporisers (low resistance, draw-over types) are usually placed in the inspiratory limb, which also reduces contamination of liquid agent by condensed water vapour, which otherwise occurs readily if vaporisers are placed in the expiratory limb as exhaled gases are moist.

9.10.3   The Universal F Circuit

This system is basically a circle, but the inspiratory and expiratory tubes to and from the patient are within each other for a distance (so it is like a coaxial circle) (Figure 9.19). There is less circuit drag (it is less bulky) at the patient end than with the conventional circle. More heat conservation is possible (counter current exchange).

9.10.4   Considerations When Using Rebreathing Systems

9.10.4.1   Anaesthetic Agent Concentration
With rebreathing systems, because the FGF from the anaesthetic machine is diluted by exhaled gases and the other gases within the system before being inspired by the patient, it is difficult to know exactly what concentrations of oxygen, nitrous oxide and inhalation agent the animal does inspire with each breath, unless these are measured.

9.10.4.2   Time Constants
The rate of change of anaesthetic agent concentration in rebreathing systems is proportional to the fresh gas inflow from the anaesthetic machine, and inversely proportional to the volume of the system.

Figure 9.19 F circuit (first described by Dr Fukunaga from Japan).

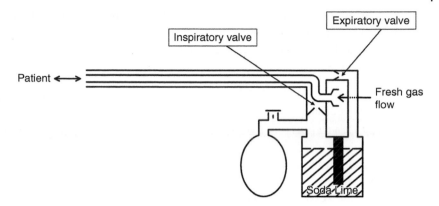

$$\text{Time constant of the system} = \frac{\text{Volume of breathing system}}{\text{Fresh gas inflow}}$$

If we change the vaporiser setting (in order to change the anaesthetic concentration in the system) without changing FGF or patient uptake:

- After one time constant, the change in anaesthetic agent concentration in the system can be expected to be 63.2% complete.
- After two time constants, the change is 86.7% complete.
- After three time constants, the change is 95% complete.
- After four time constants, the change is 98.1% complete.
- **After five time constants**, the **change is 99.33% complete**.

You need to allow at least three, and preferably five, time constants for 'equilibration'.

From this, you will see that if you want a more rapid change (increase or decrease) in anaesthetic concentration in the system, you will have to increase the FGF, and/or change (increase or decrease) the dial setting on the vaporiser by more than what you actually want to achieve, but then you must remember not to leave it like this for too long or you could end up delivering too much or too little anaesthetic agent to your patient.

If you need to reduce the anaesthetic agent concentration within the system rapidly, the vaporiser is switched off, the bag can be 'dumped' (i.e. emptied by expressing its contents out through the pop-off valve), and the oxygen flush control activated to fill the system with oxygen (and/or the oxygen flowmeter turned up, but this may be too slow to refill the system quickly enough for the patient's next breath). The bag often requires dumping more than once because even with the vaporiser switched off, the exhaled gases from the patient will contain some volatile agent, and the carbon dioxide absorbent can also harbour volatile agents. (Oxygen delivered from the 'oxygen flush' valve bypasses the vaporiser.)

9.10.4.3 Carbon Dioxide Absorbents

Soda lime is the most familiar carbon dioxide absorbent. Classically, soda lime consists of:

- **calcium hydroxide** (80 + %)
- **hygroscopic sodium hydroxide and/or potassium hydroxide as 'activators'**
- kieselguhr or silica as **'hardeners'** to **reduce dust formation,** which:
  - increases resistance in the canister
  - may also cause caking of granules (granules become clumped together by the dust), which can increase channelling and reduce absorption efficiency
  - may enter the rest of the breathing system where it can settle out to cause, e.g. one-way valve malfunction or increase the likelihood of leaks around the absorber canister gasket
  - may enter the patient's respiratory tract where it can cause caustic burns
- 14–20% added **water** (to help the reactions get going)
- a pH indicator dye
  - The two common dyes are ethyl violet, where the granules begin 'white' and change colour to purple as they are exhausted, and Clayton yellow (also known as Titan yellow), where the granules start off bright pink, and turn off-white as they are exhausted. After the end of an anaesthetic, some granules may appear to regenerate (i.e. change colour back to their starting colour), which might be confusing. This is because active chemicals (hydroxide ions) from the centre of the granules can diffuse to the surface, diluting the carbonate and causing reversal of the pH change, with apparent rejuvenation of the soda lime. However, because the amount of useful soda lime is much reduced, the soda lime very quickly changes colour back to its 'exhausted' colour at the next use. Exhausted

('spent') soda lime granules are harder and more difficult to crumble than fresh granules. The reactions that occur between carbon dioxide and soda lime can be summarised as follows:

$$CO_2 + H_2O \rightarrow H_2CO_3$$
$$H_2CO_3 + 2NaOH \rightarrow Na_2CO_3 + 2H_2O + HEAT$$
$$Na_2CO_3 + Ca(OH)_2 \rightarrow CaCO_3 + 2NaOH$$

1 kg of soda lime is said to be able to absorb 250 l of carbon dioxide

Note that the **activator is regenerated**, and that **heat** and **water** are produced. More water is produced that is used in the initial reaction; in fact, for every mole of carbon dioxide absorbed, 1 mole of water is produced. This reaction is exothermic, and the soda lime canister will feel warm when CO_2 absorption is taking place. Large animal (e.g. horse) canisters are often made of metal to help heat-dissipation as otherwise the patients may sometimes become hyperthermic. The **pH change** results in a colour change in the indicator dye.

Soda lime is caustic, so suitable precautions should be taken when handling it: according to health and safety rules, gloves, goggles, and a mask should be worn. Due to its caustic nature, soda lime will cause crazing of perspex absorber canisters and can add to the corrosion of breathing system components, which is also facilitated by breakdown products of some of the inhalation agents, such as hydrofluoric acid that is a degradation product of halothane (despite its 'stabiliser' thymol).

Other types of CO_2 absorbents have been produced (see Chapter 8 on inhalation agents). One of these was **baralyme**, but barium containing products were removed from the market by 2005. Baralyme consisted of 80–85% calcium hydroxide, and 11–20% barium hydroxide octahydrate (i.e. it had its own water of crystallisation; the water content was about 11–16%) with either no, or only a small quantity of, strong base activator because barium hydroxide acted as an activator. No hardeners were necessary. The indicator dye changed from pink to a blue/grey colour with exhaustion of the granules. One kg baralyme absorbed around 270 l of carbon dioxide.

Other, newer CO_2 absorbents also contain much less of, or even exclude, the classic strong base activators, which is important when considering possible interactions between volatile agents and CO_2 absorbents resulting in the production of compound A, formaldehyde, methanol, and carbon monoxide (see Chapter 8). Although tending to be more expensive, lithium hydroxide-based absorbents are available for medical use, some incorporating lithium chloride as a catalyst. They do not react with volatile anaesthetic agents even when desiccated, however, they are corrosive and need careful handling.

The optimum **granule size** for all absorbents is about 1.5–5 mm diameter. Soda lime is often sold according to '**mesh size**'; this is the number of holes per square inch of the mesh. In the UK, the common mesh size is 3–10; in the USA, the common mesh size is 4–8.

The absorber canister should be large enough to contain an air space between granules that is equivalent to, or greater than, the tidal volume of the patient.

When standard absorbent (mesh size 4–8ish) is used, the **intergranular space constitutes about 50% of the canister's volume.** This means that ideally the **canister should have a capacity ≥2 times the tidal volume.**

Efficiency of carbon dioxide absorption depends upon:

- The freshness and composition of the absorbent
- The available surface area for absorption, which itself depends upon:
  - canister size, shape, design (baffles etc.), and filling
  - granule size, shape, and propensity to form dust, which determine the intergranular volume
  - the presence of any channelling
- The contact time between granule surfaces and the gases, which depends upon the physical features of the breathing system, the patient's respiratory characteristics (tidal volume, breathing rate), and the FGF

Signs of carbon dioxide absorbent exhaustion include:

- Colour-change; the operator should be aware of the expected colour-change. It is not always reliable because of apparent regeneration (see earlier). Absorbent should be replaced before all the granules have changed colour
- The absorber canister does not feel warm when in use (but this may be somewhat dependent upon patient size, temperature and the FGF used)
- Increased inspired (and possibly also end tidal), carbon dioxide tension noted on capnography
- Clinical signs of hypercapnia displayed by the patient, i.e. increased breathing rate/depth, increased heart rate and possibly blood pressure (due to sympathetic stimulation), and bright pink mucous membranes (due to vasodilation)

9.11 Rebreathing Systems Compared with Non-rebreathing Systems

9.11.1 Advantages

- Rebreathing of respired gases, once the carbon dioxide has been removed, allows conservation of heat and moisture in those respired gases, which are also enhanced by the chemical reaction of carbon dioxide and the absorbent (e.g. soda lime).

- Economical because relatively small quantities of oxygen and anaesthetic gases and vapours are required.
- Less wastage and also less pollution (still must scavenge, although negligible requirement for scavenging if 'closed' system use).
- Can easily ventilate the patient's lungs.

9.11.2 Disadvantages

- Historically, rebreathing systems were thought to provide relatively high resistance to breathing because of the carbon dioxide absorbent, reversing pressure swings (and also reversing gas flow in To and Fro systems), and one-way valves, especially if condensation builds up on them (circle systems). The resistance due to the carbon dioxide absorbent, however, appears to be small, i.e. it has been estimated that the resistance offered by a full absorber canister at 60 l/min flow (the peak inspiratory flow [approx. 3–5 × minute ventilation] in a 70 kg person), is ≤1 cmH$_2$O. Reversing gas flows (in To and Fro systems), and reversing pressure swings and one-way valves (in circle systems), however, can provide more resistance to breathing. Modern valve technology has reduced the resistance offered by one-way valves, but care must be taken to ensure that condensation does not build up and affect their function. Furthermore, high FGFs tend to reduce the resistance to inspiration but increase resistance to expiration; and vice versa. Overall, the resistance in modern non-coaxial circle systems is said to be slightly greater than that found in the non-coaxial non-rebreathing systems, but somewhat less than that found in coaxial circles and co-axial non-rebreathing systems (e.g. Bain).
- Bulky circle Y-piece increases circuit drag in circle system.
- Bulky Waters' canister with short connecting tube to the patient's ETT increases circuit drag with the To and Fro.
- Beware apparatus dead space. This increases during use with the To and Fro system as CO$_2$ absorbent is exhausted; and some old circles have relatively large apparatus dead space in their Y-pieces.
- CO$_2$ absorbent can be expensive and requires changing regularly.
- Inhalation of CO$_2$ absorbent dust is possible with To and Fro systems.
- Channelling of gases around absorbent granules may also occur, especially with To and Fro systems, leading to inefficient carbon dioxide absorption.
- Circles are more complex and harder to clean than To and Fro systems.
- Normally these systems (and the patient's lung FRC) are denitrogenated (which takes some time) before attempting to use low flows, so rebreathing systems are less useful for short procedures.
- Can scavenge, but scavenging tubing increases the bulk and circuit drag, especially with the To and Fro system.
- Care must be taken if nitrous oxide is to be administered, as this may build up in concentration in the system, resulting in dilution of oxygen and the delivery of a potentially hypoxic gas mixture to the patient.
- We do not know the inspired anaesthetic concentration or the inspired oxygen and nitrous oxide concentrations, unless we use expensive equipment to measure them.
- When used in 'low flow' mode, these systems make poor use of expensive precision out-of-circuit vaporisers. Precision vaporisers also have poorer accuracy when flow rates below 0.25–0.5 l/min are used.
- Anaesthetic concentration is slower to change after the vaporiser setting is altered, unless larger changes are made to the vaporiser dial setting and FGF is also increased (see time constants, above).
- Other gases (e.g. nitrogen, methane, hydrogen, acetone), can accumulate in the system under true low flow conditions.
- You must ensure minimal leaks from the system components if you are trying to achieve true low flow anaesthesia; and gases sampled for sidestream capnography must be returned to the system if using low flow anaesthesia.
- Circle and To and Fro systems are more expensive to buy than non-rebreathing systems, although cheaper disposable (and possibly re-usable) versions are now available.
- Beware using low flows on hot days (especially with To and Fro systems as the large heat source [CO$_2$ absorber canister] is nearer the patient) because of the risk of hyperthermia and even heat stroke.

9.12 Scavenging

In 1989, the United Kingdom Control of Substances Hazardous to Health (COSHH) Code of Practice was approved by the Health and Safety Commission, under section 16 of the Health and Safety at work Act (1974). The COSHH regulations require an employer to protect employees by:

- Performing risk assessments for procedures requiring the use, storage, and handling of 'chemicals'
- Producing 'local rules', standard operating procedures, and contingency plans, for how to use, handle, and store 'chemicals' with minimum risk; including how to prevent/control exposure
- Providing control measures, including regular examination, testing, and servicing of equipment involved

- Monitoring workplace exposure regularly
- Providing information and training for employees
- Providing health surveillance

Inhalation anaesthetic agents are regulated by these COSHH guidelines. Occupational exposure standards (OESs) were set (in 1996) for each agent, and are expressed as 8 hour time weighted averages (8 hour TWAs [time weighted averages]):

- Nitrous oxide = 100 ppm
- Halothane = 10 ppm
- Isoflurane = 50 ppm
- Sevoflurane = 60 ppm

In the USA and European countries other than the UK, these limits tend to be lower, for example the limit for N_2O is 25 ppm and the limits for halothane and isoflurane are 2 ppm (and suggested to be <0.5 ppm if N_2O is in use). In the USA, the National Institute for Occupational Safety and Health (NIOSH), which was set up under the Occupational Safety and Health Act (OSHA), is a federal agency responsible for prevention of work-related injuries and illnesses, and sets legally enforceable Occupational Exposure Limits (OELs). To reduce exposure to these agents, we must therefore 'remove' waste anaesthetic gases from the workplace environment by 'scavenging'.

Halothane, isoflurane, sevoflurane, and desflurane (halogenated compounds) can be adsorbed onto activated charcoal (which, if heated, will elaborate these agents back into the atmosphere). Activated charcoal canisters are available and have minimal resistance, so can be used to scavenge from any anaesthetic breathing system. The canisters weigh 1,300 g when 'new', but must be discarded when they weigh 1,400 g (i.e. when they are 'full'). However, **activated charcoal does not remove nitrous oxide**. The only way of removing N_2O from the operating environment is to duct it away to the outside atmosphere, where it is a greenhouse gas (and contributes to global warming), causes ozone depletion (it is degraded by ultraviolet light to reactive radicals), and reacts with water to form nitric acid, therefore acid rain.

9.12.1 Scavenging Can Be Passive or Active

Passive systems duct the waste gases (which are vented from the anaesthetic breathing system via the pop-off valve) away either into a ventilation shaft that then must not recirculate air into any other room in the building, or into an activated charcoal canister (but this will not remove nitrous oxide).

Active systems require an extractor fan or vacuum pump, and then gentle suction is applied to the pop-off valve so that waste gases are sucked away.

All scavenging systems require some **safety features** though, or else there may be too much negative pressure applied to the system (especially in the case of active systems), or too much positive pressure applied (especially in the case of passive systems, e.g. if the tubing becomes kinked, it is like the pop-off valve being closed tight). Positive and negative pressure safety devices should be included, examples are given below (Figures 9.20 and 9.21).

For passive systems (Figure 9.20), the positive pressure valve usually activates at about 10 cmH₂O; and the negative pressure valve usually activates at about −0.5 cmH₂O. These protect the anaesthetic breathing system (and therefore the patient) from excessive positive and negative pressures. The bag acts as an indicator of over- or under-pressure, by observing its size. Should the bag expand or collapse too much, then the valves should operate to ensure patient safety.

For active scavenging systems (Figure 9.21), the bottom of the receiver is open to the air, and so if over- or under-pressure occurs, air/gases move through the open end; hence, the term *air-brake*.

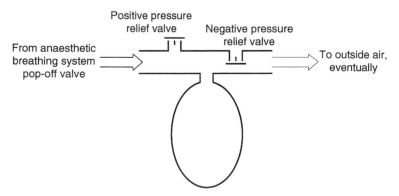

Figure 9.20 Passive scavenging 'receiver' system with safety valves.

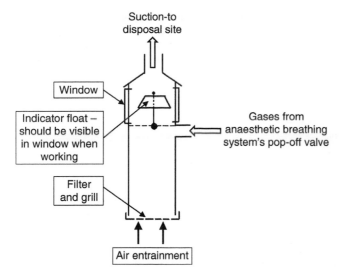

Figure 9.21 Active scavenging receiver system, often called a Barnsley receiver as it was first developed in a hospital in Barnsley, Yorkshire, UK.

9.12.2 Reducing Exposure to Anaesthetic Gases in the Workplace

- Reduce the number of inhalation (mask or chamber) inductions of anaesthesia performed.
- Use cuffed ETTs.
- Use more injectable agents.
- Use lower flows (rebreathing systems) where possible.
- Regularly check anaesthetic breathing systems for leaks.
- Fill vaporisers with their keyed-filling devices to reduce spillage.
- Where possible, fill vaporisers at the end of the day, and preferably, in a fume cupboard or well-ventilated area.
- Make sure the scavenging devices work (e.g. activated charcoal requires changing when it becomes 'saturated').
- Connect the patient's ETT to the anaesthetic breathing system before anaesthetic gases are delivered (i.e. turn on the oxygen first, then connect patient's ETT to breathing system, then finally turn on N$_2$O and vaporiser as required).
- Ideally flush/purge the patient's anaesthetic breathing system with oxygen (switch off all other anaesthetic gases/vapours) before disconnecting from the system to change patient position, or at the end of surgery. Alternatively, a 'bung' can be placed over the patient end of the breathing system after disconnection to reduce atmospheric pollution. Such disposable 'bungs' are often supplied with the anaesthetic breathing systems and may be able to be purchased separately, depending upon the manufacturer.

- Ensure the recovery area is well ventilated (once a patient is disconnected from the anaesthetic breathing system, and even after its trachea is extubated, the recovering patient continues to exhale some anaesthetic gases, which are very difficult to 'scavenge').
- The operating and recovery areas and staff should be monitored for exposure to anaesthetic gases and vapours at regular intervals.
- The operating room and recovery area should be well ventilated; 15 air changes per hour is the minimum suggested.

9.13 Endotracheal Tubes (ETTs) and Supraglottic Airway Devices (SGADs)

Different types of ETTs are available (Figures 9.22 and 9.23), and they can be made from different materials, such as red rubber, siliconised rubber (silastic or polymethylsiloxane), or various types of plastic (e.g. polyvinyl chloride (PVC) and polyurethane) or siliconised plastic; but no longer latex. Plasticisers (softeners) such as phthalates may be added to PVC to produce softer tubes, but there have been recent concerns over the potential carcinogenicity of phthalates.

Armoured tubes are reinforced with a spiral of either metal or nylon to prevent kinking and compression; these are useful for patients requiring extreme head/neck positions such as neck flexion for cerebrospinal fluid sampling. Some tubes are made with more of a curvature than others, often determined by the material they are made from. Some of the stiffer plastic and PVC tubes will actually soften if placed in warm (clean, preferably sterile) water first which may facilitate (after shaking dry) a less traumatic tracheal intubation. Tubes are typically either **cuffed** or **uncuffed** (see below), whereas **Cole pattern tubes** are shaped with a 'shoulder' that seats onto the rima glottidis. A newer design uses, instead of a cuff, a series of six flexible **silicone baffles** to create an airway seal, whilst at the same time enabling escape of gases from the lungs should excessive pressure build up (Safe-Seal™). Tubes can also be coated in flexible metal tape to give them some protection against the use of lasers (high heat energy sources near a high oxygen source is recipe for a fire).

Tubes are manufactured according to certain standards and all materials must undergo irritancy and toxicity testing. A 'Z79-IT' marking on older tubes denotes implant testing, but newer tubes should have a CE marking.

The **internal diameter** (in millimetres) of the tube is used to describe the **tube size**. However, the material from which it is made and whether it is cuffed or not,

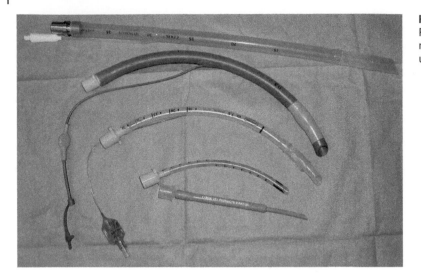

Figure 9.22 Different types of endotracheal tube. From the top: silicone rubber cuffed tube; red rubber (Magill) cuffed tube; PVC cuffed tube; PVC uncuffed tube; Cole pattern tube.

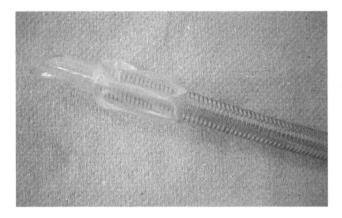

Figure 9.23 Armoured tube (see metallic spiral which prevents tube from kinking).

determine its outer diameter, which is actually what determines whether it will fit into the animal's airway or not.

It is important to try to **use the largest tube possible,** but **without causing trauma** to the animal's airway, because this ensures the minimum resistance to breathing. Resistance is proportional to length, but inversely proportional to the fourth power of the radius, so the internal diameter affects resistance much more than length. When considering resistance, the ETT may be responsible for the site of greatest resistance within the 'endotracheal tube-anaesthetic breathing system' combination. Using the largest diameter tube possible also means that the cuff (if present) will only need minimal inflation to effect a seal, which reduces the intra-cuff pressure (especially for the low volume, high pressure cuffs) and helps prevent tracheal mucosal injury (see below).

Tube length should be such that there is not a great excess protruding from the animal's mouth because this adds apparatus 'dead space' and encourages rebreathing; but neither should a massive length be inserted so far down the trachea that one mainstem bronchus is intubated and the other totally occluded (this can cause hypoxaemia very quickly). The **proximal end** of the tube should ideally **lie at the incisor arcade** and the **distal tip** of the tube should **lie somewhere between the larynx and the carina, but ideally in the proximal 1/3rd of the trachea below the cricoid ring**. The tube tip should not be positioned such a short distance through the larynx that when the cuff is inflated, the vocal cords may be traumatised. In those species with an eparterial (tracheal) bronchus (especially pigs which have relatively short tracheas), it is important to try not to occlude the entrance to this with the tube/cuff. Some tubes come with a small side-hole near the tip (the so-called **Murphy eye**) to give some protection against occlusion of a bronchus; or occasionally, the ETT can lie awkwardly within the trachea so that its open tip is obstructed against the tracheal wall, so the Murphy eye protects against this too.

Alternatives to traditional ETTs are various **Supraglottic Airway Devices** (SGADs). The first of these was the **laryngeal mask airway** (LMA, or Brain airway). Now available in several guises, it basically consists of a tube connected to a soft, inflatable cushion which provides a peri-laryngeal seal to secure the airway (Figure 9.24). Sometimes the seal provided is not very good, and a patent airway cannot be assured if laryngospasm occurs. LMAs have been used in rabbits, cats, and dogs. Very little skill is said to be required to place them as the larynx does not need to be visualised.

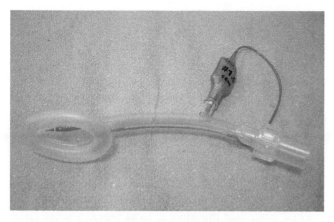

Figure 9.24 Laryngeal mask airway (sometimes referred to as a 'Brain airway', named after its designer). The photograph shows the cuff, which seats around the epiglottis/laryngeal inlet, inflated.

More recently, however, veterinary-specific versions of the human i-gel™ SGAD have been manufactured for cats and rabbits: the **v-gel**™ (Figure 9.25). These use soft ana-tomically-preshaped silicone to form an anatomically-precise seal around the airway, whilst at the same time, blocking the proximal oesophagus, with the cat version also including an inflatable cushion to improve the seal should this be necessary, e.g. for artificial ventilation. Both cat and rabbit versions come in six different sizes and can be placed rapidly and atraumatically. They offer much lower resistance to breathing than conventional ETTs because the tubing proximal to the glottis is wider. Capnography is recommended to help confirm correct placement and ensure continued correct position through-out the procedure (and the devices are made with an

(a)

(b)

(c)

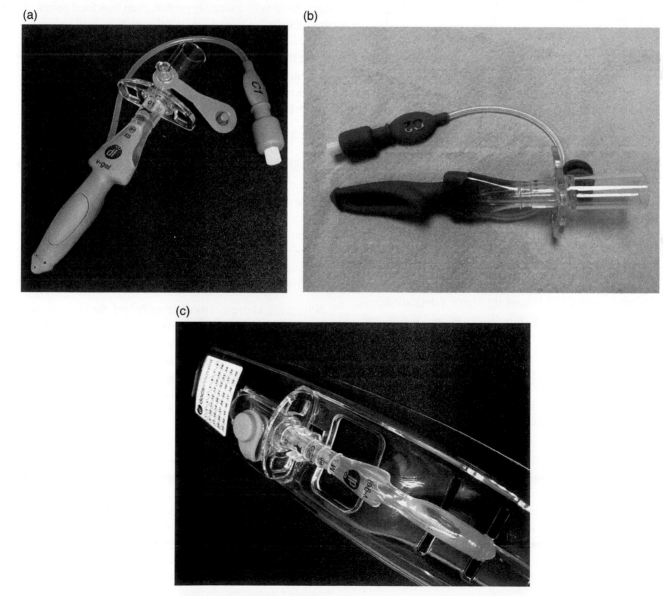

Figure 9.25 Cat v-gel showing dorsal aspect with inflatable 'cushion' and integral capnography sampling port (a); cat v-gel showing ventral aspect with laryngeal seating (b); rabbit v-gel with integral gas sampling port, shown here in its re-sterilisation tray to facilitate tracking the number of re-sterilisation cycles: maximum recommended is 40 (c).

integral gas-sampling port to facilitate this). Artificial ventilation can be provided at peak inspiratory pressures of up to 15 cmH$_2$O with v-gels. Although some protection against oesophageal reflux/regurgitation and aspiration is provided, complete protection is not guaranteed especially if there is likely to be a large quantity of refluxed/regurgitated material.

9.13.1 Cuffs

Cuffs are inflatable sleeves near the distal (patient) end of the tube and are usually made of the same material as the tube itself. Manufacturers must adhere to certain standards regarding cuff size and location on the tube. Cuffs should inflate symmetrically and should not herniate over the tip of the tube or the Murphy eye (if one is present) during normal use.

Cuffs (or shoulders or baffles) should:

- Provide an air-tight seal between the tube and the tracheal wall, which helps prevent material from the pharynx entering the distal trachea, and also reduces leakage of gases to the atmosphere during artificial ventilation
- Help to keep the tube tip in a more central position within the trachea to reduce the chance of tube-tip occlusion and also to minimise trauma of the tracheal wall by the tube tip

Uncuffed tubes were traditionally favoured for cats because the inner diameters of cuffed tubes tended to be relatively small because of the extra bulk of the cuff material. This is much less of a problem now because of better manufacturing processes and materials.

There remain, however, potential problems when using cuffed tubes, especially in cats that have a delicate dorsal tracheal ligament that can be easily ruptured by over-zealous cuff inflation. Tracheal damage/rupture is also a risk when the patient's position requires changing during anaesthesia (e.g. for dental work or multiple radiographs) because the trachea can 'move around' the tube (if the ETT is not disconnected from the breathing system first); common sites of tracheal damage being at the location of the tube tip and/or cuff.

Cuffs can be:

- Low volume, high pressure (e.g. those of red rubber tubes)
- Medium volume, medium pressure (e.g. those of silastic [siliconised rubber] tubes)
- High volume, low pressure (e.g. those of plastic tubes, in which the cuffs can be inflated to aim to provide a seal within the trachea without stretching the wall of the cuff itself)

When deflated, cuffs can present either a smooth, low profile (cuffs of red rubber and silastic tubes) or they can be quite bulky (those of plastic tubes). Low-profile cuffs inflate with a smooth profile and tend to distort the tracheal contour, whereas the high-volume, low-pressure ('floppy') cuffs tend to conform to the tracheal contour during inflation (unless they are fully or over-inflated). Low-volume, high-pressure cuffs also tend to have a relatively small area of contact with the tracheal wall, which can be subjected to high pressures, possibly resulting in focal pressure-necrosis, if the tube is in place for prolonged periods of time. Floppy cuffs should inflate with a larger area of contact with the tracheal wall, thus minimising focal pressure points, and reducing the risk of tracheal damage if used for prolonged periods of time. However, these bulky, floppy cuffs, as well as causing more trauma during intubation/extubation, often inflate with a wrinkly profile, such that focal points of contact with the trachea may still result in focal pressure-points; and the channels between the folds or wrinkles may reduce the quality of airway seal, allowing materials from the pharynx to enter the trachea and potentially causing leaks during artificial ventilation.

To inflate a cuff safely:

- Confirm that the tube is in the trachea (see below).
- Then connect the tube to the anaesthetic breathing system of choice and set the oxygen flow to the desired rate.
- Close the pop-off valve on the breathing system and gently squeeze the bag whilst simultaneously gently inflating the cuff.
- When no further gas can be heard, or detected by stethoscope, leaking around the tube, the cuff is adequately inflated.
- It is important to open the pop-off valve again.

Whilst the above protocol is sufficient for low-volume, high-pressure cuffs, it is also recommended to measure the intra-cuff pressure, especially when using tubes with high-volume, low-pressure cuffs. It is very difficult to determine the pressure in the cuff just by feeling the 'pilot balloon', but manometers can be used. Intra-cuff pressure is not very representative of tracheal wall pressure for low-volume, high-pressure cuffs because high intra-cuff pressures are required to inflate the poorly compliant cuffs regardless of cuff contact with the tracheal wall. For high-volume, low-pressure cuffs, however, provided the cuff is not stretched/over-inflated, the intra-cuff pressure approximates the pressure exerted on the tracheal wall. Some tubes are now manufactured with pressure-relief devices within the pilot balloon (e.g. Lanz™ pressure-regulating valve); these can also be very useful if nitrous oxide is to be used (see below). Intra-cuff pressures should ideally be measured regularly during long procedures as patient muscle tone will change, as may compliance of the cuff material as it warms up.

Pressures in excess of around 25 cmH$_2$O, exerted laterally on the tracheal wall, can reduce mucosal perfusion (in normovolaemic, normotensive patients), and cause tracheal mucosal ischaemia/necrosis that may lead to later stricture formation. In the shorter term, a diphtheritic membrane of necrotic/granulation tissue may form and sometimes such a flap or tube ('tracheal cast') of tissue can later (some time after tracheal extubation) act like a valve and can totally obstruct the animal's trachea, which is life-threatening. (See Further Reading for further details on obstructive fibrinous tracheal pseudomembrane formation.)

The cuff is usually inflated with air, but if you are supplying oxygen and nitrous oxide to your patient, because nitrous oxide can partition into air-filled spaces, the cuff volume/pressure can increase over time. Some people prefer to use sterile saline or water to prevent this, or a mixture of N$_2$O and oxygen in the same ratio as that to be delivered to the patient.

9.13.2 Aids to Tracheal Intubation

A laryngoscope is commonly used to aid endotracheal intubation. Various blades (e.g. straight, curved) are available, and for right-handed or left-handed use (see Further Reading for more details). When used correctly, at least in human anaesthesia, the tip of the blade of a laryngoscope should be used to depress only the base of the tongue (the blade tip being placed in the vallecula; the 'pocket' between the tongue base and ventral surface of the epiglottis). In veterinary anaesthesia, however, on occasion the blade tip may be used to gently depress the tip of the epiglottis to help visualise the glottis. Soft flexible bougies (tube-introducers/exchangers/guides) can also be used to aid the correct and gentle placement of an ETT within the trachea, either by increasing or decreasing the curvature of the tube or, following placement of the blunt tip of the bougie just through the glottis, by enabling the tracheal tube to be 'railroaded' over it. Topical lidocaine may be useful.

Occasionally, pharyngotomy or transmylohyoid incisions are required to re-direct ETTs should their oral presence be problematic and should nasotracheal intubation not be a viable alternative (See Chapter 41).

9.13.3 Problems with Airway Devices

- Malposition, e.g. placement into the oesophagus or placement into one bronchus. Capnography can help determine successful placement of ETTs and SGADs, but beware the addition of extra apparatus dead space, especially with smaller patients.
- Injury to oral, pharyngeal, laryngeal, or tracheal tissues.
- Laryngospasm may occur upon laryngoscopy/attempted tracheal intubation; this is less likely with careful placement of a SGAD. The risk of laryngospasm can be reduced by either topical application of lidocaine onto the rima glottidis, or intravenous administration of lidocaine before attempts to place an ETT or SGAD.
- Autonomic nervous system stimulation. Although commonly there is a sympathetic ('pressor') response to laryngoscopy and tracheal intubation (increased heart rate and blood pressure), occasionally vagal reflexes occur with dramatic bradycardia (even asystole), and hypotension. It is worth someone having a finger on the pulse (or monitoring the ECG), if possible, during placement of an ETT. Such haemodynamic responses are usually less marked during insertion of SGADs.
- Increases in intra-ocular pressure (IOP) and intra-cranial pressure (ICP) can occur during laryngoscopy and endotracheal intubation, mainly associated with the pressor response (see above), but this can be exacerbated if gagging/coughing are elicited. Increases in IOP have been found to be less marked with insertion of SGADs than ETTs.
- Unseen disconnection between the tube and its connector, possibly resulting in inhalation of the tube. All airway devices (ETTs and SGADs) should be securely tied in place once in position. Secure the tube, not just its connector. Beware iatrogenic alteration of atlantoaxial compression in certain breeds when the ETT tie is secured behind the occipital protruberance.
- Unplanned extubation is a problem encountered when the tube is poorly fixed in position.
- Tubes may become kinked or occluded by external compression, although this is less likely if using armoured tubes.
- Epiglottic retroversion can occur during 'blind' placement of ETTs (e.g. in horses) or SGADs. The consequences of this are uncertain, but problematic insertion of an ETT or seating of an SGAD may occur.
- Tubes can be bitten, and fragments can be inhaled.
- Tube breakage has been reported in silicone tubes that had become brittle; although biofilm formation was considered a factor, the processes of cleaning, re-sterilisation, and storage of tubes are also important.
- Tubes can become occluded with mucus or other debris (or by 'light' patients biting down on them).
- Tube occlusion can occur due to excessive cuff inflation causing 'collapse' of the tube itself (but this is unlikely with armoured tubes).
- The bevel at the end of the ETT may abut the tracheal wall and occlude the tube, especially if the cuff inflates eccentrically. A Murphy eye can be a useful safety feature in case of this complication.

- The ETT lumen may be occluded if the cuff herniates over the tip of the tube. A Murphy eye may, or not, help in this situation, depending upon its location and patency.
- If the animal's position must be changed during anaesthesia, ideally you should disconnect the anaesthetic breathing system from the patient's ETT before moving the animal. (First turn off the anaesthetic agent delivery and dump the bag contents out through the pop-off valve and into the scavenging system before you disconnect the patient to reduce theatre pollution.) If you do not disconnect the tube, then the chances are that the ETT might be forced to rotate around inside the animal's trachea when the animal's position is changed; and you can now imagine the bevelled tip carving its way through the tracheal mucosa. This can easily happen in cats, whose tracheas are not very forgiving, and tracheal tears can result.
- Excessive cuff pressures for prolonged periods of time can cause tracheal mucosal injury.
- Insufficient/ineffective seal and protection of the airway can result in aspiration and/or inadequate artificial ventilation.
- Dislodgment of SGADs can occasionally result in obstruction of the airway, although this is much less likely with the use of the anatomically-specific v-gels.
- Over-inflation of LMA cuffs can reduce the effectiveness of the airway seal and allow aspiration.
- Neuropraxias (lingual, hypoglossal, recurrent laryngeal) can occur and are thought to be associated with excessive cuff inflation pressures, particularly LMA cuffs, causing focal ischaemia in the supra- and peri-laryngeal regions.
- Use of LMAs with inflatable cuffs can cause undue compression of the base of the tongue, resulting in lingual cyanosis. The advent of the anatomically-specific v-gels has reduced this complication.
- In cats, the use of spring-loaded mouth gags (as an aid to tracheal intubation or to guard against bite-damage to the tube) can, if excessive jaw opening is maintained for any length of time, cause transient or even permanent post-anaesthetic blindness, due to compression of the maxillary arteries that can result in both retinal and cerebral ischaemia. It is worth noting that SGADs can be placed without the need to visualise the larynx and also have an integral 'bite-guard' (hard plastic connector).
- In rabbits, access to the mouth for dental procedures may be restricted with the bulkier proximal v-gel than with a narrower ETT, and movement/dislodgement of the SGAD may occur with the multiple position changes that may be necessary for the dental procedure itself.

Tube placement can be checked by:

- Direct observation of correct placement (with the aid of a laryngoscope).
- Detection of breaths exiting the tube during exhalation (by feeling them or by using a wisp of cotton wool that will move in the stream of each breath).
- Observation of condensation forming on the inside of the tube during exhalation if it is made of clear material; a cold glass microscope slide or dental mirror can also be used to detect condensation.
- Use of a purpose-made thermistor to detect the warmth of the expired gases (e.g. Apalert™).
- Use of capnography to measure the CO_2 content of the exhaled gases.
- Observation of the bag of the anaesthetic breathing system, which should deflate and inflate slightly with each inspiration and expiration, respectively.
- Detection of chest inflation (by observation or stethoscopy) when the bag of the breathing system is gently squeezed (the valve is first closed to do this); beware as occasionally this can look promising, but the patient's stomach is being inflated. It is a bad habit to press on the animal's chest to enforce an exhalation as this may encourage gastro-oesophageal reflux/regurgitation with all its repercussions (oesophagitis, choanal inflammation and later stricture formation in both these structures, increased risk of aspiration pneumonitis).
- Palpation of the neck may aid detection of inadvertent oesophageal intubation as two firm 'tubes' will be palpated (the trachea and the oesophagus, this latter with a fairly rigid ETT within it), rather than just one (the trachea).

9.14 Tracheal Extubation

Usually the cuff is deflated before the tube is gently withdrawn. Occasionally, if there is worry that some fluid, blood or debris may be near the larynx, the tube can be withdrawn with the cuff still partially or, more rarely, fully, inflated (see Chapter 33). The nearer the larynx any debris (sitting proximal to the cuff) can be brought up the trachea, the more likely the cough reflex is to be elicited and the airway thus protected.

During long surgery, especially when using non-rebreathing systems where cold/dry gases are being breathed, the tracheal secretions may become dry/tacky, so be aware that the ETT could become blocked, or even 'stuck' within the airway, by this 'glue'. If a tube feels 'stuck' in the trachea, some sterile saline can be trickled around the proximal tube in an attempt to soften the secretions. (If anticholinergics such as atropine have been given to the patient, the secretions will probably become drier and stickier even more quickly.)

Occasionally the cuff material may become 'bunched up' if there is some traction on the tube (e.g. circuit drag), during cuff deflation, which can cause difficulty during tube withdrawal through the larynx. It is therefore advised to ensure that there is no movement of the tube during cuff deflation; and if problems arise, cuff re-inflation and then subsequent deflation whilst ensuring the tube does not move within the airway, should solve the problem.

Lubricants can be used to ease both tube insertion and removal. Only water-soluble substances should be used, but gels can dry out and may aggravate tubes sticking within the airway as above. Some water-based lubricant sprays are now available (e.g. VetLube™). Lubricants may also help to improve the airway seal provided by the cuff, but it is important to ensure that lubricant does not obscure the Murphy eye (if present).

Further Reading

Alderson, B.A., Senior, J.M., and Dugdale, A.H.A. (2006). Tracheal necrosis following tracheal intubation in a dog. *Journal of Small Animal Practice* 47: 754–756.

Almeida, G., Costa, A.C., and Machado, H.S. (2016). Supraglottic airway devices: a review in a new era of airway management. *Journal of Anesthesia and Clinical Research* 7 (7) https://doi.org/10.4172/2155-6148.1000647.

Barton-Lamb, A.L., Martin-Flores, M., Scrivani, P.V. et al. (2013). Evaluation of maxillary arterial blood flow in anesthetized cats with the mouth closed and open. *The Veterinary Journal* 196: 325–331.

Concannon, K.T. (1996). Using low-flow anesthesia. *Veterinary Medicine* 91: 349–352.

Cook, T.M. and Howes, B. (2011). Recent developments in efficacy and safety of supraglottic airway devices. *Continuing Education in Anaesthesia, Critical Care and Pain* 11: 56–61.

Cook, T.M. and Kelly, F.E. (2015). Time to abandon the 'vintage' laryngeal mask airway and adopt second-generation supraglottic airway devices as first choice? *British Journal of Anaesthesia* 115: 497–499.

Crotaz, I.R. (2010). Initial feasibility investigation of the v-gel airway: an anatomically designed supraglottic airway device for use in companion animal veterinary anaesthesia. *Veterinary Anaesthesia and Analgesia* 37: 579–580.

Diez Bernal, S. and Iff, I. (2019). Airway management by transmylohyoid endotracheal intubation in two cats with mandibular trauma. *Veterinary Anaesthesia and Analgesia* 46: 405–406.

Gale, E., Ticehurst, K.E., and Zaki, S. (2015). An evaluation of fresh gas flow rates for spontaneously breathing cats and small dogs on the Humphrey ADE semi-closed breathing system. *Veterinary Anaesthesia and Analgesia* 42: 292–298.

Hartsfield, S.M., Gendreau, C.L., Smith, C.W. et al. (1977). Endotracheal intubation by pharyngotomy. *Journal of the American Animal Hospital Association* 13: 71–74.

Heath, R.B. (2019). Veterinary anesthesia intermediate rebreathing circuits. *Veterinary Anaesthesia and Analgesia* 46: 407–408.

Heath, R.B., Steffey, E.P., Thurmon, J.C. et al. (1989). Laryngotracheal lesions following routine orotracheal intubation in the horse. *Equine Veterinary Journal* 21: 434–437.

Hofmeister, E.H., Quandt, J., Braun, C., and Shepard, M. (2014). Development, implementation and impact of simple patient safety interventions in a university teaching hospital. *Veterinary Anaesthesia and Analgesia* 41: 243–248.

Holland, M., Snydere, J.R., Steffey, E.P., and Heath, R.B. (1986). Laryngotracheal injury associated with nasotracheal intubation in the horse. *Journal of the Veterinary Medical Association* 11: 1447–1450.

Hudson, L.N., Isaac, N.J.B., and Reuman, D.C. (2013). The relationship between body mass and field metabolic rate among individual birds and mammals. *Journal of Animal Ecology* 82: 1009–1020.

Hughes, L. (2016). Breathing systems and ancillary equipment. In: *BSAVA Manual of Canine and Feline Anaesthesia and Analgesia*, 3e (eds. T. Duke-Novakovski, M. de Vries and C. Seymour), 45–64. British Small Animal Veterinary Association.

Imai, A., Eisele, P.H., and Steffey, E.P. (2005). A new airway device for small laboratory animals. *Laboratory Animals* 39: 111–115.

Joliffe, C. (2008). Tracheal intubation in cats. *Veterinary Review* 135: 26–30.

Kazakos, G., Anagnostou, T.L., Savvas, I. et al. (2007). Use of the laryngeal mask airway in rabbits: placement and efficacy. *Lab Animal* 36: 29–34.

Mapleson, W.W. (2001). Anaesthetic breathing systems: semi-closed systems. *British Journal of Anaesthesia CEPD Reviews* 1: 3–7.

Martin-Flores, M., Scrivani, P.V., Loew, E. et al. (2014). Maximal and submaximal mouth opening with mouth gags in cats: implications for maxillary artery blood flow. *The Veterinary Journal* 200: 60–64.

Mitchell, S.L., McCarthy, R., Rudloff, E., and Pernell, R.T. (2000). Tracheal rupture associated with intubation in cats: 20 cases (1996–1998). *Journal of the American Veterinary Medical Association* 216: 1592–1595.

Moens, Y. (1988). Introduction to the quantitative technique of closed-circuit anesthesia in dogs. *Veterinary Surgery* 17: 98–104.

Niimura del Barro, M.V., Epadas, I., and Hughes, J.M.L. (2015). Breakage of two silicone endotracheal tubes during extubation. *Journal of Small Animal Practice* 56: 530–532.

Nunn, G. (2008). Low-flow anaesthesia. *Continuing Education in Anaesthesia, Critical Care and Pain* 8: 1–4.

Reiter, A.M. (2014). Open wide: blindness in cats after the use of mouth gags. *The Veterinary Journal* 201: 5–6.

Robin, E., Guieu, L.V., and Le Boedec, K. (2017). Recurrent obstructive fibrinous tracheal pseudomembranes in a young English bulldog. *Journal of Veterinary Internal Medicine.* 31: 550–555.

Sanchis Mora, S. and Seymour, C. (2011). An unusual complication of endotracheal intubation. *Veterinary Anaesthesia and Analgesia* 38: 158–159.

Saulez, M.N., Dzukiti, B., and Voigt, A. (2009). Traumatic perforation of the trachea in two horses caused by orotracheal intubation. *Veterinary Record* 164: 719–722.

Sawyer, D.C. (1984). Canine and feline endotracheal intubation and laryngoscopy. *The Compendium on Continuing Education for the Practising the Veterinarian* 6: 973–982.

Scrivani, P.V., Martin-Flores, M., Van Hatten, R., and Bezuidenhout, A.J. (2014). Structural and functional changes relevant to maxillary arterial blood flow observed during computed tomography and nonselective digital subtraction angiography in cats with the mouth closed and opened. *Veterinary Radiology & Ultrasound* 55: 263–276.

Skarbek, A. and Borland, K. (2019). Supraglottic airway devices: use in veterinary medicine. *Companion Animal* 24: 145–149.

Steffey, E.P. and Howland, D. (1977). Rate of change of halothane concentration in a large animal circle anesthetic system. *American Journal of Veterinary Research* 38: 1993–1996.

Stiles, J., Well, A.B., Packer, R.A., and Lantz, G.C. (2012). Post-anesthetic cortical blindness in cats: twenty cases. *The Veterinary Journal* 193: 367–373.

Trim, C.T. (1984). Complications associated with the use of the cuffless endotrahceal tube in the horse. *Journal of the Veterinary Medical Association* 185: 541–542.

Wagner, A.E. and Bednarski, R.M. (1992). Use of low-flow and closed-system anesthesia. *Journal of the American Veterinary Medical Association* 200: 1005–1010.

Recommended Books

Al-Shaikh, B. and Stacey, S. (eds.) (2013). *Essentials of Anaesthetic Equipment*, 4e. Philadelphia, USA: Churchill Livingstone, Elsevier.

Davey, A.J. and Diba, A. (eds.) (2012). *Ward's Anaesthetic Equipment*, 6e. Philadelphia, USA: Elsevier Saunders.

Dorsch, J.A. and Dorsch, S.E. (2008). *Understanding anesthesia equipment*, 5e. Philadelphia, USA: Lippincott, Williams and Wilkins, Wolters Kluwer Health.

Ehrenwerth, J., Eisenkraft, J.M., and Berry, J.M. (eds.) (2013). *Anesthetic Equipment, Principles and Applications*, 2e. Philadelphia, USA: Elsevier Saunders.

Haider, G., Lorinson, K., Lorinson, D., Auer, U. (2019). Development of a clinical tool to aid endotracheal tube size selection in dogs. *Veterinary Record* doi: 10.1136/vetrec-2018-105065

Kim, YJ., Lee S, Jung, J., Jung, H., In, S., Chang, J., Chang, D., Fahie, M. (2020). Atlantoaxial bands in small breed dogs: influence of external pressure by the endotracheal tube tie. *Journal of Small Animal Practice* 61: 163–169.

Self-test Section

1 Which component offers the highest resistance to breathing?
   A Tubing within the breathing system
   B One-way valves within the breathing system
   C CO_2 absorbent within the breathing system
   D The endotracheal tube

2 Which of the following non-rebreathing systems is most efficient during spontaneous ventilation?
   A Ayre's T-piece
   B Jackson Rees modified Ayre's T-piece
   C Lack
   D Bain

10

Anaesthetic Machines, Vaporisers, and Gas Cylinders

LEARNING OBJECTIVES

- To be able to describe the functions of an anaesthetic machine.
- To be able to define a gas and a vapour.
- To be able to describe cylinder safety features.
- To be able to outline how high-pressure gases and vapours are safely administered to patients at much lower pressures.
- To be able to describe the basic construction and function of vaporisers.

10.1 Definitions

- Gases supplied to or through the anaesthetic machine include: oxygen, nitrous oxide, medical air, and carbon dioxide
- A **gas** is strictly the name given to a substance present in the gaseous phase when at a temperature (usually room temperature) above its critical temperature
- A **vapour** is the name given to a substance present in the gaseous phase when at a temperature below its critical temperature
- The **critical temperature** is that temperature above which a gas cannot be liquefied, no matter how much it is compressed
- The **critical pressure** is the pressure required to liquefy a gas at its critical temperature

10.2 Cylinders

In the UK, Europe, North America, and many other countries, medical gases are considered as medicinal products and are therefore subject to regulations regarding their safe production, storage, and use. Table 10.1 summarises information about the physical properties and cylinder filling pressures for commonly used medical gases in the UK.

10.2.1 Cylinder Construction

Molybdenum steel cylinders are most commonly used, being relatively light for their strength. **Aluminium** cylinders are available for magnetic resonance imaging (MRI) use (molybdenum steel cylinders are strongly attracted by the magnetic field), but cannot be filled to the same high pressures as molybdenum steel cylinders. **Composite** cylinders are also now available, consisting of steel or aluminium 'liners' surrounded by Kevlar™, carbon fibre or fibreglass in epoxy resin, in a 'hoop-wrap' configuration. They are very strong, yet lightweight, and can withstand high pressures.

Cylinders come in a variety of sizes and have different valve fitments for releasing their contents (e.g. pin-index, bull nose, handwheel, or integral valves). Examples for the UK are given in Table 10.2.

10.2.2 Cylinder and Pipeline Colours

In the UK, cylinder shoulders and pipelines are colour-coded (Table 10.3) according to the International Standard ISO 32 and British/European Standard BS EN 1089 part 3. In 2012, the European Industrial Gas Association position paper EIGA PP-01 was adopted by the British Compressed Gases Association and Medicines and Healthcare products Regulatory Agency, such that by 2025, all compressed gas cylinders intended for medical use in the UK will have white

Veterinary Anaesthesia: Principles to Practice, Second Edition. Alexandra H. A. Dugdale, Georgina Beaumont, Carl Bradbrook, and Matthew Gurney.
© 2020 John Wiley & Sons Ltd. Published 2020 by John Wiley & Sons Ltd.
Companion website: www.wiley.com/go/dugdale/veterinary-anaesthesia

Table 10.1 Basic cylinder data.

Cylinder contents	State of contents	Critical temperature. (°C)	Cylinder pressure (full)	Saturated vapour pressure (SVP)
Oxygen	Compressed gas	−118	13 700 kPa	N/a
Nitrous oxide	Saturated vapour above liquid	+36.5	SVP until no more liquid remains to provide saturated vapour	4000 kPa
Carbon dioxide	Saturated vapour above liquid	+31	SVP until no more liquid remains to provide saturated vapour	5000 kPa

Table 10.2 Cylinder size and valve fitments (UK).

Content	Size C	Size D	Size E	Size F	Size HX	Size G	Size J
Oxygen	Pin index	Pin index	Pin index	Bull nose	Integral	Bull nose	Pin index, side-spindle
Nitrous oxide	Pin index	Pin index	Pin index	Handwheel	Not available	Handwheel	Not available
Carbon dioxide	Pin index	Not available	Pin index	Handwheel	Not available	Not available	Not available

Cylinder size increases from A to J; sizes A and H are not used for medical gases.

Table 10.3 Cylinder and pipeline colour.

Cylinder contents	Colour in UK	Colour in USA
Oxygen	White shoulders (and body [black body will become white body with new regulations])	Green (shoulders and body)
	White pipelines	Green pipelines
Nitrous oxide	French blue shoulders (blue body will become white body with new regulations)	French blue (shoulders and body)
	French blue pipelines	French blue pipelines
Air	Black and white 'quartered' shoulders (grey body will become white body with new regulations)	Yellow
	Black pipelines	Yellow pipelines
Carbon dioxide	Grey shoulders (grey body will become white body with new regulations)	Grey

bodies that will bear the name of the contents in large letters. Until 2025, cylinders with both old and new body colour schemes will be in circulation. In many European countries and Canada, cylinders (shoulders) are also coloured according to ISO 32; but in the USA, cylinder (shoulder) colours follow the NFPA 99 and CGA C-9 standard guidelines.

10.2.3 Cylinder Information

Cylinder necks are engraved/stamped with the chemical formula of the contents, the tare (empty) cylinder weight (for nitrous oxide and carbon dioxide), and the test pressure (TP) and date of testing. Colour- and shape-coded plastic collars between the cylinder neck and valve stem identify when the next test is due (see below). Although cylinder colour is commonly relied upon to identify the contents of a cylinder, the correct method of identification of cylinder contents is to read the label.

The **label** should state:

- The name of the contents, its chemical symbol, and product specification
- The batch number, including details of filling plant, fill date, and expiry date (which facilitates cylinder rotation in the hospital)
- Cylinder contents (litres)
- Maximum cylinder pressure
- Product licence number
- Cylinder size code
- Hazard warning diamonds
- Directions for use, storage, and handling

10.3 Pressure Units

- 1 Atmosphere = 760 mmHg (at sea level) = 1.01 bar = 10 13.25 mbar = 14.7 psi
- 1 Atmosphere = 101.325 kPa = 1033.6 cmH$_2$O
- Therefore: 760 mmHg ≈ 101 kPa ≈ 1034 cmH$_2$O
- 1 mmHg ≈ 0.133 kPa ≈ 1.36 cmH$_2$O
- 1 kPa ≈ 10.2 cmH$_2$O ≈ 7.5 mmHg ≈ 10 mbar
- 1 cmH$_2$O ≈ 0.74 mmHg

10.4 Gases in Cylinders

10.4.1 How Do We Get Pure Oxygen for Cylinders?

Oxygen is 'extracted' from cooled and liquefied air by fractional distillation. Oxygen for medical use can be supplied in either a cooled liquid form or a compressed gaseous form. Liquid oxygen can be stored in either huge vacuum flasks (vacuum insulated evaporators) as part of a cryogenic liquid system, as commonly seen in human hospitals, or, on a smaller scale, in liquid cylinder installations, as in some larger veterinary hospitals. Compressed gaseous oxygen is stored and supplied in cylinders of various sizes. Cylinders may then be directly attached to anaesthetic machines, or, for busier practices and hospitals, banks of cylinders can be attached to manifolds in order to supply piped oxygen to numerous locations within the facility (theatres, intensive care, kennels etc.).

10.4.2 What If Oxygen Cylinders Are Not Available?

Oxygen concentrators (alternatively called pressure-swing adsorbers) can be used (Figure 10.1). These consist of two chambers, each with a filter, a heat exchanger (to cool the compressed gases), and a compressor. The compressor drives filtered air into one of the chambers, where a zeolite (hydrated aluminium silicate) filter adsorbs nitrogen; the 'air' remaining in the chamber, under some degree of compression, is then fairly pure oxygen (i.e. 92–95% oxygen is achievable, the main contaminant is argon). After some time, when the 'filter' is deemed 'full', the second chamber is used, and a vacuum is applied to the first chamber to help release the nitrogen back into the atmosphere and regenerate the zeolite. Small units are capable of delivering 5–8 l/min after a few minutes of 'warm-up'. These can be used to supply oxygen to an individual anaesthetic machine or to supply supplemental oxygen in a cage-side manner to usually a single patient.

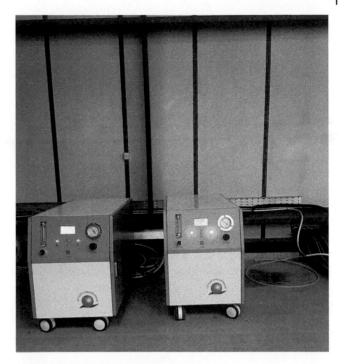

Figure 10.1 An oxygen concentrator manifold comprising two units.

Larger oxygen concentrators can be used to supply piped oxygen (up to around 80 l/min), for small hospitals, but a back-up bank of oxygen cylinders should be available.

10.4.3 How Is Nitrous Oxide Manufactured?

Nitrous oxide is produced when ammonium nitrate is thermally decomposed at 240 °C. Cylinders are partially filled with liquid nitrous oxide, above which the saturated vapour develops a pressure of 4400 kPa. Because saturated vapour pressure (SVP) varies with temperature, cylinders are partially filled according to the **filling ratio**, that is, the weight of added liquid nitrous oxide (and its vapour), divided by the weight of water the cylinder could hold if completely filled. The filling ratio is 0.75 in temperate climates, whereas it is 0.67 in tropical climates, in order to avoid build-up of excessive pressure within the cylinders in hotter operating temperatures.

10.4.4 Entonox

Entonox is a 50% : 50% mixture of gaseous oxygen and gaseous nitrous oxide. Entonox cylinders are filled to 13 700 kPa. They are initially partially filled with liquid nitrous oxide, through which compressed oxygen is bubbled resulting in evaporation of the liquid nitrous oxide so that a purely gaseous mixture results. This is called the **Poynting (or overpressure) effect**. When gases are mixed, their critical temperatures and pressures can change. With entonox, the critical temperature of nitrous oxide becomes a so-called **pseudocritical temperature** of around −6 °C; hence, at normal room temperatures, the nitrous oxide component should remain as a gas. If, however, a cylinder of entonox is exposed to temperatures below −6 °C (at a pseudocritical pressure of 11 700 kPa), the nitrous oxide component can liquefy, leaving an oxygen-rich gas above oxygen-poor liquid nitrous oxide. This separation, called **lamination**, can be reversed by re-warming and shaking or repeatedly inverting the cylinder to re-mix the cylinder contents. Should the cylinder be used without re-warming and re-mixing, a relatively high oxygen concentration is initially delivered to the patient, but as gases are withdrawn and the liquid then evaporates, a mixture of gas of decreasing oxygen content and increasing nitrous oxide content is delivered to the patient, risking delivery of a hypoxic mixture.

10.5 Cylinder Safety

Cylinders undergo **pressure/leak testing** (hydraulic testing and internal inspection) at regular intervals: every 10 years for steel cylinders and every 5 years for composite cylinders. The dates of the test are stamped into the cylinder neck and the TP engraved on the valve block (usually around 22 000 kPa, i.e. at least 50% higher than the expected normal working/service pressure). The plastic collars (which are shape- and colour-coded) denote the date of the next test due. Each time a cylinder is due to be refilled, it is visually inspected (internally and externally) for evidence of corrosion and physical impact/distortion. Flattening, bending, and impact testing is performed on one randomly-chosen cylinder every hundred, as are tensile tests, where one in a hundred cylinders is cut into strips for testing.

Cylinders should be **stored upright** to avoid damage to the valves. Cylinders that contain liquid (N_2O, CO_2) should always be used in an upright position to prevent liquefied gas entering the valve outlet, which may cause freeze-burns or damage equipment. Cylinders must be stored in such a way that they are **restrained safely** and cannot fall over. Usually they are held into wall-mounted brackets by chains or rings, or they can be placed into a rack (vertically or horizontally).

Cylinders should be stored in a **well-ventilated area, ideally away from**:

- Flammable substances, oil, grease etc.
- Heat sources (including direct sunlight)
- High voltage sources
- Drains (where grease or dense vapours/gases may collect)

- Dampness (to prevent corrosion)
- Corrosive chemicals
- Tarmac or asphalt 'floors'
- Areas where smoking is allowed

Cylinders should be labelled 'Full', 'In use', or 'Empty' as appropriate, and full cylinders should be stored away from empty cylinders. The stock of stored cylinders should be rotated so that the 'oldest' ones are used first.

Cylinder valves are protected by disposable, tamper-proof, plastic **dust covers** when they are delivered. These prevent dirt and grease getting into the valves, which, as well as preventing proper 'seating' to the attachment device (e.g. pin index yoke, bull nose fitting) and therefore causing leaks, could also be dangerous, as grease in the presence of oxygen, or indeed nitrous oxide, venting under high pressure, can cause explosions. Both oxygen and nitrous oxide can support combustion. For fire, a fuel (e.g. blob of grease), a source of ignition (e.g. the heat given out by rapidly expanding oxygen [gases decompress as they leave the cylinder]), and something to support the combustion (e.g. oxygen) are required. Valves should always be opened slowly. It used to be recommended that all cylinders were briefly opened to the air ('cracked') before being connected, to ensure that any dust or grime on the valve would be blown away so that it would not get pushed into the regulator, pressure gauge, or anaesthetic machine. Care must be taken, however, when 'cracking' cylinders; they must be firmly secured and care should be taken that the venting gases do not contact bare skin as freeze-burns may be sustained.

Bodok seals (non-combustible neoprene rubber discs bonded to an aluminium rim) are used to help make a gas-tight seal between pin-index type cylinder valves and their attachments (e.g. cylinder yoke/regulator). For bull nose cylinder valves, the regulator attachment should have a non-combustible 'O' ring to help ensure a good seal. Whenever cylinders are connected to yokes/pressure regulators, **hydrocarbon-based lubricants must never be used** to improve the seal or fit.

Cylinder valve blocks should be **engraved with the chemical symbol** of the cylinder contents. Cylinder valve blocks should also have **high pressure relief devices** so that at high temperatures, the contents are safely vented to the atmosphere. In the USA, such pressure relief devices are usually a plug of fusible (relatively low melting point) material within the valve block; in the UK, the **fusible material** (Wood's metal) is used between the valve and the cylinder neck.

Compressed gases are dry:

- To protect the cylinders from corrosion
- To protect the cylinder valves, regulators, and pressure gauges from icing, which can cause blockage and damage (including 'explosion')

Because liquid nitrous oxide evaporates to maintain the SVP above the liquid within the cylinder, the latent heat of vaporisation necessary for this evaporation is 'taken' from the cylinder and its surroundings. Hence the cylinder will feel cold to the touch, and you may see condensation of water vapour or even a thin layer of frost, develop on the outside of the cylinder (up to the liquid level), especially on cold days and at high rates of demand for nitrous oxide evaporation.

As gases leave their highly compressed state in cylinders, they expand, the pressure reduces and they 'cool' if the process is adiabatic. Usually, however, heat energy can be 'taken' from the surroundings so that the process is isothermal, especially if the rate of gas flow is not too fast. Nevertheless, gases from cylinders are 'cold' (relative to our patients) and dry, and this can lead to problems if used for prolonged time periods, as the patient's respiratory tree can be a source of heat and moisture loss and should not be desiccated (see Chapters 20 and 9). See Chapter 8 on inhalation agents for details about how the cylinder content of nitrous oxide can be calculated from cylinder weight and N_2O density or molecular mass.

10.5.1 Pin Index Safety System

The Pin Index Safety System (PISS) helps to ensure that only the correct cylinder can possibly be attached to its correct cylinder yoke (Figure 10.2), as protruding pins on the yoke attachment correspond with the arrangement of pin holes on the cylinder's valve block. There are seven possible positions for pin holes on the valve block, which are used in various combinations for the different gases (Figure 10.3). The corresponding pins are 6 mm long and 4 mm in diameter except pin 7, which is slightly wider. The seventh hole lies in the centre of the arc between positions 3 and 4, and is the only position used for entonox.

Note that bull nose fittings are size-coded for each gas.

10.5.2 Down-Regulation of Pressure

How do we reduce the high pressure of compressed gas in a cylinder down to something more user-friendly? We need a pressure-reducing valve, also called a **pressure regulator** (Figure 10.4).

Pressure regulators not only **reduce cylinder pressure** to something much more safe and workable, but **also keep the outlet gas at a constant pressure.** This is important, because, especially for oxygen, a true compressed 'gas', the initially high cylinder pressure falls linearly (at constant temperature) as the cylinder empties. For nitrous oxide, the cylinder pressure (the SVP of N_2O) only starts to fall once all the liquid N_2O has evaporated.

Two-stage regulators are capable of producing even more finely regulated constant outlet pressure.

(a)

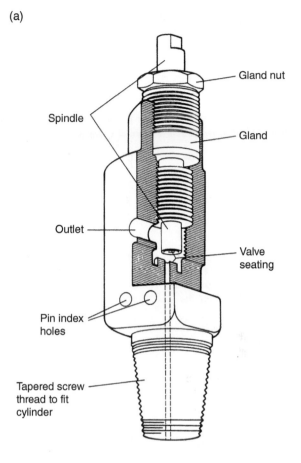

(b)

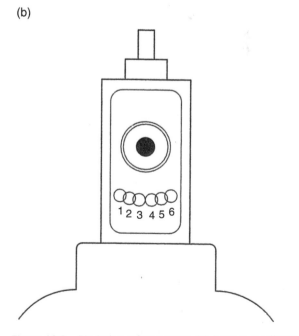

Figure 10.2 Pin index safety system. (a) A cut-away diagram through a pin index cylinder valve block. *Source:* Reproduced from Davey et al. (1992a) with permission from Elsevier. (b) Possible pin index hole positions. *Source:* Reproduced from Al-Shaikh and Stacey (2002a) with permission from Elsevier.

(a)   (b)

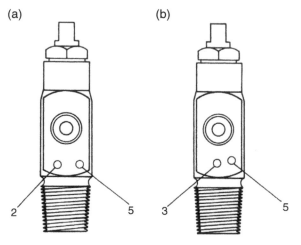

Figure 10.3 (a) Pin hole positions on O_2 cylinder (e.g. size E) valve block. (b) Pin hole positions on N_2O cylinder (e.g. size E) valve block. *Source:* Reproduced from Davey et al. (1992b) with permission from Elsevier.

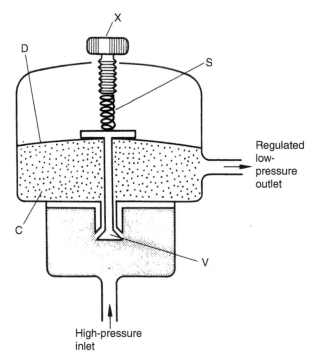

Figure 10.4 The functional parts of a pressure regulator. D, diaphragm; S, spring; C, low pressure chamber; V, valve seating; X, adjustment screw. *Source:* Reproduced from Davey et al. (1992c) with permission from Elsevier.

Regulators are gas-specific.

In the UK, cylinder pressures are regulated down to pipeline pressures of 420 kPa (c. 60 psi). In the USA, cylinder pressure is regulated down to 350 kPa (c. 50 psi) pipeline pressure. Such pipeline pressures then supply the anaesthetic machine.

The anaesthetic machine may be constructed so as to 'carry' its own gas cylinders, and therefore needs regulators and pressure gauges for each attached cylinder; and/or it may be supplied by 'piped gases' from a distant cylinder or bank of cylinders.

For anaesthetic machines that can carry cylinders *and* accept piped gases, the pressure to which the cylinders are regulated is usually a little (about 5 kPa) lower than the pipeline pressure, so that gases are preferentially drawn from the piped gas supply (higher pressure). The piped gases are therefore used preferentially, so any cylinder gases (if the cylinders are left turned 'on' by accident) should remain available in an emergency, e.g. should the piped gas supply fail.

10.6 Piped Gas Supplies

If the operating theatre has a piped gas supply, then gases are carried there from, usually, a bank of (i.e. more than one) cylinders placed somewhere distant to the operating theatre. The cylinders in each bank (there is usually one 'in use' bank, one 'full/reserve' bank, and sometimes an additional 'emergency' bank) are attached to a manifold. Non-return valves prevent flow of gases between cylinders. Each manifold includes a pressure regulator and pressure gauge and supplies, via a non-return valve, the main pipeline for that particular gas or vapour (e.g. O_2 or N_2O). The **pipes are made of degreased copper alloy** and are of a diameter to suit the demand envisaged. They terminate in special terminal outlets, usually some form of self-closing 'socket', in the operating theatre.

To access the piped gas supply, another pipeline is required, usually a flexible hose, to duct the gases to the anaesthetic machine. The **flexible (and antistatic) gas hoses** that are used have the following features:

- They are colour-coded, e.g. in the UK, white = oxygen; blue = nitrous oxide; black = medical air.
- They are permanently attached at one end (the equipment or outlet connector) to the anaesthetic machine via gas-specific non-interchangeable screw thread (NIST) fittings in the UK, where a small probe (within a nut) is profiled according to its specific gas. NIST is perhaps a misleading name as the nuts have the same internal diameter and thread, but the nuts cannot be tightened unless the gas-specific probes can be completely engaged. A similar system, called the diameter index safety system (DISS), is used in the USA, wherein the probe configuration is also gas-specific (the shoulder of the nipple varies in diameter and is gas specific). Note that UK and USA fittings are not interchangeable.
- They have an 'indexed' (i.e. gas-specific) probe or collar at the other end (the supply or inlet connector) that fits into a complementary self-closing 'socket', usually in the

(a)

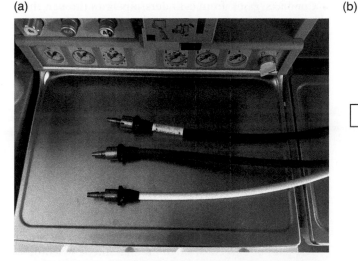

(b)

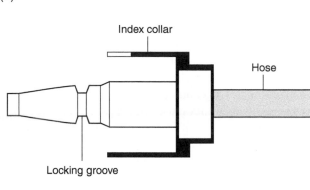

Index collar

Hose

Locking groove

Figure 10.5 Schrader probes on an anaesthetic workstation (a): black, medical air; blue, nitrous oxide; white, oxygen; and a Schrader probe schematic (b). Note that it is the collar which is important for the safety of the system. The collar varies in size between different gas hoses (a), so that you cannot plug the wrong probe into the wrong socket/pipeline supply. *Source:* Schematic reproduced from Al-Shaikh and Stacey (2002) with permission from Elsevier.

form of a quick connect/release arrangement, which is either wall-mounted or located on a ceiling boom or at the end of a pendant dangling from the ceiling. Such inlet connectors and their respective sockets are usually of the Schrader type in the UK, wherein the collar (around the probe), prevents connection to the wrong gas supply (Figure 10.5).

10.7 Pressure Gauges

Pressure gauges are necessary so that pipeline and cylinder pressures can be measured and monitored. For compressed gases such as oxygen, the cylinder pressure will decrease as the cylinder empties (Boyle's Law); but for a full nitrous oxide cylinder, which contains saturated vapour above liquid, the pressure within the cylinder remains constant (at its SVP) until all the liquid in the cylinder has evaporated, after which the pressure will finally fall. SVP is affected by temperature (see later) but small daily temperature fluctuations are likely to have little influence inside an operating theatre.

There are many different ways of measuring pressure, e.g. the 'U' tube manometer containing either water or mercury, the aneroid barometer and the mercury sphygmomanometer. These can be used for measuring relatively low pressures, but something more robust is required for measuring the high pressures of compressed gases and vapours contained within cylinders. Many high-pressure gauges work on the principle of the Bourdon pressure gauge (Figure 10.6).

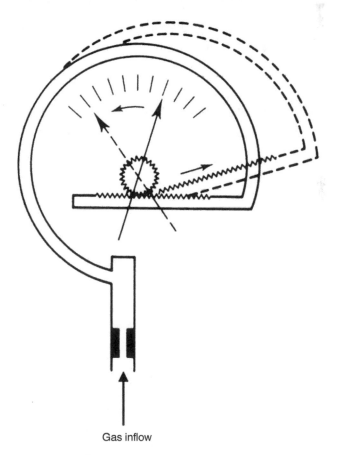

Gas inflow

Figure 10.6 Bourdon gauge. *Source:* Reproduced from Davey et al. (1992c) with permission from Elsevier.

The Bourdon gauge consists of a curved flattened tube, such that when pressurised gases enter it, the tube expands, and the curvature is partially straightened out. This moves the rack and pinion and so the pointer can move over the scale. There is a constrictor at the entrance to the gauge to protect it from sudden pressure surges. The gauge registers the cylinder pressure above atmospheric pressure, i.e. the gauge is 'zeroed' at atmospheric pressure. This is because once the cylinder contents have reduced to atmospheric pressure, gases can no longer flow out of the cylinder. (Remember that for gases to flow, they must follow a path from an area of high pressure to an area of lower pressure down a gradient; so if no pressure gradient exists, no gas flow can occur.)

If gases are piped to theatre, there is usually a low-pressure alarm. This usually sounds once the manifold pressure falls to 7–8 bar, allowing some time to change banks before the supply fails.

10.8 The Anaesthetic Machine

An anaesthetic machine can be anything from a pneumatic (i.e. function dependent upon pressurised gas supplies), wheel-about trolley or wall-mounted station to complex electrical, mechanical, and pneumatic multi-component workstations (sometimes called anaesthetic care stations), which usually also incorporate electronic monitoring devices and ventilators. Equine anaesthetic machines are normally co-mounted onto a movable trolley along with a large animal circle.

The anaesthetic machine:

- Conducts 'gases' from cylinders/pipelines through their respective flowmeters.
- Then conducts the gases through a 'back bar', on which a vaporiser can be mounted (if vaporiser out-of-circuit/circle [VOC] type of vaporiser).
- Then conducts these gases/entrained vapour to the common gas outlet (CGO), from where they can be delivered to a patient via an anaesthetic breathing system mounted on the CGO (Figure 10.7).

The CGO, where the anaesthetic breathing system is attached, may be incorporated into a 'Cardiff swivel': i.e. where, the CGO connector swivels to help position the breathing system so that it is less prone to being damaged by proximity to the patient trolley.

The path of oxygen through an anaesthetic machine is shown in Figure 10.8.

The anaesthetic machine can be thought of as consisting of three different parts, each subjected to different gas pressures.

The **high pressure part** includes those parts which receive gas at cylinder pressure (if the machine has cylinder yokes), i.e.:

- Each cylinder yoke (which normally includes a filter and a unidirectional valve)
- Each cylinder pressure regulator
- Each cylinder pressure gauge

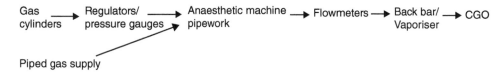

Figure 10.7 Flow of gases through the anaesthetic machine.

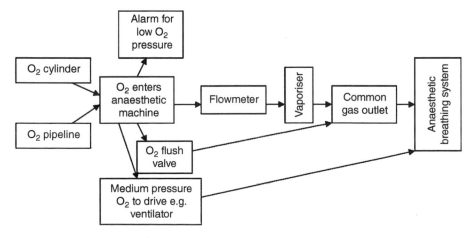

Figure 10.8 The path of oxygen through an anaesthetic machine.

The **intermediate pressure part** includes those parts that receive gases at lower, relatively constant, pressure, from pipelines, or downstream from anaesthetic machine-mounted cylinder regulators, i.e.:

- If the machine can receive piped gases; then the piped gas inlets and their pressure gauges (which normally include filters and one-way valves)
- The pipework of the anaesthetic machine itself (downstream of the cylinder or pipeline inputs)
- Medium pressure gas outlets (only oxygen), often in the form of mini-Schrader sockets (which can supply 'drive' gas to, e.g. a ventilator)
- The 'low oxygen pressure' or 'oxygen failure' alarm
- The oxygen flush valve
- All the flowmeter needle valves

The **low pressure part** includes those components distal to the flowmeter needle valves whose working pressure is around 1–10 kPa above atmospheric pressure, i.e.:

- The flowmeter tubes
- The back bar and vaporiser
- The anaesthetic machine 'check valves': the over-pressure valve (works at around 35 kPa [=350 cmH$_2$O]), and under-pressure valve, if present, which are usually sited within the CGO
- The CGO which usually incorporates a non-return valve

10.8.1 Unidirectional Valves

These are usually found in cylinder yokes and pipeline inputs to:

- Prevent gas ingress or egress (to or from the anaesthetic machine), when cylinders or pipelines are 'empty' or not attached
- Allow change of cylinders, when the anaesthetic machine is in use, without gases leaking to the atmosphere
- Prevent trans-filling between gas sources, e.g. when cylinders (or cylinders and piped supply) are at different pressures. Although pressure regulators try to ensure that the regulated pressure is fairly constant, it will fall when the cylinders are nearly empty

10.8.2 Safety Features of Anaesthetic Machines

These may vary between manufacturers, and veterinary anaesthetic machines are often cheaper to buy because they have fewer safety features. Safety features should include:

- An oxygen failure alarm; something that makes a loud noise when the oxygen supply pressure is falling.

- An emergency oxygen flush device, often labelled 'O$_2$+'. These can usually be activated regardless of whether the master switch of an electrically-enabled machine is turned ON or OFF.
- A back bar high pressure relief valve, which prevents pressure build up in the back bar, and therefore protects flowmeters and vaporisers. Usually activated at around 35 kPa (above atmospheric pressure).
- A back bar negative pressure valve, which allows air ingress should problems with gas supply occur and the patient make inspiratory efforts (see below).
- Most modern anaesthetic machines have a stop on the oxygen flowmeter control, preventing it from being turned off completely, but rather ensuring a residual mandatory minimum flow of around 50–250 ml/min. This itself, however, cannot guarantee against the delivery of a hypoxic gas mixture to the patient.

An **oxygen failure alarm** (older machines have devices based on the Ritchie whistle) should be fitted and meet certain standards:

- Must require only oxygen to operate it, and be activated when the oxygen pressure falls to c. 200 kPa.
- Must be audible, at least 60 dB at 1 m from the anaesthetic machine, and be of at least seven seconds duration, or, preferably, must not be able to be silenced until the oxygen supply is restored.
- Must be linked to a gas shut-off device, such that at least one of the following happens:

  – All gases being delivered to the patient via the CGO, except air and oxygen, are shut off.
  – There is a progressive decrease in flow of all other gases whilst oxygen flow is maintained at the pre-set proportion, until the oxygen fails altogether, at which point the supply of all other gases is shut off from the patient.
  – Pathways are established between the atmosphere and the anaesthetic machine, such that air can be entrained through a negative pressure valve (so the patient is not denied some form of oxygen supply), and anaesthetic gases are vented to the atmosphere.

The Ritchie whistle sounded when the oxygen pressure fell to about 250 kPa and continued to sound until the oxygen pressure fell to about 40 kPa, but at an oxygen pressure of about 200 kPa, all gases being delivered to the patient were diverted away from the patient and vented to the atmosphere through the high pressure relief valve, causing a second droning/whistling type of sound; and an air-intake (negative pressure relief) valve could then be activated, also causing another whistling/droning sound with each inspiration.

The **emergency oxygen/oxygen flush valve** is supplied by oxygen at c. 420 kPa, such that when activated, the oxygen flow created through the CGO of the anaesthetic machine (bypassing the flowmeters and vaporiser), is around 45 l/min (minimum 35 l/min and usually not exceeding a maximum of 75 l/min). This can be used to purge an anaesthetic breathing system of anaesthetic vapour and N_2O in an emergency situation. It should be protected from accidental activation and on modern machines, it should not be able to be locked in an 'on' position.

10.9 Flowmeters

These consist of tapered glass or plastic tubes, which are calibrated according to the gas they convey. They are operated by means of a needle valve, which is opened/closed by a knob (anticlockwise to open; clockwise to close). An indicator 'float' within the tube is used to 'read off' the flow against the calibrations etched or painted on the tube (Figure 10.9). If the indicator is a bobbin, then the flow is read from the top of the bobbin. If the indicator is a ball, then the flow is read from the middle (equator) of the ball.

Some bobbins are designed to rotate within the tubes (rotameters), and therefore have an upper 'rim' (wider than the body of the bobbin), with slanted grooves ('flutes'), cut into it which enable rotation of the bobbin in a gas stream. A spot marker is usually painted onto the side of a rotating bobbin to visualise its rotation. Such bobbins may also be 'skirted'.

Poiseuille's equation is important when considering the flow of fluids and gases through tubular, annular, or orifice structures. It takes two forms depending upon whether the flow is laminar or turbulent:

$$\textbf{Laminar flow} = \frac{\text{Pressure gradient} \times \pi \times \text{radius}^4}{8 \times \eta \times \text{length}}$$

where η = viscosity.

$$\textbf{Turbulent flow} \; \alpha \; \frac{\sqrt{\text{Pressure gradient} \times \text{radius}^2}}{\sqrt{\rho} \times \text{length}}$$

where ρ = density.

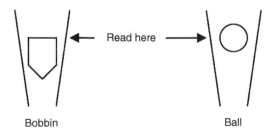

Figure 10.9 Different types of 'indicator floats', usually made of glass or aluminium.

In flowmeter tubes, at low flows when the indicator float is nearer the bottom of the tube, the annular shaped gap around the float is relatively tubular (definition of a tube is when the length exceeds the diameter); and flow is governed by viscosity because flow tends to be more laminar. At higher flows when the float is higher up, the annular shaped gap around the float is more like an orifice (i.e. diameter > length), and flow is more turbulent, so density becomes more important.

These flowmeters are called **variable area, constant differential pressure flowmeters** because the variation in size of the gap maintains a constant differential pressure across the float and the float position can be used to indicate the gas flow.

Flowmeter tubes are calibrated individually, with their indicator floats, and with the gas in question being dry and at a specific temperature and pressure near to those of the expected operating range (e.g. room temperature [c. 18–25 °C] and sea level pressure). Flowmeters are not calibrated from zero but are calibrated from the lowest accurate flow.

Several designs of flowmeters exist. Sometimes you may find two flowmeter tubes in series, so called **cascade flowmeters**, controlled by one knob, where the first tube has smaller graduations (e.g. calibrated up to 1 l/min), and the second, larger graduations; note that gas flow is read from the highest indication. You may also come across a unique design: **expanded range; dual scale**, where there is one flowmeter tube with two floats and two scales, so that one float is calibrated against the larger graduations, and the other against the smaller.

The oxygen flowmeter should have a recognisably different knob, in size, colour, and 'feel' compared to the control knobs of the other gas flowmeters. The oxygen flowmeter knob should be bigger, with a chunkier fluted edge, and it should stick out further than all other control knobs to enable it to be more quickly identified. In the UK, it should be coloured white, or sometimes is a black knob with a white face; whereas in the USA, it is coloured green.

10.9.1 Problems with Flowmeters

10.9.1.1 Flowmeter Tube Not Vertical
Flowmeters are usually designed to work in an upright position, so if tilted, the indicator may stick against the side of the tube, and the 'annular' gap around the float becomes complex in shape, so that it may read inaccurately.

10.9.1.2 Float Sticks to the Sides of the Tube or to the Tube 'Stops' at the Top or Bottom of the Tube
Floats may stick to the side of the tube if the tube is tilted, or if there is dirt, grease, or static within the tube. Dirt can change the weight of the float, and change the internal

'shape' of the flowmeter tube, leading to inaccuracies. Floats may also stick to the tube stops at the bottom or top of the tube, usually because of dirt or static. Compressed gases should be filtered as they are 'released' from cylinders, or as they enter the anaesthetic machine from pipeline supplies. Some flowmeter tubes are coated (inside and out), with a very fine layer of an antistatic/conducting material (e.g. gold) to relay any static electricity safely to earth.

10.9.1.3 Float Not Spinning in Gas Flow

Floats (usually bobbins) that are designed to spin or rotate in the gas flow (flowmeters can then be called rotameters) may fail to rotate, and therefore may give an inaccurate measurement of the flow. This is usually a consequence of them sticking to the inside of the tube because of dirt or static (see above).

10.9.1.4 Cracked Flowmeters

Oxygen should be the last gas to enter the common manifold. The **flowmeters** of the anaesthetic machine are usually **arranged in a bank**, from which each supplies a **common manifold**. Oxygen should be the last gas to enter this manifold, to reduce the risks of a hypoxic mixture of gases being delivered to the patient should there be any cracks in the tubes.

Historically, in the UK, the oxygen flowmeter is positioned to the left of all others because Mr. Boyle who first pioneered the 'anaesthetic machine' was left-handed. This could, however, cause problems because the oxygen flowmeter is the first to deliver gases into the common manifold, and if there are leaks in the other flowmeter tubes, then a hypoxic gas mixture could be relayed to the patient. In the USA, the oxygen flowmeter is placed to the right of all the others, from where it has no problem in being the last flowmeter to supply the common manifold. In the UK, modifications to the common manifold have now made it possible for **oxygen to enter the common manifold last** (Figures 10.10 and 10.11).

Anti-hypoxia (hypoxic guard) devices, which aim to ensure that no less than 25% oxygen is delivered through the CGO, can be: mechanical (e.g. the 'Link 25' system, which uses a mechanical interlink in the form of a chain, to link the nitrous oxide control valve to that of oxygen), pneumatic (e.g. the Pneupac ratio system, which uses a ratio mixer valve), or electronic (some machines incorporate

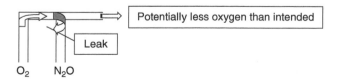

Figure 10.10 Old flowmeter system.

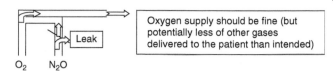

Figure 10.11 Newer flowmeter system.

a paramagnetic oxygen analyser to sample gases leaving the flowmeter block, which sounds an electronic alarm and interrupts the nitrous oxide supply should the oxygen percentage fall below the acceptable minimum of 25%). Note that these devices do not take account of other gases that may be delivered from the flowmeter block, such as medical air or carbon dioxide; and if delivering low fresh gas flows to circle systems, there is a risk that a hypoxic mixture of gases may develop within the circle even with 25% oxygen leaving the CGO.

10.9.1.5 Electronically-Controlled Gas Flows and Mixtures

Some modern anaesthetic workstations, e.g. the General Electric Healthcare (formerly Datex Ohmeda) Aisys (**A**naesthetic **I**ntegrated **Sys**tem) care station, do not use manually-controlled needle valves and flowmeters for the primary determination of the fresh gas mixture leaving the CGO, but rather use electronics to control the individual gas flows and final mixture of gases leaving the CGO (including anaesthetic agent concentration, see below). In the GE Healthcare Aisys care station, a screen displays 'electronic flowmeter representations' to facilitate visualisation of the relative gas flows (Figure 10.12).

10.10 Vaporisers

Downstream from the flowmeter manifold, on the anaesthetic machine 'back bar', is the vaporiser mounting, if the **V**aporiser is to be used 'Out-of-Circuit' (**VOC**). Let us now consider some of the important features of vaporisers.

Figure 10.13 shows the basic construction of a vaporiser. Inflow gas ('fresh gas' from the anaesthetic machine flowmeters) is split into two streams on entering the vaporiser. One stream flows through the bypass channel and the other, smaller stream, passes through the vaporising chamber to 'collect' anaesthetic agent vapour whilst on its travels. The two gas streams then re-unite before leaving the vaporiser.

The vaporising chamber is designed so that the gas leaving it (the 'carrier' gas), is always fully saturated with vapour before rejoining the bypass gas. This should be achieved despite changes in gas flow and some temperature fluctuations (see below for temperature compensating devices).

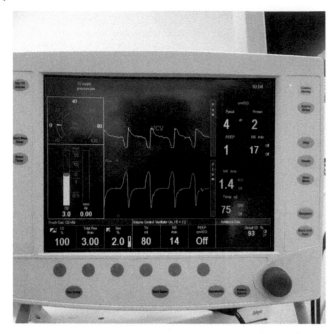

Figure 10.12 Electronic flowmeter display of the GE Healthcare Aisys anaesthesia care station, showing 3 l/min oxygen flow and no medical air flow (bottom left panel); also note 2% sevoflurane is being delivered, and there is an indicator to show that the sevoflurane Aladin™ cassette vaporiser is half full. *Source:* Image courtesy of Paul MacFarlane.

Within the vaporising chamber, saturation of carrier gas with vapour is facilitated by increasing the surface area of contact between the carrier gas and the liquid anaesthetic agent, usually by means of wicks and baffles incorporated into the vaporising chamber. The desired output concentration is obtained by adjusting the percentage control dial, which alters the 'splitting ratio' of the inflow gas, so that more, or less, gas is diverted into the carrier gas stream. Temperature compensating devices can also affect the splitting ratio (see below).

10.11 Vaporisation of Volatile Anaesthetic Agents

This depends upon:

- Agent volatility (boiling point)
- Temperature of the liquid agent at which vaporisation is expected to occur
- Temperature of the gas in contact with the liquid agent

- Flow of gas over/past/through the liquid agent
- Surface area of contact between the gas and the liquid agent

10.11.1 Agent Volatility

There is nothing we can do to alter this. Table 10.4 shows that most of the agents we use have a boiling point above normal room temperature, so these agents are liquid at room temperature. Note, however, that desflurane has a much lower boiling point. We will come back to consider this agent, and why it needs a special vaporiser, later.

10.11.2 Agent Temperature

If we have a liquid agent in a vaporising chamber, then as it vaporises, heat is required (i.e. the latent heat of evaporation/ vaporisation). This heat is 'taken' from the liquid agent remaining, and from the immediate environment of the liquid agent (i.e. the material of the vaporisation chamber in which the liquid is placed and the gas in contact with the liquid).

If the vaporisation chamber is made of a material with a low specific heat capacity and low thermal conductivity (i.e. effectively a thermal insulator), then the temperature of the liquid agent will drop as the agent evaporates, and its evaporation rate will slow down as its temperature drops further and further away from its boiling point. If, however, the vaporisation chamber is made of a material of high specific heat capacity (i.e. it can hold a lot of thermal energy), and high thermal conductivity (i.e. can conduct heat quickly), then it acts as a very good heat source; and its rapid conduction of heat means that the temperature of the liquid agent is unlikely to drop very much during vaporisation, so that the vaporisation rate should be unaffected as vaporisation proceeds.

Table 10.4 Volatile agent boiling points.

Agent	Boiling point (°C)
Halothane	50.2
Isoflurane	48.5
Sevoflurane	58.5
Desflurane	23.5

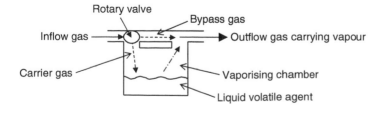

Figure 10.13 Basic vaporiser construction. The rotary valve alters the proportion of gas diverted through the vaporising chamber.

Temperature, by affecting vaporisation, affects the SVP; the cooler, the lower the SVP; the warmer, the greater the SVP. Remember that the **boiling point** of a liquid is the **temperature at which its SVP equals atmospheric pressure**.

Within the vaporisation chamber, the vapour should always be 'saturated' (Figure 10.14). The carrier gas then becomes saturated with vapour before it rejoins the bypass gas. The 'mixed' gases that leave the vaporiser then carry a concentration of vapour determined by the splitting ratio of the original fresh gas into the carrier and bypass gas flows. For example, when a halothane vaporiser concentration dial is set at 2%, the gases leaving the vaporiser consist of 2% halothane by volume and 98% other (entraining) gases. The 2% halothane is then responsible for exerting 2% of the total (i.e. atmospheric) pressure; 2% of 760 mmHg is equal to 15.2 mmHg.

Halothane's SVP at standard room temperature is 243 mmHg. Thus, halothane evaporates within the vaporiser until a SVP of 243 mmHg is created. If all the gas entering the vaporiser was diverted through the vaporisation chamber, so that all the gas leaving the vaporiser was fully saturated with halothane, then halothane would make up 243/760 (i.e. 32%), of the mixed gas composition leaving the vaporiser. Now 32% halothane is far too much to anaesthetise anything safely. We more usually need concentrations in the order of 1–3%.

Let us imagine that we have a fresh gas flow of 2 l/min heading towards our vaporiser, and we want it to deliver a halothane concentration of 1%, so we set its concentration dial at the 1% calibration. How can we calculate how much of the gas flow is diverted through the vaporisation chamber?

If total gas flow entering, and later leaving, the vaporiser is 2 l/min; and the output is set at 1%; then in every 100 ml of gas leaving the vaporiser, there must be 1 ml halothane and 99 ml of other gases. So in one minute, in the 2 l of gas leaving the vaporiser, there must be 20 ml halothane and 1980 ml other gases.

Now, within the vaporisation chamber, where the vapour is fully saturated with halothane, halothane exerts 32% of the total pressure (see above), so there is 32 ml halothane in every 100 ml of 'gas' in this chamber (i.e. every 100 ml consists of 32 ml halothane and 68 ml other gases). Or, put another way, each 1 ml halothane is accompanied by 2.125 ml of other gases. So, in order for 20 ml halothane to leave the vaporiser every minute, it must be carried in/accompanied by 42.5 ml (20 × 2.125) of other gases.

If 20 ml halothane and an accompanying 42.5 ml of other gases leave the vaporisation chamber every minute, but a total of 2000 ml must leave the whole vaporiser, we can see that 1937.5 ml/min (2000 – [20 + 42.5]), of gases must bypass the vaporisation chamber; and only 62.5 ml/min constitutes the carrier gas flow.

Old vaporisers that consisted of glass bottles were poor heat sources, so vaporisation slowed as cooling occurred. Water baths could be used to try to maintain vaporiser temperature. However, the newer vaporisers are made of metals with high specific heat capacity and high thermal conductivity (e.g. copper).

10.11.3 Temperature of Gas

The warmer the temperature of the gas into which we expect vaporisation to occur, the less hindrance there is to vaporisation (because it is less dense); although the material of the vaporising chamber (and its temperature) usually has the greater influence in practice. See also below under temperature compensation devices.

10.11.4 Gas Flow

Vaporiser output at very low, and very high, gas flows can be inaccurate (see later).

10.11.5 Surface Area of 'Contact'

If the surface area of contact between the volatile liquid and its 'carrier gas' can be increased, then vaporisation will be more efficient. The surface area of contact can be increased by: incorporating wicks into the vaporisation chamber; by using cowls and baffles to direct and redirect the gases to flow nearer the surface of the liquid; or by bubbling the agent through the liquid.

10.11.5.1 How Much Liquid Anaesthetic Agent Does a Vaporiser Use per Hour?

In 1993, Ehrenwerth and Eisenkraft gave the following formula:

$$3 \times \text{fresh gas flow}\left(1/\min\right) \times \text{concentration dial setting}\left(\%\right)$$
$$= \text{ml liquid used per hour}$$

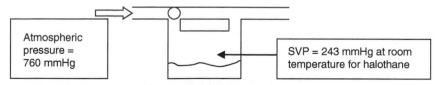

Figure 10.14 Saturated vapour fills the vaporisation chamber.

10.11.5.2 How Much Vapour Does 1 ml of Liquid Agent Produce?

For halothane, isoflurane, sevoflurane, and desflurane, whose molecular weights are around 200 g/mol and whose densities are between 1.5 and 1.9 g/ml, applying Avogadro's law enables us to determine that 1 ml of liquid agent yields about 200 ml of vapour. This illustrates why tipping over a vaporiser and contaminating its bypass channel is so dangerous.

10.12 Classification of Vaporisers

We can classify vaporisers according to their features as documented above, e.g.:

- Position? Vaporisers-in-circuit/circle (VIC) or VOC? Depends upon their internal resistance.
- How is the splitting ratio determined? For example: variable bypass (determined by vaporiser setting); 'measured flow' (operator-determined, e.g. copper kettle, where the operator had the two flows [bypass and carrier gases] to determine separately); 'dual-circuit' (e.g. desflurane vaporisers).
- What method of vaporisation is employed? For example: flow-over; bubble-through; gas/vapour blend (e.g. desflurane).
- Temperature compensation? For example: automatic; manual (copper kettle, where the operator had to vary the gas flows if the temperature changed); or not an issue because the vaporiser is heated to a constant temperature (e.g. desflurane vaporiser).
- Calibration? Yes, agent specific; or no.

10.12.1 Internal Resistance of Vaporisers

You will appreciate from the comments in the above paragraph, that if the inside of a vaporiser is cluttered with lots of wicks and baffles, then it presents a high resistance to the passage of gases through it. This is not such a problem if the vaporiser is seated on the back bar of an anaesthetic machine, where gases under some pressure (a little above atmospheric), are effectively 'pushed' through the vaporiser. In fact, vaporisers situated on the anaesthetic machine back bar, 'outside' the anaesthetic breathing system (e.g. **VOC**), are called 'high resistance' or **plenum type vaporisers**. However, some anaesthetic breathing systems, notably the Stephens circle and the similar Komesaroff circle, have special 'low resistance' vaporisers that sit 'in' the circle itself, so are called **VIC**.

These in-circuit vaporisers must offer **low resistance** to gas flow because gases flowing 'through' them are driven by the patient's respiratory efforts. They are usually positioned in the inspiratory limb to reduce contamination of their liquid anaesthetic agent contents by condensed water vapour (and much water vapour is present in the exhaled gases in the expiratory limb). They are often called **draw-over** vaporisers, as the patient's inspiratory effort 'draws' the gases through them, and over the liquid agent within them. Their 'output', in terms of anaesthetic agent concentration, tends to be much less accurate than that of plenum type vaporisers, and because of their simple construction, their temperature compensation is often poor, but they are not subject to quite the same continuous high flows, and of 'cold and dry' gases (from cylinders) as plenum type vaporisers. Draw-over vaporisers are subjected to the patient's respiratory flows, which are variable depending upon the stage of the respiratory cycle, although the gases within circle systems (whether VIC or VOC), should be warm and moist.

10.12.2 Variable Bypass

'Fresh gases' from the flowmeter manifold enter the anaesthetic machine back bar and travel towards the vaporiser. If the vaporiser is turned 'on', then some of the fresh gas flow is diverted through the vaporisation chamber of the vaporiser; the proportion being dependent upon the concentration set on the vaporiser's dial. Thus, the fresh gases entering the vaporiser are effectively split into two streams, the bypass stream and the carrier gas stream.

The splitting ratio is primarily determined by the vaporiser concentration dial, but the temperature compensation device may also affect it (see below).

10.12.3 Method of Vaporisation

Usually **flow-over**, i.e. the carrier gas literally flows over the surface of the liquid within the vaporisation chamber and over the surface of soaked wicks there. Baffles are often also incorporated. The old fashioned 'copper kettle' vaporiser had to have two gas supplies (the 'bypass' gas and the 'carrier' gas) for which the anaesthetist had to calculate the flows. The carrier gas was introduced into the vaporising chamber via a sintered bronze or glass element, so that the gas was **bubbled through** the liquid agent.

10.12.4 Temperature Compensation

We have already discussed the advantages of using a good heat source for the construction material of a vaporiser (e.g. large mass of copper), which provides a degree of temperature stabilisation, but even then, there can be variations in output, especially at high gas flows. Therefore, additional temperature compensating devices are usually incorporated to ensure that vaporiser output is what is selected on the concentration dial, over a wide range of gas flows. Note that in the Tec series of vaporisers, the term **Tec** means **te**mperature **c**ompensated.

Temperature compensation devices have been automated and usually utilise a bimetallic strip or other variable expansion technology to act as a temperature sensitive valve. With a **bimetallic strip (or similar) device**, as the temperature decreases during vaporisation (especially at high fresh gas flows), the bimetallic strip bends away from the vaporiser inlet channel, which encourages more gas to flow through the vaporisation chamber, so that vaporiser output, in terms of concentration of anaesthetic agent in the total gases leaving the vaporiser, remains constant, despite the agent's SVP falling with falling temperature (Figure 10.15).

With an ether-filled copper bellows device, expansion or contraction of the aneroid bellows with temperature changes helps to determine the proportion of gas diverted through the vaporisation chamber. With cooling, the bellows shrinks, and the bypass flow is restricted so that more gas is forced through the vaporisation chamber (Figure 10.16).

Temperature compensation mechanisms have a **limited range** over which they work best; for most vaporisers, this is between 10–18 °C and 35–40 °C. Outside these temperatures, the SVP of the agents may vary too much for vaporiser output to be accurate.

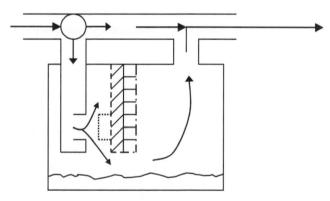

Figure 10.15 Temperature compensation achieved with variable curvature of bimetallic strip.

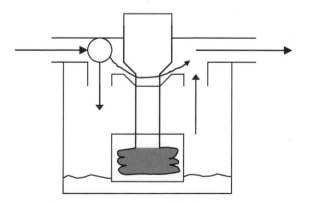

Figure 10.16 Temperature compensation achieved by variable expansion of ether-filled copper bellows.

10.12.5 Agent Specific Calibration

Each modern vaporiser is calibrated at standard temperature and pressure for the specific volatile agent for which it is intended. Calibration is also preformed over a range of gas flows.

The old copper-kettle vaporiser was not agent specific, but was also not calibrated. The anaesthetist had to calculate what flows were needed to send: (i) directly to the patient and (ii) through the vaporiser (remember that this vaporiser required two separate gas flows), in order to achieve the desired output concentration of the chosen agent at the temperature of the vaporiser at the time. The vaporiser consisted of a huge mass of copper to try to prevent cooling-related inaccuracies.

The SVP for halothane (243 mmHg), is very similar to that for isoflurane (238 mmHg). Because of their similarity, theoretically either agent could be used in either vaporiser, and the concentration delivered would be roughly correct. Enflurane (SVP 175 mmHg) and sevoflurane (SVP 160–170 mmHg) are also similar in volatility. However, it is very bad practice to fill a vaporiser intended for one agent with another (this is only possible if the vaporiser does not have the keyed-filler system), without cleaning it, recalibrating it, and re-labelling it in between.

Furthermore, liquid halothane comes with its less volatile stabiliser, thymol. Thymol does not vaporise easily, so gets left behind, and eventually it 'clogs up' wicks and the inner working parts of halothane vaporisers, which may affect vaporiser output. This is one reason why vaporisers require servicing/cleaning at least annually. It is also suggested that halothane vaporisers be completely drained (and the liquid drained, be discarded) every two weeks to slow down this clogging.

10.13 Other Features of Vaporisers

10.13.1 Effects of Ambient Atmospheric Pressure

Because SVP depends only upon temperature, and not pressure, the **atmospheric pressure itself has little effect on vaporiser output**. For example, at 760 mmHg atmospheric pressure, if the concentration dial is set at 1%, then the output partial pressure of halothane will be 1% of 760 mmHg (=7.6 mmHg). However, if the atmospheric pressure is 380 mmHg, and if the temperature has not changed, then halothane's SVP is still 243 mmHg, and the vaporising chamber contains $243/380 \times 100 = 64\%$ halothane. Although the dial says 1%, the output is actually 2%; but 2% of 380 mmHg = 7.6 mmHg, which again is the partial pressure exerted by halothane in the gases leaving the vaporiser. As it is the partial pressure of halothane in the lung alveoli, and thereby the brain, that determines whether the patient remains anaesthetised, we should not need to alter the vaporiser setting at all (unless the temperature also changes). You will recall that the MAC value is expressed in terms of percent of 1 standard (760 mmHg) atmospheric pressure.

If atmospheric pressure changes, then this equation can be used to determine the new vaporiser output:

$$\text{New vaporiser output in terms of vol\%} = C \times \left(P / P'\right)$$

where C is the vaporiser setting in vol%; P is the atmospheric pressure at which vaporiser was calibrated (standard atmospheric pressure); P' is the new atmospheric pressure.

Note that very wide variations in temperature and pressure may affect vaporiser output secondary to their effects on flow. Changes in temperature and pressure can affect gas viscosity and density, which can affect gas flow and the accuracy of flowmeters.

10.13.2　Tilt Protection

Most of the older vaporisers do not have any means of protecting the bypass gas channel from contamination by liquid agent should the vaporiser accidentally be tilted. Therefore, following accidental tilting, such vaporisers should be drained as fully as possible and then purged with a fresh gas flow (oxygen) of 5 l/min, with the concentration dial set at 5%, for at least 30 minutes (remember to scavenge). Note that different makes of vaporiser may have different instructions for this. This ensures that no liquid agent can possibly remain in the bypass, because if this were the case, a patient could receive a dangerously high percentage of anaesthetic agent.

Some of the newer vaporisers do have anti-tilting devices, e.g. the Tec 3 series are supposed to be able to withstand tilting of up to 90°, whereas the Tec 4 and 5 series should withstand tilting of up to 180°, but their manufacturers suggest you do not trust these tilt-protection devices, and still suggest emptying and purging the vaporiser should tilting occur.

10.13.3　Intermittent Back-pressure ('Pumping') Protection

Especially when positive pressure ventilation is necessary (and also when the oxygen flush valve is activated), the pressure exerted on the anaesthetic breathing system can be transmitted back to the anaesthetic machine back bar, and therefore the vaporiser. If gases that have left the vaporiser are forced to flow backwards and flow through the vaporisation chamber again, they can 'pick up' even more of the volatile agent, so the concentration of agent delivered to the patient can be much higher than originally intended. Most anaesthetic machine back bars now have pressure 'surge-protectors', in the form of constrictors, and some have one-way, non-return valves at the CGO. Most vaporisers also now have some kind of back-pressure protection, e.g. one-way check-valves or high resistance internal pathways. All of these modifications can reduce the pumping effect.

10.13.4　Carrier Gas Flow and Composition

Most modern vaporisers are designed so that their output is virtually independent of fresh gas flows over a range from c. 250 ml/min up to c. 15 l/min. Very slow flows (the gases need a bit of momentum to 'push' the relatively heavy vapour out of the vaporiser), and very fast gas flows (vaporisation in the vaporising chamber cannot keep pace with fast gas flow, so the vapour may not reach a fully saturated condition in the vaporisation chamber), tend to be associated with reduced output.

Plenum vaporisers are designed to work with carrier gas flows at more stable flows than draw-over vaporisers, which are subject to a wide variation in flows, e.g. from nil (during an end-expiratory pause), up to peak inspiratory flows (which can be about three to five times minute ventilation, so about 20 l/min for a 25 kg dog).

The gas composition, in terms of its temperature, its viscosity and density, and its chemical properties, can affect vaporiser output. For example, nitrous oxide will dissolve, to some extent, in liquid anaesthetic agents. When nitrous oxide flow is first turned on, this dissolution into the liquid anaesthetic agent will effectively reduce the volume of carrier gas passing through the vaporisation chamber, and thus will reduce vapour output. However, this is only a transient effect, as the amount of dissolved nitrous oxide soon reaches equilibrium with that in the carrier gas. The dissolution of nitrous oxide into the liquid anaesthetic agent may also slightly reduce its vaporisation (and SVP) by changing its chemical properties (and also somewhat diluting it). (Volatile anaesthetic agents also diffuse into/through plastic and rubber components of anaesthetic breathing systems and can be adsorbed into, as well as chemically-degraded by, carbon dioxide absorbents – see Chapter 8.)

10.13.5　Gas Flow Direction

If a vaporiser is erroneously connected 'back-to-front', higher vapour concentrations than those 'dialled up' may be delivered.

10.13.6　Liquid Level – How Full?

Most vaporisers work best when filled to the correct 'level'. Too empty, and they cannot produce accurate output; too full and the wick may be totally submerged, thus reducing the surface area available for evaporation, so output may again not be optimal. Also, if the vaporiser is too full, there is a risk of liquid agent escaping into the bypass channel which is very dangerous. Vaporisers usually have a 'sight-glass' that has 'empty' and 'full' markers, and vaporisers work best when the liquid level is between these two levels.

When vaporisers are filled, they should be turned 'off' (except the desflurane vaporiser, see later). If they are turned 'on' whilst gases are flowing through them, the gases will try to bubble out through the filler port, which as well as being wasteful and messy, leads to local environmental pollution. If a vaporiser is turned 'on' during filling, when gases are not flowing, there is a risk of over-filling it, with subsequent problems as mentioned above.

10.13.7 Vaporiser Filling

Some vaporisers have a funnel-shaped filling port, where liquid agent is literally poured in. Newer vaporisers have some kind of agent-specific filling device, the design of which depends upon the manufacturer. One well-known **keyed-filler system** is the **Fraser-Sweatman safety system**. These keyed filler devices are in the form of agent-specific vaporiser-filling nozzles that are geometrically coded (keyed) at both ends to fit, firstly the collar on the bottle of agent, and secondly the filling port of the agent's vaporiser (by way of an agent-specific 'groove' that docks into the filling port of the correct vaporiser). Another system is the **Easy-fill system** whereby the agent bottles are manufactured with an integral agent-specific filling spout that is compatible with the port on the vaporiser's filling block. (Easy-Fill bottle adapters are also available, which fit only the correct bottle collar.)

All fillers are also colour-coded according to agent:

- Red for halothane
- Purple for isoflurane
- Yellow for sevoflurane
- Blue for desflurane

These keyed-filling devices also reduce spillage of liquid agent, eliminate the problem of air-locks, and help prevent over-filling of vaporisers.

10.13.8 Discolouration of Agent

Some vaporisers incorporate plastic spacers between paper wicks, and these can react with the liquid anaesthetic agent, which causes discoloration (yellowy-brown), but apparently without any significant consequence to vaporiser output.

10.13.9 Corrosion

Halothane requires a stabiliser/preservative, thymol, to reduce its degradation. The more fluorinated an agent, the less 'reactive' it is, so isoflurane, sevoflurane, and desflurane do not need stabilisers/preservatives as such. However, sevoflurane is bottled in plastic or lacquered aluminium and has water added to reduce its degradation.

One of sevoflurane's potential breakdown products (within its supply bottle) is hydrofluoric acid (although inclusion of a little water as a Lewis base 'preservative' usually prevents this). Hydrofluoric acid is very corrosive (it can etch glass), so the vaporiser material should be as robust as possible. Corrosion of the anaesthetic breathing system components can also occur.

10.13.10 Vaporiser Mounting on the Back Bar

Vaporisers can be permanently mounted onto an anaesthetic machine back bar, usually by 'conical'/tapered (so-called 'cage-mount') fittings. Alternatively, they can be detachably mounted, usually onto some quick-release type of mounting, e.g. the 'select-a-tec' system. This consists of two protruding 'male' docking port valves on the back bar and compatible 'female' docking port recesses on the vaporiser mounting bracket. Once the male and female ports have been 'married', i.e. the vaporiser is 'seated' on the back bar, it must then be 'locked' in place by turning a lever. The vaporiser must be locked into its position before any gas can flow through it. With the older Tec 3 series vaporisers, gas could flow through the vaporiser 'head' (i.e. though the bypass) as soon as the vaporiser was locked on, even before its concentration dial was actually turned 'on'. With the newer Tec 4 and 5 series vaporisers, the vaporiser must be locked onto the back bar and the concentration dial turned 'on' before any gas can flow through it.

10.13.11 Vaporiser Interlock (Exclusion) Systems

Historically, hospital anaesthetists occasionally used more than one vaporiser simultaneously, and they used to follow certain rules, such as which vaporiser was placed upstream. However, this is no longer considered good practice, but many anaesthetic machines still have back bar 'positions' available for more than one vaporiser. So, if more than one vaporiser is mounted on an anaesthetic machine (e.g. two vaporisers are attached all the time, but you only want to use one), there is the potential for inadvertently administering more than one inhalational agent to the patient, e.g. if the previous anaesthetist forgot to turn off his/her chosen vaporiser at the end of that anaesthetic and you now turn on a different vaporiser.

In order to try to prevent this dangerous situation, interlock (vaporiser exclusion) systems were introduced. These tend to function so that if two vaporisers are mounted next to each other, and one is turned on, a small rod (or rods) protrude/s sideways from it, which locate/s into the adjacent vaporiser, thus preventing it from being turned on because of immobilisation of the equivalent rod movement on that vaporiser.

10.14   Safety Features of Vaporisers

- Keyed and colour-coded filling devices (ensure correct agent and prevent over-filling)
- The 'low' position of the filling port prevents over-filling and prevents spillage into the bypass
- Vaporisers must be locked into place before they can be turned on
- The safety interlock system prevents the use of more than one vaporiser at any one time
- Anticlockwise turn 'on'; all modern vaporisers are now the same in this respect
- Most vaporisers incorporate a locking lever or button, which prevents movement of the concentration dial (to turn it 'on'), until this lever/button is depressed/unlocked. Most modern vaporisers also must be turned 'on' before gases can flow through them.

10.15   Desflurane Vaporiser

Desflurane's SVP is about 664 mmHg at room temperature, which means that it is very volatile; in fact, it is almost at its boiling point at room temperature, and small fluctuations in room temperature can greatly affect its vaporisation. In order to 'control' the vaporisation of this agent accurately, the liquid agent must be held at a constant temperature, so that its SVP is constant. This can only be achieved by using a special vaporiser, which boils the liquid agent and then heats its vapour to 39 °C, at which its SVP is 1500 mmHg.

The archetypal Tec 6 desflurane vaporiser works as follows. It consists of a thermostatically controlled agent reservoir, which holds about 400 ml of liquid agent. It is heated (requires electrical supply, and has battery backup) to a temperature of 39 °C. At this temperature, the SVP of desflurane is 194 kPa (1500 mmHg). When vapour is required, a valve opens and pure vapour (under some pressure) is allowed to leave the reservoir. This 'high' pressure vapour passes through an electronic pressure regulator, which reduces its pressure to around 1–2 kPa above atmospheric pressure (i.e. the sort of pressure that is normally found in a plenum type vaporiser). From this pressure regulator, the vapour is then, according to the dialled up percentage, 'fed into' a carrier gas stream, which has been 'regulated' to a similar pressure, and then the 'blended' gas flow can leave the vaporiser.

The vaporiser requires a 5–10 minutes warm-up time to reach its operating temperature. It cannot be turned on until it is ready. It is the one vaporiser that you can fill whilst it is in use; at dial settings of 8% or less, but not at the higher settings (it delivers up to 18%). This is necessary because turning off a desflurane vaporiser in order to fill it might allow the patient to wake up because it is an agent of very low blood solubility. Desflurane bottles are plastic-coated, to help them withstand the high pressures generated by evaporated liquid agent at a range of room temperatures.

10.16   Cassette Type Vaporisers

These are found in machines such as the General Electric Healthcare (formerly Datex-Ohmeda) Aisys (Anaesthesia Integrated System) anaesthetic care station (Figure 10.17). Only one vaporiser can be locked into the 'active' bay at any one time, agent identification being through colour-coding, agent name, an agent-specific keyed-filling device and an agent-specific sequence of magnets housed within the casing of the vaporiser. These cassette type vaporisers are of the plenum type. The flow of fresh gases through the vaporiser and operation of the proportional control valve (splitting the flow between bypass and carrier channels) being determined electronically so that the desired concentration of agent is accurately delivered in the gases leaving the CGO.

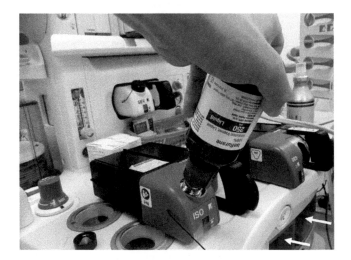

Figure 10.17 Isoflurane Aladin™ cassette vaporiser being filled. Note the desflurane Aladin cassette vaporiser (blue), adjacent to the isoflurane vaporiser; both these vaporisers, once filled, are then returned to their 'storage' bays (white arrows) until use. Note here the sevoflurane Aladin cassette vaporiser (yellow) in the 'active' bay. *Source:* Image courtesy of Paul MacFarlane.

10.17   VIC: Stephens Circle and Komesaroff Machine

If we apply the principles of vaporiser classification to VIC, what do we find?

- The splitting ratio is determined by the concentration dial position (although 'calibrations' are 'rough', see below).
- The method of vaporisation is flow-over. Wicks may be included to enhance vaporisation of the less volatile agents, but they also increase resistance. Wicks must be metal (so provide some temperature compensation ability too), as cloth wicks tend to become saturated by condensed water vapour.
- They have no temperature compensation devices. They are made of glass and their output varies with gas flow.
- The anaesthetic agent concentration within the circle will decrease if the fresh gas flow entering the circle is increased because additional entry of 'cool' 'fresh' gases (which are not carrying anaesthetic agent) will tend to reduce vaporisation and dilute out the anaesthetic-laden gases already within the circle (especially at faster flows as vaporsation cannot keep up due to lack of temperature compensation).

- They have no accurate calibrations. Their output can be increased by turning the dial to a higher value, e.g. the Goldman vaporiser has one dial setting for off, and three positions for on: 1–3.
- They are designed for use within an anaesthetic breathing system, usually in the inspiratory limb of a circle type system. They have low internal resistance to enable patient breathing efforts to move gases through them, hence they are called draw-over vaporisers. When the vaporiser is within the circle, the patient can regulate its own anaesthetic depth. For example, if the level of anaesthesia becomes too deep, then the animal breathes more slowly, and less gas is drawn over the liquid agent in the vaporiser. Couple this with the fact that the vapour already present within the circle is getting diluted by the continuing inflow of 'cold' fresh gas from the anaesthetic machine, and you will see that anaesthesia will 'lighten'. Conversely, if the animal is too light, it will tend to breathe faster (unless it breath-holds), so more gases are drawn through the vaporiser, and the vapour concentration within the circuit increases, so anaesthesia deepens. This sort of 'feedback' control system, however, is over-ridden if you apply artificial ventilation.

These systems can take a bit of getting used to, and patients tend to regulate their depth of anaesthesia to a deep plane.

References

Al-Shaikh, B. and Stacey, S. (eds.) (2002). Medical gas supply. In: *Essentials of Anaesthetic Equipment*, 2e, 1–13. Elsevier.

Davey, A., JTB, M., and Ward, C.S. (eds.) (1992a). The continuous flow anaesthetic machine. In: *Ward's Anaesthetic Equipment*, 3e, 94–112. Elsevier.

Davey, A., JTB, M., and Ward, C.S. (eds.) (1992b). The supply of anaesthetic gases. In: *Ward's Anaesthetic Equipment*, 3e, 32–38. Elsevier.

Davey, A., JTB, M., and Ward, C.S. (eds.) (1992c). Physical principles. In: *Ward's Anaesthetic Equipment*, 3e, 1–19. Elsevier.

Further Reading

Alibhai, H. (2016). The anaesthetic machine and vaporisers. In: *BSAVA Manual of Canine and Feline Anaesthesia and Analgesia*, 3e (eds. T. Duke-Novakovski, M. de Vries and C. Seymour), 24–44. Gloucester, UK: BSAVA Publications.

Ambrisko, T.D. and Klide, A.M. (2006). Evaluation of isoflurane and sevoflurane vaporizers over a wide range of oxygen flow rates. *American Journal of Veterinary Research* 67: 936–940. ***(Discusses the potential problems of vaporisers being calibrated with air, yet being used with oxygen.).***

Boumphrey, S. and Marshall, N. (2011). Understanding vaporizers. *Continuing Education in Anaesthesia, Critical Care and Pain* 11: 199–203.

Clutton, E. (1995). The right anaesthetic machine for you? *In Practice* 17: 83–88.

Dosch, M.P. (2016). The anesthesia gas machine. www.udmercy.edu/crna.agm.

Eales, M. and Cooper, R. (2007). Principles of anaesthetic vaporizers. *Anaesthesia and Intensive Care Medicine* 8: 111–115.

Hartsfield, S.M. (1994). Practical problems with veterinary anaesthesia machines. *Journal of Veterinary Anaesthesia* 21: 86–98.

Peyton, J. and Cooper, R. (2007). Anaesthetic machines. *Anaesthesia and Intensive Care Medicine* 8: 107–111.

Sinclair, C.M., Thadsad, M.K., and Barker, I. (2006). Modern anaesthetic machines. *Continuing Education in Anaesthesia, Critical Care and Pain* 6: 75–78.

Books

Al-Shaikh, B. and Stacey, S. (2013). *Essentials of Anaesthetic Equipment*, 4e (eds. B. Al-Shaikh and S. Stacey). London, UK: Elsevier.

Aston, D., Rivers, A., and Dharmadasa, A. (2014). *Equipment in Anaesthesia and Critical Care: A Complete Guide for the FRCA* (eds. D. Aston, A. Rivers and A. Dharmadasa). Oxford, UK: Scion Publishing.

Davey, J.A. and Diba, A. (2012). *Ward's Anaesthetic Equipment*, 6e (eds. A.J. Davey and A. Diba). London, UK: Saunders Elsevier.

Dorsh, J.A. and Dorsch, S.E. (2008). *Understanding Anesthesia Equipment*, 5e (eds. J.A. Dorsch and S.E. Dorsch). Pennsylvania, USA: Lippicott, Williams and Wilkins.

Ehrenwerth, J., Eisenkraft, J.B., and Berry, J.M. (2013). *Anesthesia Equipment: Principles and Applications*, 2e (eds. J. Ehrenwerth, J.B. Eisenkraft and J.M. Berry). Pennsylvania, USA: Elsevier Saunders.

Rose, G. and McLarney, J.T. (2014). *Anesthesia Equipment Simplified* (eds. G. Rose and J.T. McLarney). New York, USA: McGraw Hill Education.

Self-test Section

1 The high pressure part of the anaesthetic machine includes which of the following?
    A The cylinder yokes
    B The oxygen alarm
    C The oxygen flush/emergency oxygen valve
    D The flowmeter block

2 For gases flowing through flowmeters, which of the following statements is **false**?

    A At low flows, the indicated flow depends more upon the viscosity of the gas than its density.
    B Temperature affects both the density and viscosity of gases and so can affect flowmeter accuracy.
    C The pressure difference across the indicator varies with the internal diameter of the flowmeter tube.
    D Turbulent flow occurs at shorter, wider constrictions.

11

Anaesthetic Machine Checks

Various checks should be performed before an anaesthetic machine is used.

- If required, ensure the anaesthetic machine is plugged into an electrical power supply and that the **master switch is turned on**.
  - Modern anaesthesia workstations usually require that an electrical master switch be turned 'on' before flowmeters can be activated (see below).
- Ensure that there is **sufficient oxygen** and other gases in the available cylinders or piped hospital supply.
  - The chemical contents of each cylinder should be checked according to the chemical name on its label (do not rely on the cylinder colour).
  - Cylinders beyond their expiry date should not be used.
  - All cylinder valves should be able to be opened, i.e. the correct cylinder spanner/key should be available. (Cylinder valves should not be closed so tightly that they cannot be opened.)
  - Once any gas cylinders for immediate use (e.g. O_2, N_2O, medical air) have been turned 'on', listen/feel carefully for **leaks** around the cylinder valves and throughout the anaesthetic machine's plumbing, if accessible. Special non-combustible (usually soapy) leak detection fluid is available.
  - If there is a piped gas supply to the operating theatre, check that the **non-interchangeable probes** of the gas hoses are inserted into their respective **sockets** (these are of the Schrader type in the UK). Once in place, give each probe a gentle tug (the **tug test**) to ensure that it has engaged correctly into the socket.
  - Note that in modern anaesthesia workstations, once the master switch has been turned on and an oxygen supply has been provided (piped supply connected, or cylinder attached and opened), a mandatory minimum oxygen flow (50–250 ml/min) is usually established.

- Check that the **flowmeters** are functional. Ensure that the indicator floats can move throughout the whole range of their scales and check that the floats do not stick either to the sides of the flowmeter tubes, or to the 'stops' at the top and bottom of the flowmeter tubes. Rotameter floats should rotate when gases are flowing.
  - Note that when there is a mandatory minimum oxygen flow, it will not usually be possible to turn the oxygen flow fully 'off'.
- Check that there is a **vaporiser** available for the volatile agent of choice and only use vaporisers that are 'in date' with respect to their servicing. The vaporiser may be permanently plumbed into the back bar of the anaesthetic machine (on cage-mount fittings), or 'removable' (i.e. quick-release mounting). Using some oxygen flow, check for leaks around cage-mount connections or from around quick-release seatings. With quick-release mounted vaporisers, check for leaks both before and after mounting the vaporiser and locking it into position. Leak tests should also be performed with the vaporiser turned both 'off' and 'on' (remembering to scavenge the waste gases). Turn the oxygen flow 'off', or to its mandatory minimum flow once these leak tests are completed.
- Ensure that the vaporiser can be turned 'on' and that the concentration dial can be turned throughout its full range of concentrations. (Halothane vaporiser flow-splitting valves [actuated by turning the concentration dial] were notorious for become sticky through deposition of the non-volatile 'stabiliser', thymol.)
- Ensure that the vaporiser is full, and with the correct agent, and that there is sufficient spare supply of volatile agent.

Before attempting these next checks, make sure that the vaporiser and any nitrous oxide flow are turned 'off' to reduce theatre contamination.

Veterinary Anaesthesia: Principles to Practice, Second Edition. Alexandra H. A. Dugdale, Georgina Beaumont, Carl Bradbrook, and Matthew Gurney.
© 2020 John Wiley & Sons Ltd. Published 2020 by John Wiley & Sons Ltd.
Companion website: www.wiley.com/go/dugdale/veterinary-anaesthesia

- With just oxygen flowing, feel for gas exiting through the common gas outlet (CGO) of the anaesthetic machine. Ideally an oxygen analyser should be used to confirm that this gas is indeed oxygen.
- With oxygen still flowing, briefly occlude the CGO, and watch the O_2 flowmeter indicator float. It should 'fall' (with the increased back pressure created, which also increases the gas's density). If the CGO occlusion is maintained for a little longer, the **high (positive) pressure relief valve** (if fitted) should be activated and gases should be heard escaping from the anaesthetic machine back bar (usually near the CGO). If the float fails to 'fall', there may be a leak somewhere in the back bar.
- Preferably with the oxygen flow turned 'off' (or to its mandatory minimum flow), check that the **emergency oxygen flush valve** is functional.
- To check the **oxygen failure device**, the O_2 cylinder/ pipeline supply must first be turned 'off'/disconnected, respectively. Then turn 'on' (or 'up', for machines with a mandatory minimum flow), the O_2 flow to drain oxygen from the machine, and watch the O_2 pressure gauge register a fall in O_2 pressure. An audible alarm should sound once the pressure falls to around 200 kPa. Remember to re-establish the O_2 supply, i.e. re-open the oxygen cylinder or plug the oxygen hose back into the piped supply, before starting an anaesthetic.
- To perform a **negative pressure leak test on the anaesthetic machine**, you need a rubber squeezy suction bulb. With all flowmeters and vaporiser (if present) turned 'off' (the master switch may need to be turned 'off' to stop mandatory minimum oxygen flow), attach the pre-squeezed (i.e. empty) suction bulb to the CGO and wait for at least 10 seconds. This effectively applies a gentle vacuum to the low pressure parts of the anaesthetic machine. If there are any leaks, the bulb will 'fill' easily. If not, the bulb will stay empty. This test should also be repeated with the vaporiser turned 'on', but with no gases flowing. The bulb should not fill. When the test is complete, the master switch should be turned back 'on' to re-enable the flowmeters and re-establish the mandatory minimum oxygen flow.
- To check if the **negative pressure (air inlet) valve** is working, greater negative pressure needs to be applied than for the negative pressure leak test above. With all flowmeters turned 'off' (and the master switch turned 'off' on machines with mandatory minimum oxygen flow), a tube (e.g. an endotracheal tube) can be connected to the CGO, and by sucking on the free end of the tube, sufficient negative pressure can be created to perform the test, which should activate the back bar negative pressure relief valve, which will be heard 'squeaking'. Not all veterinary machines have this safety feature.

When the test is complete, the master switch should be turned back 'on' to re-enable the flowmeters and re-establish the mandatory minimum oxygen flow.

- The **anaesthetic breathing systems** should also be tested. Turn the oxygen flow to, e.g. 2 l/min.

For all the breathing systems, if the patient's end of the system is occluded and the 'pop-off' valve is closed (or for a Jackson Rees modified Ayre's T-piece, the open end of the bag is occluded), ensure that the system/bag fills. If the bag is then squeezed gently, any leaks may be detected. (Note that some newer 'pop-off' valves have a high pressure release port, which usually operates at around 30 cmH$_2$O for human paediatric valves and around 60 cmH$_2$O for human adult valves.) Then ensure that all 'pop-off' valves are opened again so that the systems are ready, and not dangerous, for use.

With Bain systems, it is important to establish that the inner tube is intact, or else there is a risk of causing excessive rebreathing of exhaled gases. The simplest way to do this is to set the oxygen flow to, say, 2 l/min and then to occlude the end of the inner (fresh gas supply) hose at the patient's end of the system. The flowmeter float should fall (due to back-pressure/increased gas density), and the anaesthetic machine's back bar high pressure relief valve may activate.

Another way of testing anaesthetic breathing systems for leaks is to use a manometer. Circle systems often have manometers incorporated into their design. Manometers can be purchased for other breathing systems. Small leaks can be very important for circles where 'low flow' anaesthesia may be practised because even small gas leaks can represent a significant wastage/loss from the system. If the patient's end of the breathing system is temporarily occluded, and the pop-off valve closed, the system can be 'filled' using oxygen flow until the pressure registered on the manometer reads about 30–40 cmH$_2$O. The oxygen flow is then turned 'off' (the master switch must be turned 'off' on machines with a mandatory minimum flow), and the pressure registered on the manometer is monitored: If there are no leaks, the measured pressure should not change. If there are leaks, then the pressure will fall. The leak rate can be most easily determined in machines where there is no mandatory minimum oxygen flow by turning the O_2 flowmeter 'on' and adjusting the oxygen flow until the pressure reading remains constant. **Leaks of more than 100 ml/min are not acceptable for a circle system if 'low flow' anaesthesia is planned**. Common sites for leaks in circles are around the valves and around the absorber canister. Once the leak tests have been completed, it is important to open any breathing system pop-off valves.

The oxygen flow should also be turned 'off', or back to the mandatory minimum flow (the master switch must be turned back 'on').

The **waste anaesthetic gas scavenging and disposal system** should be checked (e.g. adequate, but not excessive, suction should be available for active systems; the weight of active charcoal canisters should be checked for passive systems).

Once the anaesthetic machine and anaesthetic breathing systems have been checked, it is important to check the functioning of any **ventilator and monitoring equipment** that might be required.

All the **ancillary equipment** (endotracheal tubes, laryngoscopes, suction, etc.), **drugs, and fluids** necessary should also be available, including an emergency drugs box.

12

Local Anaesthetics

LEARNING OBJECTIVES

- To be able to describe the basic pharmacology of local anaesthetic agents in terms of their chemical structure, including the two types of molecular linkage, and their mechanism of action at voltage sensitive sodium channels.
- To appreciate the possible order of blockade of mixed nerves.
- To be able to discuss the features of the two main groups of local anaesthetics (amide- and ester-linked) that affect onset and duration of action, tissue penetration, and toxicity.
- To be able to describe the clinical effects of toxicity.
- To be able to discuss the different routes of application/administration of local anaesthetic agents.

12.1 Mechanism of Action

Local anaesthetics are weak bases, which reversibly 'block' voltage-gated sodium channels; and thereby prevent membrane depolarisation. They may also block various other ion channels (e.g. HCN channels), and have other actions, such as anti-inflammatory effects (see below).

Voltage-gated sodium channels exist in various conformational 'states', and pass through at least these different states as the membrane potential changes:

- Resting (or 'rested-closed')
- Open or activated
- Inactivated (or 'inactivated-closed') or desensitised

The channels may change between states as shown in Figure 12.1.

Local anaesthetics **preferentially block the inactivated and open/activated channels,** but not the resting state (i.e. $I > O >> R$); and because their dissociation from the channel takes longer than their association with it, they tend to stabilise sodium channels (and therefore the membrane) in a non-excitable, non-conducting state. Sodium channels are transmembrane 'pores', formed by at least one α and one or two β membrane-spanning protein subunits.

Because of this voltage-gated sodium channel blockade, local anaesthetics are able to inhibit membrane depolarisation, and therefore the development and transmission of electrical currents within 'excitable' tissues, notably neurons and muscles (especially cardiac muscle). The ease of blockade of electrical impulses (block of sodium currents) depends upon the sodium channel density in the tissue concerned, the 'state' of the channels, and how well 'insulated' they are from the applied local anaesthetic.

For example, if we apply local anaesthetic to a mixed spinal nerve, the nerve consists of several types of nerve fibres; some are myelinated (with variable thickness of myelin sheath depending upon nerve type), and some are unmyelinated nerves with just loose Schwann cell covering. The different types of nerve fibres conduct currents at different velocities. The velocity of conduction is primarily dependent upon the fibre diameter. Smaller diameter fibres have higher resistance to current passage, and so slower transmission velocity. Smaller diameter fibres also usually have a relatively smaller absolute number of sodium channels per unit of membrane length, so the 'size' of sodium current generated is limited, which also limits the conduction velocity. Unmyelinated nerves are very susceptible to local anaesthetic action because:

- There is minimal 'insulation', thus allowing the polar local anaesthetic molecules easy access to the nerve membranes.
- They are usually small diameter fibres, so that the overall number of sodium channels per unit length of fibre is small, so complete conduction blockade is accomplished easily by low doses of local anaesthetic.

Veterinary Anaesthesia: Principles to Practice, Second Edition. Alexandra H. A. Dugdale, Georgina Beaumont, Carl Bradbrook, and Matthew Gurney.
© 2020 John Wiley & Sons Ltd. Published 2020 by John Wiley & Sons Ltd.
Companion website: www.wiley.com/go/dugdale/veterinary-anaesthesia

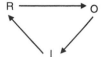

Figure 12.1 Voltage-gated sodium channels may change between the states of resting (R), open (O) and inactivated (I) in the direction of the arrows.

Myelinated nerve fibres use 'saltatory' conduction, whereby current 'jumps' from one node of Ranvier to the next, and because of this, only three successive nodes need to be blocked by local anaesthetic to effect total conduction block in the fibre. Nodes are not insulated by myelin, and therefore are more susceptible to block by local anaesthetics than the internodal parts of the nerve fibre. Although there tends to be a high density of sodium channels at nodes, sufficient channels *may* actually be blocked more easily at three successive nodes of a myelinated nerve fibre than along a sufficient length of non-myelinated nerve fibre, to block conduction. Therefore, sometimes, myelinated fibres appear to block more easily than unmyelinated fibres. The order of blockade of the fibres also depends upon their frequency of 'use' or firing (see below).

The quoted order of blockade of a mixed nerve is usually:

1) **Preganglionic sympathetic** B fibres (poorly myelinated).
2) **Post-ganglionic sympathetic** C fibres; also **temperature** and **pain** fibres (C and Aδ fibres). (C fibres are unmyelinated; Aδ fibres are poorly myelinated.)
3) **Touch** (discriminatory), **deep pressure**, **muscle spindle sensory** fibres (flower spray endings). (Myelinated Aβ fibres).
4) **Motor fibres to muscle spindles** (myelinated Aγ fibres).

5) **Proprioception** (myelinated Aα fibres), and **somatic motor** fibres (myelinated Aα fibres); also **muscle spindle sensory** fibres (annulospiral endings) (myelinated Aα fibres), and **sensory fibres of Golgi tendon organs** (myelinated Aα fibres).

When myelinated fibres block before unmyelinated fibres, it may be partly because of 'use-dependent' (or 'frequency of firing'-dependent) blockade. That is, those fibres that are more active have more channels in a state that can be blocked by local anaesthetic agents (remember I > O >> R). So Aδ fibres (fast pain; incisional pain) may block before C fibres (slow pain), and sometimes Aα fibres seem to block first, if these fibres are more inherently active (see later). Clinically, we should therefore expect a more effective blockade where pain is already present, although this is difficult to demonstrate.

Some texts describe the effects of differential nerve blockade as follows. If the local anaesthetic is applied to a mixed peripheral nerve at **X**, its differential effects spread out in 'wavefronts' (Figure 12.2).

In large mixed nerves, those fibres on the 'outside' of the nerve are blocked first (the **mantle effect**). These usually supply the more proximal parts of a limb, whilst distal parts are supplied by nerves lying deeper within the mixed nerve. Hence, limbs tend to become 'blocked' from proximal to distal, and the block wears off in the reverse sequence so that sensation to the toes blocks last and returns first.

12.2 Chemical Structure of Local Anaesthetic Agents

Although a number of drugs possess 'local anaesthetic-like' activity and 'membrane stabilising' properties (e.g. phenothiazines, pethidine, ketamine, atropine, α2 agonists

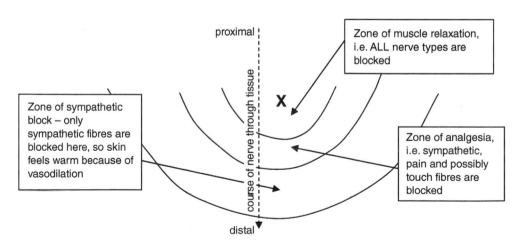

Figure 12.2 Zones of desensitisation following local anaesthesia of a peripheral nerve at X.

and antagonists, antihistamines, anticonvulsants, and beta blockers), the local anaesthetics that we use specifically to block nerve conduction have a common chemical structure:

Aromatic group ----- Intermediate link ----- Amino group
(lipophilic)   (hydrocarbon chain)   (hydrophilic)

The amino group most often consists of a tertiary amine, except:

- Prilocaine, which has a secondary amine instead.
- Benzocaine, which does not have a tertiary amine group and so cannot exist in the ionised (RNH^+) form.

The nature of the **intermediate link** (i.e. whether it contains an ester or an amide group) defines the two broad sub-groups of local anaesthetic agents:

- the ester-linked group ($-C(=O)-O-C-$)
- the amide-linked group ($-NH-C(=O)-$)

The distance between the lipophilic and hydrophilic groups is important, and for best activity, must be 6–9 Angstroms (i.e. 4–5 atoms).

Most local anaesthetics are prepared as racemic mixtures of R and S enantiomers, but lidocaine is achiral.

Local anaesthetics, although weak bases with low water solubility, can be formulated as hydrochloride salts, which dissolve readily in water at pH 4–7. The commonly used local anaesthetic agents have pKa values between 7.6 and 8.9 (see below). Within the body (both extracellular and intracellular fluids), most local anaesthetic agents are therefore fairly well ionised. Both the **ionised and unionised forms** of the local anaesthetic are ultimately **important** for sodium channel blocking activity (Figure 12.3). Both forms exist according to the following equilibrium, where RN is the tertiary amine

form (free base), and RNH^+ is the quaternary N^+ state (ionised state).

$$RN + H^+ \leftrightarrow RNH^+$$

The **pH of the commercially available formulations is acidic** (e.g. the hydrochloride 'salt' of lidocaine has pH 6.5), and thus increases the amount of drug in the ionised form. After injection into tissues, the physiological pH is more alkaline (about 7.4), and the acidity of the injected solution is easily buffered (so raising the pH of the injectate), so that an increase in the unionised lipophilic form is favoured.

The ionised form (RNH^+) can block sodium channels from the 'outside' of the cell membrane, whilst the unionised (RN) form easily crosses cell membranes. The unionised form (RN) can block sodium channels from 'within' the membrane; and once inside the cell, where the intracellular pH is slightly more acidic than the extracellular fluid, an increase in ionised form is favoured. The ionised form (RNH^+) can now also 'block' sodium channels from the 'inside' of the cell membrane.

As we have seen, RN can 'block' channels from 'within' the membrane; and this hydrophobic blocking action is non-frequency-dependent (non-use-dependent), whereas hydrophilic channel blocking by RNH^+, whether from inside or outside the membrane, is frequency-dependent.

Benzocaine cannot exist in the ionised form, and possibly just blocks channels from 'within' the membrane.

12.2.1 Ester-linked Local Anaesthetics (Benzoic Acid Derivatives)

- Cocaine
- Procaine
- 2-chloroprocaine
- Benzocaine
- Tetracaine (Amethocaine)
- Cinchocaine (Dibucaine)

12.2.1.1 Properties of the Amino-esters

- Poor tissue penetration.
- Short duration of action because rapid metabolism (hydrolysis), by tissue and plasma esterases/cholinesterases (most of which are produced by the liver, e.g. butyrylcholinesterase, also known as pseudo-cholinesterase). Beware recent organophosphate treatment. Cocaine is the exception because it undergoes only hepatic metabolism. Note that cerebrospinal fluid (CSF) contains no esterases, so accidental intrathecal injection produces very long duration of effects.

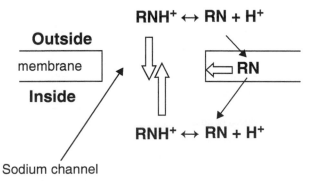

Figure 12.3 Sites of action of local anaesthetic agents at excitable membranes. Open arrows denote channel 'blocking'. RN is the tertiary amine form (free base), and RNH^+ is the quaternary N^+ state (ionised state).

- Possibly less chance of toxicity because of rapid metabolism (short duration of action).
- Possibly responsible for causing allergic reactions. One of the metabolites is para-amino benzoic acid (pABA), which is implicated in various allergic/hypersensitivity reactions. Also, pABA antagonises the actions of trimethoprim potentiated sulphonamides.

12.2.2 Amide-linked Local Anaesthetics (Aniline Derivatives)

- Lidocaine (lignocaine)
- Mepivacaine
- Bupivacaine (& laevo-bupivacaine)
- Ropivacaine
- Prilocaine

12.2.2.1 Properties of the Amino-amides

- Good tissue penetration.
- Longer duration of action (compared to amino-esters), as slower elimination by hepatic metabolism (amidase enzymes). Metabolites are subsequently excreted in urine. There is minimal excretion of the parent compound into urine and bile.
- Slower elimination may increase risk of toxicity.

- Possible allergic reactions because of methylparaben (methyl parahydroxybenzoate), which is commonly included as a preservative and can be broken down to pABA.
- Other complications are that prilocaine, especially the R isomer, is metabolised to ortho-toluidine, which oxidises haemoglobin (causing the formation of methaemoglobin). Methaemoglobinaemia may occur with prilocaine toxicity. Excessive use of EMLA cream (see later), of which prilocaine is one component, can also result in such toxicity.

12.3 Physicochemical Properties of Local Anaesthetics

Tables 12.1 and 12.2 summarise the physicochemical properties of local anaesthetic agents and how they relate to their clinical effects.

12.3.1 Key Characteristics

- The dissociation constant (**pKa**) that partly determines **onset** of action.
- **Lipid solubility** that partly determines **potency**.
- **Protein binding** that partly determines **duration** of action.

Table 12.1 Physicochemical properties of commonly used local anaesthetic agents.

	pKa	Onset	Relative lipid solubility	Toxicity	Relative potency	Protein binding	Duration of action
Procaine	8.9	Slow	1	Very low	1	6%	Short
Tetracaine	8.5	Slow	200	Medium	8	75%	Long
Lidocaine	7.9	Fast	150	Medium	2	65%	Intermediate
Prilocaine	7.9	Fast	50	Low	2	55%	Intermediate
Mepivacaine	7.6	Fast	50	Low	2.5	75%	Intermediate
Bupivacaine	8.16	Moderate	1000	High	8	95%	Long
Ropivacaine	8.1	Moderate	400	Medium	6	95%	Long

Table 12.2 Relationship between physicochemical properties and clinical effects.

Physicochemical characteristic	Correlate
pKa	Speed of onset
Tissue penetrance	Speed of onset
Vasodilator potential	Duration of action (Potency? Toxicity?)
Lipid solubility	Potency (toxicity?) Onset (and duration?) of action
Protein binding	Duration of action (Toxicity?)
Chemical linkage	Affects metabolism (duration of action)
Frequency/use-dependent blockade	Sensori-motor dissociation/discrimination

pKa is defined as the pH at which half the drug is present in the unionised form and half in the ionised form. *Speed of onset of block is proportional to the concentration of the unionised form outside the neuronal membrane.* Those local anaesthetic agents with pKa values near body pH (such as lidocaine) offer a faster onset of action (compared to bupivacaine) because relatively more RN is present. In fact, more equal amounts of RN and RNH$^+$ are present, and whilst extracellular RN concentration is important for speed of onset of block, both forms are ultimately necessary for local anaesthetic activity. Interestingly 2-chloroprocaine has a high pKa (8.7), yet a very rapid onset, so it is believed that 'tissue penetrance' also has a role (see information on concentration effect below, as often relatively high concentration [c.3%] solutions of 2-chloroprocaine were used that would also hasten onset of block). **Tissue penetrance** depends upon a number of factors: degree of ionisation (pKa, local pH), fat solubility, ease of molecular diffusion (molecular size, concentration gradient), and addition of dispersers. If the tissue is inflamed, it tends to have a lower (more acidic), pH, and therefore tends to reduce the amount of unionised form present and delays the onset of block.

Warming the local anaesthetic solution can lower the pKa (because dissociation constants are affected by temperature), and therefore hasten the block onset by increasing the amount of RN available to diffuse into the nerve. Warming the solution is also said to reduce the stinging often perceived on initial injection. However, **cooling** of nerves results in a reduction in conduction velocity, and therefore potentiation of the anaesthetic effect.

Alkalinising the solution before injection can also alter the pH of the solution to nearer the drug's pKa, favouring more equal amounts of ionised and unionised forms, and also reducing stinging on injection; but care must be taken not to over-alkalinise the solution as precipitation can occur. Alkalinisation usually involves addition of a small amount of bicarbonate:

To 1 ml lidocaine 2% add 0.1 ml of an 8.4% sodium bicarbonate solution

To 1 ml bupivacaine 0.5% add 0.01 ml of an 8.4% sodium bicarbonate solution

Sometimes, instead of hydrochloride salts, salts of carbonic acid are available (i.e. carbon dioxide is 'added' to the solution to increase its acidity and favour RNH$^+$ formation and increase solubility in aqueous solution). The idea behind this is that once injected into tissues, excess CO_2 is supposed to enter cells rapidly, thereby creating a more acidic intracellular environment and a less acidic extracellular environment, which favours formation of RN outside the cell, but RNH$^+$ inside the cell, with the result of a rapid onset of block. This addition of carbonic acid/CO_2 is called **carbonation.**

The onset of block can also be hastened by application of a higher concentration of local anaesthetic solution (but beware toxicity). This is simply via the **concentration effect**. That is, the more drug that is applied, the more RN and RNH$^+$ forms are present, and the faster the onset of block. Hence, *topical* local anaesthetics are often prepared in higher concentrations than those intended for *injection.*

Local anaesthetic agents have inherent vasoactive properties. The response may depend on dose, e.g. low doses resulting in vasoconstriction and higher doses resulting in vasodilation, but the different drugs, and their different enantiomers, may also have different actions; and actions in different species may be different. E.g.:

- Cocaine is a potent vasoconstrictor.
- Procaine causes mild vasodilation.
- Tetracaine (amethocaine) causes mild vasodilation.
- Lidocaine (has no enantiomers as it is achiral) causes vasodilation.
- Racemic mepivacaine lacks vasodilator activity (or may cause slight vasoconstriction).
- S-bupivacaine causes less vasodilation than R-bupivacaine and the racemic mixture; when the racemic mixture is applied, only mild vasodilation results.
- Ropivacaine has vasoconstrictor properties.
- The vasodilatory (and other cardiovascular) effects of lidocaine and bupivacaine at toxic doses can be reversed by lipid emulsion (see below).

If the local anaesthetic causes vasoconstriction, then systemic absorption is delayed, and the duration of block is prolonged. If it causes vasodilation, then systemic absorption is more rapid and the duration of block is shortened. The degree of vascularity at the site of application/administration will also influence duration of activity.

Cocaine is a potent vasoconstrictor because it inhibits monoamine (including catecholamine) re-uptake by 'uptake 1', and it inhibits monoamine oxidase, so it enhances monoaminergic neurotransmitter concentration at, e.g. sympathetic nerve terminals. It also stimulates central adrenergic pathways by which it can produce dependence.

Vasoconstrictors are commonly added to local anaesthetic agents with inherent vasodilator activity (e.g. lidocaine). **Epinephrine** (adrenaline) is the most common vasoconstrictor used, although various other agents, including **phenylephrine,** have also been used. If epinephrine is used, in order for it to remain stable in solution (long shelf life), the pH of the solution must be quite acidic. Most commercially available local anaesthetic solutions already have a slightly acidic pH (pH 6.5–7.2). The pH of commercially available lidocaine hydrochloride 1 and 2% plain solutions is around 6.4–6.6, whereas that of lidocaine 1 or 2% solutions with epinephrine is around 4–4.5. For plain bupivacaine 0.25 and 0.5% solutions, the pH is around 5.6–5.8. Increasing the acidity (to about pH 4–5) to keep epinephrine stable, further enhances the formation of the RNH^+ form of the local anaesthetic, and delays block onset, but this effect is negated by the vasoconstrictor (alpha 1 agonist) effect (of epinephrine) on the neural vasculature, which keeps a high concentration of local anaesthetic in the vicinity of the administered local anaesthetic. Epinephrine also has some 'local anaesthetic'-type activity of its own, which may help to enhance the block, although epinephrine does not appear to produce sensory or motor block by itself. Epinephrine may, however, induce neural ischaemia and the resulting metabolic changes may affect ion channels (beware also this mechanism of potential neurotoxicity), and it may have action at neuronal alpha 2 adrenoceptors with resultant effects on neuronal ion (especially potassium) channels. When included in local anaesthetic solutions at concentrations less than 5 µg/ml, epinephrine has not been associated with any major adverse systemic cardiovascular events. In people, however, the inclusion of low concentrations of epinephrine in local anaesthetic preparations has also been used to facilitate the early detection of inadvertent intravascular injection because of the minor cardiovascular sequelae (heart rate, blood pressure, and ECG changes).

Vasoconstrictors reduce the systemic absorption of local anaesthetics from their sites of application. By maximising the 'amount' (concentration) of a local anaesthetic at its application site, a more rapid onset of block is achieved. Reduction in systemic absorption also prolongs the duration of block and reduces the chance of systemic toxicity.

The addition of epinephrine to bupivacaine makes little difference because racemic bupivacaine has no appreciable vasodilator effect at clinically appropriate doses, is highly lipid soluble and highly protein (including sodium channel)-bound, and thus tends to have a long duration of action almost regardless of local vasomotor tone.

Basic drugs, such as local anaesthetic agents, prefer to **bind** to globulins, especially **α1-acid glycoprotein**, whereas acidic drugs prefer to bind to albumin. Acid–base disturbances may alter the degree of protein binding and the degree of ionisation of local anaesthetics, and may alter their pharmacokinetics and pharmacodynamics.

Sensorimotor dissociation/discrimination refers to the ability of some local anaesthetics to preferentially block sensation, whilst leaving motor nerve conduction undisturbed. The drug's pKa may be partly responsible for differential sensory/motor block, as the amount of drug present in the unionised form (more fat-soluble) will partly determine how easily it can cross nerve sheaths and neuronal membranes, so nerve fibres with different degrees of myelination are differently susceptible to block. It is normally expected that sensory fibres are blocked 'first' in preference to motor fibres (see above).

Sensorimotor discrimination may also be associated with the phenomenon of use-dependent or frequency-dependent blockade of sodium channels; whereby the nerves in which sodium channels are most active are more susceptible to blockade. Under general anaesthesia, the patient should not be moving voluntarily, so motor fibres are quiet and therefore relatively resistant to block, but sensory fibres are stimulated by surgery and should be more susceptible to block. Local anaesthetics tend to take longer to dissociate from sodium channels than they do to block them in the first place, so that spatial and temporal summation of effect can also occur.

Lidocaine and bupivacaine are very good at producing this sensorimotor dissociation. However, there may be more to this phenomenon yet to be discovered. For example, perhaps the sodium channels of sensory and motor nerves are differentially sensitive to certain local anaesthetics, or may be the interchange of sodium channels between their various states is different between different nerve types and differently affected by different local anaesthetics.

Some ester-linked local anaesthetics used to be available with added **hyaluronidase (a disperser)**. This was supposed to speed onset of block (by enhancing tissue penetration) and increase the spread of anaesthesia, thus increasing the likelihood of successful nerve blockade. However, duration of block was also reduced because systemic absorption was enhanced, and enhanced absorption could increase the risk of toxicity.

Other additives may be included. **Preservatives** such as sodium metabisulphite or methylparaben are commonly added. It is often recommended to use preservative-free solutions for neuraxial anaesthesia due to the potential neurotoxicity of such agents. The addition of **glucose** to local anaesthetic solutions can alter their density (baricity), which may be used to influence their spread within the CSF. Hypo-, iso-, and hyper-baric formulations are available. The density of CSF in dogs, cats, and horses is about 1.010 so that 1% lidocaine, 0.5% bupivacaine, and 1% ropivacaine are slightly hypobaric.

An α2 agonist may also be included with the local anaesthetic agent for performing local blocks, with three potential mechanisms of boosting the resultant analgesia/anaesthesia: systemic absorption and subsequent systemic analgesia; local vasoconstriction, which may hasten the onset and prolong the duration of the block (see 'concentration effect' above); and, by reducing the I_h repolarisation current activity, the duration of block may also be prolonged (see Chapter 4).

There has been much recent interest in the use of **dexamethasone**, either included with the local anaesthetic agent for performing a local block or given IV at the time of the local anaesthetic block. A recent editorial sheds interesting light on whether or not the analgesia is enhanced (see Further Reading).

12.3.2 Toxic Doses

Toxic doses depend upon the species; the block performed; vascularity of the area infiltrated; whether the local anaesthetic solution includes epinephrine, hyaluronidase, and preservatives; and patient factors such as health status, but are of the order of:

- **Lidocaine: toxic dose ≥ 4–6 plain (−10 with epinephrine) mg/kg; safe dose ≈ 2–3 mg/kg without epinephrine (4–7 mg/kg with epinephrine)**
- **Procaine: toxic dose ≥ 5 plain (−10 with epinephrine) mg/kg; safe dose ≈ 4 mg/kg without epinephrine (8 mg/kg with epinephrine)**
- **Mepivacaine: toxic dose ≥ 4–6 mg/kg; safe dose 2–3 mg/kg**
- **Bupivacaine: toxic dose > 2 mg/kg; safe dose ≈ 1–2 mg/kg**
- **Ropivacaine: toxic dose > 3 mg/kg; safe dose ≈ 1.5–3 mg/kg**
- **Prilocaine: toxic dose > 6 mg/kg; safe dose 2–4 mg/kg**
- **Tetracaine: toxic dose > 4 mg/kg; safe dose 2–3 mg/kg**

Regarding the above doses, it is probably wise to err on the low side, **especially for cats**. Whether they are 'more sensitive' or just easier to overdose because of their small size is undetermined.

If you are going to perform more than one block (e.g. spray cat's larynx with lidocaine [2–4 mg/spray] before tracheal intubation, then perform a brachial plexus block with lidocaine), beware the total dose of lidocaine used. If you want to use different local anaesthetics (e.g. lidocaine for one block and bupivacaine for another), beware the **cumulative toxicity** effects. Keep the individual drug doses below their respective toxic doses in order to avoid cumulative toxicity.

12.3.3 Adverse Reactions and Toxicity

12.3.3.1 True Allergic Reactions

These are more likely after use of ester-linked local anaesthetics because the allergic reactions are related to pABA production from their hydrolysis. However, methylparaben can be used as a preservative for amide-linked local anaesthetics and its metabolism can also lead to pABA production.

12.3.3.2 Local Tissue Injury/Neurotoxicity

Local tissue injury or neurotoxicity can occur due to:

- Preservatives.
- Vasoconstrictors (if 'end arteries' are vasoconstricted, then distal tissue ischaemia/necrosis can occur).
- Nerve injury (either due to direct trauma from the needle tip, or secondary to ischaemia, which occurs especially following sub-perineurium [intrafascicular] injection of local anaesthetic solution which then causes occlusion of the vasa nervorum); usually transient neural/neuromuscular dysfunction. (Never inject if you encounter resistance.)
- Needle injury to blood vessels, with haematoma formation. (Beware coagulopathies.)
- Introduction of infection. (Use good aseptic technique.)
- In high concentrations, local anaesthetics act like detergents and can cause irreversible damage to nerves (detergent effect on both myelin sheaths and neuronal cell membranes), so be careful what concentrations you choose, especially for intrathecal injection.

12.3.3.3 Systemic Toxicity

Systemic toxicity may occur due to the 'membrane stabilising' actions of these drugs on excitable brain and myocardial cells. It depends upon the blood concentration of the agent and its affinity for sodium channels in nerves, myocardium, and skeletal muscle cells. It may follow:

- Absolute overdose
- Inadvertent intravascular injection
- Individual sensitivity (Different species may also be differentially sensitive to different local anaesthetics)

Plasma concentration depends upon:

- Total dose given
- Rate of absorption (local tissue vascularity, vasoactivity of the drug, addition of vasoconstrictors)
- Distribution to tissues (occurs in proportion to their relative perfusion, so brain, heart, and vital organs receive large proportions of the amount absorbed)
- Metabolism and elimination: plasma esterases (for esters, except cocaine), or hepatic metabolism (for amides)

Progressive depression of the CNS and the cardiovascular system occurs as plasma concentration of the local anaesthetic agent increases (Figure 12.4). Usually CNS signs are seen first: depressed consciousness, convulsions, and apnoea. Serious cardiovascular effects usually occur secondarily to hypoxaemia (follows apnoea) or after intravenous injection of a large dose of bupivacaine (cardiotoxicity). The ratio of the dose required to produce cardiovascular collapse to that required to induce seizures,

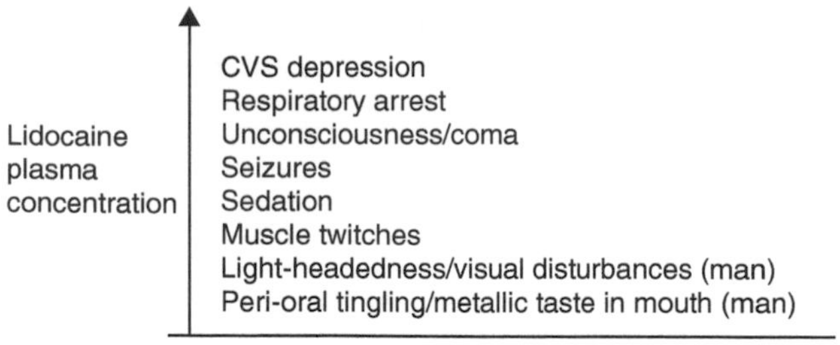

CVS depression
Respiratory arrest
Unconsciousness/coma
Seizures
Sedation
Muscle twitches
Light-headedness/visual disturbances (man)
Peri-oral tingling/metallic taste in mouth (man)

Lidocaine plasma concentration

Figure 12.4 Typical systemic toxicity described for lidocaine.

the so-called **CC/CNS ratio** is used to compare agents. Bupivacaine has a CC/CNS ratio of 2.0 compared with 7.1 for lidocaine.

As the plasma concentration of lidocaine increases (Figure 12.4), the signs of systemic toxicity progress from sedation, through seizures to depression, unconsciousness, and coma to respiratory arrest and cardiovascular collapse. When local/regional blocks are performed under general anaesthesia, cardiovascular changes the most noticeable signs of toxicity.

Inadvertent intrathecal injection can lead to hyperacute CNS toxicity and secondary cardiorespiratory depression. All the local anaesthetics have similar toxic : therapeutic ratios for CNS toxicity, but the seizure threshold varies for each drug and species. Cardiovascular depression is not usually seen until the plasma concentration reaches around three times the seizure threshold plasma concentration. However, bupivacaine prolongs cardiac conduction and increases the chance of re-entrant arrhythmias at concentrations only slightly above those of the seizure threshold. Cats also appear to be particularly sensitive to cardiovascular depression with systemically administered lidocaine.

Local anaesthetics may prefer to block cardiac sodium channels over neuronal or skeletal muscle sodium channels (perhaps because of use-dependency/intrinsic higher affinity/different inactivation properties), but they can block a variety of voltage- and ligand-gated ion channels. Bupivacaine, with its extremely great ability to bind proteins, slows the recovery of cardiac sodium channels much more than lidocaine, and is therefore much more arrhythmogenic. Bupivacaine may also bind to (and inhibit) a mitochondrial enzyme, carnitine acylcarnitine translocase, which is important for fatty acid oxidation and ATP generation in the heart, such that bupivacaine effectively blocks cardiac mitochondrial oxidative phosphorylation.

Local anaesthetic cardiovascular toxicity is classically described to follow three phases in humans: initial tachycardia and hypertension, intermediate myocardial depression and hypotension, and finally a terminal phase that involves widespread peripheral vasodilation, severe hypotension, and cardiac arrhythmias (tachycardic arrhythmias, bradycardic arrhythmias, and asystole). In dogs and cats, heart rate may not change much, but direct myocardial depression can lead to severe hypotension.

Treatment for local anaesthetic systemic toxicity (most usually seen as cardiovascular toxicity) is **lipid emulsion** (20% Intralipid™) administered intravenously as a bolus of 1.5 ml/kg over 1 minute, followed by a continuous infusion of 0.25–0.5 ml/kg/min (i.e. 15–30 ml/kg/h), with up to two extra 1.5 ml/kg boluses (at 5 minutes intervals) if required, until resolution of signs or until the maximum total dose of 12 ml/kg (for 20% lipid emulsion) has been administered. Lipid toxicity can occur at higher doses, although the clinical signs of this may not be recognised in anaesthetised animals, but include: dyspnoea, pyrexia, seizures, coma, coagulation abnormalities, and hepatic dysfunction. Other side effects of lipid rescue include facial pruritus, pancreatitis, and corneal lipidosis. The exact 'lipid rescue' mechanism of action is unknown, but local anaesthetics may be 'drawn' into the 'lipid sink' and away from tissues, and the lipid also provides fatty acids that may help restore cardiac metabolism and cardiomyocyte energy supply (which is inhibited by bupivacaine). Bretylium may be required should lipid rescue not be effective with the maximum safe dose of lipid emulsion.

Beware hepatic dysfunction that results in both reduced amide-linked local anaesthetic metabolism and reduced ester-linked local anaesthetic metabolism (because of reduced plasma/pseudo-cholinesterase production).

Organophosphate treatment results in inhibition of neuromuscular junction acetylcholinesterase and pseudocholinesterase, so expect prolonged action of ester-linked local anaesthetics, and possibly increased chance of toxicity.

Some people are poor producers of plasma cholinesterase, or they produce atypical plasma cholinesterase. A test of plasma cholinesterase activity is available for man, called the **dibucaine test**. (Dibucaine [cinchocaine is its recommended international non-proprietary name] is the cardiotoxic local anaesthetic used with quinalbarbital, for euthanasia, in Somulose™ and is an ester-type local anaesthetic.) The test results are expressed as the Dibucaine number, which represents the percentage inhibition of that patient's plasma cholinesterase by cinchocaine.

12.3.3.4 Methaemoglobinaemia

Methaemoglobinaemia can be seen following the use of high doses of prilocaine. The R-enantiomer especially is metabolised to ortho-toluidine (o-toluidine), which is responsible for oxidation of the haem iron in haemoglobin from the ferrous state to the ferric state (i.e. haemoglobin becomes methaemoglobin). Cats are said to be especially susceptible to this, so also beware excessive application of EMLA cream. Methaemoglobinaemia has also been reported following benzocaine administration.

12.3.3.5 Bupivacaine and Cardiotoxicity

The R-enantiomer is more cardiotoxic than the S-enantiomer (also known as laevo-bupivacaine). S-bupivacaine has similar local anaesthetic potency to R-bupivacaine and there are only small differences in intrinsic affinity and stereoselectivity of both isomers for the sodium channels of skeletal muscle and heart muscle, but overall the S-isomer may bind proteins (including sodium channels) slightly less well, which may partly explain its reduced cardiotoxicity. Laevo-bupivacaine (S-bupivacaine) is available commercially as 'Chirocaine™'.

12.3.3.6 Chondrotoxicity

All local anaesthetics can cause damage to cartilage, more so in osteoarthritic joints than 'normal' healthy joints. Toxicity is drug-, concentration-, and exposure time-dependent and may also be related to the preservatives and acidic pH of most commercially available solutions. Mitochondrial dysfunction, apoptosis, and necrosis appear to be involved in the mechanism/s of toxicity. Ropivacaine appears to be less chondro toxic than mepivacaine, which is less chondrotoxic than lidocaine, which is slightly less chondrotoxic than bupivacaine.

12.3.3.7 Nerve Damage

Injury to the nerve is a potential risk of local anaesthetic techniques. Injections made external to the epineurium (which surrounds a peripheral nerve) are considered perineural, whereas those made beneath the epineurium, i.e. intraneural, can be either extrafascicular or intrafascicular, depending upon whether the perineurium is broached. Deposition of local anaesthetic beneath the epineurium of a mixed nerve, but not broaching the perineurium, and thus made into the fascia/fat between nerve fascicles (extrafascicular), is potentially less damaging than injecting beneath the perineurium of individual nerve fascicles (intrafascicular) and into the endoneurial connective tissue.

The *aim is to deposit the solution around the nerve (perineural)* and not inject into the nerve (intraneural, either extra- or intrafascicular). If resistance is encountered during injection, the needle should be redirected. Techniques such as electro-neuro-location and ultrasound guidance are intended to reduce such risks. With ultrasound visualisation it is possible to document intraneural injection. Whilst some authors report no adverse effects from this, safe practice teaches us not to inject into nerves.

12.3.3.8 Myotoxicity

The problem of myotoxicity and subsequent myodegeneration (with occasional poor recovery or even non-recovery of muscle function), as a consequence of local/regional nerve blockade, has recently been highlighted in a human review. As for chondrotoxicity, myotoxicity shows a drug-, concentration-, and exposure duration-dependency, with bupivacaine the most commonly implicated local anaesthetic. The mechanism of toxicity (apoptosis/necrosis) is thought to be via disruption of intracellular calcium homeostasis in skeletal muscle.

12.4 Uses of Local Anaesthetics

12.4.1 Dilution of Local Anaesthetic Solutions

Sometimes a less concentrated solution of local anaesthetic is required, e.g. for performing nerve blocks or wound infiltration in small patients. Local anaesthetic solutions can be diluted to achieve this; the best diluent is sterile normal saline as it is slightly acidic and tends to preserve the pH of the parent solution. Bear in mind, however, that the greater the local anaesthetic concentration, the more effective the block.

12.4.2 Mixtures of Local Anaesthetic Solutions

Mixture of a quick-onset, short-duration local anaesthetic with a longer-onset, prolonged duration local anaesthetic has often been suggested to give the advantage of a rapid onset of block with prolonged duration. However, this may not actually happen because mixing of short- and long-acting local anaesthetics:

- dilutes each agent: the reduced concentration can slow the speed of onset of the block and may reduce its intensity
- changes the pH of the mixture: this may affect the onset time
- reduces the dose of each agent that can be given (because of cumulative toxicity): this will decrease the block duration

For example, a 1 : 1 (by volume) mixture of 2% plain lidocaine (pH 6.42) and 0.5% plain bupivacaine (pH 5.55), results in a solution of 1% lidocaine and 0.25% bupivacaine with a pH of 6.38. Compared with the parent solutions, the new pH of the mixture may very slightly slow lidocaine's onset, yet slightly hasten the onset of bupivacaine block; but the reduced concentration of both can slow the onset of both. Overall, the onset of block might be slightly slower than expected from lidocaine alone and the duration of block may be shorter than expected from bupivacaine alone, prompting some authors to suggest that there is little clinical advantage to using such mixtures.

12.4.3 Surface or Topical Application

- Mucous membranes (e.g. larynx for endotracheal intubation; bovine teat canals; bull nose pre-insertion of bull ring if bilateral infra-orbital nerve blocks are not possible).
- Conjunctiva or cornea.
- Skin: patches are now available that result in only very low systemic absorption although documentation of analgesia from these is yet to be demonstrated in animals.
- Synovial or intra-articular.
- Interpleural.
- Intra-abdominal for peritoneal 'splash block' (e.g. dogs with pancreatitis or even post ovariohysterectomy or other coeliotomy).
- Topical application to a wound (even including into a fracture site), including 'splash' blocks.

12.4.4 Non-specific Infiltration

- Line block/reverse 7 (or inverse L) block/field block/ring block.
- Intratesticular injection pre-castration improves analgesia under general anaesthesia and reduces volatile anaesthetic requirements.
- Incisional/wound infiltration (e.g. via 'soaker' catheters) can be used in surgical incisions, e.g. thoracotomy and coeliotomy incisions and after total ear canal ablation.

12.4.5 Specific Nerve Blocks: 'Local / Regional' Blocks

- Limbs; prior to limb surgeries (especially in small animals where blocks commonly anaesthetise proximal limb structures); also commonly used for more distal limb structures during horse lameness work-ups.
- Heads; regional anaesthesia (see Chapters 13 and 16).
- Intercostal block.
- Paravertebral block.
- Epidural (extradural) block.
- Intrathecal (true spinal/subarachnoid) block.

12.4.6 Intravenous Regional Anaesthesia (IVRA) – Bier's Block

- Another type of 'regional' block.

12.4.7 Systemic Administration

- By IV infusion (only lidocaine, without epinephrine).

12.5 Some of the Local Anaesthetics Available

12.5.1 Procaine

Available as a 5% solution with epinephrine (adrenaline). It is the only local anaesthetic licenced for use in farm animals in the UK. Procaine is an ester-linked local anaesthetic, therefore has relatively poor tissue penetration (so be as accurate as possible with injection sites when performing nerve blocks). It has a slowish onset of action and short duration of effect, and is associated with occasional allergic reactions. Beware concurrent use of trimethoprim potentiated sulphonamides for treatment of infection, as the pABA produced may reduce antibiotic effectiveness. Although procaine inherently causes some vasodilation, the veterinary licenced product contains the vasoconstrictor epinephrine which helps to hasten the onset, and prolong the duration of effect. When administered systemically by IV infusion, procaine has analgesic properties (studies in man), but this route is not licenced in animals (and the preparation containing epinephrine should not be used for IV infusion).

12.5.2 Lidocaine (Formerly Lignocaine)

Commonly available as 1 and 2% solutions (with or without epinephrine [adrenaline]) for injection, 2–4% solutions for topical application/spray, 2–5% gels and ointments for topical application and a 5% patch. Lidocaine was the first amide-linked local anaesthetic to be produced commercially. It is not a chiral compound; it does not exist in different isomeric forms. It has a quick onset of action with good tissue penetration (causes local vasodilation unless epinephrine is added) and a duration of effect of about 1 hour (2 hours with epinephrine). A greater reliability of nerve blocks is usually observed because of its greater tissue penetrance, so you do not need absolute accuracy when performing nerve blocks. It demonstrates frequency-dependent (use-dependent) block, so some sensorimotor discrimination is observed. Sometimes nerve root (radicular) irritation can occur after neuraxial administration, especially with higher concentration solutions (probably due more to its detergent effect on nerve membranes than any preservatives present). Like other local anaesthetic agents, the unionised form can cross the placenta, and once in the foetus (which is more acidic than the dam), it can 'ion-trap' there, so beware foetal toxicity.

Other properties of lidocaine are that it is:

- Antiarrhythmic/proarrhythmic.
- Anticonvulsant/pro-convulsant.

- Analgesic (and allows MAC reduction) when administered systemically in low doses, but may not reduce the stress response to anaesthesia/surgery.
- Prokinetic (enhances gut motility) at least where gut motility is already compromised (e.g. colic cases); mechanism of action uncertain, but, besides a small direct action on the intestinal smooth muscles, is possibly secondary to its analgesic and anti-inflammatory effects.
- Anti-inflammatory (reduces inflammatory mediator production/action; has vasodilator properties; reduces white blood cell margination and has anti-thrombotic effects; reduces inflammation-induced increases in vascular permeability. It is often said to prevent the 'no-reflow' phenomenon during reperfusion subsequent to tissue ischaemia, by preserving/enhancing capillary patency).

The use of lidocaine in or near wounds/surgical incisions has been hotly debated as some surgeons believe it reduces wound healing (possibly via its anti-inflammatory effects) and enhances tissue infection (also by its anti-inflammatory effects). However, most authors believe that it causes no ill effects; and in fact, the analgesia is beneficial. One study in rabbits certainly showed no difference in speed of wound healing or strength of healing/healed tissue and several studies document no effect on infection rates.

12.5.2.1 Some Lidocaine Preparations Available for Topical Use

- **Xylocaine gel** (2% lidocaine = 20 mg/ml)
- **Xylocaine ointment** (5% lidocaine)
- **Xylocaine spray** (10 mg lidocaine per 'dose')
- **Xylocaine 4% solution** (lidocaine solution for topical application)
- **Intubeaze™** (Dechra) = 2% lidocaine spray; each spray delivers 0.1–0.2 ml (i.e. 2–4 mg of lidocaine HCl). Be careful with how many sprays you deliver to the larynx of a kitten before you intubate its trachea (toxic dose '>2–3 mg/kg). Some veterinarians prefer to dilute a 2% solution of lidocaine and deliver it via a small syringe (attached to an IV cannula) for producing local anaesthesia of the larynx in tiny patients.

12.5.3 Mepivacaine

An amide-linked local anaesthetic agent, and the 'parent' of bupivacaine. Causes minimal overall effect on vascular tone. It has a slightly slower onset than lidocaine, a slightly longer duration, and is slightly more potent. It causes minimal tissue 'reaction' (vascular tone effects), and therefore is preferred for local nerve blocks in horses over lidocaine as it does not produce large weals at injection sites. Reported to be less chondrotoxic that lidocaine and bupivacaine.

12.5.4 Bupivacaine

An amide-linked local anaesthetic available in solutions of 0.5, 0.25, and 0.125%. It is a derivative of mepivacaine. Bupivacaine has longer side chains than mepivacaine, is more lipid soluble, and has greater protein binding. Its higher pKa means a slower onset, but its higher lipid solubility and protein binding mean higher potency and longer duration of action. Addition of epinephrine (adrenaline) makes little difference to the duration of action (see above). Bupivacaine demonstrates frequency-dependent block and sensorimotor discrimination similar to (slightly better than) lidocaine, but sometimes the block is more patchy. *It is four times as potent as lidocaine for myocardial depression, but 16 times as potent as an arrhythmogen.* Bupivacaine crosses the placenta less than lidocaine, possibly due to it being more highly protein bound. Laevo-bupivacaine (Chirocaine) is less cardiotoxic (see above).

12.5.4.1 Liposome-Encapsulated Bupivacaine (Nocita™)

By encapsulating bupivacaine in multivesicular liposomes, the drug becomes an extended release formulation with a duration of action of 72 hours. The liposomes have a honeycomb-like structure, made up of nonconcentric lipid bilayers, that creates chambers to contain the bupivacaine. Nocita is licenced for wound infiltration post-canine cruciate surgery in the USA and also for nerve blocks specific for onychectomy in cats. Adverse reactions are reported as discharge from the incision, incisional inflammation, and vomiting. This product should not be used concurrently with other amide local anaesthetics due to the risk of cumulative toxicity. There are anecdotal reports of Nocita being used for dental nerve blocks.

12.5.5 Ropivacaine

Ropivacaine is an amide-linked local anaesthetic with a similar pKa to bupivacaine (8.1). It is available in solutions of 1, 0.75, 0.5, and 0.2%. For calculating appropriate doses, the same volume of 0.75% ropivacaine can be used as would have been used for 0.5% bupivacaine. It has properties somewhere between bupivacaine and mepivacaine. Slightly quicker onset than bupivacaine (despite similar pKa and lower lipid solubility, so may be a concentration effect phenomenon too) with slightly shorter duration (slightly less protein binding). Less lipid soluble than bupivacaine, therefore slightly less potent. Possibly causes mild inherent vasoconstriction. Marketed as the S-enantiomer only. Less cardiotoxic than racemic bupivacaine. Of all the local anaesthetics, ropivacaine is probably the least chondrotoxic, but all are chondrotoxic in a drug-, time-, and concentration-dependent manner.

12.5.6 EMLA™ Cream

Eutectic Mixture of Local Anaesthetics. This is an emulsion of prilocaine and lidocaine bases, which forms a constant melting point (eutectic) mixture, of lower melting point than either of the constituents. The pH of the mixture is 9.4, so that the unionised forms (RN) of both agents are favoured, hence increasing absorption across the relatively fatty skin or mucosa. One study documented less reaction to IV cannula placement after 60 minutes compared to 30 minutes. It is absorbed more rapidly across the mucosa, but is not supposed to be administered by this route (in case a toxic dose is given).

12.5.7 Prilocaine

This is an amide-linked local anaesthetic with very low toxicity because its absorption is relatively slow, yet its metabolism is very rapid. This, in theory, should reduce the potential for systemic toxicity, but metabolism, especially of the R-enantiomer, produces ortho-toluidine, which can oxidise haem iron and cause methaemoglobinaemia. Prilocaine can be used for diagnostic local nerve blocks and produces very little local tissue 'reaction' (i.e. very little swelling is observed because of minimal effect on local vasomotor tone).

12.5.8 Tetracaine (Formerly Amethocaine)

An ester-linked local anaesthetic especially for topical anaesthesia of the conjunctiva/cornea. Available as 0.5 and 1% solutions. It stings for 30 seconds or so after first application and may stimulate lacrimation, so wait for that sensation to pass and the 'block' to work before continuing with ocular surface examination or surgery. Also available as a topical anaesthetic (4% gel) for skin application as Ametop™ and may be preferred to EMLA™ cream prior to venepuncture because it acts more rapidly and produces less local vasoconstriction, thus aiding vessel identification.

12.5.9 2-Chloroprocaine

An ester-linked local anaesthetic. Has a rapid onset of action despite a high pKa, possibly because it has good 'tissue penetrance'. It has a short duration of action due to rapid hydrolysis, and therefore a relatively low risk of toxicity. There used to be some concerns that after use for IVRA, it caused thrombophlebitis; and after epidural use, neurotoxic effects were seen, but this is now thought to have been due to one of the anti-oxidants (e.g. sodium bisulphite) included in the preparation.

12.5.10 Proxymetacaine

A topical local anaesthetic for ocular administration, usually available as a 0.5% solution, e.g. Ophthaine™.

Further Reading

Best, C.A., Best, A.A., Best, T.J., and Hamilton, D.A. (2015). Buffered lidocaine and bupivacaine mixture – the ideal local anesthetic solution? *Plastic Surgery* 23: 87–90.

Butterworth, J., Cole, L., and Marlow, G. (1993). Inhibition of brain cell excitability by lidocaine, QX314 and tetrodotoxin: a mechanism for analgesia from infused local anesthetics? *Acta Anaesthesiologica Scandinavica* 37: 516–523.

Cassutto, B.H. and Gfeller, R.W. (2003). Use of intravenous lidocaine to prevent reperfusion injury and subsequent multiple organ dysfunction syndrome. *Journal of Veterinary Emergency and Critical Care* 13: 137–148.

Chambers, W.A. (1992). Peripheral nerve damage and regional anaesthesia. *British Journal of Anaesthesia* 69: 429–430.

Christie, L.E., Picard, J., and Weinberg, G.L. (2015). Local anaesthetic systemic toxicity. *BJA Education* 15: 136–142.

Cuvillon, P., Nouvellon, E., Ripart, J. et al. (2009). A comparison of the pharmacodynamics and pharmacokinetics of bupivacaine, ropivacaine (with epinephrine) and their equal volume mixtures with lidocaine used for femoral and sciatic nerve blocks: a double-blinded randomized study. *Anesthesia and Analgesia* 108: 641–649.

Desai, M., Albrecht, E., and El-Boghdadly, K. (2019). Perineural adjuncts for peripheral nerve block. *BJA Education* 19: 276–282.

Dumoulin, M. and Oosterlinck, M. (2017). Local anaesthetics: more than meets the eye. *The Veterinary Journal* 228: 13–14.

Dzikiti, T.B., Hellebrekers, L.J., and van Dijk, P. (2003). Effects of intravenous lidocaine on isoflurane concentration, physiological parameters, metabolic parameters and stress-related hormones in horses undergoing surgery. *Journal of Veterinary Medicine. A, Physiology, Pathology, Clinical Medicine* 50: 190–195.

Hollmann, M.W. and Durieux, M.E. (2000). Local anesthetics and the inflammatory response. *Anesthesiology* 93: 858–875.

Hussain, N., McCartney, C.J.L., Neal, J.M. et al. (2018). Local anaesthetic-induced myotoxicity in regional anaesthesia: a systematic review and empirical analysis. *British Journal of Anaesthesia* 121: 822–841.

Jeng, C.L., Torrillo, T.M., and Rosenblatt, M.A. (2010). Complications of peripheral nerve blocks. *British Journal of Anaesthesia* 105: i97–i107.

Kitagawa, N., Oda, M., and Totoki, T. (2004). Possible mechanism of irreversible nerve injury caused by local anesthetics: detergent properties of local anesthetics and membrane disruption. *Anesthesiology* 100: 962–967.

Lascelles, B.D.X., Rausch-Derra, L.C., Wofford, J.A., and Huebner, M. (2016). Pilot, randomized, placebo-controlled clinical field study to evaluate the effectiveness of bupivacaine liposome injectable suspension for the provision of post-surgical analgesia in dogs undergoing stifle surgery. *BMC Veterinary Research* 12: 168. https://doi.org/10.1186/s12917-016-0798-1.

Marhofer, P. and Hopkins, P.M. (2019). Dexamethasone in regional anaesthesia: travelling up a blind alley? *Anaesthesia* 74: 969–972.

O'Flaherty, D., McCartney, C.J.L., and Ng, S.C. (2018). Nerve injury after peripheral nerve blockade- current understanding and guidelines. *BJA Education* 18: 384–390.

Picard, J. and Meek, T. (2006). Lipid emulsion to treat overdose of local anaesthetic: the gift of the glob. *Anaesthesia* 61: 107–109.

Piper, S.L. and Kim, H.T. (2008). Comparison of ropivacaine and bupivacaine toxicity in human articular chondrocytes. *Journal of Bone and Joint Surgery* 90: 986–991.

Rioja Garcia, E. (2015). Local anesthetics. In: *Veterinary Anesthesia and Analgesia, the Fifth Edition of Lumb and Jones* (eds. K.A. Grimm, L.A. Lamont, W.J. Tranquilli, et al.), 332–354. Iowa, USA: Wiley Blackwell.

Robertson, S.A., Sanchez, L.C., Merritt, A.M., and Doherty, T.J. (2005). Effect of systemic lidocaine on visceral and somatic nociception in conscious horses. *Equine Veterinary Journal* 37: 122–127.

Rosenberg, P.H., Veering, B.T., and Urmey, W.F. (2004). Maximum recommended doses of local anesthetics: a multifactorial concept. *Regional Anesthesia and Pain Medicine* 29: 564–575.

Savvas, I., Papazoglou, L.G., Kazakos, G. et al. (2008). Incisional block with bupivacaine for analgesia after celiotomy in dogs. *Journal of the American Animal Hospital Association* 44: 60–66.

Swain, A., Nag, D.S., Sahu, S., and Samaddar, D.P. (2017). Adjuvants to local anesthetics: current understanding and future trends. *World Journal of Clinical Cases* 5: 307–323.

Van Oostrom, H. and Knowles, T. (2018). The efficacy of EMLA cream for intravenous catheter placement in client-owned dogs. *Veterinary Anaesthesia and Analgesia* 45: 604–608.

Vasseur, P.B., Paul, H.A., Dybdal, N., and Crumley, L. (1984). Effects of local anesthetics on healing of abdominal wounds in rabbits. *American Journal of Veterinary Research* 45: 2385–2388.

Weinberg, G., Ripper, R., Feinstein, D.L., and Hoffman, W. (2003). Lipid emulsion infusion rescues dogs from bupivacaine-induced cardiac toxicity. *Regional Anesthesia and Pain Medicine* 28: 198–202.

Willatts, D.G. and Reynolds, F. (1985). Comparison of the vasoactivity of amide and ester local anaesthetics: an intradermal study. *British Journal of Anaesthesia* 57: 1006–1011.

Video of bupivacaine intoxication in rat and treatment with intralipid: https://lifeinthefastlane.com/intralipid-myth-or-miracle.

Self-test Section

1 Which of the following is least chondrotoxic?
   A Bupivacaine
   B Ropivacaine
   C Mepivacaine
   D Lidocaine

2 Describe the steps you would take in response be to a suspected intravenous injection of bupivacaine?

13

Local Anaesthetic Techniques for the Head
Small Animals

LEARNING OBJECTIVE

- To be familiar with nerve blocks for dental, ocular, aural, and other surgical procedures of the head

---

13.1 Introduction

The facial nerve (cranial nerve VII) only supplies motor innervation to the muscles of facial expression. If we want to block sensation, we must therefore concern ourselves with branches of the trigeminal nerve (cranial nerve V) (Figure 13.1).

13.1.1 Dental Blocks

For dental work, the two nerves that require blocking are the maxillary nerve for the upper dental arcade and the inferior alveolar branch of the mandibular nerve for the lower arcade. These nerves can be blocked at different sites.

13.1.1.1 Maxillary Nerve Block
Blocks the maxillary branch of the trigeminal nerve, including its pterygopalatine branch. Figures 13.2–13.5 show possible sites of injection to block the maxillary nerve within the pterygopalatine fossa, near the site where the pterygopalatine branch leaves it and before the maxillary nerve enters the maxillary foramen as the infraorbital nerve. Deposition of local anaesthetic within the pterygopalatine fossa usually affects the pterygopalatine branch of the maxillary nerve, and therefore usually also blocks the palatine and nasal nerves.

13.1.1.1.1 Structures Blocked
Nose (nasal planum and most of bridge of nose), upper lip, upper teeth, palate, maxilla, ipsilaterally.

13.1.1.1.2 Site for Nerve Block
Approaches are either extra-oral or intra-oral and include: sub-zygomatic (Figure 13.2), maxillary tuberosity (caudal to the last molar) (Figure 13.3), retrograde, via the infraorbital canal (Figure 13.4), and transorbital (Figure 13.5). Site for

local anaesthetic deposition is in the pterygopalatine fossa between the rostral alar foramen and the maxillary foramen (entrance to the infraorbital canal). Several superior alveolar (dental) branches arise from the nerve, both just before it enters, and within, the infraorbital canal.

13.1.1.1.3 Method

- Needle: 23–25 g, 1″.
- Dose for dogs >20 kg: 1–3 ml lidocaine 2% ± epinephrine, or 1–3 ml ropivacaine 0.75%, or 1–2 ml bupivacaine 0.5%. Dose for cats and small dogs: 1–2 ml lidocaine 1% ± epinephrine, or 1–2 ml ropivacaine 0.5%, or 1–2 ml bupivacaine 0.25%. If bilateral blocks are required, beware the total dose of local anaesthetic used.

Sub-zygomatic, Extra-oral Approach (Figure 13.2)
The needle is inserted percutaneously, at 90° to the skin surface and in a medial direction, just below the ventral border of the zygomatic arch, and, for medium-sized dogs, about 0.5 cm caudal to a perpendicular line dropped from the lateral canthus of the eye (pro rata for other patient sizes). The needle is then advanced into the pterygopalatine fossa, aiming slightly rostrally. If bone is touched, the needle should be withdrawn by 1–2 mm. Aspirate before injection to check that the needle has not penetrated a blood vessel.

Maxillary Tuberosity, Intra-oral Approach (Figure 13.3)
The needle is inserted intra-orally caudal/caudo-lateral to the last molar and the maxillary tuberosity, aiming for the maxillary foramen (slight rostral angle). Insert the needle tip no deeper than the root apices of the last molar, which is usually around 15–20 mm in medium-large dogs and 5–10 mm in cats and small dogs. Take care to avoid globe puncture.

Veterinary Anaesthesia: Principles to Practice, Second Edition. Alexandra H. A. Dugdale, Georgina Beaumont, Carl Bradbrook, and Matthew Gurney.
© 2020 John Wiley & Sons Ltd. Published 2020 by John Wiley & Sons Ltd.
Companion website: www.wiley.com/go/dugdale/veterinary-anaesthesia

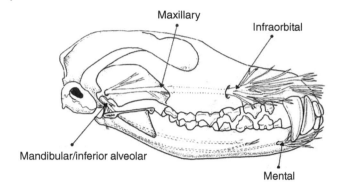

Maxillary

Infraorbital

Mandibular/inferior alveolar

Mental

Figure 13.1 Nerves relevant to dental and oral surgery.

(b)

(a)

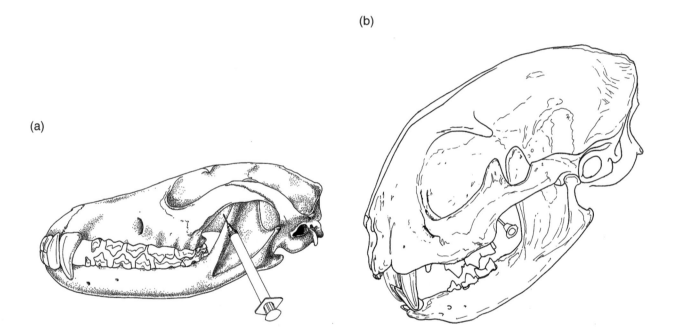

Figure 13.2 Sub-zygomatic approach to the maxillary nerve for dog (a) and cat (b).

Figure 13.3 Maxillary tuberosity, intra-oral approach to the maxillary nerve.

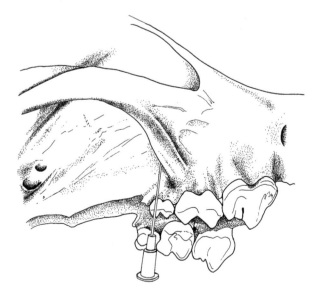

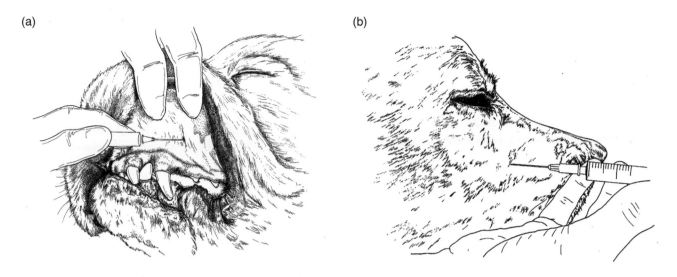

Figure 13.4 Infraorbital canal, intra-oral approach (a) and extra-oral approach (b) to the maxillary nerve.

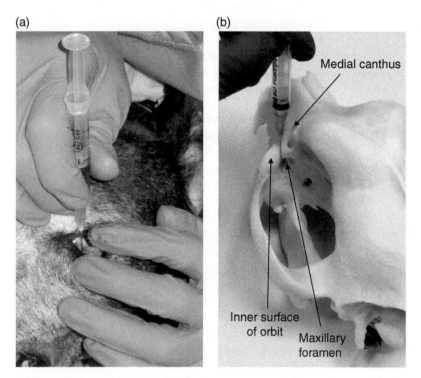

Figure 13.5 Transorbital approach to maxillary nerve block: (a) gentle retropulsion of the globe facilitates needle placement; (b) shows vertical orientation of needle about 5 mm lateral to the medial canthus. *Source:* Image reproduced with kind permission from Langton & Walker (2017).

Infraorbital canal, Extra- or Intra-oral Approach (Figure 13.4)
A needle or, preferably, intravenous cannula is inserted into the infraorbital canal from the infraorbital foramen, taking care not to cause excessive damage to the nerve. The needle/cannula is advanced to the level of the maxillary foramen, which is premeasured as roughly to the level of the lateral canthus of the eye in mesaticephalic and dolichocephalic breeds, but take care not to advance the catheter beyond the medial canthus of the eye in brachycephalic breeds to reduce the chance of globe puncture.

Transorbital Approach (Figure 13.5)
Whilst gently retropulsing the globe 'through the eyelid' (i.e. using the eyelid for protection of the eye), a needle can

be inserted ventrolaterally to the medial canthus of the eye, just inside the ventral orbital rim, aiming for the maxillary foramen that is located a few mm ventrally.

13.1.1.2 Infraorbital Nerve Block
Blocks the infraorbital nerve (a branch of the maxillary nerve), where it leaves the infraorbital canal at the infraorbital foramen (Figures 13.6 and 13.7).

13.1.1.2.1 Structures Blocked
Upper lip, nose (nasal planum and roof of nasal cavity), and skin rostroventral to infraorbital foramen, ipsilaterally. If the nerve is blocked where it exits the infraorbital foramen, teeth are unlikely to be desensitised unless local anaesthetic diffuses into the infraorbital canal. A maxillary block is preferred for dental extractions.

13.1.1.2.2 Site for Nerve Block
Where the infraorbital nerve exits the infraorbital foramen. The infraorbital foramen is located approximately midway between the rostrodorsal border of the zygomatic arch and the ipsilateral canine root tip, although its location also depends upon the patient's nose length (Figure 13.6). In

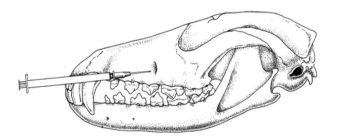

Figure 13.6 Infraorbital nerve block in a dog.

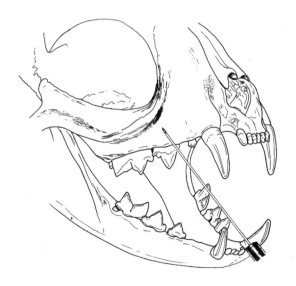

Figure 13.7 Infraorbital nerve block in a cat.

cats and brachycephalic dogs, the foramen is located much closer to the rostral end of the zygomatic arch. In cats (Figure 13.7), the foramen lies very close to the globe and a sub-zygomatic maxillary nerve block is often preferred to reduce the chance of accidental globe puncture and injection of local anaesthetic into the eyeball.

13.1.1.2.3 Method
- Needle: 22–25 g, 5/8–1″ (depends upon patient size).
- Dose for dogs >20 kg: 0.5–1 ml lidocaine 2% ± epinephrine, or 0.5–1 ml ropivacaine 0.75%, or 0.5–1 ml bupivacaine 0.5%.
- Dose for cats and small dogs: 0.25–0.5 ml lidocaine 1% ± epinephrine, or 0.25–0.5 ml ropivacaine 0.5%, or 0.25–0.5 ml bupivacaine 0.25%.
- Bilateral block will be required for surgery on both sides of the nasal bridge or nasal planum. Beware the total dose of local anaesthetic used.

The needle can be inserted intra-orally (i.e. the lip can be reflected up) or extra-orally (through the skin). The needle tip is inserted about 0.5 cm rostral to the bony lip of the foramen, and then advanced gently towards the foramen but should not be inserted into the foramen. Aspirate before injection to ensure the needle is not in a blood vessel.

13.1.1.3 Inferior Alveolar Nerve Block – At the Mandibular Foramen
Blocks the inferior alveolar nerve, which is the continuation of the mandibular nerve after the auriculotemporal, buccal, and lingual branches have left the mandibular nerve root. Occasionally, attempts to block the inferior alveolar nerve will also successfully block the lingual nerve that is sensory to the rostral two thirds of the tongue and this may result in self-trauma, such that bilateral blocks should only be undertaken with caution and use of shorter-acting local anaesthetic agents in advised (see below).

13.1.1.3.1 Structures Blocked
Lower teeth, mandible, skin, and mucosa of lower lip, ipsilaterally.

13.1.1.3.2 Site for Nerve Block
Where the inferior alveolar nerve enters the mandibular canal at the mandibular foramen (Figures 13.8 and 13.9).

13.1.1.3.3 Method
- Needle: 21–23 g, 1″ or longer (depending upon size of patient).
- Dose for dogs >20 kg: 1–2 ml lidocaine 2% ± epinephrine, or 1–2 ml ropivacaine 0.75%, or 1–1.5 ml bupivacaine 0.5%.
- Dose for cats and small dogs: 0.5–1 ml lidocaine 1% ± epinephrine, or 0.5–1 ml ropivacaine 0.5%, or 0.5–1 ml bupivacaine 0.25%.

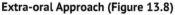

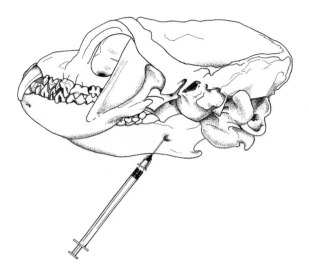

Figure 13.8 Extra-oral approach to the inferior alveolar nerve at the mandibular foramen.

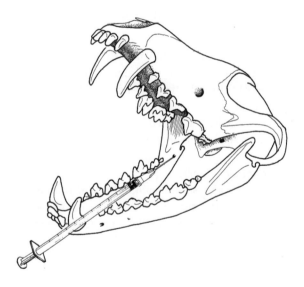

Figure 13.9 Intra-oral approach to the inferior alveolar nerve at the mandibular foramen.

Figure 13.10 Mental nerve block.

Extra-oral Approach (Figure 13.8)

The lip of the mandibular foramen can just about be palpated; this is more difficult in bigger dogs and those with a pronounced medial pterygoid muscle (e.g. Rottweilers, Mastiffs, and bull terrier types). The needle can then be inserted percutaneously at the vascular notch on the ventral border of the lower angle of the jaw, and advanced against the medial side of the mandible, directed towards the foramen. In a 25 kg dog, this would mean inserting the needle approximately 1.5 cm rostral to the angular process of the mandible, and the foramen is approximately 1.5 cm vertically up from the lower edge of the mandible. Aspirate before injection. Ensure the injected local anaesthetic forms a bleb within the fascia surrounding the nerve between the medial aspect of the mandible and the muscle.

Intra-oral Approach (Figure 13.9)

The needle is inserted intra-orally into the fascia overlying the nerve, whilst the operator attempts to palpate the mandibular foramen, which lies on the medial surface of the mandible roughly half-way between the last molar and the angular process of the jaw. Palpation of the foramen can be difficult in small patients where an extra-oral approach is often preferred.

With bilateral blocks, occasionally both lingual nerves can also be blocked. Each lingual nerve branches off just before the inferior mandibular alveolar nerve enters the mandibular foramen. If this happens, the animal may have trouble feeling its tongue and may traumatise or bite it, especially during recovery from anaesthesia. For this reason, lidocaine is recommended for bilateral blocks as the effect will be shorter.

13.1.1.4 Mental Nerve Block

Blocks the mental nerves which are the terminal, extra-osseous branches of the inferior alveolar nerves of the mandibular division of the trigeminal nerve. The middle (biggest) mental foramen can be hard to palpate, but can be located just about level with (slightly rostral to) the second premolar, near the apex of the root of the canine tooth, and at about the mid-point of the dorso-ventral 'height' of the mandibular ramus at this site (Figure 13.10).

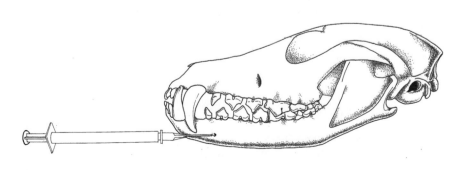

13.1.1.4.1 Structures Blocked

Lower lip and chin rostral to the site of the block, ipsilaterally. If the nerves are blocked where they exit the mandibular foramen, teeth are unlikely to be desensitised unless local anaesthetic diffuses into the mandibular canal.

13.1.1.4.2 Site for Nerve Block

Where the middle mental nerve exits the mandibular canal from the middle mental foramen. The middle mental foramen is biggest of the mental foramina in dogs and carries the largest of the mental nerves.

13.1.1.4.3 Method

- Needle: 21–23 g, 5/8″.
- Dose for dogs >20 kg: 0.5–1 ml lidocaine 2% ± epinephrine, or 0.5–1 ml ropivacaine 0.75%, or 0.5–1 ml bupivacaine 0.5%.
- Dose for cats and small dogs: 0.25–0.5 ml lidocaine 1% ± epinephrine, or 0.25–0.5 ml ropivacaine 0.5%, or 0.25–0.5 ml bupivacaine 0.25%.

The needle is inserted either percutaneously or intra-orally after folding down the lip (although the labial frenulum can be a nuisance), judging the position of the foramen from the second premolar (if present). Aspirate before injection. Bilateral blocks are required, e.g. for surgery on the bilateral fleshy part of the chin.

13.1.1.5 Palatine Nerve Block

Desensitises the mucosa of the hard palate. Does not anaesthetise the teeth. Bilateral blocks are required for a cleft palate repair. Inject halfway between the midline (of the roof of the mouth) and the teeth, at the level of the fourth premolar, bilaterally. Ensure careful aspiration as the palatine artery runs in close apposition. (Block of the maxillary nerve within the pterygopalatine fossa usually also blocks the palatine nerves.)

13.1.1.5.1 Method

- Needle: 25 g, 5/8″.
- Dose for dogs >20 kg: 0.2 ml lidocaine 2% ± epinephrine, or 0.2 ml ropivacaine 0.75%, or 0.2 ml bupivacaine 0.5%.
- Dose for cats and small dogs: 0.1 ml lidocaine 1% ± epinephrine, or 0.1 ml ropivacaine 0.5%, or 0.1 ml bupivacaine 0.25%.

13.1.1.6 Other Techniques

See Chapter 41 on dental considerations.

13.1.2 Ocular Blocks

13.1.2.1 Ophthalmic Nerve Block

Aims to block the ophthalmic division of the trigeminal nerve, but may also block the maxillary nerve. Some people consider this block to be a sub-zygomatic approach to performing a type of retrobulbar block.

13.1.2.1.1 Structures Blocked

Eye, orbit, conjunctiva, eyelids, forehead skin. Some of the lower eyelid is supplied by the zygomatic nerve, which is a branch of the maxillary nerve, and in performing this block, you may also block the maxillary nerve.

13.1.2.1.2 Site for Nerve Block

In the pterygopalatine fossa, but now aiming for the orbital fissure, where the ophthalmic branch of the trigeminal nerve leaves the cranial vault. The orbital fissure lies slightly further rostrally than the rostral alar foramen, but caudal to the maxillary foramen.

13.1.2.1.3 Method

- Needle: 23 g, 1–1.5″.
- Dose for dogs >20 kg: 2 ml lidocaine 2% ± epinephrine, or 1–2 ml ropivacaine 0.75%, or 1–2 ml bupivacaine 0.5%.
- Dose for cats and small dogs: 1 ml lidocaine 1% ± epinephrine, or 1 ml ropivacaine 0.5%, or 1 ml bupivacaine 0.25%.

The nerve block is performed similarly to the maxillary nerve block (i.e. aim under the ventral border of the zygomatic arch), but this time as near as possible 'on' the perpendicular line dropped from the lateral canthus of the eye. The needle is directed caudomedially and very slightly dorsally. Aspirate before injection.

13.1.2.2 Retrobulbar Block

Deposition of local anaesthetic *within* the cone of muscles supplying the globe (**intraconal**) blocks cranial nerves II, III, IV, V (ophthalmic and maxillary branches), and VI (Figure 13.11).

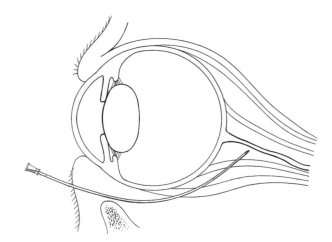

Figure 13.11 Retrobulbar, intraconal block.

13.1.2.2.1 *Structures Blocked* This block **desensitises** the eye, the eyelids, and most of the upper face. Some eyelid tone may remain from palpebral (cranial nerve VII) motor innervation to the orbicularis oculi muscle, and a palpebral block may be required. There are several potential risks with the retrobulbar block (see below), so it is often reserved for enucleations. This block was fashionable at one time to reduce the vagal oculocardiac reflex occasionally seen with ocular traction or pressure during eye surgery, but the actual performance of the block may itself stimulate this reflex.

13.1.2.2.2 *Method*

- Needle: 21–23 g, slightly curved and flexible, 3″.
- Dose for dogs >20 kg: 1–2 ml lidocaine 2% ± epinephrine, or 1–2 ml ropivacaine 0.75%, or 1–2 ml bupivacaine 0.5%.
- Dose for cats and small dogs: 0.5 ml lidocaine 1% ± epinephrine, or 0.5 ml ropivacaine 0.5%, or 0.5 ml bupivacaine 0.25%.

Many variations of technique are reported in the literature. The simplest is a 1-point injection. One technique involves using a pre-curved needle that is inserted slightly medial to the lateral canthus (10 o'clock for right eye; 2 o'clock for left eye) just below the dorsal orbital rim, and carefully advanced under the roof of the orbit around and behind the eyeball, taking care not to puncture it. Alternatively, a straight needle can be inserted slightly lateral to the medial canthus just inside the ventral orbital rim (5 o'clock for right eye; 7 o'clock for left eye), and advanced along the floor of the orbit to approach the point of the muscular cone, but with this technique, there is a greater risk of the needle tip penetrating the optic nerve sheath beneath which lies cerebrosoinal fluid (CSF); intrathecal injection of local anaesthetic will result in direct central nervous system (CNS) toxicity.

The needle can be inserted through the eyelid (i.e. a transpalpebral approach), but most people prefer to gently retract the eyelid and then insert the needle into the conjunctival fornix. A little topical local anaesthetic (e.g. proparacaine, proxymetacaine, tetracaine) may be instilled into the conjunctival sac to desensitise the conjunctiva first. Aspirate before injection. Signs of a successful block are a mydriatic pupil, reduced lacrimation, exophthalmos, and a centrally positioned eye.

If a retrobulbar block is contra-indicated (infection; neoplasia), a local soak block can be performed after enucleation whereby absorbable collagen sponge is soaked with 1–2 ml bupivacaine 0.5% and left in situ.

13.1.2.2.3 *Potential Complications*

- Damage to globe
- Damage to optic nerve (less of a concern for enucleations)
- Damage to ocular blood supply (less of a concern for enucleations)
- Retrobulbar haemorrhage
- Increased retrobulbar, and therefore intra-ocular, pressure due to: the volume of local anaesthetic injected which tends to proptose the eye, and any retrobulbar haemorrhage
- Injection of local anaesthetic into the CSF within the optic nerve meningeal sheath (see immediate signs of CNS toxicity)
- The oculocardiac reflex may occur as the block is performed
- Seeding of neoplastic cells

13.1.2.3 Peribulbar Block

This forms an alternative to the retrobulbar block, but in the peribulbar block technique, local anaesthetic is deposited *outside* the cone of muscles supplying the globe (**extraconal**).

Local anaesthetic is injected at four equal points on the clock face (or you can think of it like North, East, South, and West), so as to encircle the globe. Nerves blocked include the long (from ophthalmic [II] nerve) and short (from ciliary ganglion) ciliary nerves, the extraconal branches of the ophthalmic and maxillary (V) nerves, and the motor nerves to the extra-ocular muscles (III, IV, and VI). Using a straight (or only slightly curved) needle, which is kept tangential to the globe, and ensuring the needle tip is inserted no deeper than the equator of the globe, the local anaesthetic is deposited outside the cone of extra-ocular muscles. Gentle pressure is then applied to the globe for around 10 minutes to help disperse the local anaesthetic. The needle can be passed transcutaneously or transconjunctivally (topical conjunctival anaesthesia is required first). Palpebral block (motor block) may also be necessary, although the relatively large volume of local anaesthetic used for this block (compared to the retrobulbar block) may result in sufficient diffusion to block the palpebral nerve. Complications include transiently increased intra-ocular pressure, peribulbar haemorrhage, globe perforation, and chemosis, especially as the overall volume of local anaesthetic used can be greater than that used for the retrobulbar technique. Ideally, try to keep the volume to around 0.1–0.5 ml (depending upon patient size) at each injection site using diluted solutions for smaller patients where indicated.

A **periconal** variant of the peribulbar technique has also been described in people and rabbits, in which local anaesthetic is deposited more posteriorly than the equator of the eye (see further reading).

There is much debate about the difference between the retrobulbar and peribulbar techniques as there is actually no intermuscular fascia between the intraconal and extraconal compartments, and therefore deposited local anaesthetic will diffuse easily between the two compartments.

13.1.2.4 Sub-Tenon Block (Parabulbar Block)

The sub-Tenon block (Figure 13.12), represents another alternative to the retrobulbar block and with possibly fewer complications than the peribulbar block. Tenon's capsule is the dense, fibroelastic connective tissue layer that envelops the posterior part of the globe. The sub-Tenon (epi-scleral 'space') block requires a small incision to be made, firstly through the conjunctiva (topical local anaesthetic can be applied first) about half way between the limbus and the fornix, and then through Tenon's capsule so that a curved blunt cannula can be passed in the plane between the capsule and the sclera so that the cannula's tip lies beyond the globe's equator in the virtual, epi-scleral 'space'. Local anaesthetic solution (1–2 ml per average dog) is then injected to block the nerves as listed for the retrobulbar block. The main complication is conjunctival haemorrhage, which is usually easily controlled as the site of haemorrhage is easily visualised. Chemosis is another common occurrence, but is usually transient. Note that the eyelids are not desensitised and sometimes complete akinesia of the eye is not achieved.

13.1.2.5 Infiltration Anaesthesia

Infiltrative blocks can be used for anaesthesia of the eyelids. Anaesthetic is infiltrated in a diamond shape around the orbital rim to desensitise the eyelids. The areas desensitised are: medial canthus and medial parts of upper and lower eyelids innervated by the infratrochlear nerve (ophthalmic V); middle-to-lateral part of upper eyelid innervated by the frontal nerve (ophthalmic V); lower eyelid and lateral canthus innervated by the zygomaticofacial nerve (branch of zygomatic nerve, itself a branch of maxillary V). The lateral part of the upper eyelid also receives some innervation from the zygomaticotemporal nerve (in the dog and cat, this is a branch of the zygomatic nerve, itself a branch of maxillary V). In dogs and cats, the lacrimal nerve

(usually a branch of ophthalmic V, but occasionally a branch of maxillary V) may not always supply innervation to the lateral portion of the upper eyelid.

13.1.2.6 Palpebral Nerve Block

The palpebral nerve, a continuation of the auriculopalpebral nerve (a branch of facial VII), provides motor innervation to the eyelids and can be blocked to reduce blinking activity and blepharospasm during surgery. It must only be used alongside other methods of anaesthesia/analgesia as the palpebral block itself does not produce desensitisation. The palpebral nerve is palpated as it runs superficially across the highest point of the dorsal aspect of the zygomatic arch.

13.1.2.6.1 Method

- Dose for dogs >20 kg: 0.25–0.5 ml lidocaine 2% ± epinephrine, or 0.25–0.5 ml ropivacaine 0.75%, or 0.25–0.5 ml bupivacaine 0.5%.
- Dose for cats and small dogs: 0.25 ml lidocaine 1% ± epinephrine, or 0.25 ml ropivacaine 0.5%, or 0.25 ml bupivacaine 0.25%.

13.1.2.7 Topical Anaesthesia

Used for ophthalmic examination. Commonly used agents are proxymetacaine or tetracaine.

Proxymetacaine 0.5%/1.0%: onset 1 minute, duration 25–55 minutes. Maximal effect at 15 minutes.

Tetracaine 0.5%/1.0%: onset and duration of action not reported.

All topical local anaesthetics are reported to delay healing of corneal ulcers.

13.1.3 Auricular Blocks

The **great auricular nerve** (originating from spinal segmental nerves Ce1 and Ce2) and the **auriculotemporal nerve** (branch of mandibular V) can be blocked for aural procedures such as total ear canal ablation (TECA) (Figure 13.13).

In the authors' experience, the following technique has been successful and resulted in less inadvertent vascular puncture than another technique which has recently been described by Stathopoulos (see Further Reading). The vertical ear canal is palpated. The auriculotemporal nerve lies superficially just cranial to the vertical ear canal and the great auricular nerve lies superficially caudal to the vertical canal.

To block the auriculotemporal nerve, direct the needle tip towards the base of a 'V' formed by the zygomatic arch and the rostral edge of the vertical ear canal. Note the proximity of the facial nerve to the auriculotemporal nerve

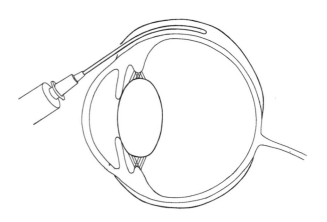

Figure 13.12 Sub-Tenon block.

(b)

(a)

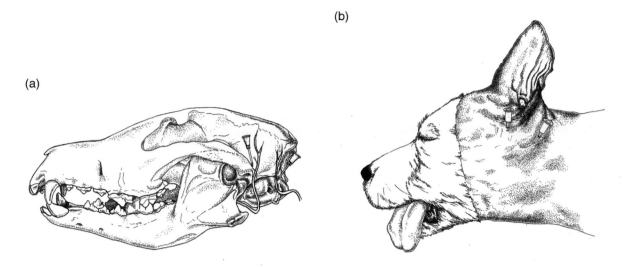

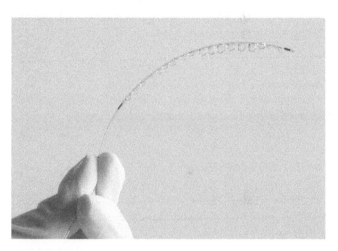

Figure 13.13 Auriculotemporal (rostral site) and great auricular (caudal site) nerve blocks; showing nerves in relation to skull (a); and 'skin surface' view (b).

here, especially the auriculopalpebral branch, which may also be inadvertently blocked (ptosis may be seen post-operatively).

To block the great auricular nerve, a needle can be passed just ventrally to the wing of the atlas (Ce1), aiming for, and perpendicularly to, the caudal aspect of the vertical ear canal (although this depends somewhat upon the position of the animal's head relative to its neck). Alternatively, a needle can be inserted on the caudal aspect of the vertical ear canal so that its tip lies where a line drawn from along the lateral aspect of the wing of the atlas would intersect a line drawn along the caudal aspect of the vertical ear canal.

For a TECA, local anaesthetic can be injected along the proposed surgical incision sites rostral and caudal to the vertical ear canal, to improve the chance of successful blocks. This may result in facial nerve paralysis (which is also a potential complication of the surgery), but any inadvertent effect from the local anaesthetic should only be transient. Alternatively, a local anaesthetic soak can be performed prior to closure of the surgical wound. A wound 'soaker' catheter can also be placed into the incision for either intermittent injection or continuous infusion of local anaesthetic to prolong post-operative analgesia (Figure 13.14).

Figure 13.14 A wound soaker-catheter. *Source:* Courtesy of Vygon Vet.

- Dose for dogs >20 kg: 1–2 ml lidocaine 2% ± epinephrine, or 1–2 ml ropivacaine 0.75%, or 1–2 ml bupivacaine 0.5%.
- Dose for cats and small dogs: 0.25 ml lidocaine 1% ± epinephrine, or 0.25 ml ropivacaine 0.5%, or 0.25 ml bupivacaine 0.25%.

Further Reading

Aguiar, J., Chebroux, A., Martinez-Taboada, F., and Leece, E.A. (2015). Analgesic effects of maxillary and inferior alveolar nerve blocks in cats undergoing dental extractions. *Journal of Feline Medicine and Surgery* 17: 110–116.

Campoy, L., Read, M.R., and Peralta, S. (2015). Canine and feline local anesthetic and analgesic techniques. In: *Veterinary Anesthesia and Analgesia, Fifth Edition of Lumb and Jones* (eds. K.A. Grimm, L.A. Lamont, W.J. Tranquilli, et al.), 827–856. Iowa, USA: Wiley-Blackwell.

De Vries, M. and Putter, G. (2015). Perioperative anaesthetic care of the cat undergoing dental and oral procedures. *Journal of Feline Medicine and Surgery* 17: 25–36.

Gracis, M. (2013). The Oral cavity. In: *Small Animal Regional Anesthesia & Analgesia*, 1e (eds. L. Campoy and M.R. Read), 119–140. Iowa, USA: Wiley Blackwell.

Giuliano, E.A. and Walsh, K. (2013). The eye. In: *Small Animal Regional Anesthesia & Analgesia*, 1e (eds. L. Campoy and M.R. Read), 103–118. Iowa, USA: Wiley Blackwell.

Kushnir, Y., Marwitz, G.S., Shilo-Benjamini, Y., and Milgram, J. (2018). Description of a regional anaesthesia technique for the dorsal cranium in the dog: a cadaveric study. *Veterinary Anaesthesia and Analgesia* 45: 684–694.

Langton, D.C. and Walker, J.J.A. (2017). A transorbital approach to the maxillary nerve block in dogs: a cadaver study. *Veterinary Anaesthesia and Analgesia* 44: 173–177.

Milella, L. and Gurney, M.A. (2016). Dental and oral surgery. In: *BSAVA Manual of Canine and Feline Anaesthesia and Analgesia*, 3e (eds. T. Duke-Novakovski, M. de Vries and C. Seymour), 272–282. Gloucester, UK: BSAVA Publications.

Najman, I.E., Ferreira, J.Z., Abimussi, C.J.X. et al. (2015). Ultrasound-assisted periconal ocular blockade in rabbits. *Veterinary Anaesthesia and Analgesia* 42: 433–441.

Najman, I.E., Meirelles, R., Ramos, L.B. et al. (2015). A randomized controlled trial of periconal eye blockade with or without ultrasound guidance. *Anaesthesia* 70: 571–576.

O'Morrow, C. (2010). Advanced dental local nerve block anesthesia. *Canadian Veterinary Journal* 51: 1411–1415.

Palte, H.D., Gayer, S., Arrieta, E. et al. (2012). Are ultrasound-guided ophthalmic blocks injurious to the eye? A comparative rabbit model study of two ultrasound devices evaluating intraorbital thermal and structural changes. *Anesthesia and Analgesia* 115: 194–201.

Reuss-Lamky, H. (2007). Administering dental nerve blocks. *Journal of the American Animal Hospital Association* 43: 298–305.

Shilo-Benjamini, Y. (2019). A review of ophthalmic local and regional anesthesia in dogs and cats. *Veterinary Anaesthesia and Analgesia* 46: 14–27.

Shilo-Benjamini, Y., Pascoe, P.J., Wisner, E.R. et al. (2017). A comparison of retrobulbar and two peribulbar regional anaesthetic techniques in dog cadavers. *Veterinary Anaesthesia and Analgesia* 44: 925–932.

Stathopoulou, T.R., Pinelas, R., Haar, G.T. et al. (2018). Description of a new approach for great auricular and auriculotemporal nerve blocks: a cadaveric study in foxes and dogs. *Veterinary Medicine and Science* 4: 91–97.

Viscasillas, J., Seymour, C.J., and Brodbelt, D.C. (2013). A cadaver study comparing two approaches for performing maxillary nerve blocks in dogs. *Veterinary Anaesthesia and Analgesia* 40: 212–219.

Self-test Section

1 True or False? The lacrimal nerve is usually a branch of the ophthalmic division of the trigeminal nerve.

2 True or False? Inadvertent lingual nerve block is a complication of the maxillary nerve block.

3 True or False? The retrobulbar block involves extraconal deposition of local anaesthetic.

14

Local Anaesthetic Techniques for the Limbs

Small Animals

LEARNING OBJECTIVES

- To be familiar with the main techniques for limb analgesia in small animals.

14.1 Use of Local Anaesthetics

- Neuraxial anaesthesia and analgesia: epidural (extradural) or true spinal (intrathecal/subarachnoid)
- Local/regional anaesthesia: individual nerve blocks or plexus blocks (perineural administration)
- Ring blocks
- Intravenous regional anaesthesia (IVRA)
- Intralesional: wound, fracture site, or incisional infiltration (asepsis must be maintained)
- Intra-articular

Although neuraxial or local/regional anaesthesia can provide excellent analgesia for surgery under general anaesthesia, a good working knowledge of anatomy is required, especially for performing perineural infiltration of local anaesthetic agents. Approaches have been described for blockade of individual nerves of the thoracic and pelvic limbs and are outlined below (and see Further Reading). As a reduction in stress biomarkers has been demonstrated when successful local/regional anaesthetic techniques have been employed, they should be provided wherever possible.

14.2 Nerve Location and Ultrasound

Accurate deposition of the local anaesthetic agent is key to a successful block, but, at the same time, nerve damage should be avoided. The use of an electrical nerve stimulator/locator (electro-neuro-locator, or ENL, Figure 14.1) and ultrasound

(US) can assist with this, improving safety and accuracy. The ENL is a current generator that is preferably used with an insulated needle. The current is conducted down the insulated needle so that it emanates only from the tip of the needle. A higher current (1.0 mA) is initially used to search for a nerve that also has a corresponding motor reflex, e.g. the sciatic nerve. The motor response to stimulation of the sciatic nerve is dorsal extension or plantar flexion of the digits. Once this motor response is seen, the current is decreased to around 0.4 (0.2–0.5) mA in a step-wise fashion, observing decreasing twitch strength. At currents below 0.2–0.3 mA, there should be no twitch, meaning that the needle is *near* the nerve but not *in* the nerve (although ultrasound visualisation of the injection combined with assessment of injection pressure are suggested to better help guarantee against intraneural injection). The current can then be turned back up, just enough to visualise the motor response once again, and it should then be noted that the twitch disappears (the Raj test) after injection of (0.1)–0.5–1 ml of local anaesthetic due to both physical displacement of the needle from the nerve by the injectate and a change in electrical conductivity around the nerve following the injection.

With ultrasound, acoustic windows have been described for many blocks. The needle (which may also be an insulated stimulating needle attached to an ENL) should be inserted in-plane with the transducer so that its tip can be visualised continuously. Once its tip is located near the nerve to be targeted, a small volume of anaesthetic is injected first to verify correct tip location. Although originally it was thought that deposition of local anaesthetic circumferentially

Veterinary Anaesthesia: Principles to Practice, Second Edition. Alexandra H. A. Dugdale, Georgina Beaumont, Carl Bradbrook, and Matthew Gurney.
© 2020 John Wiley & Sons Ltd. Published 2020 by John Wiley & Sons Ltd.
Companion website: www.wiley.com/go/dugdale/veterinary-anaesthesia

(a)

(b)

(c)

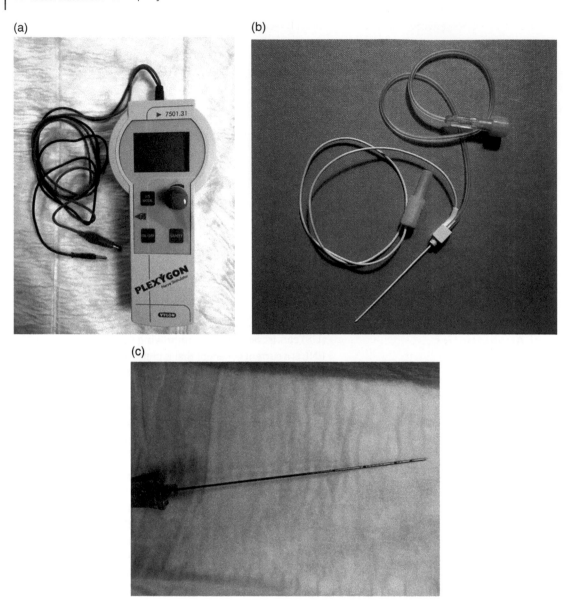

Figure 14.1 Electro-neuro-locator (a); insulated stimulating needle with injection port and extension set (b); insulated needle showing graduations and surface etching to improve visualisation during ultrasonography (c).

around the nerve (visualised as a doughnut of solution [black] around the hyperechoic nerve) would produce the best block, a recent study has suggested that deposition 'above' or 'below' the nerve is likely to be as effective. One useful advantage of US over the use of ENL alone is that it can be used to identify blood vessels, which can then be avoided.

14.3 Neuraxial Anaesthesia

14.3.1 Intrathecal/Subarachnoid/'True Spinal' Anaesthesia/Analgesia

Intrathecal injections, where the injectate actually enters the CSF surrounding the spinal cord, are less commonly

performed than epidural (extradural) injections. Table 14.1 highlights some of the features of the two types of neuraxial anaesthesia/analgesia.

Many local anaesthetic solutions (lidocaine 1%, bupivacaine 0.5%, and ropivacaine 1%) are slightly **hypobaric** (less dense than CSF) in horses, dogs, and cats (CSF specific gravity is around 1.010 in these species), and so if inadvertently injected into the CSF, the best ploy to avoid cranial spread to the brain is actually to tip the animal 'head-down', or at least, do not tip it 'head-up'. Lidocaine 2% is **isobaric** with CSF (i.e. both have specific gravity of 1.010). Special **hyperbaric** local anaesthetic and opioid solutions (usually containing glucose) are available for intrathecal injections (e.g. 'heavy lidocaine') so that patient

Table 14.1 Comparison of true spinal (intrathecal) and epidural (extradural) techniques.

Feature	Extradural	Subarachnoid (intrathecal)
Injection made into	Epidural fat	CSF
Volume/dose of injectate	Rel. high	Rel. low
Speed of onset	Rel. slow	Rel. fast
Duration (depends on drug characteristics)	Rel. long	Rel. short
Potential errors	Injection into CSF Injection into subdural 'space'	Injection into epidural fat Injection into subdural 'space'
'Headache'	No	Yes (postdural puncture)
Risk of toxicity	Could inject IV or into CSF	Rapid spread to brain in CSF
Effects of patient positioning after injection	Not very position-sensitive (i.e. gravity can affect spread in epidural space, but the effect is not huge)	Position-sensitive, i.e. gravity and baricity (density) of injectate greatly affect spread in CSF
Reliability of block	Not brilliant	Much better

positioning can utilise gravity to direct the spread of the injected solution. Morphine and methadone tend to be hypobaric, but when diluted in normal saline or glucose solutions, may become iso- or hyper-baric respectively. Hyperbaric bupivacaine 0.5% is advised at a dose of 0.25 mg/kg (0.05 ml/kg) for spinal anaesthesia.

14.3.2 Epidural (Extradural) Anaesthesia/Analgesia

Drugs are administered outside the dura mater, hence the terms extradural or epidural. The term *epidural* is a hybrid of both Greek (*epi*) and Latin (*dura*) words, whereas the term *extradural* is derived purely from Latin words and is therefore more etymologically correct. Indications are: for tail, hindlimb, perineal, pelvic, abdominal, or thoracic surgery; to provide pain relief for acute pancreatitis; and to provide analgesia in cats with aorto-iliac thrombosis. Local anaesthetic injected extradurally reduces sympathetic tone to the hind end of the animal (promotes vasodilation), which may be beneficial in cats with aortic thromboembolism in addition to the analgesia afforded.

Gravity can influence the epidural spread of drugs as can the injectate dose (volume), the amount and distribution of fat within the epidural space, and the pressure within the epidural space. In most normal subjects, at least in the standing or sternal positions, there is a **slight negative pressure in the caudal epidural space**, although the pressure in the epidural space is influenced by the intrathoracic and intra-abdominal pressures too. The greatest negative pressure in the epidural space is usually in the thoracic segment, so that cranial spread of injectate tends to be encouraged (from more caudal injection sites).

Nevertheless, the block occurs earliest and is most intense at the site of injection.

When an extradural injection has been performed, even if the drug travels rostrally within the epidural space, it cannot enter the brain from the epidural space because the epidural space is non-existent at the site of the cisterna magna (Ce1–Ce2), since the periosteum and dura mater fuse to form one layer. Extradural injections, however, especially if large volumes are injected rapidly, can result in transient increases in extradural pressure and secondary increases in intracranial pressure with accompanying decreases in spinal cord and cerebral blood flows. Such rapid changes in pressure have been suspected to be the root cause of bradycardia and arrhythmias following extradural (and also intrathecal) injection, although a change in autonomic balance to vagal dominance and stimulation of various vagal/vasovagal reflexes have also been suggested.

14.3.2.1 Terminology
- **Caudal**, **low**, or **posterior** are terms sometimes applied to the extradural technique where the animal retains the motor function of its hindlimbs.
- **Cranial**, **high**, or **anterior** are terms applied to the technique where the animal loses control of its hindlimbs.

The distinction in terminology depends upon the quantity of drug injected, not the site of injection. The commonest injection sites are lumbo-sacral and sacro- (or inter-) coccygeal. The sacro-/inter-coccygeal site may be preferred for perineal surgery or tail surgery as it may result in less motor blockade of the pelvic limbs, and it can be useful to facilitate urethral catheterisation in sedated cats suffering from urethral obstruction.

14.3.2.2 Injection Sites

For the **lumbo-sacral approach**, the craniodorsal iliac spines are located by palpation. If an imaginary line is drawn between these, it should intersect the dorsal spinous process of the last (7th) lumbar vertebra. Slightly caudal to the dorsal spinous process of the 7th lumbar vertebra, a 'dip' can be palpated between it and the first of the smaller sacral dorsal processes; this is the Lu7-Sa1 interspace. The lumbo-sacral space can be located by placing the thumb and middle finger on the craniodorsal iliac spines and then forming a triangle with the index finger (Figure 14.2). The spinal needle is inserted in the midline and perpendicularly to this space (Figures 14.3 and 14.4).

The exact injection site differs slightly for cats and dogs (Figures 14.3 and 14.4). For dogs, due to the shape of the dorsal spinous processes, aim in the centre of the Lu7-Sa1 interspace. For cats, due to the shape of the dorsal spinous processes, aim in the caudal third of the Lu7-Sa1 interspace.

The spinal cord terminates as the conus medullaris at about vertebrae Lu6-Lu7 in most dogs, whereas it terminates at around Sa1-Sa3 in cats. The meningeal sac (containing CSF) continues slightly further caudally than the conus

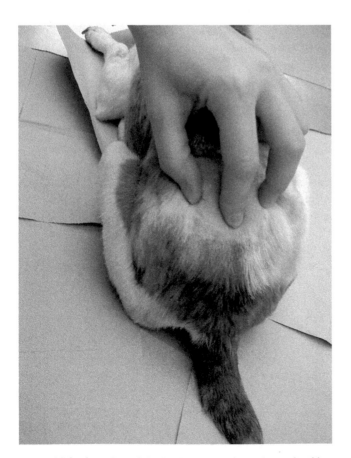

Figure 14.2 Location of the lumbo-sacral space determined by forming a triangle with the thumb and first two fingers.

medullaris of the spinal cord, but in most dogs, it terminates at about Lu7-Sa1. The caudal termination of the meningeal sac (containing CSF) continues further caudally in cats than in dogs. It is therefore more possible to perform a true spinal (intrathecal) injection in cats, even when attempting to perform only an epidural (extradural) injection.

For sacro-/inter-coccygeal extradural injections, the needle should be inserted in the midline of the most mobile joint, either the sacro-coccygeal space or first inter-coccygeal space, which can be ascertained by moving the tail up and down. The needle is advanced at a 30–45° angle cranially. At this site, there should be no risk of inadvertent intrathecal injection, but blood vessels may be damaged resulting in bleeding or the potential for intravascular injection.

14.3.2.2.1 Animal Positioning for Epidural Injection

Patients are usually placed in either sternal or lateral recumbency under sedation or general anaesthesia. In sternal recumbency, the Lu7–Sa1 interspace is easiest to palpate with the hindlimbs 'frog-legged' beneath the animal because this relieves tension in the supraspinous ligament (Figure 14.5a). Once the space has been located, then the hind legs can be drawn forwards (Figure 14.5b). Although this makes the Lu7–Sa1 interspace harder to palpate because it tenses the dorsal supraspinous ligament (and also interspinous ligament), it is supposed to enable a better 'popping sensation' to be felt as the, additionally tensed, interarcuate ligament (ligamentum flavum) is penetrated. In lateral recumbency, the hindlimbs can be drawn forwards, and the forelimbs may also be drawn backwards to help arch the spine and facilitate identification of the correct interspace and injection (Figure 14.6). The area of the injection site must be clipped and aseptically prepared.

14.3.2.2.2 Technique

As the needle is inserted (bevel directed cranially), it will first pass through the skin; then the subcutaneous fat; then the dorsal supraspinous ligament; then the interspinous ligament; and finally, the interarcuate ligament (also called the ligamentum flavum) (Figure 14.7). It is on passing through this interarcuate ligament with the needle that a 'popping' sensation can usually be felt.

Once the needle is in position, observe for a few seconds to ensure that no blood or CSF issues from the hub, and then aspirate to check again for blood or CSF. If bleeding is observed, then you may prefer to abandon the technique as, not only is intravascular injection a risk, but it also becomes difficult to discern whether CSF is also present. Unless the animal has a coagulation abnormality, it is unlikely that it will suffer any untoward effects from a small amount of haemorrhage. If CSF is observed, the technique can either be abandoned, or converted to a true

Figure 14.3 Slightly different needle insertion sites in the lumbo-sacral space for dogs (a) and cats (b). *Source:* Reproduced from Flecknell and Waterman-Pearson (2000) with permission from Elsevier.

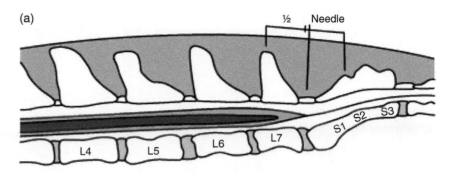

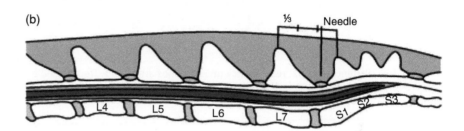

Figure 14.4 Location of lumbo-sacral needle placement site for dog. *Source:* Reproduced from McKelvey and Hollingshead (2003) with permission from Elsevier.

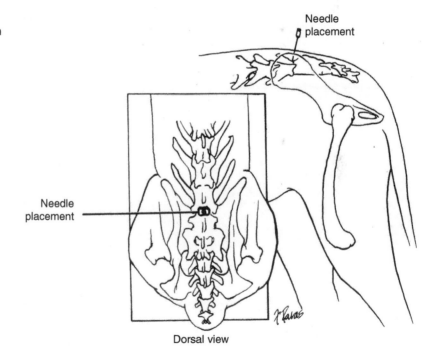

Dorsal view

spinal (intrathecal) technique, but you must reduce the prepared doses to about one quarter, or less.

If the needle penetrates the intervertebral space too deeply, the needle tip may grate against the bony floor of the vertebral canal or even embed into an intervertebral disc. If this occurs, the needle should be withdrawn slightly before attempting injection. There are two vertebral venous sinuses that lie on the floor of the vertebral canal, and a central spinal artery also lies ventrally, whereas dorsally, there are paired lateral spinal arteries. The result is that there is an increased risk of penetrating a blood vessel if the needle tip travels deeper within the vertebral canal. Also, the deeper the needle penetrates the vertebral canal, the more likely it is to come into close proximity with the cauda equina nerves. The 'tail waggle' that ensues can be used as a sign of correct needle placement, but the needle should be withdrawn slightly before attempting injection to try to avoid nerve damage.

(a)

(b)

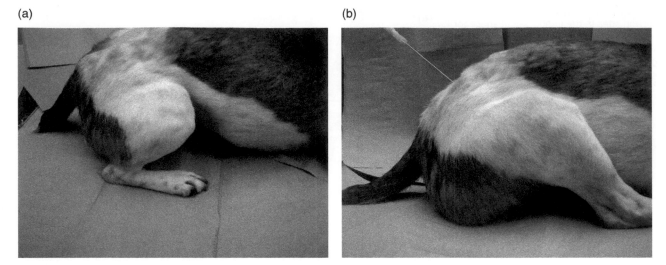

Figure 14.5 Patient in sternal recumbency. (a) Hindlimbs are initially frog-legged to facilitate identification of lumbo-sacral space, then (b) drawn forwards to tense the interarcuate ligament to improve the sensation of the needle 'popping through' into the epidural space.

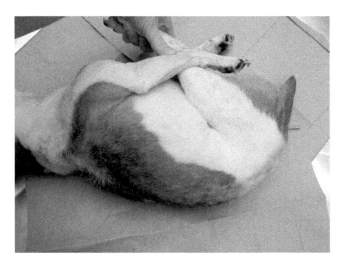

Figure 14.6 Position used to tense the interarcuate ligament for lumbo-sacral injection, with the patient in lateral recumbency.

After confirmation that the needle tip is correctly positioned within the epidural space, the injection is made over at least 30–60 seconds. Rapid extradural injection of cold drugs can produce a shivering response with increased respiratory rate and depth, known as **Durrans' sign** (the mechanism for this is uncertain). It is therefore preferable to warm the injectate (e.g. by holding the syringe in a warm hand for a few minutes) before injection. After the injection has been completed, the animal can be positioned in dorsal recumbency so as to use gravity to encourage block of the sensory nerves (which lie dorsally), and if analgesia on only one side is required, the animal can be laid on that

side. This allows 'gravity assist' to help the injected drug reach the site of interest.

It is good practice to monitor heart and breathing rates during extradural injection of drugs. As well as increased rate and depth of breathing, bradycardia and arrhythmias have also been reported during injection, possibly related to rapid injection. Rapid injection also increases the speed of vertebral vascular absorption and increases the risk of systemic toxicity. It is also advisable to ensure IV access (cannula), before the injection is performed. Not only can the depth of anaesthesia lighten during injection, requiring further doses of anaesthetic agents to be administered, but other drugs and fluids may need to be administered by this route should an emergency arise.

14.3.2.3 Why Use Spinal Needles?

Spinal needles have three features that help in their particular function and use:

- A short bevel makes them 'relatively blunt' so that if nerves are 'hit', the needle tends to push between nerve fibres as it penetrates the nerve, rather than transect them. This relative bluntness is also believed to enhance the 'popping' sensation on penetrating the ligamentum flavum.
- A notch in the hub tells you which way the bevel is orientated.
- A stylette reduces the chance of needle-blockage with a plug of skin/subcutaneous tissue/ligament/bone or intervertebral disc.

Commonly used needle sizes are shown in Table 14.2, although **needle length can be predicted in dogs**: i.e.

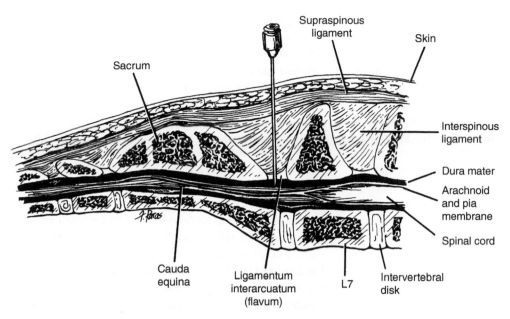

Figure 14.7 The structures traversed during needle placement for extradural injection. *Source:* Reproduced from McKelvey and Hollingshead (2003) with permission from Elsevier.

Table 14.2 Commonly used needle sizes for lumbo-sacral extradural injections.

Animal size (kg)	Needle gauge	Needle length
<5	25	1″
5–10	22	1.5″
10–45	22 or 20	2–2.5″
>45	22 or 20	3.5″

depth from the skin to the neuraxial space at the lumbo-sacral site is calculated by:

$$13.00 + (2.63\,\text{Body Condition Score}) + (0.69\,\text{Body Mass})$$

where BCS is scored out of 9 and body mass is in kilogrammes, giving a result in millimetres.

14.3.2.4 How Can You Tell If the Needle Tip Is in the Epidural Space?

A **definite 'popping' sensation** and a sudden loss of resistance to needle advancement may be felt as the needle penetrates the ligamentum flavum (Figure 14.7).

There is sudden loss of resistance to injection during needle entry into the epidural space and thereafter, lack of resistance to injection of a test dose. For example, a 5 ml syringe (ideally a low-friction syringe) filled with 3 ml sterile saline and 1 ml air is attached to the spinal needle and gentle pressure is applied to the syringe plunger as the needle is advanced into the epidural space.

(When the syringe is attached to the spinal needle, the air floats to form a cushion above the saline; therefore, the air is less likely to be injected when the patient is lying in sternal recumbency than in lateral recumbency.) A sudden loss of resistance to injection accompanies the needle tip entry into the epidural space. The injection should then be possible with minimal resistance and the air cushion should not be compressed. You may even find that, because of the slight negative pressure in the epidural space, the injectate tends to be sucked in.

The **hanging drop technique (Gutierrez's sign)** relies on the usual slight negative pressure within the caudal epidural space. Using a styletted needle, the tip of the needle/stylette assembly is inserted through the skin and subcutaneous tissues. The stylette is then removed and a drop of sterile saline is applied to the open needle hub before the needle is advanced further. Upon entry of the needle tip into the epidural space, the bleb of saline should be sucked in due to the slight negative pressure. This test is successful in 80% of dogs in sternal recumbency. It is not easy to perform when the patient is in lateral recumbency, and at least in goats, lateral recumbency may reduce the negativity of the epidural pressure at the lumbo-sacral site. An alternative for lateral recumbency is the **running drip method** whereby the epidural needle is connected to an infusion set with the line open; when the epidural space is entered, the fluid should run freely.

The **'whoosh' test** has also been described, where air is injected, and auscultation is performed over the spine, cranial to the injection site, with a stethoscope or Doppler flow probe. Better, however, is the **'swoosh' test**, in which, ideally, ultrasound imaging (superior to using a stethoscope or Doppler ultrasound probe) is used to visualise the turbulence that is caused within the 'epidural space' of the vertebral canal when the actual liquid solution of chosen drug/s is injected.

Use of a **nerve locator** has been described to locate the epidural space. The motor response desired is movement of the tail at a current of 0.3 mA. This can identify penetration of the interarcuate ligament, but not dural penetration, so it can be difficult to confirm epidural versus intrathecal needle tip location, the latter of which is more of a risk in cats.

Ultrasound has been described in cats and dogs to identify both epidural and intrathecal deposition of injectate. Ultrasound has also been used in dogs to distinguish epidural from intrathecal needle placement at the more cranial injection site of Lu5/Lu6.

14.3.2.5 Contra-indications
14.3.2.5.1 Relative
- Obesity makes it difficult to find landmarks.
- Pelvic (or lower lumbar spine or lumbo-sacral) injuries may distort the local anatomy.
- Pre-existing neuropathies may make it difficult to distinguish worsening of a prior condition from neural damage caused by the technique.
- Hypovolaemia; local anaesthetics may exacerbate hypotension because they can block sympathetic fibres, causing vasodilation, and may also block cardio-accelerator fibres, preventing any possible compensatory reflex tachycardia.

14.3.2.5.2 Absolute
- Coagulopathies may result in unlimited and uncontrollable haemorrhage.
- Infection, especially skin infection at the proposed injection site or even other distant foci of infection, including bad periodontal disease, risks local or haematogenous spread of infection to the injection site.
- Raised intracranial pressure is often cited as an absolute contraindication in humans because injection into the epidural space can cause further increases in intracranial pressure, albeit usually only transient.

14.3.2.6 Complications
- Hypotension. Local anaesthetics deposited extradurally around the caudal part of the spinal cord result in sympathetic block to the caudal end of the animal with resulting peripheral vasodilation, a relative hypovolaemia, and therefore hypotension. If the block spreads far enough cranially, the sympathetic cardio-accelerator fibres are also affected, resulting in inhibition of a reflex

tachycardia that would otherwise help to offset the hypotension. Hypotension tends to be worse in animals that are already hypovolaemic or shocky. If necessary, hypotension can be treated with IV fluids and vasopressors. Ideally, intravenous access should be secured before extradural injection of local anaesthetic is performed; and some people will give a 'bolus' of IV fluids before extradural injection is performed to offset this hypotension. *Autonomic blockade is suggested to extend for two spinal cord segments further cranially than sensory block, which itself is said to extend for two spinal segments more cranially than motor block.*

- Pelvic limb ataxia; this is less of a worry for small animals than large animals (e.g. cattle), which may 'do the splits', and where recumbency itself may cause problems for the animal and for the proposed surgical procedure.
- Very far cranial spread may block the intercostal and phrenic (Ce 5, 6, 7) nerves, resulting in hypoventilation or even apnoea.
- Horner's syndrome, due to cranial migration of local anaesthetic (to spinal segments Th1-Th3), has also been reported, and is due to blockade of sympathetic fibres to the face and eye. It appears to be more likely in obese or pregnant animals both of which conditions tend to encourage cranial spread of injectate.
- Unintended dural puncture; this is more common in cats and careful observation for CSF should be undertaken following needle placement.
- Hypothermia; is more common in smaller animals and is due to local anaesthetics causing peripheral vasodilation in caudal parts, which facilitates heat loss, and motor blockade of large muscle groups that prevents shivering thermogenesis.
- There may be increased bleeding at the surgical site due to vasodilation. This may be a nuisance for surgery.
- Signs of local anaesthetic toxicity (e.g. CNS depression and cardiorespiratory depression) can follow inadvertent intrathecal injection or intravascular injection; or very rapid systemic absorption.
- Introduction of infection (meningitis/osteomyelitis/neuritis).
- Spinal cord/nerve damage (following needle insertion [rare]; or secondary to haemorrhage, or introduction of infection, or use of high concentrations of local anaesthetics or due to preservatives or other adjuncts).
- Urinary (and faecal) retention can follow the neuraxial administration of local anaesthetics or indeed opioids.
- Pruritus is occasionally associated with neuraxially-administered opioids. The mechanism is uncertain, but appears to involve opioid receptor-mediated effects because it can be suppressed with naloxone. This is unlike the histamine release-associated pruritus that can

accompany systemically-administered opioids, which is related to their ability to stimulate mast cells (and basophils) to degranulate and can be treated with antihistamines. See Further Reading.

- There have been some reports of poor hair regrowth or white hair growth at the site of injection. The cause is uncertain, but may be more associated with hair clipping and aseptic skin preparation than related to neuraxial anaesthesia.
- Poor results. Extradural drug delivery can never be guaranteed to work because of individual animal differences, etc. Patchy blocks are more common after too rapid injection, or if the injectate is very cold, or if previous extradural injections have been given and scar tissue has formed within the epidural space. Unilateral blocks may also result after an extradural catheter is placed if its tip lies to one side.
- Inadvertent injection into the potential subdural 'space' (between the dura mater and arachnoid mater) may result in perceived block failure, but block onset is delayed with wider spread of sensory block than expected, usually with minimal motor block but with profound sympathetic block and subsequent hypotension, and cephalad spread can result in ventilatory failure and CNS toxicity.

14.3.2.7 Drugs and Doses

Drugs should be preservative-free and sterile. **Dilution of drugs is best done using sterile saline for local anaesthetics and sterile water for opioids.** The commonly used drugs and doses shown in Table 14.3 are suitable for injection at the lumbo-sacral site and will provide adequate analgesia up to the first or second lumbar segmental nerves (Lu1/2). Doses can be increased (doubled) to provide analgesia up to the fourth or fifth thoracic segmental nerves (Th4/5), but beware toxicity, especially with local anaesthetic agents in cats.

It is generally agreed that, for injection at the lumbo-sacral site, a **drug volume of 0.2 ml/kg gives sufficient spread for pelvic limb surgery, i.e. up to Lu3/Lu4** (origin of the femoral nerve). To provide **anaesthesia of the abdomen, >0.2 ml/kg (even up to 0.6 ml/kg)** local anaesthetic is required and 'mls of injectate per cm of crown-rump length' is often cited in preference to 'mls of injectate per kg body weight'. Some authors advocate **not to exceed 1 ml injectate per 5–7 kg body weight**, and **not to inject more than 6 ml maximum for any dog**, however using the crown-rump length calculation gives volumes in excess of these (see work by Otero in Further Reading). An increase in adverse cardiovascular effects is seen with higher volumes of local anaesthetics, so caution is warranted.

Recent research in cadavers has demonstrated that for the same injectate volume, whether the injection was made at the lumbo-sacral or sacro-coccygeal site, there was an equivalent cranial spread. Therefore, it appears that injectate volumes may not need to be increased when administered at the sacro-coccygeal site compared with the lumbo-sacral site for the same desired cranial spread.

A lower dose/volume of drug/s is, however, usually sufficient for sacro-/inter-coccygeal administration where only perineal or tail anaesthesia/analgesia is required, e.g. usually 0.1–0.2 ml/kg. Lidocaine gives the most rapid onset and so is recommended for facilitating urethral catheterisation in cats with urethral obstruction.

Extradural injection of 'low doses' of local anaesthetics (e.g. 0.05 ml/kg bupivacaine 0.5%) should produce minimal motor fibre blockade, but animals may still become recumbent because some of the nerves involved in the maintenance of postural muscle tone, through spinal reflex arcs (e.g. innervation of muscle spindles and Golgi tendon organs) may be blocked. Higher doses of local anaesthetics will more than likely produce hindlimb motor block, and

Table 14.3 Commonly used drugs and doses for extradural injection.

Drug	Dose	Onset time (min)	Duration (h)
Lidocaine	2–3 mg/kg	5–10	1–2 (2 with epinephrine)
Bupivacaine	1 mg/kg	15–20	4–8(+)
Ropivacaine	1.5 mg/kg	10–15	4–6(+)
Morphine	0.1 mg/kg	20–60+	16–24
Buprenorphine	5–15 μg/kg	60	16–24
Methadone	0.1 mg/kg	30	4
Morphine + bupivacaine	0.05–0.1 mg/kg + 0.5–1 mg/kg	15	16–24

in people, decrease or loss of the patellar tendon reflex (Westphal's sign) is used to determine whether the block has been successful.

With combinations of lidocaine and bupivacaine, the doses of each are reduced (e.g. half and half) to avoid administering a toxic cumulative dose. Epinephrine may be included with local anaesthetics to prolong the duration of block, and possibly enhance their speed of onset, by 'localising' injected drug to the injection site, and perhaps, through adding a little 'local anaesthetic' like action of its own.

For opioids, the less fat soluble they are, the slower their onset of effect and the longer their extradural duration of action (the slower their systemic absorption). Morphine is less lipophilic than methadone and so has a slower onset and longer duration of action when used epidurally. Morphine at 0.1 mg/kg may provide adequate analgesia up to Th4/5; increasing the dose to 0.2 mg/kg is more likely to provide adequate analgesia up to this level and possibly to Th2 without systemic side effects. Thus, neuraxial techniques can provide analgesia for abdominal or thoracic surgery/pain. However, epidural morphine 0.1 mg/kg is more effective for thoracotomy when administered at the thoracic level, versus lumbo-sacral (see Further Reading).

Extradurally-administered opioids are rarely solely sufficient for surgery (e.g. in a sedated animal) because although they provide excellent analgesia against C fibre pain (slow, burning, second, protopathic pain), they provide poor analgesia against Aδ fibre pain (fast, sharp, incisional, first, epicritic pain). In order to perform surgery under extradural analgesia, a local anaesthetic or an α2 agonist is required. Although α2 agonists produce analgesia similar to opioids, they also have local anaesthetic effects and are systemically absorbed, resulting in sedation, so caution is advised if α2 agonist sedation has already been administered.

If opioids alone are administered extradurally, then the animal should remain standing and ambulatory because motor nerve blockade does not occur (although mild ataxia and occasionally myoclonus have been reported after extradural morphine, possibly due to some local anaesthetic activity of the opioid itself or due to effects on spinal reflex arcs).

The addition of local anaesthetics to morphine has been shown to facilitate morphine's antinociceptive effect in rats. It therefore makes sense to combine these two drug classes.

Remifentanil should not be administered by the neuraxial routes because glycine is included in the preparation. Glycine is a CNS inhibitory neurotransmitter, but is also a co-agonist at NMDA receptors.

Ketamine (preservative free, and especially, just the S-isomer) is now available for use by the extradural route, either alone or in combination with other drugs, but is not yet licenced for this use in veterinary species.

The α2 agonists medetomidine and dexmedetomidine have been used epidurally in dogs, although one study reported demyelination of oligodendrocytes in rabbits with dexmedetomidine. A dose of 5 μg/kg medetomidine did not show advantage over morphine 0.1 mg/kg in dogs undergoing cruciate surgery, although isoflurane sparing effects have been noted with 10–20 μg/kg. Systemic absorption and, therefore, systemic analgesia, however, may be partly responsible for this observation. Dexmedetomidine 4 μg/kg combined with bupivacaine 1 mg/kg increased time to return of motor function compared to morphine/bupivacaine, but also showed a shorter time to return to urination. Currently, however, these drugs are not available as preservative-free formulations. If they are to be used, a new (previously unbroached) bottle should be used. Due to their slight local anaesthetic activity, α2 agonists can produce, not only sensory block, but also some ataxia because of motor nerve blockade. Furthermore, their systemic absorption can lead to sedative and myorelaxant effects, which may also manifest as ataxia.

14.3.2.8 Factors Affecting Cranial Spread of Anaesthesia or Analgesia

These include:

- Patient size
- Patient age
- Patient conformation, including obesity
- Increased intra-abdominal pressure (e.g. pregnancy, gastric dilation, extreme obesity)
- Dose (mass) of drug injected. The same mass of drug administered in different volumes gives similar sensory blockade
- Volume of drug injected – but see above as this tends to be related to drug dose
- Physico-chemical properties of the injected solution (e.g. density, viscosity, temperature; inclusion of epinephrine)
- Direction of needle bevel
- Rate of injection (injection 'pressure') – equivocal

Overall, with extradural injections, it has been said that it is neither the volume, nor the concentration of injectate, nor even the rate of injection ('pressure' of injection), that influence cephalad spread of analgesia/anaesthesia, but the actual mass (dose) of drug given. The volume and concentration of injectate are, however, related to the dose. For example, injection of 0.4 ml/kg bupivacaine 0.25% resulted in more cardiovascular effects than 0.2 ml/kg of 0.25% bupivacaine in dogs.

Anaesthesia/analgesia may be less 'patchy' if a lower volume/higher concentration of drug is injected more slowly, and warming the injectate to body temperature may also help. One of the problems with extradural drug administration is that the efficacy is difficult to guarantee.

For unilateral hindlimb procedures, keeping the surgical limb in a dependent position for 5–10 minutes after the injection may improve the block on that side. One study showed increased spread of methylene blue dye on the dependent side after such a manoeuvre.

Use decreased doses with old, pregnant, and obese animals because:

- Old animals have more fibrous tissue blocking intervertebral foramina, so extradurally injected drugs can travel, and produce effects, further cranially.
- Pregnant animals tend to have engorged vertebral blood vessels due to the higher intra-abdominal pressure. This means that there is a relative reduction in the amount of space available within the spinal canal and, therefore, a relatively smaller extradural space. The high intra-abdominal pressure (gravid uterus) also pushes more soft tissues into the intervertebral foramina, which may partly block the foramina (as with older animals), further reducing the space available within the spinal canal. Progesterone also hastens the onset of local anaesthetic blockade, presenting another reason to reduce doses.
- Obese animals tend to have more fat in their extradural spaces, again relatively reducing the extradural space capacity. Severe obesity also increases intra-abdominal pressure. Although some authors recommend using the occiput-coccygeal length for calculation of local anaesthetic volumes, it is probably more important to dose according to lean body mass.

14.3.2.9 Proposed Sites of Drug Action After Extradural Injection

Drugs can be absorbed systemically from the epidural 'space', so consideration of their systemic effects/side effects should be made. Furthermore, if systemic administration of the same/same class of drug is proposed, then be aware of the total doses used.

After injection into the epidural 'space' the drug can:

- Escape from the epidural space/vertebral canal via the intervertebral foramina to effectively produce a 'high paravertebral block'.
- Be absorbed into the vertebral venous sinuses (and produce a systemic effect).
- Be absorbed into epidural lymphatics (and produce a systemic effect).

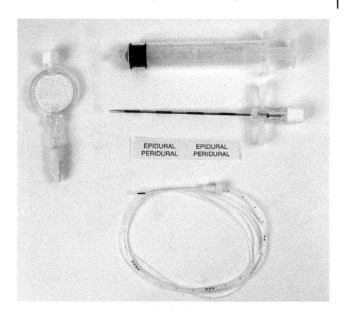

Figure 14.8 Mini epidural kit. *Source:* Image courtesy of Vygon Vet.

- Cross the dura mater and arachnoid mater and enter the CSF, from where it can slowly enter the spinal cord and spinal nerve roots across the pia mater.

14.3.2.10 Epidural Catheters

For prolonged anaesthesia/analgesia, an epidural catheter can be placed using a commercially available kit (Figure 14.8). This includes a Tuohy needle with a bevel that facilitates cranial advancement of the catheter. The catheter is placed at the lumbo-sacral junction and advanced to a level where the analgesia is desired. Catheters can be left in situ for several days provided that strict aseptic technique is observed. Opioids and/or local anaesthetics are administered on an intermittent basis, although some authors recommend continuous delivery via a syringe driver.

14.4 Regional Anaesthesia for the Thoracic Limb

14.4.1 Brachial Plexus Block (At Axillary Level)

The area blocked is from the elbow region distally. The nerves blocked are the radial, median, ulnar, musculocutaneous, and axillary (Figure 14.9), which originate from Ce6-Th1.

14.4.1.1 Landmarks and Technique

Point of shoulder (acromion and greater tuberosity of humerus). The animal is best positioned in lateral recumbency.

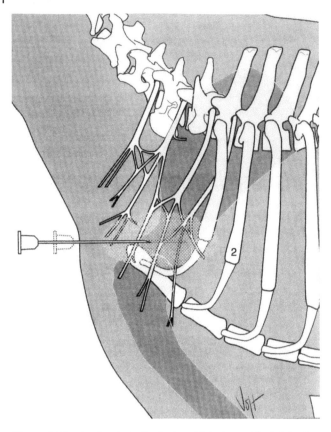

Figure 14.9 Anatomical site for brachial plexus block injection. *Source:* Reproduced from Muir et al. (2007) with permission from Elsevier.

Table 14.4 Nerves and corresponding motor responses for electro-neuro-location (thoracic limb).

Nerve	Motor response
Radial	Extension of the carpus and digits (also elbow extension)
Ulnar	Flexion of the carpus and digits (deep digital flexors)
Median	Flexion of carpus and digits (superficial and deep digital flexors)
Musculocutaneous	Elbow flexion

The region around and especially medial to the shoulder joint and medially to the cranial border of the scapula should be clipped and aseptically prepared. A needle of suitable length is then inserted medial to the shoulder joint, staying on the medial aspect of the scapula, but staying outside the chest. The needle is advanced parallel to the vertebral column, aiming for the costochondral junction of the first rib. Aspiration, to be sure the needle tip is not in a blood vessel, is performed prior to injection of a small aliquot of the total volume; the remainder is injected as the needle is withdrawn, aspirating before each subsequent injection (Figure 14.9). An assistant can be helpful to 'elevate' the scapula/shoulder.

Using an electrical nerve locator to 'identify' branches of the brachial plexus (electro-neuro-location) can greatly improve the chance of successful block (see Further Reading and Table 14.4). Ultrasound guidance will also aid identification of the nerves to be blocked and, visualisation of the spread of injected local anaesthetic may help to reduce the total injectate volume required (see Further Reading for more information on the various approaches).

The chosen needle size depends upon the size of the dog or cat. For larger dogs, a 7.5–10 cm needle may be required,

and some operators prefer to use spinal needles because their relative bluntness reduces the potential to cause nerve (and possibly blood vessel) damage. Needle gauge should be around 21–23 g.

14.4.1.2 Dose of Local Anaesthetic
- Bupivacaine 1–2 mg/kg; onset around 20–30 minutes, duration c. 6–8 hours ++.
- Lidocaine c. 3 mg/kg; onset around 10–20 minutes, duration c. 1–2 hours (nearer 2 hours if lidocaine with epinephrine is used).

The local anaesthetic solutions commercially available (2% lidocaine, 0.5% bupivacaine, and 0.75% ropivacaine) can be diluted with sterile saline in order to increase the volume of injectate and increase the spread of local anaesthetic. A good final injectate volume would be about 0.4 ml/kg.

14.4.1.3 Potential Complications
- Pneumothorax
- Large haematomas
- Inadvertent intravascular injection of local anaesthetic with subsequent signs of local anaesthetic toxicity (convulsions, respiratory, and cardiac depression)
- Brachial plexus damage with ensuing neuritis, paresis, or paralysis (may be permanent)
- Introduction of infection into the axilla
- Paraesthesias (e.g. abnormal sensation, 'itching'). This may worry the animal (as may loss of sensation in the limb) during onset of block (if not under general anaesthesia) and during recovery from the block
- Residual block can sometimes last up to 24 hours, so slight motor impairment may be noticeable for this time. The reason for this is uncertain, but it may follow subperineurium, extrafascicular deposition of local anaesthetic. This can result in, not only neural ischaemia (secondary to compression of the vasa nervorum), which itself enhances nerve conduction block, but also the

delayed systemic absorption of local anaesthetic from this site tends to prolong its duration of effect.

Ultrasound guidance combined with electrical nerve stimulation can also be used to help position a catheter for intermittent or continuous infusion of local anaesthetic to help provide intra- and post-operative analgesia (Figure 14.10).

14.4.2 Brachial Plexus Block; Subscalenic Approach

Figure 14.11 outlines the sites for the common approaches to brachial plexus block at three different levels. This approach is somewhat intermediate between the axillary and cervical paravertebral approaches. (See Further Reading.)

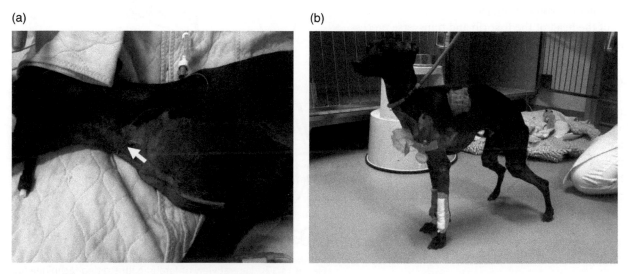

(a) **(b)**

Figure 14.10 Repeated or continuous infusion of local anaesthetic at the site of the left brachial plexus was enabled in this patient by ultrasound- and electro-neuro-location-guided placement of an epidural catheter, which was held in position with a Chinese finger-trap suture (white arrow) prior to radial and ulnar osteotomies (a); and post-operatively with dressing pulled down to reveal a filter attached to the catheter (b).

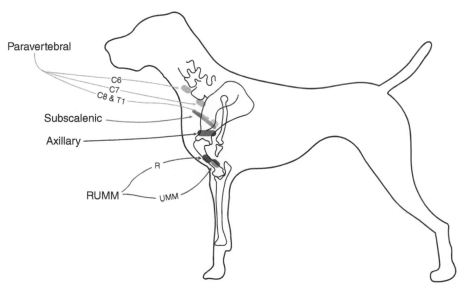

Figure 14.11 Approaches described for thoracic limb nerve blocks. *Source:* Image reproduced with kind permission from Portela et al. (2018b).

14.4.3 Cervical Paravertebral Block

This technique targets the nerves (Ce6-Th1) where they emerge from the spinal cord, so blocks more proximally than the brachial plexus block at axillary level, i.e. the shoulder and brachium are included (Figure 14.11). Palpation of the vertebrae is essential, so the technique is somewhat limited to animals of an ideal (or thin) body condition score. The block is easier to perform with an electrical nerve locator to aid identification of the relevant nerves.

14.4.3.1 Landmarks and Technique

Palpation of the head of the first rib and transverse process of Ce6 is essential. Retract the scapula to make this easier. The needle is advanced towards the head of the first rib and caudally off the back of the rib to block Th1, to a depth of approx. 5–10 mm. The needle is then directed forwards off the cranial border of the rib head to a similar depth to block Ce8. Moving cranially, palpate the transverse process of Ce6 and direct the needle off the caudal border to block Ce7, then move off the cranial border to block Ce6. A volume of 0.5–1.0 ml should suffice for each site. Use of an electrical nerve locator certainly enhances the accuracy of this technique.

14.4.3.2 Potential Complications

- Pneumothorax
- Haematoma
- Inadvertent intravascular injection
- Nerve damage
- Unilateral phrenic nerve paralysis (temporary) if landmarks are not accurate/depending upon the degree that branches of Ce6–Ce8 contribute to the phrenic nerve
- Transient Horner's syndrome
- Epidural spread of local anaesthetic
- Block failure

14.4.4 Radial, Ulnar, Musculocutaneous and Median (RUMM) nerve Block

Blockade of these nerves in the mid-humeral region, after they leave the brachial plexus, provides anaesthesia distal to the elbow. The radial nerve is easily palpated over the lateral aspect of the distal third of the humerus (Figure 14.12). A volume of 0.05–0.1 ml/kg local anaesthetic is adequate. The ulnar and median nerves lie in close apposition on the medial aspect of the distal third of the humerus, caudal to the brachial artery (Figure 14.13). The musculocutaneous nerve lies cranial to the artery. A volume of 0.05–0.1 ml/kg for each site (musculocutaneous and median/ulnar) is recommended. Following poor results from palpation-only techniques, both electro-neuro-location (Table 14.4) and ultrasound-guided techniques have been described.

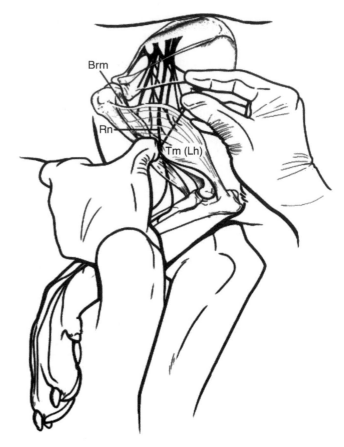

Figure 14.12 Lateral view of forelimb illustrating technique for radial nerve block. Tm (Lh), lateral head of triceps muscle; Brm, brachialis muscle; Rn, radial nerve. *Source:* Reproduced from Trumpatori et al. (2010).

14.5 Regional Anaesthesia for the Pelvic Limb

Anaesthesia of the entire pelvic limb can be achieved with perineural anaesthetic administration around the main nerves of the lumbo-sacral plexus, Lu4-Sa2, which are the femoral (Lu4-Lu6) and sciatic (Lu6-Sa2) nerves plus the lateral cutaneous femoral (Lu3-Lu5), obturator (Lu4-Lu6), and the caudal cutaneous femoral (Lu7-Sa2) nerves (Figure 14.14 and Table 14.5).

14.5.1 Femoral Nerve Block

The femoral nerve arises primarily from the 4th, 5th, and 6th lumbar segmental nerves and forms part of the lumbar plexus, which lies within the psoas compartment, before emerging from the iliopsoas muscle, strictly as the saphenous nerve, to lie on the cranial aspect of the femoral artery, which can be palpated in the femoral triangle. The femoral nerve has both sensory and motor components, whereas the saphenous is purely sensory.

Several approaches are described to the femoral/saphenous nerve as detailed below.

14.5.1.1 Inguinal Approach to Femoral/Saphenous Nerve Block

The femoral (saphenous) nerve is blocked within the femoral triangle where is lies along the cranial border of the femoral artery – the artery is easily palpated and acts as the main landmark. The nerve lies relatively superficially. Once the femoral artery has been palpated, a needle is carefully inserted perpendicularly to the skin so that its tip lies just at the cranial border of the artery and around 0.05–0.1 ml/kg local anaesthetic is then deposited (after careful aspiration to guard against intra-arterial injection). Usually only the saphenous nerve is blocked, but, depending upon how proximal the block is performed within the femoral triangle, the spread of local anaesthetic injected and individual variation of nerve branching, the block may extend proximally enough to block the femoral nerve itself (i.e. it may extend to the psoas compartment, which may also result in obturator nerve block). A volume of 0.1 ml/kg bupivacaine 0.5% has been shown to produce a block of 8–10 hours duration in dogs.

Use of an ENL (stifle extension is the expected motor response to nerve stimulation) can be helpful, but the block can be performed without. Ultrasound can also be used with insertion of the needle through the sartorius muscle to target the femoral/saphenous nerve.

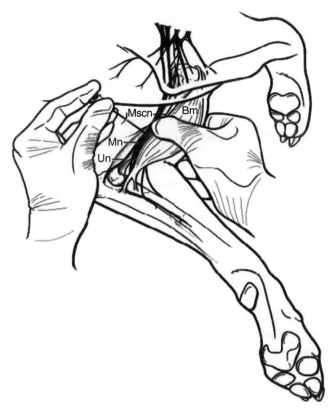

Figure 14.13 Medial view of forelimb illustrating technique for ulnar, musculocutaneous, and median nerve blocks. Bm, biceps brachialis muscle; Un, ulnar nerve; Mscn, musculocutaneous nerve; Mn, median nerve. *Source:* Reproduced from Trumpatori et al. (2010).

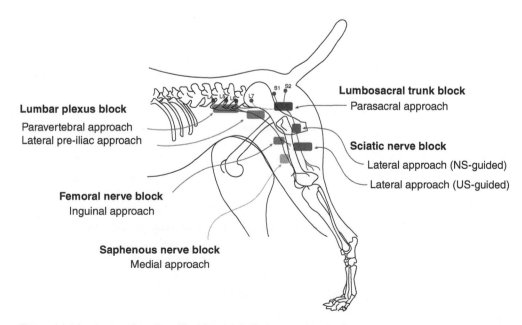

Figure 14.14 Approaches described for pelvic limb nerve blocks. *Source:* Image reproduced with kind permission from Portela et al. (2018a).

Table 14.5 Nerves and corresponding motor responses for electro-neuro-location (pelvic limb).

Nerve	Motor response
Sciatic – peroneal	Hock flexion
	Digital extension
Sciatic – tibial	Stifle flexion
	Hock extension
	Digital flexion
Femoral	Stifle extension

14.5.1.1.1 Potential Complications

- Vascular puncture (keep at least one finger on the femoral artery near the injection site and aspirate prior to injection)
- Intraneural injection/nerve damage
- Block failure

14.5.1.1.2 Mid-thigh Approach to Saphenous Nerve Block

Requiring US guidance for this approach, the saphenous nerve is targeted at a mid-thigh site, distal to the femoral triangle. As the saphenous nerve is sensory only, its blockade will not interfere with the animal's ability to weight-bear. A volume of 0.1 ml/kg bupivacaine 0.5% is recommended for a duration of action of 8–10 hours.

14.5.1.1.3 Potential Complications

- Inadvertent intravascular injection
- Intraneural injection/nerve damage
- At this level, saphenous nerve block will always miss any obturator contribution to the medial genicular nerve, resulting in potential partial block of the stifle
- Block failure

Whichever approach is chosen for a femoral/saphenous nerve block, it is usually performed in conjunction with a sciatic nerve block for anaesthesia of the stifle and distal limb (see below). In a percentage of dogs, however, the medial genicular nerve (which originates from the saphenous nerve) receives a contribution from the obturator nerve. The obturator nerve is not usually blocked by the inguinal or saphenous approaches to the femoral/saphenous nerve, but both the femoral and obturator nerves should be blocked when a psoas compartment (lumbar plexus) block is performed (see below). An inguinal approach to the femoral/saphenous nerve (plus sciatic nerve block), however, was shown to provide comparable analgesia to epidural anaesthesia in dogs undergoing stifle surgery.

14.5.2 Obturator Nerve Block

The obturator nerve also arises from the fourth to sixth lumbar segmental nerves. In dogs, in addition to innervating the caudal aspect of the hip and stifle joints, it can sometimes contribute to the medial genicular nerve (branch of saphenous nerve) to help supply the medial aspect of the stifle joint. Ultrasound visualisation can be used to block the obturator nerve where it emerges, ventrally from the obturator foramen, and courses ventrally along the caudal aspect of the pectineus muscle.

The obturator nerve can, however, be blocked by performing a psoas compartment block, which also blocks the femoral nerve more proximally. Although this can be attempted using a dorsal (paravertebral) or lateral pre-iliac approach, these techniques are most suited to at least electrical nerve-stimulator-guidance and/or ultrasound-guidance (see below and Further Reading).

14.5.3 Lumbar Plexus Block (Also Known as the Psoas Compartment Block)

The lumbar plexus is located within the iliopsoas muscle and contains six nerves: the iliohypogastric, ilioinguinal, genitofemoral, lateral cutaneous femoral, femoral, and obturator nerves. It is recommended to use an ENL for these blocks.

14.5.3.1 Lateral Pre-iliac Approach

With the patient in lateral recumbency, the needle insertion point is just cranial to the wing of the ilium at the level of the sixth lumbar vertebra. To find the insertion point, one line is drawn perpendicularly 'down' (from the dorsal midline), from the dorsal spinous process (or transverse process) of the sixth lumbar vertebra; a second line is drawn, parallel to the vertebral column, cranially, from the most cranial part of the iliac crest, which is often the cranial ventral iliac spine. Where these two lines intersect represents the needle insertion site. The needle is inserted at an angle of 30–45° to the skin, pointing caudally and parallel to the long axis of the spine. It is advanced, carefully, through iliocostalis lumborum epaxial muscle and into the psoas compartment. An electrical nerve locator is used, and the motor response is contraction of the quadriceps femoris muscle and stifle extension. A volume of 0.2 ml/kg bupivacaine 0.5% is recommended in cats and dogs.

14.5.3.2 Parasagittal Paravertebral Approach

With the patient in lateral recumbency, the needle is advanced parasagittally (perpendicularly to the dorsum of the animal) at the level of fifth to sixth lumbar vertebral interspace, through the epaxial musculature and then into the hypaxial iliopsoas muscle. If the fifth lumbar vertebral transverse process is contacted, the needle is walked off in a caudal direction and advanced to enter the iliopsoas muscle. An electrical nerve locator is used, and the motor response is contraction of the quadriceps femoris muscle and stifle extension. A volume of 0.4 ml/kg bupivacaine 0.5% is recommended.

Alternatively, the three spinal segmental nerves that comprise the femoral nerve (Lu4, Lu5, and Lu6) can be blocked separately, paravertebrally, using a smaller volume of local anaesthetic for each nerve root (0.4 ml/kg bupivacaine 0.5% divided between the three).

14.5.3.2.1 Potential Complications
- Vascular puncture
- Abdominal penetration
- Abdominal viscus puncture
- Block failure

14.5.4 Sciatic Nerve Block

The sciatic nerve arises from the last two lumbar and first two sacral segmental nerves (Lu6-Sa2), and cascades over the greater ischiatic notch of the ischium to pass between the greater trochanter of the femur and the ischial tuberosity of the pelvis.

There are three approaches to the sciatic nerve: the lateral approach, the para-sacral approach, and the trans-gluteal approach. If using an ENL, the desired motor response is digital flexion or extension. Contractions of biceps femoris or hamstring muscles is not an acceptable end point. Block success has been demonstrated by increased perfusion index in the distal limb (see Further Reading).

14.5.4.1 Potential Complications
- Vascular puncture
- Intraneural injection/nerve damage
- Rectal puncture (with the dorsal para-sacral approach)
- Block failure

14.5.4.2 Lateral Approach
This is the easiest approach to perform and does not require an ENL or US, although ENL guidance can help verify correct needle placement. If an imaginary line is drawn between the femoral greater trochanter and ischial tuberosity, then a needle inserted, with slight cranial inclination from perpendicular to the skin, 1/3rd the distance along this line from the greater trochanter, and usually no deeper than 1–2 cm (depending upon the size of the patient), should enable deposition of 0.05–0.1 ml/kg local anaesthetic in the vicinity of the nerve before it branches into its separate tibial and peroneal divisions. Aspirate first to avoid inadvertent intravascular injection. Using US, both divisions of the sciatic nerve can be visualised slightly further distally to the above injection site, and a needle, introduced in plane with the US transducer, can be visualised, after insertion on the caudal aspect of the limb, between the biceps femoris and semitendinosus muscles, and perineural deposition of local anaesthetic observed.

14.5.4.3 Para-sacral Approach
Requires ENL guidance. A line drawn from the cranial dorsal iliac spine to the ischial tuberosity is divided into thirds with the injection site being at the junction of the cranial and middle third. The needle is inserted perpendicularly to the skin on the animal's dorsum, in a parasagittal plane, and advanced under ENL guidance whilst looking for the desired response to nerve stimulation. After aspiration, to guard against inadvertent intravascular injection, a volume of 0.05–0.1 ml/kg local anaesthetic is injected.

14.5.4.4 Trans-gluteal Approach
Best performed using US or at least an ENL, but not yet fully evaluated clinically. A first line is drawn between the ischial tuberosity and the cranial dorsal iliac spine and divided into thirds. A point at the junction of the middle and caudal thirds is marked. Then a further line is drawn, parallel to the vertebral column from the cranial dorsal iliac spine extending caudally. Finally, a third line is drawn from the point marked on first line and perpendicular to it to intersect the second line. The needle insertion point then lies half-way along this final line. The needle is introduced in a cranioventral direction (60° angle to the vertical, parallel to the animal's long axis), and inserted through the superficial gluteal muscle just cranial to the sacrotuberous ligament, until it just touches the ischium. Early studies reported the necessity to use relatively large volumes of local anaesthetic, which resulted in very prolonged block durations.

14.6 Regional Techniques Relevant to Thoracic and Pelvic Limbs

14.6.1 Ring Blocks

Local anaesthetic agents can be injected to encircle the area of interest, e.g. before digit amputation (as an alternative to performing digital nerve blocks). It is important to exclude epinephrine from the local anaesthetic solution if encircling an appendage or other structure whose perfusion may be compromised by the inclusion of a vasoconstrictor. **Do not inject through inflamed or infected tissues.**

14.6.2 Digital Nerve Blocks

Each digit is supplied by two sets of axial and abaxial digital nerves: the dorsal and the palmar or plantar. If the digit is imagined in cross-section at its base, and viewed as a clock face, these run at the 10 o'clock, 2 o'clock, 4 o'clock, and 8 o'clock positions. Local anaesthetic (total volume 1–2 ml, depending upon patient size) is injected using a small gauge needle, axially and abaxially, just above and below the medial and lateral mid-points.

14.6.3 Intravenous Regional Anaesthesia (IVRA; Bier's Block)

This is an excellent technique to provide distal limb anaesthesia and analgesia. A superficial vein may be cannulated distal to where the tourniquet is to be placed. The distal limb is then usually exsanguinated using either an Esmarch bandage (be careful not to dislodge the cannula during Esmarch bandage placement or unwrapping after the tourniquet is placed) or by holding the limb above heart level for five minutes. The tourniquet is placed proximal to the site of interest. The Esmarch bandage (if one was placed), is then unwrapped.

Lidocaine (usually without epinephrine) is then injected into the vein either via the pre-placed cannula or 'off the needle'. The safe dose of lidocaine is 2–3 mg/kg, but it can be diluted in sterile normal saline if necessary. At least 10 minutes should be allowed for onset of anaesthesia/analgesia.

Tourniquets can be safely placed on the limbs of small animals for up to two hours, and anaesthesia/analgesia persists for as long as the tourniquet is in place. A bloodless surgical field and the reduced potential for blood loss can be advantageous. The tourniquet should not be released for at least 20 minutes to avoid the sudden delivery of a relatively large dose of local anaesthetic (and perhaps vasoconstrictor) into the circulation which increases the risk of systemic toxicity. When the tourniquet is finally released, sensation returns within 5–15 minutes; the animal should be monitored closely for signs of systemic local anaesthetic toxicity and other problems that can follow occlusion of limb perfusion, i.e. ischaemia and reperfusion (e.g. hypotension and arrhythmias).

Neither bupivacaine nor ropivacaine should be used because of the risk of escape into the systemic circulation and cardiotoxicity.

14.6.3.1 Dose
For a 25 kg dog, 2–5 ml of 1% lidocaine is used, preferably without epinephrine so as to enhance the extravascular tissue distribution of the local anaesthetic and hasten the onset of block.

The mechanisms and sites of action of IVRA are disputed, but appear to involve almost immediate blockade of sensory nerve terminals and then a slightly delayed block of small diameter nerve fibres, and possibly even larger nerve trunks, probably because local anaesthetic is transported to the nerves in the vasa nervorum. Neural ischaemia, secondary to tourniquet application, may also result in some deterioration of nerve conduction, which may enhance anaesthesia/analgesia; but tourniquet application itself can be painful. It is usual to inject the local anaesthetic agent as distally in the limb as possible and also in a distal (toewards) direction if possible. Anaesthesia/analgesia spreads proximally and distally from the injection site with the digits usually becoming blocked last.

14.6.3.2 Potential Complications
- Inadequate anaesthesia/analgesia (tourniquet not tight enough or insufficient local anaesthetic was injected or insufficient time was allowed for the local anaesthetic to work).
- Inadvertent systemic local anaesthetic toxicity (tourniquet not tight enough).
- Ischaemic damage to structures distal to the tourniquet (rare).
- Pain after removal of tourniquet (possibly due to ischaemia or reperfusion). (Tourniquet application itself can be quite a noxious stimulus and can result in the 'tourniquet effect': typically observed as hypertension and possibly also tachycardia following sympathetic stimulation. This may even last for as long as the tourniquet is in applied.)
- Hypotension/arrhythmias after tourniquet removal (due to reactive hyperaemia/vasodilation in ischaemic limb with or without reabsorption into the general circulation of products of anaerobic metabolism including K^+ and free radicals). Rare if the tourniquet is only in place for <2 hours.
- Difficulty in identifying a suitable vein; usually only a problem if local inflammation or cellulitis is present. (Cellulitis is a relative contra-indication to the use of this technique; others being local skin infection, vasculitis, and compound fractures [which complicate Esmarch bandage application and may also affect limb perfusion].)

14.6.4 Intra-articular Analgesia

In the small animal peri-operative setting, intra-articular analgesia can be a part of the intra-operative analgesia regimen during arthroscopies or arthrotomies. Local anaesthetic may be injected before the joint is opened and may be repeated, with or without opioid, at the end of surgery after the joint is closed once again. Although some chemical synovitis may ensue, the reaction is no worse than following instillation of normal saline. However, there are increasing worries about the possible chondrotoxic effects of intra-articular local anaesthetic agents, the mechanisms of which are as yet unknown, but may be related to the local anaesthetic agent itself, the concentration of the solution and overall 'dose', the pH of the solution, the presence of preservatives and/or vasoconstrictors, the duration of exposure of the cartilage to the agent, etc. (see Further Reading). Ropivacaine appears to be the least chondrotoxic.

The most severe cases of chondrotoxicity in people have been related to repeated/prolonged infusion of bupivacaine using 'pain pumps'. Evidence in rabbits shows that chondrocyte viability returns with time and that saline also affects chondrocyte viability in the short term.

14.6.4.1 Doses Quoted for Stifle and Elbow Injection in Dogs

- Ropivacaine 0.75 mg/kg (equivalent to 0.1 ml/kg of a 0.75% solution)
- Morphine 0.1 mg/kg (diluted with saline to 0.1 ml/kg)

- For arthroscopy, any local anaesthetic injected pre-surgery will be washed from the joint by continuous lavage during surgery. Mepivacaine gives 20 minutes of anaesthesia in this context; lidocaine can be expected to behave similarly.

Various other agents have been used in humans. Clonidine (an α2 agonist) has been administered at 1 μg/kg; neostigmine, ketamine and various other novel agents have also been tried, with some success. Even normal saline itself has been shown to provide some analgesia.

References

Flecknell, P. and Waterman-Pearson, A. (eds.) (2000). Management of postoperative and other acute pain. In: *Pain Management in Animals*, 81–145. London: W.B. Saunders.

McKelvey, D. and Hollingshead, K.W. (eds.) (2003). Special techniques. In: *Veterinary Anesthesia and Analgesia*, 3e, 286–314. St. Louis, Missouri: Mosby, Elsevier.

Muir, W.W., JAE, H., Bednarski, R.M., and Skarda, R.T. (eds.) (2007). Local anesthesia in dogs and cats. In: *Handbook of Veterinary Anesthesia*, 4e, 118–139. St. Louis, Missouri: Mosby, Elsevier.

Portela, D.A., Verdier, N., and Otero, P.E. (2018a). Regional anesthetic techniques for the pelvic limb and abdominal wall in small animals: a review of the literature and technique description. *The Veterinary Journal* 238: 27–40.

Portela, D.A., Verdier, N., and Otero, P.E. (2018b). Regional anesthetic techniques for the thoracic limb and thorax in small animals: a review of the literature and technique description. *The Veterinary Journal* 241: 8–19.

Trumpatori, B.J., Carter, J.E., Hash, J. et al. (2010). Evaluation of a midhumeral block of the radial, ulnar, musculocutaneous and median (RUMM block) nerves for analgesia of the distal aspect of the thoracic limb in dogs. *Veterinary Surgery* 39: 785–796.

Further Reading

Adami, C. and Gendron, K. (2017). What is the evidence? The issue of verifying correct needle position during epidural anaesthesia in dogs. *Veterinary Anaesthesia and Analgesia* 44: 212–218.

Ballantyne, J.C., Loach, A.B., and Carr, D.B. (1988). Itching after epidural and spinal opiates. *Pain* 33: 149–160.

Bauquier, S.H. (2012). Hypotension and pruritus induced by neuraxial anaesthesia in a cat. *Australian Veterinary Journal* 90: 402–403.

Blass, C.E. and Moore, R.W. (1984). The tourniquet in surgery. A review. *Veterinary Surgery* 13: 111–114.

Campoy, L. (2008). Fundamentals of regional anesthesia using nerve stimulation in the dog. In: *Recent Advances in Veterinary Anesthesia and Analgesia: Companion Animals* (eds. R.D. Gleed and J.W. Ludders). Ithaca, New York: International Veterinary Information Service (www.ivis.org Document number A1416.0408).

Campoy, L. and Mahler, S.P. (2013). The pelvic limb. In: *Small Animal Regional Anesthesia & Analgesia*, 1e (eds. L. Campoy and M.R. Read), 199–226. Iowa, USA: Wiley Blackwell.

Campoy, L. and Read, M.R. (2013). The thoracic limb. In: *Small Animal Regional Anesthesia & Analgesia*, 1e (eds. L. Campoy and M.R. Read), 141–166. Iowa, USA: Wiley Blackwell.

Castineiras, D., Viscasillas, J., and Seymour, C. (2015). A modified approach for performing ultrasound-guided radial, ulnar, median and musculocutaneous nerve block in a dog. *Veterinary Anaesthesia and Analgesia* 42: 659–661.

Chabel, C., Russel, L.C., and Lee, R. (1990). Tourniquet-induced limb ischemia: a neurophysiologic animal model. *Anesthesiology* 72: 1038–1044.

Dalrymple, P. and Chelliah, S. (2006). Electrical nerve locators. *Continuing Education in Anaesthesia, Critical Care and Pain* 6: 32–36.

Day, T.K., Pepper, W.T., Tobias, T.A. et al. (1995). Comparison of intra-articular and epidural morphine for analgesia following stifle arthrotomy in dogs. *Veterinary Surgery* 24: 522–530.

Dawkins, M. (1963). The identification of the epidural space: a critical analysis of the various methods employed. *Anaesthesia* 18: 66–77.

De Conno, F., Caraceni, A., Martini, C. et al. (1991). Hyperalgesia and myoclonus with intrathecal infusion of high-dose morphine. *Pain* 47: 337–339.

Deloughty, J.L. and Griffiths, R. (2009). Arterial tourniquets. *Continuing Education in Anaesthesia, Critical Care and Pain* 9: 56–60. *(Excellent review of physiological effects of tourniquets and complications of their use; based on their use in man.).*

Dias, R.S.G., Soares, J.H.N., DdeSe, C. et al. (2018). Cardiovascular and respiratory effects of lumbosacral epidural bupivacaine in isoflurane-anesthetized dogs: the effects of two volumes of 0.25% solution. *PLoS One* 13 (4): 18.

Duke-Novakovski, T. (2016). Pain management II: local and regional anaesthetic techniques. In: *BSAVA Manual of Canine and Feline Anaesthesia and Analgesia*, 3e (eds. T. Duke Novakovski, M. de Vries and C. Seymour), 143–158. Gloucester, UK: BSAVA Publications.

Fettes, P.D.W., Jansson, J.-R., and Wildsmith, J.A.W. (2009). Failed spinal anaesthesia: mechanisms, management and prevention. *British Journal of Anaesthesia* 102: 739–748. *(This review, based on humans, reminds us that intrathecal/true spinal blocks can also sometimes fail.).*

Ferreira, J.P. (2018). Epidural anaesthesia-analgesia in the dog and cat: considerations, technique and complications. *Companion Animal* 23: 628–636.

Ganesh, A. and Maxwell, L.G. (2007). Pathophysiology and management of opioid-induced pruritus. *Drugs* 67: 2323–2333.

Garcia-Pereira, F. (2018). Epidural anaesthesia and analgesia in small animal practice: an update. *The Veterinary Journal* 242: 24–32.

Gatson, B.J., Garcia-Pereira, F.L., James, M., Carrera-Justiz, S., Lewis, D.D. (2016). Use of a perfusion index to confirm the presence of sciatic nerve blockade in dogs. *Veterinary Anaesthesia and Analgesia* 43: 662–669.

Grocott, H.P. and Mutch, W.A.C. (1996). Epidural anesthesia and acutely increased intracranial pressure. *Anesthesiology* 85: 1086–1091.

Gurney, M.A. and Leece, E.A. (2014). Analgesia for pelvic limb surgery. A review of peripheral nerve blocks and the extradural technique. *Veterinary Anaesthesia and Analgesia* 41: 445–458.

Heavner, J.E., Rosenberg, P.H., Kytta, J., and Hassio, J. (1987). Multiple mechanisms involved in intravenous regional anesthesia. *Veterinary Surgery* 16: 321.

Iff, I., Larenza, M.P., and Moens, Y.P.S. (2009). The extradural pressure profile in goats following extradural injection. *Veterinary Anaesthesia and Analgesia* 36: 180–185.

Iff, I., Valeskini, K., and Mosing, M. (2012). Severe pruritus and myoclonus following intrathecal morphine administration in a dog. *Canadian Veterinary Journal* 53: 983–986.

Jones, R.S. (2001). Epidural analgesia in the dog and cat. *The Veterinary Journal* 161: 123–131.

Keates, H.L., Cramond, T., and Smith, M.T. (1999). Intraarticular and periarticular opioid binding in inflamed tissue in experimental canine arthritis. *Anesthesia and Analgesia* 89: 409–415.

Khan, Z., Munro, E., Shaw, D., and Faller, K.M.E. (2019). Variation in the position of the conus medullaris and the dural sac in adult dogs. *Veterinary Record* 185: 20. https://doi.org/10.1136/vr.105279.

Leung, J.B.Y., Rodrigo-Mocholi, D., and Martinez-Taboada, F. (2019). In-plane and out-of-plane needle insertion comparison for a novel lateral block of the radial, ulnar, median and musculocutaneous nerves in cats. *Veterinary Anaesthesia and Analgesia* 46: 523–528.

Lillie, P.E., Glynn, C.J., and Fenwick, D.G. (1984). Site of action of intravenous regional anesthesia. *Anesthesiology* 61: 507–510.

Low, J., Johnston, N., and Morris, C. (2008). Epidural analgesia: first do no harm. *Anaesthesia* 63: 1–3. *(Discusses the pros and cons of epidural anaesthesia with respect to the stress response and outcome after, in particular, abdominal [gastrointestinal tract] surgery.).*

Mahler, S.P. and Adogwa, A.O. (2008). Anatomical and experimental studies of brachial plexus, sciatic and femoral nerve-location using peripheral nerve stimulation in the dog. *Veterinary Anaesthesia and Analgesia* 35: 80–89.

Marhofer, D., Karmakar, M.K., Marhofer, P. et al. (2014). Does circumferential spread of local anaesthetic improve the success of peripheral nerve block? *British Journal of Anaesthesia* 113: 177–185.

O'Hearn, A. and Wright, B.D. (2011). Coccygeal epidural with local anesthetic for catheterization and pain management in the treatment of feline urethral obstruction. *Journal of Veterinary Emergency and Critical Care* 21: 50–52.

Otero, P.E. and Portela, D.A. (2019). *Small Animal Regional Anesthesia*, 2e. Buenos Aires: 5m Publishing.

Otero, P., Tarragona, L., Ceballos, M., and Portela, D. (2009). Epidural cephalic spread of a local anesthetic in dogs: a mathematical model using the column length. Proceedings of the 10th World Congress of Veterinary Anaesthesia Glasgow, Scotland, pp. 125. *(See also Figure 14.29 in: Small Animal Regional Anesthesia and Analgesia (2013) Eds: Campoy L, Read M. Wiley-Blackwell.)*

Otero, P.E., Verdier, N., Ceballos, M.R. et al. (2014). The use of electrical stimulation to guide epidural and intrathecal needle advancement at the L5-L6 intervertebral space in dogs. *Veterinary Anaesthesia and Analgesia* 41: 543–547.

Otero, P.E., Verdier, N., Zaccagnini, A.S. et al. (2016). Sonographic evaluation of epidural and intrathecal injections in cats. *Veterinary Anaesthesia and Analgesia* 43: 652–661.

Ranger, M.R.B., Irwin, G.J., Bunbury, K.M., and Peutrell, J.M. (2008). Changing body position alters the location of the spinal cord within the vertebral canal: a magnetic resonance imaging study. *British Journal of Anaesthesia* 101: 804–809.

Romano, M., Portela, D.A., Breghi, G., and Otero, P.E. (2016). Stress-related biomarkers in dogs administered regional anaesthesia or fentanyl for analgesia during stifle surgery. *Veterinary Anaesthesia and Analgesia* 43: 44–54.

Salinas, F.V. (2003). Location, location, location: continuous peripheral nerve blocks and stimulating catheters. *Regional Anesthesia and Pain Medicine* 28: 79–82.

Son, W.G., Jang, M., Yoon, J. et al. (2014). The effect of epidural injection speed on epidural pressure and distribution of solution in anesthetized dogs. *Veterinary Anaesthesia and Analgesia* 41: 526–533.

Szarvas, S., Harmon, D., and Murphy, D. (2003). Neuraxial opioid-induced pruritus: a review. *Journal of Clinical Anaesthesia* 15: 234–239.

Szucs, S., Morau, D., Sultan, S.F. et al. (2014). A comparison of three techniques (local anesthetic deposited circumferential to vs. above vs. below the nerve) for ultrasound guided femoral nerve block. *BMC Anesthesiology* 14: 6. https://doi.org/10.1186/1471-2253-14-6, https://bmcanesthesiol.biomedcentral.com/articles/10.1186/1471-2253-14-6.

Steagall, P.V.M., Simon, B.T., Teixeira Neto, F., and Luna, S.P.L. (2017). An update on drugs used for lumbosacral epidural anesthesia and analgesia in dogs. *Frontiers in Veterinary Science* 4: 68.

Tsui, B.C., Wagner, A., and Finucane, B. (2004). Electrophysiologic effect of injectates on peripheral nerve stimulation. *Regional Anesthesia and Pain Medicine* 29: 189–193. *(Explains the Raj test.)*.

Tucker, G.T. and Boas, R.A. (1971). Pharmacokinetic aspects of intravenous regional anesthesia. *Anesthesiology* 34: 538–549.

Tuominen, M. (1996). Spinal needle tip design – does it make any difference? *Current Opinion in Anaesthesiology* 9: 395–398.

Vesovski, S., Makara, M., and Martinez-Taboada, F. (2019). Computer tomographic comparison of cranial spread of contrast in lumbosacral and sacrococcygeal epidural injections in dog cadavers. *Veterinary Anaesthesia and Analgesia* 46: 510–515. *(Useful graph outlining cranial spread according to volume injected; similar to Otero et al. 2009.).*

Vettorato, E., Bradbrook, C., Gurney, M. et al. (2012). Peripheral nerve blocks of the pelvic limb in dogs: a retrospective clinical study. *Veterinary and Comparative Orthopaedics and Traumatology* 25: 314–320.

Viscasillas, J., Sanchis-Mora, S., Hoy, C., and Alibhai, H. (2012). Transient Horner's syndrome after paravertebral brachial plexus block in a dog. *Veterinary Anaesthesia and Analgesia* 40: 104–106.

Webb, S.T. and Ghosh, S. (2009). Intra-articular bupivacaine: potentially chondrotoxic? *British Journal of Anaesthesia* 102: 439–441.

Self-test Section

1 What motor responses are seen with nerve stimulation of the radial nerve?
   A Carpal extension and digit flexion
   B Carpal extension and digit extension
   C Carpal flexion and digit flexion
   D Carpal flexion and digit extension

2 What is Gutierrez's sign?
   A Increased rate and depth of breathing during epidural injection
   B Reduced or absent patellar tendon reflex (knee-jerk) after epidural with local anaesthetic
   C Hanging drop technique as used to define entry of the needle tip into the epidural space

15

Miscellaneous Local Anaesthetic Techniques

Small Animals

LEARNING OBJECTIVES

- To be familiar with local anaesthetic techniques for the chest and abdomen.

15.1 Truncal Blocks

15.1.1 Intercostal Nerve Block

15.1.1.1 Indications
- Thoracotomy
- Rib fractures and flail chest
- Chest drainage

See also Chapter 48 on respiratory emergencies.

15.1.1.2 Site
A neurovascular bundle is associated with the caudal border of each rib (Figure 15.1) and lies deep to the external and internal intercostal muscles. Once the intercostal nerve leaves the intervertebral foramen, it runs parallel to the rib giving off cutaneous branches.

There is much **overlap of the segmental innervation** of the chest wall, so that **at least two, and preferably three, 'segments' cranial and caudal to, and including the intercostal site where anaesthesia is needed, should be blocked.** For example, for insertion of a chest drain, the tube should enter the thoracic cavity at about intercostal space 7 or 8. Thus intercostal nerve blocks should be performed for intercostal nerves 5–9 or 6–10. For lateral thoracotomy, the surgical incision is usually made at about intercostal space 4, so that intercostal nerves 2, 3, 4, 5, and 6 should be blocked.

15.1.1.3 Technique
Needle: 23–25 g, 5/8–1″. Doses: Lidocaine 1–2% (± epinephrine); 3 mg/kg (plain) to 7 mg/kg (with epinephrine) for dogs; nearer 2 mg/kg (plain) to 4 mg/kg (with epinephrine) for cats; or bupivacaine 0.25–0.5%, 1 mg/kg for dogs and cats. Lidocaine anaesthesia only lasts one to two hours, whereas bupivacaine anaesthesia lasts four to eight hours.

A mixture combining lidocaine (≤2 mg/kg) for rapid onset with bupivacaine (≤1 mg/kg) for prolonged duration of effect can be used, but mixing of local anaesthetics does not necessarily produce these clinical benefits. Beware total doses of local anaesthetics used, especially if planning to perform other blocks too, e.g. an interpleural block. As a guide, about 0.25–1 ml of local anaesthetic solution is injected at each site, depending upon the animal's size.

Aiming perpendicularly to the body wall, the needle is slid off the caudal border of the rib, and proximally, as near to the intervertebral foramen as possible (i.e. as proximally along the intercostal nerve as possible, so as to block most of its cutaneous, muscular and pleural branches). Aspiration before injection reduces the risk of inadvertent intravascular injection.

The nerve blocks can be performed during surgery (commonplace during thoracotomies) as the nerves are easily visualised just beneath the parietal pleura by the surgeon. Better pre-emptive analgesia is, however, provided by performing the nerve blocks before the surgical incision is made.

Analgesia is usually excellent and is provided without respiratory depression. In conjunction with high dose extradural morphine (0.2 mg/kg), excellent analgesia is produced for thoracotomies, especially sternal splits, without respiratory depression; see Chapter 14. Bupivacaine has been reported to provide up to 16 hours analgesia in this context.

Veterinary Anaesthesia: Principles to Practice, Second Edition. Alexandra H. A. Dugdale, Georgina Beaumont, Carl Bradbrook, and Matthew Gurney.
© 2020 John Wiley & Sons Ltd. Published 2020 by John Wiley & Sons Ltd.
Companion website: www.wiley.com/go/dugdale/veterinary-anaesthesia

cranial   caudal

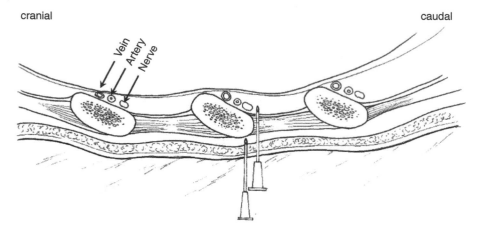

Figure 15.1 The intercostal nerves are closely associated with the caudal borders of the ribs.

15.1.1.4 Potential Complications

Complications are usually associated with poor technique and include:

- Pneumothorax
- Haemothorax
- Lung damage

15.1.2 Interpleural (Intrapleural or Pleural) 'block'

15.1.2.1 Indications

- Analgesia following thoracotomy
- Analgesia for thoracostomy tube: during in-dwelling, peri-drainage, pre-removal
- Analgesia for rib fractures or chest wall trauma
- Analgesia for neoplastic conditions of the chest wall, pleura or mediastinum
- Analgesia for painful abdominal (especially cranial abdominal) conditions (e.g. pancreatitis, cholecystectomy, renal surgery)

Some clinicians prefer repeating intercostal blocks in conscious patients in preference to repeating pleural instillation of local anaesthetics. Transient stinging accompanies the injection of local anaesthetics, although it can be reduced a little by adding sodium bicarbonate and warming the solution (see below and Chapter 12).

To 1 ml bupivacaine 0.5%, add 0.01 ml of 8.4% sodium bicarbonate

To 1 ml lidocaine 2%, add 0.1 ml of 8.4% sodium bicarbonate

15.1.2.2 Mechanisms

Exactly how instillation of local anaesthetic solutions into the pleural 'space' produces such widespread analgesia is not fully understood. It is thought that there is diffusion of

local anaesthetic through the parietal pleura (and possibly through the diaphragm) to effectively produce multiple thoracic intercostal (and cranial lumbar paravertebral) blocks with desensitisation of the thoracic (and cranial lumbar) sympathetic chain and the splanchnic (sympathetic) nerves. There could also be rapid systemic absorption from the huge 'surface area' of the pleura with a resultant analgesic effect similar to that following intravenous administration.

15.1.2.3 Technique

Local anaesthetic solution can be instilled through an in-dwelling chest drain. Otherwise, a catheter or chest tube may be placed into the pleural space either percutaneously, or under direct view (e.g. before closure of a thoracotomy incision). If drainage of viscous material (e.g. purulent fluid) from the pleural space is not required, then small gauge catheters that utilise the Seldinger technique (and which are otherwise more suited to drainage of air from the chest) can be used for instillation of local anaesthetic into the pleural space.

15.1.2.4 Dose of Local Anaesthetic

If local anaesthetic has already been used, e.g. if an intercostal nerve block has already been performed, keep in mind the total doses. Lidocaine is commonly used topically in cats to desensitise the larynx for tracheal intubation. If this was done within the previous hour, that lidocaine is still 'on board', so calculate doses accordingly.

Bupivacaine is favoured for its longer duration of action. The toxic dose is said to be ≥2 mg/kg, so that 1 (−2) mg/kg is a commonly chosen dose. If using more than one type of local anaesthetic, be aware of cumulative toxicities. Bupivacaine 1 mg/kg q 6–8 hours is a commonly used dose.

Depending upon the patient's size, between 1 and about 10 ml of total volume can be instilled. Stock local anaesthetic solutions can be diluted with sterile saline. Some operators will gently roll the animal onto the side that requires most analgesia for several minutes after instillation of the local anaesthetic.

15.1.2.5 Potential Complications

- Interpleural catheter-related complications (see chest drain complications in Chapter 48, e.g. pneumothorax, infection, pleural effusion).
- Phrenic nerve block; beware of causing bilateral diaphragmatic paralysis.
- Vagosympathetic trunk 'nerve block'; unwanted autonomic nervous system effects may develop.
- Although there are fears of cardiotoxicity with interpleural local anaesthetics (especially bupivacaine), following pericardectomy, one study reported that after thoracotomy for pericardectomy, when bupivacaine (1.5 mg/kg) and lidocaine (1.5 mg/kg) were injected interpleurally, only a mild detrimental effect on cardiac output was noted with no arrhythmias.

The optimal approach for analgesia for thoracotomy is a combination of systemic opioid and NSAID complemented with extradural morphine, interpleural, and intercostal blocks. The erector spinae plane block may also be a useful addition in future (see below).

15.1.3 Erector Spinae Plane Block

Potentially useful for providing analgesia for thoracic, abdominal, spinal, and possibly also neck and pelvic pain/ procedures. Preliminary canine cadaver studies using ultrasound guidance show some promise, but optimal doses and injection volumes remain to be determined.

15.1.4 Transverse Abdominus Plane (TAP) Block

The TAP block has been described in cadavers and clinical cases. The lateral abdominal wall consists of three muscle layers: the external abdominal oblique, internal abdominal oblique, and transversus abdominis. This technique, performed bilaterally, can provide analgesia for a midline celiotomy incision and aims to block the ventral branches of segmental nerves Th9-Lu3 within the TAP between the internal abdominal oblique and transversus abdominis muscles. Distribution of local anaesthetic needs to be extensive to cover all nerves and a subcostal and midabdominal approach have been described. With ultrasound guidance, the local anaesthetic solution can be seen spreading along the plane between the muscle layers, this being known as hydrodissection. A relatively large volume is required and no one technique, with respect to injection

site/s and injectate volume, has yet gained overall popularity. That said, several options have been reported:

- Subcostal approach: the US transducer is positioned parallel to the costal arch. Bupivacaine 0.5%, 2 mg/kg is diluted fourfold to 0.125% with saline, and hydrodissection is observed during injection of the solution to ensure block of a more extensive area.
- A two-site technique with both a subcostal and midabdominal approach using 0.3 ml/kg bupivacaine 0.25% per site.
- One study using 1 mg/kg bupivacaine 0.5% diluted in 2% lidocaine to a volume of 1.5 ml per site in cats (resulting in total doses of 2 mg/kg bupivacaine and 4–12 mg/kg lidocaine for animals between 3 and 5 kg) demonstrated low pain scores and low analgesic requirements post-ovariectomy. Even at such large doses, no local anaesthetic toxicity was reported, possibly because of the slow systemic absorption from the fascial plane.

The TAP block only offers analgesia to the muscle layers and parietal peritoneum, and newer techniques aim to offer some visceral analgesia in addition.

15.1.4.1 Potential Complications

- Peritoneal deposition of local anaesthetic
- Block failure (especially at the ventral midline such that a rectus sheath block [see chapter 33] may be complementary)

15.1.5 Quadratus Lumborum Block

Segmental nerves Th12-Lu3 run in the sub-lumbar area between the quadratus lumborum and the psoas muscles, and, along with the sympathetic nerves that join the ventral branches, innervate the abdominal wall and viscera. The quadratus lumborum block is reported to provide both somatic and visceral analgesia (and has been suggested to provide an indirect paravertebral block, or 'paravertebral by proxy'). It is an ultrasound-guided approach at the level of Lu1/Lu2. Early reports suggest effective anaesthesia post-ovariohysterectomy in dogs and further studies are underway.

15.1.6 Incisional Block

Infiltration of local anaesthetic subcutaneously along the proposed line of incision (Figure 15.2) affords anaesthesia pre- and post-incision. For a mid-line celiotomy, lidocaine 4 mg/kg can be infiltrated five minutes prior to incision. At the end of the procedure, bupivacaine can be infiltrated to provide a longer duration of anaesthesia. (To further extend bupivacaine's duration of action, the liposome encapsulated formulation can be used, but this product should not

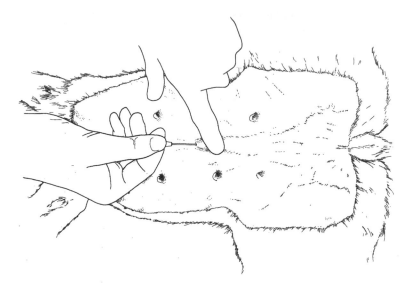

Figure 15.2 Incisional block; an initial injection of local anaesthetic enables subsequent injections (along the line of proposed incision) to be made into already desensitised tissues.

be used concurrently with other amide local anaesthetics due to the risk of cumulative toxicity.) Interestingly, one study reported no additional advantage of incisional bupivacaine in addition to intraperitoneal bupivacaine for post-operative analgesia in dogs undergoing ovariohysterectomy under general anaesthesia (acepromazine and morphine for premedication, propofol for anaesthetic induction, and isoflurane for anaesthetic maintenance; carprofen was administered SC just after endotracheal intubation).

15.1.7 Intraperitoneal 'block'

Instillation of local anaesthetic solution into the peritoneal cavity can form part of a multi-modal analgesic approach for abdominal surgery/painful conditions. Doses/volumes are not yet clearly defined and care must be taken not to exceed toxic doses (beware if multiple local/regional techniques are performed), but, for bupivacaine (longer-acting agents are usually preferred), are in the order of 2 (−4) mg/kg for dogs and 1 (−2) mg/kg for cats.

15.1.8 Other Techniques

Techniques affording useful analgesia for abdominal and chest surgery/pain include epidural (extradural) and intrathecal techniques (see Chapter 14). Anaesthesia of the perineum can be achieved by epidural techniques, but there has also been recent interest in bilateral ultrasound-guided pudendal nerve blocks for cats undergoing perineal urethrostomy (see Further Reading). Large surgical and clean traumatic wounds may lend themselves to the use of wound soaker catheters for intermittent or continuous delivery of local anaesthetic (see Chapter 13).

15.2 Anaesthesia for Castration or Spay

Intratesticular lidocaine has been shown to reduce isoflurane requirements during castration (0.5–1.0 ml per testicle), although had no effect on post-operative pain scores. In addition to intratesticular deposition, local anaesthetic can also be infused around the spermatic cord as well as at the site of incision. A recent knowledge summary in cats has highlighted that the benefit of intratesticular lidocaine only becomes apparent when full mμ agonist opioids are not included in the anaesthetic technique. The literature is confusing in dogs: one study showed a benefit of intratesticular lidocaine (premedication included morphine) for intra-operative antinociception, whereas another showed no benefit of intratesticular lidocaine/bupivacaine (premedication included morphine) on post-operative pain. Whilst sacro-coccygeal epidural lidocaine or intratesticular lidocaine in cats provided similar intra-operative antinociception to systemic methadone, the post-operative analgesia was, not surprisingly, of shorter duration with both local anaesthetic techniques.

For ovariectomy or ovariohysterectomy, mesovarian (ovarian pedicle) injection of local anaesthetic appears to provide no advantage over an anaesthetic protocol which includes a pure mμ agonist opioid, at least in dogs. Intraperitoneal local anaesthetic, possibly combined with incisional block, may, however, help provide post-operative analgesia.

15.3 Pancreatitis

Analgesia for these cases can present quite a challenge, not the least because many of these animals have other co-existent diseases. NSAIDs can be a worry with respect to gastrointestinal tract ulceration. Corticosteroids may be contra-indicated, as, in addition to gastrointestinal side effects, they have been known to promote the development of pancreatitis. Opioids, such as morphine, have often been considered contra-indicated, because morphine may cause vomiting (usually only after the first dose though), and there has been the worry that full mu receptor agonist opioids may encourage constriction of the bile duct and pancreatic duct sphincters (although this is less of a problem for dogs than for cats and humans as dogs do not have a true sphincter of Oddi). Although pethidine is useful (it is spasmolytic for these sphincters), it is short acting and painful on intramuscular injection, so that the patient will soon become averse to repeated injections. Buprenorphine or butorphanol may be less of a problem than morphine for these sphincters, but the analgesia they afford is of a lesser quality. Therefore, continuous infusions of opioids such as methadone or fentanyl are often the mainstay of analgesia with these cases.

Additional strategies include:

- Extradural morphine: reduces systemic side effects, and therefore reduces sphincter problems
- Interpleural local anaesthetic administration
- Combined interpleural and intraperitoneal local anaesthetic administration (or consider other truncal blocks)
- Continuous intravenous lidocaine infusion
- Occasional boluses or continuous intravenous infusion of ketamine

Further Reading

Adami, C., Angeli, G., Haenssgen, K. et al. (2013). Development of an ultrasound-guided technique for pudendal nerve block in cat cadavers. *Journal of Feline Medicine and Surgery* 15: 901–907.

Adami, C., Daver, T., Spadavecchia, C., and Angeli, G. (2014). Ultrasound-guided pudendal nerve block in cats undergoing perineal urethrostomy: a prospective, randomized, investigator-blind, placebo-controlled clinical trial. *Journal of Feline Medicine and Surgery* 16: 340–345.

Bernard, F., Kudnig, S.T., and Monnet, E.M. (2006). Hemodynamic effects of interpleural lidocaine and bupivacaine combination in anesthetized dogs with and without an open pericardium. *Veterinary Surgery* 35: 252–258.

Best, C.A., Best, A.A., Best, T.J., and Hamilton, D.A. (2015). Buffered lidocaine and bupivacaine mixture – the ideal local anesthetic solution? *Plastic Surgery* 23: 87–90.

Bubalo, V., Moens, Y.P.S., Holzmann, A., and Coppens, P.C. (2008). Anaesthetic sparing effect of local anaesthetic on the ovarian pedicle during ovariohysterectomy in dogs. *Veterinary Anaesthesia and Analgesia* 35: 537–542.

Campoy, L., Read, M.R., and Peralta, S. (2015). Canine and feline local anesthetic and analgesic techniques. In: *Veterinary Anesthesia and Analgesia, the Fifth Edition of Lumb and Jones* (eds. K.A. Grimm, L.A. Lamont, W.J. Tranquilli, et al.), 827–856. Iowa, USA: Wiley Blackwell.

Conzemius, M.G., Brockman, D.J., King, L.G., and Perkowski, S.Z. (1994). Analgesia in dogs after intercostal thoracotomy: a clinical trial comparing intravenous buprenorphine and interpleural bupivacaine. *Veterinary Surgery* 23: 291–298.

Cuvillon, P., Nouvellon, E., Ripart, J. et al. (2009). A comparison of the pharmacodynamics and pharmacokinetics of bupivacaine, ropivacaine (with epinephrine) and their equal volume mixtures with lidocaine used for femoral and sciatic nerve blocks: a double-blinded randomized study. *Anesthesia and Analgesia* 108: 641–649.

Dravid, R.M. and Paul, R.E. (2007). Interpleural block – part 1. *Anaesthesia* 62: 1039–1049.

Drozdynska, M., Monticelli, P., Neilson, D., and Viscasillas, J. (2017). Ultrasound-guided subcostal oblique transversus abdominis plane block in canine cadavers. *Veterinary Anaesthesia and Analgesia* 44: 183–186.

Fausak, E., Rodriguez, E., Simle, A. et al. (2018). Does the use of intratesticular blocks in cats undergoing orchiectomies serve as an effective adjunctive analgesic? *Veterinary Evidence* 3 (4) http://dx.doi.org/10.18849/ve. v3i4.160.

Fernandez-Parra, R., Zilberstein, L., Fontaine, C., and Adami, C. (2017). Comparison of intratesticular lidocaine, sacrococcygeal epidural lidocaine and intravenous methadone in cats undergoing castration: a prospective, randomized, investigator-blind clinical trial. *Veterinary Anaesthesia and Analgesia* 44: 356–363.

Ferreira, T.H., St James, M., Schroeder, C.A. et al. (2019). Description of an ultrasound-guided erector spinae plane block and the spread of dye in dog cadavers. *Veterinary Anaesthesia and Analgesia* 46: 516–522.

Huuskonen, V., Hughes, L.J.M., Banon, E.E., and West, W. (2013). Intratesticular lidocaine reduces the response to surgical castration in dogs. *Veterinary Anaesthesia and Analgesia* 40: 74–82.

Kalchofner Guerrero, K.S., Campagna, I., Bruhl-Day, R. et al. (2016). Intraperitoneal bupivacaine with or without incisional bupivacaine for postoperative analgesia in dogs undergoing ovariohysterectomy. *Veterinary Anaesthesia and Analgesia* 43: 571–578.

McKenzie, A.G. and Mathe, S. (1993). Interpleural local anaesthesia: anatomical basis for mechanism of action. *British Journal of Anaesthesia* 76: 297–299.

Portela, D.A., Verdier, N., and Otero, P.E. (2018). Regional anesthetic techniques for the pelvic limb and abdominal wall in small animals: a review of the literature and technique description. *The Veterinary Journal* 238: 27–40.

Portela, D.A., Verdier, N., and Otero, P.E. (2018). Regional anesthetic techniques for the thoracic limb and thorax in small animals: a review of the literature and technique description. *The Veterinary Journal* 241: 8–19.

Ribotsky, B.M., Berkowitz, K.D., and Montague, J.R. (1996). Local anesthetics: is there an advantage to mixing solutions? *Journal of the American Podiatric Association* 87: 487–491.

Skouropoulou, D., Lacitignola, L., Centonze, P. et al. (2018). Perioperative analgesic effects of an ultrasound-guided transversus abdominis plane block with a mixture of bupivacaine and lidocaine in cats undergoing ovariectomy. *Veterinary Anaesthesia and Analgesia* 45: 374–383.

Steagall, P.V.M., Benito, J., Monteiro, B., Lascelles, D., Kronen, P.W., Murrell, J.C., Robertson, S., Wright, B., and Yamashita, K. (2020). Intraperitoneal and incisional analgesia in small animals: simple, cost-effective techniques. *Journal of Small Animal Practice* 61: 19–23.

Stevens, B.J., Posner, L.P., Jones, C.A., and Lascelles, B.D. (2013). Comparison of the effect of intratesticular lidocaine/bupivacaine vs. saline placebo on pain scores and incision site reactions in dogs undergoing routine castration. *The Veterinary Journal* 196: 499–503.

Self-test Section

1 For an intercostal block, how many 'segments' cranial and caudal to the site of 'injury' should be blocked.

2 Between which abdominal muscles is the transversus abdominis plane located?

3 Describe a multimodal analgesia approach for management of a dog with flail chest.

16

Local Anaesthetic Techniques

Horses

LEARNING OBJECTIVES

- To be familiar with local/regional anaesthetic techniques for the horse's head.
- To appreciate which nerves supply motor and sensory innervation to the head.
- To be familiar with the technique of epidural (extradural) anaesthesia.

16.1 Equine Limb Nerve Blocks

Concerning limb analgesia, similar techniques to those in small animals, or indeed cattle, can be applied to horses. However, the most common reason for requiring limb analgesia is for lameness evaluation. A recent review of the evidence suggests that, should sedation be required, the shortest acting α2 agonist (xylazine) *may* be used, but, because of its analgesic actions, care should be exercised when interpreting subtle changes, particularly in mild forelimb lameness, in these sedated (and analgesed) animals. The reader is referred to orthopaedic texts for specific diagnostic equine limb perineural blocks. Table 16.1 compares the commonly available local anaesthetics.

For evaluation of lameness, diagnostic nerve blocks are initially performed distally in the limb before progressing to more proximal blocks, and a medium-acting local anaesthetic drug is chosen, commonly **mepivacaine** (Carbocaine™, Intra-Epicaine™). If mepivacaine is not available, then often the next favoured choice is **prilocaine**, another amide-linked local anaesthetic that also causes minimal effect on vasomotor tone and minimal weal formation at injection sites.

The long duration of action of bupivacaine renders it less suitable for diagnostic nerve blocks, but often more suitable for peri-operative analgesia of the distal limb. More proximal limb nerve blockade, however, can compromise recovery quality because the patient effectively has a 'dead leg'.

Intra-articular analgesia with local anaesthetic agents and/or opioids can be performed in standing or anaesthetised horses. Ropivacaine is the least chondrotoxic of the agents.

16.2 Head Blocks

These can provide local/regional anaesthesia of the eyes and periocular structures, the teeth and associated tissues, the paranasal sinuses, and soft tissue and bony structures of the head, including the ears. All these techniques can be used to provide part of a balanced anaesthetic and analgesic technique in horses undergoing standing surgery (with sedation – see Chapters 28 and 31), or surgery under general anaesthesia. Figure 16.1 shows useful anatomical landmarks and positions of the various nerve foramina. Appropriate aseptic preparation of injection sites should always be performed.

16.2.1 Infraorbital Nerve Block

After exiting the cranial vault at the round foramen (within the pterygopalatine fossa), the maxillary nerve gives rise to the zygomatic and pterygopalatine nerves before entering the infraorbital canal at the maxillary foramen. Just before entering, and within the infraorbital canal, caudal, middle, and cranial superior alveolar (dental) nerve branches arise

Veterinary Anaesthesia: Principles to Practice, Second Edition. Alexandra H. A. Dugdale, Georgina Beaumont, Carl Bradbrook, and Matthew Gurney.
© 2020 John Wiley & Sons Ltd. Published 2020 by John Wiley & Sons Ltd.
Companion website: www.wiley.com/go/dugdale/veterinary-anaesthesia

Table 16.1 Comparison of commonly available local anaesthetic drugs for diagnostic nerve blocks.

	Lidocaine	Prilocaine	Mepivacaine	Ropivacaine	Bupivacaine
Onset (min)	5–10 min	10–15 min	**10–15 min**	10–20 min	15–20 min
Duration (h)	1 h without epinephrine; 2 h with epinephrine	1–2 h without epinephrine; 1–2.5 h with epinephrine	**c. 2 h**	3–5 (+) h	4–8 (+) h
Vasomotor effects	Causes local vasodilation resulting in weals at injection sites (often interpreted as 'tissue reaction' because areas where local anaesthetic is injected often look swollen), therefore not first choice	Little overall effect; little local weal formation, so can be used for limb nerve blocks without causing transient unsightly swellings. Might need to be more accurate with placement of blocks, because poorer tissue penetration than lidocaine, hence usually second choice to mepivacaine	No overall effect on vascular tone; little local swelling/weal formation, so tends to be the preferred agent for limb nerve blocks	Marketed as the S-enantiomer alone which produces little overall effect on vascular tone, perhaps mild vasoconstriction	The racemic mixture produces little overall effect on vascular tone
Maximum recommended dose	2–3 mg/kg (without epinephrine) (4–7 mg/kg with epinephrine)	2–4 mg/kg (without epinephrine) 4–8 mg/kg (with epineprhine)	2–3 mg/kg	1–3 mg/kg	1–2 mg/kg
% solution available	1 and 2% with or without epinephrine	1, 2, 4% with or without epinephrine	2%	0.2, 0.5, 0.75, 1%	0.25, 0.5 and 0.75%
Relative doses (volumes) for injection	1 ml of 2%	1 ml of 4%	1 ml of 2%	1 ml of 0.75%	1 ml of 0.5%

from the infraorbital nerve. The infraorbital nerve leaves the infraorbital canal at the infraorbital foramen.

16.2.1.1 Sites of Block

1) Where infraorbital nerve emerges from infraorbital foramen (Figure 16.1).
2) Within infraorbital canal.

16.2.1.2 Structures Desensitised

1) The upper lip, the nostril, the roof of the nasal cavity, and the skin of the face rostroventral to the foramen, ispilaterally.
2) As above, plus the incisors, the canine, and possibly the first one to two cheek teeth (with their associated gum and bone), and some more skin towards the medial canthus of the eye.

16.2.1.3 Technique

The infraorbital foramen lies about halfway along, and slightly dorsal to, a line between the rostral end of the facial crest and the naso-incisive notch; and it is partly covered by the thin strap-like levator nasolabialis superioris muscle, which, if reflected upwards a little, facilitates palpation of the bony rim of the foramen. Using the thumb and first two fingers can help locate the foramen by forming a shallow triangle: with the thumb on the rostral end of the facial crest and the middle finger at the nasoincisive notch (to form the base of the triangle), the index finger tip locates the foramen at the apex of a very shallow triangle.

The dental (alveolar) nerves supplying the ipsilateral incisors, canine, and first few cheek teeth arise from the

infraorbital nerve within the infraorbital canal. In order to block these, local anaesthetic must be infiltrated about 2–4 cm retrogradely into the canal. Holding digital pressure at the infraorbital foramen both during, and for several (up to 60) seconds after injection, may assist retrograde spread, and retention of the injectate within the canal.

Once the foramen is located and after clipping and aseptic preparation of the skin, a 20–23 g needle can be inserted, either with its tip at the opening of the foramen for the first technique or advanced carefully into the canal by about 2–4 cm for the second technique. The latter can be quite painful, so the horse will usually require sedation. Furthermore, a small bleb of local anaesthetic can be injected subcutaneously prior to needle placement to reduce the chance of the horse suddenly reacting. Aspirate to avoid inadvertent intravascular injection before injection of about 5 ml of local anaesthetic. Excessive injection pressure should be avoided, especially for the intracanal technique as it may signal intraneural injection or even needle tip placement into the bony wall of the infraorbital canal.

16.2.2 Maxillary Nerve Block

16.2.2.1 Site of Block

The site of maxillary nerve blockade is within the pterygopalatine fossa, between where the pterygopalatine nerve branches off the maxillary nerve and where the maxillary nerve enters the infraorbital canal through the maxillary foramen. The block can be performed in the sedated or anaesthetised patient.

16.2.2.2 Structures Desensitised

All the ipsilateral teeth, most of the paranasal sinuses and nasal cavity in addition to: the upper lip, the nostril, and the skin of the face, as for the infraorbital nerve block within the infraorbital canal. The dorsal nasal concha, caudal nasal septum, and rostral part of the frontal sinus, however, receive sensory innervation from the ethmoidal nerve, which is a branch of the nasociliary nerve, which is itself a branch of the ophthalmic division of the trigeminal nerve. Local anaesthetic spread in the pterygopalatine fossa may be insufficient to block the ophthalmic division of the trigeminal nerve and an ethmoidal nerve block may be required.

16.2.2.3 Technique

The pterygopalatine fossa can be accessed from laterally, by variations of a sub-zygomatic approach, or retrogradely (through the infraorbital canal), or from dorsally (via the supraorbital fossa). For all approaches, sedation may be required in the standing animal, and placing a bleb of subcutaneous local anaesthetic at the proposed site of needle insertion, prior to performance of the actual block, will

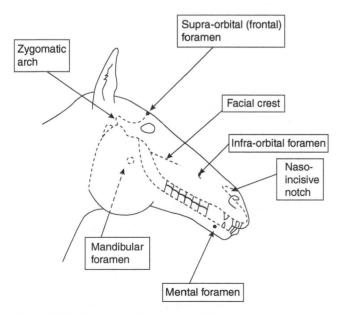

Figure 16.1 Anatomical landmarks of the horse head.

reduce patient reaction. Sufficient time (also dependent upon which local anaesthetic agent is used) should be allowed for the block to take effect. Complications include haematoma formation, exophthalmos, bulging of the supraorbital fossa, transient blindness, and, more rarely, intravascular injection that might result in high concentrations of local anaesthetic entering the cavernous sinus causing, usually transient, signs of central nervous system (CNS) toxicity with collapse/seizures.

16.2.2.3.1 Sub-zygomatic, Lateral Approaches

1) The perpendicular approach. A 10 cm long (spinal) needle, 20–23 g is inserted perpendicularly just beneath the zygomatic arch (trying to avoid the transverse facial neurovascular bundle by inserting the needle, usually just above the transverse facial artery, but sometimes, depending upon individual variation, just below it), and slightly caudal to the lateral canthus of the eye, but remaining rostral to the vertical ramus of the mandible. (The site for needle insertion beneath the zygomatic arch can be determined on an imaginary line drawn perpendicular to one along the dorsal contour of the face, and that crosses the lateral canthus.) The needle is advanced perpendicularly, and slightly ventrally, into the pterygopalatine fossa through the masseter muscle and through the extra-periorbital fat body until it contacts the palatine bone (after which the needle should be withdrawn 1–2 mm before injection is attempted). Aspiration is important (to check that a blood vessel has not been inadvertently punctured) before injection of about 10 (−20) ml of local anaesthetic. This injection technique (especially if performed more rostrally, beneath the mid orbital region) is now known to be associated with a high risk of vascular puncture and its complications therefore include haemorrhage, especially from the deep facial vein or maxillary artery, which can result in substantial haematoma formation with exophthalmos and bulging of the supraorbital fossa. The deep facial vein is continuous with the cavernous sinus and inadvertent injection of a large volume of local anaesthetic into this vein can result in almost immediate CNS toxicity and seizures or collapse. The periorbital fascia is dense enough to prevent spread of local anaesthetic into the intra-periorbital compartment (which contains the globe, extra-ocular muscle cone and associated nerves and vasculature), such that the eye and its associated structures should not be affected by the block. A slightly ventral injection angle will also help to avoid penetration of the intra-periorbital compartment. Should the optic nerve be affected, temporary blindness will result; beware with bilateral blocks. The total insertion depth of the needle averaged 6.5–7 cm in one study in mature horses (see below for comparison).

2) The extra-periorbital fat body injection technique is similar to above except the needle is inserted to a lesser depth and therefore the technique is associated with fewer complications. A Tuohy spinal needle is recommended to enable better 'feel' as the needle is advanced. A loss of resistance is said to be felt as the needle pops through the internal fascia of the masseter muscle and into the extra-periorbital fat body, at which point it is advanced a further 2–3 cm so that its tip lies within the extra-periorbital fat body, but should remain sufficiently distant from the palatine bone to avoid close proximity to major blood vessels. Injection of 10 (−20) ml local anaesthetic at this site apparently allows sufficient spread to block the maxillary nerve and its pterygopalatine branch (despite the needle tip usually being further from the nerves than with the above technique), but with a greatly reduced risk of puncturing the deep facial vein or maxillary artery and its branches (deep palatine and infraorbital arteries). The periorbital fascia is dense enough to prevent spread of local anaesthetic into the intra-periorbital compartment (which contains the globe, extra-ocular muscle cone, and associated nerves and vasculature) such that the eye and associated structure should not be affected by the block. A slightly ventral injection angle helps to avoid puncture of the intra-periorbital compartment. The total insertion depth of the needle averaged 4.5–5 cm in one study in mature horses (see above for comparison).

3) The angled, oblique, or caudo-lateral approach. This is another variation of the sub-zygomatic technique that was first described for diagnostic analgesia in headshakers and has also been variously called the posterior ethmoidal nerve block or the caudal nasal nerve block. The posterior ethmoidal nerve, also called the caudal nasal nerve, is a branch of the maxillary nerve just before it enters the maxillary foramen. Therefore, this is really another technique to block the maxillary nerve within the pterygopalatine fossa, including its pterygopalatine branch (or at the very least, the caudal nasal nerve which derives from this) before it enters the infraorbital canal through the maxillary foramen. In this technique, a 9-cm needle (for mature horses) is inserted ventral to the narrowest part of the zygomatic arch (above or below the transverse facial artery), angled obliquely, rostro-medially and ventrally, so the tip is pointed towards the contralateral upper sixth cheek tooth, and inserted until the tip contacts bone or the needle is fully inserted. A minimum of 5 ml of local anaesthetic is injected after aspirating to check that no blood vessels have been inadvertently punctured.

Complications for this approach are similar to the first described technique above.

4) Ultrasound guidance for performance of the maxillary nerve block within the pterygopalatine fossa has been described for both horses and donkeys and can improve accuracy of the block whilst reducing complications, especially when performed using a needle guidance positioning system. Furthermore, a reduced volume of local anaesthetic is often sufficient.

16.2.2.3.2 The Retrograde Approach

The retrograde approach via the infraorbital foramen deposits local anaesthetic into the infraorbital canal to encourage its retrograde spread to the maxillary foramen. This approach avoids the vascular structures within the pterygopalatine fossa and also the intra-orbital, periocular structures, and should, therefore, be associated with fewer complications. Tuohy needles of about 8–10 cm length and 19 g are preferred for mature horses, and with their anti-coring curved tips are potentially minimally traumatic to the nerve, blood vessels, and the walls of the infraorbital canal. The infraorbital canal tends to be elliptical in cross-section (with the long axis of the ellipse in the dorsoventral direction) and somewhat serpentine in shape (although the exact course of the canal may vary with age). Needle placement into the ventral aspect of the infraorbital canal via the ventral part of the infraorbital foramen, followed by gentle advancement, often requiring re-direction/rotation to accommodate any curvature of the canal (especially 4–5 cm into the canal), appears to be most successful. Digital pressure over the infraorbital foramen both during, and for several seconds after injection, may help retain the injectate within the canal and facilitate its retrograde spread. Excessive injection pressure should be avoided, as it may signal intraneural injection or even needle tip placement into the bony wall of the infraorbital canal. Occasionally, the needle tip may penetrate the bony wall of the canal, which may result in epistaxis and failure of the block, but apparently without long-term consequences. Sedation may be necessary. Placing a subcutaneous bleb of local anaesthetic at the site of needle entry, prior to performance of the actual block, also reduces patient reaction. Digitally displacing the levator nasolabialis superioris and the infraorbital nerve 'upwards' helps to locate the needle into the ventral part of the infraorbital foramen and canal. An injection volume of around 10 ml of local anaesthetic has been suggested.

16.2.2.3.3 The Dorsal, Supraorbital Approach

This dorsal approach to the pterygopalatine fossa, via the supraorbital fossa, aims to block the maxillary nerve. A 7–10 cm spinal needle is inserted at the most medial rim of the supraorbital fossa, aiming to pass medially to the cone of extra-ocular muscles and towards the maxillary tuberosity so

that local anaesthetic is deposited into the pterygopalatine fossa near to the maxillary nerve. However, this approach is similar to one described for performing retrobulbar anaesthesia, which makes it unsurprising that retrobulbar block is reported as a 'complication' of this technique. To help reduce the chance of this, should dorsal rotation of the globe be observed during needle placement, then the needle should be withdrawn and re-directed. The ophthalmic nerve may also be blocked by this technique, which may be useful as block of one of its branches, the ethmoidal nerve, improves desensitisation of the paranasal sinuses and nasal structures.

16.2.3 Ethmoidal Nerve Block

The ethmoidal nerve is a branch of the nasociliary nerve that itself derives from the ophthalmic division of the trigeminal nerve. It provides sensation to the dorsal nasal concha, the caudal part of the nasal septum and the rostral part of the frontal sinus. The techniques described above for blocking the maxillary nerve within the pterygopalatine fossa may be sufficient to also block this nerve, but full sino-nasal desensitisation cannot always be guaranteed and a separate ethmoidal nerve block may be required (and although topical local anaesthetic can also be applied to the sino-nasal mucosa, the subsequent desensitisation may not be as effective or long lasting). Recent research has defined the anatomical landmarks for needle positioning to achieve such a block. The injection site is at a palpable notch at the rostromedial aspect of the supraorbital fossa – where the caudal aspect of the zygomatic process of the frontal bone emerges from the frontal bone, caudal and medial to the orbit. The needle is inserted at this site, making an angle of 110° to the sagittal plane and also 110° to the transverse plane. The insertion depth is around 6 cm for a mature horse. Injection (after initial aspiration to reduce the risks of inadvertent intravascular or intrathecal injection) of 5 ml of local anaesthetic is suggested with some local anaesthetic being deposited during withdrawal of the needle. Retrobulbar block is a 'complication' of this technique.

16.2.4 Supraorbital/Frontal Nerve Block

16.2.4.1 Site of Block

The supraorbital nerve is a branch of the ophthalmic division of the trigeminal nerve. It emerges from the supraorbital foramen that lies roughly halfway between the medial and lateral canthi, and about 1 cm 'above' the bony upper rim of the orbit (Figure 16.1).

16.2.4.2 Structures Desensitised

The middle two-thirds of the upper eyelid and the forehead skin. Note that the medial and lateral canthi themselves are not desensitised. Some motor block of levator palpebrae superioris also occurs (i.e. branches of the oculomotor nerve [III] are also blocked). A useful block to perform when inserting subpalpebral lavage systems.

16.2.4.3 Technique

Once the foramen has been located by palpation, a 23–25 g, 5/8″ needle is inserted (through aseptically prepared skin) so as to deposit 1–3 ml local anaesthetic: initially subcutaneously at the entrance to the foramen, and then subsequently ≤1 cm into the foramen. Aspiration is important prior to injection to check the needle has not penetrated the frontal artery or vein. The use of longer needles risks popping through into the orbit and possibly damaging the eyeball. In flighty horses, attaching the needle to an extension set (with integral Luer-lock for security), and then to the syringe, enables distant injection and reduces the chance of operator injury should the patient suddenly move its head.

16.2.5 Infratrochlear, Zygomatic, and Lacrimal Nerve Blocks

These nerve branches supply sensation to the rest of the periorbital region:

- **Infratrochlear nerve** is a branch of the ophthalmic division of the trigeminal nerve. It supplies sensation to the medial canthus, nictitans, lacrimal duct region, medial parts of upper and lower eyelids, and a small sector of facial skin 'fanning out' from the medial canthus.
- **Lacrimal nerve** is also a branch of the ophthalmic division of the trigeminal nerve. It supplies sensation to the lateral canthus, the lateral quarter of the upper eyelid, and a tiny segment of skin between the lateral canthus and the base of the ear.
- **Zygomatic (zygomaticofacial) nerve** is a branch of the maxillary division of the trigeminal nerve. It supplies sensation to the middle-lateral two-thirds of the lower eyelid and a small sector of skin 'fanning out' from the ventral eyelid margin.

16.2.5.1 Sites for Blocks

All of these nerves can be blocked as they cross the orbital rim, but their exact location can be tricky to find. The infratrochlear nerve can be blocked at the tiny bony notch located just dorso-lateral to the medial canthus on the upper orbital rim. The lacrimal nerve is blocked just dorso-medial to the lateral canthus on the upper orbital rim. The zygomatic nerve is blocked medial to the lateral canthus along the lower orbital rim; its position is sometimes described as being almost at the mid-point of the ventral

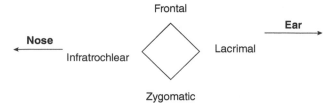

Figure 16.2 Representation of location of peri-orbital nerves.

orbital rim. The peri-orbital nerves can be thought of as forming four points of a diamond (Figure 16.2).

If unsure of the location of these nerves, local anaesthetic can be infiltrated all the way around the orbital rim. The suggested dose is 0.5–1 ml of local anaesthetic per 1 cm of skin or tissue to be desensitised. The combination of all four blocks is called a **diamond block.**

16.2.6 Mental Nerve Block

16.2.6.1 Sites of Block

1) Where the mental nerve emerges from the mental foramen (Figure 16.1).
2) Within the mandibular canal.

16.2.6.2 Structures Desensitised

1) The lower lip rostral to the foramen, ipsilaterally.
2) As above, plus incisors, canine, and possibly the first one to three cheek teeth and their associated gum and bone.

16.2.6.3 Technique

The mental foramen lies at the level of the caudal third of the interdental space ('bar of the mouth' or diastema), slightly hidden under another strap-like muscle called the depressor labii inferioris, which can be reflected 'upwards' to facilitate palpation of the foramen. The nerves supplying the lower teeth arise from the inferior alveolar nerve within the canal. In order to desensitise the ipsilateral incisors, canine, and possibly first three cheek teeth, local anaesthetic should ideally be deposited up to 2–5 cm retrogradely into the canal from the mental foramen. The mental foramen can be approached percutaneously (extra-orally), or transmucosally (intra-orally). It is located ventral to the commissure of the lips.

Horses may require sedation. Placing a subcutaneous bleb of local anaesthetic at the proposed needle insertion site may also reduce patient reaction during subsequent performance of the block.

16.2.6.3.1 Percutaneous Technique

A 20–22 g, 1–3″ hypodermic or 4″ Tuohy needle is inserted percutaneously (after aseptic preparation of the site) so that its tip lies at the entrance to the mental foramen for the first technique; or so that the needle tip can then be advanced, gently, retrogradely, at least 1–2 cm into the rostral part of the canal for the second version of the technique. Aspiration before injection is important to avoid inadvertent intravascular injection. About 3–5 ml of local anaesthetic is usually sufficient for the first technique, but up to 10 ml may be required to ensure success for the second. For the intracanal technique, digital pressure over the mental foramen both during, and for several seconds after, injection may help retain the injectate within the canal and facilitate its retrograde spread. Excessive injection pressure should be avoided, especially for the intracanal technique as it may signal intraneural injection or even needle tip placement into the bony wall of the mandibular canal. For the intracanal technique, the needle tip may occasionally penetrate through the wall of the canal so that local anaesthetic is inadvertently injected into the adjacent mandibular cancellous bone.

16.2.6.3.2 *Intra-oral Technique*

Deflection of the lower lip enables insertion of a hypodermic or Tuohy needle from about 1 cm rostral to the mental foramen in order to deposit local anaesthetic either at the entrance of the foramen, or within the mandibular canal, after the needle tip is inserted at least 1–2 cm retrogradely into the mandibular canal. One study using different injectate volumes for an intracanal technique, suggested that 10 ml of injectate resulted in sufficient retrograde spread within the canal to reach the site of the fourth premolar, but that digital pressure over the foramen during and for a few seconds after injection made little difference to retention and retrograde spread of injectate within the canal.

16.2.7 Mandibular Foramen (Inferior Alveolar Nerve) Block

16.2.7.1 Site of Block

Where the inferior alveolar nerve enters the mandibular foramen on the medial aspect of the vertical ramus of the mandible (Figure 16.1). This can be technically challenging and is easier to perform if the patient is sedated or under general anaesthesia.

16.2.7.2 Structures Desensitised

All ipsilateral lower teeth and associated mandibular bone in addition to the lower lip and skin, as mentioned for the intramandibular canal technique for mental nerve block. Using the extra-oral techniques, especially with larger volumes of injected local anaesthetic, it is common to also block the lingual nerve, which branches off the mandibular nerve before it enters the maxillary foramen as the inferior alveolar nerve. Lingual nerve block and subsequent desensitisation of the hemi-tongue can result in self-trauma such

that bilateral mandibular foramen block is cautioned against because the resulting trauma can be more severe. Shorter acting local anaesthetics and restricting the volume injected may help to guard against this complication, but if there are any concerns, the horse's tongue should be examined for trauma the following day, and subsequently, if thought necessary. In the published reports, no clinical signs associated with tongue trauma had been reported by the owners and healing was uneventful, so it is possible that this complication is under-recognised.

16.2.7.3 Technique

The mandibular foramen lies on the medial aspect of the mandible. Its position can be approximated where a line drawn along the occlusal surface of the premolar cheek teeth (rostral to the curve of Spee) is intersected, at 90° by another line drawn down from the lateral canthus of the eye. A recent study has shown that the actual position of the foramen is normally very slightly dorsal and caudal to the intersection of these lines. Sufficient time should be allowed for the block to take effect (which also depends upon which local anaesthetic agent is chosen).

16.2.7.3.1 *Extra-oral Approaches*

1) Ventral, vertical approach. A bleb of local anaesthetic may be injected subcutaneously at the proposed needle insertion site to reduce the chance of patient movement during performance of the actual block. A 10–15 cm spinal needle is inserted at the ventromedial aspect of the horizontal ramus of the mandible, so as to follow the imaginary line dropped from the lateral canthus, and advanced vertically, dorsally, keeping as close to the inner aspect of the mandible as possible. The insertion depth is judged against another needle of the same length (that is placed on the lateral aspect of the cheek, in the same orientation, with its tip at the proposed foramen site) so that the tip of the inserted needle lies at the required depth to reach the mandibular foramen. Injection of 10–15 ml local anaesthetic is then performed after initial aspiration to check for inadvertent vascular puncture.

2) Caudoventral, angled approach. The needle can be inserted at the angle formed where the horizontal and vertical mandibular rami meet, and advanced rostrodorsally, close to the medial aspect of the mandible, towards the medial canthus of the ipsilateral eye, until the needle tip reaches the proposed site of the mandibular foramen, as determined by intersection of the lines mentioned above (and using another needle of the same length to help judge insertion depth) or until the lip of the foramen is contacted by the needle tip. Injection of 10–15 ml local anaesthetic is then performed after initial aspiration to check for inadvertent vascular puncture.

3) Caudal approach. The needle is inserted at the caudal border of the vertical ramus of the mandible and advanced rostrally, keeping close to the medial surface of the mandible, along the imaginary line extended from that drawn along the occlusal surface of the pre-molar cheek teeth, until the predetermined site of the mandibular foramen is reached (using a perpendicular line dropped from the lateral canthus, as previously described). Injection of 10–15 ml local anaesthetic is then performed, after initial aspiration to check for inadvertent vascular puncture.

4) Caudal, angled approach. The needle can be inserted on the caudal border of the mandible, about 3 cm below the temporomandibular joint, in the slight depression between the ear base and the wing of the atlas, and advanced rostroventrally along the medial side of the mandible. The head can be turned slightly away from the operator to facilitate this technique. Injection of 10–15 ml local anaesthetic is then performed after initial aspiration to check for inadvertent vascular puncture.

16.2.7.3.2 Intra-oral Approach

Using specially designed equipment, a curved needle (attached to a syringe and extension set which enables distant injection) is inserted: firstly into the mucoperiosteum just behind the third mandibular molar, at a site slightly 'above' its occlusal surface, enabling injection of 1 ml local anaesthetic submucosally to facilitate advancement of the needle for the actual nerve block, and then, subsequently, the needle is advanced until it contacts the rostral edge of the angle of the mandible and it is then rotated so that its tip slides down the medial surface of the mandible, staying close to the bony surface, for about 35 mm, at which position, its tip should lie at the mandibular foramen and distal to where the lingual branch leaves the mandibular nerve. A small volume of only around 5 ml of local anaesthetic should be sufficient to block the inferior alveolar nerve at its entrance to the mandibular foramen using this technique, whilst leaving the lingual nerve unaffected.

16.2.8 Palpebral Nerve Block/Auriculopalpebral Nerve Block

Figure 16.3 shows the three different sites for this nerve block. The auriculopalpebral nerve is a branch of the facial nerve (cranial nerve VII) and is therefore **only motor**. The auriculopalpebral nerve is motor to several of the peri-ocular superficial muscles, especially the orbicularis oculi muscle, which can contract so tightly in horses that it can make examination of the eye almost impossible. This nerve block can therefore facilitate eye examination when tight blepharospasm is present. However, if you want to do anything painful to the peri-ocular structures, the ocular surface, or the globe, some form of sensory block is required. Instillation of topical local anaesthetic into the conjunctival sac may suffice, e.g. for removal of a grass seed from the conjunctival sac.

Combining an (auriculo-) palpebral block with a supraorbital nerve block goes a long way to reducing tight closure of the eyelids in horses with very painful corneal lesions or uveitis because the supraorbital nerve block also blocks some motor innervation to upper eyelid muscles (e.g. levator palpebrae superioris).

This block does, however, reduce blinking, so be aware of corneal drying and further foreign body accumulation if the patient is in a dusty environment.

16.2.8.1 Site/s of Block

- In the triangular depression where a line along the ventral border of the zygomatic arch intersects with a vertical line drawn up from the caudal border of the vertical ramus of the mandible (the cross in Figure 16.3).
- In the triangular depression where a line along the dorsal border of the zygomatic arch transects a vertical line drawn up from the caudal border of the vertical mandibular ramus (the line with a circle at its end in Figure 16.3).
- Where the palpebral nerve crosses the dorsal margin of the zygomatic arch; roughly halfway between the eye and the ear, just about at the highest point of the zygomatic arch and slightly on its medial aspect. The nerve is palpable as a tiny band crossing the zygomatic rim. A block performed at this site is more correctly called a palpebral nerve block rather than an auriculopalpebral nerve block as no ear droop will be produced (the arrow in Figure 16.3).

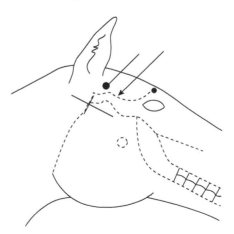

Figure 16.3 Sites for (auriculo-) palpebral nerve block. See text for details.

16.2.8.2 Technique

Choose one of the above sites for injection. A 22–25 g, 1″ needle and 1–5 ml of local anaesthetic are required.

16.2.9 Retrobulbar Block

This is most usually performed to enable enucleation and can be performed in sedated (standing), or anaesthetised patients. Similar techniques to those described for small animals can be used (see Chapter 13) and the same precautions and complications apply.

16.2.9.1 Site/s of Block

Local anaesthetic (10–20 ml) is deposited within the cone of muscles that surround the globe, in what is described as an intraconal technique, with a view to blocking cranial nerves II, III, IV, V (ophthalmic and maxillary), and VI. The globe, eyelids, and most of the upper face should be desensitised, but to produce eyelid akinesis, a palpebral block (VII) will be required. Sufficient time (at least 10–15 minutes and dependent upon which local anaesthetic is used) should be allowed to elapse for the block to take effect.

A successful block is demonstrated by exophthalmos, reduced lacrimation, mydriasis, and a central, akinetic eye – but these may not be obvious in a badly diseased eye.

16.2.9.2 Technique

Many variations of technique are reported in the literature.

1) Trans-orbital approaches. Several techniques have been described, but the simplest is a 1-point injection. The site of this single injection can also vary. One technique involves using a pre-curved needle that is inserted slightly dorso-medial to the lateral canthus (10 o'clock for right eye; 2 o'clock for left eye), just below the dorsal orbital rim, and carefully advanced under the roof of the orbit, around and behind the eyeball, taking care not to puncture it. Alternatively, a straight needle can be inserted slightly ventro-lateral to the medial canthus, just inside the ventral orbital rim (5 o'clock for right eye; 7 o'clock for left eye), and advanced along the floor of the orbit to approach the point of the extra-ocular muscular cone (conus ocularis); but with this technique, there is a greater risk of the needle tip penetrating the optic nerve sheath beneath which lies CSF; intrathecal injection of local anaesthetic will result in direct CNS toxicity. Depending upon the pathology present, the needle can be inserted through the eyelid (i.e. a transpalpebral approach) or the eyelid can be retracted to enable needle insertion into the conjunctival fornix. A little topical local anaesthetic (e.g. tetracaine, proxymetacaine) may be instilled into the conjunctival sac to desensitise the conjunctiva first. The approaches described below do not involve injections into the structures immediately surrounding the ocular surface.

2) Dorsal, supra-orbital fossa approach. A 10-cm spinal needle is inserted, vertically, ventrally into the supra-orbital fossa just caudal to the dorsal orbital rim (i.e. supraorbital process of the frontal bone). As the needle is advanced (aiming for the apex of the extra-ocular cone of muscles), the globe is watched after the globe rotates upwards and then resumes its original position, this signals that the needle has entered the extra-ocular muscle cone, and injection of 10–20 ml of local anaesthetic (with prior aspiration) can now be made slowly. With this technique, the eyelids may not be desensitised because the ophthalmic and maxillary nerves may not become well blocked, therefore a diamond block can be a useful adjunct. One report using ultrasound for this technique demonstrated promising results, but needs to be repeated in clinical cases.

3) Lateral approach. Less favoured. Somewhat reminiscent of the Peterson block used in cattle, this technique involves advancing a 10–15 cm needle beneath the zygomatic arch, caudal to the lateral canthus, and fairly perpendicularly into the pterygopalatine fossa with a slight dorsal angle (compared with the slight cranioventral angulation as used for the maxillary nerve block). As the needle is advanced into the extra-ocular muscle cone, lateral deviation of the globe may be noted, at which point needle advancement should stop and 10–20 ml of local anaesthetic is injected, after initial aspiration to reduce the risk of inadvertent intravascular injection. Maxillary nerve block may also be achieved.

Potential complications include: reduced blinking, proptosis and increased intraocular pressure may cause further damage to the globe (less of a concern if enucleation is to be performed), stimulation of the oculocardiac reflex may actually occur during injection of the local anaesthetic behind the eye (although once the block has taken effect, this reflex should be abolished), damage to the globe (which also risks spread/seeding of infection or tumour to adjacent tissues), damage to blood vessels behind the eye with potential inadvertent intravascular injection and/or haematoma formation, damage to the optic nerve (less of a worry if enucleation is to be performed), inadvertent injection of local anaesthetic into the cerebrospinal fluid within the meningeal sheath that surrounds the optic nerve (potentially leading to signs of CNS toxicity, although these may be less obvious in animals under general anaesthesia).

16.2.10 Other Techniques for Ocular Desensitisation

A *four-point peribulbar* (extraconal) technique and a *sub-Tenon* approach are also possible in horses and follow the same principles as described for small animals, but using larger volumes of local anaesthetic (see Chapter 13).

16.2.11 Great Auricular and Internal Auricular Nerve Blocks

These can provide desensitisation of the pinna and external ear canal for minor surgical procedures.

16.2.11.1 Sites of Blocks

The great auricular nerve is a branch of the second (and possibly also the first) cervical segmental nerve and supplies the caudal aspect of the pinna. It can be palpated on the caudal aspect of the pinna at its base as a small band that can be felt to 'slip' under the finger.

The internal auricular nerve branches off the facial nerve soon after the latter emerges through the stylomastoid foramen. Though normally only motor, it appears that this nerve is sensory to the inner aspect of the pinna and external auditory meatus. (In small animals, the auriculotemporal nerve, arising from the mandibular division of the trigeminal nerve, very close to the emergence of the facial nerve, is considered to supply sensory innervation to the internal aspects of the ear canal.) The internal auricular nerve can be located where it passes through the auricular cartilage at a small notch, which is palpable, laterally, at the base of the auricular cartilage.

16.2.11.2 Technique

Where the great auricular nerve can be slipped under the finger, 1–2 ml of local anaesthetic is deposited subcutaneously using a 23 g 5/8″ needle.

Where the internal auricular nerve passes through the notch in the lateral base of the auricular cartilage, 1–2 ml local anaesthetic is deposited after directing the needle tip into the notch using a 23 g 5/8″ needle.

16.2.12 Paravertebral Block

This can be performed in horses to provide flank anaesthesia.

16.2.12.1 Landmarks and Sites of Block

A vertical line drawn up from the caudal border of the last rib, locates the transverse process of the third lumbar vertebra. Judging the horizontal distance between the second and third lumbar transverse processes gives you an estimate of the distance between the first and second lumbar transverse processes.

Spinal segmental nerves **Th18, Lu1, and Lu2** can be blocked paravertebrally either off, and just (about 1 cm) below and above, the cranial borders of the first, second, and third lumbar transverse processes, or off (and just below and above) the cranial edge of the transverse process of the first lumbar vertebra (for Th18) and then the off (and just below and above) the caudal edges of the first (for Lu1) and second (for Lu2) lumbar transverse processes, similarly to cattle (see Chapter 33). For each spinal segmental nerve, the ventral branches and sympathetic chain are blocked by injection just below the intertransverse ligament, and the dorsal branches are blocked by injection just above the intertransverse ligament.

16.2.12.2 Technique

Sedation is usually required. Injection sites should be prepared aseptically and small blebs of subcutaneous local anaesthetic at the proposed needle insertion sites (roughly half-way along the transverse processes from the dorsal midline) help to reduce muscle spasm upon subsequent placement of paravertebral needles. Paravertebral needles, long spinal needles, or the stylettes from long over-the-needle catheters (at least 10 cm long, about 20 g) are used, and about 30–40 ml local anaesthetic for each nerve (25–30 ml for the ventral branches and 10 ml for the dorsal branches). If a bleb of local anaesthetic is placed in the needle hub, it can help detect inadvertent entry into the peritoneal cavity as, in a standing animal, the dorsal peritoneal cavity is usually under negative pressure, so the bleb gets sucked into the needle. Should this happen, the needle should be withdrawn slightly until no further negative pressure is appreciated.

Nerve location by electrical stimulation to aid performance of the paravertebral block has recently been described. This enabled smaller volumes of local anaesthetic to be used and also avoided potential inadvertent blockade of the third lumbar segmental nerve, which can result in potentially dangerous ipsilateral hindlimb weakness. The use of ultrasound to help locate the segmental nerves responsible for innervation of the lumbar spine in horses has been described (see Further Reading), but has not yet been reported for performing paravertebral block for flank anaesthesia. See also Chapter 14 on small animals.

16.2.13 Caudal Epidural (Extradural) Analgesia/Anaesthesia

This is a useful technique to provide desensitisation of the perineum, tail, and caudal intrapelvic viscera whilst hopefully maintaining locomotor function of the hindlimbs. Sedation may be required.

16.2.13.1 Location of Site

The commonest injection site is the first coccygeal interspace. This space is located by 'pumping' the tail up and down and feeling for the most obvious/most moveable interspace (usually Co1–Co2; but occasionally Sa5–Co1). The site is usually about 1–2 cm cranial to the first tail hairs. Aseptic preparation of the injection site is of paramount importance. Placing a subcutaneous bleb of local anaesthetic at the proposed needle insertion site can help reduce patient reaction on subsequent introduction of the epidural needle. The needle itself is then inserted in the midline, either perpendicularly to the croup or at about 30° (as if aiming up the vertebral canal).

Various techniques can be used to help ensure correct position of the needle within the epidural space, including sudden loss of resistance after the ligamentum flavum is penetrated, followed by aspiration of a hanging drop of sterile saline (as there is normally negative pressure in the caudal epidural space), and minimal resistance to injection with no appreciable compression of an air bubble included in the syringe. (See Chapter 14 for further explanation of these techniques.)

Sometimes, upon advancement of the needle through the ligamentum flavum, it is easy to advance the needle so as to embed its tip in the floor of the vertebral canal. If this occurs, there will be high resistance to any attempted injection and the needle should be withdrawn 1–2 mm before further attempts to ascertain its position are made. If styletted spinal needles are not used, coring of tissue is possible (especially if the needle is advanced into the floor of the vertebral canal) and the tip of the needle may become blocked. Never apply excessive pressure whilst trying to insert the needle as it has been reported that it is possible for the needle to pass between the vertebrae and into the rectum below.

After local anaesthetic is injected, signs of a successful block include relaxation of the anal sphincter, lack of response to gentle needle-prick of the perineum and a flaccid tail. For further information, see notes on cattle (Chapter 33) and small animal (Chapter 14) extradural injection techniques and Further Reading.

16.2.13.2 What to Inject for an Average 500 kg Horse to Avoid Hindlimb Motor Block

Use preservative-free preparations where possible, and especially if multiple doses are to be administered. Table 16.2 summarises commonly used drugs and combinations.

- 5–10 ml lidocaine 2%. Onset 5–10 minutes and may take up to 20 minutes for full effect to develop (sometimes a little longer than for cattle where it normally takes about 5 minutes, possibly because there is usually more fat in the epidural space of horses than of dairy type cattle). Duration 1–2 hours.
- 5–7 ml mepivacaine 2%. Onset 10–20 minutes. Duration 2+ hours.
- 0.17 mg/kg xylazine, made up to 10 ml in normal saline. Onset 15–20 minutes. Duration 2–4 hours. (Or, 0.25 mg/kg xylazine in 8 ml normal saline: onset 10–15 minutes; duration 3+ hours.) Beware systemic absorption and sedation.
- 0.17 mg/kg xylazine + 0.22 mg/kg lidocaine (without epinephrine). Onset 5–10 minutes. Sweating in perineal region accompanies onset of analgesia. Duration 5 hours. Duration longer than either agent alone, possibly due to some vasoconstriction due to the xylazine, but also perhaps due to its local anaesthetic-like activity.
- Detomidine 60 µg/kg, diluted to final volume of 10 ml. Onset 10–15 minutes. Duration 2–3 hours. Despite this being a relatively more potent dose of detomidine than the above mentioned 0.17–0.25 mg/kg xylazine (at least if administered intravenously), the duration of analgesia is less than that after xylazine, possibly due to more rapid systemic absorption. Xylazine may have more vasoconstrictive action due to its greater α1 agonist actions, so delaying absorption.
- Morphine 0.1 mg/kg, made up to final volume 10 ml. Onset 1–4(+) hours. Duration 17 up to 24 hours. Analgesia extends cranially to at least the first lumbar segment. (Morphine 0.2 mg/kg assures analgesia up to ninth thoracic segment; onset is slightly quicker, and duration slightly longer at this higher dose). Occasionally pruritus (usually focal/segmental) follows the neuraxial administration of opioids; the effect is believed to be opioid receptor-mediated as naloxone can antagonise it. (See Further Reading and also Chapter 14.)
- Morphine 0.05–0.1 mg/kg + detomidine 30 µg/kg made up to final volume of 10 ml. Onset c. 20 minutes. Duration 12–24 hours.

16.2.14 True Spinal/Subarachnoid/Intrathecal Anaesthesia/Analgesia

The reader is referred to anaesthetic texts for the best techniques and drug doses (see Further Reading).

16.2.15 Bilateral Block of the Pudendal Nerves, Their Superficial and Deep Perineal Branches, and the Caudal Rectal Nerves

Although a technique similar to that performed in cattle (involving per rectum palpation of needle placement) has been described in horses (see Further Reading), the

Table 16.2 Drug doses for epidural (extradural) injection for a typical 500 kg horse.

Drug	Volume	Onset	Duration
Lidocaine 2%	5–10 ml	5–10 min	1–2 h
Mepivacaine 2%	5 ml	10–20 min	2 h
Xylazine 0.17 mg/kg	Can dilute to 10 ml in saline	15 min	2–5 h
Detomidine 60 μg/kg	Can dilute to 10 ml in saline	15 min	2–3 h
Morphine 0.1 mg/kg	Can dilute to 10 ml in saline or sterile water	1–4 h	17–24 h
Morphine 0.05–0.1 mg/kg + Detomidine 30 μg/kg	Can dilute to 10 ml in saline	20 min	17–24 h

pudendal nerves can be blocked more distally as they course around the ischial arch. Bilateral blockade of the pudendal nerves, their perineal branches (which arise proximal to the ischial arch), and the caudal rectal nerves (which arise slightly more proximally than the perineal nerves) should desensitise the perineum, anus, rectum, and penis, external lamina of prepuce, and scrotal skin (not testicles) in males, or the vulva, vagina, cervix, distal urethra, and caudal udder in females. This is a useful technique to anaesthetise the penis and cause its extrusion in males so that examination and surgery can be performed, or in females to reduce straining after vaginal trauma. Sedation is usually required.

The perineal area should be thoroughly cleaned and aseptically prepared. The ischial arch should be palpable. A 3″ 22 g needle is inserted on either side of midline, about 2.5 cm above the ischial arch and 2.5 cm lateral from the midline. Local anaesthetic (5 ml) is then injected subcutaneously, bilaterally, at the needle insertion sites to block the superficial perineal nerves, which also reduces patient reaction when the pudendal block is performed in the standing, sedated patient. On each side, the needle can then be advanced ventromedially until it contacts the floor of the ischial arch, just lateral to the midline, and 10 ml of local anaesthetic is then injected (after aspiration) to block each pudendal nerve. Before each needle is completely withdrawn, it can be redirected cranio-dorsally about 1 cm and a further 5 ml of local anaesthetic injected, to ensure block of the deep perineal and caudal rectal nerves.

The block is usually effective within 5–10 minutes. Using a short-acting local anaesthetic in males reduces the problems of prolonged penile protrusion and dependent oedema that may lead to paraphimosis. Occasionally the needles may penetrate the penile tissue, but this has not been reported to have had any serious consequences.

16.2.16 Other Blocks/Techniques

To accompany dental surgery, topical local anaesthetic gels (e.g. prilocaine gel) can be applied to the gingiva. Other supplementary techniques, commonly used in people and which may be applicable, include periodontal (intraligamentary) anaesthesia and supra-periosteal injection (see Chapter 41 for more details).

Intratesticular local anaesthetic (commonly lidocaine or mepivacaine) should be administered during castration whether this is performed as a standing procedure or under general anaesthesia. Rapid distribution of local anaesthetic occurs to the spermatic cord because of the high rate of testicular lymph flow found in all species studied to date, which means that the peak anaesthetic effect is likely to occur within 3–10 minutes of injection (after which time, the block also wanes rapidly). Local anaesthetic deposited into the testicle does not spread to the cremaster muscle itself or to the skin incision site, but should result in block of visceral afferent fibres in the spermatic cord. Deposition of further local anaesthetic at the incision site should help reduce the reaction to skin incision.

During standing laparoscopic surgery for ovariectomy or cryptorchidectomy, local anaesthetic may be deposted into the mesovarium (reported to provide better antinociception than intra-ovarian injection) or into the testicle and/or mesorchium (prior to surgical transection of the ovarian pedicle or spermatic cord), respectively, to provide extra antinociception for the surgery.

For truncal anaesthesia, a variety of techniques may be possible: e.g., an ultrasound-guided transversus abdominal plane (TAP) block has been investigated in pony cadavers, ultrasound-guided rectus sheath catheter placement has also been described in pony cadavers, and, more recently, a bilateral caudal intercostal block has been described for use in horses undergoing laparotomy.

Variations of the TAP block have become commonly adopted for various veterinary species but, depending upon the exact sites and volumes of deposition of local anaesthetic, may not achieve full abdominal wall and ventral midline anaesthesia. This is also found in humans, such that TAP blocks are commonly combined with rectus sheath blocks to ensure complete analgesia of the ventral midline, both cranial and caudal to the umbilicus. TAP blocks and quadratus lumborum blocks, alongside several techniques for achieving 'paraspinal/intercostal' blocks are, however, now believed to be just indirect ways of achieving paravertebral spread ('paravertebral block by proxy'). Moreover, the human literature suggests that truncal blocks that provide a combination of somatic and visceral/sympathetic chain blockade (i.e. only guaranteed by true paravertebral techniques) are superior (better at preventing persistent post-operative pain) to those that achieve only somatic block. It therefore appears that such techniques require further evaluation and refinement before their widespread use in veterinary clinical cases.

16.2.17 Continuous Intravenous Infusion of Lidocaine

This is becoming increasingly used as a component of 'balanced anaesthesia' for its analgesic effects. It can also be used to form a part of a 'balanced analgesic' regimen. See Chapters 3, 6, 28, and 30.

Further Reading

Abass, M., Picek, S., Garzon, J.F.G. et al. (2018). Local mepivacaine before castration of horses under medetomidine isoflurane balanced anaesthesia is effective to reduce perioperative nociception and cytokine release. *Equine Veterinary Journal* 50: 733–738.

Baldo, C.F., Almeida, D., Wendt-Hornickle, E., and Guedes, A. (2018). Transverse abdominal plane block in ponies: a preliminary anatomical study. *Veterinary Anaesthesia and Analgesia* 45: 392–296.

Bardell, D.B., Iff, I., and Mosing, M. (2010). A cadaver study comparing two approaches to perform a maxillary nerve block in the horse. *Equine Veterinary Journal* 42: 721–725.

Bird, A.R., Morley, S.J., Sherlock, C.E., and Mair, T.S. (2018). The outcomes of epidural anaesthesia in horses with perineal and tail melanomas: complications associated with ataxia and the risks of rope recovery. *Equine Veterinary Education* https://doi.org/10.1111/eve.12911.

Burford, J.H. and Corley, K.T. (2006). Morphine-associated pruritus after single extradural administration in a horse. *Veterinary Anaesthesia and Analgesia* 33: 193–198.

Caldwell, F.J. and Easley, K.J. (2012). Self-inflicted lingual trauma secondary to inferior alveolar nerve block in three horses. *Equine Veterinary Education* 24: 119–123.

Carpenter, R.E. and Byron, C.R. (2015). Equine local anesthetic and analgesic techniques. In: *Veterinary Anesthesia and Analgesia, the Fifth Edition of Lumb and Jones* (eds. K.A. Grimm, L.A. Lamont, W.J. Tranquilli, et al.), 886–911. Iowa, USA: Wiley Blackwell.

Caruso, M., Schumacher, J., and Henry, R. (2016). Peripheral injection of the ethmoidal nerve of horses. *Veterinary Surgery* 45: 494–498.

Costache, I., Pawa, A., and Abdallah, F.W. (2018). Paravertebral by proxy – time to redefine the paravertebral block. *Anaesthesia* 73: 1185–1188.

De Cozar, M.J. (2019). Can I give alpha-2 agonists for blocking and accurately assess the horse's lameness once blocked? *Equine Veterinary Education* 31: 111–112.

Duarte, P.C., Paz, C.F.R., Oliveira, A.P.L. et al. (2017). Caudal epidural anesthesia in mares after bicarbonate addition to a lidocaine-epinephrine combination. *Veterinary Anaesthesia and Analgesia* 44: 943–950.

Du Toit, N. (2015). Which nerve blocks will help me with a tooth extraction? *Equine Veterinary Education* 27: 275–276.

Eckert, R.E., Griffin, C.E., Cohen, N.D., and Marx, S. (2019). Investigation into intraoral approach for nerve block injection at the mental foramen in the horse. *Equine Veterinary Education* 31: 328–334.

Farstvedt, E.G. and Hendrickson, D.A. (2006). Intraoperative pain responses following intraovarian or mesovarian injection of lidocaine in mares undergoing standing laparoscopic ovarietcomy. *Journal of the American Veterinary Medical Association* 227: 593–596.

Gingold, B.M.C., hassen, K.M., Milloway, M.C. et al. (2018). Caudal intercostal block for abdominal surgery in horses. *Veterinary Record* 183: 164–165.

Goodrich, L.R., Nixon, A.J., Fubini, S.L. et al. (2002). Epidural morphine and detomidine decreases postoperative hindlimb lameness in horses after bilateral stifle arthroscopy. *Veterinary Surgery* 31: 232–239.

Grosenbaugh, D.A., Skarda, R.T., and Muir, W.W. (1999). Caudal regional anaesthesia in horses. *Equine Veterinary Education* 11: 98–105.

Grubb, T.L., Reibold, T.W., and Huber, M.J. (1992). Comparison of lidocaine, xylazine and xylazine/lidocaine for caudal epidural analgesia in horses. *Journal of the American Veterinary Medical Association* 201: 1187–1190.

Haga, H.A., Lykkjen, S., Revold, T., and Ranheim, B. (2006). Effect of intratesticular injection of lidocaine on cardiovascular responses to castration in isoflurane-anesthetized stallions. *American Journal of Veterinary Research* 67: 403–408.

Hagag, U. and Tawfiek, M.G. (2018). Blind versus ultrasound-guided maxillary nerve block in donkeys. *Veterinary Anaesthesia and Analgesia* 45: 103–110.

Harding, P.G., Smith, R.L., and Barakzai, S.Z. (2012). Comparison of two approaches to performing an inferior alveolar nerve block in the horse. *Australian Veterinary Journal* 90: 146–150.

Hebbard, P. (2014). TAP block nomenclature. *Anaesthesia* 70: 105–106.

Henry, T., Pusterla, N., Guedes, A.G.P., and Verstraete, F.J.M. (2014). Evaluation and clinical use of an intraoral inferior alveolar nerve block in the horse. *Equine Veterinary Journal* 46: 706–710.

Hermans, H., Veraa, S., Wolschrijn, C.F., and van Loon, J.P.A.M. (2019). Local anaethetic techniques for the equine head, towards guided techniques and new applications. *Equine Veterinary Education* 31: 432–440.

Iff, I., Mosing, M., Lechner, T., and Moens, Y. (2010). The use of an acoustic device to identify the extradural space in standing horses. *Veterinary Anaesthesia and Analgesia* 37: 57–62.

Joyce, J. and Hendrickson, D.A. (2005). Comparison of intraoperative pain responses following intratesticular or mesorchial injection of lidocaine in standing horses undergoing laparoscopic cryptorchidectomy. *Journal of the American Veterinary Medical Association* 229: 1779–1783.

Kalchofner, K.S., Kummer, M., Price, J., and Bettschart-Wolfensberger, R. (2007). Pruritus in two horses following epidurally administered morphine. *Equine Veterinary Education* 19: 590–594.

Levine, J.M., Levine, G.J., Hoffman, A.G., and Bratton, G. (2008). Comparative anatomy of the horse, ox and dog: the brain and associated vessels. *Compendium for Continuing Education for the Practising Veterinarian*: Equine April 2008: 153–164.

McCoy, A.M., Schaefer, E., and Malone, E. (2007). How to perform effective blocks of the equine ear. Proceedings of the 53rd Convention of the American Association of Equine Practitioners (December 2007). Orlando, Florida. 397–398.

Moon, P.F. and Suter, C.M. (1993). Paravertebral thoracolumbar anaesthesia in 10 horses. *Equine Veterinary Journal* 25: 304–308.

Morath, U., Luyet, C., Spadavecchia, C. et al. (2013). Ultrasound-guided retrobulbar nerve block in horses: a cadaveric study. *Veterinary Anaesthesia and Analgesia* 40: 205–211.

Nannarone, S., Bini, G., Vuerich, M. et al. (2016). Retrograde maxillary nerve perineural injection: a tomographic and anatomical evaluation of the infraorbital canal and evaluation of needle type and size in equine cadavers. *The Veterinary Journal* 217: 33–39.

Newton, S.A., Knottenbelt, D.C., and Eldridge, P.R. (2000). Headshaking in horses: possible aetiopathogenesis suggested by the results of diagnostic tests and several treatment regimes used in 20 cases. *Equine Veterinary Journal* 32: 208–216.

O'Neill, H.D., Garcia-Pereira, F.L., and Mohankumar, P.S. (2014). Ultrasound-guided injection of the maxillary nerve in the horse. *Equine Veterinary Journal* 46: 180–184.

Rawlinson, J.E., Bass, L., Capmoy, L. et al. (2018). Evaluation of the equine mental foramen block: cadaveric and in vivo injectate diffusion. *Veterinary Anaesthesia and Analgesia* 45: 839–848.

Rieder, C.M., Zwick, T., Hopster, K. et al. (2016). Maxillary nerve block within the pterygopalatine fossa for oral extraction of maxillary cheek teeth in 80 horses. *Pferdeheilkunde* 32: 587–594.

Roberts, V.L.H., Perkins, J.D., Skarlina, E. et al. (2013). Caudal anaesthesia of the infraorbital nerve for diagnosis of idiopathic headshaking and caudal compression of the infraorbital nerve for its treatment, in 58 horses. *Equine Veterinary Journal* 45: 107–110.

Robertson, S.A., Sanchez, L.C., Merritt, A.M., and Doherty, T.J. (2005). Effect of systemic lidocaine on visceral and somatic nociception in conscious horses. *Equine Veterinary Journal* 37: 122–127.

Santos, L.C. and Gallacher, K. (2017). Nerve stimulation-guided thoracolumbar paravertebral block for flank laparotomy in a horse. *Veterinary Anaesthesia and Analgesia* 44: 187–188.

Schumacher, J., Bratton, G.R., and Williams, J.W. (1985). Pudendal and caudal rectal nerve blocks in the horse – an anesthetic procedure for reproductive surgery. *Theriogenology* 24: 457–464.

Skarda, R.T. and Muir, W.W. (1996). Comparison of antinociceptive, cardiovascular and respiratory effects, head ptosis and position of pelvic limbs in mares after caudal epidural administration of xylazine and detomidine hydrochloride solution. *American Journal of Veterinary Research* 57: 1338–1345.

Staszyk, C., Bienert, A., Baumer, W. et al. (2008). Simulation of local anaesthetic nerve block of the infraorbital nerve within the pterygopalatine fossa: anatomical landmarks defined by computed tomography. *Research in Veterinary Science* 85: 399–406.

Stauffer, S., Cordner, B., Dixon, J., and Witte, T. (2017). Maxillary nerve blocks in horses: an experimental comparison of surface landmark and ultrasound-guided techniques. *Veterinary Anaesthesia and Analgesia* 44: 951–958.

Sysel, A.M., Pleasant, R.S., Jacobson, J.D. et al. (1997). Systemic and local effects associated with long-term epidural catheterisation and morphine-detomidine administration in horses. *Veterinary Surgery* 26: 141–149.

Tremaine, W.H. (2007). Local analgesic techniques for the equine head. *Equine Veterinary Education* 19: 495–503.

Tremain, H. (2019). Local analgesia techniques for dental and head procedures in horses. *In Practice* 41: 165–176.

Vandeweerd, J., Desbrosse, F., Clegg, P. et al. (2007). Innervation and nerve injections of the lumbar spine of the horse: a cadaveric study. *Equine Veterinary Journal* 39: 59–63.

Wilmink, S., Warren-Smith, C.M.R., and Roberts, V.L.H. (2014). Accuracy of needle placement in diagnostic local analgesia of the maxillary nerve for investigation of trigeminally mediated headshaking in horses. *Veterinary Record* https://doi.org/10.1136/vr.102518.

Self-test Section

1   The internal auricular nerve is a branch of which cranial nerve?

   A   Ophthalmic branch of trigeminal
   B   Maxillary branch of trigeminal
   C   Mandibular branch of trigeminal
   D   Facial nerve

2   Which vein, which contains no valves so that flow can be bi-directional to aid brain cooling, communicates with the cavernous sinus at the base of the brain?

17

Muscle Relaxants

LEARNING OBJECTIVES

- To be able to discuss the indications and contra-indications for use of neuromuscular blockers (NMBs).
- To be able to describe the basic neuromuscular junction (NMJ) structure and function.
- To be able to compare and contrast depolarising and non-depolarising NMBs.
- To be able to discuss how the degree of neuromuscular block can be monitored.
- To be able to discuss how the depth of anaesthesia can be monitored during neuromuscular blockade.
- To be able to discuss the considerations for 'reversal' of the block and recognise any complications.
- To be aware of the influence of other drugs/conditions on the degree of neuromuscular block.

17.1 Introduction

17.1.1 Why Use Neuromuscular Blockade (Muscle Relaxation)?

- To **facilitate surgery**: fracture reduction, thoracic surgery, deep abdominal surgery, or ophthalmic surgery where the operating field must remain as still as possible.
- To **facilitate artificial ventilation** (i.e. manual or mechanical ventilation, which is usually provided in the form of positive pressure ventilation). Not all patients that require artificial ventilation require muscle relaxation because by simply ventilating their lungs a little more than they would for themselves, we can reduce their blood CO_2 tension to reduce their ventilatory drive, and so we can 'capture' control of their ventilation. However, some patients continue to 'fight the ventilator', which can cause problems (e.g. during thoracotomy where the lungs should not be inflating as the surgeon incises into the chest cavity), or simply be a nuisance.
- As **part of a balanced anaesthetic technique**, it may be especially useful in high risk cases, where the 'muscle relaxation' component of general anaesthesia can be provided with an NMB, but choose one with minimal side effects and a duration to suit your need. You must be able to monitor the depth of anaesthesia in any paralysed patient.
- For **endotracheal intubation**, especially in humans and occasionally cats or pigs (these species are prone to laryngospasm).

17.1.2 How Can We Relax Muscles?

There are several ways to achieve muscle relaxation (of striated muscles):

- Reduce the requirement for reflex or voluntary muscular activity, e.g. general anaesthesia results in reduced muscular activity.
- Interfere with reflexes that control postural muscle strength. Benzodiazepines and guaiphenesin inhibit these reflexes at spinal cord level.
- Block motor nerve conduction. Local anaesthetics can achieve this.
- Block acetylcholine synthesis (or choline re-uptake), or storage in vesicles or vesicle transport in the motor nerve terminal.
- Block acetylcholine release from motor nerve terminals, e.g. botulinum toxin prevents vesicles of acetylcholine from fusing with the nerve membrane for exocytosis.
- Block the action of acetylcholine on the post-synaptic (muscle) membrane. This is achieved with NMBs.

Veterinary Anaesthesia: Principles to Practice, Second Edition. Alexandra H. A. Dugdale, Georgina Beaumont, Carl Bradbrook, and Matthew Gurney.
© 2020 John Wiley & Sons Ltd. Published 2020 by John Wiley & Sons Ltd.
Companion website: www.wiley.com/go/dugdale/veterinary-anaesthesia

- Prevent muscle contraction. Inhalation agents affect calcium channels, so reduce calcium entry and produce a degree of muscle weakness. Dantrolene interferes with excitation-contraction coupling by inhibiting calcium release from the sarcoplasmic reticulum.

17.1.3 Choice of Muscle Relaxant

Choice of muscle relaxant is influenced by:

- Anaesthetic and surgical requirements
- Speed of onset of action required
- Duration of action required
- Potential side effects

17.1.4 Contra-indications to Muscle Relaxation

- Inability to ventilate the patient's lungs adequately
- Inability to be able to judge and monitor the depth of anaesthesia adequately
- Inability to assess the degree of neuromuscular blockade and its reversal

17.2 Centrally Acting Muscle Relaxants

Centrally acting skeletal muscle relaxants do not act specifically at the peripheral NMJs.

17.2.1 Guaiphenesin

Guaiphenesin (guaifenesin; glyceryl guaiacolate [GG]; glyceryl guaiacolate ether [GGE]) is a propanediol derivative of wood tar. (See Chapter 33 on ruminant anaesthesia, and also Chapter 31 on field anaesthesia techniques for horses.)

Guaiphenesin inhibits reflex arc internuncial neuronal relay in the spinal cord and brainstem, and thus tends to reduce postural muscle strength. It crosses the blood–brain barrier and placenta. It causes minimal interference with the animal's ability to breathe when used at the normal doses. It has some sedative properties (possibly due to actions within the reticular formation) with minimal cardiovascular depressant side effects (mild hypotension), but it is irritant to vascular endothelium and to tissues, especially if transvascular or extravascular deposition occurs. It has some antitussive action, but is also an expectorant.

A 10% solution is currently commercially available that can be diluted in dextrose-saline (0.18% saline, 4% glucose) down to a 5% solution if required. Homemade solutions were used prior to the advent of the commercial solution. These were variously solubilised in dextrose, water, or saline to try to reduce guaiphenesin's side effects of tending to cause thrombosis (especially with concentrations >10% and if infused rapidly under pressure) and haemolysis (especially with solutions of concentrations >15% (horses) or >5% (cattle), which exclude stabilising substances). Glucose or fructose have been included as 'stabilisers' to try to protect erythrocytes from osmotic damage/haemolysis. Commercial products tend to include glucose and are often solubilised in N-methyl pyrrolidone (an organic solvent also used as a paint stripper, which has the potential to be irritant itself).

The dose required is 30–100 + mg/kg. The lethal overdose is in excess of around 300–400 mg/kg. It is metabolised in the liver and the metabolites are excreted in the urine. Although fairly rapidly metabolised, it has the potential to be cumulative. One metabolite, catechol (or at least a compound with cross-reactivity to catechol) may be responsible for most of the side effects. Doses exceeding 150–180 mg/kg will produce side effects of some cardiorespiratory depression (with hypotension, occasional arrhythmias, and altered, often apneustic, breathing patterns with an overall reduction in minute ventilation), paradoxical muscle rigidity, and central nervous system (CNS) excitement reactions/seizure-like activity.

Not used in small animal practice.

17.2.2 Benzodiazepines

Benzodiazepines (e.g. diazepam and midazolam) are also described as centrally acting skeletal muscle relaxants because they also inhibit internuncial neurotransmission in the spinal cord and brainstem via actions at benzodiazepine binding sites (predominantly located on $GABA_A$ and glycine receptors). Again, this results in postural muscle weakness, without any real inhibition of respiratory muscle function, however, in large doses, they will cause some cardiorespiratory depression.

Benzodiazepines are metabolised in the liver and there are some active metabolites from diazepam's metabolism. Benzodiazepines can produce some anxiolysis and sedation, but are also capable of causing paradoxical CNS excitement reactions too, possibly due to the phenomenon of disinhibition (over-inhibition of inhibitory neurotransmission, resulting in uncontrolled excitement). This is more common in mature animals when used alone. These drugs can also cross the placenta.

17.3 Neuromuscular Blocking Agents

These are the true, peripherally acting, skeletal 'muscle relaxants'. These drugs do not provide analgesia, sedation, or hypnosis, and because they 'paralyse' all skeletal muscles, including the respiratory muscles, artificial ventilation is necessary to keep the patient alive.

These are **all quaternary ammonium compounds** with at least one N^+ that **can interact with the α subunits of the post-synaptic nicotinic acetylcholine receptors** (NAChRs) of the NMJ, to block neuromuscular transmission.

Each nicotinic (N) acetylcholine receptor consists of 5 glycoprotein subunits which span the post-synaptic membrane. Normal adult NMJ NAChRs consist of two α subunits, one β subunit, one δ subunit, and one ε subunit. Foetal NAChRs and extra-junctional NAChRs consist of two α subunits, one β, one δ, and one γ subunit.

Normally, two acetylcholine molecules must bind simultaneously, one to each of the two α subunits, for channel activation to occur, so two acetylcholine (ACh) molecules are required for one channel to open. Activation of the channel results in conformational change and opening of a 'pore', a non-specific cation channel, through which sodium (and calcium) can move into, and potassium can move out of, the muscle cell.

At the NMJ (Figure 17.1), the post-synaptic muscle membrane at the 'motor end plate' is highly folded. This helps to increase the area of 'contact' (across a narrow synaptic cleft), between the pre- and post-synaptic cells. The folded postjunctional membrane has most NAChRs concentrated on the shoulders of its folds, but the crypts are also important as they harbour much acetylcholinesterase that is necessary to destroy the transmitter, acetylcholine, once it has done its job. Acetylcholine is hydrolysed by this enzyme, and the choline that is formed can be taken up again by the prejunctional nerve terminal, and recycled to form further acetylcholine.

17.3.1 Pre-synaptic Receptors

There may be nicotinic, muscarinic, and even adrenergic pre-junctional receptors. These may be involved in positive and negative feedback loops for enhancing, or diminishing, transmitter release, respectively. Some presynaptic receptors result in mobilisation of ACh from distant reserve stores to the readily releasable stores. The prejunctional (neuronal) NAChRs may differ from the post-junctional (muscle) NAChR; and some of them may be similar to those found in autonomic ganglia. It is important to note that some of these pre-junctional receptors may also be blocked by our neuromuscular blocking drugs (see later).

17.3.2 Post-synaptic Receptors

Can be junctional or extrajunctional. Extrajunctional receptors are up-regulated (increased in number ± sensitivity):

- If denervation of the muscle occurs
- With extensive burn injuries
- If disuse of muscle occurs

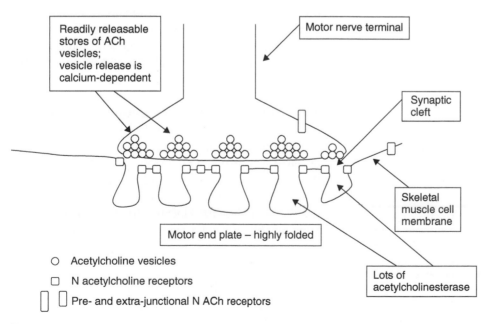

Figure 17.1 The neuromuscular junction.

Denervation and burns result in up-regulation of receptors throughout the post-synaptic muscle membrane, whereas disuse results in up-regulation of receptors in the perijunctional area only. Although both junctional and extra-junctional receptors can be affected by neuromuscular blocking drugs, only those receptors in or near the NMJ can participate in normal neuromuscular transmission. The normal channel 'open' time is about 1 ms for junctional receptors, but much longer for extra-junctional receptors (partly related to reduced proximity of acetylcholinesterase).

In order for successful neuromuscular transmission to occur, 5–20% of motor end plate NAChRs must be 'open' so that an all-or-none muscle action potential can be generated (5–20% is quoted because NMJs vary in sensitivity.) Therefore, there are many 'spare' receptors; and these spare receptors offer a large 'margin of safety to neuromuscular transmission', which forms the basis of our clinical monitoring of neuromuscular blockade.

The large number of spare receptors make neuromuscular block by non-depolarising agents more difficult, whereas they make block by depolarising agents much easier.

Quantal release of ACh occurs spontaneously, and randomly, and each quantal packet contains insufficient ACh for a muscle action potential to be generated, but sufficient for some depolarisation of the motor end plate, which can be recorded by electro-physiological techniques as a 'mini end-plate potential' (MEPP). If several quanta are released simultaneously, then MEPP summation occurs, but a muscle action potential is only generated when the end plate is depolarised sufficiently to reach its threshold potential.

17.3.3 Order of Blockade of Muscle Activity

The commonly quoted order of blockade of muscle activity for the dog is shown in Figure 17.2. Recovery from, or reversal of, neuromuscular blockade tends to follow the reverse order, but not always exactly. The order of muscle relaxation and recovery also depends upon local muscle blood flow (to deliver the NMB, and take it away) and temperature (which affects metabolism and physiological current generation). A recent study using rocuronium in

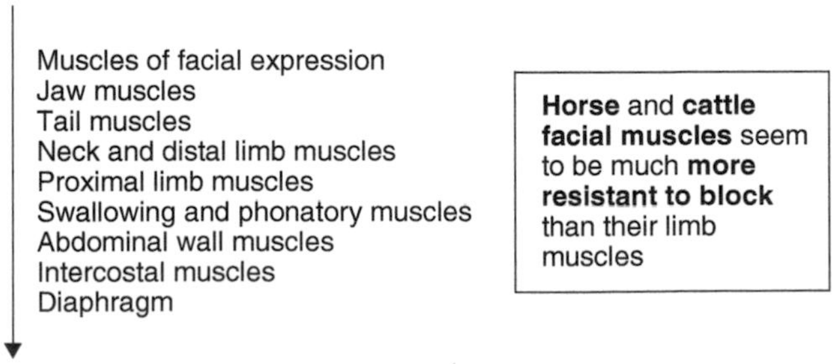

Muscles of facial expression
Jaw muscles
Tail muscles
Neck and distal limb muscles
Proximal limb muscles
Swallowing and phonatory muscles
Abdominal wall muscles
Intercostal muscles
Diaphragm

Horse and **cattle facial muscles** seem to be much **more resistant to block** than their limb muscles

Figure 17.2 The normal sequence of muscle block quoted for the dog.

dogs demonstrated that laryngeal muscle activity took longer to return than pelvic limb muscular activity. So, although in theory, it is possible to titrate neuromuscular block to get relaxation of, e.g. the extra-ocular muscles for eye surgery, whilst maintaining respiratory muscle function, in practice, this is very difficult to do, as patients can respond quite individually to the NMBs. Therefore, you should always be prepared to provide artificial ventilation.

17.3.4 Development of NMBs

The South American Indians used 'arrow poison' to dart their prey, which they could then catch because they were immobilised. The highly ionised compound cannot be absorbed via the gastrointestinal tract, so the eater cannot suffer from the same poison. They used an extract, which we call 'curare', primarily from the leaves and bark of a tropical climbing plant/liana called *Chondrodendron tomentosum*. (*Strychnos toxifera* is another liana from which similar compounds can be derived.) Later, this was purified, and the active substance was called d-tubocurarine. Muscle relaxation was demonstrated to be reversible, as animals were shown to recover as long as their ventilation was supported. Muscle relaxants gained a place in balanced anaesthesia, but because d-tubocurarine, and later succinylcholine, were found to have many unwanted side effects, the race started to try to discover newer and better drugs that did not cause massive histamine release, and did not have too much activity at autonomic ganglia or cardiac muscarinic acetylcholine receptors.

Drug development was also driven by two important aspects of muscle relaxation for humans. Firstly, that neuromuscular block should be rapid in onset, to allow rapid tracheal intubation (to 'secure the airway' and protect the patient's lungs against aspiration); and secondly, that it should be of short duration (in case tracheal intubation is unsuccessful), so that the patient can regain respiratory muscle function as soon as possible (i.e. can almost cope without needing their lungs to be ventilated). Succinylcholine is rapid in onset and has a short duration of action in humans, but it has a number of side effects, so the search was also on for a drug that had rapid onset but short duration and fewer side effects. Although there are several neuromuscular blocking drugs available for use in humans, this discussion will focus on the ones that you may use in veterinary species.

17.3.5 Types of Neuromuscular Blocking Drugs Available

- Non-depolarising NMBs
- Depolarising NMBs

All contain at least one quaternary ammonium group and are highly ionised. Therefore, they are restricted to the extracellular fluid (ECF); they do not cross the blood–brain barrier or the placenta. Because they are restricted to the ECF, their volume of distribution is almost equal to the ECF volume. These drugs do bind proteins, however, and can be around 50% protein-bound in plasma.

Where two quaternary ammonium groups exist, the distance between them is important for their activity (because they interact with the two α subunits of the NAChR). If the length of carbon chain between the two N^+ groups is 10 carbon atoms, then the compound will favour interaction with the muscle-type NAChR of NMJs; whereas if there are only six carbon atoms in the chain, the compound will prefer the neuronal-type NAChR of autonomic ganglia.

17.3.5.1 Non-depolarising NMBs

Non-depolarising NMBs fall into two broad groups:

- The aminosteroids
- The benzylisoquinoliniums

Non-depolarising NMBs are classically thought to act by competing with acetylcholine at the NMJ, where they bind to NAChRs but without causing their 'activation'. Because of the enormous safety margin for neuromuscular transmission (lots of 'spare receptors'), at least 75% of these NAChRs must be blocked by these competitive antagonist non-depolarising NMBs, for any degree of neuromuscular block to be detected, and upwards of 92% NAChR occupancy by non-depolarising NMBs is required for complete block of neuromuscular transmission. (There is some variation, between muscles, of NMJ sensitivity to neuromuscular block.)

The benzylisoquinoliniums are sometimes referred to as the leptocurares (long spindly molecules), and are generally susceptible to hydrolysis by non-specific plasma esterases or to spontaneous Hofmann elimination (at normal body temperature and pH). This contrasts with the aminosteroids, or pachycurares (stumpy fat molecules), which are more resistant to such attack and are instead metabolised by the liver and are more likely to have active metabolites and be cumulative. Metabolites, and some unchanged parent compound, are then excreted in the urine or bile.

The benzylisoquinoliniums are generally more likely to evoke histamine release.

Onset of block is thought to be dependent upon swamping as many NAChRs as possible, so high doses of NMBs tend to be given for rapid onset of block. However, with the more 'potent' non-depolarising NMBs, smaller doses will produce a good degree of neuromuscular block, but the onset of block then tends to be delayed because only a small dose is administered. Overall:

$$\text{Time to onset of block} \propto 1/\text{dose}$$

17.3.5.1.1 Cardiovascular Effects of Non-depolarising NMBs

- Cardiac muscarinic receptor effects (due to receptor block).
- Autonomic ganglia nicotinic receptor effects (due to receptor block).
- Histamine release (as a group, the aminosteroids tend to be more acidic and are less likely to stimulate histamine release than the benzylisoquinoliniums).

The autonomic margin of safety This is the dose difference between that necessary for neuromuscular blockade and that to produce circulatory effects. Vecuronium and cis-atracurium have the widest safety margins. Overall, there is considerable variation between drugs and species, and even between individuals. The prevailing autonomic tone and administration of other drugs may also influence the outcome.

17.3.5.1.2 Characteristics of Incomplete Non-depolarising Neuromuscular Block

Non-depolarising NMBs are competitive antagonists and compete with ACh for post-synaptic NAChRs. Features of non-depolarising block include:

- Slow onset of block compared to depolarising block (because lots of NAChRs have to be blocked).
- No initial muscle fasciculations.
- 'Fade' is demonstrable after tetanic, train-of-four (TOF) stimulation or double-burst stimulation (DBS).
- Post-tetanic potentiation occurs.
- Block is enhanced by other non-depolarising NMBs.
- Block is reversible with anticholinesterases.
- If the post-synaptic muscle is stimulated directly, it will contract.

What is 'fade'? *Fade* refers to the unsustained muscle tension developed by a muscle when incomplete non-depolarising neuromuscular block exists and a supramaximal electrical stimulus (usually a tetanic stimulus or several individual stimuli in quick succession, like TOF) is applied to the motor neuron supplying the muscle under study (Figure 17.3). The electrical stimulus must be supramaximal in order to recruit all the nerve fibres of the motor neuron so that all motor units receive an input.

Why does fade occur with non-depolarising NMBs? Fade is thought to represent a problem with the normal pre-synaptic transmitter recycling, mobilisation, and release. There are pre-synaptic autoreceptors that are involved in both positive and negative feedback of transmitter release. Pre-synaptic NAChR (subtype α3β2) blockade by non-depolarising NMBs can reduce normal ACh

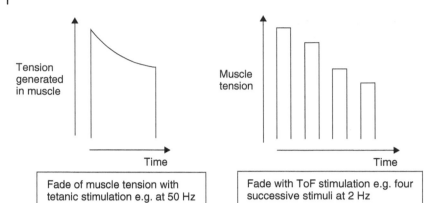

Figure 17.3 Representation of 'fade'.

mobilisation and release. Pre-synaptic (possibly nicotinic) receptor blockade may reduce choline re-uptake, and therefore slow the synthesis of ACh. Pre- and post-synaptic receptors/ion channels may also be susceptible to nonspecific 'open channel block', e.g. by the NMB (especially if it is present in high concentration), and possibly even by ACh itself.

With depolarising block (phase I), fade is minimal (and usually said not to occur because clinically significant fade is not apparent) because succinylcholine does not inhibit the pre-synaptic NAChR ($\alpha3\beta2$ subtype) and may affect pre-junctional receptors to enhance transmitter release.

Fade seems to be very variable with TOF stimulation patterns in horses, whereas it is more predictable with tetanic stimulation patterns.

Post-tetanic potentiation This is normally seen as an increase in the muscle tension developed after a period of tetanic stimulation in normal 'non-blocked' muscle. It is thought to occur because of pre-synaptic events, including increased choline re-uptake and enhanced ACh resynthesis (following the large release of transmitter during the tetanic stimulation) and mobilisation of ACh stores from distant reserve stores to the readily releasable stores. Some degree of post-tetanic potentiation remains during partial non-depolarising block, but is not seen during phase I depolarising block. This may be because any enhanced pre-synaptic transmitter release (by the depolarising blocker), occurring at onset of block, has diminished the pre-synaptic stores, or that during phase I block, any further ACh release only serves to reinforce (enhance) the depolarising block.

17.3.5.1.3 Some Non-depolarising NMBs
Aminosteroids include d-tubocurarine, pancuronium, vecuronium, rocuronium. **Benzylisoquinoliniums** include atracurium, cisatracurium, and mivacurium. Table 17.1

summarises some details of commonly used non-depolarising NMBs. These NMBs can be administered by continuous infusion, e.g.:

- Vecuronium: loading dose 0.1 mg/kg IV; then infusion at 0.1 mg/kg/h but titrate as necessary to just maintain one twitch of TOF.
- Rocuronium: Loading dose 0.5 mg/kg IV; infusion 0.2–0.6 mg/kg/h.

NMBs can be categorised according to their onset and duration of action.

Onset
- Rapid: succinylcholine (<1 minute)
- Medium–rapid: rocuronium (one to two minutes)
- Medium: atracurium, vecuronium, mivacurium (one to three minutes)
- Slow: pancuronium (three to five minutes)

Duration
- Ultra–short acting: e.g. succinylcholine (e.g. two to three minutes, but depends upon species)
- Short acting: mivacurium (10–20 minutes)
- Intermediate acting: atracurium, vecuronium (15–40 minutes)
- Long acting: pancuronium (40+ minutes)

If prolonged neuromuscular block is required, e.g. longer than that produced after a single dose of agent, then top-up doses (of around a quarter to a half of the original dose) can be given, or continuous infusions can be administered. Top-up doses are usually given when, e.g. one or more twitches return in response to TOF stimulation or, the first or second response to DBS returns. With continuous infusions, the infusion rate is usually tailored to keep, e.g. just the first twitch response to TOF stimulation or DBS present.

Table 17.1 Features of common non-depolarising neuromuscular blockers.

Drug	First dose (mg/kg)	Onset (min)	Duration (min)	Renal excretion	Biliary excretion	Hepatic metabolism	Histamine release
Atracurium	0.1–0.25	1–3	20–45	Not significant	Not significant	Not significant	Yes
Vecuronium	0.05–0.1	1–3	15–30	15–25%	40–75%	20–30%	No
Pancuronium	0.07	3–5	40–70	80%	5–10%	10–40%	No
Rocuronium	0.35	1–2	20–60	10–25%	50–70%	10–20%	No?
Mivacurium	0.08	1–2–3^a	12–20	Not significant	Not significant	Not significant	Yes

^{a} Depends upon species.

17.3.5.1.4 Pancuronium

A bisquaternary aminosteroid compound. Few side effects, but it can block cardiac muscarinic receptors and cause tachycardia. No histamine release. No autonomic nervous system (ANS) ganglionic effects. Excreted almost entirely unchanged into the urine, therefore potentially cumulative in patients with renal failure.

17.3.5.1.5 Vecuronium

A monoquaternary derivative of pancuronium. Comes as a dry powder that must be reconstituted with water and then has a shelf life of 24 hours in daylight and room temperature. Very few side effects. No ANS ganglion effects, no cardiac muscarinic receptor effects. No histamine release (although sporadic cases of 'anaphylaxis' reported in humans). Very wide autonomic safety margin. Can be used for infusion, but some of its metabolites may have some activity, so possibly slightly cumulative. Not much renal excretion compared to pancuronium, but it is extensively metabolised in the liver; so it is possibly safer in patients with a degree of renal failure, but beware patients with poor hepatic function.

17.3.5.1.6 Rocuronium

Monoquaternary aminosteroid, closely related to vecuronium, but less potent (so tends to be given in higher doses, therefore faster onset [advantage for man] but also longer duration). More stable in aqueous solution than vecuronium; shelf life three months. Few side effects, but more cardiovascular effects: you may observe heart rate and blood pressure changes, and histamine release is more likely than with

vecuronium (rocuronium can cause anaphylaxis in people). Narrower autonomic safety margin than vecuronium. Much less hepatic metabolism than vecuronium (more biliary and urinary excretion), so less likely to produce active metabolites; less cumulative and possibly better suited to long infusions.

17.3.5.1.7 Atracurium

A bisquaternary benzylisoquinolinium compound. The commercially available solution actually consists of several (about 10) isomers, and must be refrigerated until use because of spontaneous degradation at room temperature. Atracurium has a unique elimination pathway. It undergoes spontaneous chemodegradation in plasma (at normal body temperature and pH) by 'Hofmann elimination', independently of hepatic or renal function (therefore useful if hepatic or renal disease). It is also susceptible to non-specific esterase hydrolysis in plasma (Figure 17.4). It is a useful NMB for continuous infusions as it is non-cumulative.

Laudanosine (a product of atracurium chemodegradation) has neurotoxic activities in rats (causes convulsions) because, unlike the parent compound, it can cross the blood–brain barrier. (Laudanosine requires renal excretion for its clearance from plasma.) However, there have been no reports of CNS problems in dogs, cats, or horses. Atracurium can cause histamine release, but has no ANS ganglion effects or cardiac muscarinic effects. It has a wide autonomic safety margin. The commercially available solution is acidified to minimise the likelihood of spontaneous degradation *in vitro*. Storage at room temperature results in a reduction in potency of the order of 5% every 30 days.

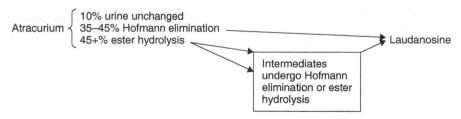

Figure 17.4 Elimination pathways for atracurium.

17.3.5.1.8 Cis-atracurium

Purified form of one of the 10 stereoisomers of atracurium; the cis-cis isomer. More potent than atracurium, therefore the dose required is smaller so the onset of block is longer and the duration of block is shorter. Much less histamine release than atracurium. Wider autonomic safety margin than atracurium. In contrast to atracurium, non-specific plasma esterases do not seem to be involved in metabolism of cisatracurium. Most of it is degraded by Hofmann elimination, with some (15%) excreted unchanged in the urine. Although potentially more laudanosine produced per mg of cis-atracurium administered compared with atracurium, overall laudanosine production is less because a smaller dose is given (it is more potent).

17.3.5.1.9 Mivacurium

A bisquaternary benzylisoquinolinium. Actually exists as three stereoisomers, two of which are 'active'. This molecule has the wrong shape for Hofmann elimination, so **undergoes plasma ester hydrolysis by plasma cholinesterase**. (Plasma cholinesterase is also known as pseudocholinesterase or butyrylcholinesterase.) The rate of hydrolysis depends upon plasma mivacurium concentration, and therefore increasing the dose administered does not prolong the duration of block. Causes some histamine release. No effects at ANS ganglia or cardiac muscarinic receptors. Beware genetic- or organophosphate-induced reduction in plasma cholinesterase activity as the block can then be prolonged. Onset of block appears quicker in cats than in humans.

17.3.5.2 Depolarising NMBs

17.3.5.2.1 Succinylcholine (Suxamethonium) Chloride

Succinylcholine is the only depolarising NMB in clinical use. Succinylcholine consists of two acetylcholine molecules back to back. One molecule of succinylcholine can then result in interaction with the two α subunits of one NAChR, to produce channel activation/opening. This results in generation of muscle action potentials and muscle contractions, seen as inco-ordinated muscle fasciculations. The onset of effect after administration of succinylcholine is rapid because the drug only needs to interact with 5–20% of post-synaptic NAChRs to produce its block. However, unlike the situation with normal neuromuscular transmission whereby the acetylcholine (ACh) transmitter is rapidly broken down, succinylcholine is not hydrolysed by acetylcholinesterase, and can sit on the NAChR for longer, maintaining the channel in its open state. This sustained depolarisation results in post-synaptic membrane refractoriness (because voltage sensitive [voltage-gated] sodium channels in the peri-junctional area become refractory to stimulation), and hence neuromuscular block.

Succinylcholine must diffuse away from the NMJ into the ECF or blood, where it is relatively slowly hydrolysed by plasma/pseudocholinesterase (produced by the liver) to succinylmonocholine (which has a tiny amount of activity), which is then even more slowly broken down by either acetylcholinesterase or plasma cholinesterase to succinic acid and choline. Some succinylcholine is broken down by alkaline hydrolysis, and a small amount may be excreted in the urine unchanged.

The amounts, affinities, and efficacies of pseudocholinesterase vary among species, so that the duration of action of succinylcholine varies among species in addition to being somewhat dose-dependent. For example, humans, cats, and pigs are relatively resistant to succinylcholine block, which therefore only lasts about two to five minutes after large-ish doses. Dogs and horses have intermediate sensitivity, and ruminants are much more sensitive and block with relatively small doses can last around 15–20 minutes. The activity of pseudocholinesterase can be tested with the ester-linked local anaesthetic agent dibucaine (cinchocaine) in the dibucaine test (see Chapter 12). Table 17.2 outlines the species-dependent doses and durations of activity of succinylcholine.

Beware recent treatment with organophosphates as the inhibition of pseudocholinesterase can prolong the block (and increase the chances of a phase II block developing, see below).

Cardiovascular effects Succinylcholine can also interact with other nicotinic, and even muscarinic, ACh receptors, e.g. in autonomic ganglia and at post-synaptic parasympathetic nerve terminals (e.g. in heart and gut). Bradycardia and hypotension are seen in some species, whereas tachycardia and hypertension are seen in others. Bradycardia and hypotension are believed to result from direct cardiac muscarinic cholinergic receptor stimulation with negative inotropic and negative chronotropic effects. Tachycardia and hypertension are believed to follow activation of nicotinic cholinergic receptors in autonomic ganglia. Histamine

Table 17.2 Succinylcholine in different species. Onset of block is within 30–60 seconds.

Species	Dose (mg/kg)	Duration (min)
Dog	0.1–0.3	10–20
Cat	0.5–1	2–6
Pig	0.5–2	2–3
Horse	0.04–0.15	4–1 0
Ruminants	0.02	15 ++

release may also occur, resulting in vasodilation and hypotension (usually with some degree of reflex tachycardia).

Problems with succinylcholine

- Species differences in plasma cholinesterase (pseudocholinesterase/butyrylcholinesterase), and therefore in duration of block.
- Myalgia (muscle pain) after fasciculations; and even muscle damage, e.g. both extensor and flexor muscles are stimulated to contract simultaneously so muscle fibres may tear.
- Release of K^+, phosphate, and myoglobin from damaged muscle cells (beware arrhythmias, kidney damage).
- Malignant hyperthermia trigger in pigs, dogs, humans, horses, cats.
- Transient increase in intra-ocular pressure during fasciculations of extra-ocular muscles.
- Transient increase in intragastric pressure during abdominal muscle fasciculations.
- In burns patients, with increased numbers of extrajunctional receptors that are responsive to succinylcholine, these channels can remain open for a relatively long time (are often called 'leaky'), and so ionic movements continue for longer. Hyperkalaemia may result.
- Burns patients and those with denervation or disuse have upregulation of extrajunctional receptors, and therefore are more susceptible to depolarising block, but are more resistant to non-depolarising block (because more of these 'spare' receptors need blocking).
- Beware recent treatment with organophosphate compounds that can result in prolonged block.
- Occasional histamine release.
- Succinylcholine should be kept in the refrigerator as it undergoes spontaneous hydrolysis, which is more rapid at room temperature.

17.3.5.2.2 Characteristics of Incomplete Depolarising Neuromuscular Blockade

Initial depolarising block (Phase I block) There is rapid onset of initial depolarisation with muscle fasciculations, then neuromuscular block ensues.

The features of phase I block:

- Shows no 'fade' with tetanic stimulation, TOF stimulation or DBS
- Shows no post-tetanic potentiation
- Can be enhanced by anticholinesterases (which allow an increase in the local ACh concentration)
- Direct stimulation of the post-synaptic muscle cell does not elicit contraction

With prolonged action of the drug (seen as an individual response especially in dogs, or following large doses or many top-up doses), the 'blocked' NAChRs may become 'desensitised', and/or the 'pores' that they form when 'open' may become 'blocked' by the physical presence of drug in the ion channel (called 'open channel block'). Once this happens (exact mechanism unknown), the post-synaptic membrane can repolarise, and the neuromuscular block then takes on the characteristics of a non-depolarising block (see below).

Desensitisation block (Phase II block) The features of phase II block:

- 'Fade' can be demonstrated
- Post-tetanic potentiation occurs
- Block can now be reversed with anticholinesterases
- Direct muscle stimulation results in contraction

The development of phase II block and its reversibility with anticholinesterases is not predictable, but it commonly follows a single dose of succinylcholine in dogs.

Other terms you may hear are 'dual block' (or 'raised-threshold' block), which may occur as receptor desensitisation takes place and the membrane potential is returning towards normal, but remains somewhat refractory to stimulation.

17.3.6 Monitoring of Patients

17.3.6.1 Monitoring Anaesthetic Depth in a Paralysed Patient

Anaesthetic depth is monitored, mainly by looking at signs from the ANS:

- Heart rate
- Blood pressure
- Sweating
- Salivation
- Lacrimation
- Defecation/urination (possibly anal tone). The anal sphincter has an internal smooth muscle part, and an external striated muscle part; only the latter is affected by NMBs.
- Some voluntary motor movements may be possible. Because we rarely produce a 100% block and different muscles have different sensitivies to neuromuscular blockade, there is the potential for some movement. This may be a tongue curl or a paw movement. Aγ motor neuron NMJs tend to be blocked first (so that postural muscle strength/tone is lost first), whereas Aα fibre NMJs may be more resistant to allow occasional voluntary movement despite seemingly adequate block.

17.3.6.2 Monitoring Neuromuscular Blockade

What follows below relates mainly to the non-depolarising agents. We have already determined that in order for any degree of muscle weakness or relaxation to become apparent, we must block at least 75% of post-synaptic NAChRs with a non-depolarising NMB. Complete relaxation requires at least 92% receptor occupancy. Normally, between 75 and 85% receptor blockade is sufficient for good surgical conditions.

Simply monitoring muscle tone, we can assess:

- **Diaphragmatic movements** (i.e. the animal 'fights the ventilator') as the block wears off. This is easier to 'see' with capnography (e.g. 'curare clefts'; see Chapter 18).
- You may note a decrease in **chest compliance** during ventilation when the chest muscles 'tone up' as the block wears off (compliance may be measured by the use of spirometry).
- **Jaw tone** increases as the block wears off.
- **Eye position** alters as the block wears off (i.e. in dogs, a relaxed central eye rotates forwards and downwards if anaesthetic depth is at a surgical plane).
- **Reflex activity** returns as the block wears off, e.g. palpebral reflexes and limb withdrawal reflexes return.

We can, however, monitor the degree of neuromuscular block more precisely than this. For effective neuromuscular blockade, we must block most of the normal neuromuscular transmission so we can only 'measure' what remains. This is where all those spare receptors are useful to help us measure the degree of neuromuscular blockade. Now, if we apply an electrical stimulus to the motor nerve of a muscle whose action ('twitch response') we can 'observe', we can gauge the muscle response: e.g. for the peroneal nerve we observe digital extension or hock flexion; for the ulnar nerve, we observe digit and carpal flexion; for the dorsal buccal branch of facial nerve, we observe muzzle (orbicularis oris) twitch. As the degree of neuromuscular block is increased, we expect to see less muscle movement as a result of electrical stimulation of the motor nerve.

The electrical stimulus applied (by the peripheral nerve stimulator, Figure 17.5) must be 'supramaximal' in order to recruit all the nerve fibres to the motor unit of our attention. Usually supramaximal stimuli are of the order of 50 mA minimum (some say up to 100 mA). By convention, the **n**egative electrode is placed directly over the **n**erve to be stimulated, whereas the **p**ositive electrode is placed more **p**roximally along the course of the nerve.

It is good practice to apply a supramaximal tetanic (50 Hz) stimulus for two to five seconds before assessing response to nerve stimulation by our chosen stimulus pattern. This 'stabilisation' technique ensures that all nerve fibres of the motor unit are recruited, and that the

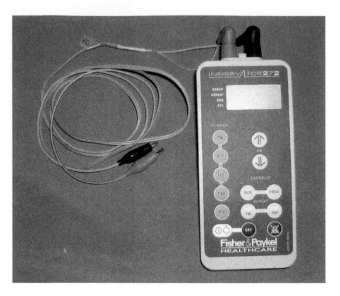

Figure 17.5 Fisher & Paykel Innervator 272™ peripheral nerve stimulator with positive (red) and negative (black) electrodes attached for peripheral nerve stimulation by single twitch (TW), tetanic (TET), train-of-four (TOF) or double-burst stimulation (DBS). The unit can also provide a post-tetanic count (PTC), which can also help determine depth of neuromuscular block.

maximum possible 'baseline' muscle response is evoked in response to the nerve stimulation. This must be done before neuromuscular blocking drugs are given, so that when the block wears off, or is reversed, we know what the maximum response should be. Otherwise things can get quite confusing because it can appear that recovery to more than 100% of baseline response is possible. Such enhanced evoked mechanical response after repeated indirect motor nerve stimulation is referred to as the 'staircase phenomenon'. The mechanism is not fully understood, but recruitment of previously inactive nerve fibres, increase in local blood flow, and increased phosphorylation of the regulatory light chains of myosin (which effectively increases the muscle's sensitivity to calcium) may be involved. If using TOF or DBS (rather than a single tetanic stimulus), each set of four or two stimuli, respectively, incorporates its own control, so that precise determination of a true baseline measurement is not always necessary for clinical cases, whereas it may be more crucial for research studies. Nevertheless, the duration and type of nerve stimulation before NMB administration can also hugely influence the measured onset and duration of NMB effect. To reduce variation between studies, it has therefore been suggested that tetanic preconditioning, using a two- to five-second tetanic (50 Hz) stimulus, be applied to shorten the time required to achieve baseline stabilisation as this particular technique has led to the least variation in results.

When we apply a stimulus to a peripheral nerve, we can:

- Observe the visual twitch response.
- Palpate the 'tactile' twitch response.
- Transduce the mechanical 'twitch' response: force transduction measures the evoked tension in the muscle (mechanomyography); acceleration transduction measures the evoked acceleration of the moving part (acceleromyography); deformation of a material may be measured using a piezoelectric polymer and mechanosensor (kinemyography; Datex Ohmeda M-NMT module).
- Measure the electrical response of the muscle: electromyography (EMG).
- Measure the low frequency sounds created during muscle contractions using special microphones. Originally called acoustic myography, but now called phonomyography. Very easily applicable in the clinical situation as it can be applied to any muscle, even those from which it would otherwise be difficult to record force of contraction or acceleration (e.g. peri-ocular facial muscles).

Because our visual and tactile acuity is not good, especially when trying to compare a response to one seen five minutes previously, various techniques can be used to increase our chances of detecting changes. These involve different modes of applying our electrical stimulus.

Electrical stimuli can be applied:

- In **single discharges (TW)**, giving individual twitch (TW) responses, which can be repeated when the observer requires or automatically at 0.1–1 Hz frequency.
- In a **TOF pattern**, giving T1, T2, T3, and T4 responses, which can also be repeated when the observer requires or automatically at intervals of 10 seconds (Figure 17.6).
- In a **DBS pattern**, giving D1 and D2 responses, repeated as necessary or automatically at intervals of 10 seconds (Figure 17.6).
- As a **tetanic stimulus (TET)** (e.g. for one to five seconds), which can be repeated as required.

The responses to single stimuli are not easy to assess or compare. With TOF, DBS, and TET, we can see 'fade'; and with TOF and DBS, we can compare the response to the final stimulus with that to the first during the same time frame of stimulation (see **TOF ratio** and **DBS ratio** below).

If fade exists, we may see or feel (or, better, measure) that the last twitch in the TOF, or the response to the second short burst with DBS, is less obvious than the first. (If a depolarising NMB was used, we can only see that the overall twitch response magnitude is less, compared to the pre-block twitch response; as fade does not occur, at least with phase I block.) Figure 17.7 shows the differing muscle twitch responses with TOF stimulation following various degrees of block with a non-depolarising NMB.

Figure 17.6 Two different forms of electrical stimulation: train-of-four stimulation (TOF) and double-burst stimulation (DBS).

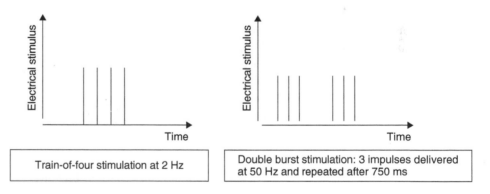

Train-of-four stimulation at 2 Hz

Double burst stimulation: 3 impulses delivered at 50 Hz and repeated after 750 ms

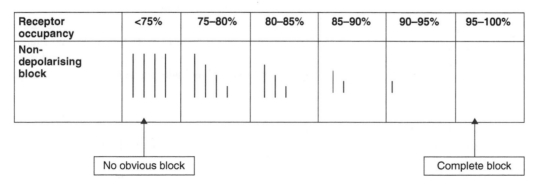

Receptor occupancy	<75%	75–80%	80–85%	85–90%	90–95%	95–100%
Non-depolarising block						

No obvious block

Complete block

Figure 17.7 Muscle twitch responses recorded with train-of-four (TOF) stimulation (with non-depolarising NMB).

With TOF stimulation:

- The last (fourth) twitch is all but abolished with just over 75% receptor blockade by non-depolarising blocker.
- The third and second (as well as fourth) twitches are all but abolished with c. 85–90% receptor block.
- The first twitch (as well as the second, third, and fourth) is all but abolished with c. 92 + % receptor blockade.

The twitch response to single electrical stimuli (TW) reflects events at the post-junctional membrane, whereas the responses to TET, TOF, or DBS reflect events at the pre-synaptic membrane too.

The stimulated nerve impulses result in ACh release at the NMJ, which competes with the non-depolarising NMB for NAChRs; but depolarising neuromuscular blockade is non-competitive because succinylcholine results in membrane refractoriness (phase I block) to any released ACh (at least whilst phase I block lasts).

You may hear of the **TOF ratio**. This is the ratio of the response to the fourth stimulus (i.e. fourth twitch 'height'), compared to the response to the first stimulus (i.e. first twitch 'height'). If the TOF ratio is ≥0.7, it is almost impossible to detect fade visually. We can only really detect TOF ratios of <0.4–0.5 visually or even palpably. Because it is considered that adequate recovery of muscle function after block wears off (or is reversed), requires a TOF ratio of at least 0.7, and our ability to detect TOF ratios of ≥0.7 is almost impossible, then the DBS technique was devised. With this technique, possibly because of the larger responses, we can appreciate visually and palpably a **DBS ratio** (last response compared to first) of 0.67. Interestingly, a recent study showed that there was a 50% success rate in visually identifying fade of 0.7 by both TOF and DBS, with DBS having a slight advantage at greater degrees of fade (deeper levels of block; smaller ratios). At lesser degrees of fade (shallower block; greater ratios), although TOF appeared to have a slight advantage over DBS, success rates were less than 50% with both techniques. It is, however, now believed that for a patient to be able to breathe adequately on its own, and maintain adequate laryngeal and pharyngeal protective reflexes (to protect the airway from, e.g. aspiration), a TOF ratio of ≥0.9 is necessary. Hence, most modern devices used to monitor neuromuscular blockade include some means of transducing the twitch response to peripheral nerve stimulation to give an objective, quantitative measure (instead of subjective, qualitative estimations).

17.4 Factors Affecting Neuromuscular Block

17.4.1 Drugs

17.4.1.1 Volatile Anaesthetic Agents
These enhance neuromuscular block in a dose-dependent fashion. Different volatile agents may affect different NMBs differently; e.g. for vecuronium and succinylcholine, isoflurane enhances the block more than halothane.

There may be several mechanisms for this, including alteration of regional muscle blood flow (e.g. isoflurane is a potent vasodilator), calcium channel blockade (pre-synaptically to reduce transmitter release, and post-synaptically to reduce muscle response/contraction), and CNS depression (to reduce overall muscle tone).

17.4.1.2 Injectable Anaesthetic Agents
These have minimal effects.

17.4.1.3 Antibiotics
Tetracyclines, macrolides, aminoglycosides, polymixin B, metronidazole (not penicillins or cephalosporins or trimethoprim potentiated sulphonamides [TMPS]) may block (non- specifically) both pre- and post-junctional calcium channels. This results in both reduced ACh release and reduced response to ACh.

17.4.1.4 Local Anaesthetics
These inhibit nerve conduction, synaptic transmission and skeletal muscle excitation-contraction coupling. Remember that ester-linked local anaesthetics can also compete with succinylcholine and mivacurium for metabolism by plasma cholinesterase, so succinylcholine and mivacurium block could potentially be prolonged (although unlikely at clinical doses).

17.4.1.5 Diuretics
Diuretics shrink the ECF volume, so reduce the volume of distribution of these compounds and enhance their actions by effectively increasing their concentration, but they also increase glomerular filtration rate (GFR) and renal excretion. Diuretics may also cause electrolyte changes that may affect neuromuscular blockade (see below).

17.4.1.6 Antidysrhythmics and Anticonvulsants
Local anaesthetics, beta blockers, calcium channel blockers, barbiturates, and phenytoin may all reduce pre-synaptic ACh release.

17.4.1.7 Dantrolene

Dantrolene blocks neuromuscular excitation–contraction coupling and enhances neuromuscular block.

17.4.1.8 Corticosteroids

These increase choline-acetyl-transferase activity, and so increase transmitter availability, helping to reverse non-depolarising block, but enhancing depolarising block.

17.4.1.9 Lithium Compounds (e.g. Anticonvulsants)

Lithium compounds inhibit cholinesterase activity, so prolong depolarising (and possibly mivacurium), neuromuscular block, but reduce the potency and duration of non-depolarising block.

17.4.1.10 Metoclopramide

This inhibits cholinesterase activity and so enhances the duration of depolarising (and possibly mivacurium) block, but reduces the potency and duration of non-depolarising blockers.

17.4.1.11 Organophosphate Compounds

These inhibit acetylcholinesterase and pseudocholinesterase, and so increase ACh availability at NMJs, and reduce metabolism of succinylcholine and mivacurium. They prolong depolarising and mivacurium block, and reduce the potency and duration of non-depolarising (bar mivacurium) block. They may increase the chance of phase II block developing with succinylcholine.

17.4.1.12 Electrolytes

17.4.1.12.1 Mg^{2+}

ECF hypermagnesaemia enhances non-depolarising block (reduces pre-synaptic transmitter release and post-synaptic membrane responsiveness), and may shorten depolarising (and mivacurium) block due to enhancement of plasma cholinesterase (pseudocholinesterase) activity.

17.4.1.12.2 K^+

Acute increase in extracellular potassium causes depolarisation (the equilibrium potential becomes less negative) of membranes (pre- and post-synaptic), and thus antagonises non-depolarising block (by enhancing ACh release), but enhances depolarising block. Acute decrease in ECF potassium causes hyperpolarisation (the equilibrium potential becomes more negative), and thus increases the resistance to depolarising block (by decreasing ACh release), but enhances non-depolarising block.

17.4.1.12.3 Ca^{2+}

Hypocalcaemia reduces ACh release and muscle response, so enhances non-depolarising block. Hypercalcaemia enhances ACh release and may weakly antagonise non-depolarising block.

17.4.2 Other Factors Affecting Neuromuscular Block

17.4.2.1 pH

Respiratory and metabolic perturbations may affect different NMBs differently. Acidosis slows, and alkalosis speeds up, Hofmann elimination, but such pH changes are unlikely to have much effect over the range of pH compatible with life (possibly because pH changes affect ester hydrolysis in an opposite way to how they affect Hofmann elimination i.e. acidosis speeds up, and alkalosis slows, ester hydrolysis). Respiratory acidosis has been shown to prolong the action of some non-depolarising NMBs (e.g. atracurium and vecuronium); and respiratory alkalosis antagonises them. Metabolic alkalosis has been shown to prolong block by pancuronium.

17.4.2.2 Temperature

Has variable effects. Hypothermia can slow the circulation and metabolism and alter drug pharmacokinetics. Mild hypothermia tends to antagonise non-depolarising blocks (action potential duration is increased, so more ACh is released), but deep hypothermia enhances non-depolarising block (reduces ACh release and delays drug elimination). Onset of block is also delayed if circulation is slowed, so beware overdosing in cold animals.

17.4.2.3 Age

Receptor types at NMJs, ECF volume, and metabolic capacity all change with age. Neonates are 'mini-myasthenics' and have an increased sensitivity to non-depolarising NMBs (least noticeable with atracurium), but are relatively resistant to succinylcholine. They also have a relatively large ECF, so can be easy to overdose at first; but elimination (hepatic/plasma cholinesterase) is often slower so that drug action can be prolonged. Geriatrics also have increased sensitivity to non-depolarising NMBs (least noticeable with atracurium) due to reduction in ECF volume (relative increase in body fat, e.g. sarcopaenic obesity), reduction in hepatic and renal blood flow and function, and NMJ changes.

17.4.2.4 Gender

Females tend to be more susceptible to NMBs than males because they have relatively more body fat, so have relatively less ECF volume (therefore they have a smaller volume of distribution for the drugs).

17.4.2.5 Obesity

Obese patients have a relatively low ECF, so are more susceptible to neuromuscular block; but also tend to have higher plasma cholinesterase, so are actually slightly more resistant to succinylcholine and mivacurium.

17.4.2.6 Hypovolaemia

Reduction in ECF volume, of any cause, can increase susceptibility to neuromuscular block.

17.4.2.7 Pregnancy

Pregnancy increases blood volume, and therefore ECF volume, but decreases plasma cholinesterase activity. Pregnant animals may seem relatively resistant to non-depolarising blockers at first, although their action may then be prolonged. They are more susceptible to prolonged block with succinylcholine (and mivacurium).

17.4.2.8 Liver Disease

Reduced plasma cholinesterase increases sensitivity to succinylcholine and also mivacurium. Reduced hepatic metabolism of aminosteroids delays their elimination. If generalised oedema, (due to hypoproteinaemia), and therefore increased ECF volume accompanies the hepatic disease, then patients may initially seem more resistant to neuromuscular block, but then drug elimination takes longer. Most problems are seen with infusions or multiple doses.

17.4.2.9 Kidney Disease

Certain NMBs (gallamine, pancuronium, pipecuronium) are excreted almost entirely unchanged in the urine, so beware prolonged action if renal function is poor. (Plasma cholinesterase may be reduced too.)

17.4.2.10 Diabetes Mellitus

Duration of action of vecuronium and rocuronium are shorter in diabetic dogs, whereas the duration of action of atracurium is unaffected. In humans, the opposite seems to be the case for the aminosteroid NMBs. In people, the diabetic polyneuropathy that can accompany both type 1 and 2 diabetes mellitus, even when subclinical, can require higher supramaximal currents for nerve stimulation, and can also delay recovery from non-depolarising NMBs, which also predisposes these patients to residual neuromuscular block. The reason/s for the discrepancy is/are unknown, but diabetic dogs may also be Cushingoid or receive exogenous corticosteroids that have been shown to antagonise the effects of non-depolarising agents. Other pharmacokinetic factors may also be involved (altered volume of distribution, hepatic enzyme induction, or altered renal clearance), but blood glucose control does not seem to be directly involved.

17.4.2.11 Burns

Increased susceptibility to succinylcholine block (increase in number of NAChRs), but increased resistance to non-depolarising block.

17.4.2.12 Myotonia

Increased susceptibility to succinylcholine.

17.4.2.13 Myasthenia

Increased susceptibility to non-depolarising block (fewer functional receptors) and increased resistance to succinylcholine.

17.4.2.14 Denervation/Disuse

Increased sensitivity to succinylcholine (more receptors), but increased resistance to non-depolarising NMBs.

17.4.2.15 Genetic Susceptibility

Genetic susceptibility to malignant hyperthermia has been reported in the following so far: humans, horses, dogs, pigs, cats, and rats.

17.5 Reversal of Non-depolarising Neuromuscular Blockade

During partial (incomplete) non-depolarising neuromuscular block, if the amount/availability of ACh in the synaptic cleft can be increased, then the block can be antagonised, and muscular strength can be restored because the extra ACh competes with and displaces the blocker from some of the receptors.

The amount of ACh in the synaptic cleft can be increased by:

- Repetitively stimulating the motor nerve (tetanic stimulation) in the hope of mobilising ACh stores for release at the nerve terminal.
- Using anticholinesterase drugs, which inhibit cholinesterase enzymes (particularly acetylcholinesterase at NMJs).

17.5.1 Anticholinesterases

These are classified according to how they inhibit acetylcholinesterase:

- Reversible inhibition, e.g. edrophonium forms a reversible electrostatic attachment to the enzyme's anionic site.
- Reversible formation of carbamyl esters, e.g. carbamate insecticides such as neostigmine, physostigmine, pyridostigmine are hydrolysed by the enzyme, which itself

becomes carbamylated (at the esteratic site) in the process. The carbamate–enzyme bond then has a half-life of about 30 minutes for dissociation, compared with 40 microseconds for dissociation of the acetylated enzyme (which occurs during 'normal' destruction of ACh), and so the enzyme is effectively out of action for a considerable time.

- Irreversible inactivation by phosphorylation, e.g. the organophosphate insecticides.

Neostigmine also inhibits plasma cholinesterase (butyrylcholinesterase), and can also delay recovery from succinylcholine and mivacurium.

17.5.1.1 Actions of Anticholinesterase

Anticholinesterases act by more than just enzyme inhibition. They have at least two actions:

- Acetylcholinesterase inhibition. In the absence of a previously administered NMB (which otherwise offers some protection, due to the substantial post-synaptic NAChR occupancy persisting for some time even after complete [clinical] neuromuscular block reversal), the increased ACh availability at the NMJ due to acetylcholinesterase inhibition could lead to a depolarising type block itself. (See Further Reading.)
- Pre-synaptic effects. The drugs themselves (or the increase in ACh they cause in the synaptic cleft) act on pre-synaptic receptors to result in antidromic action potentials in the nerve terminals and repetitive firing of motor nerve terminals (resulting in increased ACh release).
- Drugs with quaternary N^+ groups may also be able to act on post-synaptic NAChR, and therefore these enzyme inhibitors may also have some neuromuscular blocking activity; but usually this requires very high (possibly non-clinical) doses.

The enzyme acetylcholinesterase has an 'active site' that is optimally targeted by molecules of certain structures (Figure 17.8). We can see how the enzyme's natural substrate, acetylcholine, 'fits' (Figure 17.9). Enzyme inhibitors are therefore based on the idea that they should be alternative/competitive substrates for the enzyme. There is an optimal 'length' between the quaternary N^+ and the ester linkage of these enzyme inhibitors so that these groups are complementary to the different parts of the active site of the enzyme.

The pharmacological effects of anticholinesterases are due to:

- An increase in ACh availability at the NMJ
- An increase in ACh availability at the autonomic ganglia
- An increase in ACh availability at the post-synaptic parasympathetic nerve terminals (e.g. heart, gastrointestinal tract, respiratory tract)

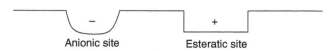

Figure 17.8   Acetylcholinesterase's esteratic site and nearby anionic site.

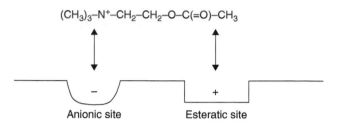

Figure 17.9   Interaction of acetylcholine with acetylcholinesterase.

Therefore, an increase in nicotinic cholinergic receptor activity and in muscarinic cholinergic receptor activity may be observed when these anticholinesterases are administered. Muscarinic effects are evoked by lower concentrations of ACh than those required for production of nicotinic effects at autonomic ganglia and NMJs, but reversal of neuromuscular blockade requires the nicotinic effects, so we cannot avoid producing muscarinic effects, which are therefore a nuisance.

Unwanted muscarinic effects include:

- Bradycardia (even bradyarrhythmias/asystole), and possibly hypotension
- Salivation and increase in other GI secretions
- Miosis
- Lacrimation
- Hyperperistalsis (defecation)
- Urination
- Bronchoconstriction and increased respiratory tract mucus secretion

The expression of these muscarinic effects, however, can be prevented by the concurrent administration of **anticholinergics (antimuscarinics)** such as atropine or glycopyrrolate, which leave the nicotinic (NMJ) effects undisturbed. See Chapters 4, 25, and 28 for more information about anticholinergics, which have their own side effects.

17.5.2 Factors Determining Reversal

Reversal of neuromuscular block depends upon:

- Which NMB was administered.
- The 'depth' of neuromuscular blockade at which reversal is being attempted.
- Which anticholinesterase is chosen and the dose given.

- The chosen 'end point' for 'successful' reversal of neuromuscular block, e.g. a certain TOF ratio (usually ≥0.95) or the ability to breathe spontaneously and with adequate tidal volume. Normal tidal volume is around 10–20 ml/kg; or a baseline measurement of the patient's actual tidal volume may have been taken (e.g. with spirometry or a Wright's respirometer) so that post-reversal tidal volume can be compared with the pre-neuromuscular block value to judge adequacy of reversal. (In humans, the ability to sustain a head-lift, blow out a match, or hand-grip strength can be assessed, but our patients are not so co-operative.)

Note that peripheral chemoreceptors have nicotinic and muscarinic acetylcholine receptors, and are responsible for sensing blood O_2 and CO_2 tensions. The sensitivity of these peripheral chemoreceptors is reduced by some neuromuscular blocking agents (e.g. vecuronium, atracurium), especially to oxygen (reducing the hypoxic drive to breathing), such that not all respiratory depression is due to respiratory muscle paralysis. (But the central chemoreceptors, which are most important for driving the ventilatory response to CO_2, are protected from NMBs by the blood–brain barrier.)

17.5.3 How to Judge Adequacy of Reversal

After reversal drugs have been administered, it is important to observe the patient to ensure that reversal is adequate, paying particular attention to respiratory function. Even in the presence of strong evoked muscle responses to peripheral nerve stimulation, the ability to breathe may be inadequate. **Do not re-awaken the animal from anaesthesia until you are sure that it is not still paralysed.**

To judge adequacy of breathing:

- Observe the patient's respiratory efforts. Does the chest movement look good or pathetic?
- Observe the capnograph trace for its 'form' and for the end tidal carbon dioxide ($ETCO_2$) value as you try to wean the animal off artificial ventilation. The animal should be able to maintain a normal capnograph waveform; and adequacy of its ventilation can be judged by its $ETCO_2$ value, i.e. hypoventilation results in increasing $ETCO_2$ values (unless the patient's spontaneous tidal volume is so small that CO_2 can hardly be exhaled, in which case, one artificially induced or assisted breath will reveal hypercapnia).
- Measure the patient's tidal volume, e.g. using spirometry or a Wright's respirometer. Normal tidal volume during quiet breathing is around 10–20 ml/kg. This can be especially useful if values can be compared to baseline (pre-NMB).

- One can measure the negative pressure that the animal can generate for/on inspiration, by transiently occluding the endotracheal tube, and measuring the inspiratory effort with a manometer/aneroid pressure gauge. Horses are normally able to generate −10 to −25 cmH$_2$O pressure; dogs, around −5 cmH$_2$O.

If it appears that the first dose of reversal drug/s was not enough, then more can be given, usually after about five to seven minutes.

17.5.4 When Should You Reverse Neuromuscular Block?

Before you 'awaken' the animal from its anaesthetic. It is generally taught that non-depolarising neuromuscular block should only be reversed when signs of spontaneous recovery from blockade are observed (whilst the animal is still under general anaesthesia), e.g. when the twitch responses to nerve stimulation re-appear/increase or the animal starts to breathe for itself. This author likes to see the return of at least two, and preferably all four, twitches to TOF stimulation even though 'fade' may still be apparent. This is because too early reversal (when the degree of neuromuscular block is 'deep') may just result in excessive ACh activity at the NMJ that can cause desensitisation (± 'open channel block') of the post-synaptic membrane, which may complicate monitoring of neuromuscular blockade and eventual reversal of the block.

Phase I depolarising blockade cannot be reversed by the use of anticholinesterases (see notes above); and although phase II block may be reversible with anticholinesterases, its reversibility is not predictable, and it may not always be easy to assess if and when phase I block changes character and becomes phase II block.

17.5.5 Should You Always Reverse Non-depolarising Neuromuscular Block?

If one dose of NMB was administered at the beginning of surgery, and that surgery continued for several hours, and there is no reason to assume that the animal cannot metabolise/eliminate the chosen drug, and you are happy that it can breathe adequately on its own (measure tidal volume, or assess end tidal [or arterial blood] carbon dioxide tension over several minutes when the animal is breathing spontaneously, and observe that the animal is capable of keeping these within 'normal' limits), then reversal should not be necessary as there appears to be no significant residual neuromuscular blocking activity. However, some people will still administer a dose of reversal agent just to be absolutely sure.

17.5.6 Problems with Reversal

If there are problems with reversal, e.g. if the animal does not seem to recover from neuromuscular blockade:

- Check its temperature (remember the effects of hypothermia).
- Check for acid–base disturbances, especially respiratory acidosis that happens if an animal hypoventilates (which it may do if the block is inadequately reversed); respiratory acidosis can prolong the duration of block.
- Check for electrolyte disturbances.
- Is the depth of anaesthesia too deep?
- Did you use neuromuscular-block-potentiating antibiotics?
- Are the animal's lungs being hyperventilated inadvertently? If the animal is hypocapnic, then it has very little drive to breathe.
- Is there any chance that the animal has undiagnosed renal, hepatic or underlying muscle disease?

17.5.7 Residual Blockade

This may occur even when visual or tactile assessment suggests that recovery from neuromuscular block is complete. The presence of residual blockade may have consequences for the patient, in particular, poor strength within the upper airway musculature (pharyngeal as well as laryngeal), and has been associated with worse outcomes in human anaesthesia. To avoid residual block in the recovery period, quantitative assessment of the TOF ratio must be performed.

17.5.8 Recurarisation

This occurs when neuromuscular block has apparently been successfully reversed and the patient is breathing well, but, sometime later, the patient seems to become reparalysed despite no further muscle relaxant drugs being given. Potential causes of this phenomenon include:

- Reversal agent has shorter half-life than NMB and it was administered when the degree of neuromuscular block was 'deep'.
- Enterohepatic recirculation of NMB (many NMBs are at least partly excreted unchanged into bile).
- Receptors may become 'desensitised' to NMBs for a while, but with time become sensitive again; so, for NMBs with long half-lives, reblock can occur.
- Inadvertent administration of NMBs, e.g. when residual NMB within fluid lines or connectors is flushed into the patient's vein.

17.5.9 Drugs Used to Reverse Non-depolarising Neuromuscular Block

1) An **anticholinesterase** (e.g. neostigmine or edrophonium).

   Neostigmine may have fewer pre-synaptic effects than edrophonium, but also inhibits plasma cholinesterase (pseudocholinesterase/butyrylcholinesterase). Edrophonium may be a better inhibitor of acetylcholinesterase than neostigmine. Edrophonium and neostigmine may not be equally effective for reversal of atracurium (edrophonium is possibly better) and vecuronium (neostigmine is possibly better).

2) Possibly plus an **anticholinergic antimuscarinic** (e.g. atropine or glycopyrrolate).

   The best way to administer an anticholinesterase and an anticholinergic is so that reversal of neuromuscular block is produced with no/minimal changes in heart rate. To this end, the 'onset' (and duration) of action of the two drugs should be matched as far as possible.

Atropine and edrophonium are well matched. They have similar pharmacokinetics, and, when given together, their onset times are matched (both relatively quick), and they both have relatively short durations of action. However, it seems that in the clinical situation, the duration of action of edrophonium is little different from that of neostigmine, possibly because although its interaction with the enzyme is brief, it is a repeatable interaction. The reader is referred to the Further Reading section for an excellent discussion of the possible reasons for the observed paradoxical effects of edrophonium and atropine in sheep.

Glycopyrrolate and neostigmine are well matched. Both have slightly slower onset times and are long-acting.

Interestingly, many books still recommend the administration of the anticholinergic first, followed a little later by the anticholinesterase, to minimise the risk of causing bradycardia (which is perhaps more detrimental than the tachycardia that you may see initially after the anticholinergic). In reality, both the anticholinesterase and the anticholinergic can be administered simultaneously, slowly intravenously, whilst monitoring the heart rate and rhythm carefully.

In horses (and humans), edrophonium seems to have very few muscarinic effects, and therefore very few cardiovascular side effects, so inclusion of an anticholinergic is not always necessary, i.e. edrophonium can be used on its own safely. In horses, it is useful not to have to give anticholinergics as these can reduce gut motility and have been blamed for causing post-operative colic. Edrophonium has, however, not been readily available, at least in the UK, in the recent past.

17.6   Doses for Dogs (and Cats)

After vecuronium, either of these combinations:

- Neostigmine   (0.08 mg/kg) + atropine   (0.04 mg/kg) slowly IV.
- Neostigmine   (0.08 mg/kg) + glycopyrrolate   (0.01–0.02 mg/kg) slowly IV.

After atracurium:
Edrophonium 0.1–0.5 mg/kg (possibly + atropine [0.04 mg/kg]) slowly IV.

17.7   Doses for Horses

After atracurium, at c. 0.1 mg/kg, edrophonium alone can be administered at 0.1 mg/kg; up to 0.5 mg/kg if necessary.

17.7.1   Sugammadex

Sugammadex is a gamma cyclodextrin compound. Cyclodextrins are cyclic oligosaccharides that can encapsulate lipophilic molecules such as steroidal compounds. Being water soluble, cyclodextrins can allow lipophilic compounds to be solubilised in water. Sugammadex is specially sized and shaped so that one rocuronium molecule fits into the cavity of its ring, aided by electrostatic interaction between the negatively charged side chains of the cyclodextrin interacting with the positively charged quaternary nitrogen groups of the rocuronium, which locks the neuromuscular blocking molecule in place. This 'lock' is irreversible once made, and therefore further access of bound rocuronium to NAChRs is prevented, and dissociation of rocuronium from NAChRs is encouraged when the local rocuronium concentration falls; hence, reversal of neuromuscular block is achieved. The complex (1 sugammadex + 1 rocuronium) is filtered by the glomerulus and excreted in urine. Sugammadex can also bind other aminosteroid NMBs, e.g. vecuronium (also in a 1 : 1 ratio), but with much less affinity than rocuronium. Sugammadex, however, will not encapsulate the benzylisoquinoliniums as their shape/structure does not 'fit the hole in the doughnut'.

Sugammadex has no direct cholinergic effects, so there is no need to administer an anticholinergic compound alongside it, which therefore avoids the unwanted effects of both anticholinesterase and anticholinergic drugs. Sugammadex reverses profound neuromuscular block by rocuronium, and is three times faster than using an anticholinesterase. Sugammadex has been investigated in dogs and been found to reverse profound rocuronium or vecuronium neuromuscular blockade; and in horses, to reverse profound rocuronium

block. Unlike anticholinesterases, sugammadex is safe to give in the presence of 'deep' rocuronium block because it does not increase the local acetylcholine concentration at the NMJ. In people, sugammadex can cause hypersensitivity reactions ranging from mild (urticaria, sneezing) to full-blown anaphylaxis.

17.7.1.1   Alfaxalone

Alfaxalone is solubilised in 2 alpha-hydroxypropyl beta cyclodextrin. This beta cyclodextrin is doughnut-shaped and the central cavity is a hydrophobic place where the lipophilic neurosteroid, alfaxalone, can be carried. Alfaxalone does not fit into the central cavity of sugammadex, and rocuronium does not fit the central cavity of 2 alpha-hydroxypropyl beta cyclodextrin.

17.8   Notes

17.8.1   Fumarates

Gantacurium is an ultra-short acting non-depolarising neuromuscular blocking agent belonging to a new class of NMBs: the fumarates (or olefinic [double-bonded] isoquinolinium diesters). Gantacurium itself is a chlorofumarate; an asymmetric enantiomeric (single isomer) olefinic isoquinolinium diester of chlorofumaric acid. It is inactivated by two spontaneous processes, neither of which involve the liver or kidneys. The first of these involves a rapid chemical degradation that involves adduction to L-cysteine at the central olefinic double-bond. L-cysteine adduction involves the replacement of a chlorine with L-cysteine that results in the formation of a heterocyclic ring within the overall structure, rendering it inactive as an NMB. The second process is a slower destruction, of both the adduct and the parent compound, by pH-dependent (alkaline) ester hydrolysis in plasma. If block is very profound, exogenous L-cysteine can be administered to hasten block reversal.

CW002, an analogue of gantacurium, is also a fumarate non-depolarising NMB compound but lacks chlorine at the fumarate double-bond and is symmetrical. Like gantacurium, however, it can also be inactivated by L-cysteine-adduction, but the process appears to be pH-dependent and is slower than for gantacurium, making it an intermediate-acting NMB. Similarly to gantacurium, if neuromuscular block is very profound, exogenous L-cysteine can be administered to hasten its reversal.

Gantacurium and CW002 appear to be associated with few autonomic side effects and minimal histamine release.

Gantacurium and CW002 have been investigated as alternatives to succinylcholine in humans. Whilst CW002 is not yet available for clinical use, gantacurium has been investigated in the cat to facilitate tracheal intubation.

CW011, another analogue of gantacurium, is a non-halogenated olefinic isoquinolinium diester NMB with slower degradation by endogenous L-cysteine adduction, and is therefore intermediate-acting. Little clinical information is currently available.

17.8.1.1 Calabadions

In conjunction with the continued development of new muscle relaxants, new antagonists such as **calabadion 1** and **2** are in development to allow reversal to be performed at any time point. These compounds are acyclic members of the cucurbit[n]uril family of so-called 'molecular containers', and, by being flexible and able to expand their 'cavities', they can encapsulate both the aminosteroidal and the larger benzylisoquinolinium NMBs. These calabadions are rapidly excreted by the kidneys to appear in the urine, presumably still containing their captured NMB targets.

Both calabadion 1 and 2 can reverse vecuronium, rocuronium, and cisatracurium even at deep levels of neuromuscular blockade. Interestingly, calabadion 1 has also been shown to form inclusion complexes with local anaesthetics in aqueous solution *in vitro*, so may provide another means of treating local anaesthetic toxicity in the future.

Further Reading

Andersson, M.L., Moller, A.M., and Wildgaard, K. (2019). Butyrylcholinesterase deficiency and its clinical importance in anaesthesia: a systematic review. *Anaesthesia* 74: 518–528.

Armendariz-Buil, I., Lobat-Solores, F., and Aguilera-Celorrio, L. (2016). Diabetes mellitus and neuromuscular blockade: a review. *Journal of Diabetes and Metabolism* 7 https://doi.org/10.4172/2155-6156.1000678.

Bradbury, A.G. and Clutton, R.E. (2016). Are neuromuscular blocking agents being misused in laboratory pigs? *British Journal of Anaesthesia* 116: 476–485.

Bowdle, A., Bussey, L., Michaelsen, K., Jelacic, S., Nair, B., Togashi, K., and Hulvershorn, J. (2020). A comparison of a prototype electromyograph vs. a mechanomyograph and an acceleromyograph for assessment of neuromuscular blockade. *Anaesthesia* 75: 187–195.

Clutton, R.E. and Glasby, M. (2008). Cardiovascular and autonomic nervous effects of edrophonium and atropine combinations during neuromuscular blockade antagonism in sheep. *Veterinary Anaesthesia and Analgesia* 35: 191–200.

De Boer, H.D. and Carlos, R.V. (2018). New drug developments for neuromuscular blockade and reversal: gantacurium, CW002, CW011 and calabadion. *Current Anesthesiology Reports* 8: 119–124.

Fuchs-Buder, T., Schreiber, J.-U., and Meistelman, C. (2009). Monitoring neuromuscular blockade: an update. *Anaesthesia* 64 (Suppl 1): 82–89.

Haga, H.A., Betternberg, V., and Lervik, S. (2019). Rocuronium infusion: a higher rate is needed in diabetic than nondiabetic dogs. *Veterinary Anaesthesia and Analgesia* 46: 28–35.

Hoffmann, U., Grosse-Sundrup, M., Elkermann-Haerter, K. et al. (2013). Calabadion: a new agent to reverse the effects of benzylisoquinoline and steroidal neuromuscular-blocking agents. *Anesthesiology* 119: 317–325.

Hunter, J.M. (2017). Reversal of residual neuromuscular block: complications associated with perioperative management of muscle relaxation. *British Journal of Anaesthesia* 119 (Suppl.1): i52–i62.

Hunter, J.M. (2018a). Optimising conditions for tracheal intubation: should neuromuscular blocking agents always be used? *British Journal of Anaesthesia* 120: 1150–1153.

Hunter, J.M. (2018b). Qualitative monitoring is inadequate for reliably determining full recovery from neuromuscular block whatever the protocol used. *British Journal of Anaesthesia* 121: 499–500.

Jones, R.S., Auer, U., and Mosing, M. (2015). Reversal of neuromuscular block in companion animals. *Veterinary Anaesthesia and Analgesia* 42: 455–471.

Khirwadkar, R. and Hunter, J.M. (2012). Neuromuscular physiology and pharmacology: an update. *Continuing Education in Anaesthesia, Critical Care and Pain* 12: 237–244.

Kopman, A.F., Kumar, S., Klewicka, M.M., and Neumann, G.G. (2001). The staircase phenomenon: implications for monitoring of neuromuscular transmission. *Anesthesiology* 95: 403–407.

Lee, C. (2009). Goodbye suxamethonium! *Anaesthesia* 64 (Suppl.1): 73–81.

Lee, G.C., Iyengar, S., Szenohradszky, J. et al. (1997). Improving the design of muscle relaxant studies: stabilization period and tetanic recruitment. *Anesthesiology* 86: 48–54.

Lien, C.A. (2011). Development and potential clinical impact of ultra-short acting neuromuscular blocking agents. *British Journal of Anaesthesia* 107 (S1): i60–i71.

Lundstrom, L.H., Duez, C.H.V., Norskov, A.K. et al. (2018). Effects of avoidance or use of neuromuscular blocking agents on outcomes in tracheal intubation: a Cochrane systematic review. *British Journal of Anaesthesia* 120: 1381–1393.

Martin-Flores, M., Cheetham, J., Campoy, L. et al. (2015). Effect of gantacurium on evoked laryngospasm and duration of apnea in anesthetized healthy cats. *American Journal of Veterinary Research* 76: 216–223.

Martin-Flores, M., Sakai, D.M., Campoy, L., and Gleed, R.D. (2018). Survey of how different groups of veterinarians manage the use of neuromuscular blocking agents in anesthetized dogs. *Veterinary Anaesthesia and Analgesia* 45: 443–451.

Martin-Flores, M., Sakai, D.M., Tseng, C.T. et al. (2019). Can we see fade? A survey of anesthesia providers and our ability to detect partial neuromuscular block in dogs. *Veterinary Anaesthesia and Analgesia* 46: 182–187.

Martyn, J.A.J., Fagerlund, M.J., and Eriksson, L.I. (2009). Basic principles of neuromuscular transmission. *Anaesthesia* 64 (Suppl.1): 1–9.

Naguib, M. and Kopman, A.F. (2018). Neostigmine-induced weakness: what are the facts? *Anaesthesia* 73: 1055–1066.

Rodney, G., Raju, P.K.B.C., and Ball, D.R. (2015). Not just monitoring: a strategy for managing neuromuscular blockade. *Anaesthesia* 70: 1105–1118.

Sakai, D.M., Zornow, K.A., Campoy, L. et al. (2018). Intravenous rocuronium 0.3 mg/kg improves the conditions for tracheal intubation in cats: a randomized, placebo-controlled trial. *Journal of Feline Medicine and Surgery* 20: 1124–1129.

Zafirova, Z. and Dalton, A. (2018). Neuromuscular blockers and reversal agents and their impact on anesthesia practice. *Best Practice in Research and Clinical Anaesthesiology* 32: 203–211.

Note that the whole supplement of *Anaesthesia*, volume 64, supplement 1 (2009) is devoted to neuromuscular block and its reversal.

Self-test Section

1   Sugammadex can encapsulate which of the following neuromuscular blocking agents?
    A Succinylcholine (suxamethonium)
    B Atracurium
    C Rocuronium
    D Mivacurium

2   List the qualitative and quantitative methods that exist to monitor the depth of neuromuscular block.

18

Monitoring Animals during General Anaesthesia

LEARNING OBJECTIVES

- To be able to discuss why patient monitoring is necessary.
- To be able to monitor the physiological status of an anaesthetised patient and its depth of anaesthesia using both unsophisticated methods (senses, stethoscopes) and more sophisticated monitoring devices: both non-invasive and invasive.
- To be familiar with common problems associated with monitoring devices.

18.1 Introduction

> **To monitor is to observe continually; it is the measure of an anaesthetist!**
> **If you do one thing, then do no harm.**

Monitoring should start from pre-operative patient assessment and should continue right the way through recovery. Monitoring a patient's physiological status provides warning signals when things go wrong, which enables early intervention, and, hopefully, aversion of trouble. Monitoring involves making measurements and comparing these against standard reference 'normal' values or ranges of values. This requires not only some means of making the measurements, but also some knowledge of the normal values, which may differ between species and circumstances.

18.2 Aims of Monitoring Physiological Status

- To maintain the function of certain body organ systems as close to physiological normality as possible.
- To maintain an adequate 'depth' of anaesthesia (not too deep or light) under different levels of surgical stimulation during a procedure.
- To promote patient safety. Horses, especially, suffer a high risk of morbidity and mortality under general

anaesthesia (GA): complication/death rate of 1 in 100 (all cases) to 1 in 200 (healthy), compared to 1 in 900 for cats, and 1 in 1,800 for dogs (healthy animals).
- To ensure safety of personnel (and patient) by maintaining adequacy of antinociception/analgesia and unresponsiveness of the patient to surgical stimuli.
- For potential legal implications, it is important to keep accurate and complete records of events during an anaesthetic.

18.3 How to Monitor the Patient's Status

Never underestimate the human senses (sight, smell, hearing, and touch), and our powers of data interpretation and integration which can be put to good effect to monitor anaesthetised patients. Modern equipment can, however, help us, often by providing earlier warning signals than we alone can detect, thus buying us a little more time to sort things out so that we can hopefully prevent a critical incident; but machines should never be solely relied upon.

18.4 What Should Be Monitored

- Central nervous system (CNS)
- Cardiovascular system (CVS)
- Respiratory system
- Temperature

Veterinary Anaesthesia: Principles to Practice, Second Edition. Alexandra H. A. Dugdale, Georgina Beaumont, Carl Bradbrook, and Matthew Gurney.
© 2020 John Wiley & Sons Ltd. Published 2020 by John Wiley & Sons Ltd.
Companion website: www.wiley.com/go/dugdale/veterinary-anaesthesia

- Neuromuscular function
- Renal function
- Metabolic status; haematological and biochemical variables may, occasionally, require monitoring
- Coagulation status may require monitoring in some circumstances

18.4.1 Monitoring the CNS

All agents that induce a state of GA depress the CNS to a greater or lesser extent. Traditionally, anaesthetists have utilised the various reflexes of the CNS to help them assess the level of CNS responsiveness, and, from that, judge the depth of anaesthesia.

18.4.1.1 Assessment of Reflexes

- **Palpebral reflex:** check both eyes, if possible; becomes refractory with over-stimulation; affected if irritants such as hair, blood, or surgical scrub enters the eyes.
- **Corneal reflex:** in most species, it is present until deep/surgical levels of anaesthesia (although sometimes persists in the horse). Regular touching of the cornea, whilst tear production is depressed, can damage the cornea.
- **Gag reflex and jaw tone.** Laryngeal and pharyngeal reflexes may persist in pigs and cats until deeper planes of anaesthesia than in other species.
- **Limb withdrawal reflexes.**
- **Perineal reflex (anal tone).**
- **Righting reflex:** often used for exotics.

18.4.1.1.1 Assessment of Eye Position, Movement, Lacrimation

In horses, ruminants, dogs, and cats, the eyes can also reflect the level of CNS depression via globe position, palpebral reflex, presence of spontaneous nystagmus, and lacrimation. There is some variation among species, e.g. horses tend to maintain a slow palpebral reflex under deeper planes of anaesthesia than do dogs. Globe position in horses, however, can be unreliable and one eye may assume a different position from the other, which is also confusing.

Globe position in dogs, cats, and ruminants is much more reliable. In dogs and cats, the globes tend to rotate ventromedially (forwards and downwards) as anaesthesia deepens towards the surgical planes, but the globes then become central (with loss of palpebral reflex and lacrimation) if anaesthesia deepens further.

In cattle, the globes rotate ventrally as anaesthesia progresses from light planes to surgical planes (Figure 18.1), and then they rotate back to a central position with greater depth of anaesthesia. As anaesthesia lightens, the globes follow these excursions in the exact reverse order.

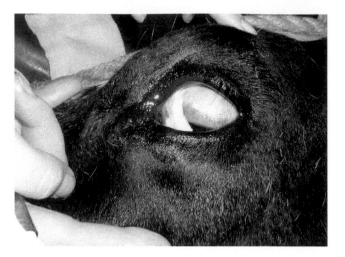

Figure 18.1 Ventral rotation of the globe during 'surgical' plane of anaesthesia in a cow.

18.4.1.2 Assessment of Autonomic Nervous System Activity

The activity of the autonomic nervous system can also be used to help us gauge anaesthetic depth. If an animal is 'too light', the sympathetic nervous system tends to be stimulated and catecholamines are released, which tend to cause an increase in heart rate and/or blood pressure. Small animals and ruminants tend to show increases in both heart rate and blood pressure, whereas horses more commonly show only increases in blood pressure, without very obvious changes in heart rate.

Occasionally, however, when animals are 'too light', and painful surgical stimulation occurs, vagal reflexes may be stimulated, resulting in a fall in blood pressure and heart rate. This occurs because the animal has effectively 'fainted' (i.e. vasovagal syncope). Although it seems counterintuitive, the plane of anaesthesia needs deepening. Animals may 'vagal' in this way near the end of surgery, when anaesthesia has been lightened in anticipation of surgery completion – a technique that is best avoided to prevent this response Always assess other signs of anaesthetic depth, such as eye reflexes and jaw tone, to help guide an appropriate response.

Also, be aware of other factors that may influence autonomic tone, such as hypovolaemia, drug administration, and dysautonomias.

18.4.1.3 Electroencephalography (EEG)

A more sophisticated way of monitoring the CNS under anaesthesia is EEG. This requires specialised machinery and interpretation of recorded data. The high cost and difficulty of interpretation preclude this form of monitoring from routine veterinary use at the moment.

EEG is the recording of electrical activity of the cortical areas of the brain, using the 'nearest' location for electrodes (i.e. on the scalp). The EEG consists of spontaneous and evoked activity. The complex waveform of the raw EEG can be analysed by Fourier transformation into its component parts. The different frequencies are delta (<4 Hz), theta (4–8 Hz), alpha (9–13 Hz), and beta (>13 Hz).

During consciousness, the raw EEG data (i.e. before Fourier transformation) is said to be 'desynchronised' and usually consists of low-amplitude, high-frequency components (e.g. alpha and beta waves). With anaesthesia, initially, there may be an increase in beta activity, but alpha activity is suppressed. As anaesthesia deepens, lower frequency, higher amplitude rhythms (theta and delta) appear, and the EEG becomes progressively more synchronised. With further increase in anaesthetic depth, periods of little or no EEG activity may be recorded (isoelectric = flat line), separated by bursts of activity: This is often described as the phase of 'burst suppression'. As depth increases still further, the EEG eventually becomes quiescent (i.e. isoelectric).

In addition to anaesthetic drugs, other factors can affect the EEG such as hypoxia, hypercapnia, extreme hypocapnia (cerebral ischaemia secondary to cerebral vasoconstriction), hypothermia, and extreme hypotension (poor perfusion).

18.4.1.3.1 Interpretation of EEGs

Raw EEG data is hard to interpret, especially in real time. Therefore, fast Fourier analysis of the different frequencies is performed, with further analysis of how these change with segments of time called epochs. This can be variously displayed:

- **Power spectrum analysis.** Epochs of 2–16 seconds undergo Fourier analysis, then power (i.e. amplitude squared) is plotted against frequency for each epoch.
- **Compressed spectral array.** Power/frequency graphs are smoothed and sequential epochs are stacked up to give a mountain range appearance.
- **Density modulated spectral array.** Each epoch is represented by a line of dots of different sizes (density) according to power at that frequency.

Spectral edge frequency (SEF) is defined as the frequency below which a certain percentage of the total power of the EEG is located. This is usually 50, 80, or 95%; hence MF (**median frequency or SEF50**), SEF80, or SEF95. Shifts in SEF can help to determine drug (anaesthetic/hypnotic and analgesic/antinociceptive) effects, and it may be that MF varies differently to SEF95.

Brainstem evoked responses (potentials) disappear later than spontaneous EEG activity under anaesthesia. These include auditory, visual, (somato-)sensory, (somato-) motor, and autonomic. Some are finding some place in the race to discover a better way of monitoring anaesthetic depth in man. Others, such as BAER (brainstem auditory evoked potentials), and ERG (electroretinography), are used for assessing animals for deafness, or some forms of blindness, respectively.

Bispectral index (BIS) measures correlation of the phase between different frequency components of the EEG, and, at present, uses human algorithms and human EEG data. BIS values correlate fairly well with degrees of sedation/hypnosis in man, but depend very much upon which sedative/anaesthetic drug/s is/are being administered. BIS is measured on a scale from 0 (isoelectric) to 100 (awake). BIS has been investigated in various veterinary species, although its reliability is yet to be established, and therefore its use in the clinical setting remains unsupported.

18.4.2 Monitoring the CVS

Pre-operative assessment of CVS function is important. Figure 18.2 outlines the factors involved in determining **tissue oxygen delivery** (maintenance of which is the ultimate goal of the anaesthetist), many of which can be monitored.

It is important to monitor the CVS in animals under GA, not only because many anaesthetic agents have profound effects on the CVS, but also because many disease states and surgical procedures also have profound influences on the CVS. Although, ultimately, we are concerned with maintaining oxygen delivery to the tissues, both a functioning respiratory system and a functioning CVS are required to achieve this.

As oxygen delivery to the tissues depends primarily upon the cardiac output and the oxygen content of arterial blood, ideally we should be monitoring these, however, this is not so easy in the clinical situation; and a global figure for cardiac output may not help us to know, e.g. how well the left retina or right kidney are being perfused.

$$\text{Cardiac output} = \text{Stroke volume} \times \text{Heart rate}$$

$$\text{Cardiac output} = \frac{\text{Mean arterial pressure} (-\text{Central venous pressure})}{\text{Systemic vascular resistance}}$$

If we cannot measure **cardiac output**, but wish to measure what has sometimes been called the 'next best thing' (i.e. mean arterial blood pressure; MAP), we can combine these equations to derive an expression for MAP as follows:

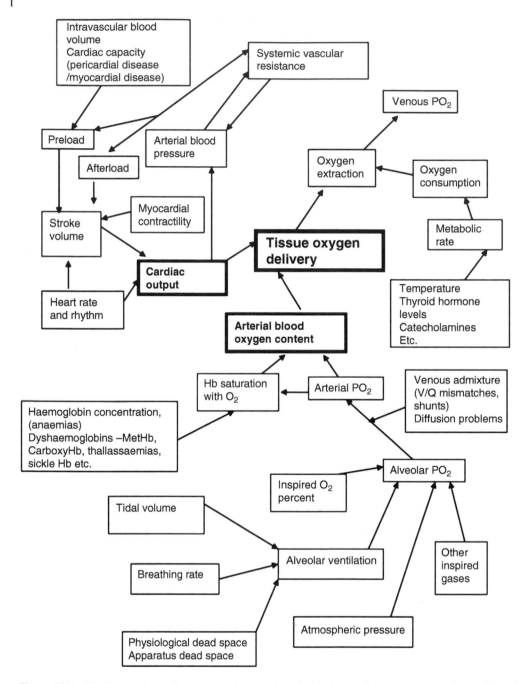

Figure 18.2 Cardiovascular and respiratory factors that should be considered for measuring and monitoring.

$$\textbf{MAP} = \textbf{Heart rate} \times \textbf{Stroke volume} \times$$
$$\textbf{Systemic vascular resistance}$$

Although **MAP** can be measured much more easily, it is only one determinant of cardiac output and cannot tell us much about actual tissue perfusion, except that we can have a number for the 'driving pressure' behind the potential blood flow. For most tissues to be able to autoregulate their blood flow, they require the MAP to be of the order

of at least 60–70 mmHg (and no more than around 150–160 mmHg). The perfusion pressure for a tissue is given by MAP minus intracompartmental pressure. For muscles, where the intracompartmental pressure may reach 30–40 mmHg during recumbency, a perfusion pressure of at least 30–40 mmHg is required for maintenance of muscle perfusion and oxygen delivery.

Heart rate is also an important determinant of cardiac output, and of MAP; and again, at least we can measure heart rate relatively easily. The other variables in the equations are much harder to measure in a clinical situation.

The **Bezold-Jarisch (B-J) reflex** (a vaso-vagal reflex, see also Chapter 19), resulting in profound bradycardia and hypotension, can be caused by the following:

- Acute massive hypovolaemia (decompensating, shocky animals); high epidural with local anaesthetic that results in massive vasodilation of hind end of animal, and also blocks sympathetic cardioaccelerator fibres, thus preventing reflex tachycardia that would otherwise try to offset the fall in blood pressure.
- Sudden critical obstruction to venous return such as compression of vena cava by rolling a heavily pregnant animal quickly into dorsal recumbency.
- 'Emotional' causes, e.g. patient 'awareness' during light anaesthesia.

Arrhythmias can be associated with poor ventricular filling (especially tachyarrhythmias where the heart has less time to fill in between beats) and poor ventricular emptying (because of in-co-ordinated contractions), and so can lead to a reduction in cardiac output.

18.4.2.1 Cardiac Output Measurement

Cardiac output measurement is currently mainly a research tool for vets due to the expense of the equipment. Techniques include:

- **Thermodilution cardiac output:** requires intracardiac catheterisation (e.g. Swan-Ganz catheter). Cardiac output is inversely proportional to the area under the temperature/time curve. Often said to be the 'gold standard' technique.
- **Indicator dye dilution cardiac output:** where cardiac output is the quantity of dye injected divided by the area under the concentration/time curve.
- **Lithium dilution cardiac output:** does not require intracardiac catheterisation. Cardiac output is the quantity of lithium injected divided by the area under the concentration/time curve. The lithium sensor, however, may be affected by some drugs, e.g. xylazine and synthetic catecholamines.
- **Fick principle cardiac output:** follows the principle that oxygen uptake by the lungs equals the oxygen added to the pulmonary blood. Therefore, cardiac output equals oxygen uptake divided by the arterial-to-venous blood oxygen content difference.
- **Total or partial CO_2 rebreathing cardiac output:** is a noninvasive technique and requires the application of mechanical (usually positive pressure) ventilation. Total CO_2 rebreathing cardiac output uses a form of the Fick equation, but in place of oxygen measurements, it uses

CO_2. Therefore, cardiac output equals CO_2 production divided by venous- to-arterial CO_2 content difference. Partial CO_2 rebreathing methods use a differential form of this CO_2 Fick equation.

- **TOE** (trans-oesophageal echocardiography): uses Doppler ultrasonography to measure blood velocity in the descending aorta. Although the aortic root would be a better place to measure this, it is not easy to obtain a steady image of this or the ascending aorta. The velocity-time integral of blood flow through the descending aorta is multiplied by the aortic cross-sectional area to give the volume flow rate of blood (related to the stroke volume). This is multiplied by the heart rate to give an estimation of cardiac output, and can give beat-to-beat information. (Note slight 'error' as only the descending aorta is imaged.) A canine-specific oesophageal Doppler probe has been developed and allows measurement of stroke volume and other flow indices during anaesthesia (CardioQ™). This may prove a useful additional monitoring tool during anaesthesia for sick patients in the future, although currently its cost and challenge to correctly position its probe and interpret its measurements may limit its use.
- **Bullet method:** uses echocardiography and considers the heart to be shaped like a bullet; long and short axis views of the heart are obtained and the dimensions are compared in systole and diastole to assess the change in 'volume', and therefore cardiac output.
- **Pulse contour integrated continuous cardiac output:** uses pulse plethysmography to define the 'shape' (contour) of a peripheral arterial pulse which is then 'calibrated' against a measurement of cardiac output (often using the lithium dilution technique). In between fairly regular calibrations, the pulse contour can then be used to calculate the beat-to-beat cardiac output. More recently, a system of predicting cardiac output continuously (beat-by-beat) from arterial pulse contour analysis (using an algorithm based on the Pressure Recording Analytical Method [PRAM], and requiring no prior calibration) has become available to vets for clinical use (MostCare^UP™). Its applications and limitations are currently being investigated.
- **Thoracic electrical bio-impedance,** and impedance cardiography. The reader is referred to specialised texts.

18.4.2.2 Assessment of Intravascular Volume Status and Response to a Fluid Bolus Challenge

Newer dynamic assessment methods are based upon the magnitude of variation in arterial blood pressure with respiratory cycles, most usually determined during positive pressure ventilation. The use of the Masimo™ technology's pleth(ysmographic) variability index (PVI) offers a convenient method to make this assessment in veterinary patients.

PVI measures the change in perfusion index (PI) over time across multiple, complete respiratory cycles and is displayed as a percentage from 0 to 100%. PI is the ratio of pulsatile to non-pulsatile (static) blood flow in a peripheral tissue bed and is also given as a percentage. Changes in PVI may reflect changes in the CVS such as vascular tone, patient blood volume, and intrathoracic pressure. There are studies in dogs showing that this may be a useful method to assess likelihood to respond to fluid bolus therapy when hypotensive during anaesthesia, and therefore the likelihood of hypovolaemia. Mechanical ventilation is, however, required to make a valid assessment. Current literature suggests that a hypotensive patient with a PVI more than 15% is likely to be a fluid-responder, and therefore a crystalloid fluid bolus may be administered and the PVI reassessed (if a responder, the PVI should reduce). Patients with PVI values below 15% are unlikely to respond to (further) fluid challenges, and so if they are hypotensive, other interventions are required to improve arterial blood pressure, e.g. vasopressor or inotropic support.

18.4.2.3 Heart Rate and Rhythm Monitoring

It is important to monitor the heart rate because it gives us some indication of cardiac output and also of the autonomic tone. The assessment of heart rhythm, by electrocardiography (ECG), is also important for the evaluation of any arrhythmias. Methods of monitoring the heart rate and rhythm are given below.

18.4.2.3.1 *Palpation of the Apex Beat*

Advantages are that no equipment is necessary, minimal skill is required, and it is non-invasive. Disadvantages are that access may be limited in some cases, e.g. a patient under drapes, and accurate assessment of arrhythmias is difficult.

18.4.2.3.2 *Auscultation*

- **Precordial stethoscopy:** the advantage is that you can use a conventional stethoscope. Disadvantages are that access may be limited and interpretation of arrhythmias may be difficult.
- **Oesophageal stethoscopy** is very useful; advantages are that it uses simple cheap equipment and can monitor respiration rate at the same time. Figure 18.3 shows an oesophageal stethoscope. The disadvantage is that interpretation of arrhythmias may be difficult.

18.4.2.3.3 *Electrocardiography*

Essential for the accurate diagnosis of arrhythmias. **Not reliable for basic monitoring** because **only gives information about the electrical activity of the heart in**

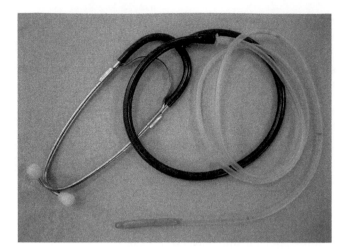

Figure 18.3 Oesophageal stethoscope (three sizes available).

terms of rate and rhythm. The ECG **cannot tell us if the heart is actually beating,** and if so, how well it is pumping blood around the body, e.g. pulseless electrical activity can occur where the ECG looks completely normal but the myocardium does not contract. Advantages are that it allows monitoring of electrical activity of the heart and early detection of arrhythmias. Disadvantages are that it gives no information on cardiac output and requires adequate knowledge of cardiology for accurate interpretation.

18.4.2.3.4 *Echocardiography*

Echocardiography in the form of trans-oesophageal echo (TOE) is being used increasingly in human anaesthesia to image the heart's performance in real time, and also to measure cardiac output on a beat-to-beat basis. Technology has not yet been developed in all veterinary species (a canine probe is available) due to cost and differences in chest shape and heart/oesophageal alignment.

18.4.2.3.5 *Palpation of the Pulse*

This assesses pulse rate, rhythm, and quality/character. The best sites for palpation of arterial pulses may vary between the various veterinary species. Peripheral and more central pulses can also be compared. Sites for pulse palpation include:

- Femoral arteries (considered central) all animals.
- Brachial arteries (considered central) in birds and large animals.
- Lingual arteries (peripheral) in dogs.
- Palatine arteries (peripheral) in horses (Figure 18.4).
- Transverse facial arteries (peripheral) in horses.
- Mandibular and mandibular facial arteries (peripheral) in horses, ruminants, and pigs.
- Branches of caudal auricular arteries (peripheral) in all animals.

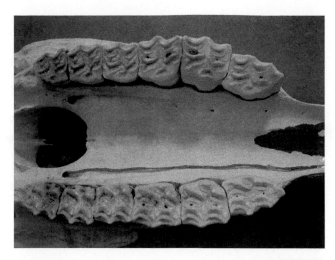

Figure 18.4 The course of one of the paired palatine arteries is shown in this horse skull with string. Either artery may be palpated during anaesthesia.

- Dorsal pedal and palmar metacarpal arch arteries (peripheral) in dogs and cats.
- Dorsal/lateral metatarsal arteries (peripheral) in horses.
- Median (middle) coccygeal (caudal) arteries (peripheral) in horses and cattle.

When you palpate a pulse, you should be assessing three factors:

- 'Pulse pressure': the difference between the systolic and diastolic pressures. A pulse of 120/80 mmHg may feel similar to a pulse of 80/40 mmHg, but the mean pressures would be very different (see below).
- 'Mean pressure': can be guesstimated by how easy it is to occlude the arterial pulse by digital pressure and by assessing how 'full' or 'turgid' the artery feels between the pulses, but high degrees of vasomotor tone can fool you.
- 'Character' of the pulse, e.g., we may describe a pulse as 'bounding', when a large difference between systolic and diastolic pressures exists. This is common in conditions such as aortic valvular insufficiency.

Pulses can be difficult to palpate in very small animals and exotics, but some other techniques may detect them more easily, e.g. pulse oximeters or Doppler blood flow probes.

18.4.2.3.6 Pulse Oximeters and Doppler Flow Probes

Pulse oximeters and Doppler flow probes can give an indication of pulse rate; and you may see (from the plethysmograph trace) or hear (with Doppler) if arrhythmias are present.

18.4.2.4 Arterial Blood Pressure Measurement

In many cases, it is useful to be able to measure arterial blood pressure, rather than relying on subjective assessment from pulse pressure palpation, and there are a number of methods available to do this. MAP can be derived from systolic (SAP) and diastolic (DAP) arterial pressures as follows:

$$MAP = \frac{\left(SAP - DAP\right)}{3} + DAP$$

18.4.2.4.1 Indirect and Non-invasive Techniques

Sphygmomanometry An appropriately sized inflatable cuff/bladder, the pressure in which is measured by a mercury or aneroid manometer, is placed proximally on a limb (or tail-base) and inflated until blood flow to the distal appendage is occluded. Then the cuff/bladder is deflated slowly (optimal deflation rate has been determined to be around 2 mmHg per heart beat over a wide range of heart rates [40–120 beats/min] in people), and the return of pulsatile blood flow in an artery distal to the cuff is detected by palpation, auscultation (stethoscopy), by Doppler-shifted ultrasound (which detects either arterial wall motion [Doppler kineto-arteriography, which is seldom used in modern instruments], or red cell movement [and therefore blood flow] within the artery, producing an audible signal) (Figure 18.5), or even pulse oximetry (if an appropriately sized/shaped and unpigmented distal appendage tissue bed is available).

When using a **Doppler** blood flow probe, the cuff/bladder pressure at which the returning blood flow is first detected (first audible 'pulse' sounds; and manometer needle starts to flick in time with the pulse) is usually taken as the systolic pressure. The diastolic pressure is more difficult to determine as it depends upon a more subjective interpretation (no further changes in 'pulse' sounds; manometer needle ceases to flick). The mean pressure is calculated from the systolic and diastolic pressures using the equation above.

Advantages are: it is a relatively simple technique; it is non-invasive; pulse rate and rhythm can also be monitored; it can be used in the face of slow heart rates; arrhythmias and low blood pressures and the equipment is inexpensive. **Disadvantages** are: it is labour-intensive; thick hair or fat can interfere with measurement (hair must be clipped away or a glabrous site chosen, and ultrasound coupling gel is required to improve signal acquisition); the technique is usually used to measure only 'systolic' pressure and only intermittent measurements are possible.

When using Doppler ultrasound flow probes, the apparent systolic pressure determined may be slightly less than the actual systolic pressure: often the accuracy of readings is given as within ±10 mmHg of the true systolic pressure. For cats, some people advocate adding 14.7 mmHg to the Doppler pressure reading obtained, to give a more accurate

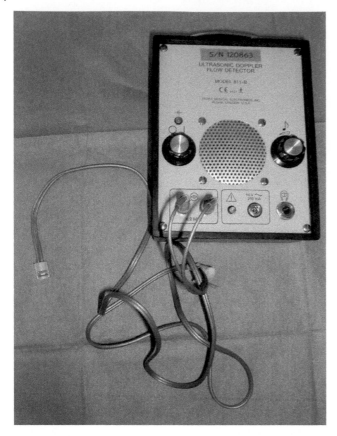

Figure 18.5 Doppler ultrasound blood flow probe. Blood flowing towards the transducer increases the frequency of the reflected waves (e.g. incident waves have a frequency of 2 MHz, whereas reflected waves have a frequency of 2.25 MHz; the difference is 250 Hz, which is in the audible range).

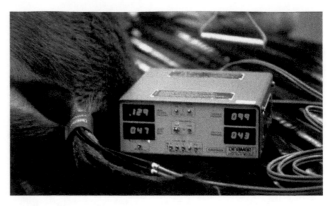

Figure 18.6 Oscillometric non-invasive blood pressure monitor; cuff placed on donkey's tail-head. Note that the pulse rate is also displayed, in addition to systolic, diastolic, and mean pressures.

systolic pressure, or even take the Doppler readings as being closer to mean arterial pressure than the systolic pressure. In reality, the measured 'Doppler blood pressure' is usually somewhere between the actual mean and systolic pressures, but the degree of error is difficult to predict, and indeed in numerous studies, the Doppler method has failed to meet the American College of Veterinary Internal Medicine (ACVIM) validation criteria.

Oscillometric Devices These are automated versions of the sphygmomanometry technique. An inflatable bladder (often referred to as the cuff) (with or without a covering sleeve) of appropriate size (see below) is placed on an appendage (limb or tail) (Figure 18.6). The machine then cyclically inflates and deflates the cuff, and sensors detect pressure changes in the cuff during its deflation as pulsatile flow returns to the appendage. These changes in cuff pressure, as pulsatile flow returns are used to determine systolic (at maximal rate of increase in oscillation size), mean (at maximal oscillation amplitude) and diastolic (at maximal decrease in oscillation size or disappearance of oscillations) pressures. Pulse rate is usually also determined: the displayed value should be confirmed to be the same as actual pulse rate before blood pressure readings are accepted.

Advantages are: it is noninvasive; minimally labour-intensive; and most machines can be programmed to take readings every 1–10 minutes. **Disadvantages** are: the equipment tends to be expensive; does not work well in the presence of arrhythmias, slow pulse rates or low blood pressures; tends not to work well with hairy or fat appendages or in animals less than about 7 kg; gives only intermittent readings that are retrospective by the time the machine displays the values (we really prefer real time and beat-to-beat information); and can give erroneous values, although the trend in readouts should reflect the real situation. MAP values are the most accurate.

Larger 'cuffs' generally consist of a rubber bladder (the business part) within a protective sleeve of material, whereas smaller 'cuffs' tend to be made of plastic, e.g. polyvinyl chloride (PVC) and do not require further protection. The terms *cuffs* and *bladders* tend to be used interchangeably. There may be one or two hoses connected to the cuff/bladder, depending upon whether inflation/deflation and pressure measurement require independent ports.

For best results, the cuff/bladder width should be c. 0.4 (0.2–0.6) times the circumference of the appendage. For rubber bladders, the length of the inflatable bladder should be c. 0.8–1 times the circumference of the appendage, but plastic cuffs must be able to encircle the appendage in order to fasten.

Ideally, the cuff should be placed on an appendage at the same level as the heart. If the cuff is positioned on an appendage below heart height, falsely high pressure readings will be obtained. If the cuff is positioned on an appendage above heart height, falsely low pressure readings will be obtained. Values can, however, be corrected to true heart height (a 10 cm height difference is approximately equal to a 7.4 mmHg pressure difference). When only trends in blood pressure are required, the uncorrected values may be used. It is important, however, not to mix corrected and uncorrected values.

If the **cuff is too narrow or too loose, falsely high readings** will be obtained. If the cuff is **too wide or too tight, falsely low readings** will result.

High Definition Oscillometric (HDO) Devices Highly sensitive oscillometric devices display the detected cuff pressures on a computer screen so the operator can visualise the reading in real time, enabling arrhythmias and artefacts to be detected and readings to be discounted in such circumstances. Most HDO devices can repeat measurements every 1–10 minutes. This technique may improve the success of achieving readings in smaller patients, although HDO has not always been shown to meet the ACVIM validation criteria for all measured pressures when compared with invasive arterial blood pressure measurements in studies in dogs and cats, both conscious and during anaesthesia.

Plethysmography As a byproduct of how a pulse oximeter determines the saturation of haemoglobin with oxygen, pulsatile blood flow is measured. This information can be displayed in waveform as a plethysmograph (a 'pulse volume graph') (Figure 18.7), or as a visual 'signal strength' indicator (e.g. in the form of a stack of little bars that light up; the more that light up, the stronger the signal), and some monitors may display a message such as 'weak signal strength'. Although not quantitative in these display forms, the qualitative information obtained about arterial blood pressure can be very useful. Note that PVI assessment is currently available with Masimo technology (see above).

18.4.2.4.2 Direct (Invasive) Techniques

The actual blood pressure value recorded from different arteries will vary because of their different sizes and distances (number of branches) from the aortic root, which affects their compliance (more peripheral arteries tend to be 'stiffer'). This 'distal pulse amplification' results in increasing systolic, very slightly decreasing diastolic, but almost unchanging (very little decrease) mean arterial pressure in arteries with increasing distance from the aorta.

It is important to **measure pressure against a reference level** (level of the heart; often the sternal manubrium is used as a landmark), so devices to measure/record pressure need to be **zeroed to atmospheric pressure at this level**.

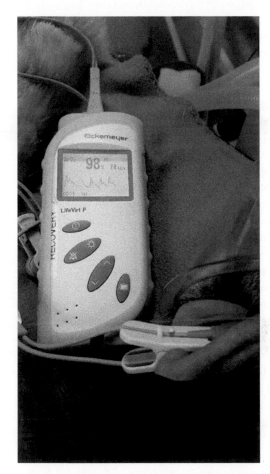

Figure 18.7 LifeVet P™ portable pulse oximeter displaying the pulse rate (74), oxygen saturation of arterial blood haemoglobin (SpO$_2$ 98%), and the plethysmograph ('pulse volume') trace.

After an arterial cannula is placed, it is connected via non-compliant extension tubing (containing heparinised saline or heparinised glucose) to a pressure transducer device that converts the arterial pulse into a numerical value with or without a pulse waveform display. Pressure transducers can be any of the following:

Saline Filled 'U' Manometer

This is similar to how we measure central venous pressure (CVP), but needs to be quite 'tall' as arterial pressures are expected to be much higher than venous pressures. MAP values can be determined fairly accurately, but not systolic and diastolic because of excessive inertia of the fluid column that damps the fluid meniscus swing between systolic and diastolic pressures.

Aneroid Manometer

The inner workings of the aneroid manometer must be protected from arterial blood and other fluids, so an air column, or a 'pressure veil™' (a rubber glove-finger in a plastic case/syringe barrel), is incorporated (Figure 18.8). In either case, once the system has been 'primed' (i.e. filled with heparinised fluid, but leaving an air column [<10 cm] between the fluid and the manometer), and also pressurised so that the manometer needle reads more than the expected systolic arterial pressure), the fluid–air interface is positioned at heart level to zero the manometer to atmospheric pressure at heart level, before finally opening the three-way tap so that the pulsating arterial blood communicates directly with the fluid column and manometer. Only MAP can be determined because the needle movements between systolic and diastolic pressures are damped by the inertia in the system.

Electronic Pressure Transducer

Most commonly a strain gauge is used, whose deformation is detected as a change in electrical resistance (measured using a Wheatstone bridge), which is subsequently converted into a pressure signal. Numerical pressure values are given, usually alongside a waveform display. The transducer must be zeroed to atmospheric pressure at the level of the heart (Figure 18.9). If the transducer is positioned above heart level, the values measured are falsely low; if positioned below heart level, the values measured are falsely high.

Damping and resonance are important considerations for electronic pressure transducers. An arterial waveform can be described in terms of Fourier analysis as a complex sine wave, composed of its fundamental frequency (the pulse rate) and a series of (at least the first 10) harmonics. The strain gauge in the transducer and

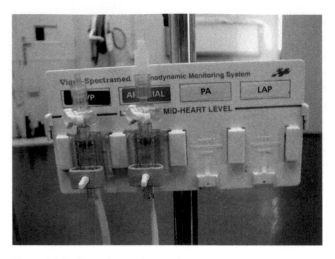

Figure 18.9 Two electronic pressure transducers mounted so that their height can be adjusted for zeroing to atmospheric pressure at the level of the heart.

the fluid-filled catheter and extension tube (the hydraulic coupling), constitute the catheter-tubing-transducer system which can undergo simple harmonic motion when subjected to a pressure pulse and this may affect the accuracy of the measured pressure. Resonance in the system results in over-estimation of pressures whereas damping in the system results in under-estimation of pressures.

The resonant frequency of the catheter-tubing-transducer system must be greater than the frequency of oscillations to which it is responding or else the signal may be distorted by resonance. For example, the higher harmonics of arterial waveforms of dogs lie in the region of 20 Hz, so a system with a resonant frequency of 30–40 Hz should work well. The dynamic response of a catheter-tubing-transducer system depends upon:

- The fundamental frequency of the input signal (expected pulse rate).
- The resonant (natural) frequency of the catheter-tubing-transducer system.
- The degree of damping present in the catheter-tubing-transducer-system.

The natural frequency of a system is that at which it resonates. For the catheter-tubing-transducer system this should be of the order of at least 10 times the fundamental frequency of what is being measured.

Natural frequency

$$= 1/(2\pi) \times \sqrt{\frac{(\text{Stiffness of diaphragm})}{(\text{Mass of oscillating fluid and diaphragm})}}$$

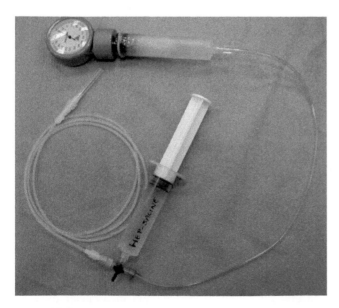

Figure 18.8 Pressure veil™ attached to aneroid manometer.

The most important factors are:

- Length and diameter of catheter/extension tubing.
- Density of fluid within catheter/extension tubing.
- Continuity of fluid column within catheter/extension tubing.

The extension tubing should have low compliance, and ideally non-compliant tubing should be used. Short stiff extension tubing can increase the resonant frequency of the system, but beware using long extension tubing where low pulse rates are expected. The hydraulic coupling should be a continuous fluid column. Blood clots in the system (usually at the catheter end) increase damping. Small air bubbles increase resonance whereas large air bubbles increase damping.

The catheter-tubing-transducer system damping can be checked by performing a fast-flush test with the following possible results:

- **Under-damping** is indicated by excessive oscillation ('thrilling') of the pressure response before stabilising (Figure 18.10). Damping factor << 0.7.
- **Excessive damping** is indicated by a slow decline in pressure and the absence of an overshoot (Figure 18.11). Damping factor > 1.0.
- **Critical damping** is said to exist where there is 'just' no overshoot; the damping factor is 1.0 (Figure 18.12).
- **Optimal damping**, when the waveform should show minimal distortion due to resonance and minimal distortion due to phase shift (caused by excessive damping), is present when the pressure overshoot is limited to 6–7% of the initial pressure displacement: the damping factor is 0.6–0.7 (ideally 0.64) (Figure 18.13).

It is usual to aim for slight under-damping so that, as long as the natural frequency of the system is high enough, the advantages of detail and responsiveness outweigh the potential problems of resonance. With use, some increase in damping is inevitable (by the occasional air bubble or blood clot in the system), so starting with a slightly under-damped system gives more 'room' for damping to occur before the system becomes over-damped.

Mean arterial pressure is the most accurate value because:

- Excessive damping results in underestimation of the systolic pressure, yet over-estimation of diastolic pressure.
- Excessive resonance in the system tends to over-estimate systolic pressure and under-estimate diastolic pressure.

18.4.2.4.3 Why Measure Arterial Blood Pressure, Especially Directly?

Most tissues and organs can autoregulate their perfusion, although the degree to which this occurs depends upon the organ/tissue: coronary, cerebral, and renal circulations show excellent autoregulation; skeletal muscle and splanchnic circulations show moderate autoregulation; skin shows very little autoregulatory capacity. Autoregulatory ability, however, depends upon the body maintaining arterial blood pressures within a 'normal' range. Different tissues and organs have slightly different **autoregulatory thresholds** (and ranges) of arterial blood pressure over which autoregulation works best, but the organs and tissues that we worry most about are the kidneys (especially small animals) and skeletal muscles (especially horses). For 'normotensive' patients, if we maintain MAP ≥60–70 mmHg (and ≤around 150–160 mmHg), then autoregulation should be maintained. We also like to see DAP >40 mmHg, as below this, coronary perfusion (which occurs, at least to the left ventricle, mainly during diastole, and therefore depends upon DAP) may become compromised. Monitoring arterial blood pressure also assists us in monitoring anaesthetic depth, but values should be interpreted in light of other measured variables, especially cardiorespiratory variables (see Chapter 19).

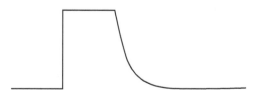

Figure 18.12 Critical damping.

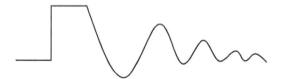

Figure 18.10 Under-damping.

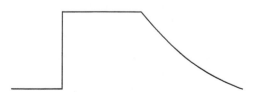

Figure 18.11 Excessive damping.

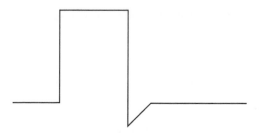

Figure 18.13 Optimal damping.

The **arterial pressure waveform** can also give us more information than just systolic, mean and diastolic blood pressures, but beware over-interpretation. The area under the systolic part of the curve can tell us about the stroke volume, and therefore cardiac output (but the incisure on the downslope of a peripheral arterial waveform is not a true 'dicrotic notch' [unlike that on an aortic pressure waveform], and therefore is not indicative of the end of systole, but rather depends upon the summation of reflections of the arterial pressure wave); the rate of change of pressure over time on the upstroke can tell us about myocardial contractility (but also depends upon local vascular tone); a steep downslope and low incisure occur with low systemic vascular resistance (SVR), whereas a high downslope incisure is present with high SVR; hypovolaemia is suggested by a narrow wave with a low downslope incisure, and large changes in e.g. peak systolic pressure (i.e. >12–13% 'systolic pressure variation' [SPV], or 'pulse pressure variation' [PPV]) when positive pressure ventilation is applied.

18.4.2.4.4 Potential Complications of Arterial Catheterisation

- Trauma
- Haematoma
- Emboli (air or thrombi)
- Infection
- Necrosis of distal tissues (if a functional end artery is cannulated and then becomes thrombosed)
- Damage to peri-arterial structures e.g. veins, nerves, parotid ducts, etc.

18.4.2.4.5 Advantages and Disadvantages of Direct Arterial Blood Pressure Measurement

Advantages of direct arterial blood pressure measurement include: real time 'beat-to-beat' information may be obtained; accurate values should be obtained; and it provides arterial access for sampling arterial blood for blood gas analysis. The pressure waveform itself can also give extra information.

Disadvantages of direct arterial blood pressure measurement are: a little skill is required and the above listed complications may occur (rare).

18.4.2.5 CVP Measurement

CVP gives a measure of the ability of the heart to cope with the volume of blood being returned to it. It indicates a balance between the cardiac output and the venous return. Clinical examination can provide you with an impression of CVP, e.g. check jugular filling and emptying with the head/body in normal position. Jugular vein distension is present with increased CVP.

CVP measurement is invasive and requires catheterisation of the jugular (more rarely the femoral/medial saphenous) vein, so that the tip of the catheter lies, ideally, in the right atrium (but beware creating arrhythmias if the catheter tickles the heart), or at least in the intrathoracic portion of the cranial (or caudal) vena cava. The catheter is attached to a 'U' tube manometer or an electronic pressure transducer via an extension tube, and either device should be zeroed to atmospheric pressure at the level of the right atrium (tricuspid valve). Normal values are around 0–10 cm H_2O for standing animals.

CVP (waveform shown in Figure 18.14) gives us a guide to 'how full' the circulation is, and can be used as a rough guide to whether the patient is hypovolaemic, normovolaemic, or hypervolaemic, but is influenced by several factors (see below). CVP, a 'static' assessment of intravascular volume status, has largely been superseded in human medicine by dynamic indices of fluid-responsiveness, which are beginning to be introduced into veterinary medicine, at least in tertiary veterinary referral hospitals. These dynamic indices, often ascertained during positive pressure ventilation, include evaluations of arterial pressure plethysmographs such as SPV, pulse pressure variation (PPV), and the pleth(ysmographic) variability index (PVI, see above), and various ultrasonographically-obtained measures such as aortic flow peak velocity variation and caudal vena cava distensibility index (see Further reading).

18.4.2.5.1 Factors Influencing CVP

- Heart chamber filling (beware myocardial and pericardial problems).
- Stage of heart cycle (systole/diastole).
- Intrathoracic pressures: CVP varies with stage in the respiratory cycle (inspiration/expiration), and is also affected by pleural space disease and positive pressure ventilation. It is best measured during the end-expiratory pause, ensuring no positive end expiratory pressure (PEEP).

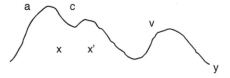

Figure 18.14 Typical CVP waveform. **a,** atrial contraction; **c,** tricuspid valve cusps displaced back into right atrium (during ventricular contraction); **v,** end of ventricular contraction, distortion of right atrium and atrial filling from vena cava; **x descent,** atrial relaxation +/− ventricular contraction pulling down on A-V valve ring; **x′ descent,** atrial relaxation +/− ventricular contraction pulling down on A-V valve ring; **y descent,** opening of tricuspid valve and emptying of blood into ventricle. In **horses,** a positive **h** wave may occur shortly after the y descent and is thought to be due to the continued filling of the right atrium during diastasis.

- Intra-abdominal pressure (beware bloat, colics, and gastric dilation/volvulus).
- The patient's position (e.g. standing, head down, dorsally recumbent).

Overall, serial measurements (trends) are much more useful than single readings, but must be taken under the same conditions and patient position.

18.4.2.6 Peripheral Perfusion Assessment
18.4.2.6.1 Blood Lactate Measurement
Serial measurements of blood lactate concentration can be extremely useful. **Arterial lactate reflects net body lactate balance.** Venous blood can also be used, although venous lactate is influenced by the net lactate balance of the specific portion of the circulation drained by that vessel. Venous lactate values tend to be slightly lower than arterial blood values because of lactate uptake by tissues and also the slightly lower pH of venous blood tends to favour lactate uptake by red blood cells via their monocarboxylate transporters (see Chapter 22).

18.4.2.6.2 Systemic P(a-v)O₂ Difference
Tissue oxygen extraction may be influenced by perfusion (cardiac output), metabolic rate, and any interference with the ability to utilise oxygen (see Chapters 22 and 26).

18.4.2.6.3 Urine Output (and Specific Gravity)
Can help to determine the adequacy of circulating blood volume and peripheral tissue (including kidney) perfusion, but also provides information about renal function/dysfunction. **Normal urine output is 1–1.5 ml/kg/h.**

18.4.2.6.4 Core-Peripheral Temperature Gradients
The core-periphery temperature gradient is **normally of the order of 2–4 °C,** but a larger gradient than this (cool periphery) is associated with poor peripheral perfusion and is seen, e.g. in hypovolaemia/shock states.

18.4.2.6.5 Mucous Membrane Colour and Capillary Refill Time (CRT)
Mucous membrane colour and CRT can also be a guide to the state of the circulation and peripheral perfusion, but a dead animal can have a normal CRT (≤2 seconds) because of backflow of blood from both the venous and arterial sides of the capillary. Some drugs and disease states also influence CRT, therefore interpret CRT in conjunction with other clinical findings; never rely on it solely, although a CRT of >4 seconds is probably significant. (Note: To assess CRT properly, the mucous membrane should be blanched for a good 5 seconds first.)

18.4.2.7 Other Assessments of the CVS: Blood Work
18.4.2.7.1 Haematological Analyses
Analyses such as packed cell volume (PCV), total solids (TS), and haematological profiles only provide information about the constituents of blood at a particular time and should be carried out before anaesthesia if thought necessary. Occasionally it may be necessary to track changes in PCV, haemoglobin concentration, and TS during long surgical procedures, e.g. where much fluid therapy support is required or high blood loss is encountered.

18.4.2.7.2 Coagulation Assessments
Coagulation profiles are usually performed pre-operatively where there are concerns of coagulopathies but, intra- or post-operative assessments may be required in unforeseen circumstances. There are an increasing number of patient-side (point-of-care) devices to help quantify some aspects of coagulation (prothrombin time (PT), activated partial thromboplastin time (aPTT), and viscoelastometry), which may help to guide more immediate therapies.

18.4.2.7.3 Biochemical Analyses
Determinations of renal or hepatic function and checking glucose or electrolyte balance is normally done pre-operatively, but sometimes it is useful to be able to track, e.g. changes in electrolytes or glucose, during a long surgical procedure.

18.4.3 Monitoring the Respiratory System

Pre-anaesthetic evaluation of the respiratory system forms an important part of overall patient assessment.

In order to deliver oxygen (and anaesthetic agents) to the tissues (including the brain), we need a delivery system (the CVS), and a transport medium (blood) that can carry gases and exchange them efficiently at a gas/liquid interface (which, for terrestrial animals means the lungs, which must be ventilated).

The simplest way to monitor the respiratory system is by observing:

- Breathing rate
- Breathing rhythm
- Tidal volume/depth of each breath
- Mucous membrane colour

$$\text{Minute ventilation} = \text{breathing rate} \times \text{tidal volume}$$

Minute ventilation is also called *minute respiratory volume.*

18.4.3.1 Breathing Rate Monitoring
- **Observe or palpate the chest wall** (difficult in draped animals).
- **Observe movements of reservoir/rebreathing bag** in the anaesthetic breathing system.
- With some circle systems, you can **see the valves move,** or **hear the clicking** of the valves as they open and close.

- Sometimes you can **see water vapour, cyclically condensing/evaporating at the endotracheal (ET) tube connection.**
- **Oesophageal stethoscopy** can be used to detect breath sounds. **Advantages:** cheap and simple; can also monitor heart rate. **Disadvantages:** sometimes breaths are difficult to hear, especially in small patients with small tidal volumes.
- **Apalerts™** (apnoea alerts) use thermistors housed in the ET tube connector to measure the temperature difference between inspired and expired gases to determine breathing rate.
- **Breathing rate is often displayed by monitors of end tidal carbon dioxide tension.**
- **Some ECG machines can display breathing rate** (baseline wandering due to breathing movements is converted into breathing rate using changes in thoracic impedance).

18.4.3.2 Tidal Volume Measurement

The tidal volume is very difficult to determine accurately from mere observations of patient chest or reservoir/rebreathing bag movement. It can be measured by devices such as the Wright's respirometer, spirometers, or pneumotachometers/tachographs.

18.4.3.3 Mucous Membrane Colour

This can tell us a little about blood oxygenation, but also gives information about tissue perfusion. Note: A 'slow' circulation can have increased peripheral oxygen extraction, and so the tissues look more 'blue'. Mucous membrane colour is very subjective and may depend upon many other factors, such as background lighting, drug administration, and vasomotor tone.

- **White** mucous membranes are associated with anaemia or intense tissue vasoconstriction.
- **Yellow** mucous membranes are associated with jaundice. Beware the starved horse – because it has no gall bladder, and therefore bile secretion is continuous, there will be increased unconjugated bilirubin in its blood during starvation, so mucous membranes look yellowy; also beware the horse with a lot of carotene in its diet (carrots, fresh grass) as mucous membranes will look more orangey yellow too.
- **Grey/purple/cyanotic** mucous membranes are associated with poor tissue oxygen delivery (poor cardiac output or insufficient oxygen to meet the tissue's demands). **Cyanosis is generally not observed until there is at least 5 g/dl of deoxyhaemoglobin present** (therefore it is impossible to detect in anaemic patients with <5 g/dl of Hb in the first place).

- **Navy blue** mucous membranes are said to be associated with excess nitrous oxide administration (accompanied by [or perhaps due to], hypoxia/cyanosis).
- **Cherry red** mucous membranes are associated with carbon monoxide poisoning (i.e. large amounts of carboxyhaemoglobin).
- **Muddy brown** mucous membranes are associated with methaemoglobin, where the haem iron is oxidised, and therefore with nitrite poisoning (especially large animals), paracetamol poisoning (especially cats), or excessive doses of prilocaine local anaesthetic.
- **Brick red/brown/cyanosed** mucous membranes are all associated with systemic inflammatory response syndrome/sepsis and endotoxaemic states.

18.4.3.4 Monitoring the Efficiency of Ventilation

Requires some means of measuring gaseous exchange at the lungs.

- The gold standard is to measure **arterial blood gas tensions** (see Chapter 21).
- The second best is to measure **end tidal carbon dioxide tension.**
- Some information can be gained from measurement of the saturation of haemoglobin with oxygen by **pulse oximetry**, but high inspired oxygen concentrations can impair the detection of hypoventilation.

18.4.3.4.1 Blood Gas Analysis

Best method to determine how well oxygenated the blood is, but gas exchange at the lungs, ventilation, and pulmonary perfusion (i.e. cardiovascular function) are all involved, i.e. the cardiovascular and respiratory systems are inextricably linked. Arterial blood gas analysis tells us how well the blood is oxygenated at the lungs. Venous blood gas analysis tells us how much oxygen remains in the blood after tissues have been perfused, and thus depends upon original uptake of oxygen in the lungs, tissue perfusion, and peripheral extraction of oxygen, and so reflects pulmonary and cardiovascular statuses and tissue metabolism. The 'ideal' mixed venous blood is that taken from the pulmonary artery. Blood gas analysis also tells us the acid–base status of the patient and helps us to determine the cause (respiratory and/or metabolic) of any perturbations (see Chapter 21).

The total amount of oxygen carried in a certain volume of blood depends upon:

- Amount of functional haemoglobin in that blood.
- Percentage saturation of that Hb with O_2 (SpO_2 if derived from a pulse oximeter; SaO_2 if calculated by a blood gas analyser).
- Amount of O_2 dissolved in physical solution in the blood (plasma), i.e. PaO_2.

The total oxygen content/carriage of 100 ml of blood (CaO_2) is given by the following equation.

$$CaO_2 = \left(\left[Hb\right] \times \%satn \times 1.34\right) + \left(PaO_2 \times 0.003\right)$$

where: [Hb] = haemoglobin concentration in g/dl; % satn = percentage saturation of haemoglobin with oxygen (SpO_2 or SaO_2), but expressed as a decimal; 1.34 = Hüfner's constant, which may be quoted as anything from 1.31 to 1.39 ml/g. It is the oxygen carrying capacity of haemoglobin, and equals the number of ml of oxygen actually bound to 1 g of haemoglobin under standard conditions (standard atmospheric pressure and 37 °C). Finally, 0.003 = Ostwald solubility coefficient and equals the number of ml of oxygen carried by 100 ml (i.e. 1 dl), of plasma for each 1 mmHg PO_2.

We try to ensure adequate tissue oxygen delivery in our anaesthetised patients.

$$\textbf{Tissue oxygen delivery} = \textbf{Cardiac output} \times \textbf{CaO}_2$$

$$\textbf{Tissue oxygen delivery} = \left(\textbf{Heart rate} \times \textbf{stroke volume}\right) \times \textbf{CaO}_2$$

18.4.3.4.2 Capnography/Capnometry

Why measure end tidal CO_2 ($ETCO_2$) tension? Note that some machines measure $ETCO_2$ percentage rather than tension (partial pressure). Alveolar CO_2 tension normally equilibrates with pulmonary capillary CO_2 tension by the time the pulmonary capillary blood has 'traversed' the alveolar bed. Pulmonary capillary blood comes from pulmonary arterial blood, and pulmonary arterial blood was the systemic venous blood returning to the heart in the venae cavae. Systemic venous blood has relatively low oxygen tension and high carbon dioxide tension. Pulmonary capillary blood, after undergoing gaseous exchange in the alveoli, becomes pulmonary venous blood, and returns to the left side of the heart, to be pumped out through the aorta. Hence, pulmonary venous blood (which has been oxygenated and has given up some of its CO_2) becomes systemic arterial blood.

The alveolar CO_2 tension, measurable as end tidal CO_2 tension, should therefore reflect the systemic arterial CO_2 tension. So, we could say, **ETCO$_2$ tension reflects the systemic arterial CO$_2$ tension.**

$ETCO_2$ tension also gives us an idea of the efficiency of alveolar ventilation (as long as cardiac output and metabolic rate remain unchanged), because of the relationship:

$$\textbf{Alveolar CO}_2 \textbf{ tension} \propto \frac{1}{\textbf{Alveolar ventilation}}$$

There is normally some dilution of the ideally ventilated and perfused alveolar gases with alveolar dead space gases (which have not undergone any gaseous exchange), so that the $ETCO_2$ tension is often slightly less (1–5 mmHg difference in man and small animals) than the actual alveolar (and therefore systemic arterial) CO_2 tension. In horses, this difference can be much greater (10–15 mmHg because of greater ventilation/perfusion mismatches). Occasionally, 'inverse gradients' occur (i.e. $ETCO_2$ tension is greater than alveolar CO_2 tension), usually at very slow breathing rates, and when alveoli empty 'unevenly' with, e.g. pulmonary disease.

Whenever $ETCO_2$ tension is measured, it is useful to take the occasional arterial blood sample to determine the arterial CO_2 tension ($PaCO_2$), to compare with the $ETCO_2$ tension. The trend in $ETCO_2$ values (i.e. if values increase or decrease) is usually reliable, although (especially for horses), the actual values of $ETCO_2$ and $PaCO_2$ may differ quite considerably.

The normal value for systemic arterial CO_2 'tension' (or 'partial pressure') is around 35–45 mmHg (and often towards the lower end [32–35 mmHg] for cats), and so values should be similar for $ETCO_2$ tension. However, under anaesthesia, when most patients hypoventilate to some degree because of respiratory depression, these values may increase. It is usual to aim to maintain the values for $PaCO_2$ (and $ETCO_2$) tension between 35 and 60 mmHg. Below 20 mmHg (you are probably hyperventilating the animal), cerebral blood vessel vasoconstriction can be severe enough to compromise cerebral oxygen delivery; and current recommendations are to try to avoid $ETCO_2$ tensions below about 35 mmHg. Above 60 mmHg, blood pH starts to become more acidic (see Chapter 21), which may compromise myocardial function; and although the high CO_2 stimulates sympathetic nervous system activity, which may be useful, it may also result in an increased incidence of cardiac arrhythmias.

Capnometry/capnography techniques measure the amount of CO_2 (commonly by infrared [IR] absorption spectrometry) in gases continuously sampled from near the ET tube connector, and usually determine the breathing rate as well as the $ETCO_2$ tension (or percentage). $ETCO_2$ tension reflects systemic arterial CO_2 tension. Continuous monitoring is either by sidestream (including microstream) or mainstream techniques.

Sidestream sampling requires gases to be 'withdrawn' from the anaesthetic breathing system near/at the ET tube connector (low dead space connectors are available for patients <5 kg), usually at a rate of about 200 ml/min. This sampling rate may be a problem in smaller patients where it may be close to the minute ventilation. Although some machines allow selection of slower sampling rates for smaller patients, this may compromise signal quality, so microstream or mainstream sampling may be preferable.

Sampled gases then reach the measuring chamber (with a slight delay, so the information is slightly historical), where their IR absorption is compared to a standard, before the result is displayed, either numerically, e.g. by a needle-gauge capnometer (=capnometry), or in graphic form as either a time or a trend capnogram (=capnography) (Figures 18.15 and 18.16, respectively). Water vapour must be removed before the sample reaches the measuring chamber, as H_2O interferes with IR absorption by CO_2. The volume of gases removed from the anaesthetic breathing system should either be scavenged or returned to the system (especially where low flow techniques are used as such gas sampling can constitute a significant proportion of the

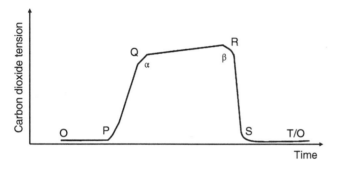

Figure 18.15 Typical capnograph trace (called a time capnogram) from high speed (75 cm/min) recording of single breath. Inspiratory segment, R to T (=**phase 0**); expiratory segment, O to R (includes the end expiratory pause so it may be difficult to define the exact end of expiration); anatomical dead space gases exhaled, O to P (=**phase I**); mixture of dead space and alveolar gases exhaled, P to Q (=**phase II**); pure alveolar gases exhaled, Q to R = alveolar plateau (=**phase III**); ETCO2 reading is taken at R; occasionally a sharp upswing (**phase IV**) may be noted at the end of the plateau, especially if the plateau is flat, this is usually a sign of reduced thoracic compliance; **α angle** = angle between phase II and phase III (tells of ventilation/perfusion status of the lungs); **β angle** = angle between phase III and descending limb of inspiratory segment, R to S (helps assess extent of rebreathing).

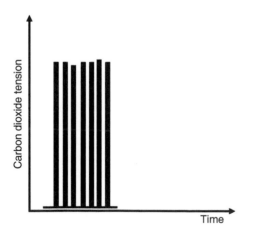

Figure 18.16 A trend capnogram; obtained when recording speed is slow (25 mm/min). Each bar represents one breath.

gases delivered to the breathing system), at a point distant from where the sampling is occurring.

Microstream sampling is a form of sidestream sampling, but where the IR emitter source is not a 'hot' black body as used in conventional machines, but a 'cold' molecular correlation spectroscopy source wherein IR emission is generated by a radiofrequency discharge (as used in gas lasers), with resultant emission of a very narrow range of IR wavelengths (4.20–4.25 μm), highly specific for CO_2 (and unaffected by other gases). This reduces the pathlength required in the sampling cell, and therefore reduces the sampling cell size (to 15 μl), which reduces the gas sampling rate required to only 50 ml/min without compromising response time or accuracy. Special microbore sampling lines (Filterline™) incorporate hydrophobic filters and Nafion™ tubing (to eliminate water), and the low dead space airway sampling adapter contains multiple, variously orientated, hydrophobic, small sampling ports at the midline of the expected gas flow path, which reduce the risk of sampling line occlusion.

Mainstream sampling requires an ET tube in-line sampling chamber/adapter with a sensor/analyser, which contains the necessary 'machinery' to analyse the CO_2 content of the gases in real-time, again by IR absorption spectroscopy. There is virtually no time delay in displaying the results. A heating element contained within the sensor prevents water vapour interference. Sampling chamber/adapters used to be very delicate, but modern versions are more durable, and disposable (single-use) versions are now available, eliminating the need for cleaning and sterilisation between patients. Furthermore, low dead space 'neonatal' sampling chamber/adapters are now available. Finally, modern sensors are also more lightweight, and their wires are less heavy than first-generation mainstream analysers, thus producing less drag on the ET tube. Mainstream analysers tend to give more accurate results than sidestream analysers because there is no need for a sampling line in which dispersion of gases can occur. There is also no need for extra scavenging and no concern where low flow techniques are used because no gases are removed from the breathing system. Time capnograms or trend capnograms can again be displayed.

Monitoring ETCO2

ETCO2 values depend upon:

- Rate of production of CO_2 (depends upon metabolic rate, which depends upon, e.g. temperature, thyroid hormones, catecholamines, malignant hyperthermia).
- Alveolar ventilation (e.g. if alveolar ventilation decreases, then alveolar CO_2 increases, and therefore the ETCO2 value increases).

- Cardiac output, and therefore pulmonary (alveolar) perfusion. For example, if cardiac arrest or massive pulmonary embolism occurs, alveolar perfusion ceases, so alveolar gases equilibrate with inhaled gases (if ventilation continues, e.g. by mechanical ventilation) so the $ETCO_2$ value decreases. Monitoring $ETCO_2$ values can be a useful indicator of return of 'a circulation' when resuscitation from cardiac arrest is performed.

Therefore, monitoring $ETCO_2$ values tells us about metabolism, ventilation, and circulation. It can also provide us with useful information about our anaesthetic breathing system:

- Is the ET tube in the airway or the oesophagus?
- Is the ET tube patent?
- Is the ET tube too long (protruding out from the patient's incisor arcade), resulting in increased apparatus dead space and rebreathing of CO_2? (Alternatively, over-long ET tubes can result in endobronchial intubation, also resulting in hypercapnia and also hypoxaemia.)
- Is the soda lime working or is there rebreathing of CO_2 because the soda lime is exhausted? Most capnometers and capnographs will enable you to determine if the inhaled CO_2 is too high.
- Are the one-way valves in the circle system working or is there rebreathing of CO_2?
- Is the fresh gas flow (FGF) high enough with non-rebreathing systems or is there some rebreathing of CO_2-laden gases?

Interpretation of $ETCO_2$ Values

Because the $ETCO_2$ value depends upon at least three factors, we must be careful how we interpret it. The $ETCO_2$ value accurately reflects $PaCO_2$ only when:

- There are no major ventilation/perfusion mismatches (no major shunts or dead space problems) or major diffusion problems.
- The tidal volume is adequate to displace the alveolar gases to the point of sampling.
- A cuffed ET tube is used, so that there are no leaks, and no 'dilution' of the sample (which needs aspirating into the sampling line by a small pump, with sidestream sampling), with entrained air.
- The FGF is not so excessive as to dilute the sample.
- The sampling rate is not so excessive as to interfere with the patient's ventilation, or dilute the end tidal sample with fresh gases or dead space gases.
- There are no major 'time constant' differences between different parts of the lungs to ensure that the $ETCO_2$ value reflects the 'majority situation'. Different lobes of the lungs often have different inflation and deflation

rates (reflected by 'time constants', where a time constant equals lung lobe volume divided by the rate of flow into or out of that lobe). With disease or atelectasis (e.g. under anaesthesia, especially horses), there can be large differences in time constants between different lobes of the lungs.

With small patients like cats, a number of the above points are not always adhered to; a better sampling position may be nearer the carina rather than at the 'proximal' end of the ET tube, but this would require a special modification of the ET tube.

If $ETCO_2$ value is increasing, look out for:

- Increased CO_2 inhalation: suggests either i) rebreathing (check for increased apparatus dead space, e.g. due to long portion of ET tube projecting externally beyond incisor arcade, or large internal volume of ET tube connectors/HMEs/sampling adapters; and check anaesthetic breathing system for faulty one-way valves, exhausted soda lime, and insufficient FGF); or ii) inadvertent delivery of CO_2 into the fresh gases. (An HME is a heat-and-moisture exchanger, which also may include a microbial filter [HMEF] and is sited between the ET tube and the anaesthetic breathing system, and may contain a sampling port for sidestream capnography.)
- Increased CO_2 production: suggests increased metabolism, perhaps because the patient is too 'lightly' anaesthetised, malignant hyperthermia is developing, the patient is seizuring, a thyroid storm is developing, or there is a phaeochromocytoma.
- Decreased CO_2 excretion: suggests hypoventilation (perhaps because the patient is too 'deep' (see also Chapter 19).
- Endobronchial intubation (so that one lung is bypassed). An increase in $PaCO_2$ and a decrease in PaO_2 are seen on blood gas analysis.

If $ETCO_2$ value is decreasing, look out for:

- Increased CO_2 excretion: suggests hyperventilation, perhaps because of over-zealous mechanical ventilation or the patient is becoming too 'light' (see also Chapter 19).
- Decreased CO_2 production: suggests lowered basal metabolic rate, perhaps with deep anaesthesia, hypothermia, or hypothyroidism.
- Decreased cardiac output: possible cardiac arrest or pulmonary embolism (air/thrombus/fat/bone marrow).
- Disconnection, blockage, or leaks in sampling system, or the ET tube cuff may have become deflated.

Figure 18.17 summarises the interpretations for commonly observed time capnograms.

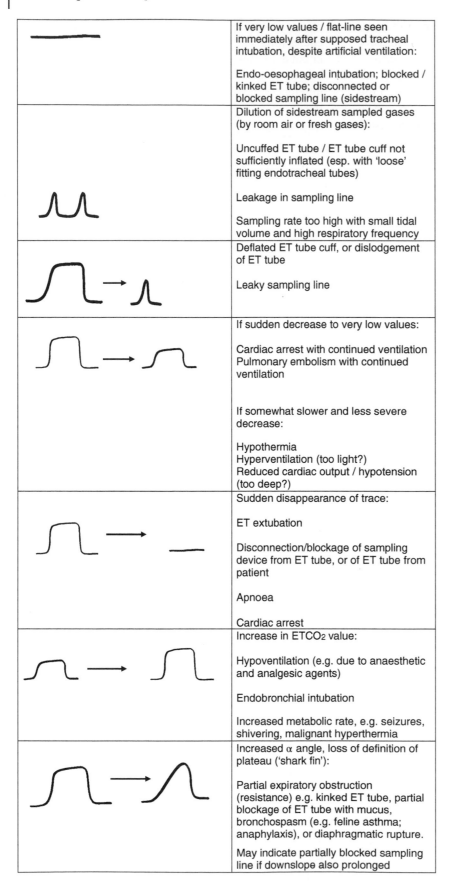

	If very low values / flat-line seen immediately after supposed tracheal intubation, despite artificial ventilation: Endo-oesophageal intubation; blocked / kinked ET tube; disconnected or blocked sampling line (sidestream)
	Dilution of sidestream sampled gases (by room air or fresh gases): Uncuffed ET tube / ET tube cuff not sufficiently inflated (esp. with 'loose' fitting endotracheal tubes) Leakage in sampling line Sampling rate too high with small tidal volume and high respiratory frequency
	Deflated ET tube cuff, or dislodgement of ET tube Leaky sampling line
	If sudden decrease to very low values: Cardiac arrest with continued ventilation Pulmonary embolism with continued ventilation If somewhat slower and less severe decrease: Hypothermia Hyperventilation (too light?) Reduced cardiac output / hypotension (too deep?)
	Sudden disappearance of trace: ET extubation Disconnection/blockage of sampling device from ET tube, or of ET tube from patient Apnoea Cardiac arrest
	Increase in ETCO$_2$ value: Hypoventilation (e.g. due to anaesthetic and analgesic agents) Endobronchial intubation Increased metabolic rate, e.g. seizures, shivering, malignant hyperthermia
	Increased α angle, loss of definition of plateau ('shark fin'): Partial expiratory obstruction (resistance) e.g. kinked ET tube, partial blockage of ET tube with mucus, bronchospasm (e.g. feline asthma; anaphylaxis), or diaphragmatic rupture. May indicate partially blocked sampling line if downslope also prolonged

Figure 18.17 Interpretation of common capnogram waveforms.

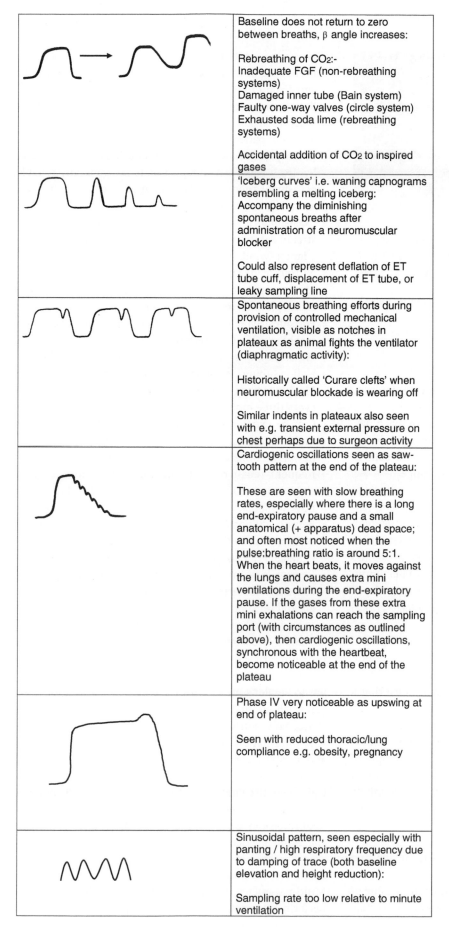

	Baseline does not return to zero between breaths, β angle increases: Rebreathing of CO_2:- Inadequate FGF (non-rebreathing systems) Damaged inner tube (Bain system) Faulty one-way valves (circle system) Exhausted soda lime (rebreathing systems) Accidental addition of CO_2 to inspired gases
	'Iceberg curves' i.e. waning capnograms resembling a melting iceberg: Accompany the diminishing spontaneous breaths after administration of a neuromuscular blocker Could also represent deflation of ET tube cuff, displacement of ET tube, or leaky sampling line
	Spontaneous breathing efforts during provision of controlled mechanical ventilation, visible as notches in plateaux as animal fights the ventilator (diaphragmatic activity): Historically called 'Curare clefts' when neuromuscular blockade is wearing off Similar indents in plateaux also seen with e.g. transient external pressure on chest perhaps due to surgeon activity
	Cardiogenic oscillations seen as saw-tooth pattern at the end of the plateau: These are seen with slow breathing rates, especially where there is a long end-expiratory pause and a small anatomical (+ apparatus) dead space; and often most noticed when the pulse:breathing ratio is around 5:1. When the heart beats, it moves against the lungs and causes extra mini ventilations during the end-expiratory pause. If the gases from these extra mini exhalations can reach the sampling port (with circumstances as outlined above), then cardiogenic oscillations, synchronous with the heartbeat, become noticeable at the end of the plateau
	Phase IV very noticeable as upswing at end of plateau: Seen with reduced thoracic/lung compliance e.g. obesity, pregnancy
	Sinusoidal pattern, seen especially with panting / high respiratory frequency due to damping of trace (both baseline elevation and height reduction): Sampling rate too low relative to minute ventilation

Figure 18.17 (Continued)

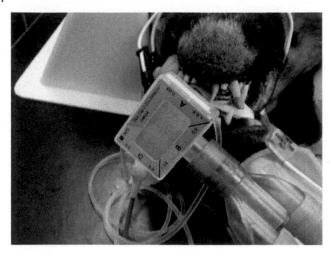

Figure 18.18 Colorimetric CO_2 detector (Easy-Cap II™) being used for a dog.

Advantages

- Non-invasive and continuous.
- Can reduce the frequency for arterial blood gas analysis.
- Real-time signal with mainstream analysers.
- Breathing rate also displayed by most modern machines.
- Very useful when having to ventilate the patient's lungs, as ventilation can be tailored, almost breath by breath, to keep the $ETCO_2$ value within the desired range.
- Colorimetric devices are useful to determine tracheal versus oesophageal intubation (Figure 18.18). The pH-sensitive chemicals last about two hours, so they can only be used for relatively short procedures to determine breathing rates and only give a limited range of colours between purple (no CO_2) and bright yellow (a maximum of 5 % $ETCO_2$). Trade names include: Nellcor Easy-Cap II and Pedi-Cap for larger (>15 kg) and smaller (<15 kg) animals, respectively.
- Many machines will also give values of inspired and expired O_2 tensions (called oxygraphy), which is useful when using low flow anaesthesia, medical air, or nitrous oxide where there is always the danger of delivering a hypoxic mixture of gases to your patient.
- Some machines may also display information about the inhaled anaesthetic agent in use, e.g. its inspired concentration, its end tidal concentration, and the multiple of that agent's MAC value being administered to the patient (also warnings can be given when you are potentially delivering very high anaesthetic agent concentrations).

Disadvantages

- Sampling delay with sidestream analysers means that displayed data are slightly historical.
- Sidestream sampling can remove a significant volume of gases from the anaesthetic breathing system. These may

be scavenged, but if low flow techniques are used, it is preferable to return them to the breathing system at a site distant to the gas sampling site.

- Sidestream analysers, in particular, can be inaccurate when high sampling rates (around 200 ml/min) are used for small patients with small tidal volumes, yet high respiratory frequencies (leading to dilution of sampled gases by 'fresh gases'). Although trends are generally reliable, occasional arterial blood gas analyses may be helpful if the sampling rate cannot be reduced (e.g. to 50 ml/min).
- Occasionally, respiratory secretions may block sidestream sampling lines or obscure mainstream sampling adapter 'windows'.
- Nitrous oxide and oxygen can interfere with carbon dioxide measurement (through 'collision-broadening'), although most modern analysers are less affected.
- For sidestream analysers, sampling lines must be impermeable to CO_2 (e.g. Teflon).
- Water traps or special water-permeable sampling line (e.g. Nafion tubing), must be used with sidestream analysers.
- Machines need to be re-calibrated from time to time (e.g. every three months).
- Can be expensive. The adapters and sensors of earlier mainstream analysers tended to be prone to damage, but newer versions are more robust, reducing the need for frequent repair or replacement. Furthermore, cheaper single-use mainstream sampling chamber/adapters are now available, eliminating the costs of re-sterilisation.
- Beware addition of dead space to the anaesthetic breathing system, with both sidestream and mainstream analysers, although low dead space adapters are now available for both.
- Beware 'drag' on the anaesthetic breathing system by, especially, mainstream analysers, although modern adapters and sensors are much less bulky than earlier versions.

18.4.3.4.3 Volumetric Capnography

In volumetric capnography, waveforms of CO_2 tension are plotted against integrated flow or volume, in a manner similar to Fowler's method for the single breath test for nitrogen washout, in order to measure anatomical/airway dead space. Volumetric capnograms can be interpreted to provide information not only about $ETCO_2$ tension, but also about mixed expired CO_2 tension and CO_2 elimination. Furthermore, they can provide information about anatomical, and with calculations (using, e.g. the Enghoff-modified Bohr equation), physiological [anatomical + alveolar] and total [physiological + apparatus] dead space; and the dead space and alveolar components of the tidal volume.

18.4.3.4.4 Spirometry

Multi-parameter monitors may also have the capability to perform spirometry. This monitoring modality allows for the measurement of a number of variables associated with ventilation, including:

- Tidal volume (expired and inspired)
- Minute volume
- Compliance (respiratory system, C_{rs})
- Airway pressures

Spirometry is based on the principle of measuring laminar gas flow through a fixed resistance with the use of two Pitot tubes (facing in opposite directions within the gas flow) that are connected to pressure transducers. The pressure difference between the two Pitot tubes is proportional to the square of the flow rate. From this, tidal volume, and subsequently, minute respiratory volume, may be measured. It also allows the displaying of pressure/volume and flow/volume loops that can aid in the diagnosis and management of various ventilatory disturbances.

18.4.3.4.5 *Pulse Oximetry*

This determines the degree of saturation of haemoglobin with oxygen. From the haemoglobin/oxygen dissociation curve, you will recall how oxygen tension of arterial blood (PaO_2), is related to haemoglobin saturation with oxygen (SaO_2) by a sigmoid curve (so shaped because of the co-operative binding characteristics of oxygen with the 4 haem groups in each haemogblobin molecule). On the slope part of the curve, a large fall in saturation follows a small decrease in PaO_2.

Pulse oximetry is based on two principles:

- **Pulse photoplethysmography:** changing volume of a tissue bed (due to arterial pulsation) can be measured by change in light absorption.
- **Spectrophotometric oximetry:** deoxyhaemoglobin and oxyhaemoglobin absorb different wavelengths of light differently; they have different absorption spectra. Oxyhaemoglobin looks red because it reflects red light and absorbs blue light; deoxyhaemoglobin looks blue because it reflects blue light and absorbs red.

Beer–Lambert's law defines how light absorbance increases with the concentration of an absorbing/attenuating substance within a medium (Beer), and also increases with the pathlength for light travel (Lambert).

$$\textbf{Absorbance} = \textbf{e.L.c}$$

where L is the pathlength, c is the concentration of the absorbing substance in the medium and e is the molar extinction coefficient.

Pulse oximeters have either transmittance or reflectance 'probes' (the things we clip onto the tongue [if transmittance (Figure 18.19)] or place into the oesophagus or cloaca [if reflectance]). Both types of probes contain light emitting diodes (LEDs) that shine light of red and IR wavelengths alternately (at an alternating frequency of 770–1000 Hz) through or into the chosen tissue bed (tongue, toe, ear, cloaca/rectum/oesophagus). A receiver (opposite the emitter if a transmittance probe, or set at an angle to the emitter if a reflectance probe) then receives the signal after it has traversed the tissue bed in question.

The signal received has a 'constant' part ('background') that is due to non-pulsatile tissue (venous blood, muscle, bone) and an 'alternating' part that is due to the pulsatile arterial flow. The machine then 'discounts' the constant background signal, paying attention to only the pulsatile signal. The ratio of red to IR light absorption of this pulsatile, arterial signal is then used to determine the percentage saturation of the haemoglobin with oxygen. That is, SpO_2 values, indicative of 'fractional' saturation of haemoglobin with oxygen (i.e. dyshaemoglobins cannot be accounted for when only two wavelengths are used; see below), are determined from R values (see Figure 18.20), where R is the ratio of pulsatile absorption at 660 nm (red)

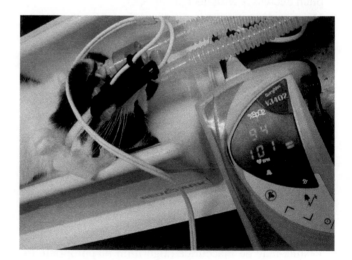

Figure 18.19 V3402™ pulse oximeter with transmittance probe attached to cat's tongue.

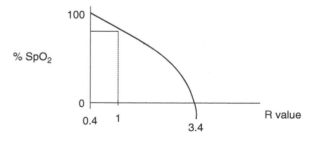

Figure 18.20 Pulse oximetry algorithm for determination of percentage SpO_2 value.

to pulsatile absorption at 940 nm (IR). Most machines use an algorithm based on human haemoglobin, but validated for dog, horse, pig, cow, and cat haemoglobin, from which they can 'read off' (calculate), a saturation value (Figure 18.20) for any given R value.

Note that **if R equals 1,** the pulse oximetry **SpO_2 reading will be 85–87%;** and with a poor signal: noise ratio, the R value tends towards 1, so beware.

Pulse oximetry readings are generally fairly accurate (within 5%) between saturations of 70–100%. Values below 70% are extrapolated (<70% means big trouble).

Advantages

- Noninvasive.
- Continuous.
- Pretty quick response time (only slight lag between actual pulse and reading being displayed), but the more peripheral the tissue bed/artery chosen, the longer the time from events happening at the aorta to reach the peripheral circulation.
- Many machines will display a pulse rate too, and each pulse may be accompanied by an audible 'beep', whose pitch decreases with decreasing SpO_2.
- Many machines will give an idea of signal strength, perhaps in the form of a series of illuminated bars (Figure 18.19); the more bars that are illuminated, the better the signal strength, and therefore, possibly, the better the signal (pulse) quality, or in the form of a pulse plethysmograph (i.e. a pulse volume graph) that can give extra information, similar to that displayed by an arterial pressure wave (Figure 18.7).
- No need for re-calibration.
- Decreases the necessity for multiple arterial blood gas analyses.
- Relatively cheap.

Disadvantages

- Results may be inaccurate (algorithm inappropriate for species in which it is used; or poor signal detection; see below).
- Can be quite a 'late' indicator of trouble (i.e. PaO_2 can decrease markedly for only a slight fall in SpO_2) (see notes on blood gas analysis in Chapter 21).
- Signal strength indicators only tell of tissue perfusion at the site of the probe (Figure 18.19).

Signal detection/acquisition may be a problem, e.g.:

- Hypotension
- Hypovolaemia (peripheral vasoconstriction)
- Hypothermia (peripheral vasoconstriction)
- Drugs (e.g. α2 agonists), and catecholamines (perhaps too 'light') may cause peripheral vasoconstriction

- Slow heart rates and also very rapid heart rates (beware use in rabbits and exotic species in which the heart rates can exceed the maximum readout of some monitors)
- Arrhythmias
- Venous pulsations, especially in A-V anastomoses (e.g. in skin), may be a nuisance
- Other pigments in skin or blood (dyes; bilirubin [little effect in modern analysers]; carboxyhaemoglobin [SpO_2 tends to over-read: beware animals from recent house fires with smoke or carbon monoxide inhalation]; methaemoglobin [SpO_2 tends to read 85%])
- Anaemia (pulse oximetry needs at least some haemoglobin to be present)
- Patient movement
- Poor probe positioning (causing 'optical shunt', later called the penumbra effect) results in readings tending towards a value of 85–87% because of poor signal: noise ratio
- Excessive fat or hair at probe site
- Very thin tissue beds (too much light transmitted or reflected, so poor signal-to-noise ratio)
- Extraneous light (especially fluorescent tubes). If high 'noise' compared to signal strength, then reading tends to c. 85–87%

Masimo Pulse Co-oximetry Technology

Pulse co-oximetry monitors utilise multiple wavelength spectrophotometry (extra light wavelengths in addition to red and IR, which are the only two wavelengths used in traditional pulse oximeters), to allow more accurate SpO_2 measurement in the presence of abnormal haemoglobins, such as carboxy- and met-haemoglobin. By utilising pulse co-oximetry, in addition to SpO_2 ('functional' saturation of haemoglobin with oxygen; where the dyshaemoglobins, carboxy- and met-haemoglobin, can be accounted for and excluded), this technology allows for the measurement of a number of additional indices including: haemoglobin concentrations (total, carboxy- and met-haemoglobin concentrations), oxygen content, a peripheral perfusion index (PI), and a pleth variability index (PVI), which quantifies respiratory variations in the plethysmograph curve. Masimo signal extraction technology also facilitates greater accuracy in states of hypoperfusion and movement.

18.4.4 Gas and Agent Monitoring

18.4.4.1 Oxygen Meters

Routinely used by medical anaesthetists to help verify that oxygen is delivered through the common gas outlet of anaesthetic machines. Oxygen measurement devices may also be incorporated into other gas analysers, e.g. alongside capnography and volatile anaesthetic agent monitoring. Different technologies are used to measure oxygen:

galvanic cells, polarographic cells (Clark electrodes), and paramagnetic techniques.

18.4.4.2 Anaesthetic Agent Monitors

Volatile anaesthetic agents and nitrous oxide can also be measured in the gases inspired and expired by patients. Again, different technologies exist. IR absorption spectrometry is probably the commonest technique used, but other technologies are available, e.g. ultraviolet absorption, mass spectrometry, and Raman scattering. Methane in exhaled gases from the patient can interfere with some IR absorption devices, depending upon the wavelengths used, and can cause falsely elevated readings for the volatile anaesthetic agents. It is advisable to check the machine's specification before use, especially in horses and ruminants. Some aerosol propellants (e.g. HFA 134a [hydrofluoroalkane (1,1,1,2-tetrafluoroethane)], used in asthmatic inhalers) may also interfere with volatile agent monitoring by IR absorptiometry as their IR absorption spectra overlap those of the halogenated volatile anaesthetic agents.

18.4.5 Monitoring the Neuromuscular System

Most of the time, we do not monitor the neuromuscular system as such, except, e.g. when testing the presence/strength of limb withdrawal reflexes or when certain electrolyte imbalances may affect neuromuscular activity (muscle twitches/seizures). However, when we use peripherally acting neuromuscular blocking agents to effectively 'paralyse' our patients, then it is important to monitor the degree of neuromuscular block for two reasons:

- To ensure adequate neuromuscular blockade when it is needed (e.g. for surgery).
- To ensure adequate return of neuromuscular function when 'paralysis' is no longer required (i.e. when the animal recovers from anaesthesia it must now be able to breathe and move for itself). See Chapter 17 on muscle relaxants for further explanation.

18.4.6 Temperature Monitoring

Temperature is commonly measured with thermometers (expansion type, e.g. mercury in glass), thermistors, or thermocouples. True core temperature is measured in the pulmonary artery during the end-expiratory pause, and is best approximated by deep oesophageal temperature. Rectal temperature may be a poor substitute (especially with faeces present), but is the most commonly used and least invasive site. If the tympanic membrane is intact and the ear canal 'clean', radiant heat (IR) from the tympanic membrane can be measured over a very short time (c. five seconds) by a thermopile (collection of thermocouples), but the best results are obtained with devices which are specifically designed for the ear of the particular species in question.

Temperature can be helpful in assessing the cardiovascular status of animals (i.e. cold extremities or increased core-periphery temperature gradients may be present in shock states). Temperature is also vitally important to monitor in anaesthetised animals, especially in 'small' animals with a large surface area : volume ratio. Anaesthesia generally lowers the metabolic rate and reduces muscle activity/shivering ability (and therefore reduces heat production), and depresses the 'thermostat' in the hypothalamus of the CNS, reducing the patient's ability to thermoregulate. Many of the drugs we use during anaesthesia also cause peripheral vasodilation, and thereby enhance heat loss. This is exacerbated by us clipping large patches of fur (reducing insulation), then using copious volumes of scrub solution, and then surgical spirit (wetting the animal and enhancing evaporative cooling). Hypothermia can be a real problem in very young and small animals. Preventing heat loss is easier than re-warming an animal. See Chapter 20.

Some degree of hypothermia is common in many of our anaesthetised patients and can be one of the causes of a prolonged recovery. **Ideally, an animal's rectal temperature should be back to 37.0 °C before it leaves recovery to return to its kennel.**

Hyperthermia can also be a problem. Beware malignant hyperthermia (see especially Chapter 35), but also, on hot days, if using rebreathing systems (which retain/produce heat and moisture [soda lime reaction with CO_2 is exothermic and produces some water]), and if a heat and moisture exchanger is also used, and the theatre is not air-conditioned, and the operating lights are producing massive amounts of heat, the patient may become hyperthermic.

18.4.7 Monitoring the Renal System

As many anaesthetic agents can cause hypotension, and some may impair/alter renal function, it is important to consider the kidneys. As mentioned earlier, urine output can be measured (normally ~1–1.5 ml/kg/h). This requires bladder catheterisation and initial emptying, to achieve a 'baseline'. Urine production can then be measured, and samples taken for dipstick analysis, and, in particular, specific gravity determination. Although we tend not to routinely monitor urine output during anaesthesia, it can be affected by a number of factors during anaesthesia and plays an important role in the intensive care setting.

The stress response to anaesthesia includes an increase in anti-diuretic hormone (ADH) secretion, and so we can expect a reduction in urine output during, and for some time after, GA. Some drugs (e.g. α2 agonists) can also affect urine output (see Chapters 4 and 28 on sedatives), and whether the patient receives IV fluids during anaesthesia can also influence urine output.

Thus, whilst not routinely monitoring urine output under anaesthesia, we do things during anaesthesia with the kidneys in mind. For example, we like to have some idea of MAP (we know that most anaesthetic agents will depress blood pressure to some degree) as autoregulation of tissue blood flow (including the kidneys) only occurs over a range of blood pressures (from a MAP of ~60–70 mmHg up to ~150–160 mmHg for 'normal' patients). If renal perfusion cannot be autoregulated, then the renal cells with the highest metabolic requirements become compromised and 'damaged', particularly the most metabolically active renal tubular epithelial cells. During anaesthesia, IV fluids, positive inotropes, and vasopressors may be necessary to help to support blood pressure. The administration of IV fluids to support the circulation in patients with pre-existing hypovolaemia, is a must. In some circumstances, drugs such as sodium nitroprusside (vasodilator) may be required to counter hypertension that may develop during surgery for, e.g. thyroid tumours or phaeochromocytomas.

We also consider carefully the use of, e.g. imaging contrast agents and NSAIDs. Contrast agents can be nephrotoxic, and NSAIDs can further compromise renal blood flow in the presence of hypotension and can lead to renal medullary/papillary necrosis and acute renal failure.

18.5 Multiparameter Monitors

Electronic devices are now becoming widely available that enable monitoring of several variables in one unit, thereby improving convenience (Figure 18.21).

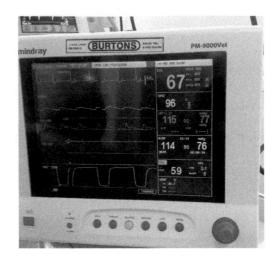

Figure 18.21 The screen display of a Mindray PM-9000Vet™ multiparameter monitor showing, from the top, ECG, pulse oximetry, direct arterial blood pressure, non-invasive blood pressure (numerical values in white), capnography, and temperature (bottom right). Anaesthetic agent monitoring was not available on this particular unit, although the necessary modules are available for this model.

18.6 Summary

These notes provide a brief outline of the ways in which animals under anaesthesia can be monitored. They are by no means exhaustive, but illustrate the potential available. Not all of these methods are applicable to every case; sometimes it can take longer to instrument an animal in order to monitor its status than it can to perform the surgery (e.g. cat castration); so judgement should be exercised on a case-by-case basis.

Further Reading

Ansari, B.M., Zochios, V., Falter, F., and Klein, A.A. (2016). Physiological controversies and methods used to determine fluid responsiveness: a qualitative systematic review. *Anaesthesia* 71: 94–105.

Berkenstadt, H., Friedman, Z., Preisman, S. et al. (2005). Pulse pressure and stroke volume variations during severe haemorrhage in ventilated dogs. *British Journal of Anaesthesia* 94: 721–726.

Bilbrough, G. (2003). Critical care monitoring of small animal patients. *In Practice* 25: 542–549.

Bilbrough, G. (2006). A practical guide to capnography. *In Practice* 28: 312–319.

Briganti, A., Evangelista, F., Centonze, P. et al. (2018). A preliminary study evaluating cardiac output measurement using pressure recording analytical method (PRAM) in anaesthetized dogs. *BMC Veterinary Research* 14: 72. https://doi.org/10.1186/s12917-018-1392-5.

Bucci, M., Rabozzi, R., Guglielmini, C., and Franci, P. (2017). Respiratory variation in aortic peak blood velocity and caudal vena cava diameter can predict fluid responsiveness in anaesthetised and mechanically ventilated dogs. *The Veterinary Journal* 227: 30–35.

Caney, S. (2007). Non-invasive blood pressure measurement in cats. *In Practice* 29: 398–403.

Cannesson, M., Le Manach, Y., Hofer, C.K. et al. (2011). Assessing the diagnostic accuracy of pulse pressure variations for the prediction of fluid responsiveness: a "Gray zone" approach. *Anesthesiology* 115: 231–241.

Carr, A.P., Duke, T., and Egner, B. (2008). Blood pressure in small animals: part I: hypertension and hypotension and an update on technology. *European Journal of Companion Animal Practice* 18: 135–142.

Celeita-Rodriguez, N., Teixeira-Neto, F.J., Garofalo, N.A. et al. (2019). Comparison of the diagnostic accuracy of dynamic and static preload indexes to predict fluid responsiveness in mechanically ventilated, isoflurane anaesthetised dogs. *Veterinary Anaesthesia and Analgesia* 46: 276–288.

Cerejo SA, Teixeira-Neto FJ, Garofalo NA, Pimenta ELM, Zanuzzo FS, Klein AV (2020) Effects of cuff size and position on the agreement between arterial blood pressure measured by Doppler ultrasound and through a dorsal pedal artery catheter in anesthetized cats. *Veterinary Anaesthesia and Analgesia* 47, 191–199.

Chambers, D., Huang, C., and Matthews, G. (2015). *Basic Physiology for Anaesthetists* (eds. D. Chambers, C. Huang and G. Matthews). Cambridge University Press.

Chan, E.D., Chan, M.M., and Chan, M.M. (2013). Pulse oximetry: understanding its basic principles facilitates appreciation of its limitations. *Respiratory Medicine* 107: 789–799.

Chappell, D., Jacob, M., Hofmann-Kiefer, K. et al. (2008). A rational approach to perioperative fluid management. *Anesthesiology* 109: 723–740.

Colman, Y. and Krauss, B. (1999). Microstream capnography technology: a new approach to an old problem. *Journal of Clinical Monitoring* 15: 403–409.

Corley, K.T.T., Donaldson, L.L., Durando, M.M., and Birks, E.K. (2003). Cardiac output technologies with special reference to the horse. *Journal of Veterinary Internal Medicine* 17: 262–272.

Coutrot, M., Joachim, J., Depret, F. et al. (2019). Noninvasive continuous detection of arterial hypotension during induction of anaesthesia using a photoplethysmographic signal: proof of concept. *British Journal of Anaesthesia* 122: 605–612.

Cross, M. and Plunkett, E. (2014). *Physics, Pharmacology and Physiology for Anaesthetists: Key Concepts for the FRCA*, 2e. Cambridge, UK: Cambridge University Press.

Deflandre, C.J.A. and Hellebrekers, L.J. (2008). Clinical evaluation of the Surgivet V60046, a non-invasive blood pressure monitor in anaesthetized dogs. *Veterinary Anaesthesia and Analgesia* 35: 13–21.

Desai, N. and Garry, D. (2018). Assessing dynamic fluid-responsiveness using transthoracic echocardiography in intensive care. *BJA Education* 18: 218–226.

Dyson, D. (2007). Indirect measurement of blood pressure using a pulse oximeter in isoflurane anesthetized dogs. *Journal of Veterinary Emergency and Critical Care* 17: 135–142.

Esper, S.A. and Pinsky, M.R. (2014). Arterial waveform analysis. *Best Practice & Research Clinical Anaesthesiology* 28: 363–380.

Fielding, C.L. and Stolba, C.N. (2012). Pulse pressure variation and systolic pressure variation in horses undergoing general anesthesia. *Journal of Veterinary Emergency and Critical Care* 22: 372–375.

Gelman, S. (2008). Venous function and central venous pressure: a physiologic story. *Anesthesiology* 108: 735–748.

Gonzalez, A.M., Mann, F.A., Preziosi, D.E. et al. (2002). Measurement of body temperature by use of auricular thermometers versus rectal thermometers in dogs with otitis externa. *Journal of the American Veterinary Medical Association* 221: 378–380.

Habre, W., Asztalos, T., Sly, P.D., and Petak, F. (2001). Viscosity and density of common anaesthetic gases: implications for flow measurements. *British Journal of Anaesthesia* 87: 602–607.

Hopster, K., Ambrisko, T.D., and Kaestner, S.B.R. (2017). Influence of catecholamines at different dosages on the function of the LidCO sensor in isoflurane anesthetized horses. *Journal of Veterinary Emergency and Critical Care* 27: 651–657.

Jubran, A. (2015). Pulse oximetry. *Critical Care* 19: 272. https://doi.org/10.1186/s13054-015-0984-8.

Kissin, I. (2000). Depth of anaesthesia and bispectral index monitoring. *Anesthesia and Analgesia* 90: 1114–1117.

Kronen, P. (2007). Monitoring of patients under anaesthesia. *European Journal of Companion Animal Practice* 17: 153–160.

Kwak, J., Yoon, H., Kim, J. et al. (2018). Ultrasonographic measurement of caudal vena cava to aortic ratios for determination of volume depletion in normal beagle dogs. *Veterinary Radiology and Ultrasound* 59: 203–211.

Lavadaniti, M. (2008). Invasive and noninvasive methods for cardiac output measurement. *International Journal of Caring Sciences* 1: 112–117.

Levin, P.D., Levin, D., and Avidan, A. (2004). Medical aerosol propellant interference with infrared anaesthetic gas monitors. *British Journal of Anaesthesia* 92: 865–869.

Linton, R.A.F., Band, D.M., and Haire, K.M. (1993). A new method of measuring cardiac output in man using lithium dilution. *British Journal of Anaesthesia* 71: 262–266.

Madger, S. (1998). More respect for the CVP. Editorial. *Intensive Care Medicine* 24: 651–653.

Mair, A., Martinez-Taboada, F., and Nitzan, M. (2016). Effect of lingual gauze swab placement on pulse oximeter readings in anaesthetised dogs and cats. *Veterinary Record* https://doi.org/10.1136/vr.103861.

Marik, P.E., Cavallazzi, R., Vasu, T., and Hirani, A. (2009). Dynamic changes in arterial waveform derived variables and fluid responsiveness in mechanically ventilated patients: a systematic review of the literature. *Critical Care Medicine* 37: 2642–2647.

Marik, P.E., Monnet, X., and Teboul, J.-L. (2011). Hemodynamic parameters to guide fluid therapy. *Annals of Intensive Care* 1: 1. http://annalsofintensivecare.com/content/1/1/1.

Marotto, S., Bradbrook, C., and Zoff, A. (2018). Anaesthetic complications and preparedness part 1: pre- and intra-operative complications. *Companion Animal* 23: 578–584.

Marval, P. (2006). SI units and simple respiratory and cardiac mechanics. *Continuing Education in Anaesthesia, Critical Care and Pain* 6: 188–191.

Mathis, A. (2016). Practical guide to monitoring anaesthetized small animal patients. *In Practice* 38: 363–372.

Meneghini, C., Rabozzi, R., and Franci, P. (2016). Correlation of the ratio of caudal vena cava diameter and aorta diameter with systolic pressure variation in anaesthetized dogs. *American Journal of Veterinary Research* 77: 137–143.

Menon, D.K. (2001). Mapping the anatomy of unconsciousness: imaging anaesthetic action in the brain. *Editorial. British Journal of Anaesthesia* 86: 607–610.

Miller, A. and Mandeville, J. (2016). Predicting and measuring fluid responsiveness with echocardiography. *Echo Research and Practice* https://doi.org/10.1530/ERP-16-0008.

Mosing, M., Waldmann, A.D., Raisis, A. et al. (2019). Monitoring of tidal ventilation by electrical impedance tomography in anaesthetised horses. *Equine Veterinary Journal* 51: 222–226.

Naik, B.I. and Durieux, M.E. (2014). Hemodynamic monitoring devices: putting it all together. *Best Practice & Research Clinical Anaesthesiology* 28: 477–488.

Nitzan, M., Romem, A., and Koppel, R. (2014). Pulse oximetry: fundamentals and technology update. *Medical Devices: Evidence and Research* 7: 231–239.

Noel-Morgan, J. and Muir, W.W. (2018). Anesthesia-associated relative hypovolemia: mechanisms, monitoring and treatment considerations. *Frontiers in Veterinary Science* https://doi.org/10.3389/fvets/2018.00053.

Otto, K. and Short, C.E. (1991). Electroencephalographic power spectrum analysis as a monitor of anesthetic depth in horses. *Veterinary Surgery* 20: 362–371.

Palazzo, M. (2001). Circulating volume and clinical assessment of the circulation. *Editorial. British Journal of Anaesthesia* 86: 743–746.

Pang, D., Hethey, J., Caulkett, N.A., and Duke, T. (2007). Partial pressure of end-tidal CO_2 sampled via an intranasal catheter as a substitute for partial pressure of arterial CO_2 in dogs. *Journal of Veterinary Emergency and Critical Care* 17: 143–148.

Poth, J.M., Beck, D.R., and Bartels, K. (2014). Ultrasonography for haemodynamic monitoring. *Best Practice & Research Clinical Anaesthesiology* 28: 337–351.

Rampil, I.J. (2001). Monitoring depth of anesthesia. *Current Opinion in Anaesthesiology* 14: 649–653.

Roberson, R.S. (2014). Respiratory variation in cardiopulmonary interactions. *Best Practice & Research Clinical Anaesthesiology* 28: 407–418.

Rudolff, A.S., Moens, Y.P.S., Driessen, B., and Ambrisko, T.D. (2014). Comparison of an infrared anaesthetic agent analyser (Datex-Ohmeda) with refractometry for measurement of isoflurane, sevoflurane and desflurane concentrations. *Veterinary Anaesthesia and Analgesia* 41: 386–392.

Scarabelli, S., Cripps, P., Rioja, E., and Alderson, B. (2016). Adverse reactions following administration of contrast media for diagnostic imaging in anaesthetized dogs and cats: a retrospective study. *Veterinary Anaesthesia and Analgesia* 43: 502–510.

Schauvliege, S. (2016). Patient monitoring and monitoring equipment. In: *BSAVA Manual of Canine and Feline Anaesthesia and Analgesia* (eds. T. Duke-Novakovski, M. de Vries and C. Seymour), 77–96. Gloucester, UK: BSAVA. **(Excellent resource.)**.

Shah, S.B., Hariharan, U., and Bhargava, A.K. (2015). Anaesthetic in the garb of a propellant. *Indian Journal of Anaesthesia* 59: 258–260.

Stoneham, M.D. (1999). Less is more. … Using systolic pressure variation to assess hypovolaemia. *Editorial British Journal of Anaesthesia* 83: 550–551.

Sullivan, G. and Edmondson, C. (2008). Heat and temperature. *Continuing Education in Anaesthesia, Critical Care and Pain* 8: 104–107.

Teixeira, F.J., Carregaro, A.B., Mannarino, R. et al. (2002). Comparison of a sidestream capnograph and a mainstream capnograph in mechanically ventilated dogs. *Journal of the American Veterinary Medical Association* 221: 1582–1585.

Turner, P.G., Dugdale, A., Young, I.S., and Taylor, S. (2008). Portable mass spectrometry for measurement of anaesthetic agents and methane in respiratory gases. *The Veterinary Journal* 177: 36–44.

Tusman, G., Bohm, S.H., and Suarez-Sipmann, F. (2017). Advanced uses of pulse oximetry for monitoring mechanically ventilated patients. *Anesthesia and Analgesia* 124: 62–71.

Verschuren, F., Heinonen, E., Clause, D. et al. (2005). Volumetric capnography: reliability and reproducibility in spontaneously breathing patients. *Clinical Physiology and Functional Imaging* 25: 275–280.

Ward, M. and Langton, J.A. (2007). Blood pressure measurement. *Continuing Education in Anaesthesia, Critical Care and Pain* 7: 122–126.

Watson, X. and Cecconi, M. (2017). Haemodynamic monitoring in the peri-operative period: the past, the present and the future. *Anaesthesia* 72 (Suppl. 1): 7–15.

Zoff, A., Dugdale, A.H.A., Scarabelli, S., and Rioja, E. (2019). Evaluation of pulse co-oximetry to determine haemoglobin saturation with oxygen and haemoglobin concentration in anaesthetized horses: a retrospective study. *Veterinary Anaesthesia and Analgesia* 46: 452–457.

Self-test Section

1. During surgery in a dog in dorsal recumbency, arterial blood pressure is being monitored directly from the left dorsal pedal artery via an electronic pressure transducer. The MAP measures 70 mmHg before the surgeon decides to lower the operating table by 30 cm. If the position of the pressure transducer is not also lowered, and no haemodynamic changes have occurred in the patient, what reading should now be displayed for the MAP?

2. What are the relative advantages and disadvantages of sidestream and mainstream capnography?

3. If both the lead II and lead III traces of the ECG fail to display, but lead I displays normally, which electrode is likely to have lost contact?
   A Left arm
   B Right arm
   C Left leg
   D Right leg (earth electrode)

19

Troubleshooting Some of the Problems Encountered in Anaesthetised Patients

Table 19.1 Hypertension with tachycardia. Hypertension is defined as mean arterial pressure (MAP) > 120 mmHg; the definitions of tachycardia are species-dependent.

Main causes	Action
Lightening plane of anaesthesia/nociception	Turn up vaporiser; if more urgent, consider giving top-up dose of induction agent and /or analgesic (opioid/ketamine)
Hypercapnia (increased sympathetic tone):	
• Hypoventilation	• Start positive pressure ventilation (PPV)/increase PPV if nec.
• Rebreathing (check fresh gas flow [FGF]; check one-way valves and soda lime in circles; check inner tube in Bain non-rebreathing system; could be increased dead space e.g. endotracheal tube [ETT] projecting out of mouth a long way)	• Swap anaesthetic breathing system if this is thought to be a problem
• Endobronchial intubation	• Replace/reposition ETT tube
• Increased CO_2 production (hyperthermia; thyroid storm; phaeochromocytoma)	• Appropriate treatment for these conditions
Early stages of hypoxaemia	Check SpO_2 and/or PaO_2
Drugs – sympathomimetics; anticholinergics	Check why the drugs were given in the first place
Hyperthermia/pyrexia (incl. malignant hyperthermia)	Check temperature; treat as required
Hyperthyroid – thyroid storm	Symptomatic and supportive treatment may be required
Phaeochromocytoma	Symptomatic and supportive treatment may be required
Iatrogenic intravascular volume overload (Bainbridge reflex)	Beware pulmonary oedema as another side effect of fluid overload.

Table 19.2 Hypertension with bradycardia. Hypertension is defined as MAP > 120 mmHg, the definitions of bradycardia are species-dependent.

Main causes	Action
Intravenous $α_2$ agonists	Effect is transient, so should improve within 5–10 minutes
	If very worried, can partly antagonise with IM or *slow* IV (may be off-licence) α2 antagonist, e.g. atipamezole
Can occur with raised intracranial pressure as the ischaemic CNS response is a massive stimulation of the sympathetic nervous system (often accompanied by unusual breathing patterns) = Cushing's triad	If under GA, aim to hyperventilate (PPV) so that $ETCO_2$ tension decreases to about 30–35 mmHg
Iatrogenic intravascular volume overload	Symptomatic and supportive treatment; diuretics may be indicated

Veterinary Anaesthesia: Principles to Practice, Second Edition. Alexandra H. A. Dugdale, Georgina Beaumont, Carl Bradbrook, and Matthew Gurney.
© 2020 John Wiley & Sons Ltd. Published 2020 by John Wiley & Sons Ltd.
Companion website: www.wiley.com/go/dugdale/veterinary-anaesthesia

Table 19.3 Hypotension with tachycardia. Hypotension is defined as MAP < 60–70 mmHg, the definitions of tachycardia are species-dependent.

Main causes	Action
Hypovolaemia until proved otherwise: • Absolute – haemorrhage; severe dehydration or other fluid losses • Relative (vasodilation) – sepsis/drugs (e.g. acepromazine; volatile anaesthetic agents) • Relative (redistribution) – adverse drug reactions/anaphylaxis (e.g. antibiotics, contrast agents)	IV fluid bolus/es • 5–10-20 ml/kg balanced isotonic crystalloid solution over ~15 minutes (use lowest volume for cats) Or • 2.5–5 ml/kg colloid or hypertonic saline over 10–15 minutes (use lowest volume for cats) Positive inotropes and vasopressors may be required for some types of 'shock' Adrenaline may be required for anaphylaxis
PPV with excessive Peak Inspiratory Pressure (PIP) or Positive End Expiratory Pressure (PEEP) (This can be especially a problem if animal also hypovolaemic)	Try to reduce PIP; may need to increase breathing rate to compensate for reduced tidal volume, or else $ETCO_2$ tension will increase Reduce PEEP if possible (Note: due to CO_2's variable effects on haemodynamics, hypotension may be alleviated or exacerbated by alterations in P_aCO_2)
Aorto-caval compression (supine hypotensive syndrome): Abdominal distension/pregnancy combined with dorsal recumbency	Try to tilt the animal gently towards the left side to relieve pressure on the abdominal vena cava; sometimes fluid boluses can also help, as can positive inotropes and/or vasopressors
Pneumothorax and cardiac tamponade can reduce right heart venous return, thus impairing left heart cardiac output	Hopefully these conditions would be known about before anaesthesia; emergency interventions may be required
Arrhythmias, e.g. ventricular tachycardia, may be associated with poor cardiac output	Check ECG; antidysrhythmics may be required if there is haemodynamic compromise

Table 19.4 Hypotension with bradycardia. Hypotension is defined as MAP < 60–70 mmHg, the definitions of bradycardia are species-dependent.

Main causes	Action
Large doses of α_2 agonists and opioids	Possibly consider α_2 antagonists (e.g. atipamezole); naloxone; anticholinergics; check anaesthetic depth
Vagal and vaso-vagal reflexes: • Visceral traction; gastric distension during endoscopy • Head and neck surgery, including ocular manipulation and even laryngoscopy/tracheal intubation • Occasionally seen during bronchoalveolar lavage (especially if large volumes of cold saline are used) • Extreme and acute hypovolaemia (decompensation) – sometimes this is the first, often transient, phase of an anaphylactic reaction • High epidural with local anaesthetic	• Suspend surgical manipulation if possible • Try anticholinergics (glycopyrrolate/atropine) • Cardiopulmonary resuscitation (CPR) may be appropriate • CPR/emergency treatment for anaphylactic shock may be required • IV fluid boluses or ephedrine (or other positive inotrope/vasopressor) may be required
Hyperkalaemia	Check ECG for typical changes (P waves disappearing/large spikey T waves) Check blood K^+ Calcium chloride or calcium gluconate can restore normal ECG for a few minutes; other actions may be required to lower the potassium

Hypothermia	Attempt to conserve body heat and apply active warming – but beware not to cause excessive peripheral vasodilation as this can worsen the haemodynamic status
	Check blood glucose
Severe hypoglycaemia	Check blood glucose; 0.25–1 g/kg slow IV glucose if glucose <3.5 mmol/l (do not use solutions more concentrated than 10–20% via peripheral veins)
Severe hypoxaemia	Check SpO_2 (and PaO_2/blood pH etc. if nec.)
	Symptomatic and supportive treatment as nec.
Idioventricular (ventricular escape) rhythm	Check ECG: investigate potential causes and treat as nec.
Primary heart disease; including breed-specific conditions	Requires ECG and cardiac workup.
	Treatment as required – which may include emergency external pacing before a pacemaker can be fitted

Table 19.5 Hypercapnia. Hypercapnia is defined here as $ETCO_2$ tension >60 mmHg (8 kPa).

Main causes	Action
Hypoventilation (problems with the actual movement of gases into/out of lungs):	
• Obstruction of airways/breathing system	• Check breathing system and ETT
• Poor chest wall/diaphragm movement; poor lung expansion	
– Muscle relaxation under deep GA	• Lighten GA if appropriate; start PPV
– Neuromuscular blocker (NMB) not adequately reversed	• Reverse NMB if appropriate; provide PPV as nec.
– Neuro/muscular disorders	• Check animal's presentation; provide PPV as nec.
– Poor neural control of ventilation	
○ deep GA reduces chemoreceptor sensitivity → reduced ventilatory drive	• Lighten GA if appropriate; provide PPV as nec.
○ cervical/spinal lesions interfere with phrenic/intercostal nerve activity	• Check animal's presentation; provide PPV as nec.
– Chest wall trauma/flail chest	• Check animal's presentation; provide PPV as nec.
– Increased intrathoracic pressure, e.g. pleural and/or mediastinal space filled by fat (obesity), fluid, air, viscera (diaphragmatic hernia), etc.	• Check animal's presentation; beware OBESITY; start PPV but monitor PIP carefully as this may need to be relatively high
– Increased intra-abdominal pressure, e.g. fat, foetus, fluid, flatus, faeces, tumour etc. → diaphragmatic splinting	• Check animal's presentation; start PPV, but monitor PIP carefully as this may need to be relatively high
– Increased extrathoracic or extra-abdominal pressure, e.g. surgeon/equipment leaning on animal	• Check surgeon; check for tightly cross-tied legs or tight-fitting trough/other support
– Pulmonary parenchymal disease	• Check animal's presentation; start gentle PPV
– Endobronchial intubation	• Reverse/reposition/replace ETT
CO_2 rebreathing:	
• Excessive dead space (ETT projecting out of mouth a long way?)	• Consider replacing or repositioning ET tube
• Faulty one-way valves in circle systems	• Check apparatus. Switch to new breathing system
• Exhausted soda lime in circle systems	• Switch to new breathing system if nec.
• Damaged inner tube in Bain system	• Check breathing system and replace if nec.
• Too low fresh gas flow in non-rebreathing systems	• Adjust FGF if required

(Continued)

Table 19.5 (Continued)

Main causes	Action
Increased CO_2 production (hypermetabolic states):	
• Hyperthermia	
– iatrogenic (over-efficient prevention of patient cooling!!)	– Stop patient-warming; start patient cooling
– drug reaction (some antibiotics [and opioids in cats, horses, and cattle] can cause hyperthermia without any other clinical signs)	– Stop patient warming; start patient cooling
– malignant hyperthermia	– Stop patient warming; start patient cooling (cool IV fluids; cool lavage fluids [gastric, cystic, colonic]; surface dousing with cool water/spirit and application of fans to aid evaporative cooling); stop administration of trigger, e.g. inhalation agents (brand new breathing system with high FGF and without a heat and moisture exchanger (HME) [and with activated charcoal filters] may help); IV anaesthetic agents may be required; PPV may be required; dantrolene may be required; monitor blood gases, electrolytes, lactate, and renal function in addition to temperature
• Hyperthyroidism/thyroid storm	– Symptomatic and supportive treatment
• Phaeochromocytoma	– Symptomatic and supportive treatment

Table 19.6 Hypocapnia. Hypocapnia is defined here as $ETCO_2$ tension < 30–35 mmHg (4–4.6 kPa). If $ETCO_2$ tension falls below 20 mmHg (2.7 kPa), brain perfusion becomes compromised.

Main cause	Action
Iatrogenic hyperventilation with PPV	Reduce ventilation frequency and/or tidal volume
Animals under light plane of anaesthesia/increased nociception can hyperventilate (breathe fast and/or deep) – but $ETCO_2$ tension does not usually fall below ~30 mmHg	Deepen anaesthesia (inhalation/injectable) and/or give extra analgesics if nec.
Other causes of hyperventilation ($ETCO_2$ tension not usually below ~30 mmHg) include: • Hypotension (increased ventilatory drive secondary to metabolic acidosis) • Hypoxaemia (increased ventilatory drive due to hypoxaemia and metabolic acidosis)	Usually $ETCO_2$ tension does not fall below ~30 mmHg; it is often more important to treat the underlying hypotension or hypoxaemia

Decreased CO_2 production (hypometabolic states), but $ETCO_2$ tension does not usually fall below ~30 mmHg:
• Hypothermia
• Hypothyroidism
	Symptomatic and supportive treatment as required:
	  – Check/address patient temperature and anaesthetic depth
	  – Check patient history and clinical details

A sudden dramatic decrease in $ETCO_2$ tension in the face of continued ventilation at the previous rate (which may be spontaneous or artificial), can be due to reduced pulmonary perfusion, e.g. impending or actual cardiac arrest or pulmonary embolism. Causes include: • Underlying medical conditions • Adverse drug reactions/anaphylaxis	Supportive treatment or CPR may be required
Low $ETCO_2$ tension may also be seen with capnography gas sampling problems causing sample dilution, including: • Deflated ETT cuff or loose-fitting uncuffed tube • Leaky sidestream sampling line • Too high a sampling rate (sidestream) relative to tidal volume, esp. with high breathing rates	 • Check endotracheal tube and cuff (if present) • Check sampling line • Sampling rate can be reduced in some machines; alternatively, microstream technology uses slower sampling rates without slowing the response time; mainstream sampling would be preferable if available

Very low $ETCO_2$ tension and the absence of a visible capnogram waveform may be seen with:

• Apnoea (can occur with too light a plane of anaesthesia/increased nocicpetion and breath-holding, or too deep a plane of anaesthesia and respiratory depression)	• Check patient – provide PPV and check capnogram and $ETCO_2$ tension following this
• Inadvertent oesophageal intubation or dislodgement/extubation of the endotracheal tube	• Check endotracheal tube position
• Blocked/kinked endotracheal tube	• Check endotracheal tube patency
• Disconnection between sampling site and endotracheal tube	• Check endotracheal tube position and connection to sampling device and breathing system
• Blocked sampling line (sidestream sampling)	• Check sampling line

Table 19.7 Hypoxaemia. Hypoxaemia is defined here as $PaO_2 < 100$ mmHg (13.3 kPa) and especially if <60 mmHg (8 kPa), particularly if breathing 100% O_2; and $SpO_2 < 90\%$.

Main causes	Action
Inadequate O_2 supply	Check: cylinder contents/pipeline pressure; flowmeter
Profound hypoventilation/apnoea:	
• Obstruction somewhere in anaesthetic breathing system	• May need to replace breathing system
• Airway obstruction (ETT or lower trachea/bronchi)	• May need to use suction; may need to replace ETT
• Poor chest wall movement/lung expansion	
– Weak respiratory muscles (deep GA; NMB not adequately reversed; neuromuscular disorders)	• Lighten anaesthetic depth if nec.; provide PPV as nec.; reverse NMB if appropriate
– Poor neural control of ventilation (deep GA; neck/spinal lesions)	• Check animal's presentation; lighten GA if appropriate; start PPV
– Increased intrathoracic pressure (abnormal pleural space filling, incl. obesity)	• Check animal's presentation; provide PPV as nec., but may need rel. high peak inspiratory pressure; may need to drain chest
– Diaphragmatic splinting (increased intra-abdominal pressure)	• Check animal's presentation; provide PPV as nec., but may need rel. high peak inspiratory pressure
– Increased extrathoracic or extra-abdominal pressure (equipment/people leaning on patient)	• Check surgeon; check for tightly cross-tied legs or tight-fitting trough
– Pulmonary parenchymal disease	• Check animal's presentation; provide gentle PPV; increase $O_2\%$ delivered if not already 100%
Circulatory failure (to lungs [e.g. pulmonary thromboembolus]; to whole body)	CPR may be required
In horses, ventilation-perfusion mismatch is a common cause of hypoxaemia	Increase $O_2\%$ delivered; PPV/recruitment manoeuvre/PEEP; salbutamol aerosolised into trachea; support CV function
Increased O_2 requirement/hypermetabolic states	Increase delivered $O_2\%$ if possible; treat the cause; cool pyrexic patients; re-warm if hypothermic
• Seizures/shivering/pyrexia/malignant hyperthermia	

Table 19.8 Hypothermia. Hypothermia is defined here as temperature <37 °C.

Main cause	Action
Usually iatrogenic	Attempt to re-warm using all possible ways, but warming up the room is one of the most effective methods as it slows down further heat losses and helps all your other interventions

Table 19.9 Hyperthermia. Hyperthermia is defined here as temperature >39.5 °C.

Main causes	Action
Animal may already by pyrexic (e.g. due to infection or post-ictal)	Treat the cause; consider NSAIDs, anticonvulsants etc.
Large, fat, hairy animals under GA on circle system (low-ish fresh gas flow) undergoing Magnetic Resonance Imaging	Increase FGF to circle; do not use HME; take off any insulative blankets; start cooling
Large, fat, hairy animals under GA on circle system (low-ish fresh gas flow), and under drapes etc. on hot days in theatre	Increase FGF to circle; do not use HME; start cooling beneath drapes if poss. (and turn off any heat mattresses/forced warm air 'blankets')
Drug reactions (e.g. antibiotics, opioids [cats, horses, cattle]) – can occasionally cause hyperthermia with no other clinical signs	Usually self-limiting; but stop patient warming and start patient-cooling
Malignant hyperthermia (uncontrollable and escalating hyperthermia)	Turn off any volatile anaesthetic agents (replace with IV); swap anaesthetic breathing system to new system, ideally with activated charcoal filters and with high FGF; provide PPV; provide circulatory support; start active cooling; dantrolene may be required

20

Inadvertent Peri-operative Hypothermia

LEARNING OBJECTIVES

- To appreciate the (patho-)physiological effects of hypothermia.
- To be familiar with routes and prevention of heat loss.

20.1 Introduction

Hypothermia is defined as a reduction in core body temperature, by greater than one standard deviation, below the normal mean core temperature for that species, under resting conditions, in a thermoneutral environment. For a dog, this is <37.8 °C. Hypothermia has significant consequences when core temperature falls below 34 °C for most of our veterinary homoiotherms. Note that core temperature (i.e. deep oesophageal temperature) is, on average, 0.4 °C (even up to 1.2 °C) higher than rectal temperature. There is also a circadian variation in temperature (i.e. variation of ±0.5 °C about the mean rectal temperature has been documented for dogs), and temperature is influenced by environmental factors and also the site and method of its measurement. Therefore, for measuring trends, ideally the same site and technique/instrument should be used.

Heat is a form of energy and temperature is a measure of the heat content of a body.

Homeotherm: an organism that must maintain a stable internal body temperature to survive, regardless of environmental temperature (warm- or cold-blooded).
Homoiotherm: a warm-blooded organism.

20.2 Adverse Effects of Hypothermia

Once core temperature falls to 33–35.5 °C, cardiovascular, respiratory, and central nervous system (CNS) depression become marked, and below 33 °C, mortality increases.

20.2.1 Metabolic Rate

Metabolic rate decreases by ~10% per 1 °C decrease in core temperature:

- Drug metabolism/elimination is reduced, therefore dose requirements reduce and drug overdoses may occur.
- Recovery may be prolonged because drug metabolism is reduced.
- Cell sodium pump activity is reduced; cells become oedematous and swell. Electrolyte abnormalities and pH imbalances may follow, e.g. hyperkalaemia and acidosis. May see initial hyperglycaemia.
- Contributes to organoprotection (especially CNS) of permissive/therapeutic hypothermia, e.g. following CPCR.

20.2.2 Blood Viscosity

Blood viscosity increases as PCV increases (because red cells swell, and splenic contraction tends to accompany acidosis and hypothermia). Myocardial work increases.

20.2.3 Coagulation

Blood becomes hypocoagulable as platelets sequester in blood sinusoids in liver, spleen, and bone marrow; [one stage] prothrombin time ([OS]PT) and activated partial thromboplastin time (APTT) become prolonged (enzymic activity slows with hypothermia).

Veterinary Anaesthesia: Principles to Practice, Second Edition. Alexandra H. A. Dugdale, Georgina Beaumont, Carl Bradbrook, and Matthew Gurney.
© 2020 John Wiley & Sons Ltd. Published 2020 by John Wiley & Sons Ltd.
Companion website: www.wiley.com/go/dugdale/veterinary-anaesthesia

20.2.4 CNS Activity

Depression of CNS activity reduces volatile agent requirement: MAC reduces by ~5% per 1 °C decrease in core temperature.

- Confusion <35 °C
- Unconsciousness ~30 °C
- Cessation of cerebral electrical activity <18 °C

20.2.5 Myocardial Performance

Conduction velocities are slowed, leading to the **myocardium becoming irritable** at <30 °C, predisposing to arrhythmias (especially ventricular). Heart rate slows, and **bradycardia is non-responsive to anticholinergics**. ECG changes include: S–T segment depression, T wave inversion, increased P–R interval, QRS widening, and possibly waves at the so called 'J' point: called J waves or Osborn waves (positive deflections at the end of the QRS complex) at ~30 °C. The **fibrillation threshold is said to be 28 °C**.

20.2.6 Haemodynamics

Along with bradycardia, blood pressure falls as baroreceptor sensitivity/reflexes are depressed, and cardiac output is reduced. The resultant reduced capillary perfusion promotes anaerobic metabolism and lactic acidosis. Reduced cardiac output affects inhalation agent 'uptake', effectively deepening anaesthesia; beware anaesthetic overdose as MAC is also reduced with the hypothermia-related reduction in CNS excitability and increase in gas solubilities. Glomerular filtration rate (GFR) decreases; urine production may reduce, but this is offset to some degree by diuresis subsequent to reduced sodium and water reabsorption. Renal acid/base regulating functions are depressed, promoting metabolic acidosis.

20.2.7 Peripheral Vascular Tone

Once the temperature falls below about 34–35 °C, thermoregulatory arterio-venous shunting and peripheral vasoconstriction occurs slowing heat loss but making venous/arterial access more difficult. Vasodilation occurs below 20 °C when vasoconstriction can no longer be maintained.

20.2.8 Ventilation

Chemoreceptor sensitivity/reflexes are depressed leading to hypoventilation (bradypnoea; apnoea at ~24 °C), with respiratory acidosis.

20.2.9 Mucociliary Activity

This is reduced, increasing risk of respiratory secretion accumulation and infection.

20.2.10 Post-operative Shivering

During recovery, which tends to be prolonged if the patient is hypothermic, post-operative shivering occurs (at temperatures >34 °C), increasing patient oxygen demand (which can increase by 1.5–5x in people) at a time when F_IO_2 is not usually supplemented.

20.2.11 Immune Cell Function

Immunodepression increases the risk of infection, and of metastasis of neoplastic cells. Concerns regarding delayed wound healing have been difficult to prove in veterinary studies.

20.2.12 Oxygen/Haemoglobin Dissociation Curve

Hypothermia results in a left-shift that is opposed somewhat by respiratory and metabolic acidoses. Overall, a slight left-shift prevails resulting in impeded tissue oxygen delivery, predisposing to anaerobic metabolism and exacerbation of metabolic acidosis. However, oxygen requirement is reduced because of the lowered basal metabolic rate (BMR), unless shivering occurs.

20.2.13 Blood Gas Analysis

Should we correct for patient temperature? See Chapter 21 for further discussion. Whichever technique you choose (alpha-stat or pH-stat), be consistent.

20.2.14 Death

Death occurs at ~20 °C (if preceding derangements were survived).

20.3 Peri-anaesthetic Heat Loss

Inadvertent peri-operative hypothermia is common, with moderate-to-severe hypothermia developing in 32.1% of dogs and 70.9% of cats. Mechanisms include (see also Figure 20.1):

- Metabolic rate reduces by 15–40% under general anaesthesia, with a consequent reduction in non-shivering thermogenesis (especially important in neonates).

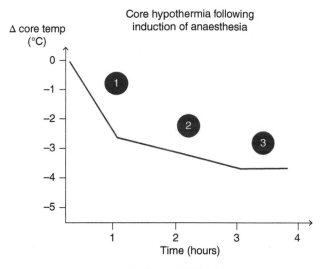

Figure 20.1 Stages of core hypothermia following induction of anaesthesia. Δ = Change in. ① = Stage 1 – redistribution. ② = Stage 2 – linear loss. ③ = Stage 3 – core temperature plateau or equilibrium. Note that for combined general and neuraxial anaesthesia, there may be no stage 3 because peripheral vasoconstriction is prevented.

- Fasting prevents the heat production associated with digestion of food and assimilation of nutrients (diet-induced thermogenesis, also known as the specific dynamic action of food).
- The lower thermoregulatory response threshold is reduced. (The normal inter-threshold range widens from about 0.4 °C to about 4 °C, due to both a decrease in the lower response threshold and an increase in the upper response threshold). A reduction in the lower thermoregulatory response threshold means reductions in both the vasoconstriction and shivering thresholds.
- Vasodilation occurs both directly (drug-induced) and indirectly (due to the lowered vasoconstriction threshold), and facilitates peripheral heat loss.
- Shivering thermogenesis is prevented both directly (most anaesthetic agents and adjuncts reduce muscle tone/produce muscle relaxation) and indirectly (due to lowered shivering threshold).
- Unconsciousness/hypnosis prevents heat seeking behaviour.

20.3.1   Stage 1: Redistribution Phase

- Redistribution of heat from the core to the peripheral compartment or 'shell' results in rapid core temperature decline. Body heat content remains unchanged. (There is normally a 2–4 °C temperature difference between the core and peripheral compartments.)
- Primarily due to vasodilation. Vasodilation may be direct (due to sedative and anaesthetic agents) and indirect (due to the lowering of the vasoconstriction

threshold). Vasoconstrictors (e.g. α2 agonists) may attenuate redistribution.
- Often ≥1.5 °C decrease in core temperature occurs within the first hour. Subsequent reductions in core temperature can amount to a further $1+$°C over the next two hours. Redistribution is the dominant cause of temperature fall over the first three hours of anaesthesia.
- Prewarming increases body heat content (not the core temperature), and reduces the core-to-periphery temperature gradient, thus slowing redistributive heat transfer and core cooling.

20.3.2   Stage 2: Linear Phase

- This slower, linear phase of temperature reduction occurs when heat loss exceeds that produced by metabolism (metabolic rate is reduced by 15–40% under general anaesthesia).
- A significant cause of core hypothermia.
- Four mechanisms: radiation (40%), convection (30%), evaporation (25%), and conduction (5%). Animals with minimal insulation (lean, high surface area : volume, or short, sparse, or absent fur) undergo more rapid heat loss, especially radiant, convective, and conductive, than the equivalent well-insulated animal (fat, low surface area : volume, or long fur or 'double/under coat').
- Passive insulation and active warming methods are most effective in this phase.

20.3.3   Stage 3: Core Temperature Plateau or Equilibration Phase

- The core temperature plateau is reached when heat production equals heat loss, and can be actively or passively maintained.
  - An active plateau occurs after thermoregulatory defences have been activated, particularly thermoregulatory vasoconstriction, which usually occurs at core temperatures of 34–35 °C (in humans). It appears that it is not just vasoconstriction diverting warm blood away from the skin to reduce cutaneous heat loss, but rather the constriction of arterio-venous shunts in the appendages, resulting in redistribution of blood, that is most important in core heat conservation.
  - A passive plateau is reached when this thermal equilibrium occurs without activation of thermoregulatory defences. With warm ambient temperatures, good insulation and/or active warming, a passive plateau can be reached at relatively warm core temperatures. With cooler ambient temperatures and less efficient insulation/warming, however, core temperature decreases to lower values, but equilibrium is still reached eventually because, although both heat loss

and heat production decrease with decreases in body temperature, they do so at dissimilar rates (heat loss slows faster/more than heat production).

- Unlikely to occur much prior to myocardial fibrillation and death in most hospital conditions (ambient temperature 18–23 °C).

20.4 Risk Factors for Development of Hypothermia

- Smaller body size (greater relative surface area)
- Young age (small size [see above]; little insulative white adipose tissue [although some species have brown fat]; immature thermoregulatory abilities [prone to hypoglycaemia, poor non-shivering and shivering thermogenesis; poor control of peripheral vascular tone])
- Advanced age (lower BMR; poorer control of peripheral vascular tone)
- Poor body condition/poor nutritional status (lack of insulative fat; lower BMR)
- Hypothyroidism
- Higher ASA status
- Prolonged anaesthesia time
- More invasive/extensive surgery (greater exposure of body cavities/surface)
- Cool environmental temperatures in 'wards' and operating theatres
- Combination of regional, especially neuraxial, anaesthesia with general anaesthesia (loss of autonomic vaso-regulation and reduced shivering)

20.5 Minimising Heat Loss

Care should be taken when employing active warming to ensure hyperthermia does not occur. Rewarming rates >1 °C/h can cause tissue damage (and vasodilation may increase intracranial pressure, reducing cerebral perfusion and potentially worsening neurological outcomes), aim instead for ~1 °C/h or, if hypothermia was more profound, then nearer 0.25–0.5 °C/h.

20.5.1 Minimise Anaesthesia and Surgical Time

Heat loss increases with anaesthesia duration. Although local anaesthetic techniques may facilitate surgery (perhaps

shortening anaesthetic time), they do produce sympathetic block in the anaesthetised tissues, where the resultant vasodilation promotes heat loss; and also motor block, which reduces shivering. This is often most noticeable with neuraxial techniques that can both increase heat loss (via vasodilation) and decrease heat production (by shivering) in a relatively large caudal part of the body.

20.5.2 Warm Environment

Beginning immediately after premedication and continuing throughout preparation for surgery, surgery itself and right through until recovery is complete, ensure a warm environment for the patient. Keeping the ambient temperature ≥23 °C is one of the most effective methods to slow the development of hypothermia but is often uncomfortable for personnel.

Patient pre-warming has been shown to be beneficial in rats and humans, but not in cats and dogs; this may, however, reflect interrupted warming rather than a failure of the principle.

20.5.3 Minimise Evaporative Losses (Especially from Alcohols)

Only clip and wet the animal when necessary. Use warm solutions where possible during surgical site preparation. Dry the patient as much as possible if wetting occurs. Rebreathing systems, especially at medium or low fresh gas flows, avoid cooling (and drying) of the respiratory tract to reduce overall heat loss. Heat and moisture exchangers (HMEs) (Figure 20.2) may be used with, especially, non-rebreathing systems.

20.5.4 Use Warm Fluids for IV Administration and Body Cavity Lavage

If possible, warm intravenous and lavage fluids to around 38 °C and try to keep IV fluids warm during their passage through giving sets (Figure 20.3). (There have been concerns in the recent human literature about aluminium release [into the fluids] from heating plates, whether 'coated' or not, which form an integral part of the disposable 'cartridges' of certain fluid-warming devices [see Further Reading].)

20.5.5 Maintain Body Heat

For all parts of the patient not required for surgical or anaesthetic access, especially limbs and tails (which are good examples of high surface area : volume body parts, from which heat loss is rapid), the following may be useful peri-operatively:

- Forced warm air 'blankets' (e.g. Bair Hugger™) (Figure 20.4) or neonatal incubators (pre- or post-anaesthesia for small individuals).

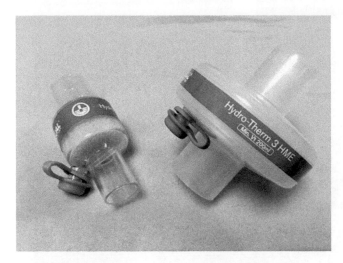

Figure 20.2 Heat and moisture exchangers (HME) may be combined with antimicrobial filters (HMEF) and are available in a range of different sizes, many with side-ports for sidestream capnography.

- Heat pads or heat mattresses (conductive or resistive) (e.g. HotDog™, Figure 20.5).
- Circulating warm water beds.
- Heat lamps.
- 'Hot hands' (beware rupture and wetting).
- Insulative/reflective blankets or wraps (cotton wool, bubble wrap, space blankets, foil).

20.6 Increasing Heat Production?

Intravenous infusions of amino acid solutions stimulate diet-induced thermogenesis and increase peripheral vasoconstriction, reducing heat loss (noradrenergic mechanisms appear to be involved), and can therefore delay the development of inadvertent intra-operative hypothermia. The extent of this, however, varies between healthy and sick (e.g. septic), patients and further investigations are required in veterinary species regarding safety and efficacy for patients of different physiological status. Intravenous caffeine is also a metabolic stimulant and has been investigated in people to aid in prevention of hypothermia, however, it also has systemic side effects.

(a)　　　　　　　　　　(b)

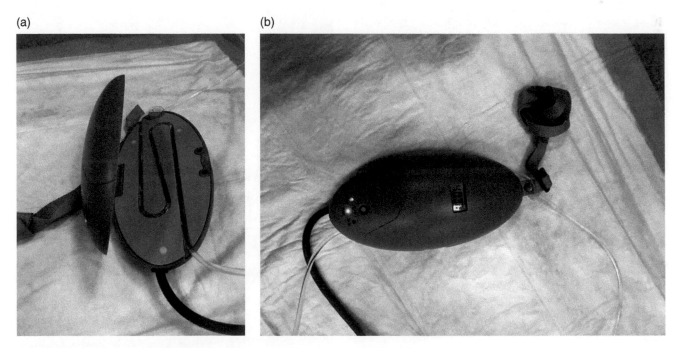

Figure 20.3 JorVet™ in-line IV fluid warmer. *Source:* Images courtesy Jo Raszplewicz.

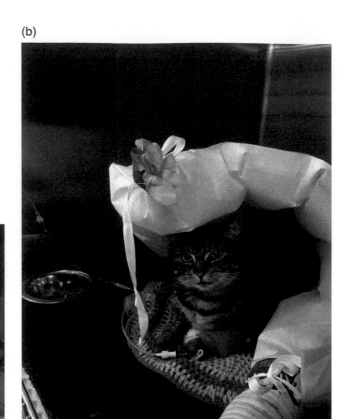

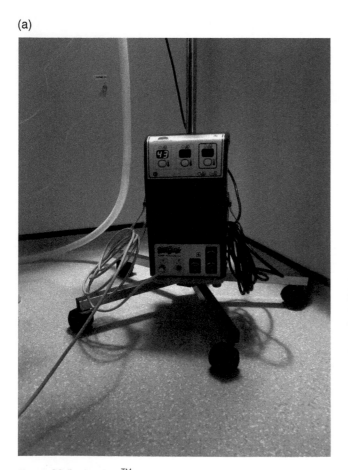

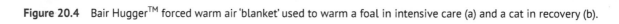

Figure 20.4 Bair Hugger™ forced warm air 'blanket' used to warm a foal in intensive care (a) and a cat in recovery (b).

(a)

(b)

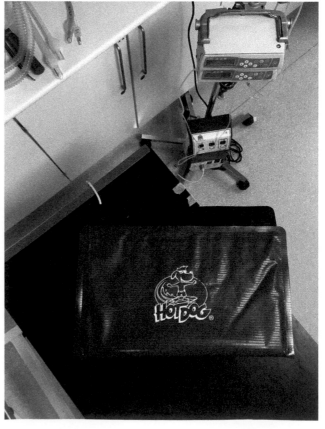

Figure 20.5 HotDog™ unit (a) and blanket (b).

Further Reading

Aarnes, T.K., Bednarski, R.M., Lerche, P., and Hubbell, J.A.E. (2017). Effect of pre-warming on perioperative hypothermia and anesthetic recovery in small breed dogs undergoing ovariohysterectomy. *Canadian Veterinary Journal* 58: 175–179.

Armstrong, S.R., Roberts, B.K., and Aronsohn, M. (2005). Perioperative hypothermia. *Journal of Veterinary Emergency and Critical Care* 15: 32–37.

Beal, W.M., Brown, D.C., and Shofer, F.S. (2000). The effects of perioperative hypothermia and the duration of anesthesia on postoperative would infection rate in clean wounds: a retrospective study. *Veterinary Surgery* 29: 123–127.

Bligh, J. and Johnson, K. (1973). Glossary of terms for thermal physiology. *Journal of Applied Physiology* 35: 941–961.

Brodeur, A., Wright, A., and Cortes, Y. (2017). Hypothermia and targeted temperature management in cats and dogs. *Journal of Veterinary Emergency and Critical Care* 27: 151–163.

Buggy, D.J. and Crossley, A.W.A. (2000). Thermoregulation, mild perioperative hypothermia and post-anaesthetic shivering. *British Journal of Anaesthesia* 84: 615–628.

Cabell, L.W., Perkowski, S.Z., Gregor, T., and Smith, G.K. (1997). The effects of active peripheral skin warming on perioperative hypothermia in dogs. *Veterinary Surgery* 26: 79–85.

Clark-Price, S. (2015). Inadvertent perianesthetic hypothermia in small animal patients. *Veterinary Clinics of North America: Small Animal Practice* 45: 983–994.

Clark-Price, S.C., Phillips, H., Selmic, L.E. et al. (2018). Effect of intraoperative infusion of amino acids on body temperature, serum biochemistry, serum insulin and recovery variables in healthy dogs undergoing ovariohysterectomy. *Veterinary Record* https://doi.org/10.1136/vr.104479.

Clutton, R.E. (2017). Limiting heat loss during surgery in small animals. *Veterinary Record* 180: 495–497.

Dix, G.M., Jones, A., Knowles, T.G., and Holt, P.E. (2006). Methods used in veterinary practice to maintain the temperature of intravenous fluids. *Veterinary Record* 159: 451–456.

Greer, R.J., Cohn, L.A., Dodam, J.R. et al. (2007). Comparison of three methods of temperature measurement in hypothermic, euthermic and hyperthermic dogs. *Journal of the American Veterinary Medical Association* 230: 1841–1848.

Horn, E.-P., Bein, B., Böhm, R. et al. (2012). The effect of short time periods of pre-operative warming in the prevention of peri-operative hypothermia. *Anaesthesia* 67: 612–617.

John, M., Ford, J., and Harper, M. (2014). Peri-operative warming devices: performance and clinical application. *Anaesthesia* 69: 623–638.

Kirkbride, D.A. and Buggy, D.J. (2003). Thermoregulation and mild perioperative hypothermia. *British Journal of Anaesthesia CEPD Reviews* 3: 24–28.

Kurz, A., Sessler, D.I., Christensen, R., and Dechert, M. (1995). Heat balance and distribution during the core-temperature plateau in anesthetized humans. *Anesthesiology* 83: 491–499.

Mayerhofer, I., Scherzer, S., Gabler, C., and Van den Hoven, R. (2005). Hypothermia in horses induced by general anaesthesia and limiting measures. *Equine Veterinary Education* 17: 53–56.

Murison, P. (2001). Prevention and treatment of perioperative hypothermia in animals under 5kg bodyweight. *In Practice* 23: 412–418.

Oncken, A.K., Kirby, R., and Rudloff, E. (2001). Hypothermia in critically ill dogs and cats. *Compendium for Continuing Education for the Practising Veterinarian* 23: 506–521.

Perl, T., Kunze-Szikszay, N., Brauer, A. et al. (2019). Aluminium release by coated and uncoated fluid-warming devices. *Anaesthesia* 74: 708–713.

Redondo, J.I., Rubio, M., Soler, G. et al. (2007). Normal values and incidence of cardiorespiratory complications in dogs during general anaesthesia: a review of 1281 cases. *Journal of Veterinary Medicine A, Physiology, Pathology, Clinical Medicine* 54: 470–477.

Rigotti, C.F., Jolliffe, C.T., and Leece, E.A. (2015). Effect of prewarming on the body temperature of small dogs undergoing inhalation anesthesia. *Journal of the American Veterinary Medical Association* 247: 765–770.

Riley, C. and Andrzejowski, J. (2018). Inadvertent perioperative hypothermia. *BJA Education* 18: 227–233.

Redondo, J.I., Suesta, P., Gil, L. et al. (2012a). Retrospective study of the prevalence of postanaesthetic hypothermia in cats. *Veterinary Record* 170: 206–209.

Redondo, J.I., Suesta, P., Serra, I. et al. (2012b). Retrospective study of the prevalence of postanaesthetic hypothermia in dogs. *Veterinary Record* 17: 374. https://doi.org/10.1136/vr.100476.

Roder, G., Sessler, D.I., Roth, G. et al. (2011). Intra-operative rewarming with HotDog resistive heating and forced-air heating: a trial of lower-body warming. *Anesthesia* 66: 667–674.

Schuster, C.J. and Pang, D.S.J. (2018). Forced-air pre-warming prevents peri-anaesthetic hypothermia and shortens recovery in adult rats. *Laboratory Animals* 52: 142–151.

Sessler, D.I. (1997). Mild perioperative hypothermia. *The New England Journal of Medicine* 336: 1730–1337.

Sessler, D.I. (2000). Perioperative heat balance. *Anesthesiology* 92: 578–596.

Sullivan, G. and Edmondson, C. (2008). Heat and temperature. *Continuing Education in Anaesthesia, Critical Care and Pain* 8: 104–107.

Swaim, S., Lee, A., and Hughes, K. (1989). Heating pads and thermal burns in small animals. *Journal of American Animal Hospital Association* 25: 156–162.

Self-test Section

1 List the four mechanisms of linear heat loss during general anaesthesia.

2 What is a safe rewarming rate (° C per hour)?

3 List at least five potentially adverse consequences of hypothermia.

21

Blood Gas Analysis

LEARNING OBJECTIVES

- To be able to describe the carriage of oxygen and carbon dioxide in the blood.
- To be able to relate haemoglobin saturation to partial pressure of oxygen in plasma.
- To be able to define pH and discuss the basic homeostasis of pH in the body.
- To be able to define pKa and explain its importance for buffering systems.
- To be familiar with the common causes of respiratory and metabolic (non-respiratory) disturbances.
- To be able to interpret blood gas results using the traditional approach (based upon the Henderson–Hasselbalch equation) and know when and how to intervene.

21.1 Introduction

Blood gas analysis helps determine:

- Blood pH
- Blood oxygenation
- Blood CO_2 carriage

Arterial blood samples are the most useful, giving information about pulmonary gaseous exchange and acid–base status. Venous samples can also tell us about acid–base status and give some indication of oxygen extraction by the tissues. Arterial and venous samples can be taken simultaneously to compare, usually the oxygen tensions, providing more information about how well the peripheral tissues are being perfused and extracting oxygen. Lithium heparin (pH-balanced) is the anticoagulant of choice, as sodium heparin affects sodium measurement, and Na^+K^+EDTA will chelate calcium and affect sodium and potassium measurement. Most manufacturers supply ready-heparinised syringes (e.g. Drihep™), for convenience and to reduce the technical problems associated with home-made heparinised syringes. Ideally, all samples should be withdrawn, as anaerobically as possible, over one to two respiratory cycles, and analysed as soon as possible or at least within 10–15 minutes. If analysis is knowingly going to be delayed, samples can be refrigerated or stored on iced water, but beware sample deterioration with prolonged, cool storage, especially for electrolytes (see Further Reading). Gentle agitation (to avoid haemolysis) by rolling the capped syringe between the palms or by inverting it several times, end-to-end, should be performed before analysis to ensure adequate mixing for a homogeneous sample.

Blood gas analysers measure three variables using three different electrodes:

- pH
- Partial pressure (or tension) of O_2 (PO_2)
- Partial pressure of CO_2 (PCO_2)

All other values given are calculated from these (using algorithms based on Sigaard-Anderson diagrams or Davenport diagrams) and include:

- Bicarbonate (HCO_3^-)
- Base excess (BE)
- Percentage saturation of haemoglobin with oxygen (SO_2)

Portable and bench-top analysers are increasingly available (Figures 21.1 and 21.2). Newer machines also measure electrolytes, glucose, and lactate amongst other variables. Some machines even allow continuous blood gas monitoring, but these are expensive.

Veterinary Anaesthesia: Principles to Practice, Second Edition. Alexandra H. A. Dugdale, Georgina Beaumont, Carl Bradbrook, and Matthew Gurney.
© 2020 John Wiley & Sons Ltd. Published 2020 by John Wiley & Sons Ltd.
Companion website: www.wiley.com/go/dugdale/veterinary-anaesthesia

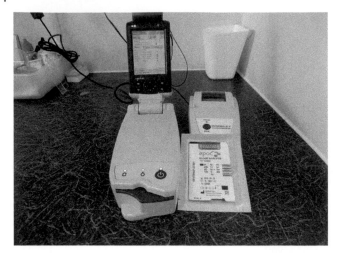

Figure 21.1 Portable analyser with printer and single-use cartridge.

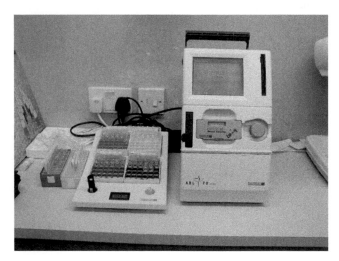

Figure 21.2 A bench-top analyser with its quality control solutions in the tray to the left.

21.2 pH

Based on the Arrhenius definition of an acid, as a substance that yields hydrogen ions when in aqueous solution, Sørensen proposed the following equation, where pH is inversely related to the H^+ ion concentration:

$$pH = \log_{10} \frac{1}{\left[H^+\right]}$$

The pH scale ranges from 0 to 14. For pure water, which dissociates into H^+ (or rather H_3O^+), and OH^- ions, at 25 °C, 7.0 is neutral pH (and therefore, <7 is defined as acidic and >7 as alkaline). Note that *neutrality* is defined as the condition of equivalent concentrations of H^+ and OH^- ions, so the pH of pure water is always 'neutral'. The pH of

pure water at neutrality (pN_w), however, is not always 7. At different temperatures, a greater or fewer number of water molecules dissociate, so that the H^+ concentration, and therefore the pH of neutrality, changes (see later). Commonly, however, we consider a pH of 7 to be neutral, pH values below 7 to be acidic, and those above 7 to be alkaline.

The term *pH buffer* describes a substance that acts to normalise a pH disturbance within a 'system'. Usually, chemical buffers are weak acids and their conjugate bases. The weak acid partially dissociates in water to produce some negatively charged ions (the base), and some H^+ ions. 'Weak' acids do not fully dissociate when dissolved in water:

$$HA \leftrightarrow H^+ + A^-$$

Note that 'strong' acids fully dissociate (ionise) in aqueous solution:

$$HA \rightarrow H^+ + A^-$$

In the body, carbon dioxide is produced during metabolism and undergoes the following reactions:

$$CO_2 + H_2O \underset{\text{anhydrase}}{\overset{\text{Carbonic}}{\longleftrightarrow}} H_2CO_3 \leftrightarrow H^+ + HCO_3^-$$

These reactions are described as equilibria because they never go to completion in either direction, hence the bi-directional arrows. Carbonic acid (H_2CO_3) is a weak acid, i.e. it does not fully dissociate in water, so it is a good compound for buffering. Although we cannot measure carbonic acid concentration, we can measure carbon dioxide tension and pH, and derive the bicarbonate concentration. Therefore, the above expression can be thought of as one equilibrium:

$$CO_2 + H_2O \leftrightarrow H^+ + HCO_3^-$$

We can apply the law of mass action and Le Chatelier's principle to this equilibrium, i.e. it can be pushed to the left or right by changes in the concentrations of any of the reactants. For example, increasing H^+ ion concentration drives the reaction towards the left, whereas decreasing H^+ ion concentration pulls the reaction to the right. Similarly, increasing CO_2 pushes the reaction to the right, whereas decreasing CO_2 pulls the reaction to the left.

Rearranging the above equation and considering pH instead of $[H^+]$ concentration, brings us to the Henderson–Hasselbalch equation:

$$pH = pK_a + \log_{10}\left(\frac{HCO_3^-}{\alpha \times P_aCO_2}\right)$$

where the pKa of the bicarbonate buffer system is 6.1; and α is the solubility coefficient for CO_2, which is 0.03 mmol/l/mmHg, or 0.23 mmol/l/kPa, at 37 °C. The generic form of the Henderson–Hasselbalch equation

is: $pH = pK_a + \log_{10}\dfrac{\left[A^-\right]}{\left[HA\right]}$

21.2.1 Regulating pH

Regulation is required because most biochemical (metabolic) reactions can only occur efficiently within a narrow pH range. The normal pH range compatible with life is 6.8–7.8; the body endeavours to tightly regulate the extracellular fluid (ECF) pH to 7.35–7.45.

21.2.1.1 Possible pH derangements

To judge the direction of any pH change, the value of 7.4 is used for arterial blood. Blood that is more acidic than normal is called **acidaemic**. Blood that is more alkaline than normal is called **alkalaemic**. Only when we know the cause of the pH perturbation (i.e. whether it is the respiratory system at fault or the non-respiratory/metabolic system) should we say that there is an **acidosis** or an **alkalosis**. For example, if the blood pH is on the acidic side of normal, and we know (from the rest of our blood gas analysis) that the respiratory system is to blame, we can say there is a **respiratory acidosis**. Strictly speaking, only blood with a pH outside the normal range is considered truly either acidaemic or alkalaemic. With this in mind, if the blood pH remains within the normal range [but varies from 7.4], an X-osis may exist without an X-aemia, but it will be appreciated that an X-aemia will always be accompanied by an X-osis; where X- = acid- or alkal-.

The following processes are responsible for pH disturbances:

- **Acidosis:** metabolic (non-respiratory) or respiratory
- **Alkalosis:** metabolic (non-respiratory) or respiratory
- **Mixed disorders:** can be additive (e.g. metabolic acidosis + respiratory acidosis) or offsetting (e.g. metabolic acidosis + respiratory alkalosis)

Examples of **causes of respiratory acidosis** are:

- Hypoventilation under anaesthesia, especially deep anaesthesia (and common in anaesthetised horses)
- Pulmonary or pleural space disease (may include very obese animals) (may be accompanied by dyspnoea and hypoxaemia)
- Neck lesions with diaphragmatic paralysis
- Respiratory obstruction, e.g. laryngeal paralysis (may be accompanied by hypoxaemia and dyspnoea)

Examples of **causes of respiratory alkalosis** are:

- Hyperventilation secondary to anaemia, or hypoxaemia (e.g. pneumonia, high altitude)
- Hyperventilation secondary over-zealous positive pressure ventilation (in anaesthetised patients)
- Hyperventilation secondary to fear/excitement
- Hyperventilation secondary to hyperthermia

Examples of **causes of metabolic acidosis** are:

- Ketoacidosis (with diabetes mellitus)
- Lactic acidosis (secondary to hypovolaemia and tissue anaerobic metabolism; also accompanies endotoxaemia)
- Prolonged diarrhoea (partly due to bicarbonate HCO_3^- loss)
- Failure of kidneys to excrete an acid load
- In ruminants, salivary buffer losses under anaesthesia (predominantly bicarbonate HCO_3^-)

Examples of **causes of metabolic alkalosis** are:

- Commonly iatrogenic after sodium bicarbonate treatment
- Can accompany acute or prolonged gastric vomiting (acid loss)
- In ruminants, can accompany abomasal acid sequestration

Regardless of the cause of the primary disturbance/s, the body will try to mount **compensatory responses**.

21.2.1.2 How Does the Body Regulate Its pH?

Three systems regulate pH:

1) *Chemical buffers in the extracellular and intracellular fluids*

   The extracellular buffers act immediately (seconds to minutes), and the intracellular buffers act next (within minutes). Chemical buffers include the bicarbonate system; the phosphate system; the ammonia/ammonium system (kidney tubules); and proteins, both extracellular and intracellular (especially haemoglobin inside red blood cells). There is also a transcellular H^+/K^+ ion exchange which aids buffering.

   Some important consequences of haemoglobin's structure and functions are:
   - The **Bohr effect:** the rightward shift of the haemoglobin-oxygen dissociation curve in tissues, i.e. increased PCO_2 and $[H^+]$ in the tissues increases binding of these to haemoglobin, so oxygen release from the haemoglobin is enhanced. At the lungs, the opposite occurs, such that oxygen uptake by haemoglobin is facilitated.
   - The **Haldane effect:** the release of oxygen from haemoglobin in tissues leaves deoxyhaemoglobin with its greater affinity for binding CO_2 and H^+ ions. At the lungs, the increased binding of O_2 to haemoglobin

and formation of oxyhaemoglobin enhances CO_2 and H^+ release.

- The above two effects are linked.
- The **chloride shift (Hamburger shift)**: in tissues, CO_2 enters red cells and O_2 is given up by haemoglobin. CO_2 is converted to carbonic acid by carbonic anhydrase with subsequent formation of H^+ and bicarbonate HCO_3^- ions. H^+ and CO_2 are more easily bound by deoxyhaemoglobin (than oxyhaemoglobin), leaving bicarbonate ions HCO_3^- free to leave the red cell. To maintain electrical neutrality, Cl^- enters red cells: the so-called chloride shift. The reverse occurs in the lungs.

2) *Respiratory system*

Changing alveolar minute ventilation regulates the blood content of CO_2, providing a coarse control in the medium term (minutes to hours).

3) *The kidneys*

The kidneys can excrete or re/absorb acids and bases. They act in the longer term (hours to days), providing fine control. The *liver and GI tract* are also important to provide substrates, e.g. glutamine, which is metabolised by renal proximal tubular cells to HCO_3^- and NH_4^+. Bicarbonate is 'regained' when NH_4^+ and various buffers (including phosphate compounds) are excreted. Although the kidneys have an important role in acid–base, water, and electrolyte balance, the gut and liver have modulatory roles.

21.2.1.2.1 How the Three pH Regulatory Systems Work

The most important chemical buffer system in the blood is the **bicarbonate buffer system**; described by the equations above. **Carbonic anhydrase** catalyses the reaction of carbon dioxide with water (to produce the weak acid, carbonic acid), and so plays a vital role in this buffer system. Other buffer systems include the phosphate buffer system and the ability of many proteins to bind H^+ ions. These chemical buffers act almost immediately when normal blood pH is disturbed.

The pKa of a chemical buffer system describes the pH at which it is half dissociated, and half undissociated; i.e. for a weak acid, where $[HA] = [A^-]$. For chemical buffers to work best, their pKa needs to be within ± 1pH unit of the pH of their normal working environment, so that (more or less) equal concentrations of the weak acid and its conjugate base are present. In such a situation, should the pH of the environment now be disturbed, the buffer system can respond (more or less) equally to either an acid or an alkaline challenge.

The bicarbonate buffer system has been extensively studied. It is an excellent buffer system in both the extracellular fluid (ECF) and intracellular fluid (ICF) because it is so abundant, despite its pKa being less than ideal for the ECF. Its pKa is 6.1; whereas normal ECF pH is ~7.4, so it is a

better buffer for the ICF where the intracellular pH is more acidic, ~6.8 (6.5–7.2). However, it is still a good buffer for the ECF because of its **abundance** and because it is an **open buffer**. That is, the amount of bicarbonate buffer available (in the ECF compartment) is not fixed, but can be varied by varying pulmonary ventilation (which changes PCO_2, which then changes the bicarbonate concentration through the above equilibria); see below. (In addition, the kidneys can affect H^+ and HCO_3^- concentrations; see below.)

If blood pH cannot be fully corrected by these chemical buffers (i.e. buffering capacity is exhausted), then the other mechanisms come into play.

The respiratory system works in the medium term to try to correct blood pH by altering blood PCO_2 (see above). The control offered by the respiratory system is somewhat 'coarse' (i.e. not perfect). This limited control is partly due to the respiratory system also being responsible for oxygenation of the patient. For example, if the patient was suffering from lactic acidosis (a metabolic acidosis), then if ventilation was increased (by breathing faster and/or deeper), more CO_2 is blown off, and a respiratory alkalosis is created which partially 'offsets' the metabolic acidosis. The extracellular pH is corrected back towards normal, even though the respiratory system has now created perturbations in PCO_2. But there is a limit to just how 'fast/deep' we can ventilate (it is tiring for the respiratory muscles to work this hard), and if PCO_2 falls below about 20mmHg, cerebral blood vessel vasoconstriction (and reduced off-loading of oxygen from haemoglobin in the tissues due to left shift of the haemoglobin-oxygen dissociation curve) can result in ischaemic brain damage. Therefore, there are natural limits to this compensatory response.

Alternatively, in the presence of metabolic alkalosis, by slowing ventilation, PCO_2 increases, creating a respiratory acidosis to offset the metabolic alkalosis. But again, the magnitude of the response is limited, e.g. reduced ventilation can result in hypoxaemia, which increases the ventilatory drive, so the response is self-limiting.

If the pH is still not returned to normal after the first two systems are activated, the kidneys finally sort things out, as long as they have adequate perfusion and kidney function is normal. The control offered by the kidneys is a long-term option, i.e. it does not occur very quickly, but provides 'fine' control and will eventually correct the pH to essentially normal.

21.3 PO$_2$ and PCO$_2$

The P represents partial pressure or tension, which are ways of expressing the concentration of a gas dissolved in a liquid. The a, v, or $\bar{v}$ (e.g. P_aO_2, P_vCO_2, $P_{\bar{v}}CO_2$) represent **arterial**, **venous**, or **mixed venous**, respectively.

21.3.1 How is CO₂ Carried in Blood?

- 70–75% is carried as bicarbonate. Carbon dioxide reacts with water, under the influence of carbonic anhydrase, to form carbonic acid, which then partially dissociates into H^+ and HCO_3^-.
- 7–10% dissolves in blood (imagine it as very tiny bubbles). This is the portion responsible for the measured PCO_2.
- 15–25% binds to proteins, especially haemoglobin, forming 'carbamino-compounds' (e.g. carbamino-haemoglobin).

21.3.2 How is O₂ Carried in the Blood?

- 98% is carried in combination with haemoglobin in the red blood cells.
- 2% is dissolved in plasma (the very tiny bubbles again). This is the portion that is responsible for the PO_2.

$$C_aO_2 = \left(1.34 \times [Hb] \times S_aO_2\right) + \left(P_aO_2 \times 0.003\right)$$

where C_aO_2 is the oxygen content (or carriage) in ml oxygen per 100 ml of arterial blood; 1.34 is Hüfner's constant (ml O_2 carried per 1 g of fully saturated haemoglobin); [Hb] is haemoglobin concentration (normally ~15 g/dl); S_aO_2 is percentage saturation of haemoglobin with oxygen (as a decimal); P_aO_2 is partial pressure of O_2 (dissolved in arterial plasma); 0.003 is the Ostwald solubility coefficient, i.e. the number of ml of O_2 carried in 100 ml blood per 1 mmHg partial pressure of oxygen, at 37 °C.

From this equation, we can see that without haemoglobin, we would be struggling for oxygen carriage as haemoglobin increases the oxygen carrying capacity of our blood by about 60 times (i.e. $1.34 \times 15 \times 0.97 = 19.5$ ml oxygen per 100 ml blood is carried by haemoglobin, versus $100 \times 0.003 = 0.3$ ml oxygen per 100 ml blood is carried in physical solution).

The sigmoid shaped haemoglobin–oxygen dissociation curve (Figure 21.3) shows how well saturated (with oxygen) haemoglobin inside red blood cells can be, for a given partial pressure of oxygen (oxygen in physical solution) in the blood's plasma. Because of the long plateau, note how the saturation of haemoglobin with oxygen only decreases by a relatively small amount (from 100% down to 90%) for a dramatic fall in P_aO_2 (e.g. from 500 mmHg down to 60 mmHg). But once the shoulder of the curve is reached, any further, even small, reductions in P_aO_2 are now accompanied by dramatic drops in saturation, e.g. once P_aO_2 falls below 60 mmHg (saturation ~90%), the saturation falls rapidly too because we are on the steep slope of the curve.

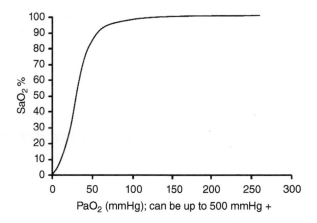

Figure 21.3 Haemoglobin–oxygen dissociation curve.

Table 21.1 Typical haemoglobin P_{50} values for various mammals (with ranges, if available).

	Haemoglobin P_{50} (mmHg)
Camel	22 (21–23)
Cat	35 (34–36)
Cow	35 (25–35)
Dog	30 (28–31.5)
Horse	24 (24–26)
Human	26.7 (26–29)
Llama	21 (17.5–22)
Pig	33 (32–34)

Hypoxaemia is often classified as mild if P_aO_2 80–90 mmHg; moderate if P_aO_2 60–80 mmHg; and severe if $P_aO_2 < 60$ mmHg.

Remember that the exact position of the curve depends upon the patient's temperature, PCO_2, and pH amongst other factors, such as the P_{50} of its haemoglobin. The **P_{50}** is the partial pressure of oxygen at which the haemoglobin is 50% saturated with oxygen (around 30 mmHg for dogs) and differs for different species and breeds (Table 21.1).

Note that P_{50} values can be age- and breed-specific.

The Hb/O₂ dissociation curve shifts to the right with:

- Low pH
- High PCO_2
- High temperature
- Lactic acidosis (e.g. exercise)
- High 2,3-diphosphoglycerate (2,3-DPG) (e.g. chronic anaemia), in species in which 2,3-DPG is an allosteric modulator of oxygen binding to haemoglobin
- Hyperchloraemia and hyperphosphataemia

The Hb/O_2 dissociation curve shifts to the left with:

- High pH
- Low PCO_2
- Hypothermia
- Foetal Hb
- Low 2,3-DPG, in species in which 2,3-DPG is an allosteric modulator of oxygen binding to haemoglobin
- Hypochloraemia and hypophosphataemia (the effect of hypophosphataemia is partly due to low 2,3-DPG)

Before we can interpret the results of blood gas analysis, we need to know the **normal ranges** of the values (Table 21.2). Note that the 'normal' values given in Table 21.2 assume that the patient is breathing room air and that its temperature is 37 °C. Reference intervals should ideally be those specific to the analyser being used. The 'normal ranges' given here are quite 'generous' to accommodate much of the published data. Most blood gas analysers assume the patient's temperature is 37 °C, unless instructed otherwise.

As a rule of thumb, to guesstimate what P_aO_2 should be if we know the inspired oxygen percentage, we can use a rough derivation of the alveolar gas equation:

$$\text{Alveolar } PO_2 \text{ (and therefore arterial } PO_2,}$$
$$\text{in an ideal world)} \propto \text{Inspired } O_2 \text{ tension}$$

$$\text{Rule of thumb : Inspired } O_2 \text{ (percentage)} \times 5 \approx P_aO_2 \text{ mmHg}$$

For example, room air has approx. 21% oxygen, so $21\% \times 5 = P_aO_2$ of 105 mmHg. Under anaesthesia with approximately 100% inspired oxygen, the expected P_aO_2 would be about 500 mmHg (although this is rarely achieved in anaesthetised horses because of ventilation/perfusion [$\dot{V} : \dot{Q}$], mismatches in their lungs).

Table 21.2 Typical blood gas values for dogs (and where values differ significantly, for horses and cats).

Variable	Arterial blood	Venous blood
pH	7.4 (7.35–7.45) (Cats 7.4 [7.3–7.45])	7.35 (7.35–7.45)
P_aO_2 (room air)	100 mmHg (90–120)	40 mmHg
P_aCO_2	40 mmHg (35–45) (Cats 31 [25–37])	45 mmHg (Cats 35–40)
HCO_3^-	21–28 mmol/l (Cats c. 18)	24–28 mmol/l (Cats c. 21)
Base excess (BE)	−5 to +5 mmol/l (Cats usually negative and may be below −6) (Adult horses not usually negative; up to c. +8)	−5 to +5 mmol/l (Cats usually negative) (Adult horses usually positive)
Hb saturation with O_2	Approx. 98%	70–75%

There are various other ways of guesstimating the efficiency of oxygenation, as outlined below.

21.3.2.1 Indices of Oxygenation

- P_aO_2/P_AO_2 ratio. If <0.85, then severe venous admixture exists.
- $P_aO_2 + P_aCO_2$. If >140 ± 20 mmHg (at sea level), and breathing room air, then ability of lungs to oxygenate the blood is normal. If <120 mmHg, then there is venous admixture or reduced efficiency of gaseous exchange in the lungs.
- P_aO_2/F_IO_2 ratio. Normal is 450–530; <300 accompanies mild lung inefficiency, <200 accompanies severe lung inefficiency.
- $P_{(A-a)}O_2$ difference. Need to use the alveolar gas equation (see below) to calculate P_AO_2, and then calculate the difference. You can guesstimate the RQ at 0.8, and use the blood gas analysis results for arterial CO_2 tension (P_aCO_2) in place of P_ACO_2. Subtract measured P_aO_2 from calculated P_AO_2 and if the result is >15 mmHg on room air, then there is reduced lung efficiency.
- Respiratory index $P_{(A-a)}O_2/P_aO_2$.
- Intrapulmonary shunt (see below).

21.3.2.1.1 The Alveolar Gas Equation
The form that we usually use is:

$$P_AO_2 = P_IO_2 - \frac{P_ACO_2}{RQ}$$

where P_AO_2 is alveolar partial pressure of oxygen; P_IO_2 is partial pressure of humidified (saturated) inspired oxygen; P_ACO_2 is alveolar partial pressure of carbon dioxide ($\approx$ systemic arterial blood CO_2 tension, P_aCO_2); RQ is respiratory quotient (normally estimated at 0.8, but can be 0.8–1.0).

$$\text{Now, } P_IO_2 = F_IO_2 \times \left(P_B - P_{H2O}\right)$$

where F_IO_2 is fraction of oxygen in inspired air; P_B is atmospheric (barometric) pressure; P_{H2O} is saturated water vapour pressure at body temperature (37 °C), which is 47 mmHg.

$$\text{So, } P_AO_2 = F_IO_2\left(P_B - P_{H2O}\right) - \frac{P_ACO_2}{RQ}$$

If we apply this to room air, then:

$$P_AO_2 = 0.21\left(760 - 47\right) - \left(40/0.8\right)$$
$$= \left(0.21 \times 713\right) - 50$$
$$= 150 - 50$$
$$\text{i.e. } P_AO_2 = 100 \text{ mmHg}$$

If gaseous exchange were ideal, arterial PO_2 (P_aO_2) would also be c.100 mmHg.

If we apply this to an animal breathing almost 100% oxygen under anaesthesia (there would probably be 1–2% anaesthetic agent present, but for the purpose of this exercise we will forget that for the moment), then:

$$P_AO_2 = 1(760 - 47) - (40/0.8)$$
$$= 713 - 50$$
$$= 663 \text{ mmHg}$$

In an ideal situation, P_aO_2 would also be 663 mmHg, so our guestimate of 500 is a bit short, but the ideal situation rarely exists in reality. (The actual atmospheric pressure will also affect the results.)

Conversion of mmHg to and from kPa

$1\text{mmHg} \approx 0.133\text{kPa}$

$1\text{kPa} = 7.5\text{mmHg}$

For example : $100\text{mmHg} = (100 \times 0.133)\text{KPa} = 13.3\text{kPa}$

$5\text{kPa} = (5 \times 7.5)\text{mmHg} = 37.5\text{mmHg}$

21.3.2.1.2 The Shunt Equation

Not all areas of lung are equally ventilated or perfused, resulting in $\dot{V} : \dot{Q}$ mismatches. In some areas of lung, perfusion may exceed ventilation. At its extreme (i.e. where perfusion occurs in areas with no ventilation), this can be considered as wasted perfusion or intrapulmonary shunt. The 'intrapulmonary shunt' ($\dot{Q}_s$) is most often discussed in terms of a calculated (intra)pulmonary shunt fraction, i.e. as the (theoretical) proportion of the total cardiac output ($\dot{Q}_t$) entering the pulmonary veins, which has not participated in gas exchange, and therefore constitutes 'venous admixture'. That is, pulmonary venous blood from 'intrapulmonary shunt' areas mixes with pulmonary venous blood from areas of lung with better ventilation/ perfusion matching, to result in some decrease of overall oxygen content and increase of overall carbon dioxide content in the mixed pulmonary venous blood, which becomes the systemic arterial blood The shunt equation uses the oxygen content of pulmonary end-capillary ($C_c'O_2$), arterial (C_aO_2), and mixed venous blood ($C_{\bar{v}}O_2$) to determine the (intra)pulmonary shunt fraction ($\dot{Q}_s/\dot{Q}_t$),

$$\frac{\dot{Q}_s}{\dot{Q}_t} = \frac{C_c'O_2 - C_aO_2}{C_c'O_2 - C_{\bar{v}}O_2}$$

Paired systemic arterial and mixed venous (pulmonary arterial) blood samples are obtained to calculate the respective oxygen contents, and the end-capillary oxygen content is calculated using the alveolar gas equation (to first determine P_AO_2 and then C_AO_2, which is a surrogate for $C_c'O_2$),

Table 21.3 Ability of increasing F_1O_2 (%) alone to correct hypoxaemia caused by intrapulmonary shunt.

Intrapulmonary shunt (%)	Shunt severity	F_1O_2 required to correct hypoxaemia (%)
<10	Normal	21%
10	Mild	30%
20	Moderate	57%
30	Moderate–severe	97%
40	Severe	Hypoxaemia not fully corrected with 100% F_1O_2
50	Severe	Increased F_1O_2 has minimal impact on P_aO_2

knowing F_1O_2 and P_aCO_2 (end-capillary blood gases should be in equilibrium with the alveoli). As obtaining a mixed venous sample requires a pulmonary artery catheter, which is associated with significant morbidity and is rarely indicated clinically, **a central venous blood sample can provide a more convenient estimate of mixed venous blood values**, but caution is advised, as simple substitution of values may lead to errors. (An alternative method, the estimated F-shunt, assumes that tissue oxygen extraction is constant and so there is a fixed arterial-to-mixed venous oxygen content difference of 3.5 ml/dl, negating the need for a pulmonary artery catheter. The expression for mixed venous oxygen content in the denominator of the above equation is therefore replaced by $[C_a O_2 + 3.5]$.) The degree of intrapulmonary shunt indicates whether increased F_1O_2 alone can correct the hypoxaemia or not (Table 21.3).

Anaesthesia, recumbency (dorsal > lateral >> sternal), and $F_1O_2 > 0.6$ all promote the development/exacerbation of atelectasis and intrapulmonary shunt. Because CO_2 is more readily diffusible than O_2, the intrapulmonary shunt fraction must approach 50% before P_aCO_2 is impacted.

21.4 Interpreting Blood Gases

When interpreting blood gas results:

- Look at the oxygenation (PO_2)
- Look at the pH and decide if it is normal or more acidic or more alkaline than normal
- Look at PCO_2 and HCO_3^-
- Check BE

21.4.1 Oxygenation (P_aO_2)

From the rule of thumb above, we can calculate the expected P_aO_2. Many horses have poor oxygenation under general anaesthesia, especially larger horses and in dorsal recumbency, because of hypoventilation, reduced cardiac output, and venous admixture ($\dot{V} : \dot{Q}$ mismatches).

P_aO_2 values below 90 mmHg (certainly in anaesthetised animals on >21% inspired oxygen) start to ring alarm bells. The levels of hypoxaemia have been described as:

P_aO_2 80–90 mmHg = mild hypoxaemia
P_aO_2 60–80 mmHg = moderate hypoxaemia
P_aO_2 < 60 mmHg = severe hypoxaemia

Once hypoxaemic, and certainly if the **P_aO_2 is below 60 mmHg**, some **interventions** must be made to try to improve it. These include:

- Increase the inspired oxygen percentage (if not already 100%). High concentrations of oxygen, however, increase resorption/absorption atelectasis, i.e. the collapse/closure of alveoli 'behind closed small airways' because of rapid absorption of relatively soluble oxygen in the absence of a more insoluble gas such as nitrogen. Some suggest we should incorporate such insoluble gases as N_2, N_2O, or He to 'splint' the alveoli open; however, this is more of a preventative strategy than a treatment when hypoxaemia already exists. Note that, from Table 21.3, if severe hypoxaemia exists because of severe intrapulmonary shunt, merely increasing the inspired oxygen percentage will have minimal effect on improving the P_aO_2.
- Institute artificial ventilation (i.e. mechanical ventilation, which is most commonly provided in the form of positive pressure ventilation [PPV]).
- Apply positive end expiratory pressure (PEEP) to try to 'splint' alveoli open and prevent them from re-collapsing between breaths, and consider an alveolar recruitment manoeuvre (both of which can have deleterious effects on blood pressure).
- Try clenbuterol IV, or perhaps better, aerosolised salbutamol intratracheally (see below). Once thought to improve oxygenation by causing bronchodilation and helping to open previously closed small airways and alveoli, these β_2 agonists are now thought to act primarily by promoting vasodilation (and thereby helping to improve V : Q matching) in areas of alveolar dead space (where ventilation is present in the absence of perfusion), and where alveoli are relatively under-perfused.
- Ensure adequate pulmonary perfusion (i.e. mean arterial blood pressure 60–70 mmHg minimum), check anaesthetic depth, and give fluid and/or inotropic and/or vasopressor support as necessary.

21.4.1.1 Clenbuterol

Clenbuterol is a β_2 agonist, and therefore is a smooth muscle relaxant (bronchodilator, uterine relaxant, vasodilator etc.). It also causes positive inotropic and positive

chronotropic effects. Tachycardia tends to occur, both in response to vasodilation (baroreflex response to hypotension), and also through direct effects on cardiac β_2 receptors. Little overall change in blood pressure results because tachycardia helps offset any vasodilatory hypotension, and the vasodilation also counters any positive inotropic tendencies towards hypertension. The tachycardia, however, increases myocardial oxygen demand (just when the oxygen supply is not all that great), and could potentially result in arrhythmias. Clenbuterol also causes sweating (due to beta adrenergic sweating and possibly secondary to peripheral vasodilation), lacrimation, and a lightening of the plane of anaesthesia. Furthermore, the muscle tremors it causes are thought to promote poorer quality recoveries from anaesthesia in horses (perhaps due to muscle soreness following the fasciculation-type activity and sweaty, slippery recovery box floors).

21.4.1.2 Salbutamol

When aerosolised and delivered into the respiratory tract during inhalation, a low dose of salbutamol results in better improvement in oxygenation and fewer side effects (less obvious tachycardia and less profuse sweating) than clenbuterol.

21.4.1.3 Artificial Ventilation

Although applying artificial ventilation techniques may help improve alveolar recruitment and may reduce alveolar CO_2 content, which also helps improve P_aO_2, it can have detrimental effects. Abnormal positive pressure within the chest reduces venous return (the venae cavae get squashed) and reduces cardiac output. This is especially problematic if the animal is already hypovolaemic (i.e. the venae cavae are already 'relatively empty'), and is exacerbated further by dorsal recumbency. Occasionally, artificial ventilation may over-inflate areas of the lung that were ventilating 'ideally' before our intervention; and this over-inflation may 'stretch' and therefore 'narrow', or even occlude, the alveolar capillaries that would otherwise have been responsible for gaseous exchange at these alveoli. Thus we can convert normal $\dot{V} : \dot{Q}$ areas of lung into/towards alveolar dead space. Additionally, we may not be able to do much to re-inflate atelectatic parts of the lung, despite our best efforts to 'recruit' alveoli in such areas of perfusion in excess of ventilation (e.g. 'intrapulmonary shunt').

21.4.2 pH

Abnormal pH can be associated with respiratory acidosis or alkalosis, metabolic acidosis or alkalosis, or a mixture of respiratory and metabolic derangements. Remember that disturbances can be acute or chronic. The body tries to make compensatory responses to correct ECF pH, so we may see compensatory (or secondary), disturbances. For example, a horse with colic and metabolic acidosis (e.g. bicarbonate loss into gut secretions that get sequestered in twisted bowel, and lactic acidosis due to both localised gut ischaemia and systemic hypovolaemia) may hyperventilate. Although this might be partly due to hypovolaemic hypotension, pain, or abdominal distension making ventilation more difficult, it could also be due to a compensatory response to the metabolic acidosis.

Therapeutic interventions should be **considered** once pH is outside the 'normal' range, and especially if **<7.1–7.2 or >>7.6** (although such levels of alkalosis are rare unless iatrogenically-induced).

21.4.3 PCO_2

This is often higher than normal in anaesthetised animals, especially large animals, because they tend to hypoventilate when anaesthetised and recumbent. Higher than normal PCO_2 and lower than normal pH is called respiratory acidosis. In order to correct this, PPV should be instituted, to help the patient to blow off more carbon dioxide.

Values of $P_aCO_2 > 60–70$ mmHg may require intervention (blood pH may approach the worrying range for acidaemia; sympathetic nervous system stimulation can elicit catecholamine-induced cardiac arrhythmias).

At the other extreme, P_aCO_2 values of <20 mmHg should be avoided because cerebral blood vessels become so constricted that brain perfusion and oxygenation can become compromised. (It is rare to see PCO_2 values so low, except with over-zealous artificial ventilation). Autoregulation of cerebral blood flow (CBF) is exquisitely responsive to P_aCO_2 (actually via the pH). This is useful when dealing with head trauma and raised intracranial pressure (ICP), because by deliberately hyperventilating these patients to P_aCO_2 of 30–35 mmHg, we reduce intracranial blood volume (at least for several hours, until the system re-adjusts itself). In accordance with the Monro-Kellie doctrine, this reduces ICP, which may be life-saving.

$$\text{Remember the equilibrium}: CO_2 + H_2O \leftrightarrow H^+ + HCO_3^-$$

If CO_2 increases, the reaction gets pushed to the right, so $[H^+]$ increases (and therefore pH decreases to more acidic values), but bicarbonate also increases. However, when the pH changes in the acidic direction, the bicarbonate buffering system becomes more efficient because the system pH is nearer to the buffer's pKa. It may seem strange that the acidity can increase even when the bicarbonate concentration (the buffer) also increases, but pH, by definition, is related only to the H^+ concentration.

21.4.4 Bicarbonate

This should increase if CO_2 increases and decrease if CO_2 decreases (see equilibrium above). Therefore, with primary respiratory disturbances, the direction of change (increase or decrease) of bicarbonate concentration should be the same as that for CO_2. If the direction of change is opposite, then something else is happening.

21.4.5 Base Excess (BE)

This relates to the buffering ability of all the chemical buffers present, including, importantly, haemoglobin; and we look at the BE value in conjunction with the pH, HCO_3^-, and the PCO_2. If the animal is short of chemical buffering ability, the deficit of chemical buffers is referred to as a 'negative base excess' (instead of 'base deficit'). Metabolic acidoses are accompanied by a negative (more negative than 'normal') base excess, whereas metabolic alkaloses are accompanied by a positive (more positive than 'normal') base excess.

21.4.5.1 Definition of BE

The base excess is the number of millimoles of acid or alkali that must be added to 1 l of blood to restore its pH to normal (7.4), after first cancelling out any perturbations in PCO_2 (and therefore secondary changes in HCO_3^-) due to respiratory causes, by equilibrating the blood sample with a PCO_2 of 40 mmHg, at 37 °C, and at the actual oxygen saturation of the patient.

Therefore, the BE value tells us of metabolic problems only (being independent of primary changes in PCO_2).

The above definition strictly refers to the actual base excess (ABE) or **BE(b)** because it tells us about the buffering capacity of whole blood (includes bicarbonate HCO_3^-, phosphate, haemoglobin, and plasma proteins, of which bicarbonate HCO_3^- and haemoglobin are the most important buffers, although not quite of equal importance). It also requires knowledge of the haemoglobin concentration of the blood, which is measured or estimated by the blood gas analyser.

However, if we wish to extend our knowledge of the blood (which is only one compartment of ECF with a small ICF compartment [the red blood cells which contain the very important buffer, haemoglobin]) to the whole of the ECF, we can assume the haemoglobin content of the blood is 'shared' between all the ECF compartments (by convention, [Hb] is divided by three for adults, or by four for neonates). The calculations result in a value that tells us about the buffering capacity of all the ECF compartments, denoted as standard base excess (SBE) or **BE(ecf)**.

BE(ecf) is often said to be the better value to use in interpretation of metabolic problems, so **from here on, BE refers to BE(ecf).**

21.4.5.2 Administering Sodium Bicarbonate

When the BE value is more negative than $-7\,mmol/l$ in arterial blood (allow more negative values for cats) (usually when also accompanied by a low pH, i.e. c. 7.1–7.2 and a low HCO_3^-), we could treat the metabolic acidosis by administering sodium bicarbonate intravenously, usually in addition to other intravenous fluid therapy. We can calculate how much HCO_3^- an adult animal needs by using the following equation:

$$\mathbf{mmol\,HCO_3^-\,required = BE \times 0.3 \times body\ weight\,(kg)}$$

One-third of the body weight is a rough estimate of the animal's ECF volume because it is the buffer deficiency of fluid in this compartment that we have measured and that we are primarily concerned with. For **neonates, 0.45** is used.

Because HCO_3^- is not an innocuous substance to give (i.e. we can cause more complications than we cure), usually **half of the calculated amount is given first**, and then the base excess is re-evaluated to determine if further doses are required. **Alternatively**, instead of using the measured BE value in the above equation, we could use either the difference between the negatively low BE value from the blood gas analysis and -5 (the low end of our 'normal range'), or even the difference between the negatively low BE value and -7 (our intervention point) in the equation, to result in lower calculated bicarbonate doses, which do not then need to be halved.

21.4.5.2.1 Problems Associated with Bicarbonate Administration

Commonly available 8.4% $NaHCO_3$ is a hypertonic fluid, so if given rapidly it has some similar effects to hypertonic (c. 7.2%) saline; these effects can also be seen, slightly less dramatically after the 4.2% solution, which is also hypertonic:

- **Haemodilution** (decreases packed cell volume [PCV], total protein, platelets, clotting factors, chloride, potassium, calcium, magnesium). Care if already anaemic, hypoproteinaemic, poor clotting ability, hypokalaemic, or hypocalcaemic. Hypokalaemia, hypomagnesaemia and hypocalcaemia add to muscle weakness (including respiratory muscles), gastrointestinal ileus, and problems for other excitable membranes (heart muscle and nerves), possibly leading to arrhythmias and seizures. Hypokalaemia also interferes with renal function (hypokalaemic nephropathy, i.e. reduced ability of kidneys to concentrate urine).

- Increases sodium (beware **hypernatraemia**).
- **Volume expansion** (beware congestive heart failure).
- **Increases PCO_2** (see equilibrium above). The animal must have adequate respiratory capacity to blow off the extra CO_2 created. Beware respiratory depression in anaesthetised animals because the extra CO_2 produced can cause a 'respiratory-type' acidosis, on top of the metabolic acidosis that you are trying to treat. The extra CO_2 can also diffuse into cells to cause intracellular acidosis and cross the blood–brain barrier to cause 'paradoxical cerebrospinal fluid (CSF) acidosis'.
- Rapid pH changes also affect electrolytes, e.g. **overcorrection of acidosis** produces an alkalosis. This results in reduced ionised calcium, due to altered buffering by albumin etc., and stimulates cellular H^+/K^+ exchange causing hypokalaemia in the ECF. Cellular HCO_3^-/Cl^- exchange may also be affected.

Bicarbonate is only really suitable to help treat metabolic acidosis where there has been bicarbonate loss. It is less appropriate where the metabolic acidosis is due to a primary gain in H^+, e.g. lactic acidosis or ketoacidosis. In all cases of metabolic acidosis, however, intravenous fluid therapy usually helps by diluting H^+ and restoring renal perfusion so that the kidneys can do their job.

Why does hypovolaemia cause lactic acidosis? When an animal is hypovolaemic, the blood pressure falls, but the body tries to maintain the blood pressure so that tissue perfusion (especially of vital organs) is maintained. The sympathetic nervous system is activated, and increased catecholamines result in peripheral vasoconstriction, which 'centralises' the blood volume to where it's needed most (the vital organs). However, peripheral tissues are now starved of oxygen and start to metabolise anaerobically, which produces lactic acid.

Bicarbonate must never be used to treat respiratory acidosis; it will only serve to worsen it (because it causes an acute increase in the PCO_2).

Bicarbonate solutions should be given slowly intravenously, e.g. give the chosen dose over 10–20 minutes, and then take another arterial blood sample for blood gas analysis 15 minutes after the bicarbonate HCO_3^- administration has been completed, to allow time for re-equilibration. Bicarbonate solutions should not be administered through the same giving sets as solutions that contain calcium (e.g. Hartmann's solution) because calcium carbonate may precipitate in the giving set, cannula or vein.

The **8.4% $NaHCO_3$ solution** commonly used for large animals seems a bit of a strange concentration, but it contains 1 mmol of HCO_3^- in every 1 ml, so it makes calculations of the volume to give really easy. Note the **4.2% solution** (0.5 mmol/ml) is administered to small animals, foals, and calves. A 1.26% solution (0.15 mmol/ml) is also available. These lower percent solutions are preferred for peripheral venous administration, whereas the 8.4% solution is reserved for central vein administration only.

21.5 Other Options

Trometamol (tromethamine, tris[hydroxymethyl]aminomethane, THAM) is an organic amino alcohol buffer (pKa 7.8 at 37 °C). Its amine combines with H^+ and is renally excreted. It does not increase CO_2 production. It does not cause hypernatraemia (but may cause hyponatraemia due to haemodilution). It is hypertonic, and causes plasma volume expansion, haemodilution, and osmotic diuresis (as effective as mannitol at reducing ICP in humans). It may enter cells, can cause respiratory depression in humans and is commonly used during (human) cardiopulmonary bypass. It is available as a 0.3 M solution, and the dose is:

$$ml\,required = BE \times 1.1 \times body\,weight\left(kg\right)$$

Carbicarb is equimolar Na_2CO_3 and $NaHCO_3$. At one time, this was favoured over $NaHCO_3$ for inclusion in practice-formulated fluids for the treatment of diarrhoeic calves and lambs, as less CO_2 is generated when it buffers H^+ from metabolic acidoses. The availability of a range of more affordable, commercially available fluids has, however, reduced the need for such practice-formulated fluids.

21.6 Temperature Compensation

21.6.1 Alpha-stat or pH-stat Management

These different strategies arose because of the development of hypothermic cardiac/neuro anaesthetic techniques in humans, e.g. for hypothermic cardiopulmonary bypass (HCPB). Temperature changes alter both the dissociation (ionisation or auto-ionisation) constant of water, and therefore water's pH of neutrality (pN_w), and the solubilities (and partial pressures/tensions) of dissolved gases. Gas solubility in polar solvents decreases as the temperature increases; the increased kinetic energy of the system leads to increased gas tensions and possible escape of gases from physical solution into the atmosphere. For patients whose temperature is not 37 °C, this causes discrepancies in dissolved gas tensions between actual patient temperature and 37 °C values.

The pN_w at 25 °C is 7.0; and at 37 °C is 6.8 (roughly the same as the intracellular pH of mammals!) because water

dissociation increases at higher temperatures. Compared to normothermia, hypothermia results in a higher value of pN_w, a lower P_aCO_2 for the same number of CO_2 molecules (due to increased solubility), and increased protein affinity for H^+.

So, as the patient cools down:

- **P_aCO_2 and [H^+] decrease (pH increases)**
- CO_2 production is also reduced because of overall reduction in metabolic rate
- Cerebral vasoconstriction (due to hypocapnia) reduces CBF
- Protein protonation is minimally affected as the increased affinity of proteins for H^+ is offset by the decreased [H^+] availability
- There is **little effect on O_2 content**, as haemoglobin contributes so much more to C_aO_2 than oxygen dissolved in physical solution (P_aO_2), but **haemoglobin affinity for O_2 increases** significantly. Although this theoretically reduces oxygen availability to mitochondria, oxygen demand (metabolic rate) is also reduced during hypothermia

Blood gas analysers measure blood gases and pH at 37 °C, unless otherwise instructed, and results may not match the actual values within the hypo-/hyper-thermic patient. There are no reference ranges for normal acid–base and blood gases at temperatures other than 37 °C so, **should we correct blood gases to the patient's actual temperature or not?**

21.6.1.1 Alpha-stat Strategy

For a buffer to be effective, its pKa must be near the pH of its operating environment and its pKa must change in an appropriate (see below) way with temperature. The best *intracellular* buffers are proteins, but only the imidazole rings of their histidine residues fulfil these criteria. **Alpha is the ratio of protonated-to-total imidazole rings**. At 37 °C and with the normal intracellular pH of 6.8, alpha ≈ 0.55, that is, roughly half of the imidazole rings are protonated, and, in this state, intracellular proteins, especially enzymes, have optimal structure and function. As temperature changes, both the intracellular and extracellular pH change, but it is important that a constant gradient for H^+ ions exists between them.

Alpha-stat strategy assumes that acid–base changes induced by temperature are appropriate and that **pH 7.4 and P_aCO_2 40 mmHg are only ideal when body temperature is 37 °C**. Therefore, blood gas results are **not corrected** to actual patient temperature; instead the blood gas sample is analysed at 37 °C and the results are interpreted against normothermic (37 °C) values, regardless of actual patient temperature. Variations from normal normothermic values (particularly PCO_2), may require interventions/treatment: the aim being to maintain a constant proportion (0.55) of ionised imidazole groups of histidine residues on intracellular proteins, thereby optimising enzyme function.

Therefore, with alpha-stat strategy, as the patient cools down:

- **Aim to maintain P_aCO_2 at 40 mmHg at 37 °C**
- During hypothermia, respiratory alkalosis develops but 'total CO_2' is unchanged
  - Total $CO_2 = (\alpha \times PCO_2) + [HCO_3^-]$; where α is the solubility coefficient for carbon dioxide, which increases as body temperature decreases
- Cerebral autoregulation and enzyme function are preserved
- The risk of cerebral overperfusion, oedema, and embolic events is reduced

21.6.1.2 pH-stat Strategy

pH-stat strategy assumes that **pH 7.4 and P_aCO_2 40 mmHg are ideal, regardless of actual body temperature**. Therefore, blood gas results are **corrected** to actual patient temperature, not 37 °C (Rosenthal formulae are used by most analysers to perform these corrections). The aim is to maintain constant pH and P_aCO_2 regardless of patient temperature. For a hypothermic patient, this requires more CO_2 molecules (increased total CO_2) to achieve the equivalent, normothermic, P_aCO_2, thereby increasing CBF, and, possibly, improving neurological outcomes.

Therefore, with pH-stat strategy, as the patient cools down:

- **Aim to maintain P_aCO_2 at 40 mmHg, regardless of actual patient temperature**
- During hypothermia, respiratory alkalosis is avoided by allowing an increase in total CO_2
- Cerebral blood flow and oxygen requirement become uncoupled: CBF increases but metabolism decreases as temperature falls
- Greater CBF increases cerebral cooling, O_2 delivery and risk of embolic events
- Intracerebral steal and hyperperfusion may occur
- Calculation of the respiratory quotient (CO_2 production ÷ O_2 consumption) is confounded

21.6.1.3 Which Is Best?

There is no clear consensus as to which strategy is 'better' or 'correct'. Mammals that undergo periodic torpor (hibernation or aestivation) utilise either strategy, depending upon species. Intermittent ventilation during torpor influences results and should be considered when determining which strategy has been employed. At least one squirrel species appears to use pH-stat to hibernate and alpha-stat to aestivate.

There is conflicting evidence for the superiority of either strategy in pigs following circulatory arrest at 18–20 °C. Dogs, humans, and pigs have higher CBF during HCPB with pH-stat management. There was no difference in outcome for human adults undergoing HCPB managed with either strategy; neurological and myocardial outcomes were improved for human neonates undergoing HCPB with pH-stat management. Human adults undergoing therapeutic hypothermia following severe acute ischaemic stroke experienced significant (>20 mmHg) increases in ICP with anisocoria during pH-stat management, that resolved when alpha-stat management was instituted. Further research is required.

A combined approach has been advocated where pH-stat is used during development of hypothermia and alpha-stat used thereafter throughout circulatory arrest and rewarming. The aim of combining strategies is to gain the benefits of increased CBF and cerebral cooling rate during instigation of therapeutic hypothermia, alongside optimised protein protonation and preserved cerebral autoregulation during reperfusion and rewarming.

Regardless of which strategy is chosen, it should be used consistently throughout the hospital (or individual case), to avoid confusion.

21.7 Other Approaches to Blood Gas Analysis

21.7.1 Anion Gap

The anion gap is represented by the difference between the commonly measured plasma cations and anions.

$$Na^+ + K^+ + \text{unmeasured cations} \left(UC\right)$$
$$= Cl^- + HCO_3^- + \text{unmeasured anions} \left(UA\right)$$

$$\textbf{Anion gap} = \left(\textbf{UA} - \textbf{UC}\right) = \left(\textbf{Na}^+ + \textbf{K}^+\right) - \left(\textbf{Cl}^- + \textbf{HCO}_3^-\right)$$

$$\text{Albumin-corrected anion gap} =$$
$$\text{anion gap} + \left(0.25 \times \left[40 - \text{actual albumin g/l}\right]\right)$$

Although in reality, in order to maintain electroneutrality, the number of cations must equal the number of anions, the above calculation results in a usual excess of cations over anions because not all anions can be easily measured, e.g. lactate, acetoacetate, beta hydroxybutyrate, phosphates, sulphates, and proteins. Normal values are 12–25 mmol/l in dogs and 13–27 mmol/l in cats.

If HCO_3^- decreases (e.g. metabolic acidosis), then another anion must increase (e.g. Cl^- or UA) to maintain electrical neutrality. The anion gap may be used to differentiate between the two common types of metabolic acidosis:

- Bicarbonate loss (e.g. diarrhoea). HCO_3^- loss is compensated for by an increase in Cl^-, so we see what's called a **normal anion gap, hyperchloraemic metabolic acidosis**.
- Accumulation of unmeasured anions (organic acid gain, e.g. diabetic ketoacidosis). The increase in organic acids (ketones) results in bicarbonate buffer consumption to maintain pH (HCO_3^- is reduced), but no change in Cl^- occurs because of the organic acid anions. Hence, we see what's called a **high anion gap, normochloraemic metabolic acidosis**.

21.7.2 Quantitative Approaches

Examples are the Fencl-Stewart approach and the ion-equilibrium theory. These approaches more critically evaluate changes in BE and can be used to calculate a 'strong ion gap', but you need to be able to measure more 'ionic' components in the blood; see Further Reading.

21.8 Examples

21.8.1 Horse Under GA, Lateral Recumbency, Arterial Sample

pH	7.28	(N = 7.35–7.45)
PCO_2	71.6 mmHg	(N = 35–45)
PO_2	254.7 mmHg	Depends upon F_IO_2
HCO_3^-	33.7 mmol/l	(N = 21–28)
BE	4.0 mmol/l	(N = −5 to +8)

Interpretation:

- Consider oxygenation first. Assuming the horse is breathing ~100% oxygen, if we apply the rule of thumb, P_AO_2 (and hopefully P_aO_2) should be $100 \times 5 = 500$ mmHg. Well it is not, but this is a horse, and values over 100 mmHg are a bonus.
- Look at the pH. There is an acidaemia.
- Look at the PCO_2. It is higher than normal, so already we could say that at least part of the acidaemia is due to a respiratory acidosis, but also look at the bicarbonate. It is high too, which is what we would expect with a primary respiratory acidosis. But to be sure, see the next point.
- Look at the BE value. It is within normal limits, so as far as we can tell this is a primary respiratory acidosis. The rise in HCO_3^- is in line with what some would call the expected metabolic compensatory response for acute respiratory acidosis (see Table 21.4).

Table 21.4 Expected compensatory changes.

Disorder	Expected compensatory responses
Metabolic acidosis	1 mmol/l ↓ in HCO_3^- → (0.7–)1(−1.3) mmHg ↓ in P_aCO_2
Metabolic alkalosis	1 mmol/l ↑ in HCO_3^- → 0.6–0.7 mmHg ↑ in P_aCO_2
Acute respiratory acidosis	1 mmHg ↑ in P_aCO_2 → 0.1–0.15 mmol/l ↑ in HCO_3^-
Chronic respiratory acidosis	1 mmHg ↑ in P_aCO_2 → 0.35–0.4 mmol/l ↑ in HCO_3^-
Acute respiratory alkalosis	1 mmHg ↓ in P_aCO_2 → 0.2–0.25 mmol/l ↓ in HCO_3^-
Chronic metabolic alkalosis	1 mmHg ↓ in P_aCO_2 → 0.5–0.55 mmol/l ↓ in HCO_3^-

What can we do about it?

- Check anaesthetic depth ('too deep' can be associated with more profound respiratory depression)
- Apply PPV

A repeat blood gas analysis about 20 minutes later gave the following results:

pH	7.37	(N = 7.35–7.45)
PCO_2	52.4 mmHg	(N = 35–45)
PO_2	352.7 mmHg	Depends upon F_IO_2
HCO_3^-	30.1 mmol/l	(N = 21–28)
BE	3.4 mmol/l	(N = −5 to +8)

Interpretation:

- Oxygenation is still OK (in fact the artificial ventilation has improved it)
- pH now just back in normal range (still slightly on 'acidic side')
- PCO_2 better, but still a little high
- HCO_3^-, down a bit, but what we expect after reducing the PCO_2
- BE still normal

These results are not quite perfect, but we have made good improvement.

21.8.2 Pony (135 kg), Colic, Under GA, Dorsal Recumbency, Arterial Sample

pH	7.13	(N = 7.35–7.45)
PCO_2	57.3 mmHg	(N = 35–45)
PO_2	209.8 mmHg	Depends upon F_IO_2
HCO_3^-	19.2 mmol/l	(N = 21–28)
BE	−11.0 mmol/l	(N = −5 to +8)

Interpretation:

- Oxygenation. Assuming ~100% inspired O_2, and applying our rule of thumb, this is OK.
- pH is lower than normal, so there is an acidaemia. Values below 7.1–7.2 are also worryingly low.
- PCO_2 is higher than normal, so there is a respiratory component to the acidaemia.
- HCO_3^- is low. If there was just a primary respiratory acidosis, we would expect HCO_3^- to be higher than normal too, so because the HCO_3^- is low, it must be being used/lost somewhere else.
- BE is very negative, so there is a deficit of buffers. This means that there is also a metabolic component to the acidaemia.

So, this is a mixed metabolic and respiratory acidosis. Before the pony was anaesthetised it may have had a slight respiratory alkalosis as a compensatory response to try to offset the metabolic acidosis, but anaesthesia has probably incurred enough respiratory depression to oppose this. What can we do?

- Check anaesthetic depth
- Address the low pH:
  - Start PPV
  - Continue IV fluid therapy
  - Administer bicarbonate (BE more negative than −7 and low pH is worrying)

The amount (mmol) of HCO_3^- required = BE × (0.3 × body weight [kg])

$=11 \times (0.3 \times 135)$		$=(11-5) \times (0.3 \times 135)$
$=445.5$ mmol	**OR**	$=243$ mmol
Halve this = c. 222 mmol		(No need to halve this)

This pony received only 200 ml of 8.4% sodium bicarbonate because sodium bicarbonate comes in bottles of 200 ml. Intravenous fluid therapy was continued and artificial ventilation was instituted. A repeat arterial blood gas analysis 30 minutes later yielded these results:

pH	7.34	(N = 7.35–7.45)
PCO_2	36.6 mmHg	(N = 35–45)
PO_2	501.8 mmHg	Depends upon F_IO_2
HCO_3^-	20.1 mmol/l	(N = 21–28)
BE	−4.5 mmol/l	(N = −5 to +8)

Interpretation:

- Oxygenation good (artificial ventilation has improved it in this case).
- pH just a little on the acidic side, but not worryingly low now.
- PCO_2 on the low side of normal (perhaps we can change the ventilator settings).
- HCO_3^- is just slightly on the low side, and just a bit lower than could be expected from the PCO_2, so the bicarbonate buffer is still slightly lacking.
- BE is within 'normal' range, but Equidae usually have BE values towards the more positive end of the range. Perhaps the extra 20 mmol of bicarbonate should have been given, but these results are fine at this stage. Another blood gas analysis should be performed after a further 30 minutes to check progress.

Further Reading

Alston, T.A. (2004). Blood gases and pH during hypothermia: the "-stats". *International Anesthesiology Clinics* 42: 73–80.

Armstrong, J.A.M., Guleria, A., and Girling, K. (2007). Evaluation of gas exchange deficit in the critically ill. *Continuing Education in Anaesthesia, Critical Care and Pain* 7: 131–134. ***(Explains more about oxygenation indices.)***

Badr, A. and Nightingale, P. (2007). An alternative approach to acid–base abnormalities in critically ill patients. *Continuing Education in Anaesthesia, Critical Care and Pain* 7: 107–111.

Bardell, D., West, E., and Senior, J.M. (2017). Evaluation of a new handheld point-of-care blood gas analyser using 100 equine blood samples. *Veterinary Anaesthesia and Analgesia* 44: 77–85.

Brandis, K. (2015). Acid–base physiology. http://www.anaesthesiamcq.com/AcidBaseBook/ABindex.php (accessed April 2019). ***(A very thorough overview of acid–base and blood gas analysis.)***

Chawla, G. and Drummond, G. (2008). Water, strong ions, and weak ions. *Continuing Education in Anaesthesia, Critical Care and Pain* 8: 108–112.

Constable, P.D. (2014). Acid–base assessment: when and how to apply the Hendesron-Hasselbalch equation and strong ion difference approach. *Veterinary Clinics of North America: Food Animal Practice* 30: 295–316.

Corey, H.E. (2003). Stewart and beyond: new models of acid–base balance. *Kidney International* 64: 777–787. ***(If you like equations you'll enjoy this.)***

Cruickshank, S. and Hirschauer, N. (2004). The alveolar gas equation. *Continuing Education in Anaesthesia, Critical*

Care and Pain 4: 24–27. *(Explains the 'full' form of the alveolar gas equation.)*.

Davis, M.D., Walsh, B.K., Sittig, S.E., and Restrepo, R.D. (2013). AARC clinical practice guideline: blood gas analysis and hemoximetry: 2013. *Respiratory Care* 58: 1694–1703.

Deane, J.C., Dagleish, M.P., Benamou, A.E.M. et al. (2004). Effects of syringe material and temperature and duration of storage on the stability of equine arterial blood gas variables. *Veterinary Anaesthesia and Analgesia* 31: 250–257. *(Interesting information on stability of samples in different syringe materials and under different storage conditions for several species.)*.

Driscoll, P., Brown, T., Gwinnutt, C., and Wardle, T. (eds.) (1997). A Simple Guide to Blood Gas Analysis. London, UK: BMJ Publishing Group.

Gonzalez, A.L. and Waddell, L.S. (2016). Blood gas analyzers. *Topics in Companion Animal Medicine* 31: 27–34.

Handy, J.M. and Soni, N. (2008). Physiological effects of hyperchloraemia and acidosis. *British Journal of Anaesthesia* 101: 141–150.

Hennessey, I.A.M. and Japp, A.G. (eds.) (2007). Arterial Blood Gases Made Easy. Philadelphia, USA: Churchill Livingstone, (Elsevier Health).

Hopper, K. and Haskins, S.C. (2008). A case-based review of a simplified quantitative approach to acid–base analysis. *Journal of Veterinary Emergency and Critical Care* 18: 467–476. *(An excellent, well written and easy to follow review with examples.)*.

Kitching, A.J. and Edge, C.J. (2002). Acid–base balance: a review of normal physiology. *British Journal of Anaesthesia CEPD Reviews* 2: 3–6.

Sirker, A.A., Rhodes, A., Grounds, R.M., and Bennett, E.D. (2002). Acid–base physiology: the 'traditional' and the 'modern' approaches. *Anaesthesia* 57: 348–356.

Story, K.A. (2004). Bench-to-bedside review: a brief history of clinical acid–base. *Critical Care* 8: 253–258.

Story, D.A. and Kellum, J.A. (2005). Acid–base balance revisited: Stewart and strong ions. *Seminars in Anaestheisa, Perioperative Medicine and Pain* 24: 9–16.

Swan, H. (1982). The hydroxyl-hydrogen ion concentration ratio during hypothermia. *Surgery, Gynecology & Obstetrics* 155: 897–912.

West, E., Bardell, D., and Senior, J.M. (2014). Comparison of the EPOC and iStat analysers for canine blood gas and electrolyte analysis. *Journal of Small Animal Practice* 55: 139–144.

Self-test Section

1 What is Sørensen's definition of pH?

2 What is the pH of neutrality of water?

3 Using the paired blood-gas results (below) taken from a normothermic cat breathing room air shortly after tracheal extubation, calculate shunt fraction, classify the degree of shunt and outline key interventions.

Arterial (coccygeal) sample		Central venous (R jugular) sample	
pH	7.449	pH	7.442
PCO_2	32.8 mmHg	PCO_2	37.3 mmHg
PO_2	78.3 mmHg	PO_2	32.6 mmHg
HCO_3^-	23.4 mmol/l	HCO_3^-	23.7 mmol/l
BE	1.1 mmol/l	BE	1.3 mmol/l
SO_2	95.5%	SO_2	64.6%
Hct	32.9%	Hct	31.3%
Hb	11.2 g/dl	Hb	10.8 g/dl

22

Lactate

LEARNING OBJECTIVES
• To be able to discuss body lactate balance. • To be familiar with the causes of hyperlactataemia and lactic acidosis.

22.1 Pathways of Lactate Metabolism

The pKa of lactic acid is 3.86 so at body pH, lactic acid is almost completely ionised to lactate anions and H^+ ions. Under normal, aerobic conditions, the H^+ ions are consumed by the production of adenosine triphosphate (ATP) during oxidative phosphorylation, this acts as a kind of acid buffering. Impairment of oxidative phosphorylation greatly promotes the development of (lactic) acidosis. **Lactate is an important molecule for cellular energy supply**, particularly when cells cannot respire aerobically.

Only the L-isomer is produced in the body. D-lactate is produced by microbes in the GI tract, from where it is absorbed and metabolised slowly. In young (usually pre-ruminant) calves, lambs, and goat kids, hyper-D-lactataemia/D-lactacidosis is a syndrome of somnolence and weakness (a 'drunken appearance') or even recumbency that may occur with or without signs of overt gastrointestinal disease such as diarrhoea and dehydration, and appears to occur secondary to ruminal or colonic microbial D-lactate production and its subsequent absorption.

Hartmann's solution contains racemic lactate (50 : 50, D : L lactate). The L-lactate is oxidised (consuming H^+ and exerting an alkalinising effect), or converted back to glucose. D-lactate is metabolised more slowly, such that exogenous racemic lactate is of theoretical concern in patients with liver disease, but not usually a problem unless there is severe hepatic failure. There has been one report of exacerbation of hyperlactataemia by Hartmann's solution in dogs with lymphoma.

Figure 22.1 shows the chemical formula for lactate. Figure 22.2 shows the main biochemical pathways involved in lactate metabolism. Glucose (or glycogen) undergoes glycolysis to pyruvate. Pyruvate is the cross-roads metabolite of glycolysis and can be metabolised to acetyl CoA (irreversible), oxaloacetate (irreversible), lactate (reversible), or alanine (reversible). The most important conversions are to:

- **Acetyl CoA (dominates under normoxic conditions)** by pyruvate dehydrogenase (PDH) and oxidised nicotinic adenine dinucleotide (NAD^+) within the mitochondrial matrix. This is an irreversible transformation. PDH is a pivotal enzyme that links and controls the flux of metabolites between glycolysis and the Kreb's cycle; its activity is regulated by several factors. (PDH is activated by PDH phosphorylase, which itself is activated by calcium and insulin. PDH is deactivated by PDH kinase, which is itself activated by ATP, reduced nicotinic adenine dinucleotide (NADH), and acetyl CoA, but inhibited by pyruvate.) Acetyl CoA feeds into the Krebs cycle, which fuels oxidative phosphorylation, when mitochondrial O_2 is sufficient.

- **L-lactate (dominates when mitochondrial O_2 is deficient)** by lactate dehydrogenase (LDH) and NADH in the cytoplasm. This is a reversible transformation. Under normal conditions only 10% of pyruvate is metabolised to lactate and the lactate : pyruvate ratio is 10 : 1.

Veterinary Anaesthesia: Principles to Practice, Second Edition. Alexandra H. A. Dugdale, Georgina Beaumont, Carl Bradbrook, and Matthew Gurney.
© 2020 John Wiley & Sons Ltd. Published 2020 by John Wiley & Sons Ltd.
Companion website: www.wiley.com/go/dugdale/veterinary-anaesthesia

There are different isoenzymes of LDH, e.g. LDH-1(4H) is found in the heart and favours lactate utilisation rather than lactate production.

Theoretically, glycolysis (O_2 independent) generates 2 ATP; oxidative phosphorylation (O_2 dependent) generates a further 36 ATP, so is more rewarding. During glycolysis, 2 NAD^+ are reduced to 2 NADH. Normal cell cytoplasmic NADH levels are low because NADH stimulates lactate production; oxidative phosphorylation is crucial for regenerating NAD^+ from NADH (glycerol-3-phosphate shuttle). In chronic or critical illness, protein catabolism is common, fuelling the production of pyruvate via alanine, and, by simple mass action, overwhelming normal oxidative pathways and increasing lactate production.

Figure 22.1 Dissociated lactic acid ($C_3H_5O_2 + H^+$): lactate is half a glucose molecule.

22.1.1 Regulation of the Basic Pathway

The pathway is regulated at multiple points (Figure 22.3):

- Epinephrine (β_2 and possible α receptor effects) stimulates glycogenolysis via increased cyclic adenosine monophosphate (cAMP) and increased activity of Na^+/K^+-ATP pumps, especially in skeletal muscles.
- Alkalosis stimulates phosphofructokinase (PFK) activity; increased pyruvate, then by mass action, overwhelms aerobic pathways and increases lactate production.
- Increased ADP : ATP ratios promote glycolysis by stimulation of PFK; and also stimulate PDH for aerobic respiration.
- High [ATP] inhibits PDH, tending to promote lactate production.
- High plasma [NADH] favours LDH activity and inhibits PDH activity, promoting lactate production.
- High [acetyl CoA] inhibits PDH, favouring lactate production. (Lack of O_2 for oxidative phosphorylation results in accumulation of acetyl CoA.)

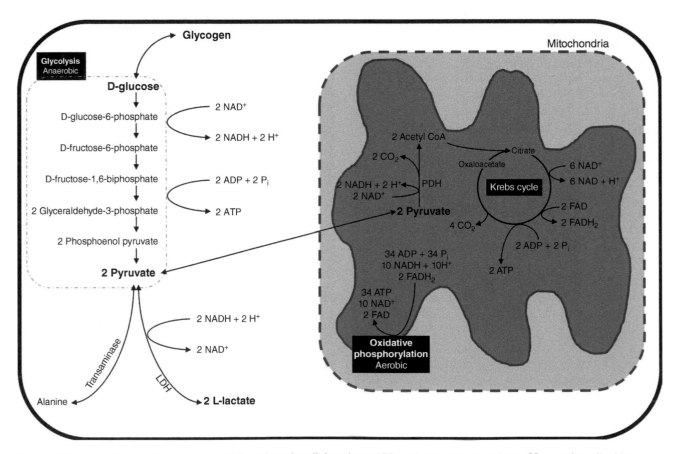

Figure 22.2 Basic biochemical pathways. ADP = adenosine diphosphate; ATP = adenosine triphosphate; CO_2 = carbon dioxide; FAD = flavin adenine dinucleotide; $FADH_2$ = fully reduced FAD (hydroquinone form); LDH = lactate dehydrogenase; NAD^+ = oxidised nicotinic adenine dinucleotide; NADH = reduced nicotinic adenine dinucleotide; PDH = pyruvate dehydrogenase; P_i = inorganic phosphate.

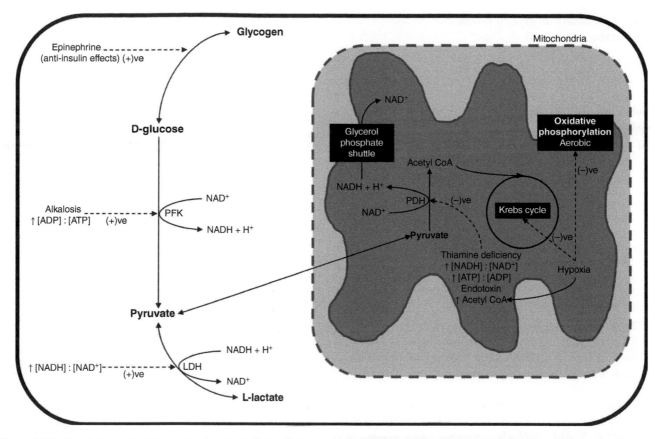

Figure 22.3 Regulation of pathways involved in lactate production and utilisation. ADP = adenosine diphosphate; ATP = adenosine triphosphate; LDH = lactate dehydrogenase; NAD^+ = oxidised nicotinic adenine dinucleotide; NADH = reduced nicotinic adenine dinucleotide; PDH = pyruvate dehydrogenase; PFK = phosphofructokinase; (+)ve = facilitation; (–)ve = inhibition.

- Thiamine is a cofactor for PDH, so deficiency, common in critical illness, results in PDH inhibition favouring lactate production.
- Gluconeogenesis results in NAD^+ production, favouring the conversion of lactate to pyruvate, fuelling further gluconeogenesis.
- Oral biguanide hypoglycaemics inhibit renal and hepatic gluconeogenesis, $[NAD^+]$ falls and [NADH] increases, promoting the transformation of pyruvate to lactate.

22.2 Lactate Balance

The overall blood lactate concentration depends upon a balance between production, consumption, excretion, and transcellular equilibrium.

Production occurs in:

- Skeletal muscles (especially white, fast fibres)
- Brain
- Adipose tissue
- Erythrocytes (also leukocytes, platelets)
- Smooth muscles
- GI tract

- Kidneys (especially medulla)
- Skin
- Retina
- (Liver, under certain conditions)
- (Lungs, e.g. with lung injury, such as acute respiratory distress syndrome [ARDS])

Consumption occurs in the:

- Liver
- Kidneys (especially cortex)
- Heart
- (Skeletal muscles)
- (Brain)

Excretion occurs via the:
- Kidneys (into urine if exceeds the high renal threshold of 6–10 mmol/l)

Transcellular equilibrium (especially erythrocytes) depends upon:

- Monocarboxylate transporters (MCTs)
- Anion exchange
- Simple diffusion of undissociated acid

22.2.1 Lactate as an End-product of Metabolism

Some tissues have no mitochondria (e.g. erythrocytes, platelets) and some have only a few (e.g. white muscle cells, some tumour cells, possibly leukocytes). These cells cannot perform (or perform only limited) oxidative phosphorylation, so glycolysis results in the production of pyruvate and/or lactate.

Erythrocytes are a special case, wherein glycolysis serves the production of 2,3-diphosphoglycerate (2,3-DPG) in species that require it for allosteric modulation of haemoglobin-oxygen carriage (see Chapter 21). The erythrocyte lactate concentration equilibrates (within minutes) with plasma lactate concentration (see above), predominantly by mono-carboxylate transporters (MCTs).

Regarding **MCTs:**

- Different types are present in different tissues
- Most common is the H^+/MCT co-transporter
- Many are stereoselective (e.g. prefer L-lactate to D-lactate)
- Monocarboxylates include lactate, pyruvate, propionate, acetoacetate, beta hydroxy-butyrate

During **anion exchange,** monocarboxylates are exchanged for Cl^- or HCO_3^-. Anion exchange is not stereoselective. **Simple diffusion** requires undissociated acid (relevant with acidaemia). It is not usually very important for lactate (pyruvate even less so), but becomes more relevant with lactic acidosis.

22.2.2 Fate of Lactate

Lactate as a fuel. Even during exercise, when muscle lactate production can be high, much is transported between cells (particularly muscle, heart, brain, and liver) and metabolised through aerobic respiration, sparing glucose, and limiting the development of lactic acidosis: this is the **lactate shuttle** and is particularly important in athletic species (e.g. humans, horses, dogs, reindeer). Lactate is oxidised to produce ATP/energy:

- Pyruvate oxidation (Krebs cycle): 336 kcal.
- Lactate oxidation (via pyruvate and Krebs cycle): 326 kcal.

Lactate as a precursor of glucose, through glucogenesis in liver and kidneys. The glucose can then be utilised by muscles to produce lactate: this is the **Cori cycle** (lactate is converted to glucose, which is converted to lactate, and so on), which also helps acid–base balance.

22.2.3 Normal Lactate Metabolism

- Basal lactate production is c. 0.8 mmol/kg/h (humans).
- Liver removes about 50–70% of lactate in blood; mainly for glucogenesis (under normal conditions).
- Renal cortex (and skeletal and cardiac muscles) convert remaining 30–50% of lactate to pyruvate for energy production via Krebs cycle.
- Urinary excretion of <5% occurs (can increase with hyperlactataemia).

22.3 Hyperlactataemia and Lactic Acidosis

The definitions of *hyperlactataemia* and *lactic acidosis* in humans are:

- Hyperlactataemia: lactate ≥2–5 mmol/l without acidaemia
- Lactic acidosis: lactate >5 mmol/l with either pH ≤7.35 or negative base excess > − 6 mmol/l

22.3.1 Causes of Increased Lactate

Either increased production and/or reduced clearance. There are two types of hyperlactataemia: A and B (non-exhaustive examples below). For comprehensive discussion of the different types of hyperlactataemia, see Rosenstein (2018).

22.3.1.1 Type A (Inadequate Tissue Oxygen Delivery; Absolute or Relative)

Type A can be the result of **decreased O_2 supply (an absolute inadequacy of tissue oxygen delivery):**

- Shock (hypovolaemic, cardiogenic, maldistributive)
- Regional hypoperfusion (tourniquet, thromboembolus, venous stasis)
- Severe hypoxaemia ($P_aO_2 \leq 30$–40 mmHg)
- Severe anaemia (PCV ≤ 10–15%, or [Hb] ≤3–5 g/dl)
- Carbon monoxide poisoning (smoke inhalation)

It can also be the result of **increased O_2 demand (a relative inadequacy of tissue oxygen delivery):**

- Increased muscular activity caused by:
  - Extreme exercise, struggling, shivering
  - Convulsions, tremors
  - Etorphine, cocaine (muscle tremors ± hypoventilation, also type B2)
- Hypermetabolic states caused by:
  - Malignant hyperthermia
  - Thyroid or catecholamine storm
  - Critical illness, systemic inflammatory response syndrome (SIRS), burns, trauma
  - Neoplasia

22.3.1.2 Type B (Impairment of Cellular Metabolism/Mitochondrial Oxygen Utilisation; No Overt Tissue Hypoxia)

Includes three subtypes: B1, B2, and B3.

Type B1 (underlying disease):

- Neoplasia (mitochondrial dysfunction, upregulated MCT, reduced clearance, also type A)
- Liver disease (lactate production > lactate consumption)
- Renal failure (lactate production > lactate consumption; ±impaired urinary excretion)
- Diabetes mellitus (oral hypoglycaemics impair gluconeogenesis; ±metabolic pseudohypoxia)
- Hyperthyroidism, phaeochromocytoma (PDH inhibition, upregulated glycolysis, hypermetabolic state, also types A and B2)
- Microcirculatory dysfunction (sepsis, maldistributive shock, also type A)
- Alkalaemia: metabolic or respiratory (increased PFK activity)
- SIRS, endotoxaemia, trauma, burns (impaired gluconeogenesis, cytopathic hypoxia, also types A and B2)
- Thiamine deficiency (PDH inhibition, critical illness)
- Alanine formation (from muscle protein breakdown, e.g. critical illness, neoplasia)
- Short bowel syndrome, diarrhoea, or other causes of increased gastrointestinal D-lactate production and its absorption)
- Malaria (impaired Hb O_2 carriage)

Type B2 (toxins, drugs):

- Glucocorticoids (PDH inhibition, upregulated glycolysis)
- Catecholamines (endogenous or exogenous), increase glycogenolysis and/or glycolysis (e.g. head injury, shock states, trauma, burns, phaeochromocytoma, iatrogenic, also type A)
- Paracetamol intoxication, salicylate intoxication (hepatic and mitochondrial dysfunction)
- Biguanide hypoglycaemics (inhibit gluconeogenesis causing decreased NAD^+:NADH)
- Cyanide (e.g. secondary to excess sodium nitroprusside treatment via complex IV inhibition)
- Sugars or sugar alcohols, e.g. fructose, lactulose, sorbitol, xylitol (upregulate glycolysis and/or impair lactate metabolism)
- Alcohols, e.g. ethanol, methanol, propylene glycol, ethylene glycol (altered NAD^+: NADH, metabolic acidosis, hepatic metabolism to pyruvate promotes lactate production)
- Endotoxin (PDH inhibition)

Type B3 (inborn errors of metabolism and mitochondrial dysfunction):
- PDH deficiency (e.g. Clumber spaniels)

22.3.1.2.1 *Example of How Hyperlactataemia/Lactic Acidosis Develops*
Sympathetic tone increases with hypovolaemia, resulting in peripheral tissue (non-vital organ) vasoconstriction and relative tissue hypoxia. Subsequent anaerobic respiration results in NADH accumulation and increased lactate production.

The hypoxic GI tract subsequently leads to bacterial/toxin translocation and endotoxaemia. Endotoxin inhibits PDH, resulting in global increases in lactate production. Endotoxin also activates leukocyte glycolysis leading to increased lactate production.

Elevated catecholamines and hyper-cytokinaemia (associated with SIRS/endotoxaemia) accelerate glycolysis. Stimulation of skeletal muscle Na^+/K^+-ATP pumps by catecholamines increases ATP utilisation and increases ADP production. Increased ADP : ATP ratios stimulate PFK to increase pyruvate production, which, by mass action, leads to increased lactate production. This is further exacerbated by increased NADH and mitochondrial dysfunction.

The liver and kidneys become producers, rather than consumers, of lactate (due to hypoperfusion and impaired function).

Do not exclusively rely on increased lactate as a marker of hypoxia because mitochondrial dysfunction (i.e. impaired oxygen utilisation) can result in increased lactate production even when tissue oxygen delivery is adequate:

- Increased lactate does not always correlate with worsening traditional indices of oxygenation
- Lactate does not always decrease when microcirculatory derangements are normalised
- Lactate does not always decrease when tissue oxygen delivery is restored or increased

22.4 Lactate Measurement

Most analysers measure only L-lactate in plasma (even if a whole blood sample is presented).

22.4.1 Enzymic Spectrophotometry

- Requires deproteinised blood
- Adds LDH in order to oxidise lactate to pyruvate in presence of NAD^+
- Light at 340 nm is used to measure resultant NADH concentration which is related to lactate concentration

22.4.2 Enzymic Amperometry (Used by Blood Gas Analysers)

- Lactate oxidase converts lactate to H_2O_2
- The H_2O_2 is oxidised at a platinum anode and produces a current proportional to the lactate concentration

- Tends to read higher than spectrophotometric method, but correction for haematocrit reduces this tendency
- Ethylene glycol interference elevates the result

22.4.3 Sample Handling

Arterial lactate reflects net body lactate balance, whereas venous lactate is influenced by the net lactate balance of the specific portion of the circulation drained by that vessel and by erythrocyte/plasma lactate equilibration. Arterial blood samples are most representative, but mixed venous or regional venous blood samples are acceptable (usually only small differences are present). Capillary blood samples are unreliable. Lactate concentrations in heparinised whole-blood samples at room temperature increase by 0.5–1.2 mmol/l in the first hour and 0.2–0.5 mmol/l/h thereafter for ≥8 hours (cats, humans).

- Samples should be analysed immediately or:
    - Store on ice (reduces cellular metabolism)
    - Precipitate proteins (reduces enzymic activity)
    - Add inhibitors of glycolysis (sodium fluoride)
- Anticoagulants have little effect
- Beware prolonged venous occlusion pre-sampling (increases lactate)
- Beware struggling during sampling (increases lactate)
- Avoid capillary blood samples

22.4.4 Normal (Adult, Resting) Lactate Concentrations

Humans: 0.3–1.3 mmol/l
Cats: 0.3–1.7 mmol/l (Rand et al. 2002)
Dogs: 0.3–2.5 mmol/l (Hughes et al. 1999)
[Beagles: 0.42–3.58 mmol/l (Evans 1987)]
Horses: c. 0.5–1 mmol/l
Rabbits: 2.1–15.2 mmol/l (Ardiaca et al. 2016)

22.5 Lactate as Possible Prognostic Indicator

Eulactataemia, or rapidly resolving hyperlacataemia, is a better predictor of survival than a single measure of hyperlactataemia is predictive of death. Hyperlactataemia is inconsistently associated with greater risk of prolonged hospitalisation and death in cat, dog, horse, and human studies. Serially measured high lactate values appear to be a more useful predictor of risk of death in dogs, horses, and humans than in cats.

Rabbits are the exception with persistently low serial lactate concentrations over 48 hours associated with a greater risk of death. **Caecotrophy is an additional source of lactate** in rabbits and may confuse the interpretation of single measurements. More research is required.

22.5.1 Human Medicine

- During in-hospital cardiac arrest and one hour after return of spontaneous circulation, blood lactate concentrations were predictive of survival.
- In trauma patients, normalisation of lactate within 24–48 hours was associated with improved survival compared with those patients with persistent hyperlactataemia during this time frame.
- Prognosis for human shock: lactate 2.5–4.9 mmol/l = mild hypoperfusion (associated with 25–35% mortality); lactate 5–9.9 mmol/l = moderate hypoperfusion (associated with 60–75% mortality); lactate >10 mmol/l = severe hypoperfusion (associated with >95% mortality); also <10% reduction in lactate concentration within two hours (associated with 41% mortality) or six hours (associated with 60% mortality).
- Lactate is more useful than cardiac output, tissue oxygen delivery, oxygen consumption, or oxygen extraction ratio to determine survival in patients with shock.
- Pyruvate also increases in states of shock/hypoperfusion, but lactate is a more sensitive predictor of outcome than pyruvate or L : P ratio.
- In early SIRS/sepsis, hyperlactataemia may reflect tissue hypoxia; early improvement of tissue oxygen delivery improves outcome.
- In established SIRS/sepsis, lactate interpretation is more complex: impaired lactate clearance and increased lactate production both occur. Increased lactate production in the absence of hypoxia is common, e.g. due to accelerated glycolysis, inhibition of PDH by endotoxin, mitochondrial dysfunction etc.
- Although dichloroacetate enhances PDH activity, and lowers blood lactate, there was no effect on haemodynamics or survival.

22.5.2 Veterinary Medicine

Cats:
- Hyperlactataemic **cats** with a ≥ 30% reduction in lactate concentration within eight hours of admission were more likely to survive than those that did not have such a marked reduction (90% vs 17% survival).
- Cat studies show a particularly inconsistent association between hyperlactataemia and risk of death.

Dogs:
- In **canine** gastric dilation/volvulus (GDV), pre-operative lactate has been used as a prognostic indicator: <6.0 mmol/l (99% survival); >6.0 mmol/l (58% survival).

- Across a range of life-threatening conditions in dogs, most (but not all) studies associated hyperlactataemia with greater risk of mortality; lower lactate concentration predicts survival better than hyperlactataemia predicts death.
- In canine trauma, lactate concentration was significantly higher in non-survivors.
- Dogs with persistent hyperlactataemia have a greater risk of death.

Horses:

- In **equine** colic, several studies have examined pre-operative blood lactate and survival and some have incorporated lactate values into a pre-operative survival score. Overall, it appears that lactate >5.5 mmol/l is associated with a poorer prognosis. Peritoneal fluid lactate was also higher in non-survivors.
- Adult horses with emergent conditions have a significantly increased odds ratio for mortality for every 1 mmol/l increase in lactate concentration at any time point (29% increase per 1 mmol/l at admission, 489% increase per 1 mmol/l at +72 hours).
- Neonatal foals with sepsis/SIRS: lower lactate at admission and after 18–36 hours treatment both correlated with survival.
- Adult and neonatal horses with persistent hyperlactataemia (± slower lactate reductions) have a greater risk of death.

Rabbits:

- Normal **rabbit** lactate concentration is very different to that of other domestic animals and humans.
- Rabbit lactate concentration may be influenced by caecotrophy, and therefore exhibits significant ultradian (i.e. throughout the day) variation. Serial samples may be of particular importance.
- In ill rabbits, a lactate increase of ≥3.3 mmol/l during the first 48 hours is associated with 95% survival at 14 days post-hospitalisation.
- Sustained, stable, low lactate (<5.5 mmol/l) was associated with rabbit death.
- In rabbits, serial lactate measurement in the first 12 hours of hospitalisation was less useful for prognostication than serial lactate measurement from 24+ hours.
- A sudden increase in lactate concentration in anorexic rabbits, with associated metabolic acidosis, is an indicator of metabolic distress.

22.5.3 Importance of Serial Lactate Determinations

These allow better evaluation of prognosis:

- Both initial blood lactate and duration of high lactate affect outcomes

- Duration of and/or failure to resolve high lactate is especially important for prognosis
- Ongoing hyperlactataemia warrants careful patient (re-) evaluation
- Hyperlactataemia (type A) should resolve within 6–12 hours of initiating treatment, with lactate concentration halving every 1–2 hours until reaching normal values

Serial measurements allow assessment of response to treatment, but be aware that initial fluid therapy may 'wash out' lactate from tissues leading to a transient increase in lactate concentration.

22.6 Other Uses of Lactate

22.6.1 Lactate in Other Body Fluids

Various fluids have been investigated:

- Peritoneal fluid has a high lactate concentration, and often higher than blood lactate, in the presence of ischaemic, septic, or malignant abdominal pathology, but there are other markers too
  - Abdominal drains increase peritoneal fluid lactate
  - In dogs, peritoneal fluid-to-blood lactate difference of >2 mmol/l has been shown to be 100% specific and sensitive for septic peritonitis; with blood-to-peritoneal fluid glucose concentration difference of >1.1 mmol/l being equally useful. In cats, whilst the blood-to-peritoneal fluid glucose difference was almost as good as in dogs for determining septic peritonitis, the lactate difference was less useful
  - Overall, in dogs and cats, blood-to- peritoneal fluid glucose difference may be a better marker than the lactate difference, for septic peritonitis
- CSF lactate reference ranges have been established in cats, dogs, horses, and humans
  - In horses, CSF lactate is increased by infectious and traumatic intracranial disease
  - In cats and dogs, increased CSF lactate is documented following intracranial trauma, but further research is required
  - In humans, CSF lactate mirrors severity of underlying disease with spinal cord fibrocartilagenous emboli, spinal cord trauma, and bacterial meningitis
- Synovial fluid lactate concentration reference ranges have been established in dogs, horses, and humans
  - In dogs and humans, elevated synovial fluid lactate is associated with septic arthroses
  - In horses, there is a poor association between synovial fluid lactate and septic arthroses
- Aqueous humour (melanoma leads to increased lactate concentration)

- Pericardial effusions (lactate concentration does not appear to be a useful discriminator between causes of effusion)
- Foetal lactate (amniotic or umbilical) has been investigated in dogs and horses with inconsistent results

22.6.2 Usefulness for Determining Viability of Skin Grafts

Using microdialysis techniques to sample chemicals produced by specific tissue beds, venous or arterial occlusion to myocutaneous flaps caused:

- Decreased glucose
- Increased pyruvate
- Increased lactate

The changes were related to flap ischaemia and the differences could differentiate between arterial and venous occlusion.

22.6.3 Role of Lactate in Neoplastic Conditions

Cancer cachexia is often associated with increased blood lactate because:

- Hypermetabolic states due to tumour products, cytokines, inflammatory mediators, etc. cause increased protein breakdown leading to increased alanine which stimulates pyruvate, and therefore lactate, production
- Tumour cells have few mitochondria, so rely more on anaerobic metabolism with more lactate production
- Tumours may outgrow their blood supply, so hypoxia limits aerobic metabolism
- Hepatic function is possibly reduced, leading, alongside altered metabolism, to increased lactate production
- With chronic illness/critical illness, thiamine becomes deficient, leading to decreased PDH activity and increased lactate production
- Intolerance to exogenous lactate develops; beware Hartmann's solution (L : D ratio 50 : 50)

22.7 Conclusions

Lactate measurements (arterial or venous):

- Form an important part of the overall assessment of haemodynamic function, especially serial values which track response to treatment
- Do not rely on lactate values (especially single determinations) alone for prognostication, although they can form a valuable part of overall patient assessment
- Rabbits do not follow the same lactate trends as other mammals

References

Ardiaca, M., Dias, S., Montesinos, A. et al. (2016). Plasmatic L-lactate in pet rabbits: association with morbidity and mortality at 14 days. *Veterinary Clinical Pathology* 45: 116–123.

Evans, G.O. (1987). Plasma lactate measurements in healthy beagle dogs. *American Journal of Veterinary Research* 48: 131–132.

Hughes, D., Rozanski, E.R., Shofer, F.S. et al. (1999). Effect of sampling site, repeated sampling, pH and PCO$_2$ on plasma lactate concentration in healthy dogs. *American Journal of Veterinary Research* 60: 521–524.

Rand, J.S., Kinnaird, E., Baglioni, A. et al. (2002). Acute stress hyperglycaemia in cats is associated with struggling and increased concentrations of lactate and norepinephrine. *Journal of Veterinary Internal Medicine* 16: 123–132.

Rosenstein, P.G., Tennent-Brown, B.S., and Hughes, D. (2018). Clinical use of plasma lactate concentration. Part 1: physiology, pathophysiology and measurement. *Journal of Veterinary Emergency and Critical Care* 28: 85–105.

Further Reading

Allen, S.E. and Holm, J.L. (2008). Lactate: physiology and clinical utility. *Journal of Veterinary Emergency and Critical Care* 18: 123–132.

Angell, J.W., Jones, G., Grove-White, D.H. et al. (2013). A prospective on farm cohort study investigating the epidemiology and pathophysiology of drunken lamb syndrome. *Veterinary Record* 172: 154.

Angell, J.W., Jones, G.L., Voigt, K., and Grove-White, D.H. (2013). Successful correction of D-lactic acid neurotoxicity (drunken lamb syndrome) by bolus administration of oral sodium bicarbonate. *Veterinary Record* https://doi.org/10.1136/vr.101536.

Astles, R., Williams, C.P., and Sedor, F. (1994). Stability of plasma lactate *in vitro* in the presence of antiglycolytic agents. *Clinical Chemistry* 40: 1327–1330.

Bonaventura, J.M., Sharpe, K., Knight, E. et al. (2015). Reliability and accuracy of six hand-held blood lactate analysers. *Journal of Sports Science and Medicine* 14: 203–214.

Bonczynski, J.J., Ludwig, L.L., Barton, L.J. et al. (2003). Comparison of peritoneal fluid and peripheral blood pH, bicarbonate, glucose and lactate concentration as a diagnostic tool for septic peritonitis in dogs and cats. *Veterinary Surgery* 32: 161–166.

Boysen, S.R., Bozzetti, M., Rose, L. et al. (2009). Effects of prednisolone on blood lactate concentrations in healthy dogs. *Journal of Veterinary Internal Medicine* 23: 1123–1125.

Christopher, M.M. and O'Neill, S. (2000). Effect of specimen collection and storage on blood glucose and lactate concentrations in healthy, hyperthyroid and diabetic cats. *Veterinary Clinical Pathology* 29: 22–28.

Corley, K.T.T., Donaldson, L.L., and Furr, M.O. (2005). Arterial lactate concentration, hospital survival, sepsis and SIRS in critically ill neonatal foals. *Equine Veterinary Journal* 37: 53–59.

Das, U.D. (2006). Is pyruvate an endogenous anti-inflammatory molecule? *Nutrition* 22: 965–972.

De Pedro, P., Wilkins, P.A., McMichael, M.A. et al. (2012). Exogenous L-lactate clearance in adult horses. *Journal of Veterinary Emergency and Critical Care* 22: 564–572.

Di Mauro, F.M. and Schoeffler, G.L. (2016). Point of care measurement of lactate. *Topics in Companion Animal Medicine* 31: 35–43.

Gladden, L.B. (2004). Lactate metabolism: a new paradigm for the third millennium. *Journal of Physiology* 558 (1): 5–30.

Henderson, I.S.F. (2013). Diagnostic and prognostic use of L-lactate measurement in equine practice. *Equine Veterinary Education* 25: 468–475.

Langlois, I., Planche, A., Boysen, S.R. et al. (2014). Blood concentrations of D- and L-lactate in healthy rabbits. *Journal of Small Animal Practice* 55: 451–456.

Lorenz, I. and Gentile, A. (2014). D-lactic acidosis in neonatal ruminants. *Veterinary Clinics of North America: Food Animal Practice* 30: 317–331.

Lorenz, I., Gentile, A., and Klee, W. (2005). Investigation of D-lactate metabolism and the clinical signs of D-lactataemia in calves. *Veterinary Record* 156: 412–415. See also correspondence from Stampfli, H. and a reply from Lorenz, I. (2005) Veterinary Record 156, 816.

McMichael, M.A., Lees, G.E., Hennessey, J. et al. (2005). Serial plasma lactate concentrations in 68 puppies aged 4 to 80 days. *Journal of Veterinary Emergency and Critical Care* 15: 17–21.

Pang, D.S. and Boysen, S. (2007). Lactate in veterinary critical care: pathophysiology and management. *Journal of the American Animal Hospital Association* 43: 270–279.

Petersen, C. (2005). D-lactic acidosis. *Nutrition in Clinical Practice* 20: 634–645.

Phypers, B. and Pierce, J.M.T. (2006). Lactate physiology in health and disease. *Continuing Education in Anaesthesia, Critical Care and Pain* 6: 128–132.

Pösö, A.R. (2002). Monocarboxylate transporters and lactate metabolism in equine athletes: a review. *Acta Veterinaria Scandinavica* 43: 63–74.

Romao, F.T.N.M.A., Pereira, P.F.V., Flaiban, K.K.M.C. et al. (2017). Intravenous administration of a polyionic solution containing 84 mEq/l of lactate resolves experimentally induced hyperchloraemic acidosis in horses. *Equine Veterinary Journal* 49: 87–93.

Rosenstein, P.G., Tennent-Brown, B.S., and Hughes, D. (2018). Clinical use of plasma lactate concentration. Part 2: prognostic and diagnostic utility and the clinical management of hyperlactatemia. *Journal of Veterinary Emergency and Critical Care* 28: 106–121.

Sachs, E.K.J., Julius, T.M., Claypool S-P, A., and Clare, M.C. (2017). Comparison of cephalic and jugular plasma lactate concentrations in sick cats: a pilot study. *Journal of Veterinary Emergency and Critical Care* 27: 193–197.

Stevenson, C.K., Kidney, B.A., Duke, T. et al. (2007). Serial blood lactate concentrations in systemically ill dogs. *Veterinary Clinical Pathology* 36: 234–239.

Szabo, S.D., Jermyn, K., Neel, J., and Mathews, K.G. (2011). Evaluation of postceliotomy peritoneal drain fluid volume, cytology and blood-to-peritoneal fluid lactate and glucose differences in normal dogs. *Veterinary Surgery* 40: 444–449.

Tennent-Brown, B.S., Wilkins, P.A., Lindborg, S. et al. (2007). Assessment of a point-of-care lactate monitor in emergency admissions of adult horses to a referral hospital. *Journal of Veterinary Internal Medicine* 21: 1090–1098.

Tennent-Brown, B.S., Wilkins, P.A., Lindborg, S. et al. (2010). Sequential plasma lactate concentrations as prognostic indicators in adult equine emergencies. *Journal of Veterinary Internal Medicine* 24: 198–205.

White, L. (2015). D-lactic acidosis: more prevalent than we think? *Practical Gastroenterology* 2015: 26–45.

Self-test Section

1 What are the broad categories of hyperlactataemia?

2 What change in lactate concentrations over time indicates a positive prognostic indicator in cats, dogs, and horses (not rabbits)?

3 What change in lactate concentrations over time indicates is a positive prognostic indicator in rabbits?

4 By how much can one expect lactate concentration to increase in a blood sample not analysed immediately, but instead, stored at room temperature (~25 °C)?

23

Fluid Therapy

LEARNING OBJECTIVES

- To be familiar with the body's water content and its distribution between the different compartments.
- To appreciate the main different types of fluid loss.
- To be able to describe the different types of fluids available (crystalloids, colloids, oxygen carriers) and be able to match these to the type/s of fluid loss/es.
- To be familiar with different routes and rates of fluid administration, and be able to choose the most appropriate.
- To be able to devise a fluid therapy plan and understand the importance of patient monitoring to assess the response to therapy.

23.1 Distribution of Fluid Within the Body

In all mammals, water makes up a significant part of the total body weight (the exact amount varies slightly with age and obesity), totalling approximately 60% or two-thirds of total body weight in mature animals. (See Chapter 37 for neonates.) Of this total, the water is distributed amongst the compartments as illustrated in Figure 23.1 and Table 23.1. It is generally considered that 1l of water weighs 1 kg as the density of water is about $1 g/cm^3$. The main division of water is between the **intracellular** and **extracellular** compartments which are separated by semipermeable cell membranes. The extracellular compartment is further subdivided, by capillary endothelium, into the **intravascular** compartment (essentially the plasma) and the **interstitial** compartment (which surrounds and bathes cells).

Total blood volume depends upon plasma volume and haematocrit (HCT), i.e. red blood cell (RBC) size and number. Total blood volume is approximately 8–9% body weight for dogs and similar for horses, i.e. plasma (5% body weight) + RBCs (4% body weight). Blood volume, however, also depends upon age, body habitus (how fat or thin), and measurement method, such that different values have been reported in the literature: e.g. it varies between 6–10% body weight (horses), 8–9% body weight (dogs), and 4.5–6.5% body weight (cats). The plasma volume itself is now considered to exist as two portions: the circulating portion and the non-circulating portion (i.e. that 'within' the endothelial surface layer (ESL), see below).

A fourth fluid compartment, the **transcellular** fluid compartment (including joint fluid, ocular fluids, cerebrospinal fluid, lymph, respiratory secretions, glandular secretions and fluid within the gastrointestinal [including bile], and urogenital tracts) accounts for only 0.6–1% of the total body water in humans, but can account for between 5 and 20% of total body water in horses and cattle, depending upon their diet. The water in skeletal components (bone and cartilage) and in transcellular fluids exchanges slowly with other compartments, so is usually ignored for fluid therapy reasons.

The distribution of water among these different compartments is governed by the osmotic gradients between them. Although water can pass freely between all compartments by osmosis, its movement is facilitated/regulated by aquaporins in many cells, e.g. kidney, brain, lens, and red blood cells. The magnesium-dependent Na^+/K^+-ATPase pump is important for maintaining osmotic gradients between intracellular and extracellular compartments.

Veterinary Anaesthesia: Principles to Practice, Second Edition. Alexandra H. A. Dugdale, Georgina Beaumont, Carl Bradbrook, and Matthew Gurney.
© 2020 John Wiley & Sons Ltd. Published 2020 by John Wiley & Sons Ltd.
Companion website: www.wiley.com/go/dugdale/veterinary-anaesthesia

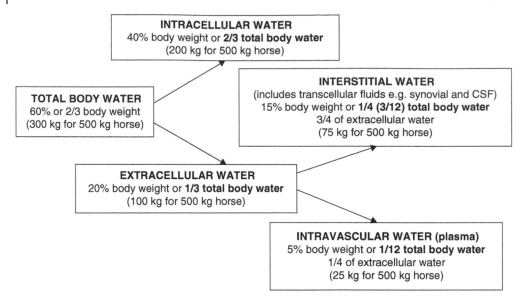

Figure 23.1 Distribution of body water.

Table 23.1 Guide to compartment volumes.

	Intracellular	Extracellular	Interstitial	Intravascular
500 kg horse	200 l	100 l	75 l	25 l
20 kg dog	8 l	4 l	3 l	1 l
5 kg dog	2 l	1 l	0.75 l	0.25 l

The **osmotically active particles** are:

- In the extracellular interstitial fluid: Na^+ and Cl^- and some protein (albumin).
- In the extracellular intravascular fluid: Na^+, Cl^- and large colloidal proteins (e.g. albumin).
- In the intracellular fluid: K^+ and proteins.

Any change to the concentration of osmotic particles within a compartment (without any change in the volume of water) will result in an alteration of the equilibrium between compartments, and therefore the ratio of distribution of water between them.

Normal plasma osmolarity is c. 280–320 mOsm/l, very little of which is provided by proteins. It can be calculated from:

$$\text{Plasma osmolarity (mOsm/l)} = 2 \times \left[Na^+\right] + 2 \times \left[K^+\right] + \left[\text{Glucose}\right] + \left[\text{Urea}\right]$$

where all values are in mmol/l.

Note that the cation concentrations are doubled to account for their associated anions, and sometimes the effect of potassium is ignored as it is usually very small. Notice what little effect plasma proteins have. Sodium ions are usually the principle governor of osmolarity, e.g. horses have plasma $[Na^+]$ c. 135 mmol/l and osmolarity c. 285 mOsm/l; dogs have plasma $[Na^+]$ c. 145 mmol/l and osmolarity c. 300 mOsm/l; cats have plasma $[Na^+]$ c. 150 mmol/l and osmolarity c. 310 mOsm/l.

Proteins in solution exert an osmotic pressure called **oncotic pressure**. However, when in plasma, since most proteins have plenty of negative charges, they also attract positively charged ions into their vicinity, thus greatly increasing their osmotic pulling power on water; this pull being described as **colloid osmotic pressure** (COP). Plasma proteins (mainly albumin) and their associated cations normally exert a COP of c. 18–25 mmHg in blood. Whilst only 0.5% of plasma osmolarity is due to albumin, albumin is normally responsible for around 75–80% of plasma COP and comprises 55–60% of the total plasma protein. See below for further expansion on this.

The tonicity of a solution or compartment refers to its ability to initiate water movement. It depends upon the number (rather than the size) of effective osmoles present that are impermeant to the surrounding solutions or compartments. **Tonicity** is therefore a measure of the **effective osmolarity** of a solution.

23.2 The Endothelial Glycocalyx

The endothelial glycocalyx (EG) forms a gel-like layer or web covering the luminal surface of vascular endothelial cells. It is comprised of membrane-bound proteoglycans and glycoproteins and various glycosaminoglycans, which may either attach to the proteogylcans or may be present within the EG as free, soluble mucopolysaccharides. The EG itself is considered inactive, but once various plasma constituents have 'bound', the active ESL is formed (which comprises the EG and bound proteins and also the subglycocalyx). The EG has a net negative charge and acts as a macromolecular sieve, excluding macromolecules greater than 70 kDa and also negatively charged molecules, red blood cells, white blood cells, and platelets. Albumin (67 kDa) binds tightly to the EG despite its net negative charge because albumin also contains some positively charged amino-acids. The endothelial cell surface glycoproteins include adhesion molecules and components of the coagulation and fibrinolytic systems. Therefore, with disruption, degradation, and/or shedding of the glycocalyx, these molecules become exposed, resulting in inflammatory cell rolling, adhesion, and diapedesis (which triggers further inflammation), and platelet aggregation and hypercoagulability. Furthermore, glycocalyx shedding results in increased vascular permeability and oedema formation. The EG also binds enzymes that scavenge free radicals, hence it plays an important anti-oxidant role in protecting the endothelium.

The ESL maintains homeostasis of the vasculature such as controlling vascular permeability and microvascular tone and it occupies a significant 'volume' within the intravascular compartment, although the EG is thinner in the microcirculation and thicker in larger vessels. The ESL is a semi-permeable membrane with respect to albumin and other plasma proteins. Presence of albumin within the EG is an important determinant of its filter function, and in disease (and also due to surgery) the transcapillary escape rate of albumin is an index of vascular permeability. The subglycocalyx layer is normally low in protein.

Understanding of the EG and ESL has led to updating of traditional ideas on Starling's equation and the theory of transcapillary fluid flux. It was previously thought that filtration of fluid at the arterial end of the capillary, primarily dependent upon hydrostatic pressure, was mostly countered by resorption at the venous end of the capillary due to greater plasma oncotic pressure than interstitial oncotic pressure, with only the excess filtered fluid being returned to the bloodstream via lymphatics. This is no longer believed to be the underlying mechanism. Instead, fluid is thought to be filtered along the whole length of the capillary, later being returned to the circulation via lymphatics. Instead of the plasma COP per se being important to oppose fluid efflux, the COP gradient across the ESL (between the protein-rich EG and protein-poor subglycocalyx) is the most important determinant in opposing fluid efflux along the whole length of the capillary. The ESL thus plays a major role in transvascular fluid shifts.

Factors promoting EG shedding and compromising its function:

- Hyperglycaemia (e.g. diabetes mellitus)
- Ischaemia (and reperfusion)
- Inflammatory mediators (SIRS, sepsis, trauma, surgery)
- Rapid IV fluid infusion (both crystalloids and synthetic colloids) and hypervolaemia (with subsequent ANP release)

Protection/restoration of the EG has been demonstrated with: N-acetyl-cysteine, hydrocortisone, sevoflurane, and anti-thrombin III.

23.3 Types of Fluid Loss

In order to implement a fluid therapy plan, it is important to determine the type of fluid loss. This is important so that the most appropriate fluid can be administered to the patient. Good history taking, thorough clinical examination, sound clinical judgement, observation, and laboratory tests can all be helpful in determining types of fluid loss.

23.3.1 Whole Blood Loss

For example, rupture of splenic haemangiosarcoma, erosion of internal carotid artery by fungal plaque in the guttural pouch, severed superficial arteries, or large veins. This fluid lost from the intravascular compartment is composed of:

- Water
- Electrolytes
- Proteins (including clotting factors)
- Red cells
- White cells
- Platelets

In the first few (four to six) hours, the composition of the remaining blood, and fluids in the other fluid compartments, does not change appreciably because pure blood loss does not result in alteration of any of the osmotic gradients between compartments acutely, so initially no huge fluid (water) shifts occur. If blood loss was significant, then after a few hours the effects of homeostatic mechanisms important for the maintenance of intravascular volume and blood pressure, such as the renin-angiotensin-aldosterone-ADH system, become more noticeable, and sodium, chloride and water are retained. These latter will distribute throughout the whole of the ECF (including the intravascular space) to cause haemodilution, i.e. the packed cell volume (PCV) will fall 4–12 hours post haemorrhage (possibly partly offset by splenic contraction). Haemodilution is promoted by altered Starling forces at the capillaries, so less interstitial fluid is formed due to lower hydrostatic pressure, yet such fluid can still be returned to the intravascular space through the lymphatics (transcapillary refill). Some albumin will be restored to the plasma from this interstitial fluid and some red blood cells may be gained from splenic stores, but new red cells will have to be made by the bone marrow, which takes three to five days. It is interesting to note that only about 40% of the total albumin is present in the intravascular space at any one time with the majority (60%) being found in the interstitial compartment.

23.3.2 ECF Loss

For example, diarrhoea, vomiting, diuresis, sweating, interstitial oedema, and intracavitary effusions (e.g. peritonitis). This is the most common type of fluid loss in clinical practice. This fluid, lost from interstitial and intravascular compartments, is composed of:

- Water
- Electrolytes (mainly Na^+ and Cl^-)

If sodium and chloride are lost in their normal ratio to water (it is common for electrolytes to be lost alongside water), then the osmotic potential of the ECF tends not to change very much. (Intravascular hypovolaemia then stimulates homeostatic mechanisms, resulting in increased sodium and water retention.) With significant losses, haemoconcentration of blood will occur, so an increase in PCV (or alternatively, HCT) and total solids (TS, or alternatively, total protein [TP]) will result, and interstitial fluid may also have a small increase in its protein concentration too. These increases in protein concentration result in tiny increases in osmotic pressure in the ECF compartment, which also favour water movement into this compartment from the ICF.

If water is lost in excess of electrolytes, then the ECF compartments become hypertonic compared to the intracellular compartment, so water moves from intracellular compartment to ECF, thus tending to offset any intravascular

hypovolaemia, but promoting intracellular dehydration. This changes the osmolarity of the cells which, in turn, is recognised in the CNS so that ADH release is promoted and thirst is stimulated until osmolarities return to normal.

If electrolytes are lost from the ECF in excess of water, the ECF compartments become hypotonic compared to intracellular compartments and then water moves into cells to swell the intracellular space, but further deplete the intravascular and interstitial spaces. CNS cells swell resulting in a reduction in ADH release.

23.3.3 Protein Rich (Even Cellular) ECF Loss

For example, some pleural and peritoneal effusions, GI sequestration, haemorrhagic gastroenteritis, protein-losing enteropathies, protein-losing nephropathies, and exudative losses with burns. Fluid is lost from interstitial and intravascular compartments, but this time is composed of:

- Water
- Electrolytes (Na^+, Cl^-)
- Proteins
- Cellular components of blood

Such fluid losses tend to have an electrolyte composition like the plasma/ECF compartment. Due to pathological processes such as inflammation, there is leakage or effusion of plasma proteins, and possibly also cellular components of blood, into the fluid. These losses (unless severely haemorrhagic), result in haemoconcentration (increased PCV or HCT), but depending upon the quantity of protein lost, the effects on plasma protein can be variable. Plasma protein has only small effects on plasma osmolarity, but if total protein (TP or TS) falls below c. 35 g/l, then oedema/ascites will develop as water is no longer easily retained in the intravascular space. As the interstitial space also becomes protein-depleted, then its osmolarity will also be slightly reduced. It is possible that these conditions may favour an increase in the movement of water into cells, and thus cellular oedema, in addition to interstitial oedema, occurs.

23.3.4 Pure Water Loss

For example, high respiratory rate (pneumonia, hyperthermia), primary water deprivation, or excessive water loss (e.g. the diuresis that occurs with diabetes insipidus). As water moves freely across all compartments, all compartments lose water. The tonicity of all compartments increases, but the remaining water distributes between the compartments in the normal ratios. All compartments show a reduction in volume alongside the increase in tonicity. This is sensed by homeostatic mechanisms so that thirst and ADH release are increased.

23.4 Response of the Body to Fluid Loss

Hypovolaemia is a reduction of fluid in the intravascular compartment (i.e. a reduced circulating volume). Intravascular volume deficits are present in all types of fluid losses. The severity of the deficit depends upon the type, magnitude, and duration of fluid loss.

Hypovolaemia can be present without dehydration (e.g. with acute haemorrhage), but dehydration cannot exist without at least some degree of hypovolaemia. Dehydration is loss of water, which affects all body compartments. When considering if a patient is dehydrated or hypovolaemic, ask yourself is this a perfusion problem and/or a hydration problem?

Clinical signs of hypovolaemia reflect the increase in sympathetic tone that is the physiological response to falling blood pressure. These are (acutely):

- Tachycardia
- Weak pulses (especially peripheral) due to vasoconstriction
- Pale mucous membranes (also due to vasoconstriction)
- Brisk capillary refill time (CRT)
- Cool extremities
- Tachypnoea

Laboratory/clinical tests that could help to confirm hypovolaemia:

- PCV (or HCT) in conjunction with TS (or TP); both increase with dehydration, whereas TS (or TP) falls slightly, but PCV (or HCT) can fall more dramatically, 6–12 hours post haemorrhage (hypovolaemia)
- High urine specific gravity and reduced urine production (<1–1.5 ml/kg/h)
- Low arterial blood pressure
- Low central venous pressure (CVP)
- Increased blood lactate

Clinical signs of dehydration (primary water deficit, but affects all fluid compartments), include:

- Thirst
- Oliguria
- Dry mucous membranes
- Reduced skin pliability
- Sunken eyes
- Depressed mentation
- Neuromuscular derangements (weakness/seizures due to hypernatraemia)

Although dehydration affects all compartments, because the intracellular compartment is by far the largest fluid compartment (in mature animals), the clinical signs associated with intracellular fluid loss are often late in onset (because of the huge reserve), but are usually clinically noticeable once the water loss associated with dehydration exceeds 5% of body mass, and become very pronounced once these losses reach 8–10% of body mass (see Table 23.2). **Laboratory tests to help confirm dehydration** include a high measured plasma Na^+ concentration, high PCV (or HCT) and TS (or TP), and increased urine specific gravity (but beware underlying diseases that can affect all of these).

23.5 Clinical Evaluation

23.5.1 History

Accurate and comprehensive history-taking can be invaluable in determining the nature and degree of fluid loss. The clinician should ask questions about normal maintenance requirements and abnormal losses:

- How much is the animal drinking? Have there been any problems with water supply or availability or the animal's ability to drink?
- How much is the animal urinating?

Table 23.2 Assessment of 'dehydration'. Note that percentages refer to percentage decreases in body mass rather than percentage losses of total body water.

Percentage reduction in body mass	Clinical signs
<5%	None
5–7%	Tacky to dry oral mucous membranes, eyes still moist, normal to mild loss of skin turgor
8–10%	Dry oral mucous membranes, eyes dull and sunken, considerable loss of skin turgor, weak rapid pulse. Oliguria, cold extremities, increased capillary refill time (CRT)
>10–12%	Very dry mucous membranes, severe eye retraction, eyes dull, complete loss of skin turgor, anuria, weak thready pulses, weak, may be recumbent, possibly reduced level of consciousness, becoming moribund
>12–15%	All above + very prolonged CRT, dying

- Has the animal been suffering from vomiting, diarrhoea, or diuresis?
- Does the animal have ascites or oedema?
- Is the animal bleeding badly? Has the animal bled?
- Has the animal been sweating profusely?

23.5.2 Clinical Examination and Laboratory Evaluation

23.5.2.1 Haemodynamic Status

- Heart (pulse) rate: tends to increase with hypovolaemia.
- Colour of mucous membranes (remember disease states such as anaemia and endotoxaemia can confuse the picture).
- CRT is not always very reliable, but tends to shorten (<1 second) in early (compensated) hypovolaemia, becoming prolonged as decompensation sets in.
- Peripheral pulse quality (pulse pressure can be estimated, very subjectively, by how easy pulses are to occlude with digital pressure): peripheral pulses become more difficult to palpate (and easier to occlude) with greater degrees of hypovolaemia. Although objective arterial blood pressure measurement is preferred, the inability to palpate peripheral and central pulses has, historically, been suggested to be associated with moderate to severe hypotension, respectively. This has recently been challenged as it has been demonstrated that peripheral pulses may remain palpable in the face of significant hypotension in both humans and dogs. Nevertheless, in the same study of dogs, the inability to palpate the metatarsal pulse had a 94% specificity (but only 33% sensitivity) to detect hypotension (defined as Doppler systolic arterial blood pressure < 90 mmHg), and femoral pulses were no longer palpable when median Doppler systolic blood pressure (SBP) had fallen to 40 mmHg. A similar study in cats reported that when metatarsal pulses were not palpable, there was an 84% likelihood of Doppler SBP being less than 75 mmHg; and when both femoral and metatarsal pulses were no longer palpable, median Doppler SBP had fallen to 30 mmHg.
- Arterial blood pressure: should be measured if possible.
- The temperature of extremities becomes cool with hypovolaemia.
- CVP: although CVP may be a useful 'static' indicator of preload, many factors can affect it (see Chapter 18), the CVP response to fluid challenges is not very predictable (some patients are 'preload-dependent responders' and others are not), and it may not always be possible to place a sufficiently long jugular or femoral venous catheter to measure it.
- Ultrasonographic measurements of caudal vena caval and descending aortic diameters, and their ratio, has shown promise as a non-invasive method to determine the volaemic status and fluid-responsiveness of patients, and has shown good correlation with a dynamic index of fluid-responsiveness, namely, systolic pressure variation in dogs. The technique, however, does require some training.
- Lactate measurement in either venous or arterial blood (little difference between them usually) can help determine the severity of hypovolaemia and reduced tissue perfusion, although serial changes in lactate are more significant.

23.5.2.2 Skin Pliability

After being raised in a pinch the skin should return rapidly to its resting position. A slower return over three to five seconds indicates 5+ % dehydration. If the skin remains in a fold, it indicates about 10–12+ % dehydration (Table 23.2). This is a very subjective test (and can be affected by, e.g. emaciation, obesity, Cushing's disease, cutaneous asthenia) and will only provide a rough guide at best. Also, if this test is being done repeatedly, then the same site should be used by the same person. Skin pliability is most useful when repeated observations are made over time to assess response to treatment.

23.5.2.3 Packed Cell Volume (or HCT)/Total Solids (or TP)

- PCV tends to increase with ECF loss and water loss.
- PCV does not immediately decrease after whole blood loss, but it takes several (>four to six) hours for the PCV, and to a lesser extent the TS, to begin to decrease.
- It should be remembered that there is an enormous variation in 'normal' PCV among individuals, so repeated samples are needed in order to provide a dynamic picture.
- In cases of pre-existing anaemia (e.g. where PCV was reduced beforehand), then the PCV could appear 'normal' (because of haemoconcentration), despite significant fluid loss. To reduce such misinterpretations, the PCV should always be interpreted alongside the TS.
- TS tends to increase with ECF loss and water loss, however, hypo- or hyper-proteinaemia can obviously obscure results. Excessive protein loss can be a problem with some conditions. At levels below 35 g/l (with albumin <20 g/l), there is a significant reduction in intravascular colloid osmotic pressure that can result in extravasation of fluid.

23.5.2.4 Urine Production and Specific Gravity

Urine production is decreased in cases of hypovolaemia where a mean arterial pressure of <60–70 mmHg causes a marked reduction in renal blood flow. Compensatory homeostatic mechanisms then cause the healthy kidney to retain water (and Na⁺) in situations of falling blood pressure. As a result, the volume of urine production decreases whilst its concentration increases. Therefore if it is possible to measure the volume of urine produced and its specific gravity (using a refractometer), an indication of fluid status can be obtained (but beware concomitant renal disease). Alongside monitoring body weight, the rate of production of urine can be used to monitor effectiveness of fluid therapy and helps to assess 'ins and outs'.

Normal urine production is 1–1.5 ml/kg/h, or 25 ml/kg/day.

Formerly, daily water requirements (normal healthy adult human) had been estimated at ~50 ml/kg/day, although current estimations are approximately 30 ml/kg/day whilst at rest and in a cool environment.

Although the value of 50 ml/kg/day may also be an over-estimate for the daily water requirement of animals, most animals live active lives and their environmental temperatures will vary. Therefore, until we learn more about the different requirements for different species under different conditions of activity and environment, a value of 50 ml/kg/day (or 2–3 ml/kg/h) is generally used.

Some people prefer to calculate maintenance requirements according to metabolic body weight (i.e. considering surface area), using the following equations, which also result in rates of around 2–3 ml/kg/h:

Cats: ml/day = 80 × (body mass [kg]$^{0.75}$)
Dogs: ml/day = 132 × (body mass [kg]$^{0.75}$)

If water requirements are around 50 ml/kg/day, then normal daily urinary water loss constitutes around 25 ml/kg/day (the 'sensible' losses), and normal daily respiratory, faecal, and skin losses constitute the other 25 ml/kg/day (the 'insensible' losses).

In animals with impaired kidney function, the compensatory mechanisms that conserve water and concentrate urine are also impaired. As a result, such animals may have either a normal or even slightly reduced specific gravity in the face of hypotension/dehydration. It is also true that animals that suffer from increased 'obligatory' water loss are more likely to suffer from hypovolaemia than 'normal' animals. For instance, an animal with polyuric renal failure will become dehydrated/hypovolaemic more quickly if it is denied access to water compared to animals with normal kidney function.

From the above and Table 23.2, it is hard to determine when an animal is <5% dehydrated, yet it may be almost dead if 15% dehydrated. If at least some of the clinical signs listed above are present, a starting point could be to guess at 10% dehydration, which is also an easy number with which to calculate the patient's fluid requirements.

23.6 Routes of Fluid Administration

23.6.1 Intravenous Route

This is the most favoured route for rapid restoration of intravascular volume. If necessary, use more than one IV cannula and always try to use the widest bore possible. Cannula care is extremely important (see Chapter 7).

It is vitally important to use the right giving sets (i.e. standard; micro-dropper or burette sets [for small dogs and cats]; blood giving sets with microfilters [for any blood products]). Burette sets are much safer for smaller animals as only the total volume required is run into the burette chamber, guarding against accidental massive fluid overload. Make sure that you are aware of the number of drops per millilitre for the type of set you use if a fluid pump is not available.

- Most standard giving sets provide 20 drops/ml.
- Micro-dropper paediatric and burette sets provide 60 drops/ml.
- Most blood giving sets provide 15 drops/ml.
- The giving sets commonly used in equine hospitals provide 10 drops/ml.

For calculating drip rates:

$$\text{Drip rate (drops/s)} = \frac{\text{Body mass (kg)} \times \text{Infusion rate (ml/kg/h)} \times \text{Drops/ml}}{3600 \text{ (s/h)}}$$

23.6.2 Intra-osseous Route

For very small patients such as neonates, venous access can be difficult to establish. In such patients, a needle can be inserted into the medullary cavity of a bone, usually the iliac crest, femoral greater trochanter, lateral humeral tuberosity, tibial crest, or even sternum, for the administration of fluids. As for intravenous cannulae, the skin should be prepared aseptically prior to placement of the needle. A styletted 20G spinal needle can be used for the procedure if intra-osseous needles are not available.

23.6.3 Intraperitoneal Route

In some circumstances, it may be necessary to administer fluids directly into the peritoneal cavity, from which they are absorbed into the circulation via the peritoneum. A bolus dose of fluid (usually an isotonic crystalloid solution) can be administered 'off the needle'. This method can be particularly useful for tiny patients, e.g. hamsters, mice, etc. The intraperitoneal route is not considered to be suitable for emergency acute volume replacement, although absorption from this site is a little quicker than from the subcutaneous site. This route is most commonly used for exotic species that tend not to have easily accessible and cannulatable superficial veins.

23.6.4 Subcutaneous Route

This is included for completeness although this is not an appropriate route for rapid large-quantity volume replacement because during acute severe hypovolaemia the perfusion to the subcutaneous tissues is much reduced, so absorption from this site is slowed. For lesser degrees of intravascular deficit, however, this route may still be used, and is often advocated for chronic renal failure cats with mild degrees of dehydration. In fact, in a recent survey, it was found that many cat owners are happy to administer fluids on a regular (even daily) basis by this route to cats with chronic renal disease.

23.6.5 Oral Route

This route is included for completeness although it is not the best route for rapid restoration of large intravascular volume deficits, especially in sick animals. Nevertheless, this route is often used in farm species. Oral rehydration therapies should supply sufficient sodium to enable restoration of ECF volume (but without causing hypernatraemia), sufficient water and other electrolytes (K^+, Cl^-, Mg^{2+}, Ca^{2+}), and something to treat acidosis if necessary. The patient's energy intake should not be forgotten, but oral rehydration therapies seldom provide sufficient on their own. Sodium can be co-transported with glucose and amino acids, so these are commonly included, in appropriate ratios to sodium, to facilitate its absorption. Glucose, glycine, and citrate can also be absorbed along with water, independently of sodium, so further aid water absorption. Glucose, glycine, alanine, glutamate (and glutamine) are also energy or protein sources and help gut epithelial cell and villus regrowth/restitution. Citrate is a bicarbonate 'sparer' and/or 'precursor' and aids correction of metabolic acidosis, although acetate used to be preferred for milk-fed animals (e.g. calves) as it was shown not to interfere with abomasal milk clotting *in vitro*. More recent work, however, has shown that oral rehydration solutions containing acetate, propionate, bicarbonate, or citrate and phosphate do not interfere with milk clotting *in vivo* in calves.

23.6.6 Rectal/Colonic Route

Occasional equine anecdotes/case reports are published regarding fluids delivered per rectum into the distal colon, from where they can be systemically absorbed. However, this route is not without its problems: rectal or colon damage; unpredictable and/or inadequate absorption; lack of knowledge regarding the best composition of such fluids, and is therefore not recommended.

23.7 Types of Parenteral Fluids

- Crystalloids
- Colloids
- Oxygen-carrying solutions (currently unavailable)
- Blood and blood products

23.7.1 Crystalloids

These are aqueous solutions made from crystalline compounds (electrolytes, sugars) and may be buffered so their pH is near that of plasma. They may be isotonic, hypotonic, or hypertonic with respect to plasma (Table 23.3). Most solutions are adjusted to be isotonic with plasma so that, *in vivo*, red blood cells do not crenate (shrink), or swell and burst. Although Hartmann's solution is listed beneath the 'isotonic' fluids in Table 23.3, once the bicarbonate ions have been 'metabolised'/utilised, then the solution is effectively hypotonic, providing water in excess of electrolytes. Glucose (dextrose)-containing solutions, although usually provided in isotonic solutions, are a good way to provide water because once the glucose has been utilised by cells, only water remains; and in fact, some metabolic water is produced in the process of glucose metabolism too. These solutions are also, therefore, effectively 'physiologically' hypotonic. Some solutions that have electrolyte compositions nearer to that of human plasma are called 'balanced' electrolyte solutions, but this term is not always used consistently and can be misleading.

Crystalloid solutions are useful for:

- ECF (including plasma) volume replacement; hypertonic crystalloids act as transient plasma volume expanders.
- Providing maintenance (water/electrolyte) requirements.
- Special occasions.

23.7.1.1 Isotonic Crystalloids

- Normal (0.9%) saline
- Ringer's solution
- Hartmann's solution (lactated Ringer's solution)
- Plasma-Lyte A
- Normosol R

Table 23.3 Characteristics of common crystalloid solutions. Note that normal plasma osmolarity = 280–320 mOsm/l; normal blood pH = 7.4.

Solution	Colloid Osmotic Pressure (mmHg)	Osmolarity (mOsm/l)	pH	(Na$^+$) (mmol/l)	(Cl$^-$) (mmol/l)	(K$^+$) (mmol/l)	(Ca^{2+}) (mmol/l)	(Mg^{2+}) (mmol/l)	Buffer (mmol/l)
Isotonic									
0.9% NaCl	0	300–308	5.0–5.7	150–154	150–154	0	0	0	0
Ringer's solution	0	309	5–7.5	147	155.5	4	2.25		23 gluconate 27 acetate
Hartmann's solution	0	273	6.5	130–131	109–111	4–5	2–3	0	28–29 lactate
Plasma-Lyte A	0	295	7.4	140	98	5	0	1.5	
Normosol R	0	295	6.6	140	98	5	0	1.5	23 gluconate 27 acetate
Physiologically hypotonic									
0.18% NaCl + 4% glucose	0	262–284	c. 4.0	30	30	0	0	0	0
5% glucose in water	0	252–278	4.0–6.5	0	0	0	0	0	0
0.45% NaCl + 5% glucose	0	432	3.5–6.5	77	77	0	0	0	0
Plamsa-Lyte 56 + 5% glucose	0	362	5.0	40	40	16	0	1.5	16 acetate
Hypotonic									
0.45% NaCl	0	154	4.5–7	77	77	0	0	0	0
Plasma-Lyte 56	0	110	5.5	40	40	13	0	1.5	16 acetate
Normosol M	0	110	5.0	40	40	13	0	1.5	16 acetate
Hypertonic									
7.2% NaCl	0	2464	c. 5.0	1232	1232	0	0	0	0
7.5% NaCl	0	2566	c. 5.0	1283	1283	0	0	0	0

23.7.1.2 Hypotonic Crystalloids
- 0.45% saline
- Plamsa-Lyte 56
- Normosol M

23.7.1.3 Physiologically Hypotonic Crystalloids
- 0.18% saline + 4% glucose
- 0.45% saline + 5% glucose
- Plasma-Lyte 56 + 5% glucose
- 5% glucose (also known as dextrose, which is the D-glucose isomer that is preferred for animal metabolism. Either anhydrous dextrose or dextrose monohydrate can be used to formulate solutions; the former yields slightly more energy per mole than the latter because it is devoid of water). This solution is also known as D5W.

23.7.1.4 Hypertonic Crystalloids
- 7.2–7.5% saline

23.7.1.5 Other Crystalloid Solutions for Special Clinical Situations Include
- Potassium chloride solutions
- Sodium bicarbonate solutions (8.4, 4.2%)
- Calcium and magnesium containing solutions
- Phosphate containing solutions
- High concentration dextrose solutions (e.g. 50% dextrose)

23.7.1.6 ECF Replacement (or 'Resuscitation') Fluids

Solutions that have a composition similar to ECF in terms of water and electrolytes are normal saline, Ringer's solution, and Hartmann's solution. Due to the concentration of sodium in these solutions being very similar to the ECF sodium concentration, these fluids are confined to the extracellular compartment. Therefore the main function of these types of fluids is to replace ECF. After these fluids are administered into the intravascular compartment, it has **traditionally** been taught that the fluid volume administered will redistribute between the intravascular (1/4) and interstitial (3/4) compartments; thus **for every 1 l of fluid administered IV, only about a quarter of this (i.e. 250 ml) remains in the intravascular space after about 30–60 minutes**.

Normal saline is not quite as closely matched to ECF as Hartmann's solution. It does not contain lactate, and with an acidic pH tends to cause a 'dilutional acidosis'. Part of the reason for this is that too much chloride is given for the body's requirements, displacing bicarbonate ions (buffer) from the ECF in order to maintain electroneutrality, and no buffer is included. Hypokalaemia is also encouraged. Normal saline is useful to help treat hyponatraemia and severe hyperkalaemia, e.g. in Addisonian cases. Historically, normal saline was advised for the treatment of hyperkalaemia associated with urethral obstruction in cats and ruptured bladder in foals. This has recently been contested as Hartmann's solution administered to cats, with experimentally-induced urethral obstruction, resulted in, not only a similar reduction in plasma potassium concentration to normal saline, but also a faster restoration of normal blood pH and without hypernatraemia or hypocalcaemia.

23.7.1.6.1 Bicarbonate Sparers or Bicarbonate Precursors?

Hartmann's solution contains lactate anions. During glucogenesis, lactate can be converted via pyruvate into glucose. For each two molecules of lactate that are required for the production of one molecule of glucose, two H^+ ions are consumed, hence lactate is said to have a 'bicarbonate sparing' effect. The oxidative metabolism of lactate and other organic anions such as acetate, propionate, gluconate, and citrate can result in the production of bicarbonate ions, and therefore these anions have also been called 'bicarbonate precursors'. Whichever the dominant mechanism for lactate, there is an overall alkalinising effect with infusion of these buffer-containing solutions.

Isotonic crystalloids that are similar to plasma in composition are less effective when used as maintenance solutions (see below) for ongoing therapy because they provide insufficient water in relation to electrolytes, but also many do not provide enough potassium (and other electrolytes), and so supplementation is required.

23.7.1.7 Hypertonic Crystalloids – Transient Plasma Volume Expanders

Most commonly hypertonic saline, with concentrations varying between 1.7 and 30% (although technically, saline solutions with NaCl concentrations greater than 0.9% are hypertonic).

23.7.1.7.1 Hypertonic Saline

The most commonly used veterinary solutions are 7.2 and 7.5% NaCl; with osmolarities of 2,464 and 2,566 mOsm/l, respectively. Hypertonic saline can be administered IV to produce a rapid, yet transient, increase in intravascular blood volume (of the order of three to four times the volume administered), and blood pressure by a number of mechanisms:

- It draws water into the intravascular space, by osmosis, primarily from the intracellular space (including red blood cells and endothelial cells, with which it comes into contact first), and, to a lesser extent, from the interstitial space. It causes a reduction in PCV, partly due to haemodilution and partly because red cells also give up some of their own water to become somewhat crenated and smaller. Although the initial increase in blood volume may be three to four times the volume administered, the effect wanes relatively rapidly as sodium accesses the whole of the extracellular fluid compartment. Osmotic equilibrium is said to be reached within about four hours, at which time it has been estimated that for every 100 ml infused, 75 ml of circulating plasma volume is gained.

- The high osmolarity of hypertonic saline independently influences the baroreflex control of sympathetic activity. It has also been suggested to cause a pulmonary-vagal reflex, followed by selective sympathetic activation, resulting in haemodynamic effects such as the venoconstriction of major capacitance vessels.

- Its hypertonicity results in direct vasodilation such that rapid administration can result in hypotension, due partly to this vasodilation and partly to the stimulation of vagal reflexes. Coronary and cerebral circulations may remain vasodilated, although the increase in blood volume may incur a postulated reflex cerebral vasoconstriction in areas where autoregulation remains intact. It **should not be administered more rapidly than 1 ml/ kg/min** to avoid significant hypotension before osmotic fluid shifts get underway.

- Its hypertonicity draws water from myocardial cells (especially if they were oedematous beforehand, e.g. in shock states), and concentrates their intracellular calcium, resulting in a further mechanism of increased inotropy, in addition to sympathetic activation and increased circulating blood volume (which increases preload). Furthermore, the increase in cardiac output may be facilitated by both a reduction in afterload due to any vasodilation (but beware during rapid administration as transient hypotension may occur); and the restoration of the transmembrane potential that may enhance the ability of cardiomyocytes to take up calcium.

Much of the published work on hypertonic saline describes its use alongside dextrans or hydroxyethyl starch solutions (colloids). The initial effect that hypertonic saline produces is only transient (30–120 minutes; in horses, its effects may last only c. 20 minutes). The inclusion of artificial colloids results in prolongation of effect rather than much extra volume expansion. The use of hypertonic saline must be followed by the administration of isotonic (or effectively hypotonic) crystalloids to replace 'borrowed' water and to provide a long-term increase in circulating volume.

A guideline dose is 4–5 ml/kg over 5–10 minutes (perhaps nearer 2–2.5 ml/kg over 5–10 minutes for cats).

Hypertonic saline can be given IV in most cases of shock, e.g. hypovolaemic or endotoxaemic, to increase intravascular volume markedly and rapidly, but, as the effects of hypertonic saline are transient, then some thought is necessary in choosing when to administer it to gain maximum benefit. For example, if hypertonic saline is given prior to anaesthetising a horse with surgical colic, it is usually administered immediately prior to anaesthesia so that the beneficial restoration of blood volume and blood pressure will be present before the cardiovascular 'insult' of anaesthetic induction. If the hypertonic saline is given too soon, then this cardiovascular advantage may be lost. The timely administration of subsequent fluids should also be considered to provide a longer lasting improvement in circulating volume and to 'pay back' the fluid drawn from the intracellular and interstitial compartments.

By 'shrinking' (i.e. 'normalising', in shock states) vascular endothelial cells (which become swollen in shock states due to reduction in sodium pump activity because of reduced ATP availability) and reducing leukocyte adhesion to endothelial cells and their activation, along with the osmotic fluid shift (which increases intravascular volume and reduces blood viscosity), and direct vasodilation (especially of arterioles), hypertonic saline can help preserve tissue perfusion and may help against ischaemia-reperfusion injury. It is an alternative to (and may have some advantages over) mannitol for traumatic brain injury (where ongoing haemorrhage can be ruled out), as it helps to restore neuronal membrane potential and endothelial Na^+/glutamate pump activity (which helps protect against the excito-toxic effects of excess glutamate release), and helps maintain blood–brain-barrier integrity. However, the use of hypertonic saline has some potential side effects:

- Hypernatraemia (it should, therefore, not be used in animals that are already hypernatraemic, although this may not always be known; but if suspicious of dehydration, then avoid). Rapid, large changes in plasma sodium can result in pontine myelinolysis (osmotic demyelination) syndromes.
- Hypokalaemia.
- Haemolysis.
- Thrombosis.
- Enhances bleeding in the face of ongoing haemorrhage because of improved haemodynamics.
- Increases the potential for re-haemorrhage, i.e. if used in cases of haemorrhagic shock, the increase in cardiac output and blood pressure after its administration may result in resumption of bleeding as the improved blood pressure may displace blood clots.

It is because of several of these problems that repeated doses of hypertonic saline are contra-indicated. Its use in small animals for acute intravascular volume resuscitation may, however, become more popular due to concerns about using artificial colloids.

23.7.1.8 Maintenance Fluids

Solutions that provide water in far greater excess of electrolytes, include:

- Dextrose-saline
- Plasma-Lyte 56 + 5% glucose
- 5% dextrose solution (D5W)

An animal's maintenance requirement is defined as the amount of water and electrolytes required to replace those lost through normal physiological processes, i.e. through respiration, perspiration, and excretion via the alimentary and urinary tracts. In the normal adult animal of ideal body condition, the estimated maintenance requirement for water is 40–60 ml/kg/day, with an average of 50 ml/kg/day or 2 ml/kg/h (although this figure is being revised for people and may be nearer 35–45 ml/kg/day). In addition to supplying water, the maintenance fluid should replace some electrolytes. Normal daily sodium requirement is around 1(−2) mmol/kg. Normal daily potassium requirement is around (1–)2 mmol/kg. Normal fluid losses are hypotonic to the ECF (but contain more potassium). However, we cannot put a solution into the vascular space that is too hypotonic, otherwise the red blood cells would swell and burst.

In the UK, we do not have a commercially available 'veterinary' fluid that has all the components that the body needs in terms of maintenance requirements. The closest options are Plasmalyte 56™ and Normosol M, although Plasma-Lyte™ 56 with 5% glucose would be an alternative maintenance solution, although it is not widely used in veterinary practice.

Ideally, we need a fluid with plenty of water, not too much sodium and chloride, but a fair bit of potassium, some magnesium, some calcium, other minerals, and vitamins. It should be noted that the amount of dextrose in the solutions described provides negligible energy at the concentrations present. For animals that cannot tolerate enteral nutrition, parenteral nutrition should be instituted as soon as possible. Parenteral nutrition is outside the scope of this chapter.

The **daily energy requirement** is c. 35 kcal/kg/day (0.15 MJ/kg/day). Note that 1 g dextrose (as the monohydrate) provides only 3.4 kcal (14.3 kJ), whereas 1 g dextrose (anhydrous) provides 3.75 kcal (15.8 kJ).

These solutions (e.g. 5% dextrose [D-glucose] in water; or 4% dextrose with 1/5th normal [0.18%] saline) are isotonic because of the dextrose ± the small amount of sodium. (Putting pure water into the bloodstream carries with it the risk of haemolysis.) Once the dextrose has been metabolised and is no longer osmotically active, only, or mainly, water remains, which can distribute freely throughout all fluid compartments as there is either no, or only a little amount of, Na^+ to trap it in the extracellular space. For each gramme of dextrose metabolised, 0.6 ml of metabolic water is also produced. Thus, if 1 l of 5% dextrose is given, then an extra 30 ml of water are generated.

These fluids are not useful for restoring circulating volume as it would require, e.g. 12 l of 5% dextrose to restore the circulating (intravascular) volume by 1 l, and by that time the red blood cells and other cells, including vascular endothelial cells, would be bursting due to water overload, and interstitial oedema would be developing. This is because the dextrose solution basically provides water, and this can freely distribute between all fluid compartments, so **only about 1/12th of the volume given IV remains in the intravascular space after 30–60 minutes**.

The solutions noted above are, however, ideal for treating primary water loss and severe hypernatraemia (see Chapter 24). They can also be used as maintenance fluids, but should contain sufficient potassium or have potassium added to them if necessary. For example, 4% glucose with 0.18% sodium chloride, supplemented with 20–30 mEq/l of potassium, is commonly used for maintenance. Or, some people alternate between, e.g. 1 bag Hartmann's solution (with K^+ supplementation to 20–30 mmol/l), followed by 2 bags of 5% dextrose (also supplemented with K^+ to 20–30 mmol/l).

23.7.1.9 Fluids for Special Occasions

These include potassium chloride and sodium bicarbonate. See also Chapters 24, 21, and 46 on electrolytes, blood gas analysis, and endocrine problems. For 50% dextrose see Chapter 44 on endocrine considerations.

23.7.1.9.1 Potassium Chloride

For supplementation of other fluids. 'Strong KCl' is the stock solution that can be added to other bags of fluids. It is a very dense (heavy) solution, so must be mixed really well once added to the fluid bag. Nothing will kill an animal quicker than to give it an overdose of K^+. The commonly available 'strong' potassium solutions are:

- 20%; 13.4 mmol K^+ in 5 ml (2.68 mmol/ml)
- 15%; 10 mmol K^+ in 5 ml (2 mmol/ml)

When fluids are supplemented with potassium for infusion, most people start by adding enough K^+ to make the final K^+ concentration between 20 and 30 mEq/l (=mmol/l). In some circumstances, it may be necessary to add more, but great care must then be taken regarding the rate of fluid administration and the maximum safe rate. See Chapter 24 on electrolytes.

Maximum safe rate for K$^+$ infusion is 0.5 mEq/kg/h. Any faster than this may put the patient in danger of acute hyperkalaemia. Never 'bolus' potassium-containing fluids.

23.7.1.9.2 Sodium Bicarbonate

See also Chapter 21 on blood gas analysis. Many disease states in animals can cause acidosis or alkalosis of varying degrees (e.g. GDV, sepsis, endotoxaemia). Acidosis is easier to treat than alkalosis. Assessment of acid/base status requires a blood gas analyser. If you do not have a means of measuring blood gases or 'total CO$_2$', then use of bicarbonate therapy can be dangerous as you have no idea how much to give.

If metabolic acidosis is due to bicarbonate loss or deficiency, then bicarbonate is an appropriate therapy to give. In most cases, however, bicarbonate therapy may not be necessary unless the pH <7.1–7.2 and the base deficit (a negative base excess) more negative than −7.0 mmol/l; i.e. fluid therapy itself may allow the homeostatic mechanisms to restore pH. If the metabolic acidosis is due to accumulation of other acids (e.g. lactic acidosis or ketoacidosis), then bicarbonate treatment may not be all that helpful, but rather the underlying cause should be treated.

If bicarbonate therapy is thought necessary, then the following formula is useful to calculate how much to give for mature animals:

$$mEq \, Bicarbonate = 0.3 \times base \, deficit \times body \, weight \, (kg)$$

Half is then administered slowly over 20–30 minutes and re-assessment is made after a further 15–30 minutes. Further doses are given as necessary. Two different concentrations of sodium bicarbonate are commonly available; 4.2 and 8.4%. Both are hypertonic with respect to plasma because of the high sodium content (i.e. the 4.2% solution has an osmolarity of 1000 mOsm/l, and the 8.4% solution has an osmolarity of 2000 mOsm/l). Normally the 4.2% (0.5 mmol/ml) solution is reserved for use in small animals and can be administered by peripheral veins, whereas the 8.4% (1 mmol/ml) solution is reserved for large animals, like horses, and should only be administered by central veins (e.g. jugular). A 1.26% (0.15 mmol/ml) solution is less commonly available. Bicarbonate solutions should not be administered concurrently through the same catheter or giving set as calcium- or magnesium-containing fluids such as Hartmann's solution because the bicarbonate and these divalent cations may precipitate out as insoluble carbonates.

Bicarbonate therapy is not a treatment for respiratory acidosis. If bicarbonate is to be given to an anaesthetised horse with a mixed metabolic and respiratory acidosis, then the respiratory component of the acidosis should be corrected first by increasing minute ventilation. Likewise, bicarbonate therapy in depressed, recumbent diarrhoeic calves should be given with caution, as it can cause a respiratory acidosis if the animals are unable to 'blow off' the extra carbon dioxide generated.

23.7.2 Colloids

Colloid solutions contain large macromolecules that cannot pass through intact capillary endothelium or cell membranes and which, when administered into the intravascular space, can therefore affect plasma COP and help to retain fluid within the intravascular compartment. The solutions can be almost iso-osmotic or hyperosmotic (also known as 'iso-oncotic' and 'hyperoncotic') with respect to plasma COP (normal is 18–25 mmHg), and they are presented in carrier electrolyte solutions, which may be either isotonic (saline, or more similar to plasma, and which may be buffered), or hypertonic with respect to plasma osmolarity (Table 23.4). Carrier solutions that contain calcium or magnesium will form insoluble precipitates if mixed with bicarbonate-containing fluids. Furthermore, solutions containing calcium should not be mixed with blood as the calcium may promote coagulation.

Colloids include:

- Synthetic colloids: gelatins, dextrans, hydroxyethyl starches
- Natural colloids: plasma, albumin
- Haemoglobin-based oxygen carrying solutions
- Blood and blood products

Colloids contain large molecules, <50–1000+ kDa. The most well-known synthetic colloids include dextrans, gelatins, and hydroxyethyl starches. Dextrans are no longer readily available. They have been withdrawn from use in many countries because of concerns regarding coaguloapthies, anaphylaxis, and renal injury associated with their use. Some details about them are given here for completeness.

23.7.2.1 Dextrans

Dextrans are macromolecular branched, neutral polysaccharides (polymers of glucose) produced by bacterial fermentation of sucrose (by *Leuconostoc mesenteroides*, a facultative anaerobe). Dextrans of molecular weights 40–70 kDa are suitable for intravenous administration. The main adverse effects of their use are anaphylactic reactions, acute renal failure (particularly with the hyperosmotic solution of 10% dextran 40), hyperglycaemia, and impaired coagulation. Allergic reactions are said to be due to naturally occurring antibodies that are cross-reactive with dextrans. Acute kidney injury (AKI), as with all colloids, is thought to be associated with one or more mechanisms.

Table 23.4 Characteristics of colloid solutions.

Solution	MWt (kDa) Ave (range)	Initial volume expansion (%)	COP (mmHg)	Osmolarity (mOsm/l)	pH	[Na⁺] (mmol/l)	[Cl⁻] (mmol/l)	[K⁺] (mmol/l)	[Ca²⁺] (mmol/l)	[Mg²⁺] (mmol/l)
Iso-osmotic colloids (in isotonic electrolyte solutions)										
6% Hetastarch	450 650	100	29–32	310	5.5	154	154	0	0	
6% Pentastarch	200	100–120	32–36	308	5.5	154	154	0	0	
6% Tetrastarch (Voluven)	130	100–130	36–38	304	4–5.5	154	154	0	0	
6% Tetrastarch (Volulyte)	130	130	36–37	283	5.7–6.5	137	110 Also acetate 34 mmol/l	4	0	1.5
Haemaccel (3.5% urea-linked gelatin)	35	70–80 (may be transiently up to 150)	25–29	293	7.3	145	145	5.1	6.25	
Gelofusin (4% succinylated gelatin)	30	80 (may be transiently up to 150)	33–35	279	7.4	154	120	0.4	0.4	
Geloplasma (3% succinylated gelatin)	30	70 (may be transiently up to 150)	26–29	273	5.8–7.0	150	100 Also lactate 30 mmol/l	5	0	1.5
4–5% Albumin	69	80	13–25	300	?	0	40	10	0	
Hyperosmotic colloids (in isotonic electrolyte solutions)										
6% Dextran 70	70	120	60–75	309–310	5.0 (3–7)	154	154	0	0	
10% Dextran 40	40	400	40	310–311	3.5–7.0	154	154	0	0	
10% Pentastarch	200	145–150	72	326	5.0	154	154	0	0	
10% Tetrastarch (Tetraspan)	130	150–200	60–74	297	4–6.5	140	118 Also 24 mmol/l acetate and 5 mmol/l malate	4	2.5	1
20–25% Albumin	69	200–400	195	1500	?	0	40	10	0	
1.3% oxyglobin in modified Hartmann's solution	200 (65–130)	Likely >100	42–43	290–310	7.8	113	113	4	?	
Hyperosmotic (in hypertonic saline)										
7.5% NaCl/20% Starch	depends upon starch type	300–400	>100	2567	Acidic	1283	1283	0	0	
7.5% NaCl/6% Dextran 70	70	300–400	62–75	2567	4.0–5.0	1283	1283	0	0	

Direct toxic effects on renal cells (i.e. uptake of colloid by the cells [vacuolisation], with subsequent water uptake, leading to cell-swelling and 'osmotic nephrosis') may occur, although is not now thought to be the main mechanism. The renal filtration of especially the smaller (40 kDa) molecules with their subsequent 'concentration' (and even precipitation), within renal tubules (intraluminal hyperviscosity), can cause obstruction and secondary renal injury. More recently, a hyperoncotic (osmotic) acute renal failure mechanism has been proposed, whereby greatly increased plasma oncotic pressure can oppose glomerular ultrafiltration enough to cause anuria, but which is reversible with appropriate fluid therapy or plasmapheresis. Coagulopathy is related to dilutional effects, dextran-mediated platelet dysfunction, decreased von Willebrand factor-factor VIII (vWF: FVIII) complex, and weakened clot strength (due to incorporation of dextran into clots). Note that adverse effects are influenced by dose, cumulative dose and time; and are also dependent upon the nature of the colloid administered (i.e. 40 kDa versus 70 kDa, its concentration and its carrier solution), and patient factors.

23.7.2.2 Gelatins

Gelatin-based colloids are derived from the chemical denaturation and hydrolysis of bovine collagen (from either skin or bone), which produces polypeptides which are smaller than gelatin itself and remain fluid at lower temperatures.

The three main types are:

- succinylated gelatins (also known as modified fluid gelatins)
- urea cross-linked gelatins
- oxypolygelatins

Their relatively low molecular weights (20–40 kDa), result in a rapid (because of the relatively large number of osmotically active particles per unit volume of fluid infused), but transient (two to three hours), volume expansion (transient because of rapid renal excretion). Adverse effects include diuresis, AKI (similar mechanisms to those proposed for dextrans), increased blood viscosity, coagulopathy (via dilutional effects, interference with platelet function and weakening of clot strength), and a generally higher rate of anaphylaxis than with other colloids. Note that adverse effects are influenced by dose, cumulative dose and time; and are also dependent upon the nature of the colloid administered (e.g. type of gelatin, concentration, and its carrier solution), and patient factors.

23.7.2.3 Starches

Starch-based colloids are derived from either waxy-maize (95% amylopectin/5% amylose) or potato (80% amylopectin/20% amylose), starches (i.e. glucose polymers), which are hydroxethylated to varying degrees; the resulting solutions being polydisperse because they contain molecules of a large range of molecular sizes. Hydroxyethylated starch (HES) solutions are therefore characterised by: their raw material source, their concentration, their molecular weight (weight-averaged or number-averaged), molar substitution (MS), substitution pattern (C2/C6 ratio), and their carrier solution. As prolonged intravascular retention time was thought to be beneficial and HES degradation depends, to some degree, upon molecular size, but especially on MS and C2/C6 ratio, the first generation HES solutions contained large molecules with high MS and high C2/C6 ratio.

For HES solutions, their molecular size is described in terms of either a weight-average (Mw, the average molecular weight) or a number-average (Mn, the total weight of polymers divided by the number of molecules). The ratio Mw/Mn gives a measure of the polydispersity of the mixture.

HES types are traditionally classified as:

- High molecular weight (450–670 kDa)
- Medium molecular weight (130–200 kDa)
- Low molecular weight (≤70 kDa)

Their *in vivo* molecular weights, however, differ from their *in vitro* Mw because plasma alpha-amylase splits larger molecules into smaller ones, and molecules <55 kDa are rapidly excreted into urine or taken up into tissues (see below). It is also of note that different species have differing plasma amylase activities: dogs have around three times, and cats around six times, the plasma amylase activity of people.

Increasing water-solubility and resistance to plasma alpha-amylase degradation (hydrolysis), is gained by substituting an increasing number of hydroxyethyl residues (in place of hydrogen atoms at the -OH side groups), at carbon atoms 2, 3, and 6, but especially C2, followed by C6, on each glucose molecule. The number of hydroxyethyl residues per anhydrous glucose subunit defines the MS, whereas the degree of substitution (DS) represents the number of substituted anhydrous glucose residues as a proportion of the total number of possible substitution sites. Based on the MS, HES solutions are characterised as hetastarches (MS = 0.7); hexastarches (MS = 0.6); pentastarches (MS = 0.5); and tetrastarches (MS = 0.4). HES types with MS 0.62–0.75 are regarded as being highly substituted, those with MS of around 0.5 as medium and those with MS ≤ 0.4 as having a low DS. Hydroxyethyl substitution, particularly at C2, confers allosteric inhibition against cleavage by plasma alpha-amylase and increases the half-life.

Adverse effects of HES solutions include coagulopathies, anaphylaxis, tissue accumulation, pruritus, AKI, and mortality. The exact adverse effects are, as with other colloids, influenced by the characteristics of the particular HES solution used (source, concentration, Mw, MS, C2/C6 ratio, and its carrier solution), and patient factors. Coagulopathies arise from several different mechanisms: dilution of plasma clotting factors and platelets; reduction of vWF: FVIII complex; accelerated fibrinogen activation and polymerisation of fibrin, followed by enhanced fibrinolysis because of reduced interaction between activated fibrin-stabilising factor and fibrin; interference with platelet GPIIbIIIa expression and activity (which binds vWF and fibrinogen), thus reduced platelet adhesion, activation, and aggregation; and increased clot fragility (because of incorporation of HES into clots that destabilises them). Although coagulopathies are less of a problem if using HES solutions with lower Mw, MS, and C2/C6 ratios (partly because of faster elimination perhaps), they may still occur.

Cellular uptake by phagocytosis (immune cells) or pinocytosis (many other cells including kidney, liver, lung, pancreas, gut, muscle, skin, nerve cells, Schwann cells, endothelial and epithelial cells), and intracellular storage of HES (leading to water accumulation, swelling and dysfunction), is common and may be responsible for organ dysfunction and pruritus. Once inside cells in lysosomes/vacuoles, degradation is slow and dependent upon alpha-glucosidase. The mechanism of pruritus is not fully understood, but may involve HES uptake into skin cells, dermal macrophages and small nerves in the skin. It does not appear to be related to histamine release as antihistamines do not alleviate it. Its onset may be delayed (one to six weeks post exposure) and it may continue for several months or years, depending upon the dose.

Although all classes of synthetic colloids can cause AKI, HES solutions have been most frequently blamed, perhaps reflecting their greater usage. It should be mentioned, however, that other factors may contribute to renal impairment, e.g. hyperchloraemia associated with the carrier solution, and daily doses in excess of those deemed safe by the manufacturers. The AKI thought to be related to HES solutions may, as with the other colloids, be due to several contributory mechanisms. Uptake of HES into renal (particularly the proximal), tubular epithelial cells results in cellular swelling and dysfunction (osmotic nephrosis); additionally, HES uptake by renal interstitial macrophages and reticulo-endothelial cells may exacerbate tubular damage through promoting inflammation. Particularly in dehydrated patients, it may be possible for smaller HES molecules, filtered by the kidney, to produce hyperviscous ultrafiltrate that may block renal tubules, resulting in secondary renal ischaemic damage. And finally, hyperoncotic/osmotic acute renal failure may occur, especially with the higher percentage solutions, as the high plasma COP can oppose ultrafiltration within the kidney, leading to oliguric/anuric acute renal failure.

The possible increased risk of mortality associated with HES solutions may be associated with coagulopathy (and increased requirement for blood or blood products), AKI and multiple organ uptake of HES that may lead to dysfunction in many organs.

Despite these adverse effects, HES solutions have been shown to have anti-inflammatory effects, although whether this is truly beneficial in cases of sepsis is debatable.

23.7.2.4 General Uses of Colloids

Colloids have been used for **intravascular volume replacement / restoration** and for **oncotic support**. In the presence of an intact vascular endothelium and functional ESL, the distribution volume of any colloid is theoretically limited to the intravascular compartment: their large molecules retain water within the intravascular space and oppose interstitial oedema formation. (It is also possible that their large macromolecules somehow incorporate into the EG and perhaps further augment the natural resistance to ultrafiltration of fluid across the capillary endothelium.) This forms the basis of the much quoted crystalloid: colloid volume requirement being c. 4 : 1 for the restoration of intravascular volume in cases of hypovolaemia where the ESL remains intact. (In comparison to colloids, crystalloids rapidly redistribute throughout the whole ECF regardless of whether the ESL is intact or not.)

In situations of ESL damage, however, the distribution volume of colloids is much greater than the intravascular space, and they behave similarly to crystalloids, such that instead of the above-mentioned c. 4 : 1 (crystalloid: colloid) volume ratio requirement for intravascular volume restoration, their advantage is much less with a crystalloid: colloid ratio nearer 1–1.5 : 1.

Although there is a little evidence that some HES molecules (particularly those around 200–250 KDa) can attenuate capillary leakage, the mechanism, magnitude, and duration of effect have yet to be conclusively demonstrated. Suggested mechanisms include reduced expression of adhesion molecules on vascular endothelium (anti-inflammatory effect), and that the HES molecules may physically plug 'holes' in leaky capillaries by becoming incorporated into the EG. Interestingly, subphysiological doses of albumin can reduce extravasation of fluid into the microcirculation (most probably by enhancing the function of the ESL) to a greater extent than HES, despite generating a lower COP (known as the COP paradox). Although colloids with high COP have been advocated to treat conditions of low COP (e.g. hypoalbuminaemia), it is the ESL, and not the plasma COP, which provides the most important oncotic gradient to oppose fluid transudation, and therefore restoring health of the ESL should become a priority. Synthetic colloids, however, may be the only products available to veterinarians to treat acute hypoalbuminaemia because, although albumin solutions may be superior to synthetic colloids, there are no cheap, readily-available, and species-specific albumin solutions available for the various veterinary species. Whenever treating hypoalbuminaemia, however, increasing plasma COP with exogenous colloids (albumin or synthetic colloids) can also suppress hepatic albumin synthesis which can further exacerbate fluid extravasation.

For all colloids, if their COP is higher than that of the plasma, not only can they limit the passage of fluid out of the intravascular compartment (if the EG is intact), but, through exerting an osmotic effect, they *may* increase intravascular volume by more than their administered volume, with water from mainly the intracellular space (red blood cells and vascular endothelial cells in the first instance), so they may be called **plasma volume expanders**. (Some authors have also suggested that water may be drawn from the ESL to augment the circulating portion of the intravascular volume.) The osmotic effect (volume expansion effect), however, depends upon the number of osmotically active particles per unit volume of solution, whereas their duration of effect (half-life in the intravascular space) depends upon the size of their osmotically active particles.

There are several colloid products available that differ by country, especially since the concerns regarding AKI (and particularly HES solutions), were highlighted in 2013. Table 23.4 outlines some of their properties. Although the various different colloids have different recommended maximum daily doses, a rough guide would be not to exceed 20 ml/kg/day where possible.

It should be noted that infusion of synthetic colloids will **affect refractometer readings** of plasma total solids. Hetastarch solutions give refractometer readings of around 4.5 g/dl; pentastarch solutions give readings of around 7.5 g/dl; tetrastarch solutions give readings of around 4.0 g/dl; 3% succinylated gelatin (geloplasma) gives readings of around 2.2 g/dl, and 4% succinylated gelatin gives readings of around 3.5 g/dl. Should large volumes of these colloids be administered, the patient's plasma TS readings will be likely to trend towards these values.

It is difficult to make specific recommendations regarding the use of synthetic colloids due to evidence in humans that the use of these substances (most evidence for HES solutions) increases the risk of AKI and the need for renal replacement therapy in critically ill or septic patients. The current Surviving Sepsis human guidelines recommend against the use of HES (and gelatin) solutions for severe sepsis and septic shock, instead suggesting the incorporation of human serum albumin (HSA) when substantial volumes of crystalloids are required (see below). One retrospective study in dogs suggests a similar risk of AKI in dogs with the use of HES solutions. Although we do not have prospective clinical trials to support this in veterinary patients it may be prudent to avoid their use in this population until further information is available. Concern also exists about their use in other conditions beyond critical illness and sepsis (e.g. for the treatment of hypovolaemia).

23.7.2.5 Albumin

Hypoalbuminaemia is a marker of disease severity and warrants attention to the underlying cause. Albumin is usually reserved for treatment of protein-losing enteropathy or nephropathy where life-threatening hypoalbuminaemia exists (<15 g/l), and in sepsis, but species-specific albumin products are generally not readily available and HSA may cause life-threatening anaphylactic reactions. Synthetic colloids therefore may be used in place of albumin (HSA) for oncotic support. See above regarding the importance of albumin for the maintenance of normal capillary permeability and the potentially beneficial effects of even subphysiological doses of albumin for helping to restore damaged ESL integrity. One problem, however, is that exogenously administered albumin or synthetic colloids will reduce the endogenous (hepatic) production of albumin. Albumin, however, is said to confer other advantages such as free radical scavenging and providing binding sites for a multitude of biochemical molecules and drugs.

The albumin deficit can be calculated by the equation below and can be replaced over several hours. Infusion is started slowly and vigilance maintained for anaphylactic reactions particularly when using non species-specific albumin products. Beware volume overload and pulmonary oedema if using solutions of 4–5%. The 20–25% solutions must be administered by central veins. If plasma is to be used instead of albumin for COP support, it has been reported that volumes as large as 40 ml/kg are required to increase albumin concentration by 1 g/dl.

$$\begin{aligned}
&\text{Dose required}\,(\mathbf{g}) \\
&= 10 \times \left(\text{desired albumin}\left[\mathbf{g/dl}\right] - \text{actual albumin}\left[\mathbf{g/dl}\right]\right) \\
&\quad \times \left(0.3 \times \text{Body weight}\left[\mathbf{kg}\right]\right)
\end{aligned}$$

23.7.2.6 Oxygen Carrying Solutions

Oxygen carrying solutions include haemoglobin (Hb)-based solutions and perfluorocarbon emulsions. Blood substitutes have gathered much attention over the last 30 years as alternatives to blood and blood products, which carry the risk of disease transmission and also immunosuppression (including increased metastasis rate in cancer patients). The first generation of Hb-based oxygen carriers (HBOCs), consisted of cross-linked Hb molecules (e.g. alpha-alpha linked or diaspirin-linked), but produced renal injury and increased mortality. Second generation HBOCs included raffinose cross-linked Hb, glutaraldehyde-polymerised Hb and polyethylene glycol conjugated (PEG-ylated) Hb. The newest generation of zero-linked polymerised haemoglobin HBOCs, however, may prove to be the safest. Haemoglobin-containing liposomes have also been developed and tend to have longer intravascular lifespans than haemoglobin-based solutions. With these, the Hb can be co-encapsulated with allosteric modulators such as 2,3-diphosphoglycerate (2,3-DPG), and metHb reductase can also be added to improve their useful lifespan.

23.7.2.6.1 Oxyglobin (Hb Glutamer 200)™

Oxyglobin™ is no longer available on the veterinary market, although it is possible that in the future similar products may replace it. Details are included here for historical interest only.

Oxyglobin was a colloidal solution containing 13 g/dl (130 mg/ml) of purified polymerised bovine haemoglobin in a modified lactated Ringer's solution, pH 7.8. The solution had a lower viscosity than blood, so could be given very much more quickly than blood if necessary. The solution was isotonic with plasma, but was slightly hyperosmotic/hyperoncotic (huge chunky highly charged molecules). It could be administered via standard infusion sets (i.e. did not require a filter), and could also be administered safely via peristaltic infusion pumps. It had a shelf-life of c. three years at room temperature although once opened, it was to be used within 24 hours because of production of metHb (i.e. oxidative damage).

Initial plasma volume expansion was up to five times the volume administered. Its half-life in the circulation was around 30–40 hours; but the duration of its oxygen-carrying effect was unknown. It was thought to provide an 'oxygen-bridge' for one to three days, e.g. until a suitable blood donor could be found.

The average molecular weight of oxyglobin was 200 kDa. Less than 5% was present as unstable dimers and tetramers, and these were rapidly excreted into the urine; hence the urine looked very red/orange (transient haemoglobinuria) for the first few hours (c. 4 hours) after dosing.

There was no need to cross-match. Multiple doses could be given, although this was not recommended. Although antibodies were raised, no antibody deposition was found in liver or kidneys, and no reduction in oxygen-carrying capacity of the repeated-dose polymerised Hb was found.

Bovine haemoglobin uses Cl^- instead of 2,3-DPG as an allosteric modulator to modify its transport of O_2, CO_2,

and H^+. (This offered another advantage over using stored blood, in which the 2,3-DPG level is often depleted so that infused red cells do not function optimally, at least immediately.) Feline haemoglobin is likewise chloride-dependent, whereas dog haemoglobin is 2,3-DPG-dependent. Horse Hb appears to be more complex; see the Further Reading.

Oxyglobin was useful for the treatment of anaemia due to:

- Haemorrhage, trauma/surgery (where concurrent hypovolaemia was likely).
- Haemolysis (immune-mediated, infectious). Patients would usually be normovolaemic (euvolaemic), so beware volume overload; administer slowly.
- Non-regenerative anaemia due to disease states such as chronic renal failure and neoplasia (again patients were probably normovolaemic, so beware volume overload).

Oxyglobin was very useful especially when blood donors were not available and there was no time to cross-match. It was, however, to be used with caution in normovolaemic states (haemolytic anaemias). Contra-indications to its use included hypervolaemic states such as congestive cardiac failure and oliguric/anuric renal failure.

P_{50}

The P_{50} is the partial pressure of oxygen (in the plasma) at which the haemoglobin is 50% saturated. The P_{50} of the oxyglobin solution was around 34–35 mmHg.

- Ruminant Hb P_{50}s are around 25–35 mmHg.
- Feline Hb P_{50} is around 34–36 mmHg.
- The P_{50} of 2,3-DPG-dependent haemoglobins (e.g. canine, human) is around 28–31 mmHg for dogs and 27 mmHg for humans.
- Horse Hb has a P_{50} of about 24–26 mmHg and is less 2,3-DPG dependent than that of the dog.
- Llamas and alpacas have Hb P_{50}s of around 17.5–22 mmHg because they are adapted to living at high altitudes.

The oxyglobin–oxygen dissociation curve lay to the right of the canine haemoglobin–oxygen dissociation curve (Figure 23.2). Thus oxyglobin was less fully saturated at low PO_2 values, or, put another way, oxyglobin was happier to give up its oxygen to tissues. Therefore oxyglobin greatly improved tissue oxygen delivery in dogs. However, this is not the whole story of why/how HBOCs improve tissue oxygen delivery, as some third generation HBOCs have P_{50} values nearer 7 mmHg (i.e. much higher oxygen affinity than native Hb), but some of these molecules also do not display co-operative binding.

Administration of HBOCs, including oxyglobin, also facilitates diffusive oxygen transfer to the tissues because

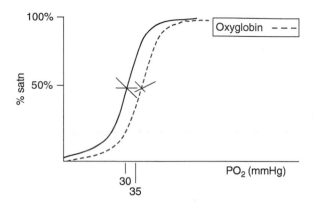

Figure 23.2 Dissociation curves for red-cell bound haemoglobin (solid line) and oxyglobin (dashed line).

they improve microcirculatory oxygen delivery. Normally, very small capillaries do not allow RBCs to pass through (Fahraeus-Lindqvist effect/plasma skimming), even though RBCs are highly deformable and can squeeze through many larger capillary beds. However, because HBOCs are not contained within red cells and the polymerised Hb is relatively smaller than RBC, there is a better chance that HBOC-containing plasma can pass through small capillaries, thus taking oxygen nearer to the cells that are likely to be most oxygen-deprived.

Consequences of Oxyglobin Administration

- Discoloration of skin, mucous membranes and sclerae for three to five days post infusion.
- Discoloration of urine (haemoglobinuria) for first four hours post infusion in healthy animals due to unstable low molecular weight polymers in the solution entering the urinary ultrafiltrate. The rest of the polymers were broken down by the reticulo-endothelial system (RES). Whilst urine was discoloured, urine dipsticks were unreliable for pH, glucose, ketones, and protein.
- PCV decreased due to haemodilution. Oxyglobin was a colloid and a potent plasma volume expander.
- Haemoglobin concentration increased (so you could not use the rule of thumb, whereby [Hb] approximately equals one-third PCV, for at least 24–48 hours).
- Total plasma protein increased.
- Pulse oximetry readings tended to become an average of red-cell Hb saturation and oxyglobin saturation.
- There was transient (24–48 hours) interference with some serum chemistries (colorimetric techniques).
- PaO_2 did not change.
- Some types of coagulation tests were affected, depending upon the methodology used. Platelet counts could be lowered by the haemodilution effects. There were concerns over dilutional coagulopathies where large volumes were given.

Hb and the Vasopressor Action of Oxyglobin As a protein, Hb is remarkable in many ways. Within the red cell environment, Hb carries O_2, CO_2, and H^+. When Hb is free in plasma, it can also perform these functions, but is less regulated. However, Hb also binds ('scavenges'), nitric oxide (NO). DeoxyHb can bind NO (termed HbNO), and oxyHb can form a nitrosothiol compound with NO (designated SNOHb).

Normally, inside RBCs, Hb does not come into close contact with vascular endothelium. But, free in plasma, as oxyglobin, it is able to contact endothelium. Capillary (and larger blood vessel), vascular endothelium produces many local modulators of vascular tone, including prostacyclin (PGI_2) a vasodilator, endothelins (vasoconstrictors), and NO (a vasodilator). Free Hb, in the form of oxyglobin, may bind the normally produced NO, and cause an overall increase in peripheral vascular tone (vasoconstriction). (Red-cell confined Hb may also have a role in NO regulation.) Such vasoconstriction, combined with plasma volume expansion, may cause problems (similar to volume over-load): high CVP, increased tissue oedema (including pulmonary), and 'congestive cardiac failure'. Because of this potential to cause volume-overload, some people were wary of administering oxyglobin. (NO-scavenging may not be the only mechanism for vasoconstriction; the low oxygen affinity [higher P_{50}] of oxyglobin may result in premature off-loading of oxygen in pre-capillary arterioles which results in autoregulatory vasoconstriction.)

Another problem in the situation of haemorrhagic hypovolaemic shock was that if oxyglobin was used to restore blood volume and oxygen-carrying capacity, especially if CVP was used to determine the end-point for infusion, then initial under-dosing (inadequate volume restoration) was possible because of the combined effects of vasoconstriction, coincident with potent plasma volume expansion. (Some authors quoted that 5 ml/kg oxyglobin was equivalent to 20 ml/kg HES solution.) With time, however, vasorelaxation occurred, which unmasked the remaining intravascular volume deficiency so further dosing was required.

23.7.3 Blood and Blood Components

Indications for transfusions include:

- Severe acute haemorrhagic shock (acute loss of >25% of total blood volume; possibly >15% if under anaesthesia)
- Haemolytic anaemia
- Aplastic anaemia
- Hypoproteinaemia
- Coagulopathies
- Thrombocytopaenia

23.7.3.1 Transfusion Triggers

In human medicine, transfusion used to be thought necessary once PCV was down to 30% and [Hb] to 10 g/dl. However, blood transfusions are expensive (in terms of resources and finances), can result in the transfer of infectious diseases, and cause immunosuppression with increased risk of tumour metastases, so this trigger has been reducing (as long as there is no accompanying cardiorespiratory disease and no evidence of impaired tissue oxygen delivery) to values around PCV 21% and [Hb] 7 g/dl. The clinical status of the patient, however, must always be borne in mind.

As far as veterinary species go, acute and chronic anaemias and different species (remember the cat has a peculiar erythron compared to the dog) may require different interventions, and each patient must be approached individually. The replacement of such arbitrary transfusion triggers with more physiological ones, e.g. markers of tissue oxygen delivery such as lactate, venous oxygen saturation, or oxygen extraction, is gradually becoming commonplace.

23.7.3.2 Some 'Rules of Thumb' Regarding Hypo-coagulation

- For clinically detectable haemorrhage to be apparent, clotting factors must be reduced to about 30% of normal.
- If clotting factor deficiencies are present, then replacement of them, up to 20–30% of what is a normal level, is usually sufficient to arrest haemorrhagic episodes.
- Platelet count $<50 \times 10^9$/l is trouble; but replacement to about 25×10^9/l can help.
- Fibrinogen ≤ 1 g/l is the critical level for haemorrhagic diatheses.
- Haemodilution with fluid therapy tends to dilute out platelets long before clotting factors become critical (as long as no clotting factor deficiency was pre-existing).

23.7.3.3 Anticoagulants/Preservatives for Blood and Blood Products

- Acid citrate dextrose (ACD) affords three weeks' storage (refrigerated). 1 ml per 7–9 ml whole blood.
- Citrate phosphate dextrose (CPD) or citrate phosphate dextrose adenine (CPD-A1) afford up to four or five weeks' refrigerated storage, respectively. 1 ml per 7–9 ml whole blood.
- Heparin: use blood immediately. Need 0.5–2 units unfractionated heparin per ml whole blood; or 5–10 units of low molecular weight heparin per ml blood.
- Other anticoagulant/preservatives are available and include CPD-SAGM (saline-adenine-glucose-mannitol), which is useful for red cell preservation (e.g. in packed red cell preparations) for refrigerated storage for up to five to six weeks.

23.7.3.3.1 Blood 'Storage Lesions'

- Decreased red cell ATP, so increased cellular rigidity/fragility; and cells are slightly swollen because membrane sodium pumps have no energy supply.
- Decreased 2,3-DPG, so oxygen dissociation curve moves to left with resultant reduced ability of haemoglobin to give up its oxygen to the tissues (Valtis-Kennedy effect). Transfused red cells regain 2,3-DPG after 24–48 hours. (Not all species have 2,3-DPG-dependent Hb though.)
- Decreased pH, so oxygen/haemoglobin dissociation curve moves to right (although overall left-shift may predominate, see above). Stored blood is poor at improving tissue oxygen delivery, at least at first.
- Increased plasma PCO_2.
- Decreased plasma PO_2.
- Increased lactate.
- Increased plasma K^+ secondary to red cell leak (as sodium pumps fail), and some haemolysis. (Especially in high K^+ red cell species and breeds: humans, horses, not normally dogs except, e.g. Japanese Akitas.)
- Increased NH_3 so beware liver disease patients.
- Decreased platelets, especially after two to three days; all gone by five days.
- Decreased labile clotting factors (after six or so hours).
- Decreased glucose.

23.7.3.4 Blood Donation Volume

Donors can safely donate up to 10% of their blood volume every four weeks, or up to 20% of blood volume not more often than every 12 weeks. Donors (preferably <8 years old), must be healthy and not anaemic. Suggested minimum weight for a dog donor is 25 kg, with minimum PCV 40%; and 4.0 kg for a cat, with minimum PCV 35%. More usually, 20% of donor blood volume is taken.

1 unit of dog blood
$$= 450 \text{ ml} \left(= 20\% \text{ blood volume for a 25 kg dog} \right)$$

1 unit of cat blood
$$= 45 \text{ ml} \left(= 20\% \text{ blood volume for a 4 kg cat} \right)$$

When taking 15–20% of donor blood volume, it is common practice to replace at least some of the volume taken with IV fluid therapy, usually with crystalloids. The desired volume of blood is usually taken over about 15 minutes.

23.7.3.4.1 Dogs

Blood volume
$$= 80 - 90 \text{ ml/kg} \left(8 - 9\% \text{ of body weight} \right)$$

Normal red cell survival is c. 120 days, although it is less than this for transfused red cells. Canine blood groups are:

- DEA 1.1
- DEA 1.2
- DEA 3
- DEA 4
- DEA 5
- DEA 6
- DEA 7
- DEA 8
- DEA 9
- DEA 10
- DEA 11
- DEA 12
- DEA 13

DEA 1.1, 1.2, and 7 are the most important (DEA 1 is the most antigenic) and the **universal donor is DEA 1.1, 1.2, and 7 negative** (with some blood banks including DEA 4 positive). Typing antisera are available for DEA 1, 4, 5, and 7.

Dogs rarely have naturally occurring alloantibodies, so the first transfusion is unlikely to cause problems. Ideally, however, cross-matching should always be performed, and must be done for dogs that have received previous transfusions. It takes between 4 and 14 days to produce antibodies after being challenged.

23.7.3.4.2 Cats

Blood volume

$$= (45) - 55 - (65) \text{ ml/kg} \left(4.5 - 6.5\% \text{ of body weight} \right)$$

Normal red cell survival is c. 75 days, although it is less than this for transfused red cells. Feline blood groups are:

- A (dominant to AB and most common).
- B (thought to be common in some breeds, e.g. Persian, British shorthair).
- AB (recessive to A; co-dominant with B).

There is **no universal donor**. Type A cats tend to have naturally occurring alloantibodies to B antigens, and type B cats have naturally occurring alloantibodies to A antigens. Type AB cats have no naturally occurring alloantibodies. Anti-A antibodies are strong haemagglutinins and haemolysins. Anti-B antibodies are weaker agglutinins and haemolysins. Cats can also have naturally occurring cold agglutinins.

More recently, the *Mik* antigen has been discovered and incompatibility can cause reactions, but the full significance of this antigen has yet to be determined.

Cross-matching should always be performed, even if the donor and recipient have compatible blood types.

Major cross – match

= donor red cells + recipient plasma

Minor cross – match

= recipient red cells + donor plasma

Should cat blood not be available, xenotransfusion, using dog's blood, *may* be performed in an emergency, and transfused red cells have a lifespan of around four days. But, future repetition of dog blood xenotransfusion in the same recipient (>4 days after initial transfusion, after which time the cat will have antibodies to canine red cells) carries a very high risk of fatal reactions.

23.7.3.4.3 Horses

Blood volume

$$= (60) - 80 - (100) \text{ ml/kg} \left(6 - 10\% \text{ body weight} \right)$$

Red cell survival time is c. 145 days, although it is less than this for transfused cells. More than 400,000 blood types are possible due to 30 different RBC antigens comprising at least eight major blood groups (A, C, D, K, P, Q, U, and T). The most immunogenic antigens are Aa from the A group and Qa from the Q group. Antigens in the C group may also be significant. There is **no universal donor,** but the preferred donor is **Aa, Ca, and Qa negative** (especially for foals suffering from neonatal isoerythrolysis). Donors (≥500 kg preferably) can give 4–8 l blood every one to three months, respectively. Geldings (or mares that have never bred) are usually preferred donors.

Cross-matching (major and minor) is advised. Blood should be transfused as soon as possible after harvesting as, with time, potassium leaks out of the RBC. The equine **erythrocyte sedimentation rate is very rapid** so that within one to two hours, plasma can be separated off.

Donkeys have blood groups B, M, and N, and also donkey factor antigen (to which horses seem naturally sensitised). This means that **donkey blood should never be given to horses**, but horse blood may (if desperate, although not advisable) be given to donkeys.

23.7.3.5 Blood Administration

- Must use giving set with in-line filter (care that this is the correct 'size', i.e. 170–200 μm, so as not to damage red cells, to ensure microthrombi do not get infused.
- Blood should be either at room temperature or preferably at 37 °C for transfusion; not cold straight from the refrigerator.
- Record recipient's baseline temperature, pulse, and respiration rates (TPR) before the start of transfusion as this makes it easier to note reactions.

- Some people like to administer an antihistamine (usually chlorphenamine, c. 0.4–0.5 mg/kg) slowly intravenously before transfusion is commenced in the hope of preventing transfusion reactions. Chlorphenamine can cause hypotension (especially if administered rapidly) and drowsiness.
- Do not administer blood through fluid lines with Hartmann's solution or other calcium-containing solutions in them because coagulation might occur in the line.
- Some peristaltic pumps will fracture the red cells; use modern blood-safe peristaltic pumps or gravity-pumps, syringe-drivers or pressure-infusors if necessary.

23.7.3.5.1 Rate of Administration

Depends upon the reason for therapy. Generally **start at ≤ 0.5 ml/kg/h**, certainly for the first 5–15 minutes to check for acute reactions. If necessary, **can then increase** up to 5–20 ml/kg/h, or faster if needed.

23.7.3.5.2 Blood Volume Requirement

It is often said that: 2.2 ml/kg of donor blood (PCV c. 40%) will raise recipient PCV by 1%, and likewise: 1 ml/kg of packed red cells (PCV c. 80–90% if not resuspended in any appreciable volume) will raise recipient PCV by c. 1%. (Note that most commercially available units of packed red cells have a PCV of around 62%.)

Therefore:

$$\text{ml donor blood required}$$
$$= \text{Desired PCV increase}$$
$$\times \left(2.2 \times \text{Recipient Body weight}\left[\text{kg}\right]\right)$$

The other formula that you may see is:

$$\text{ml donor blood required}$$
$$= \text{Recipient blood volume}$$
$$\times \frac{\left(\text{Desired PCV} - \text{Recipient PCV}\right)}{\text{Donor PCV}}$$

23.7.3.5.3 Transfusion Reactions

Can be immunologic (acute and delayed) and non-immunologic. For this reason, the transfusion should be started at 0.25–1.0 ml/kg/h for the first 15 minutes, then increased to deliver the required volume, usually over 4–6 hours. Fresh whole blood must be transfused within six hours of collection if platelets and clotting factors are required. If only red cells are required, transfusion of stored blood is sufficient and can be slower.

If a reaction occurs, stop the infusion. Perhaps try antihistamine and/or corticosteroid. If the reaction is mild, continue infusion, but at a slow/er rate. If it is severe, do not continue.

Immunologic Reactions

- Acute:
  - intravascular haemolysis, which can be fatal
- Delayed:
  - extravascular haemolysis
  - immune reactions involving other blood components, e.g. platelets or white blood cells
  - allo-sensitisation
  - transfusion-related immunomodulation (TRIM), e.g. increased metastatsis rate
  - transfusion-related acute lung injury (TRALI), a type of non-cardiogenic pulmonary oedema (see also non-immunologic reactions)

Non-immunolgic Reactions

- Hyperkalaemia (especially if large volumes of long-stored blood are given from high-K^+ red cell donors)
- Hypocalcaemia (citrate toxicity). Rare unless liver disease (and slow metabolism of citrate) or huge volumes of citrated blood are administered
- Hyperammonaemia (usually only with large volumes of long-stored blood)
- Hypervolaemia (volume overload, or transfusion associated cardiac overload, TACO)
- TRALI (immunologic mechanisms may also be involved, see above)
- Hypothermia (blood not warmed prior to infusion)
- Transmission of infectious diseases

23.7.3.5.4 Clinical Signs of Transfusion Reactions

- Agitation, restlessness, muscle tremors, change in attitude
- Nausea, vomiting, salivation
- Urticaria (especially around head), angioedema, ± pruritus
- Anaphylaxis
- Pyrexia
- Tachypnoea or dyspnoea
- Tachycardia
- Hypotension
- Seizures
- Haemolysis, jaundice, haemoglobinuria

23.7.3.6 Blood Component Therapy
23.7.3.6.1 Whole Blood

The most familiar preservative/anticoagulant is CPDA-1 (citrate, phosphate, dextrose, adenine). Commercially available blood collection bags (Baxter Fenwal) contain c. 63 ml of this preservative/anticoagulant mixture. The 'unit' of blood that can then be collected is 450 ml. (This maintains the ratio of anticoagulant: blood at 1: 7–9). Blood can be stored for up to five weeks at +4 °C (refrigerator) as long as a closed system is used for its collection. Platelets lose viability within one to five days. If aseptic technique is breached, then blood must be used within 24 hours. Filtered giving sets must always be used.

23.7.3.6.2 Packed Red Cells

Centrifugation or sedimentation can be used to help prepare these products. The red cells are then usually washed with saline (three times) and resuspended in a saline-based red cell preservative solution (e.g. SAGM), so the final PCV of commercially available units (1 unit is around 250 ml for small animals) is c. 60%. Can be administered slowly as packed red cells, especially to patients with chronic anaemic conditions that are normovolaemic. Can alternatively be further resuspended in sterile normal saline to make a less viscous solution for administration. Filtered giving sets must always be used.

23.7.3.6.3 Leukocyte-Poor Red Cells

Leukoreduction can be performed using (haem)apheresis machines and is useful if patients have antibodies to foreign white blood cells. This is more common in human medicine than veterinary medicine at the current time.

23.7.3.6.4 Fresh Frozen Plasma (FFP)

Blood must be centrifuged and plasma harvested and frozen (−18 to −20 °C) within six hours to save the labile clotting factors. FFP can be stored for up to one year (after which it is relabelled as frozen plasma and can be stored for up to a further four years). After thawing, FFP should be given within six hours to get the maximum benefit from its clotting factor content. An average 'unit' of FFP is 200 ml. It contains:

- Factors I (fibrinogen), II, V, VII, VIII, IX, X, XI, XIII (fibronectin) and von Willebrand factor
- Antithrombin III
- Alpha 1 antitrypsin
- Alpha 2 macroglobulin
- Bradykinin inhibitors
- Albumin
- Immunoglobulins

The main indications for FFP are for patients with SIRS and coagulopathies, including disseminated intravascular coagulopathy (DIC) (see Chapter 26 on shock).

23.7.3.6.5 Fresh Plasma

If plasma is harvested from blood and frozen more than six hours after its donation, many of the labile clotting factors will have degraded, and therefore it is described as just 'fresh plasma' (FP). Although FP still contains useful albumin, immunoglobulins and non-labile clotting factors (II, VII, IX, and X) large volumes are required to increase plasma proteins. For example, 40 ml/kg plasma is required to increase albumin concentration by 1 g/dl, which is a huge volume for a minimal benefit. The following equation can, however, be used for estimations of required volumes.

$$\text{ml plasma required} = \text{Recipient plasma volume} \times \frac{\left(\text{Desired TP} - \text{Recipient TP}\right)}{\text{Donor TP}}$$

For this equation, recipient plasma volume is usually taken as c. 5% of body weight (or 50 ml/kg). Despite the large volumes required, FP *may* be used to treat hypoproteinaemias of various causes but is not recommended as an effective or safe sole treatment. Frozen plasma, especially hyperimmune, is, however, useful in foals with failure of adequate (quality or quantity) colostral intake and transfer of passive immunity.

23.7.3.6.6 Purified Human Immunoglobulin

Provides 'immunotherapy'. Produced by pooling from thousands of donors. It has been used in humans in the treatment of various immune-mediated conditions, and in dogs to treat immune-mediated haemolytic anaemia, immune-mediated thrombocytopaenia, and in a case of drug-induced Stevens-Johnson syndrome, and in a cat to treat erythema multiforme. Immune-mediated (hypersensitivity etc.) reactions may occur, however, because the proteins are seen as 'foreign' by the recipient. High dose IgG given IV modulates immune-mediated diseases by several mechanisms, including:

- Excess IgG competes with receptors for the Fc portion of antibodies on mononuclear cells.
- Excess IgG may 'mop up' complement components and prevent them being involved in other immune-mediated reactions.

23.7.3.6.7 Platelet Rich Plasma (PRP)

To prepare this, blood must be kept warm after collection. Two spin cycles are necessary to concentrate the platelets into a small volume (about 55 ml). They must then be rested for an hour before being stored at room temperature (>18 °C) and slowly agitated. (PRP can also be spun again to produce 'platelet concentrate'.) **Platelets only survive for one to five days**. PRP contains about 10 000 platelets per unit. A dose of 5–10 ml/kg of PRP can increase the platelet count by 20 000/ml.

23.7.3.6.8 Cryoprecipitate

This is made by thawing FFP until it is slushy. Then it is centrifuged again so that a precipitate is obtained, which is stored at −18 to −20 °C for one year. This is called the cryoprecipitate (an average 'unit' is around 60 ml). The plasma above this is called cryopoor or cryo-supernatant (an average 'unit' is around 140 ml), and can be used for its non-labile clotting factor, albumin, and immunoglobulin content (stored at −18 to −20 °C for one year). Cryoprecipitate contains high concentrations (about 6 times those of FFP) of labile and non-labile clotting factors. In people, 2–4 ml/kg of cryoprecipitate is usually sufficient to stop a bleeding episode.

Additional Therapies   For thrombocytopaenia:

Vincristine increases platelet release from bone marrow, but these platelets may be 'immature' and poorly functional. Dose: 0.01–0.025 mg/kg IV every seven days as necessary.

For von Willebrand's disease:

Desmopressin acetate increases vW factor release from endothelium; factor VIII and vW factor then form a more stable complex in plasma. Dose: 1–4 μg/kg SC or IV (dilute in 20 ml saline and administer over 10 minutes) about 30–60 minutes before surgery **or** to a donor prior to blood collection. Effect lasts about 5 hours. **Tranexamic acid** or epsilon amino-caproic acid (which are lysine analogues and inhibitors of fibrinolysis) can also be given perioperatively to improve clot stability.

23.8   Devising a Fluid Therapy Plan

Fluid therapy goals:

- Replace like with like
- Replace volume for volume
- Replace fluids at a similar rate to that at which they are lost

23.8.1   Priority 1 Restoration of Circulating Volume

If the clinical signs and history indicate that there is a significant hypovolaemia, then the first priority of fluid therapy is to restore circulating volume as quickly as possible.

The old 'maxim' of fluid therapy is to replace like with like, and so it is important to assess the cause of hypovolaemia. How much fluid has been lost? What sort of fluid has been lost? The history and presentation of the patient may help to determine the type of fluid/s lost, but accurately working out the amount of fluid lost can be difficult. The clinical examination will help give an idea, but does not give a quantitative indication of the total amount of fluid lost. If you knew the body weight of the animal before a disease (e.g. diarrhoea) you could work out how much fluid had been lost by weighing it; assuming that body tissues are not usually gained or lost rapidly enough to effect such a major change in body weight. Then on the basis that **1 kg equals 1 l**, you can calculate the requirement, remembering that ECF is lost in the ratio of 3/4 from the interstitial space and 1/4 from the intravascular space. Remember

that the 1/4 intravascular volume deficit is your first concern to replace. Methods of working out deficit volumes using calculations based upon when the animal last drank or ate, number of vomits, and number of diarrhoea episodes and urinations are not always very practical.

Often estimation can be imprecise, but by continual reassessment and clinical evaluation during fluid therapy, e.g. monitoring heart rate, peripheral pulses, mentation, PCV/TS, skin pliability, CVP, urine output and specific gravity, and lactate, the clinician should have a reasonably clear picture of how the fluid therapy treatment is working.

How long will it take to repair the deficit? Normally **aim to replace intravascular volume deficit as quickly as possible,** then any remaining deficit can be replaced over a 12–36 hours period.

For the rapid restoration of large deficits of circulating volume, colloids, and, in some circumstances, hypertonic saline, may be advocated. If isotonic crystalloids are chosen instead to achieve the same goal, then much larger volumes are usually required. See below for more discussion on replacement rates.

In practice, you should administer the chosen fluid until the clinical signs of hypovolaemia diminish, e.g. improved mentation, heart rate trends towards normal, peripheral pulses become palpable, urine production normalises, etc. In reality, this usually means giving boluses (over 10–15 minutes) of 10–20 ml/kg isotonic crystalloids (or 2.5–5 ml/kg colloids or hypertonic saline) [use the lower end of these dose ranges for cats], and repeating (beware multiple repeats of hypertonic saline as hypernatraemia may develop) until the patient and its evaluations improve.

23.8.2   Priority 2 Replace Remaining Deficit

Once the priority of dealing with hypovolaemia has been taken care of (and hopefully tissue oxygen delivery has been restored), one can set about restoring any remaining fluid imbalances, which can be done over 12–36 hours. Note: very rapid administration of fluids results in rapid renal excretion and loss of the renal medullary concentration gradient, so-called renal medullary wash-out.

If circumstances in the practice (e.g. staffing levels) are limited, then there is nothing wrong with replacing the remaining deficit in two or three aliquots, but try to administer the fluids over as many hours as possible to allow the animal to redistribute and fully utilise the fluids administered. It may be more convenient to administer the fluids over eight hours when the patient and its IV cannula can be regularly checked than to leave it overnight, unobserved where the cannula may block or be pulled out.

Aim to restore oral fluid intake as soon as possible to reduce the complications of intravenous catheterisation and to help retain normal gut function. Commercially available electrolyte-glucose-amino acid solutions can be offered and may also be administered by naso-oesophageal tubes if deemed necessary.

Once the type of fluid deficit has been identified, the most appropriate fluid can be chosen. As stated earlier, the most common fluid lost is ECF, so Hartmann's solution can be a useful first choice. In cases of pure dehydration, however, 5% dextrose (in water) is usually preferred.

23.8.3 Priority 3 Cater for Maintenance Requirements Plus Ongoing Losses

All animals need water. The total daily water loss is made up from sensible (urinary loss, which in the healthy kidneys can be adjusted down to the minimum obligatory urine volume needed to excrete nitrogenous waste products, to conserve water) and insensible losses (inevitable losses of water, e.g. respiration, defecation, and sweating).

The normal maintenance requirement for a healthy animal is c. 2 ml/kg/h or c. 50 ml/kg/day. In practical terms, this means a 25 kg dog requires 50 ml/h or about 1.2 l/day; a 500 kg horse requires c. 1 l/h or 24 l/day.

The most suitable 'maintenance' fluids are different to the most suitable 'resuscitation/replacement' fluids. Whilst we need to maintain all the fluid compartments, the largest compartment in mature animals is the intracellular compartment as it contains the most amount of water. Intracellular fluid is very different to ECF in terms of, particularly, its Na^+, K^+, and Mg^{2+} concentrations. Also the concentrations of Na^+ and K^+ in urine are different to the ECF, e.g. urine Na^+ is 40 mmol/l (compared with c. 135–140 mmol/l in plasma) and urine K^+ is 20 mmol/l (compared with c. 4.5 mmol/l in plasma). For maintenance therapy, therefore, water, K^+, and Mg^{2+} requirements are greater than those of Na^+ (especially if the animal is not eating).

All this means that the use of Hartmann's solution or 0.9% NaCl for maintenance provides far too much Na^+ (although a healthy kidney can cope with Na^+ excess) and insufficient K^+ (but the kidney is an obligate K^+ excretor), so eventually Hartmann's solution or 0.9% NaCl will produce hypokalaemia if the animal is not eating, and may promote the development of hypernatraemia and hyperchloraemia (with metabolic acidosis). Magnesium is lost similarly to potassium, yet we are often poor at addressing our patients' magnesium requirements, and many fluids contain no magnesium. Some solutions, such as Plasma-Lyte 56 + 5% glucose, and Normosol M™, however, which contain magnesium concentrations close to normal plasma, are becoming increasingly available to veterinarians.

Otherwise, maintenance solutions can be made by adding 20–30 mEq/l potassium to 0.18% (normal/5) NaCl with 4% dextrose, or by alternating the administration of 1 'bag' of Hartmann's solution with 2 'bags' 5% dextrose, (in water) where all of these 'bags' have potassium supplemented to a final K^+ concentration of 20–30 mEq/l. (Do not exceed 0.5 mEq K^+/kg/h.)

In many cases requiring fluid therapy, however, there may also be abnormal ongoing losses (e.g. diarrhoea, exudates). Normally these ongoing losses are similar in composition to ECF and so solutions like Hartmann's solution, or similar, can be administered. Beware in all cases with large protein losses.

23.9 'Surgical Maintenance' Rates of IV Fluids for Patients under Anaesthesia

The administration of intravenous fluids to animals under anaesthesia has been justified because:

- The animal has been starved pre-anaesthesia (and often animals will not drink if they do not eat), and it is also unlikely to drink for a few hours post-surgery.
- Insensible losses continue and extra evaporative losses and mild haemorrhagic losses may be incurred during surgery.
- Arterial blood pressure often falls during anaesthesia due to the cardiovascular depressant effects (e.g. negative inotropic and vasorelaxant effects) of many of the sedative and anaesthetic agents used.
- Additional abnormal losses may be incurred such as increased urine production and sweating after α2 agonist use.

Historically, it was commonplace to provide a 'surgical maintenance rate' of five times normal maintenance for the first hour (i.e. 10 ml/kg/h; e.g. 5 l/h for a 500 kg horse), and then for the following hours this rate was reduced to 5 ml/kg/h, as long as there were no increased surgical losses. Recently, however, following medical evidence, it appears that a more conservative rate, nearer **5 ml/kg/h for dogs and 3 ml/kg/h for cats** (unless the animal was hypovolaemic before anaesthesia) should be less detrimental (in terms of potential fluid overload and tissue oedema) for a surgical maintenance rate. Also the CEPSAF study has shown increased complications with fluid therapy in cats; however, whether the fluid therapy itself was the problem (perhaps one of relative overdosage?), or just a marker of poor health, was not conclusively determined.

Fluid overload with crystalloids has potential detrimental consequences. Body weight gain is documented and is related to generalised tissue oedema. This can result in cardiopulmonary dysfunction (related to myocardial and pulmonary oedema), GI dysfunction (post-operative ileus and increased risk of anastomotic dehiscence), abdominal compartment syndrome, AKI (e.g. renal oedema within the tight renal capsule can compromise renal perfusion), hepatic dysfunction, cerebral dysfunction (may be a factor in post-op delirium), impaired haemostasis, and impaired wound healing.

23.10 Brief Notes on Fluid Therapy for Trauma/Haemorrhagic Shock

See also Chapter 26 on shock. Total blood volume for dogs is 80–90 ml/kg. Total blood volume for cats is 45–65 ml/kg.

Following (substantial) blood loss, hypovolaemic animals normally present with tachycardia, pale mucous membranes, and cool extremities. Peripheral pulses may be harder to feel. Pain and anxiety can exacerbate the tachycardia. Following acute blood loss, the PCV will not change appreciably for four to six hours. After this time interval, if no fluids are given, the PCV will gradually decrease following fluid shifts into the intravascular space from the interstitium (so-called 'transcapillary refill'); the total protein tends not to reduce much because protein (albumin) is mobilised from the interstitial space along with water.

Most healthy animals can easily withstand the acute loss of 15–25% of total blood volume. Most of these would do fine without fluid therapy as long as oral intake can be maintained. However, by giving fluids, you can reduce the chances of long-term patient morbidity (e.g. early renal problems). **Most healthy animals can survive, at least in the short term (hours), acute loss of about 40% of total blood volume**. However, these are the patients that may struggle to survive in the long term if you do not intervene with some supportive fluid therapy.

Heart rate increase, arterial ('centrally'-measured) blood pressure decrease, and CVP decrease may not become very obvious until blood loss reaches 30–40% of total blood volume. Some animals with significant hypovolaemia may present with bradycardia, which is usually a sign of decompensation.

The following ready reckoner is often quoted:

- 10–15% blood loss, replace with crystalloids
- 15–25% blood loss, replace with colloids
- >25–30% blood loss, replace with blood

Beware anaemic animals. Also, it is often stated that under anaesthesia, blood loss much over 15% of total blood volume should be replaced with blood, as patients are less tolerant of reduced tissue oxygen delivery when under general anaesthesia. This may be debatable as blood transfusion is not without its problems.

It can be hard to judge the actual volume of blood loss, but fluid therapy is aimed at correcting the clinical signs associated with hypovolaemia, and therefore high sympathetic tone. In the immediate situation, fluid therapy is aimed at reducing tachycardia and restoring the peripheral circulation (mucous membranes pinken up, extremities warm up, peripheral pulses become palpable again). Certainly within the first few hours, urine output (a good indicator of organ perfusion) should be restored, and any previously increased lactate should be returning to normal (which indicates restoration of tissue oxygen delivery and consumption). In the acute situation, hypovolaemia and the stress response (with increased ADH release) will reduce urine output, so do not necessarily expect to re-establish this within the first 60 minutes of instituting fluid therapy.

Fluid choices:

- Crystalloids: normal saline, Hartmann's solution, hypertonic saline.
- Colloids: gelatins, tetrastarch; also plasma (see below).
- Blood and blood products: fresh whole blood, stored blood, packed red cells; plasma (fresh, fresh frozen, or frozen).

With normal saline or Hartmann's solution, only about a quarter of the volume administered intravenously remains in the intravascular space after about 30–60 minutes, and then the interstitium starts to get soggy. Also, in order to maintain an increase in the circulating volume of X ml, four times X ml will need to be given, which takes a relatively long time to administer. (Dextrose-based solutions are really only a way of giving pure water into the bloodstream without lysing red cells; and such solutions partition between all fluid compartments, so are not good when trying to restore the intravascular, circulating blood volume acutely).

Colloids are, therefore, often preferred because to restore X ml of intravascular volume, only X ml of colloid solution needs to be administered (as long as the ESL is healthy). For colloids, 20 ml/kg is often suggested as a safe maximum daily dose because of the problems of possible over-expansion of plasma volume, such as haemodilutional anaemia and coagulopathy. However, manufacturers have quoted doses of nearer 30 ml/kg/day for pentastarches and 50 ml/kg/day for tetrastarches because of their supposedly lower interference with coagulation. Nevertheless, as AKI also appears related to total doses, caution would be wise. Therefore, if doses in excess of 20 ml/kg/day are seemingly required, perhaps consider why, and contemplate the use of blood products instead.

With haemorrhagic shock, fluid therapy can also begin by administering **bolus volumes of around 1/5–1/4 of the animal's normal blood volume**.

As a **very general rule for boluses**, it is **safe to start with 10–20 ml/kg crystalloids** (nearer 10 ml/kg for cats, or give slower) **or 2.5–5 ml/kg colloids** (nearer 2.5 ml/kg for cats) as your first fluid bolus, then reassess. Further boluses may be required. In emergencies, the first bolus (and also subsequent boluses, if necessary), can be administered over around 5 minutes (more rapid administration can actually [transiently] worsen hypotension). Should several boluses be required, and each bolus, or at least each successive bolus after the first, be given over 10–15 minutes, then up to 80 ml/kg crystalloids can be given in 1 hour, which is reminiscent of the 'shock dose' (i.e. 'one blood volume'), given over time (usually 'within the first hour') until a good response is observed.

Hypertonic saline behaves a little like a colloid in the first instance because of the volume expansion it causes. (Care should be taken with its administration if bleeding is uncontrolled, as further haemorrhage is promoted by the haemodynamic improvement.) However, eventually fluid shifts occur, so its final effects become more like those of normal saline although there has been some intracellular (and interstitial tissue) dehydration. It should be followed by administration of isotonic fluids, and even 'hypotonic' fluids like dextrose-containing solutions. The immediate volume expansion effect of hypertonic saline can be 'prolonged' by addition of a colloid.

All non-sanguineous fluids will cause some degree of haemodilution. Try not to let the PCV fall much below about 21–28% ([Hb] around 7–9 g/dl), or you risk reducing tissue oxygen delivery, especially if the patient is only breathing room air. Mild haemodilution, however, to a PCV of around 21–28% actually improves tissue oxygenation by reducing blood viscosity and the resistance to blood flow.

23.11 Fluids for Sepsis

With notes of caution regarding colloids, will crystalloids suffice to restore and maintain blood pressure and intravascular volume status to ensure essential organ perfusion without promoting fluid overload and the formation of oedema? The common belief that three to four times more crystalloids than colloids are needed to achieve similar hemodynamic effects is not supported by clinical observation in critically ill humans (where the ESL is unhealthy), which concurs with the results of several recent large randomised clinical trials. These trials, which compared resuscitation based on colloids or crystalloids in septic patients, found only 1–1.4 times more need for crystalloids than colloids as the maximal reported difference; a lot less than the '4 times' previously suggested. This does not mean, however, that less colloids are required, but rather that both colloids and crystalloids can similarly escape the intravascular space when leaky capillaries are present (i.e. when the ESL is no longer intact).

This highlights the need for a goal-directed approach that involves frequent reassessment of the clinical condition. Of note, in the studies this statement refers to, albumin 20% was used concurrently for treatment in these patients. Research into the role of the EG shows that it is sensitive to the effects of colloids, and synthetic colloids may have a detrimental effect on vascular integrity, whilst albumin appears to play a homeostatic role. A complementary school of thought to this suggests avoiding excessive volumes of fluids and adding vasopressor or positive inotrope therapy (see Chapter 25), if indicated, at a much earlier stage. The role of hydroscortisone in facilitating responsiveness to catecholamines and in EG protection may also warrant revisiting.

Further Reading

Adamantos, S., Boag, A., and Hughes, D. (2005). Clinical use of a haemoglobin-based oxygen carrying solution in dogs and cats. *In Practice* 27: 399–405.

Adamik, K.N., Yozova, I.D., and Regenschiet, N. (2015). Controversies in the use of hydroxyethyl starch solutions in small animal emergency and critical care. *Journal of Veterinary Emergency and Critical Care* 25: 20–47.

Alphonsus, C.S. and Rodseth, R.N. (2014). The endothelial glycocalyx: a review of the vascular barrier. *Anaesthesia* 69: 777–784.

Benton, D., Braun, H., Cobo, J.C. et al. (2014). Executive summary and conclusions from the European Hydration Institute expert conference on human hydration, health and performance. *Nutrition Reviews* 73 (S2): 148–150.

Bishop, Y. (2005). Drugs affecting nutrition and body fluids. In: *The Veterinary Formulary*, 6e, 411–413. London, UK: Bishop Y. Pharmaceutical Press. (**Discusses oral rehydration solutions**.).

Boer, C., Bossers, S.M., and Koning, N.J. (2018). Choice of fluid type: physiological concepts and perioperative indications. *British Journal of Anaesthesia* 120: 384–396.

Boscan, P., Watson, Z., and Steffey, E.P. (2007). Plasma colloid osmotic pressure and total protein trends in horses during anesthesia. *Veterinary Anaesthesia and Analgesia* 34: 275–283.

Boyd, C.J., Claus, M.A., Raisis, A.L. et al. (2019). Evaluation of biomarkers of kidney injury following 4% succinylated gelatin and 6% hydroxyethyl starch 130/0.4 administration in a canine hemorrhagic shock model. *Journal of Veterinary Emergency and Critical Care* 29: 132–142.

Brodbelt, D.C., Pfeiffer, D.U., Young, L.E., and Wood, J.L.N. (2007). Risk factors for anaesthetic-related death in cats: results from the confidential enquiry into perioperative small animal fatalities (CEPSAF). *British Journal of Anaesthesia* 99: 617–123.

Bumpus, S.E., Haskins, S.C., and Kass, P.H. (1998). Effect of synthetic colloids on refractometric readings of total solids. *Journal of Veterinary Emergency and Critical Care* 8: 21–26.

Cambournac, M., Goy-Thollot, I., Viole, A. et al. (2018). Sonographic assessment of volaemia: development and validation of a new method in dogs. *Journal of Small Animal Practice* 59: 174–182.

Cazzolli, D. and Prittie, J. (2015). The crystalloid-colloid debate: consequences of resuscitation fluid selection in veterinary critical care. *Journal of Veterinary Emergency and Critical Care* 25: 6–19.

Chappell, D., Jacob, M., Hofmann-Kiefer, K. et al. (2007). Hydrocortisone preserves the vascular barrier by protecting the endothelial glycocalyx. *Anesthesiology* 107: 776–784.

Chappell, D., Jacob, M., Hofmann-Kiefer, K. et al. (2008). A rational approach to perioperative fluid management. *Anesthesiology* 109: 723–740.

Chappell, D., Westphal, M., and Jacob, M. (2009). The impact of the glycocalyx on microcirculatory oxygen distribution in critical illness. *Current Opinion in Anaesthesiology* 22: 155–162.

Cooley, C.M., Quimby, J.M., Caney, S.M.A., and Sieberg, L.G. (2018). Survey of owner subcutaneous fluid practices in cats with chronic kidney disease. *Journal of Feline Medicine and Surgery* 20: 884–890.

Culler, C.A., Iazbik, C., and Guillaumin, J. (2017). Comparison of albumin, colloid osmotic pressure, von Willebrand factor, and coagulation factors in canine cryopoor plasma, cryoprecipitate and fresh frozen plasma. *Journal of Veterinary Emergency and Critical Care* 27: 638–644.

Culler, C.A., Balakrishnan, A., Yaxley, P.E., and Guillaumin, J. (2019). Clinical use of cryopoor plasma continuous rate infusion in critically ill, hypoalbuminemic dogs. *Journal of Veterinary Emergency and Critical Care* 29: 314–320.

Cunha, M.G.M.C.M., Freitas, G.C., Carregaro, A.B. et al. (2010). Renal and cardiorespiratory effects of treatment with lactated Ringer's solution or physiologic saline (0.9% NaCl) solution in cats with experimentally-induced urethral obstruction. *American Journal of Veterinary Research* 71: 840–846.

Davis, H., Jensen, T., Knowles, P. et al. (2013). AAHA/AAFP fluid therapy guidelines for dogs and cats. *Journal of the American Animal Hospital Association* 49: 149–159.

DiBartola, S.P. (ed.) (2012). *Fluid, Electrolyte and Acid–Base Disorders in Small Animal Practice*, 4e. Missouri, USA: Elsevier Saunders.

Doherty, M. and Buggy, D.J. (2012). Intraoperative fluids: how much is too much? *British Journal of Anaesthesia* 109: 69–79.

Driessen, B., Jahr, J.S., Lurie, F., and Gunther, R.A. (2006). Effects of isovolemic resuscitation with hemoglobin-based oxygen carrier glutamer-200 (bovine) on systemic and mesenteric perfusion and oxygenation in a canine model of hemorrhagic shock: a comparison with 6% hetstarch solution and shed blood. *Veterinary Anaesthesia and Analgesia* 33: 368–380.

Dugdale, A. (2008). Shifts in the haemoglobin-oxygen dissociation curve: can we manipulate P_{50} to good effect? *The Veterinary Journal* 175: 12–13.

Edwards, M.R. and Mythen, M.G. (2014). Fluid therapy in critical illness. *Extreme Physiology & Medicine* 3: 16. https://doi.org/10.1186/2046-7648-3-16.

Handy, J.M. and Soni, N. (2008). Physiological effects of hyperchloraemia and acidosis. *Brisith Journal of Anaesthesia* 101: 141–150.

Hart, S., Cserti-Gazdewich, C.N., and McCluskey, S.A. (2015). Red cell transfusion and the immune system. *Anaesthesia* 70 (S1): 38–45.

Hayes, G., Benedicenti, L., and Mathews, K. (2016). Retrospective cohort study on the incidence of acute kidney injury and death following hydroxyethyl starch (HES 10% 250/0.5/5:1) administration in dogs (2007–2010). *Journal of Veterinary Emergency and Critical Care* 26: 35–40.

Hollis, A. and Corley, K. (2007). Practical guide to fluid therapy in neonatal foals. *In Practice* 29: 130–137.

Hughes, D. (2000). Transvascular fluid dynamics. *Veterinary Anaesthesia and Analgesia* 27: 63–69.

Hughes, D. (2001). Fluid therapy with artificial colloids: complications and controversies. *Veterinary Anaesthesia and Analgesia* 28: 111–118.

Jahr, J.S., Akha, A.S., and Holtby, R.J. (2012). Crosslinked, polymerized and PEG-conjugated hemoglobin-based oxygen carriers: clinical safety and efficacy of recent and current products. *Current Drug Discovery Techniques* 9: 158–165.

Jungheinrich, C. (2007). The starch family: are they all equal? Pharmacokinetics and pharmacodynamics of hydroxyethyl starches. *Transfusion Alternatives in Transfusion Medicine* 9: 152–163.

Kisielewicz, C. and Self, I.A. (2014). Canine and feline blood transfusions: controversies and recent advances in administration practices. *Veterinary Anaesthesia and Analgesia* 41: 233–242.

Marik, P. and Bellomo, R. (2016). A rational approach to fluid therapy in sepsis. *British Journal of Anaesthesia* 116: 329–349.

McLean, D.J. and Shaw, A.D. (2018). Intravenous fluids: effects on renal outcomes. *British Journal of Anaesthesia* 120: 397–402.

McDevitt, R.I., Ruaux, G.C., and Baltzer, W.I. (2011). Influence of transfusion technique on survival of autologous red blood cells in the dog. *Journal of Veterinary Emergency and Critical Care* 21: 209–216.

Meneghini, C., Rabozzi, R., and Franic, P. (2016). Correlation of the ratio of caudal vena cava diameter and aorta diameter with systolic pressure variation in anesthetized dogs. *American Journal of Veterinary Research* 77: 137–143.

Morris, C., Boyd, A., and Reynolds, N. (2009). Should we really be more 'balanced' in our fluid prescribing? Editorial. *Anaesthesia* 64: 703–705. **(An excellent discussion of the dogma that surrounds 'fluid therapy'.)**.

Muir, W. (2017). Effect of intravenously administered crystalloid solutions on acid–base balance in domestic animals. *Journal of Veterinary Internal Medicine* 31: 1371–1381.

Muir, W.M. and Wellman, M.L. (2003). Hemoglobin solutions and tissue oxygenation. *Journal of Veterinary Internal Medicine* 17: 127–135.

Nappert, G. (2008). Review of current thinking on calf oral rehydration. *Cattle Practice* 16: 174–182.

Noel-Morgan, J. and Muir, W.M. (2018). Anesthesia-associated relative hypovolemia: mechaniams, monitoring and treatment considerations. *Frontiers in Veterinary Science* 5: 53. https://doi.org/10.3389/fvets/2018.00053.

Nuttall, T.J. and Malham, T. (2004). Successful intravenous human immunoglobulin treatment of drug-induced Stevens-Johnson syndrome in a dog. *Journal of Small Animal Practice* 45: 357–361.

Pries, A.R., Secomb, T.W., and Gaehtgens, P. (2000). The endothelial surface layer. *Plugers Archiv: European Journal of Physiology* 440: 653–666.

Priolo, V., Masucci, M., Spada, E. et al. (2018). Naturally occurring antibodies in cats against dog erythrocyte antigens and vice versa. *Journal of Feline Medicine and Surgery* 20: 690–695.

Reddi, B.A.J. (2013). Why is saline so acidic (and does it matter)? *International Journal of Medical Sciences* 10: 747–750.

Reineke, E.L., Rees, C., and Drobatz, K. (2016). Prediction of systolic blood pressure using peripheral pulse palpation in cats. *Journal of Veterinary Emergency and Critical Care* 26: 52–57.

Reitsma, S., Slaaf, D.W., Vink, H. et al. (2007). The endothelial glycocalyx: compostion, functions and visualization. *European Journal of Physiology* 454: 345–359.

Rhodes, A., Evans, L.E., Alhazzani, W. et al. (2017). Surviving Sepsis Campaign: International Guidelines for management of sepsis and septic shock 2016. *Intensive Care Medicine* 43: 304–377.

Santoro Beer, K. and Silverstein, D.C. (2015). Controversies in the use of fresh frozen plasma in critically ill small animal patients. *Journal of Veterinary Emergency and Critical Care* 25: 101–106.

Santry, H.P. and Alam, H.B. (2010). Fluid resuscitation: past, present and the future. *Shock* 33: 229–241.

Schmid, S.M., Cianciolo, R.E., Drobatz, K.J. et al. (2019). Postmortem evaluation of renal tubular vacuolization in critically ill dogs. *Journal of Veterinary Emergency and Critical Care* 29: 279–287.

Schortgen, F., Lacherade, J.C., Bruneel, F. et al. (2001). Effects of hydroxyethylstarch and gelatin on renal function in severe sepsis: a multicentre randomised study. *Lancet* 24: 911–916.

Schortgen, F. and Brochard, L. (2012). Withdrawing synthetic colloids in sepsis is possible and safe. *Critical Care Medicine* 40: 2709–2710.

Shah, A., Stanworth, S.J., and McKechnie, S.M. (2015). Evidence and triggers for the transfusion of blood and blood products. *Anaesthesia* 70 (S1): 10–19.

Shander, A., Javidroozi, M., Ozawa, S., and Hare, G.M.T. (2011). What is really dangerous: anaemia or transfusion? *British Journal of Anaesthesia* 107 (S1): i41–i59.

Silverstein, D.C., Aldrich, J., Haskins, S.C. et al. (2005). Assessment of changes in blood volume in response to resuscitative fluid administration in dogs. *Journal of Veterinary Emergency and Critical Care* 15: 185–192.

Soni, N. (2009). British consensus guidelines on intravenous fluid therapy for adult surgical patients (GIFTASUP) – Cassandra's view. Editorial. *Anaesthesia* 64: 235–238. **(An interesting overview of some of the controversies surrounding fluid therapy.)**.

Sparrow, R.L. (2012). Time to revisit red blood cell additive solutions and storage conditions: a role for 'omics' analyses. *Blood Transfusion* 10 (suppl.2): s7–s11.

Strandvik, G.F. (2009). Hypertonic saline in critical care: a review of the literature and guidelines for use in hypotensive states and raised intracranial pressure. *Anaesthesia* 64: 990–1003.

Van Galen, G. and Hallowell, G. (2019). Hydroxyethyl starches in equine medicine. *Journal of Veterinary Emergency and Critical Care* 29: 349–359.

Weinbaum, S., Tarbell, J.M., and Damiano, E.R. (2007). The structure and function of the endothelial glycocalyx layer. *Annual Review of Biomedical Engineering* 9: 121–167.

West, E., Pettitt, R., Jones, R.S. et al. (2013). Acid–base and electrolyte balance following administration of three crystalloid solution in dogs undergoing elective orthopaedic surgery. *Veterinary Anaesthesia and Analgesia* 40: 482–493.

Westphal, M., James, M.F.M., Kozek-Langenecker, S. et al. (2009). Hydroxyethyl starches: different products – different effects. *Anesthesiology* 111: 187–202.

Wilson, C.R., Pashmakova, M.B., Heinz, J.A. et al. (2017). Biochemical evaluation of storage lesion in canine packed erythrocytes. *Journal of Small Animal Practice* 58: 678–684.

Woodcock, T.E. and Woodcock, T.M. (2012). Revised Starling equation and the glycocalyx model of transvascular fluid exchange: an improved paradigm for prescribing intravenous fluid therapy. *British Journal of Anaesthesia* 108: 384–394.

Self-test Section

1 What is the physiological role of the endothelial glycocalyx?

2 List the current concerns regarding synthetic colloid use.

24

Electrolytes

LEARNING OBJECTIVES

- To be familiar with the causes and effects of common electrolyte imbalances.
- To be able to devise and discuss the therapeutic options.

24.1 Introduction

Fluid therapy can also be used to treat electrolyte imbalances. The main electrolytes (ions) in the body are sodium, potassium, chloride, calcium, magnesium, and phosphate. They are collectively responsible for maintaining normal cellular function, and the concentrations of these ions are normally controlled by the body's homeostatic mechanisms to within very narrow ranges. During many disease processes, the normal electrolyte balances may be disturbed when their homeostatic mechanisms become impaired or overwhelmed.

Extracellular fluid (intravascular and interstitial) contains large amounts of sodium and chloride ions, whereas the main intracellular ions are potassium, magnesium, and phosphate. The approximate distribution of these electrolytes between intracellular and extracellular fluids is summarised in Table 24.1.

Our understanding of the importance of electrolytes and electrophysiology is steadily expanding. This, along with our understanding of acid–base balance has led to the development of anion gap, strong ion difference, and strong ion gap approaches, which are all attempts to explain why electrolyte imbalances occur during metabolic disturbances (see Chapter 21 on blood gas analysis). It is outside the scope of this book to discuss electrolyte imbalances in great detail, however, the main electrolyte imbalances are briefly described below and are summarised in the tables.

24.2 Sodium

The main extracellular cation and important for maintenance of extracellular fluid (ECF) osmolarity and volume (along with chloride). Important for electrical activity in excitable cells. Involved in regulation of potassium, chloride, and bicarbonate, and therefore in acid–base balance too. Sodium imbalances are listed in Table 24.2.

When hyponatraemia or hypernatraemia is present, the following equation can be used to predict the effect of the chosen fluids to help change the blood sodium concentration by no more than 0.5 mmol/kg/h:

$$\text{Change in serum}\left[\text{Na}^+\right] = \frac{\text{Infusate}\left[\text{Na}^+\right] - \text{Serum}\left[\text{Na}^+\right]}{\left(\text{Body mass}\left(\text{kg}\right) \times 0.6\right) + 1}$$

Note that [Na$^+$] is in mmol/l. The equation therefore calculates by how much the serum sodium concentration will increase or decrease should 1 l of the chosen fluid be given. When this is known, the volume of that particular fluid to give over one hour, to ensure only 0.5 mmol/l/h increase or decrease in sodium is achieved, can then be calculated. The sodium concentrations of the various commonly used fluids can be found in Chapter 23.

Veterinary Anaesthesia: Principles to Practice, Second Edition. Alexandra H. A. Dugdale, Georgina Beaumont, Carl Bradbrook, and Matthew Gurney.
Companion website: www.wiley.com/go/dugdale/veterinary-anaesthesia

Table 24.1 Electrolyte concentrations for common species.

Electrolyte	Intracellular concentration (mEq/l)	Extracellular concentration (mEq/l)
Na^+	10–12	135–146 (human)
		136 (horse)
		144 (cattle)
		140–150 (dog)
		150–160 (cat)
K^+	140	3.5–5.5
Ca^{2+}	10	4–5.5 mEq/l ($\approx$2–2.75 mmol/l) total (human)
		2.2–2.8 mmol/l total (1.2–1.5 mmol/l ionised) (dog)
		2.0–2.6 mmol/l total (1.1–1.4 mmol/l ionised) (cat)
Mg^{2+}	40	1.5–2.5 mEq/l ($\approx$0.7–1.2 mmol/l) total
		0.9–1.2 mEq/l ($\approx$0.45–0.6 mmol/l) ionised
Cl^-	4	96–106 (human)
		100 (horse)
		103 (cattle)
		110 (dog)
		120 (cat)
Inorganic phosphates	100	1.4-2.6 mEq/l ($\approx$ 0.8–1.5 mmol/l) (human)
		0.8–1.8 mmol/l (dog)
		0.8–1.9 mmol/l (cat)

Note that values may vary slightly between laboratories.

24.3 Potassium

The major intracellular cation (about 95% of total body potassium is found within cells, with myocytes containing 60–75% of total body potassium). Important for maintenance of cell osmolarity and electroneutrality. Important for electrical activity in excitable cells. Involved in acid–base regulation. Beware blood samples taken into Na^+K^+-EDTA as potassium values will be falsely elevated. *Serum* potassium concentration can be around 0.5 mmol/l higher than *plasma* potassium concentration because potassium is released from platelets during blood clotting. If thrombocytosis is present, then serum potassium can be increased more substantially.

In the situation of acidosis, there are excess H^+ ions outside the cells. These try to enter the cells by the proton/potassium ion transcellular exchange system (Figure 24.1) by which ECF pH can be quite well buffered, but in exchange, K^+ ions must leave the cells to maintain electrochemical neutrality. The opposite happens if alkalosis exists. Although there is still much debate, it seems that respiratory acidosis has a more profound impact on ECF potassium concentration, $[K^+]$, than metabolic acidosis. With respiratory acidosis, for each 0.1 unit of pH decrease, the $[K^+]$ can increase by 0.2–1.7 mmol/l. For alkaloses, both respiratory and metabolic, with each 0.1 unit of pH increase, the $[K^+]$ tends to decrease by $\leq$0.4 mmol/l.

The potassium content of red blood cells (RBCs) varies according to the number and activity of sodium/potassium pumps in the membranes of mature RBCs, which is genetically determined (Table 24.3). 'High potassium' (HK) red cells (which lack Na^+/K^+-ATP-ase pumps) are found in humans, horses, some cattle and sheep, and certain dog breeds such as the Japanese Akitas and Shiba Inu; the others are 'low potassium' (LK) breeds. To maintain electroneutrality, the sodium content of HK RBC is lowered. Interestingly, the red cells of many species tend to be of the HK type for the first few months of life, but become LK type red cells as the animals mature. Furthermore, reticulocytes also have higher intracellular potassium concentrations. Should blood samples from HK type animals, or young animals, or those with large numbers of reticulocytes, suffer haemolysis, the potassium concentration measured will be falsely elevated. In stored blood, potassium can slowly leak from red cells as the availability of ATP declines and the pumps fail (and the red cells swell slightly as water enters, following sodium); this can lead to an increase in the plasma potassium concentration.

Table 24.2 Sodium disturbances.

Type of imbalance	Common causes	Clinical signs	Treatment
Hypernatraemia ($Na^+ > 160$–170 mmol/l in dogs; or >175 mmol/l in cats) (Associated with 'uncorrected' hyperchloraemia)	*Primary water loss*: Severe panting (high environmental temp., hyperthermia) Primary hypodipsia Water deprivation Diabetes insipidus (central or nephrogenic) *Hypotonic fluid loss*: Severe vomiting Diarrhoea Intestinal obstruction Effusions (intracavitary; burns) Chronic renal failure Osmotic diuresis (diabetes mellitus; following mannitol administration) *Excess sodium gain*: Salt poisoning Iatrogenic (hypertonic saline; sodium bicarbonate therapy) Hyperaldosteronism (Conn's syndrome or spironolactone therapy) Hyperadrenocorticism (Cushing's disease)	Severity of clinical signs is highly related to rapidity of development of hypernatraemia and its severity/increase in osmolarity. Neurological signs predominate because of changes in CNS osmolarity. Patient may be hypo-, normo-, or relatively hyper-volaemic. Irritability, confusion, dullness, lethargy, anorexia, seizures, coma Muscle weakness, myoclonus Increased thirst	Slow correction with 5% dextrose or 0.18% NaCl in 4% dextrose (4 ml/kg/h) Address the underlying cause **Rate of change of plasma sodium should not exceed 0.5 mmol/l/h** If hypernatraemia is due to pure water loss, the water deficit can be calculated by: Free water deficit (l) $= 0.6 \times$ Body Mass (kg) x $$\frac{([Na^+]_{current} - [Na^+]_{normal})}{[Na^+]_{normal}}$$ Note that the term $[0.6 \times$ Body Mass$]$ is an estimation of the total body water in mature patients. For neonates, 0.8 can be used in place of 0.6
Hyponatraemia ($Na^+ < 120$ mmol/l in dogs; or <130 mmol/l in cats) (Associated with 'uncorrected' hypochloraemia) Pseudohyponatraemia (underestimation of sodium concentration) can occur when hyperlipaemia or hyperproteinaemia are present (plasma osmolarity is normal)	*Primary water gain*: Psychogenic polydipsia *Hypotonic fluid gain*: Iatrogenic (hypotonic IV fluids, i.e. fluid low in Na) Uroabdomen SIADH (syndrome of inappropriate ADH secretion [Schwarz-Barter syndrome]: CNS disorders, prolonged positive pressure ventilation [PPV] /Positive End-Expiratory Pressure) Water excess with lesser sodium excess, e.g. congestive cardiac failure; hepatic failure; nephrotic syndrome *Excess sodium loss*: Duodenal vomiting Diarrhoea Effusions (intracavitary; burns) Severe sweating (horses) Addison's disease Diuresis *Redistribution*: Gain of other osmotic particles in ECF, e.g. hyperglycaemia, mannitol infusion Sick cell syndrome in terminally ill patients results in Na movement into cells due to reduced activity of sodium pumps	Severity of clinical signs is related to rapidity of onset of hyponatraemia and its severity/change in osmolarity (usually a decrease, but some hyperglycaemic patients may be hyper-osmolar) Neurological signs predominate. Patient may be hypo- to hyper-volaemic. Muscle weakness, tremors Restlessness, confusion, lethargy, seizures, coma Nausea and vomiting Paralytic ileus Possibly lack of thirst	0.9% NaCl (4 ml/kg/h) Hypertonic saline? Address the underlying cause **Rate of change of plasma sodium should not exceed 0.5 mmol/l/h**

Table 24.3 The potassium and sodium content of red blood cells.

Species	RBC [K$^+$] (mmol/l)	RBC [Na$^+$] (mmol/l)
Human	104–155	10–21
Swine	100–124	11–19
Sheep LK	8–39	74–121
Sheep HK	60–88	10–43
Cattle LK	7–37	72–102
Cattle HK	70	15
Horse	80–140	4–16
Dog LK	4–11	93–150
Dog HK	124	54
Cat	6–8	104–142

Table 24.4 lists potassium disturbances, whilst Table 24.5 gives the electrocardiogram (ECG) changes with potassium imbalances.

24.4 Chloride

The major ECF anion, comprising about two-thirds of total anions in ECF. Its homeostasis is closely linked with that of sodium and it is important in acid–base regulation. Measurements of serum chloride are usually corrected for possible changes in plasma free water (using a ratio of 'normal' to measured sodium concentration), so that true changes in chloride concentration can be distinguished from those occurring secondary to sodium or water changes. Table 24.6 lists chloride disturbances.

24.5 Phosphate

A major intracellular fluid anion. Organic phosphates are found mainly in cell membranes in the form of phospholipids, and hence are important for maintenance of cellular integrity. Phosphate is also important for immune function and the coagulation cascade. Inorganic phosphates are important for bone and tooth matrix (c. 85% of total body phosphates), and as intracellular compounds involved in energy metabolism (e.g. ATP, GTP), oxygen carriage by

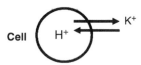

Figure 24.1 Transcellular H$^+$/K$^+$ exchange.

haemoglobin (i.e. 2,3-diphosphoglycerate [2,3-DPG]) and buffering (14–15% of total body phosphates), with only c. 1% of inorganic phosphates being found in the ECF. Of the inorganic phosphate (HPO$_4^{2-}$: H$_2$PO$_4^-$ in a ratio of around 4:1 at pH 7.4) in ECF, 10–20% is protein-bound and the remainder is either complexed (with sodium, magnesium, or calcium), or present as the free anion. The relatively small percentage of phosphate which is albumin-bound means that changes in plasma albumin concentration have little effect on phosphate concentration. The pKa of the phosphate buffer system is 6.8, facilitating its effectiveness as the most important intracellular buffer. Table 24.7 lists phosphate disturbances.

24.6 Calcium

A major cation in the body. Almost 99% of the body's total calcium is found within bones and teeth, where it is important to maintain structural integrity. Calcium is involved in maintenance of membrane integrity and permeability. It is also important for maintenance of function in excitable cells and inter- and intra-cellular signalling, and it is an important cofactor for coagulation and some inflammatory pathways (e.g. complement cascade). In plasma, calcium is present in three forms: c. 52–56% ionised ('free' and therefore biologically active); 8–10% complexed or chelated (with phosphate, bicarbonate, sulphate, citrate, or lactate); and 34–40% protein-bound (mainly to albumin). This protein binding is affected by pH, such that alkalosis tends to lead to an increase in binding (reducing the ionised fraction but without affecting the total concentration); and acidosis leads to a reduction in protein binding so that the ionised fraction increases, but, again, the total concentration remains unchanged. In intracellular fluid, most of the calcium is protein-bound or complexed so that the ionised fraction is very low because ionised calcium is highly involved in many intracellular processes.

Total and ionised calcium concentrations can be measured in blood samples. Beware samples taken into EDTA as this chelates calcium, therefore falsely lowering the value. Heparinised samples may be diluted by the anticoagulant (if present in 'liquid' form), and therefore can also result in falsely low values. Table 24.8 lists calcium disturbances.

24.7 Magnesium

About 70% of the body's total magnesium is found in bones, alongside calcium and phosphate; c. 20% is found within muscle cells and the remaining c.10% is found in other soft tissues. Almost 99% of total body magnesium is found

Table 24.4 Potassium disturbances.

Type of imbalance	Common causes	Clinical signs	Treatment
Hyperkalaemia (K^+ > 5.5 mmol/l; esp. > 7 mmol/l)	*Increased administration:* Iatrogenic (IV fluids with high K; potassium penicillin) *Reduced excretion:* Urethral obstruction Ruptured bladder (uroabdomen) Acute renal failure (anuric/oliguric) Addison's disease Severe dehydration (reduced urine output; akin to acute pre-renal failure) Repeated drainage of large volume pleural/peritoneal effusions (e.g. chylous), can result in rapid re-effusion and hypovolaemia and although ADH secretion increases, appropriately, in the face of reduced GFR, it can result in reduced renal Na^+ reabsorption and reduced K^+ excretion Near-term pregnancy in Greyhounds Drugs: NSAIDs (reduce renin and aldosterone production); ACE inhibitors (reduce aldosterone production); potassium-sparing diuretics (reduce renal potassium excretion); heparin (inhibits aldosterone secretion); trimethoprim (inhibits renal sodium reabsorption/potassium excretion in distal nephron)	(Brady)-dysrhythmias Muscle weakness, including respiratory muscles (hypoventilation), and gastrointestinal tract (resulting in ileus) Metabolic acidosis can result from stimulation of transcellular H^+/K^+ exchange	If life-threatening **arrhythmias**, give **calcium**. Hyperkalaemia makes the equilibrium ('resting') membrane potential less negative (which inactivates some Na channels); calcium raises the threshold potential and so helps to 'restore' a more normal pattern of electrical activity in the heart. However, its effects are only transient (c. 20 min), as it tends to be taken up by cells and then sequesters inside them **10% Calcium chloride: 0.1–0.2 ml/kg IV over 5–10 min** **OR** **10% Calcium gluconate: 0.5–1.5 ml/kg IV over 5–10 min (beware boron toxicity if calcium borogluconate solutions are used)** Calcium chloride 10% contains 0.68 mmol/ml or 1.36 mEq/ml of elemental calcium; whereas calcium gluconate 10% contains only 0.225 mmol/ml or 0.45 mEq/ml of elemental calcium. Calcium borogluconate 40% contains 0.9 mmol/ml or 1.8 mEq/ml of elemental calcium. Some people prefer to give calcium gluconate/borogluconate because it is harder to overdose. Note that 10 mg elemental Ca = 0.25 mmol, = 0.5 mEq Treatment can be repeated twice, but beware calcium toxicity **Dilution and diuresis** can be considered (where there is no renal impairment) **IV fluids:** Potassium-poor fluids used to be prioritised to dilute out the potassium as much as possible, but Hartmann's solution, despite containing 5 mmol/l potassium (which is, in any case, lower than the blood concentration that is being treated), is also alkalinising and so will also correct hyperkalaemia. Saline (normal or hypertonic) solutions are 'acidifying' because they tend to dilute out the body's own bicarbonate buffer and also they add a lot of chloride. Dextrose-containing solutions may be beneficial because the dextrose may stimulate insulin release, which promotes the cellular uptake of potassium. Choices are therefore: Hartmann's solution; 0.18% NaCl in 4% dextrose; or 5% dextrose. If also hyponatraemic (e.g. Addison's), then 0.9% NaCl **Diuretics:** furosemide (loop), or osmotic, which are both K^+-losing; but beware impaired renal function
Pseudohyperkalaemia (over-estimation of potassium concentration) can occur with haemolysis (with HK red cells) or thrombocytosis			

(Continued)

Table 24.4 (Continued)

Type of imbalance	Common causes	Clinical signs	Treatment
	Redistribution: Insulin deficiency, e.g. diabetes mellitus (insulin stimulates Na^+/K^+ pump activity: partly related to, and partly unrelated to, glucose uptake by cells) Drugs: beta blockers (catecholamines stimulate β receptors to increase Na^+/K^+ pump activity); digitalis glycosides (inhibit Na^+/K^+ pump activity); succinylcholine (during depolarisation, K^+ exits cells) Acidosis (metabolic or respiratory) due to transcellular K^+/H^+ exchange Massive tissue trauma/rhabdomyolysis (including trauma, burns, post-anaesthetic myopathy, malignant hyperthermia, and crush/compartmental injuries) Tumour lysis syndrome Massive intravascular haemolysis (esp. species and breeds with high K^+ inside their red cells) Reperfusion injuries (after tourniquet or thromboemboli) Hyperkalaemic periodic paralysis (Quarter horses) Anaesthesia-related hyperkalaemia in Greyhounds *Sample error:* Using EDTA tube (which contains Na^+/K^+-EDTA)		**Correct metabolic acidosis.** If you cannot measure blood gases, then guesstimate the dose of bicarbonate to be c. 1 (–2) mmol HCO_3^- per kg body weight. Administer slowly IV (over 20 min), and not into fluids containing calcium or else calcium carbonate will precipitate. Note that a pH change of 0.1 unit, can result in a change in plasma potassium concentration of 0.6 mmol/l. Giving bicarbonate to an animal with an excess of H^+ ions, results in the production of CO_2, which then must be 'blown off'. Awake animals without pulmonary disease can do this OK; but beware anaesthetised animals, whose chemoreceptors are not as sensitive as normal because the buildup of carbon dioxide can create a respiratory acidosis **Correct any respiratory acidosis:** easier under GA when an animal's lungs can be more easily ventilated. Also, if the animal is deliberately hyperventilated, at least in the short-term (more rapid and/or deep PPV breaths than 'normal'), then a respiratory alkalosis can be produced, which helps encourage H^+ ions to leave cells, and therefore K^+ ions (and also Mg^{2+} ions) to enter them **Glucose (dextrose) +/– insulin** (soluble insulin) Insulin promotes cellular uptake of glucose (by increased translocation of the GLUT 4 glucose transporter to the cell membrane), potassium (via stimulation of Na^+/K^+ pumps and inhibition of K^+ efflux), and also phosphate and magnesium, via mechanisms which have not yet been fully characterised. Can be quite a potent mechanism. Giving glucose alone stimulates endogenous insulin secretion, so that giving insulin is not always necessary, unless the patient is an insulin-deficient diabetic; but both are often given Glucose dose = 0.5–1 g/kg body weight Insulin dose = 0.2–0.5 IU soluble insulin per 1 g glucose administered The glucose/insulin mixture can be administered as one infusion; or the first half of the dose of glucose is given fairly rapidly along with the insulin; and then the second half of the glucose dose is given more slowly. Avoid excessively rapid bolus dosing with glucose, as rebound hypoglycaemia may occur (following endogenous insulin secretion), especially in young animals with less accurate glucose homeostasis Try not to administer glucose solutions of >10% by peripheral veins, as hyperosmotic solutions can be irritant and promote the development of thrombophlebitis **β2 agonists** (stimulate Na^+/K^+ pump activity), can help to internalise K^+, e.g. salbutamol can be inhaled, or terbutaline can be given IV (but be aware of the cardiovascular effects) **Cation exchange resins** can be given orally or by enema **Peritoneal dialysis** **Haemodialysis** **Mineralocorticoids** may also be considered Address underlying cause

| Hypokalaemia ($K^+ < 3.5$ mmol/l) | **Increased loss:**
Gastric vomiting (can test vomit with litmus paper)

Chronic diarrhoea

Chronic renal failure (esp. cats)

Diuresis (diabetes mellitus; post-acute renal failure; non-K^+-sparing diuretics; Cushing's disease [steroids interfere with ADH action and reduce renal PG production])

Hyperaldosteronism (Conn's syndrome; spironolactone)

Note that renal loss can be differentiated from gastro-intestinal [GI] loss by checking the fractional excretion of K^+, which is usually high (>6%) with renal loss, but low (<6%) with GI loss

Decreased intake:
Iatrogenic i.e. long-term intravenous fluid therapy or total parenteral nutrition [TPN] without K^+ supplementation

Prolonged anorexia

Redistribution:
Alkalosis

Hypomagnesaemia (i.e. reduced Na^+/ K^+ pump activity results in reduced intracellular K^+ and eventual body K^+ depletion)

Hypokalaemic periodic paralysis (Burmese cats)

Large doses of catecholamines (stimulate Na^+/K^+ pumps so that more K^+ is sequestered intracellularly)

Large doses of insulin or glucose (stimulate Na^+/K^+ pumps so that more K^+ is sequestered intracellularly) | Clinical signs depend upon rapidity of onset as well as degree of hypokalaemia

(Tachy)-dysrhythmias, hypotension

Confusion, delirium

Lethargy, apathy

Muscle weakness incl. leg (plantigrade stance), neck (ventroflexion), respiratory muscles (hypoventilation), gastrointestinal tract (ileus can result in anorexia and abdominal distension with or without constipation); bladder (detrusor atony can result in urinary retention)

Reduced ability to concentrate urine due to hypokalaemic nephropathy, which is a form of nephrogenic diabetes insipidus (due to decreased response to ADH because aquaporins are down-regulated), characterised by vacuolar changes in renal tubular epithelial cells and inflammatory interstitial changes.

Although hypokalaemia stimulates the transcellular exchange of K^+ and H^+ ions, initially lowering blood H^+ and resulting in metabolic alkalosis; chronic hypokalaemia can result in metabolic acidosis because of advancing renal insufficiency and defective renal tubular acid secretion | Oral KCl at 1 mmol/kg/day

Or oral potassium gluconate at 2.2 mmol/4.5 kg/day (divided between meals)

Include c. 30 mmol/l KCl [or potassium phosphate, if phosphate also low] in IV maintenance fluid; in some circumstances more may be added (see below) but do not exceed 0.5 mmol/kg/h potassium

For K^+ 4.1–5.0 mmol/l; add K^+ to final conc 20 mmol/l
For K^+ 3.6–4.0 mmol/l; add K^+ to final conc 25 mmol/l
For K^+ 3.1–3.5 mmol/l; add K^+ to final conc 30 mmol/l
For K^+ 2.6–3.0 mmol/l; add K^+ to final conc 40 mmol/l
For K^+ 2.1–2.5 mmol/l; add K^+ to final conc 60 mmol/l
For K^+ <2.0 mmol/l; add K^+ to final conc 80 mmol/l

See also the tables at the end of the chapter for a quick guide to potassium supplementation of commonly used crystalloid fluids
DO NOT EXCEED
0.5 mmol K^+/kg/h administration rate

Address underlying cause |

intracellularly, with only 1% being in the extracellular compartment, where it is present in one of three forms: 55% ionised ('free' and therefore biologically active); 20–30% protein (mainly albumin)-bound; and 15–25% complexed with anions. Because magnesium is not as highly albumin-bound as calcium (c. 25% compared with c. 40%), it is less affected by changes in albumin concentration. Knowledge is limited, but it appears that only about 1–2% of intracellular magnesium is present in the free ionised, and therefore active, form.

Magnesium is the natural physiological antagonist of calcium, and therefore is important in the maintenance of the normal function of excitable cells (nerve and muscle) and synapses. (It competes with calcium at synapses to affect neurotransmitter release, e.g. acetylcholine and monoamines.) It is a cofactor for many enzymes, including the ubiquitous sodium pump (magnesium-dependent Na^+/K^+-ATPase) and is therefore important in the regulation of intracellular and extracellular osmolarity. It may also have analgesic actions by its ability to inhibit activation of NMDA receptors. Table 24.9 lists magnesium disturbances.

Magnesium may have a role as a therapeutic agent in several situations besides hypomagnesaemia. Potential uses include:

- As an antidysrhythmic; especially for ventricular arrhythmias refractory to other treatments including torsades de pointes (plasma potassium should also be checked, however, as it may also be low).
- It may be useful to help treat refractory hypokalaemia (alongside potassium supplementation).
- To help treat and/or prevent hypertension and tachycardia (e.g. during surgical manipulation of phaeochromocytomas).
- To help reduce the bronchospasm associated with asthma (human).
- To help reduce or prevent reperfusion injury by reducing calcium accumulation in hypoxic cells.
- To help reduce muscle spasms in patients with tetanus.
- It has been suggested to provide analgesia by reducing activation of NMDA receptors and by inhibiting voltage-gated calcium channel activity. It has been administered IV and in combination with local anaesthetic agents, both for perineural and neuraxial administration, and has shown some promise, although some side effects have also been reported. Doses and routes of administration have not yet been accurately defined for different clinical settings and further studies are required to establish its safety.
- It has been suggested as an anticonvulsant (in pre-eclampsic women; where its action may be due to prevention of cerebral vasospasm).

Table 24.5 ECG changes with potassium imbalances.

Plasma [K⁺]	ECG disturbances
<3.5 mmol/l	Depressed ST segment; prolonged QT interval, flattened T wave; U waves (which may represent repolarisation of papillary muscles) may occur superimposed on where T wave should be '**No Pot**assium, **No T**ea'
>5.5 mmol/l	Peaked T waves; shortened Q–T interval
>6.5 mmol/l	Prolonged QRS duration
>7.0 mmol/l	Reduced P height; prolonged P–R interval
>8.5 mmol/l	No P waves; bradycardia
>9 mmol/l	Asystole; cardiac arrest; occasionally ventricular fibrillation

Table 24.6 Chloride disturbances.

Type of imbalance	Common causes	Clinical signs	Treatment
Corrected hyperchloraemia, i.e. once effects of pure water loss have been corrected for ($Cl^- > 110$ mmol/l) Pseudohyperchloraemia can be present where halides (e.g. bromide) are used for therapy as even ion selective electrodes cannot distinguish the halides	*Increased intake ($Cl^- \geq Na^+$):* Iatrogenic (e.g. normal saline, hypertonic saline, fluids with added KCl, TPN, treatment with ammonium chloride [urinary acidifier]) *Excessive loss of Na^+ relative to Cl^-:* Diarrhoea *Excessive gain of Cl^- relative to Na^+:* Renal tubular acidosis Renal failure Chronic respiratory alkalosis Metabolic acidosis	Hyperchloraemia is often associated with a tendency to metabolic acidosis Clinical signs tend to be those of a metabolic acidosis and include lethargy, weakness, tachypnoea, dyspnoea, arrhythmias and possible coma. Signs may be partly due to increased ionised calcium with the acidosis Hyperchloraemia also results in renal vasoconstriction and reduced GFR and has been associated with acute kidney injury and mortality in ICU patients	Ideally measure serum sodium concentration too Slow correction with 5% dextrose or 0.18% NaCl in 4% dextrose (4 ml/kg/h) may be appropriate Diurese (furosemide) Address the underlying cause
Corrected hypochloraemia ($Cl^- < 95$ mmol/l) Pseudohypochloraemia can occur with hyperlipaemia, which interferes with chloride measurement	*Decreased intake/absorption:* Prolonged low dietary intake Hyponatraemia (Na^+ is required for much of Cl^- absorption) Hypokalaemia (some Cl^- is absorbed with K^+) *Excessive loss of Cl^- relative to Na^+:* Vomiting (gastric or biliary) Diarrhoea Intestinal obstruction Diuresis (loop or thiazide diuretics) Chronic respiratory acidosis (bicarbonate increases, so extra chloride is lost into urine) Metabolic alkalosis (e.g. chronic vomiting, gastric dilation/volvulus [GDV], abomasal displacement) *Excessive gain of Na^+ relative to Cl^-:* Iatrogenic (sodium bicarbonate therapy)	See also notes on hyponatraemia because this may be present because of the reduced ability to reabsorb Na^+ because of Cl^- shortage Hypochloraemia is often associated with a tendency to metabolic alkalosis Clinical signs may include seizures and muscle twitches, tetany and even respiratory arrest, and may, in part, be due to changes in sodium and osmolarity as well as changes in chloride and acid/base status. Ionised calcium tends to decrease with alkalosis and may be responsible for some of the signs	Ideally measure serum sodium concentration too 0.9% NaCl (4 ml/kg/h) may be appropriate Address underlying cause

Table 24.7 Phosphate disturbances.

Type of imbalance	Common causes	Clinical signs	Treatment
Hyperphosphataemia (as yet the concentration at which clinical signs occur is not well defined)	*Physiological:* Young growing animals Post-prandial *Increased absorption/intake:* Excessive phosphate in diet Hypervitaminosis D Excessive phosphate enemas *Reduced excretion:* Pre-renal (e.g. dehydration, Addison's disease) Acute or chronic renal failure Post-renal (obstruction) Hypoparathyroidism (e.g. post bilateral thyroidectomy) *Transcellular shifts:* Tumour lysis syndrome Tissue trauma Rhabdomyolysis Haemolysis	Clinical signs are few, but hyperphosphataemia may lead to hypocalcaemia (high phosphate inhibits activation of vitamin D), and metabolic acidosis (high phosphate results in a reduction in bicarbonate) Clinical signs are usually of the neuromuscular type associated with hypocalcaemia and metabolic acidosis Hyperphosphataemia also predisposes to metastatic calcification	Dilution (IV fluids not containing phosphate) and diuresis Acetazolamide can increase urinary phosphate excretion (but can cause metabolic acidosis) Glucose or insulin administration may help Bicarbonate administration may also help Reduce absorption by oral antacid administration Check serum calcium concentration too Address underlying cause
Hypophosphataemia (mild = 0.65–0.80 mmol/l; moderate = 0.32–0.65 mmol/l; severe <0.32 mmol/l)	*Reduced absorption/intake:* Starvation/severe dietary deficiency Malabsorption Vomiting Diarrhoea Vitamin D deficiency (vit D normally increases both calcium and phosphate absorption from gut) Excessive use of antacids that bind phosphates and prevent their absorption	The anti-natriuretic and anti-diuretic effect of hypophosphataemia results in sodium and water retention and an expanded ECF, which causes tissue oedema and can contribute to congestive heart failure and impaired organ function in general	Ensure slow correction (to plasma phosphate concentration of 0.8 mmol/l), as sudden hypocalcaemia and hypomagnesaemia can accompany a sudden increase in phosphate

Increased excretion:

Diuresis (diuretics; diabetes mellitus; Cushing's disease; hyperaldosteronism [Conn's syndrome or spironolactone therapy])

Primary hyperparathyroidism (causes phosphaturia)

Transcellular shifts:

Insulin (or glucose): insulin stimulates not only glucose uptake, but uptake of electrolytes, including phosphate

Refeeding syndrome: sudden stimulation of insulin secretion possibly responsible for sudden marked reduction in glucose as well as a number of plasma electrolytes that might already have been present in low or limiting concentrations

Alkalosis (bicarbonate therapy, overzealous controlled mechanical ventilation) because alkalosis increases phosphofructokinase activity that results in increased cellular uptake of phosphate

Recovery from diabetic ketoacidosis

Weakness, ataxia

Paraesthesias

Anorexia, nausea

Disorientation/confusion

Joint and bone pain (spontaneous fractures with chronic hypophosphataemia)

Haemolysis and haemolytic anaemia (due to inadequate ATP production to maintain sodium pump activity so red cells swell and burst)

Rhabdomyolysis (due to inadequate ATP production to maintain sodium pump activity so muscle cells swell and burst); myoglobinaemia may result in acute renal failure/acute tubular necrosis

Platelet and leukocyte dysfunction

Thrombocytopaenia also exacerbates coagulation problems (prolonged clotting times may be observed)

Impaired myocardial contractility, hypotension, arrhythmias

Left shift in haemoglobin/oxygen dissociation curve (because of reduced 2,3-DPG synthesis) reduces tissue oxygen delivery in those species with 2,3-DPG-dependent haemoglobin-oxygen binding

Acute respiratory failure (impaired muscle function compounded by lack of ATP)

Seizures, coma

Sodium or potassium phosphate can be given IV for acute severe hypophosphataemia at a dose of 0.06–0.18 mmol/kg over 6 h with regular reassessment and adjustment according to response. (Monitor sodium or potassium too.) Further doses may be given. (This dose rate is equivalent to doses of around 0.25–0.5–1 mmol/kg/day)

Injectable preparations can also be given IM or SC for chronic or less severe acute hypophosphataemia

Oral preparations are preferred for mild hypophosphataemia at 0.5–2 mmol phosphate/kg/d PO

Veterinary product Foston™ contains 200 mg/ml toldimfos sodium (an organic phosphonic acid salt), which contains about 140 mg organic phosphate per ml; another injectable preparation of potassium sodium phosphate contains 2 mmol/ml phosphate; and oral tablets are available that contain 500 mg (16.1 mmol) phosphate

Address the underlying cause

Table 24.8 Calcium disturbances.

Type of imbalance	Common causes	Clinical signs	Treatment
Hypercalcaemia (total Ca >3 mmol/l; ionised calcium >1.5 mmol/l)	*Physiological:* Young animals *Idiopathic:* In cats *Increased uptake/absorption:* Excessive calcium supplementation in diet Hyperparathyroidism (esp. primary, but also secondary, and also pseudo-hyperparathyroidism, e.g. many malignancies with paraneoplastic syndrome e.g. lympho[sarco]ma, perianal adenocarcinoma) Hypervitaminosis D (some plant toxins; iatrogenic) Bone lesions (malignancy; infection) *Reduced excretion:* Addison's disease Renal failure (e.g. acute renal failure in horses) *Altered protein binding:* Acidosis results in reduced protein binding and increased ionised calcium	Polyuria/polydipsia ('renal diabetes insipidus' because Ca interferes with ADH actions) Thirst Vomiting Constipation Neuromuscular effects (twitches, stiffness to weakness, lethargy, fatigue) Bradycardia, hypertension, arrhythmias, cardiac arrest Seizures, coma Metastatic calcification, including cornea and skin and nephrocalcinosis (which may lead to renal failure: 'hypercalcaemic nephropathy') [If the product of total serum calcium concentration and serum phosphate concentration exceeds 6 mmol/l, calcium phosphate deposition in tissues becomes likely] Urolithiasis Hypercoagulability	Dilute/diurese with 0.9% NaCl (5 ml/kg/h) and furosemide (1–2 mg/kg) Bisphosphonates Corticosteroids (calciuretic) Calcitonin Trisodium edetate (chelator) Magnesium has also been suggested Sodium bicarbonate can be used in emergencies to increase blood pH, which helps to reduce the ionised calcium concentration Check other electrolytes Address underlying cause

Hypocalcaemia	Clinical signs and causes	Clinical signs	Treatment

Hypocalcaemia
(total Ca << 2 mmol/l; ionised calcium <0.8–0.9 mmol/l)
Pseudohypocalcaemia may occur with hypoalbuminaemia: although total calcium is reduced, ionised fraction is maintained normal if possible

Reduced uptake / absorption:
Dietary Ca insufficiency
Malabsorption of calcium (may occur with protein-losing enteropathies such as inflammatory bowel disease or intestinal lymphangiectasia or lymphoma)
Hypomagnesaemia (due to reduced intake, malabsorption, increased loss, e.g. vomiting, diarrhoea, diuresis, or redistribution) results in reduced parathyroid hormone (PTH) release and effect (see also next point)
Hypoparathyroidism (e.g. post bilateral thyroidectomy; hypomagnesaemia [reduces PTH release and effect]; hypermagnesaemia [may also, by competing with Ca, reduce PTH release])
Hypovitaminosis D (may be secondary to malabsorption [e.g. protein-losing enteropathies], liver disease, renal failure, hypoparathyroidism, or hyperphosphataemia)

Increased loss:
Calciuresis (hypoparathyroidism; Cushing's disease [corticosteroids inhibit Na$^+$/water reabsorption (cause pu/pd) and inhibit renal activation of vitamin D]; calciuretic and magnesiuretic diuretics such as furosemide)
Lactation (milk fever)
Sweating (horse)
Burns
Chelating agents (beware blood transfusions with excessive citrate)
Metastatic tissue calcification, e.g. with acute pancreatitis and hyperphosphataemia

Altered protein binding:
Alkalosis results in reduced ionised (active) calcium
Massive tissue trauma/rhabdomyolysis/tumour lysis syndrome – release of intracellular contents may provide further compounds which bind/chelate Ca

Clinical signs are more obvious where hypocalcaemia has occurred rapidly, and are exacerbated by hypomagnesaemia and hypokalaemia
Tachycardia, hypotension
Neuromuscular effects: twitches, spasms, and tetany may progress to weakness and paresis (sometimes see synchronous diaphragmatic flutter [thumps], rarely laryngospasm and stridor, respiratory arrest and death)
Restlessness and hypersensitivity may progress to lethargy and recumbency
Anorexia
Secondary clotting problems
Bone decalcification/defective mineralisation

10% calcium gluconate IV over 10–20 min (50–150 mg/kg, which is 0.5–1.5 ml/kg)

or

10% calcium chloride IV over 10–20 min (10–20 mg/kg, which is 0.1–0.2 ml/kg)

Once stable, further doses can be given as required, or a continuous infusion can be set up (usually the calcium solution is added to other intravenous fluids, but do not add it to bicarbonate-containing fluids because of the risk of precipitation)

For calcium gluconate, a starting rate would be around 25 mg/kg/h (0.25 ml/kg/h for a 10% solution); for calcium chloride, a starting rate would be around 5–10 mg/kg/h (0.05–0.1 ml/kg/h for a 10% solution). During infusion, regular monitoring of calcium, magnesium, phosphate and potassium is required, with adjustment of the rate as necessary.

Address underlying cause

Table 24.9 Magnesium disturbances.

Type of imbalance	Common causes	Clinical signs	Treatment
Hypermagnesaemia (total Mg > 1.2 (mild) to 2.2+ (moderate to severe) mmol/l; ionised >0.6 (mild) to 1.1+ (moderate to severe) mmol/l)	*Physiological:* Hibernation *Primary water loss:* Pure dehydration *Impaired excretion:* Acute or chronic renal failure *Excessive intake:* Iatrogenic Excessive Mg-based antacids *Redistribution:* Acidosis (similar to potassium shifts with acidosis)	Muscle weakness, incl. respiratory muscles so respiratory insufficiency possible Lethargy Hypotension (vasodilation and reduced catecholamine release) Bradycardia, cardiac dysrhythmias (similar to hyperkalaemia) Impaired coagulation Note that many of these signs may be associated with the abnormally high degree of calcium opposition.	IV calcium (50–150 mg/kg of 10% calcium gluconate; or 10–20 mg/kg of 10% calcium chloride) over 10–20 min Dilution with IV fluid therapy (0.9% saline) Diuresis Address the underlying cause
Hypomagnesaemia (total Mg < 0.45-0.7 mmol/l; ionised Mg < 0.23-0.45 mmol/l)	*Reduced intake:* Malabsorption (GI or pancreatic disease) Anorexia *Excessive loss:* Vomiting Diarrhoea Lactation Diuresis (e.g. hyperaldosteronism [Conn's syndrome; spironolactone therapy]; hyperthyroidism; chronic diabetic ketoacidosis; non-K⁺-sparing diuretics; osmotic diuretics; hypercalcaemia) *Redistribution or excessive dilution:* Iatrogenic (prolonged therapy with IV fluids or nutrition not containing Mg) Alkalosis (results in shift of magnesium into intracellular compartment, similar to potassium) Insulin, or glucose, which causes increase in insulin (both cause intracellular shift of magnesium, similar to potassium and phosphate movement) Hungry bone syndrome following bilateral parathyroidectomy for treatment of severe hyperparathyroidism (acute massive PTH depletion causes massive deposition of minerals in bone so hypocalcaemia, hypomagnesaemia and hypophosphataemia all occur) Catecholamines (cause intracellular shift of magnesium, similar to potassium movement)	Confusion, restlessness, irritability, seizures Muscle tremors, twitches, spasms, weakness (incl. ileus and dysphagia) Inappetance, weight loss Bronchoconstriction, yet respiratory muscle weakness, can cause stridor and dysphonia Hypertension (vasoconstriction), tachycardia Arrhythmias, esp. ventricular, e.g. polymorphic VPCs and torsades de pointes (ECG changes similar to hypokalaemia) Haemolysis (sodium pumps do not work well, so RBCs swell and burst) Hypercoagulability (increased platelet reactivity) Reduced ability to concentrate urine (possibly secondary to potassium-depletion) See also notes on hypokalaemia and hypocalcaemia as these may co-exist: - Hypomagnesaemia results in reduced PTH release and effectiveness, thus secondary hypocalcaemia (refractory to calcium treatment alone) is common Due to reduced sodium pump activity, the body becomes potassium depleted, hence hypokalaemia (refractory to potassium treatment alone) often co-exists	Emergency magnesium dose = 0.15–0.3 mEq/kg over 10 min Maximum magnesium dose 0.75–1.0 mEq/kg/day Note that 1 mmol of magnesium sulphate heptahydrate (MgSO₄.7H₂O), which contains 2 mEq Mg²⁺ = 246.5 mg Address the underlying cause

24.8 Guidelines for Intravenous Potassium Supplementation

24.8.1 Hartmann's Solution

Patient plasma K⁺ (mmol/l)	mmol of KCl to add to 1 l Hartmann's solution	ml of 15% KCl (2 mmol/ml) to add to 1 l Hartmann's solution	ml of 20% KCl (2.7 mmol/ml) to add to 1 l Hartmann's solution	Final [K⁺] (mmol/l)	Maximum safe infusion rate (ml/kg/h)
<2.0	75	37.5	27.8	**80**	6
2.1–2.5	55	27.5	20.4	**60**	8
2.6–3.0	35	17.5	13.0	**40**	12
3.1–3.5	25	12.5	9.3	**30**	16.5
3.6–4.0	20	10	7.4	**25**	20
4.1–5.0	15	7.5	5.6	**20**	25

Note that Hartmann's solution already contains c.5 mmol/l of K⁺.

Patient plasma K⁺ (mmol/l)	mmol of KCl to add to 500 ml Hartmann's solution	ml of 15% KCl (2 mmol/ml) to add to 500 ml Hartmann's solution	ml of 20% KCl (2.7 mmol/ml) to add to 500 ml Hartmann's solution	Final [K⁺] (mmol/l)	Maximum safe infusion rate (ml/kg/h)
<2.0	37.5	18.8	13.9	**80**	6
2.1–2.5	27.5	13.8	10.2	**60**	8
2.6–3.0	17.5	8.8	6.5	**40**	12
3.1–3.5	12.5	6.3	4.7	**30**	16.5
3.6–4.0	10	5	3.7	**25**	20
4.1–5.0	7.5	3.8	2.8	**20**	25

Note that Hartmann's solution already contains c.5 mmol/l of K⁺ (i.e. 2.5 mmol per 0.5 l).

24.9 Guidelines for Intravenous Potassium Supplementation

24.9.1 Saline or Dextrose-Saline Solution

Patient plasma K⁺ (mmol/l)	mmol of KCl to add to 500 ml SALINE solution	ml of 15% KCl (2 mmol/ml) to add to 500 ml SALINE solution	ml of 20% KCl (2.7 mmol/ml) to add to 500 ml SALINE solution	Final [K⁺] (mmol/l)	Maximum safe infusion rate (ml/kg/h)
<2.0	40	20	14.8	**80**	6
2.1–2.5	30	15	11.1	**60**	8
2.6–3.0	20	10	7.4	**40**	12
3.1–3.5	15	7.5	5.6	**30**	16.5
3.6–4.0	12.5	6.3	4.6	**25**	20
4.1–5.0	10	5	3.7	**20**	25

Note that this table can be used for other concentrations of saline, dextrose-saline, or dextrose solutions.

Patient plasma K⁺ (mmol/l)	mmol of KCl to add to 1 l SALINE solution	ml of 15% KCl (2 mmol/ml) to add to 1 l SALINE solution	ml of 20% KCl (2.7 mmol/ml) to add to 1 l SALINE solution	Final [K⁺] (mmol/l)	Maximum safe infusion rate (ml/kg/h)
<2.0	80	40	29.6	80	6
2.1–2.5	60	30	22.2	60	8
2.6–3.0	40	20	14.8	40	12
3.1–3.5	30	15	11.1	30	16.5
3.6–4.0	25	12.5	9.3	25	20
4.1–5.0	20	10	7.4	20	25

Note that this table can be used for other concentrations of saline, dextrose-saline, or dextrose solutions.

Further Reading

Aguilera, I.M. and Vaughan, R.S. (2000). Calcium and the anaesthetist. *Anaesthesia* 55: 779–790.

Borer, K.E. and Corley, K.T.T. (2006a). Electrolyte disorders in horses with colic. Part 1: potassium and magnesium. *Equine Veterinary Education* 18: 266–271.

Borer, K.E. and Corley, K.T.T. (2006b). Electrolyte disorders of horses with colic. Part 2: calcium, sodium, chloride and phosphate. *Equine Veterinary Education* 18: 320–325.

Cunha, M.G.M.C.M., Freitas, G.C., Carregaro, A.B. et al. (2010). Renal and cardiorespiratory effects of treatment with lactated Ringer's solution or physiologic saline (0.9% NaCl) solution in cats with experimentally induced urethral obstruction. *American Journal of Veterinary Research* 71: 840–846.

DiBartola, S. (2001). Disorders of sodium: hypernatraemia and hyponatraemia. *Journal of Feline Medicine and Surgery* 3: 1865–1187.

DiBartola, S.P. (ed.) (2012). Fluid, Electrolyte and Acid–Base Disorders in Small Animal Practice, 4e. Missouri, USA: Elsevier Saunders.

Dube, L. and Granry, J.-C. (2003). The therapeutic use of magnesium in anaesthesiology, intensive care and emergency medicine: a review. *Canadian Journal of Anaesthesia* 50: 732–746.

Edwards, G., Foster, A., and Livesey, C. (2008). Use of ocular fluids to aid post-mortem diagnosis in cattle and sheep. In *Practice* 31: 22–25.

Handy, J.M. and Soni, N. (2008). Physiological effects of hyperchloraemia and acidosis. *British Journal of Anaesthesia* 101: 141–150.

Macintire, D.K. (1997). Disorders of potassium, phosphorus and magnesium in critical illness. *Compendium on Continuing Education of the Practising Veterinarian: Small Animal* 19: 41–48.

McFadzean, W., Macfarlane, P., Khenissi, L., and Murrell, J.C. (2018). Repeated hyperkalaemia during two separate episodes of general anaesthesia in a nine-year-old female neutered greyhound. *Veterinary Record Case Reports* https://doi.org/10.1136/vetreccr-2018-000658.

Maloney, D.G., Appadurai, I.R., and Vaughan, R.S. (2002). Anions and the anaesthetist. *Anaesthesia* 57: 140–154.

de Morais, H.A. and DiBartola, S.P. (eds.) (2008). Volume: advances in fluid, electrolyte and acid–base disorders. *Veterinary Clinics of North America: Small Animal Practice* 38 (3): 423–753. *(Very useful resource.)*.

Rose, B.D. and Post, T.W. (eds.) (2001). Clinical Physiology of Acid–Base and Electrolyte Disorders, 5e. New York, USA: McGraw Hill.

Schaer, M., Halling, K.B., Collins, K.E., and Grant, D.C. (2001). Combined hyponatremia and hyperkalemia mimicking acute hypoadrenocorticism in three pregnant dogs. *Journal of the American Veterinary Medical Association* 218: 897–899.

Schropp, D.M. and Koviac, J. (2007). Phosphorus and phosphate metabolism in veterinary patients. *Journal of Veterinary Emergency and Critical Care* 17: 127–134.

Tappin, S. (2019). How to approach potassium and sodium abnormalities. BSAVA Companion. February 2019: 14-17. doi:10.22233/20412495.0219.14.

de Vasconcellos, K. and Skinner, D.L. (2018). Hyperchloraemia is associated with acute kidney injury and mortality in the critically ill: a retrospective observational study in a multidisciplinary intensive care unit. *Journal of Critical Care* 45: 45–51.

Wadsworth, R.L. and Siddiqhui, S. (2016). Phosphate homeostasis in critical care. *BJA Education* 16: 305–309.

Self-test Section

1. List the four main causes of hyperkalaemia, giving one or two examples in each case.

2. What are the main treatment options for hyperkalaemia?

25

Drugs Affecting the Cardiovascular System

25.1 Methylxanthines (Theophylline Derivatives)

Actions:

- Stimulate the CNS (increase reticular activating system activity), also lower the seizure threshold.
- Stimulate respiratory activity (increase sensitivity to CO_2), cause bronchodilation and enhance diaphragmatic activity.
- Stimulate cardiac activity (positive inotropy, some positive chronotropy), also lower the arrhythmia threshold.
- Diuresis: secondary to increased cardiac output, possible vasodilation, and renal tubular effects (decrease Na^+ reabsorption).
- Rheological effects: decrease RBC aggregability (increase cell flexibility) and decrease blood viscosity, also decrease platelet aggregation (decrease adhesion molecule expression).

True xanthines are adenosine **ant**agonists, and non-selective phosphodiesterase (PDE) inhibitors. They include theophylline, caffeine, aminophylline, and etamiphylline.

Pentoxifylline is another non-selective PDE inhibitor and an antagonist at adenosine 2 receptors, with vasodilatory, anti-inflammatory, and rheological effects (see Chapter 26 on Shock).

Propentofylline is an adenosine **ag**onist, with PDE inhibitor effects, and causes more vasodilation and less CNS stimulation.

25.2 Selective PDE Inhibitors (Also Called Ino-dilators)

There are several isoforms of phosphodiesterase (PDE) within the superfamily: PDE 1 to PDE 12, but these selective agents tend to target PDE 3.

Phosphodiesterase normally breaks down cAMP, so its inhibition leads to increased intracellular cAMP. In myocardial cells, this results in increased protein kinase A activity, resulting in increased intracellular ionised Ca^{2+}, and thus increased contractility (positive inotropy), whereas in smooth muscle (especially vascular), it leads to interference with translocation of Ca^{2+} into cells, resulting in relaxation (i.e. vasodilation).

PDE inhibitors:

- Bipyridine derivatives: milrinone and amrinone are PDE 3 inhibitors.
- Pyridazine derivatives: pimobendan (a benzimidazole-pyridazinone derivative) and levosimendan (a pyridazinone-dinitrile derivative).

Pimobendan is a PDE 3 inhibitor and a calcium 'sensitiser' (i.e. it increases the sensitivity of troponin for Ca^{2+} so that contractility is enhanced without the need to increase intracellular calcium concentration). It also has vasodilatory properties through being a K_{ATP} channel opener. Levosimendan is also a calcium sensitiser and a K_{ATP} channel opener (therefore is a vasodilator), but has no effects on cAMP.

- Imidazolone derivatives: enoximone is a PDE 4 inhibitor.
- Sildenafil is a PDE 5 inhibitor and is a potent vasodilator of pulmonary vasculature and the corpus cavernosum of the penis (where this isoform is mainly found).

25.3 Angiotensin I Converting Enzyme Inhibitors (ACEI)

ACE normally converts angiotensin I to angiotensin II (which is a potent vasoconstrictor and stimulates the release of aldosterone), and also breaks down bradykinin (a potent vasodilator); so that the result of ACE inhibition

Veterinary Anaesthesia: Principles to Practice, Second Edition. Alexandra H. A. Dugdale, Georgina Beaumont, Carl Bradbrook, and Matthew Gurney.
© 2020 John Wiley & Sons Ltd. Published 2020 by John Wiley & Sons Ltd.
Companion website: www.wiley.com/go/dugdale/veterinary-anaesthesia

is vasodilation, on both the arterial and venous sides of the circulation. Reduced angiotensin II also results in:

- Reduced aldosterone release (at least in the short term), so sodium and water retention are reduced.
- Reduced facilitation of sympathetic nervous system and antidiuretic hormone (ADH) activities, so adding to the hypovolaemic and hypotensive effects.

Angiotensin II promotes vascular smooth muscle proliferation and cardiac remodelling, whereas bradykinin increases prostaglandin I_2 (PGI_2) and NO, which inhibit these things. Thus ACEI also reduce the production of myotrophic factors, and therefore decrease cardiac and smooth muscle remodelling.

25.4   Digitalis Glycosides

- Inhibit Na^+/K^+-ATPase (the sodium pump, which is also upregulated in heart failure), by stabilising it in the E2-P transition state, so they increase intracellular $[Na^+]$, which in turn increases Na^+/Ca^{2+} exchange, resulting in increased intracellular $[Ca^{2+}]$, and hence positive inotropy (increased contractility).
- Sensitise baroreceptors, so that overall sympathetic tone is reduced, and parasympathetic tone is increased.
- Activate vagal nuclei, so further increasing vagal tone.
- Overall, see weak positive inotropy, which increases myocardial oxygen demand, but, myocardial oxygen demand is also reduced because of the increase in vagal activity. AV conduction is slowed, and refractory periods (at AV node) are increased due to increased vagal influences.
- Mild diuresis due to increased cardiac output.

Excellent for the treatment of atrial fibrillation. Unfortunately these agents have a low therapeutic index, therefore are often dosed according to metabolic body weight (i.e. according to body surface area) rather than actual body mass. Side effects include anorexia, vomiting, diarrhoea, arrhythmias (especially ventricular). Check $[K^+]$ also because extracellular potassium concentration increases slightly after initiation of therapy, but then, with diuresis, the total body K^+ can become depleted. Digoxin tends to be preferred over digitoxin.

25.5   Classical Anti-dysrhythmics (or Anti-arrhythmics)

- Classified (see below) by **Vaughan Williams**, with later modification of class I by Harrison.

- Under certain circumstances, all anti-dysrhythmic drugs can be pro-dysrhythmic (arrhythmogenic).
- New classification system for anti-dysrhythmics is the **Sicilian Gambit**, which is a multidimensional classification system based on pathophysiological considerations. This system identifies one or more 'vulnerable parameters' associated with specific arrhythmogenic mechanisms. It can accommodate drugs with multiple actions better than the Vaughan Williams classification. A vulnerable parameter is an electrophysiological property or event whose modification by drug therapy results in termination or suppression of the arrhythmia with minimal undesirable side effects.

Figure 25.1 shows stylised cardiac action potentials from different types of myocardial cells. The main ion currents that accompany the action potentials:

- **Phase 4** is the diastolic depolarisation phase or pacemaker potential. Spontaneous depolarisation due to Na^+ and Ca^{2+} inflow, and reduced K^+ outflow occurs in atrial and ventricular myocytes. In nodal tissue, Ca^{2+} influx and reduced K^+ efflux occur.
- **Phase 0** is the rapid depolarisation phase. Mainly Na^+ influx in atrial and ventricular myocytes; mainly Ca^{2+} influx in nodal cells.
- **Phase 1** is the early rapid repolarisation phase. K^+ efflux in atrial and ventricular myocytes.
- **Phase 2** is the slow repolarisation or plateau phase. Ca^{2+} influx (decreasing over time), with K^+ efflux (increasing over time) in atrial and ventricular myocytes.
- **Phase 3** is the rapid repolarisation phase. K^+ efflux is important in atrial and ventricular myocytes and nodal cells.

25.5.1   Class I: Sodium Channel Blockers

These do not work well in hypokalaemic patients. They work best in non-nodal tissue (nodal tissue is more dependent upon calcium entry for initiation of action potentials), where they slow conduction velocity, and result in negative

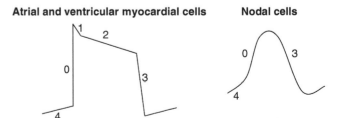

Figure 25.1   Cardiac action potentials in cardiomyocytes from different regions of the heart.

inotropy and slight negative chronotropy. They are subdivided into: Class Ia, Class Ib, and Class Ic.

25.5.1.1 Class Ia

- Moderately **depress phase 0** (slow the rate of rise of the cardiac action potential).
- **Slow conduction** to increase the action potential duration (prolong QRS interval).
- **Prolong repolarization**/refractory period (prolong QT interval) (possibly via K$^+$ channel blockade).
- Best versus ventricular arrhythmias.

Examples are procainamide and quinidine.

25.5.1.1.1 Quinidine Sulphate

Quinidine sulphate given orally, or quinidine gluconate IV, are used in the treatment of atrial fibrillation in horses, to try to convert them back into sinus rhythm. Do not use in horses with signs of congestive heart failure accompanying the atrial fibrillation. Quinidine is a Class Ia anti-dysrhythmic, but is also vagolytic (may see increase in heart rate), and an alpha blocker (causing vasodilation and hypotension).

Some of the 'side effects' of treatment with quinidine are:

- Hypotension (may see 'collapse') (due to alpha blockade ± tachycardia ± arrhythmias).
- Rapid supraventricular tachycardia (possibly due to reduction of vagal tone).
- Ventricular arrhythmias, including a particularly nasty form of multifocal (multiform/polymorphic) ventricular tachycardia called torsades de pointes.
- May see GI discomfort such as flatulence, diarrhoea, colic.
- May see upper respiratory tract obstruction/dyspnoea (possible allergic phenomenon).
- May see bizarre neurological signs, including strange behaviour, ataxia, seizures.

What can you do if problems occur during quinidine treatment?

- For hypotension: rapid IV fluids and possibly phenylephrine infusion at 0.05–3 µg/kg/min 'to effect'.
- For rapid supraventricular tachycardia, try esmolol or propranolol (0.03 mg/kg IV) or even digoxin (0.0022 mg/kg IV).
- Sodium bicarbonate (1 mg/kg IV) will rapidly reduce the concentration of free (unbound) quinidine, and thus effectively reduce its activity. (A more alkaline pH will encourage binding of quinidine to plasma proteins.)
- Magnesium sulphate (1–2.5 g/450 kg/min) has been shown to be efficacious against some forms of ventricular arrhythmias, including torsades de pointes.

- Lidocaine may also be useful against ventricular arrhythmias; try bolus 0.5 mg/kg and then onto infusion at about 25 µg/kg/min (to effect, but beware toxicity).

25.5.1.2 Class Ib
- **Mildly depress phase 0 in abnormal tissue** (i.e. mildly slow rate of rise of cardiac action potential), but no effect in normal tissue.
- Little effect on, or slight decrease of, action potential duration (little change of QRS interval).
- **Shorten repolarization**/refractory period (decrease QT interval) and can reduce re-entrant dysrhythmias.
- Best versus ventricular tachyarrhythmias.

Examples are phenytoin, lidocaine, and mexiletine.

25.5.1.2.1 Phenytoin
Phenytoin also has anticonvulsant and sympatholytic properties.

Good versus digoxin toxicity-induced arrhythmias too.

25.5.1.2.2 Lidocaine
Under some circumstances, lidocaine can be anticonvulsant, but beware systemic toxicity, where convulsions may occur. Will not work in the presence of hypokalaemia (or hypomagnesaemia).

25.5.1.2.3 Mexiletine
Mexiletine is an orally effective lidocaine analogue.

25.5.1.3 Class Ic
- **Depress phase 0** (i.e. slow the rate of rise of the cardiac action potential).
- **Slow conduction**, but have little effect on action potential duration (with almost no change [possible slight increase] in QRS interval).
- **Little effect on repolarisation** (no change in QT interval).
- Best versus ventricular arrhythmias, but can also be used versus supraventricular arrhythmias.

Examples are flecainide and propafenone.

25.5.1.3.1 Flecainide
Flecainide (a fluorinated derivative of procainamide) is associated with many side effects and can worsen heart failure.

25.5.1.3.2 Propafenone
Propafenone may be less toxic.

25.5.1.4 Class II: Beta Blockers
Beta blockers are highly protein bound, and in the face of inflammation, where acute phase proteins increase in plasma, the free concentration of drug may be reduced, leading to reduced efficacy.

- Act on **phase 4** of the cardiac action potential to **reduce automaticity** (especially SA node), and **prolong the refractory period** (e.g. prolonging AV node conduction).
- Prolong PR interval.
- No effect on QRS interval or QT interval, although sotalol may increase the QT interval.
- Are effective at nodal tissue.
- Result in **negative inotropy and negative chronotropy**.
- Best versus supraventricular arrhythmias, but also useful against ventricular arrhythmias, and best in situations of tachyarrhythmias due to high sympathetic tone.

Examples are propranolol and esmolol.

25.5.1.4.1 Propranolol

Although this can be used to treat feline hyperthyroidism and hypertrophic cardiomyopathy, beware if thromboembolic disease accompanies the cardiac problem because the slight β_2 blocking activity of propranolol will reduce vasodilation in, and distal to, clotted vessels, and may further compromise distal limb perfusion. Side effects of propranolol may include cough due to bronchospasm/bronchoconstriction (another β_2 blocking effect); beware in asthmatic cats. Propranolol often exhibits 'bradyphylaxis', i.e. an increased effect with subsequent doses, possibly due to upregulation/increased sensitivity of beta receptors.

25.5.1.4.2 Esmolol

This is much more β_1 selective, but it is very rapidly metabolised by plasma esterases, so has a very short half-life. It is therefore suited to administration 'to effect' by infusion (e.g. intra-operatively).

25.5.2 Class III: Potassium Channel Blockers

- **Prolong repolarization**/refractory period. (They have a hypothyroid like effect.)
- Prolong QT interval, with little effect on QRS interval.
- Good versus ventricular and supraventricular arrhythmias.

Examples are sotalol (also class II), bretylium (also reduces catecholamine release and so has a sort of indirect β blocking activity) and amiodarone (a benzofuran derivative). Bretylium has been reported to be effective in the treatment of bupivacaine toxicity-induced arrhythmias, although intralipid tends to be preferred now (See Chapter 12).

25.5.2.1 Class IV

Class IV is now divided into:

- Class IVa, including Ca^{2+} channel blockers (L-type).
- Class IVb, including K^+ channel openers (cromakalim; nicorandil [also a nitrate]): open K_{ATP} channels.

25.5.2.2 Class IVa

- Slow the action potential upstroke phase in AV (and SA) nodes, and prolong the PR interval. Relatively selective for AV nodal L-type calcium channels.
- Theoretical ability to prolong the action potential plateau phase in atrial, ventricular, and Purkinje tissue, but no effect on QRS interval *in vivo*.
- Best versus supraventricular arrhythmias.

They are **negative inotropes** (reduce contractility), **negative chronotropes** (reduce heart rate), **negative dromotropes** (reduce conduction velocity, especially through the AV node), but **positive lusitropes** (enhance relaxation rate [relaxation comprises both passive and active mechanisms]); and they cause vasodilation in the periphery so they reduce systemic vascular resistance and blood pressure. They also reduce the platelet release reaction (which normally enhances platelet aggregation), and may be useful in thromboembolic disorders. Because they reduce intracellular $[Ca^{2+}]$, they may provide some **cytoprotection**, especially in the face of ischaemia and reperfusion.

Classic examples are diltiazem and verapamil. The dihydropyridines include amlodipine, nifedipine, and nicardipine. **Amlodipine** is often favoured for treatment of primary systemic hypertension in cats. Nifedipine is more of a vasodilator (vascular smooth muscle relaxant), than an anti-dysrhythmic; nicardipine is similar, but with a more selective effect on coronary and cerebral vasculature.

25.5.2.3 Class IVb

- K^+ conduction is enhanced, so SA and AV nodes become hyperpolarised.
- Only used to treat supraventricular arrhythmias, except atrial fibrillation.
- Provide some protection against ischaemia via cardiac adenosine receptor actions.

Examples are adenosine, nicorandil, and cromakalim.

25.5.3 Other Anti-arrhythmics

25.5.3.1 Magnesium Sulphate

Magnesium is the natural antagonist of calcium. It is a cofactor for many enzymes, including Na^+/K^+-ATPase. It is an important intracellular ion. It competes with calcium in stimulus-secretion coupling at synapses and nerve terminals. For example, it can reduce acetylcholine release at neuromuscular junctions producing muscle weakness (including respiratory muscles); and affect neurotransmitter release at synapses in the sympathetic nervous system, resulting in sympatholytic effects. It can also enhance smooth muscle relaxation, resulting in vasodilation (hypotension), bronchodilation, and GI hypomotility. It has been shown to have anti-arrhythmic properties against some malignant forms of ventricular arrhythmias (e.g. torsades de pointes). It may interfere with coagulation.

It may reduce 'ischaemia-reperfusion/reoxygenation injury' by limiting intracellular calcium accumulation. It may have analgesic effects via its function at NMDA receptors, but this has not always been proven clinically. Its blockade of NMDA receptors, however, may afford some neuroprotection by reducing CNS excitatory glutamate activity.

25.6 Anticholinergics

For the treatment of bradyarrhythmias and bradycardias.

25.6.1 Atropine

A tertiary amine. Atropine IV has a faster onset than glycopyrrolate, and, possibly, a shorter duration of action, although this depends upon species, but c. 40–90 minutes compared with c. 2–4 hours for glycopyrrolate.

- Reduces the watery component of saliva and mucus secretions, making them more viscous and harder to clear. Also reduces tear production.
- May reduce mucociliary activity too, further compromising secretion removal.
- Slows gut motility and reduces lower oesophageal sphincter tone. GI effects usually outlast cardiovascular effects.
- Causes bronchodilation (increases dead space and may aggravate hypoventilation problems, especially under general anaesthesia).
- Crosses blood–brain barrier rapidly; causing excitation due to the 'central anticholinergic syndrome'; although excitation may in part be due to its mydriatic effect, especially in cats and horses.
- Paradoxical bradycardia is believed to occur after rapid IV administration when it is thought that the central effects (across the blood–brain barrier) occur before the peripheral effects become apparent. Some weak agonism of peripheral muscarinic receptors may contribute to the bradycardia. The eventual tachycardia may be partly due to antagonistic effects on pre-synaptic muscarinic receptors on sympathetic nerve terminals. (Acetylcholine action on these receptors normally reduces norepinephrine release.)
- Increases heart rate with little change in blood pressure.
- Increases myocardial oxygen demand too; so can be tachyarrhythmogenic.
- Contra-indicated if:
  - Pre-existing tachycardia (shock, fever).

  - Hyperthyroidism.
  - Phaeochromocytoma.
- Metabolism and elimination vary depending upon species: cats, rats, and rabbits metabolise it very quickly.

25.6.2 Glycopyrrolate (or Glycopyrronium Bromide)

Slower onset of action, therefore less useful in emergencies than atropine. Duration of action c. two to four hours.

- A synthetic quaternary ammonium compound, originally developed for antihistamine (H_2) effects.
- It reduces acidity and volume of gastric secretions more so than atropine. It reduces lower oesophageal sphincter tone and causes GI hypomotility.
- It reduces the volume of saliva and mucus secretions more so than atropine, but again they become more viscous.
- Can increase heart rate, but usually less dramatic increase than seen with atropine. Said to be less tachyarrhythmogenic.
- Supposed not to cause paradoxical bradycardia because, being a very polar molecule, does not cross the blood–brain barrier (although it may cross it slowly).
- Any paradoxical bradycardia seen may be due to some peripheral actions, as outlined above under atropine.

25.7 Other Drugs Used for Cardiovascular Support during Anaesthesia

Table 25.1 outlines the distribution of cardiovascular system adrenoceptors and Table 25.2 shows the relative activities of commonly used drugs at these receptors.

25.7.1 Positive Inotropes

25.7.1.1 Dopamine
Endogenous catecholamine, with dopaminergic agonist effects (D_1 and D_2 receptors) and adrenergic agonist effects (β and α receptors). About 25% is converted into norepinephrine in sympathetic nerve terminals.

It is often taught that different dose rates have different effects:

- With up to 2.5 μg/kg/min, D_1 and D_2 effects predominate, resulting in vasodilation (especially in renal and splanchnic beds), reduced systemic vascular resistance (possibly slightly reduced blood pressure), and enhanced cardiac output secondary to the reduced afterload. The increased cardiac output may contribute to a diuresis, which may also be due to a reduction in proximal convoluted tubule reabsorption of Na^+ (which may reduce renal tubular energy demands).

Table 25.1 Distribution of adrenergic receptors in the cardiovascular system. In the myocardium, the ratio of $\beta_1 : \beta_2$ receptors is around 60 : 40 in the atria, and nearer 85 : 15 in the ventricles.

Receptor type/location	Tissue location	Effect of stimulation
Post-synaptic α_1	Vasculature	Vasoconstriction
Post-synaptic α_2	Vasculature	Vasoconstriction
Pre-synaptic α_2	Vasculature	Decrease norepinephrine release (−ve feedback); reduction in vascular tone
Post-synaptic α_1	Cardiac	+ve inotropy especially at low heart rates (HR) (no effect on HR)
Pre-synaptic α_2	Cardiac	Decrease norepinephrine release (−ve feedback)
Post-synaptic β_2	Vasculature (especially skeletal muscles)	Vasodilation
Post-synaptic β_1	Cardiac	+ve inotropy; (+ve chronotropy); +ve dromotropy; +ve lusitropy
Post-synaptic β_2	Cardiac	+ve inotropy; +ve chronotropy. These receptors up-regulate in heart failure (i.e. when β_1 receptors down-regulate)
Post-synaptic β_2	Skeletal muscles	Increase in muscle tension generated (especially in tired muscles), ± effect on muscle spindles: these effects may be responsible for the 'tremors' seen with β_2 agonists such as clenbuterol
Post-synaptic β_2	Sweat glands	Sweating (especially horses)
Post-synaptic D_1	Renal, coronary, mesenteric vasculature	Vasodilation
Pre-synaptic D_2	CNS	Decrease norepinephrine release (−ve feedback)

Table 25.2 Relative activities of commonly used drugs at adrenergic receptors.

Drug	α_1	α_2	β_1	β_2	D
Dopamine	+ +	?	+ + + +	+ +	+ + + +
Dobutamine	+	+?	+ + + +	+ +	0
Epinephrine	+ +	+ + +	+ + + +	+ + +	0
Norepinephrine	+ + +	+ + +	+/+ +	+/−	0
Isoprenaline	−	−	+ + + +	+ + + +	0
Phenylephrine	+ +/+ + + +	?	0	0	0

- At 2.5–5 µg/kg/min, β_1 effects predominate, resulting in positive inotropy (and chronotropy). Arrhythmias may also occur.
- At infusion rates >5–20 µg/kg/min, some α_1 and α_2 activity becomes apparent, so that peripheral vasoconstriction and increased systemic vascular resistance (and afterload) occur. Blood pressure may increase as the heart is still under β agonist influence to pump harder against the increased afterload. Arrhythmias are more likely as myocardial oxygen demand is increased.

The often quoted 'renal dose' for renoprotection (increased renal perfusion, restoration of urine output) may not always hold true because different species, and different individuals within a species, express different receptor types, numbers, and sensitivities, which may also be affected by disease processes. (To improve urine output, fluid therapy and positive inotropes may be required to increase cardiac output, which secondarily increases renal perfusion and thus urine output.) Metabolism of these drugs may also be affected by other diseases.

25.7.1.2 Dobutamine

A synthetic catecholamine; an isoprenaline (isoproterenol) derivative. Has predominantly β_1 agonist activities, but also has some β_2 and α_1 actions (the latter may cause splenic contraction which can result in increased PCV). Some people suggest that dobutamine has activity at cardiac α_1 'arrhythmic' receptors.

At low to moderate infusion rates (1–5 µg/kg/min) β_1 effects predominate (i.e. positive inotropy). Positive chronotropy may also occur, but at low doses, the increase in arterial blood pressure may stimulate baroreceptor reflexes to result in bradycardias or bradyarrhythmias. Increased stroke volume (and possibly increased cardiac output), and increased blood pressure result. Overall systemic vascular resistance remains unchanged or there may be a slight reduction. Diastolic arterial pressure may fall, but systolic pressure increases so that mean pressure usually increases.

At high infusion rates (10–20 µg/kg/min), mild β_2 and α_1 activity may become apparent. You may see positive chronotropy due to β_2 and cardiac α_1 actions, but still very little change in overall systemic vascular resistance because the vasodilatory actions of β_2 agonism are 'balanced' by the vasoconstrictor effects of α_1 agonism. Tachycardias and tachyarrhythmias are more of a problem.

25.7.2 Vasopressors

25.7.2.1 Phenylephrine

Phenylephrine is a direct-acting α_1 agonist, non-catecholamine. Very high doses are said to have β effects. It is infused to effect (0.05–3 µg/kg/min) or can be given as a bolus (c. 0.01 mg/kg).

- Causes peripheral vasoconstriction, therefore increases blood pressure.
- The increased systemic vasoconstriction initially increases venous return, and, through Starling's law, increases myocardial contractility (due to increased stretch of the cardiac chambers because of increased filling). But the increase in systemic vascular resistance increases afterload on the heart and may actually reduce stroke volume, and therefore cardiac output (and therefore future venous return), even though arterial blood pressure is increased.
- Increased arterial blood pressure may cause reflex bradycardia, which may further reduce cardiac output.
- Increases myocardial oxygen demand because of increased afterload, which demands increased cardiac work.
- In cats, doses around 2 µg/kg/min may help improve cardiac output via actions on cardiac alpha receptors, but this is not the case in dogs.

25.7.2.2 Norepinephrine (Noradrenaline)

Gaining popularity amongst veterinary anaesthetists for treatment of hypotension due to vasodilation as a result of conditions such as sepsis and systemic inflammatory response syndrome (SIRS), and hypotension refractory to other treatments. Good monitoring of arterial blood pressure, ideally using the invasive method, is required, and cardiac output monitoring, when available, is the gold standard. Its dose is titrated to effect, which must be performed gradually and slowly to prevent intense vasoconstriction and a subsequent marked bradycardia and bradyarrhythmias. At low doses, has predominantly α_1 agonist effects and increased afterload may actually result in reduced cardiac output. At higher doses, has some β effects, which, through vasodilation and positive inotropy,

may help to offset the increase in afterload, therefore possibly preferable to phenylephrine (unless phenylephrine is used in conjunction with, e.g. dobutamine). Must be infused to effect (e.g. 0.05–2.5 µg/kg/min).

25.7.2.3 Vasopressin

A potent vasoconstrictor. As with all vasopressors, it is important to ensure that fluid resuscitation is provided/optimised as necessary. Norepinephrine tends to be an initial choice of vasoconstrictor, with vasopressin being reserved for refractory cases. Vasopressin also works better than catecholamines where acidaemia is present. Infusion rates of around 0.002–0.096 IU/kg/min have been reported.

25.7.3 Ino-constrictors

25.7.3.1 Ephedrine

A synthetic non-catecholamine (it is a substituted amphetamine), which has some direct, but mainly indirect, sympathomimetic actions. Reminiscent of epinephrine because it has α and β ($\beta_1 > \beta_2$) actions, with β activity predominating at lower doses, and α (especially α_1) activity predominating at higher doses. Often given as a bolus, the effects are usually short-lived (5–10 minutes), but can last longer in horses. Dose ~0.01–0.25 mg/kg, given in boluses.

In dogs, a 0.1 mg/kg bolus produced a transient increase in arterial blood pressure and cardiac output with a reflex decrease in heart rate, and an accompanying reduction in systemic vascular resistance; whereas a 0.25 mg/kg bolus resulted in increased blood pressure and cardiac output, also with a decrease in heart rate, but with an increase in systemic vascular resistance, and these effects lasted around 15 minutes.

- β_1 activity manifests as positive inotropy; and at higher doses, α activity manifests as peripheral vasoconstriction: hence it is an ino-constrictor.
- Is a MAO (monoamine oxidase) inhibitor. (It is not metabolised by either MAO or catechol-o-methyl transferase (COMT), and therefore has a relatively long duration of action.)
- Increases release of norepinephrine from sympathetic nerve terminals, but this mechanism works best after the first dose because thereafter the norepinephrine stores may not have had time to be replenished, so the phenomenon of tachyphylaxis (reduced effectiveness with subsequent doses) occurs.

25.8 Notes

Vasodilators are sometimes required: **sodium nitroprusside** is probably the most common used.

Epinephrine (adrenaline) may be considered in cases of hypotension refractory to other vasopressors or positive inotropes, although it has largely been superseded by norepinephrine (noradrenaline). At low doses, it is predominantly a β agonist (vasodilation, positive inotropy, and bronchodilation); when used at higher doses, it becomes an α agonist in addition, such that vasopressor effects are seen. Dose 0.05–1 μg/kg/min, given 'to effect'. Arrhythmias are common.

Dopexamine is a synthetic catecholamine; a derivative of dopamine. It has D_1 and $β_2$ agonist activities (with a little D_2 and $β_1$ activity). Again, there are dose-dependent results. It tends to cause a lot of vasodilation (so reduces afterload), so cardiac output is increased, but arterial blood pressure may actually fall. Inhibition of norepinephrine re-uptake may produce indirect adrenergic agonist effects (e.g. $β_1$ effects). May result in profuse sweating in horses.

Isoprenaline (isoproterenol) has $β_1$ (and some $β_2$) agonist activity. Positive inotropy and positive chronotropy result in variable effects on blood pressure.

Further Reading

Bailey, J.M. (2000). Dopamine: one size does not fit all. Editorial. *Anesthesiology* 92: 303–305.

De Backer, D., Creteur, J., Silva, E., and Vincent, J.-L. (2003). Effects of dopamine, norepinephrine, and epinephrine on the splanchnic circulation in septic shock: which is best? *Critical Care Medicine* 31: 1659–1667.

Feneck, R. (2007). Phosphodiesterase inhibitors and the cardiovascular system. *Continuing Education in Anaesthesia, Critical Care and Pain* 7: 203–207.

Filipas, M. and Vettorato, E. (2018). *How to manage hypotension under general anaesthesia*. Companion (BSAVA publication) https://doi.org/10.22233/20412495.0818.10.

Galley, H.F. (2000). Renal dose dopamine: will the message now get through? Editorial. *The Lancet* 356: 2112–2113.

Humm, K.R., Senior, J.M., Dugdale, A.H., and Summerfield, N.J. (2007). Use of sodium nitroprusside in the anaesthetic protocol of a patent ductus arteriosus ligation in a dog. *The Veterinary Journal* 173: 194–196.

Lee, Y.-H.L., Clarke, K.W., Alibhai, H.I.K., and Song, D. (1998). Effects of dopamine, dobutamine, dopexamine, phenylephrine and saline solution on intramuscular blood flow and other cardiopulmonary variables in halothane–anesthetized ponies. *American Journal of Veterinary Research* 59: 1463–1472.

Noel-Morgan, J. and Muir, W.W. (2018). Anesthesia-associated relative hypovolemia: mechanisms, monitoring and treatment considerations. *Frontiers in Veterinary Science* 5: 53. https://doi.org/10.3389/fvets.2018.00053.

Pace, C. (2019). Beginners guide to cardiac pharmacology. *The Veterinary Nurse* 10: 204–209.

Pascoe, P.J., Ilkiw, J.E., and Pypendop, B.H. (2006). Effects of increasing infusion rates of dopamine, dobutamine, epinephrine and phenylephrine in healthy anesthetized cats. *American Journal of Veterinary Research* 67: 1491–1499.

Rosati, M., Dyson, D.H., Sinclair, M.D., and Sears, W.C. (2007). Response of hypotensive dogs to dopamine hydrochloride and dobutamine hydrochloride during deep isoflurane anesthesia. *American Journal of Veterinary Research* 68: 483–494.

Ross, J.J. (2001). A systematic approach to cardiovascular pharmacology. *BJA CEPD Reviews* 1: 8–11.

Silverstein, D.C. and Santoro Beer, K.A. (2015). Controversies regarding choice of vasopressor therapy for management of septic shock in animals. *Journal of Veterinary Emergency and Critical Care* 25: 48–54.

The Sicilian Gambit: A new approach to the classification of antiarrhythmic drugs based on their actions on arrhythmogenic mechanisms (1991). The task force of the working group on arrhythmias of the European society of cardiology. *Circulation* 84: 1831–1851.

Wohl, J.S., Schwartz, D.D., Flournoy, W.S. et al. (2007). Renal hemodynamic and diuretic effects of low–dose dopamine in anesthetized cats. *Journal of Veterinary Emergency and Critical Care* 17: 45–82.

Young, L.E., Blissitt, K.J., Clutton, R.E., and Molony, V. (1998). Temporal effects of an infusion of dobutamine hydrochloride in horses anesthetized with halothane. *American Journal of Veterinary Research* 59: 1027–1032.

26

Shock, SIRS, MODS/MOF, Sepsis

LEARNING OBJECTIVES

- To be able to define shock and contextualise it as the end-stage/final common path of many possible initiating causes.
- To be able to recognise early/compensated and late/decompensated clinical presentations of shock.
- To be able to outline the pathophysiology of how systemic inflammatory response syndrome (SIRS) and multiple organ dysfunction syndrome (MODS)/multiple organ failure (MOF) can develop.
- To be able to define sepsis.
- To be able to discuss the various basic treatment options for shock states, SIRS, MODS/MOF and sepsis.
- To be able to recognise the importance of monitoring and regular patient reassessment, and of changing treatment plans as necessary.

26.1 Introduction

No matter what the inciting cause, **shock is defined as the clinical state due to inadequate cellular energy production.** It can result: from failure of the microcirculation to deliver adequate oxygen and metabolic substrates to the cells, and to remove their waste metabolic products; and/or when the cells are unable to utilise the delivered oxygen (see below). Shock, therefore, results in altered cell metabolism that increases the risk of cell death, which may progress to organ dysfunction or failure and eventual death of the patient.

Shock is the end-stage or final common path of many diseases, severe trauma, or infection. It can be thought of as a **syndrome**, a collection of clinical signs associated with these final common pathophysiological processes.

Shock has been classified according to the primary cause (e.g. haemorrhagic, anaphylactic, septic, endotoxic, neurogenic, cardiogenic) in the hope that identification of the initiating problem would help target the treatment more effectively. However, because shock is an end-stage syndrome, the clinical signs associated with it tend to be common to all its causes and it may not be so easy to diagnose the underlying cause in each case. As we will see later, a dog with gastric dilation/volvulus (GDV), of several hours'

duration may have hypovolaemic, cardiogenic, distributive, obstructive, and metabolic shock.

26.2 Main 'Types' of Shock

The main 'types' of shock (with some overlap of causes) are given below.

26.2.1 Hypovolaemic

This is an absolute deficiency of intravascular volume.

- Haemorrhagic.
- Traumatic – haemorrhage; coagulopathy of trauma.
- Severe fluid losses and dehydration.

26.2.2 Distributive/Maldistributive/Vasculogenic

Can be high or low resistance, i.e. inappropriate vasodilation or vasoconstriction can lead to maldistribution of intravascular volume.

- Sepsis/septic shock: the clinical manifestations of progressive SIRS.
- Anaphylactic shock: massive histamine release leading to vasodilation.

Veterinary Anaesthesia: Principles to Practice, Second Edition. Alexandra H. A. Dugdale, Georgina Beaumont, Carl Bradbrook, and Matthew Gurney.
© 2020 John Wiley & Sons Ltd. Published 2020 by John Wiley & Sons Ltd.
Companion website: www.wiley.com/go/dugdale/veterinary-anaesthesia

- Neurogenic shock: acute massive reduction in sympathetic tone leading to widespread vasodilation. Can follow spinal trauma or massive emotional distress (similar to the Bezold-Jarisch response resulting in vaso-vagal syncope, but with longer lasting [clinical] neuroendocrine consequences).

26.2.3 Obstructive

Impedance to venous return or cardiac output; impedance to organ perfusion.

- Cardiac tamponade; restrictive pericarditis.
- Tension pneumothorax.
- Massive pulmonary thromboembolism.
- Aorto-iliac thrombosis.
- Disseminated intravascular coagulopathy (DIC); multiple thromboses.
- Increased intra-abdominal pressure, e.g. bloat, GDV, equine tympanic colic.

26.2.4 Cardiogenic

Primary (mechanical or electrophysiological) pump failure.

- Heart failure (forward or backward), e.g. congenital or acquired heart disease.
- Myocardial depressant factors (MDF) (e.g. certain cytokines) released during SIRS can have negative inotropic effects.
- Arrhythmias (tachy- or brady-arrhythmias): disease- or drug- (including anaesthetic) induced.

26.2.5 Metabolic/Endocrine/Hypoxaemic

Factors affecting cellular respiration/metabolism, including reduced blood oxygen content, reduced metabolic substrate availability, metabolic toxins, and hormone imbalances.

- Anaemia
- Dyshaemoglobinaemia (e.g. methaemoglobinaemia; carbon monoxide inhalation and formation of carboxyhaemoglobin).
- Mitochondrial dysfunction (cyanide toxicity; endotoxins/SIRS).
- Severe pulmonary disease.
- Heatstroke.
- Malignant hyperthermia.
- Hypoglycaemia.
- Acute adrenal insufficiency in critical illness.

Figure 26.1 shows how GDV can embrace more than one type of shock. See Chapter 27 for further information.

26.3 The Final Common Path of Shock

Failure of the microcirculation to deliver sufficient oxygen and metabolic substrates to the tissues and remove their waste products may develop consequent upon one or more problems in the factors that affect O_2 supply and demand (Figure 26.2). Mitochondrial function may also be impaired by, e.g. endotoxin and certain cytokines, further exacerbating the problems. Impaired tissue oxygenation can initiate SIRS (see below).

Hypoxaemia is poor oxygenation of blood. By convention, this is usually defined as abnormally low partial pressure of oxygen in the arterial blood (PaO_2) and not by a reduction in the total oxygen carriage of arterial blood. Although this definition ignores the haemoglobin concentration and its saturation, and therefore omits the oxygen-carrying capacity of the haemoglobin present, it assumes that low PaO_2 will compromise haemoglobin saturation and therefore total oxygen content of arterial blood.

Hypoxia is poor oxygenation of tissues. It can be due to:

- Ischaemia (poor perfusion) = stagnant hypoxia.
- Poor oxygenation of blood = hypoxaemic hypoxia.
- Anaemia (poor oxygenation of blood due to inadequate haemoglobin) = anaemic hypoxia.
- Metabolic poisons that reduce the ability of cells to utilise oxygen = histotoxic or cytotoxic/cytopathic hypoxia.

Figure 26.3 demonstrates the knock-on effects of decreased cellular oxygen availability.

26.4 Responses to Shock

The body tries hard to maintain vital organ perfusion and oxygenation through activation of the sympathetic nervous system, activation of the renin-angiotensin-aldosterone system, increased antidiuretic hormone (ADH) release, and activation of the hypothalamo-pituitary–adrenal axis. Differential tissue vasoconstriction and vasodilation try to divert blood to vital organs. Fluid shifts also occur at the capillary level. Tachycardia is often observed (although bradycardia may occur in the final, decompensatory stages). Tachypnoea occurs in response to: stimulation of chemoreceptors (by their hypoperfusion/hypoxia

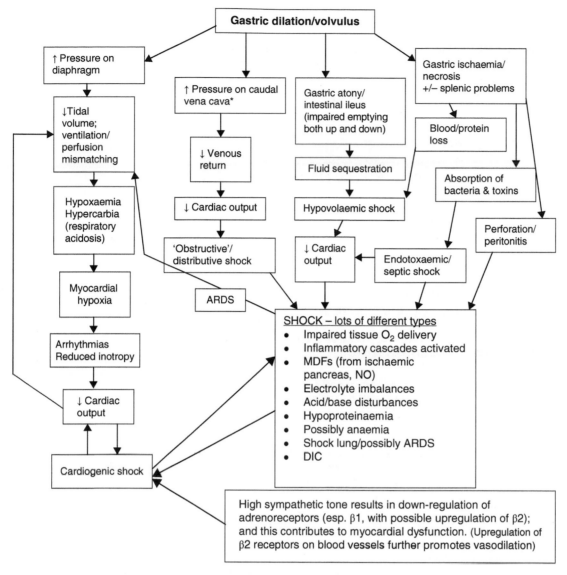

Figure 26.1 How different types of shock can co-exist. MDF, myocardial depressant factors, one of which may be nitric oxide (NO). *Compression not only of caudal vena cava, but also of hepatic portal vein causes splanchnic/renal/caudal body congestion (pooling of blood), which adds to the maldistribution of blood. ARDS (acute respiratory distress syndrome) due to pulmonary ischaemia/oedema/thromboemboli (i.e. 'shock' affects the pulmonary circulation as well as the systemic circulation).

Figure 26.2 Important players in the delivery of oxygen to the tissues. Hb, haemoglobin. Both the quality and quantity of Hb present in blood are important. Stroke volume is affected by preload, afterload, and myocardial contractility. Preload depends upon venous return (and therefore on blood volume) and cardiac chamber capacity (which can be affected by pericardial and myocardial disease). Afterload is affected by systemic vascular resistance.

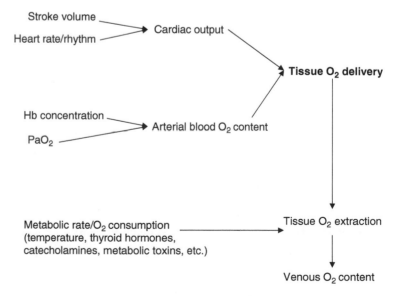

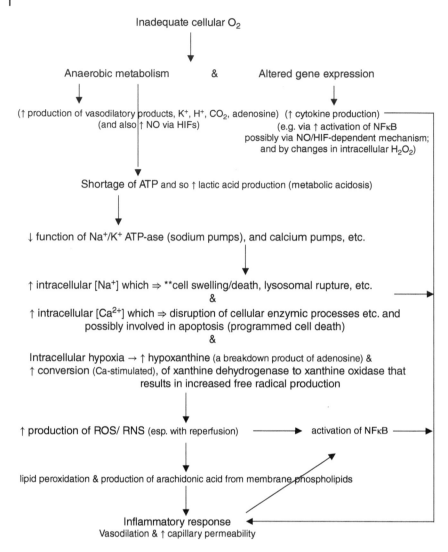

Figure 26.3 Consequences of reduced cellular oxygen availability. **Cell swelling includes capillary endothelial cells, the swelling of which further compromises tissue perfusion, and results in 'rounding up' of cells on the basement membrane, which leads to increased vascular permeability and leakage of fluid, proteins, and cells (especially inflammatory cells) into the interstitial space (causing oedema that further reduces O_2 delivery to cells). Exposure of basement membrane also exposes factors that trigger inflammatory and coagulation cascades. Mucosal 'barrier' of gut also compromised leading to bacterial translocation and endotoxaemia. Mitochondrial damage and malfunction also occur when the normal intracellular environment is disturbed. Cell death results in the release of cytosolic and nuclear components called DAMPs (damage [or danger]-associated molecular patterns) or alarmins, which can promote further inflammation and immune responses. ROS, reactive oxygen species; RNS, reactive nitrogen species; NFκB, nuclear transcription factor kappa B. HIFs (hypoxia-inducible factors) are transcription factors consisting of α and β subunits. In normally oxygenated tissues the α subunits are ubiquitinated and destroyed. In hypoxic cells, however, the α subunits can dimerise with the β subunits, and the dimers can then affect gene transcription.

and by the low blood pH with metabolic acidosis); stimulation of baroreceptors (because of their communication with the respiratory centre); and possibly in response to pain or fear.

The shock index may be helpful to determine. It is calculated as:

Shock Index = Heart rate/Systolic arterial blood pressure

where 0.9–1 is normal but >1 indicates shock.

For primary hypovolaemic shock, peripheral vasoconstriction influences the early clinical signs that include:

- Tachycardia
- (Normal to) weak peripheral pulses
- Cool extremities
- Pale mucous membranes, brisk to normal capillary refill time (CRT)

- Tachypnoea
- Reduced urine output
- Normal or only mildly subdued mentation

For primary distributive shock, peripheral vasodilation influences the early clinical signs that include:

- Fever may be present
- Tachycardia
- Pulses 'bounding' (despite hypotension)
- Warm extremities
- Brick red/hyperaemic mucous membranes, brisk CRT
- Tachypnoea
- Reduced urine output
- Normal or only slightly subdued mentation

This is the **compensatory stage**, often called the **hyperdynamic stage**. During this stage, the stress response (increased catecholamines, cortisol, glucagon, growth hormone, and possibly thyroid hormones) may result in hyperglycaemia. Insulin resistance is also a common feature. Inflammatory cells use glucose (non-insulin-dependent) as their primary energy source, which is also an acceptable energy substrate for many of the vital organs. These responses therefore help to divert energy sources to the cells which most need them. There is an overall increase in O_2/energy demand. Sympathetic nervous system and renin-angiotensin system activation and increased ADH aim to promote vasoconstriction and fluid retention.

However, if this stage continues untreated, then inflammatory mediators (e.g. cytokines, eicosanoids), the free radical NO (which is also a gasotransmitter and vasorelaxant), other free radicals and products of cellular anaerobic metabolism (e.g. K^+, CO_2, H^+, adenosine), and cell death (e.g. enzymes), can cause SIRS to progress towards MODS/MOF. Translocation of endotoxins/bacteria may also come into the picture as the gut mucosal barrier becomes compromised. Hypotension worsens. This is **the decompensatory stage**, or **hypodynamic stage**, features of which include:

- Vasodilation (especially precapillary arterioles), which worsens tissue congestion, oedema, sludging of blood flow, and microthrombi formation
- Increased vascular permeability (capillary leak syndrome [Clarkson's syndrome])
- DIC
- Negative inotropy
- Deranged cellular metabolism (increased intracellular Ca^{2+}; mitochondrial dysfunction)

For primary hypovolaemic shock, peripheral vasodilation now influences the late clinical signs that include:

- Tachycardia or bradycardia
- Peripheral pulses are poor

- Hypotension
- Mucous membranes often congested/hyperaemic/injected/icteric
- CRT prolonged, >2–3 seconds
- Glucose may be high, normal, or low
- Decreased body temperature
- Depressed mentation

For primary distributive shock, peripheral vasodilation and microvascular thromboses influence the late clinical signs that include:

- Tachycardia or bradycardia
- Peripheral pulses are weak and thready
- Hypotension
- Mucous membranes often congested/cyanotic/icteric/petechiated (DIC)
- CRT is prolonged, >2–3 seconds
- Glucose may be normal or low
- Decreased body temperature
- Depressed mentation

The rate of progression from the compensatory to the decompensatory stage depends upon the severity of the initial insult, but progression tends to be faster with distributive types of shock. (Often the picture may be a little more complicated, as more than one type of 'shock' tends to be present, e.g. endotoxin/bacterial translocation often becomes involved, after compromise of gastrointestinal [GI] tract perfusion). The decompensated stage can quickly progress to a stage refractory to treatment.

Poor prognostic indicators are:

- **Bradycardia**
- **Hypoglycaemia**
- **Hypothermia**
- **Acidosis**
- **DIC**

The physiological response to hypovolaemia/hypotension is often taught as only tachycardic; but bradycardia, which may appear 'inappropriate or paradoxical', may also occur, and tends to herald the onset of decompensation. It seems that the bradycardia may be the body's attempt to reduce O_2 requirement. Animals, especially cats that present with bradycardia, hypothermia, and hypoglycaemia, tend to have a poor prognosis, but the hyperdynamic phase appears to be rarely recognised in cats. Cats also seem more prone to becoming hyperbilirubinaemic (due to cholestasis and/or haemolysis).

The 'shock organ' is the gastro-intestinal tract in dogs, such that diarrhoea, melaena, or ileus may be noted. In contrast, the lungs are the 'shock organ' in cats, such that signs of respiratory dysfunction are more common in this species.

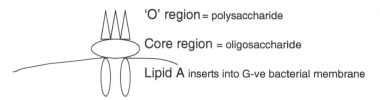

'O' region = polysaccharide

Core region = oligosaccharide

Lipid A inserts into G-ve bacterial membrane

Figure 26.4   Gram-negative bacterial endotoxin.

26.5   Systemic Inflammatory Response Syndrome (SIRS) and Multiple Organ Dysfunction Syndrome/Multiple Organ Failure (MODS/MOF)

The term SIRS describes a clinical state following exposure to infectious or non-infectious insults that can, if left untreated, progress to MODS/MOF and patient death.

26.5.1   Potential Causes of SIRS

26.5.1.1   Infectious Causes (Sepsis)
- Bacteria
- Viruses
- Fungi
- Parasites

26.5.1.2   Non-infectious Causes
- Trauma (polytrauma; major surgery)
- Inflammation (e.g. pancreatitis)
- Immune diseases
- Burns
- Heatstroke
- Hypoxaemia
- Prolonged hypovolaemia
- Neoplasia
- Components of infectious agents, e.g. endotoxins

We have already (Figure 26.3) seen how the unfavourable cellular energetics that accompany 'shock' can lead to host cell damage, resulting in the release of moieties called DAMPs (danger-associated molecular patterns, e.g. histones), which can stimulate SIRS. Below, we consider how SIRS can be triggered by endotoxin (Gram negative bacterial lipopolysaccharide [LPS]), which is considered to be a PAMP (pathogen-associated molecular pattern). Other important PAMPs include Gram positive bacterial lipoteichoic acid, peptidoglycan (murein) from both Gram positive and Gram negative bacteria, flagellin from both Gram positive and Gram negative bacteria, and fungal mannans (mannose polysaccharides). Endotoxaemia may occur with or without septicaemia. Septicaemia is often Gram negative in veterinary species, but Gram positive septicaemia can also occur.

Endotoxin is Gram-negative bacterial LPS (Figure 26.4). The lipid A region is the most important for the effects of endotoxins and is highly conserved amongst Gram negative bacteria. Endotoxin binds to lipopolysaccharide-binding protein (LBP), in the patient's blood. LBP acts as a transporter protein and helps to transfer LPS to cell membrane (especially inflammatory/immune-cell membrane) CD14 receptors. This LPS/CD14 receptor complex now interacts with a pattern-recognition receptor, Toll-like receptor 4 (TLR4), in cell membranes, which, in conjunction with another membrane protein, myeloid differentiation factor 2 (MD2), forms a receptor complex capable of activating intracellular pathways by mechanisms both dependent and independent of interaction with adaptor proteins such as myeloid differentiation factor 88, MyD88. There are two main intracellular pathways activated by MyD88-dependent mechanisms: nuclear transcription factor kappa B (NFκB) activation and activation of the mitogen-activated protein kinase (MAPK) pathway. (It is important to note that LPS signalling can also be independent of LBP, CD14, and TLR4 binding because various cell surface LPS-associated proteins [LAPs] can also act as LPS receptors.)

NFκB is an important player in the inflammatory response. It is a heterodimer that normally exists in the cytoplasm of cells bound to an inhibitory protein (inhibitor of kappa B, IκB) that renders it inactive. (The IκB alpha isoform is common in humans, whereas the beta isoform is common in horses.) Endotoxins, cytokines, and oxidants can result in separation of NFκB from IκB (through activation of Iκ kinases, which phosphorylate IκB leading to its subsequent degradation). Then, NFκB can move unhindered into the cell nucleus, where it can affect gene transcription, e.g. to result in up-regulation of COX-2 and inducible NOS (iNOS) expression.

iNOS is the inducible form of nitric oxide synthase, an enzyme that produces NO (a potent vasodilator and possibly an MDF). Constitutive NOS (cNOS), is expressed in vascular endothelial cells (eNOS) and neurons (nNOS), where NO is usually produced in small quantities. On the contrary, iNOS is expressed by vascular smooth muscle cells, hepatocytes, macrophages, and neutrophils, and NO is produced in vast quantities by iNOS. (As a free radical, NO is both a reactive nitrogen species [RNS] and a reactive oxygen species [ROS]; and it can react with other ROS, e.g. superoxide, to produce other RNS, e.g. peroxynitrite.) COX-2 is the inducible form cyclo-oxygenase that produces PGs and TXs. The NO produced by iNOS also nitrosylates and activates COX-2.

Phosphorylation of IκB can also occur independently of the Iκ kinase pathway, by a redox-regulated pathway that is controlled by intracellular H_2O_2; this pathway results in the activation of NFκB with ischaemia/reperfusion.

The result of cell 'activation' by endotoxin is the release of inflammatory mediators such as cytokines, eicosanoids (prostaglandins, thromboxanes, leukotrienes), platelet activating factor (PAF), NO, and ROS/RNS. Most of their production is stimulated through up-regulation of gene expression, e.g. NFkB is activated by endotoxin.

The majority of the clinical signs that follow significant endotoxin exposure are due to the actions of these inflammatory mediators, e.g. hypotension (due to vasodilation and fluid shifts), haemoconcentration (due to increased capillary permeability and fluid shifts), and coagulation abnormalities / DIC (vascular endothelial injury also activates endothelin signalling; endothelin is a potent vasoconstrictor and can itself activate the coagulation system). Some of the clinical signs are associated with reduced oxygen supply to the tissues. Endotoxin can also reduce the ability of cells to utilise oxygen by acting like a metabolic toxin, e.g. it reduces mitochondrial pyruvate dehydrogenase activity, resulting in an increase in lactate production, even when oxygen supply is not limiting. In the lungs, bronchoconstriction, pulmonary vasoconstriction (yet inhibition of hypoxic pulmonary vasoconstriction), thickening of the alveolar-capillary membrane (due to oedema [increased vascular permeability], and infiltration with inflammatory cells, especially neutrophils), all occur, which, alongside the accompanying hypotension, result in ventilation/perfusion mismatching and reduced pulmonary gaseous exchange (especially for oxygen, as oxygen is less soluble/diffusible than carbon dioxide). The overall result is hypoxaemia, which can exacerbate SIRS.

The body's response to endotoxin or other insults that can trigger SIRS, therefore results in the **acute phase response**: changes (regional increases or decreases) in vascular tone; increased vascular permeability; increased immune cell-adhesion to vascular endothelium that promotes further inflammatory/immune cell recruitment; activation of coagulation, kinin, and complement pathways; stimulation of the hypothalamic–pituitary axis (HPA) with development of the neuroendocrine 'stress-response'; hepatic production of acute phase proteins; negative nitrogen (protein) and energy balance; fever; and malaise.

In a 'local' setting, the integration of all these is probably important for wound healing. However, pro-inflammatory mediators and cytokines may spill over into the systemic circulation, and if they do so in sufficient quantity, then 'systemic' events occur. The systemic pro-inflammatory response is termed SIRS. Usually, the pro-inflammatory response is countered, either locally or systemically, by a compensatory anti-inflammatory response (termed the compensatory anti-inflammatory response syndrome, CARS), but if the anti-inflammatory response is insufficient, then the pro-inflammatory response gets out of hand and can become detrimental to the well-being of the animal. (Similarly, an excessive CARS can lead to detrimental immunosuppression.) The counter-regulatory responses include: a number of anti-inflammatory mediators (e.g. interleukins IL-10 and IL-13, TGF-β, protein C); suppressors of cytokine signalling (SOCS); inhibitors of activated 'signal transducers and activators of transcription' (STATs); and the heat shock response (HSR), which is a highly conserved cellular protective mechanism, whereby increased production of heat shock proteins (HSPs), and inhibition of NFκB activation, results from noxious cellular stressors such as heat, inflammation, hypoxia, or ischaemia-reperfusion injury.

An imbalance of SIRS and CARS may simply be due to overwhelming tissue injury or infection, although certain individuals may also have more difficulty with regulating their inflammatory responses (i.e. genotype appears to be important).

If unbalanced SIRS/CARS is left untreated, cellular dysfunction progresses to organ dysfunction. When compensatory mechanisms fail, organ damage occurs and MODS/MOF can become irreversible and eventually result in death of the whole organism. DIC with microvascular thrombosis is thought to play a significant part in the development of MODS/MOF, as is mitochondrial dysfunction (which is thought to occur through oxidative damage) with subsequent autophagy and depletion of mitochondrial numbers.

MODS has been defined as the potentially reversible abnormal function of at least two organ systems arising from a life-threatening physiological insult, such that homeostasis cannot be maintained without medical intervention. A dysregulated immune response is the underlying cause, but interactions among the systemic inflammatory response, the coagulation system, and the gastrointestinal tract (i.e. impaired mucosal barrier function and vast bacterial reservoir permitting toxin/bacterial translocation), appear to be important in the propagation of organ dysfunction. MODS has also been defined as the physiologic derangements of the endothelial, cardiopulmonary, renal, nervous, endocrine, and gastrointestinal systems associated with the progression of uncontrolled systemic inflammation and DIC.

Acute phase proteins increase during the acute phase reaction (N.B. see decreased albumin and decreased transferrin). They include:

- C-reactive protein (CRP)
- Complement components
- Protease inhibitors (α1 anti-trypsin, α1 anti-chymotrypsin, α2 macroglobulin, α2 anti-plasmin)
- LBP
- Serum amyloid A (SAA)
- α1 acid glycoprotein
- Clotting factors (fibrinogen, von Willebrand factor)
- Metal-binding proteins (caeruloplasmin, haemopexin, haptoglobin [transferrin usually decreases])
- Antithrombin III is reduced in many species, but is increased in cats, in which it is an acute phase protein
- Plasminogen activator inhibitor 1 (PAI-1)

26.5.2 Major Participants in the Inflammatory Response

26.5.2.1 PAF (Platelet Activating Factor)
- Activates platelets
- Increases vascular permeability
- Potent bronchoconstrictor and stimulates respiratory mucus production
- Encourages immune cell/platelet adhesion to endothelium

26.5.2.2 TNFα
- Pro-inflammatory (via NFκB): enhances production of other cytokines (ILs), PGs (via COX-2), NO (via iNOS) and adhesion molecules
- Endogenous pyrogen
- Increases endothelial and immune cell tissue factor (TF) expression (pro-coagulant)
- Reduces appetite (a cachectin [cachexin])
- Induces lethargy
- Possibly an MDF

26.5.2.3 IL-1(β)
- Pro-inflammatory (via NFκB): increases TNFα, other cytokines, NO (via iNOS), PG (via COX-2), and adhesion molecule production
- Endogenous pyrogen (leads to fever)
- Increases endothelial and immune cell TF expression
- Reduces appetite (a cachectin [cachexin])
- Possibly an MDF

26.5.2.4 IL-6
- Stimulates acute phase protein production
- Endogenous pyrogen
- May modulate IL-1 and TNFα production

26.5.2.5 IL-8
- Chemotactic (especially to neutrophils)

26.5.2.6 IL-10
- Anti-inflammatory: decreases TNFα and IL-8 production

26.5.2.7 NO (Nitric Oxide)
- Causes vasodilation (note that carbon monoxide [CO] also produces vasodilation through similar mechanism, i.e. production of cGMP)
- Increases capillary permeability
- Decreases myocardial function (possibly an MDF)
- Decreases WBC adhesion
- Decreases platelet aggregation
- Important in immunomodulation
- Affects renin release, and Na^+ and water homeostasis
- Is both a ROS and a RNS

26.6 Sepsis and Septic Shock

Nomenclature and definitions are the focus of much debate (see Further Reading). The **simplest definition of sepsis** is that it is a clinical syndrome characterised by a systemic inflammatory response to bacterial, viral, protozoal, or fungal infection that spans a continuum of severity between SIRS at one end, and septic shock (the development/persistence of hypotension despite volume replacement) at the other.

For people, sepsis is currently defined as 'life-threatening organ dysfunction caused by a dysregulated host response to infection', with septic shock being considered as 'a subset of sepsis with circulatory and cellular/metabolic dysfunction associated with a higher risk of mortality'. Both of these definitions imply an infectious cause. Note that SIRS can be associated with sepsis but also has non-infectious causes.

Definitions and clinical criteria that must be met to fulfil these definitions have not yet been universally agreed for the various veterinary species, however, criteria for the diagnosis of SIRS have been recommended.

Diagnosis of SIRS has been proposed on a basis of animals presenting with at least two (cats) or three (dogs) of the following abnormalities:

- Tachycardia or bradycardia (inappropriate/relative bradycardia appears to be more commonly found in cats than dogs)
- Tachypnoea
- Hypothermia or hyperthermia
- Leukopaenia or leukocytosis

These features, however, are non-specific and may lead to over-diagnosis. **Additional features of SIRS** include the following, although alterations in haemostatic variables (clotting times, fibrin degradation products, viscoelastic properties, etc.) are also non-specific:

- Alterations in the regulation of vasomotor tone
- Increased capillary endothelial permeability
- Coagulation abnormalities/microcirculatory dysfunction
- Anorexia
- Depression/lethargy

Illness severity scoring systems have also been applied, one promising system, at least for dogs, is the APPLE (acute patient physiologic and laboratory evaluation) fast system, which, although not able to differentiate non-infectious from infectious SIRS, appears related to prognosis.

Potential biomarkers of SIRS and sepsis have been investigated, mostly in people. Of these, CRP (an acute phase protein) may reflect the severity of the inflammatory process, but is non-specific and has a relatively long half-life. Procalcitonin (PCT) is released from stimulated monocytes/macrophages, particularly where bacterial infection is present, and has shown more promise in differentiating non-infectious SIRS from sepsis-associated SIRS. Although its role is still uncertain, PCT increases NO production via iNOS and therefore helps amplify the inflammatory response.

Cardiac dysfunction is a common consequence of systemic inflammation, at least in humans, where it has been more extensively investigated and is known as 'myocardial hibernation'. Whether protective, or indicative of poorer prognosis, is currently unknown, but cardiac biomarkers such as cardiac troponins (cTnT and cTnI) and natriuretic peptides (e.g. the N-terminal portion of pro-brain natriuretic peptide [NT-proBNP] are under investigation.

Although there is lack of a veterinary consensus definition of MODS, there is a positive correlation between the degree of organ system dysfunction and mortality. In dogs, a modified sequential organ failure (SOFA) score has been proposed in an attempt to evaluate increasing organ dysfunction.

26.6.1 Treatment for SIRS/Sepsis and MODS/MOF

The treatment goals for SIRS/sepsis and MODS/MOF are the same as those for shock. To address the cellular energy deficiency associated with shock states, the main aim is to restore tissue oxygen delivery, by trying to improve PaO_2 and cardiac output. (There remains a lot to learn about the role of cellular and subcellular dysfunction, and how to restore oxygen utilisation by the mitochondria/tissues.) In addition to this supportive care to try to preserve organ function, treatment of underlying disease processes, including source-control and antimicrobial therapy if infection is present or suspected, is also important.

Supportive treatment can be based on 'VIP':

- **V** = **v**entilation, to improve oxygenation of blood
- **I** = **i**nfusion of fluids and restoration of **i**ntravascular volume
- **P** = maintenance of myocardial **p**ump function and tissue **p**erfusion

This approach is reminiscent of the approach to cardiopulmonary cerebral resuscitation. The longer the shock-producing event is allowed to persist, the greater the consequences, and the more likely serious complications are to develop (e.g. reperfusion injury, SIRS, MODS/MOF).

26.6.1.1 Respiratory Support
26.6.1.1.1 Oxygen

Increasing the inspired O_2 concentration may help to improve the oxygenation of blood. Very rarely are our patients depressed enough (at admission) to allow endotracheal intubation (for oxygen provision and ventilation). However, placement of nasal oxygen prongs or insertion of a nasopharyngeal catheter for O_2 insufflation or use of a makeshift O_2 tent (Elizabethan collar and cling film) may be tolerated and should be beneficial.

For nasal catheters, oxygen flows of around 200 ml/kg/min can increase the inspired oxygen to around 50% (normal room air is 21%), whereas increasing the flow to around 500 ml/kg/min can increase the inspired oxygen to around 80%. Such supplementary O_2 therapy should be humidified where possible. Oxygen toxicity can develop with exposure to fractional inspired oxygen (F_IO_2) >60% for periods of time > 12–24 hours; therefore, try to reduce F_IO_2 to ≤60% as soon as possible. High airflow oxygen enrichment (HAFOE) venturi devices can offer an alternative, whereby the 'prescribed' F_IO_2 can be delivered more accurately. Serial arterial blood gas analyses are very useful in guiding oxygen supplementation.

Consider if anaemia is present: Does the patient have enough red cells and functional haemoglobin? Transfusion of blood or blood products may be appropriate. HBOCs are not currently widely available.

26.6.1.2 Circulatory Support
26.6.1.2.1 Fluids

See Chapter 23. Beware in cases of congestive cardiac failure and those with pulmonary oedema/ARDS. Hypoproteinaemic patients also warrant further consideration of fluid choices, as do those with capillary leak states.

Types of fluids:

- Crystalloids: isotonic or hypertonic
- Synthetic colloids (includes HBOCs where these are available)
- Albumin (species-specific albumin often not available)

- Plasma: fresh, fresh-frozen (or frozen); ±heparin (cofactor of antithrombin III)
- Blood: fresh or stored

Do not be afraid to change your fluid plan regularly or to use more than one type of fluid.

Routes of Administration
- Intravenous
- Intra-osseous
- Subcutaneous route is too slow
- Intraperitoneal route also slow, but may also be inappropriate for the condition (e.g. peritonitis) or the type of fluid required

Volume and Rate What are the clinical signs? Can you estimate a percentage dehydration from skin tent (increased duration of skin tent usually means between 5 and 15% dehydration), and haemoconcentration. After any acute (in the previous four to six hours) haemorrhage, the packed cell volume (PCV) and total solids (TS) will not have had time to change.

Is it important to monitor the response to treatment (Table 26.1), e.g. improvement in mentation; normalisation of heart rate, mucous membrane colour, moistness, and CRT; improvement in peripheral pulse quality and arterial blood pressure; restoration of urine output and specific gravity (SG); and closing of wide core: periphery

Table 26.1 Variables to monitor to help guide fluid therapy.

Variable	Goals of treatment
Patient mentation/responsiveness	Aim for bright, alert, responsive
Heart rate/pulse rate	Aim for >60 and <180 bpm (dog); >85 and <200 bpm (cat); 20–45 bpm (horse)
Pulse quality (central/peripheral)	Aim for strong peripheral pulses
Mucous membrane colour, moistness, CRT	Aim for pink, moist, CRT ≤2 s
Breathing rate	Aim for normal (10–40 bpm small animals; 8–16 bpm horse)
Temperature (core : periphery)	Aim for normal core or rectal temp., and temp. gradient not >3–4 °C
Skin turgor	Aim for normal
Urine output and SG	Aim for 1–1.5 ml/kg/h and SG isosthenuric (1.008–1.012, possibly up to 1.015 for cats); or up to ~1.015–1.018
CVP	Less favoured nowadays, but may still be useful. Aim for 5–10 cm H_2O (very positional, and depends a little upon intra-abdominal, pericardial, and intrathoracic pressures). Measure during end-expiratory pause
Arterial blood pressure	Aim for 60–70 mmHg mean arterial pressure
Ultrasonographic assessment of myocardial contractility	May allow assessment of inotropic state of myocardium, which may help to direct therapy
Ultrasonographic assessment of various caudal vena cava to aorta ratios (e.g. diameters) *The echocardiographic ratio of left atrial to aortic root diameter has mainly been used to determine the presence/degree of congestive heart failure, but has also gained some attention in the evaluation of relative intravascular volume status*	May help determine fluid responsiveness and direct therapy with fluids/vasopressors/positive inotropes
Blood gases and electrolytes	Aim for PaO_2 > 60–70 mmHg; and PvO_2 > 35 mmHg; pH 7.3–7.5 and normal electrolyte concentrations
Central venous oxygen saturation (blood from taken from a central venous cannula in the cranial vena cava or proximal caudal vena cava)	Aim for $ScvO_2$ > 70%
Blood glucose	Aim for normal (c. 3.5–6.5 mmol/l), but values up to renal glucose threshold (~10 mmol/l) may be tolerated. Beware hypoglycaemia.
PCV/TS	Aim for PCV >28% (can be lower if providing supplemental oxygen) and <45%; and TS >3.5 g/dl
Albumin	Aim for >2 g/dl
Hb	Aim for at least 7 (pref. 9) g/dl
Lactic acid (lactate)	A lot of influencing factors, normal <1 to ~2 mmol/l (higher in rabbits)
Body Weight	Helps monitor fluid balance ('ins' and 'outs'); and caloric intake

temperature gradients. Blood lactate concentration sometimes increases with instigation of fluid therapy (due to reperfusion), but should decrease as fluid therapy progresses.

As with all fluid therapy plans, aim to restore circulating blood volume as soon as possible; then address the deficits of the other fluid compartments; and cater for ongoing losses as well as ongoing maintenance requirements. Remember that 'volume-replacement' crystalloid fluids (e.g. normal [0.9%] saline, Hartmann's solution) are not good 'maintenance fluids'. For maintenance fluid requirements, 5% glucose (in water) or 4% glucose +1/5 normal (0.18%) saline tend to be used, but often with added K^+ and perhaps other electrolytes such as magnesium. Normosol M or Plasma-Lyte 56 with 5% dextrose are excellent choices if available. How much and how fast you administer the fluid/fluids depends upon the patient's condition, response, and the underlying cause/s of the shock. See Chapter 23.

26.6.1.2.2 Inotropes and Vasopressors

May be required for maintenance of 'normal' haemodynamic function, although sometimes a state of vasoplegia is apparent, and poor response is seen to these drugs. This may be secondary to down-regulation of both alpha and beta receptors on the vasculature and myocardium. Dobutamine, dopamine, pimobendan, ephedrine, norepinephrine, epinephrine, phenylephrine, metaraminol and methoxamine may all have a place. Vasopressin (ADH) is also sometimes administered to reduce the requirement for other vasopressors, and works in an acidic environment. It acts on V1, V2, and V3 receptors, V1 receptors being those normally responsible for vasoconstriction in the systemic circulation (but vasodilation, through an NO-mediated mechanism, in the pulmonary circulation). Vasopressin also blocks ATP-sensitive potassium channels (which are often excessively activated during shock states, leading to vasodilation), thus perhaps facilitating some restoration of vascular tone.

At one time, naloxone was suggested to reduce some of the detrimental effects of endogenous opioids (such as hypotension and gastrointestinal ileus), but no posology exists. Methylene blue, which reduces NO production (inhibits NO synthase) and therefore may help reverse some NO-induced vasodilation and decrease the production of RNS, has been used in people, but is not currently advocated for veterinary species (except for the treatment of certain poisonings where it may help to reduce the ferric state of iron in methaemoglobin back to its ferrous state).

The adrenal glands are often underactive in shock (the 'relative adrenal insufficiency of critical illness'). Supplementation with low dose corticosteroids *may* help but further evidence is required. Glucocorticoids have anti-inflammatory effects and they have permissive effects on the actions of catecholamines and help up-regulate β receptors, so may enable reduced cardiovascular support with exogenous positive inotropes and vasopressors. (ACTH stimulation test is often advised first.)

26.6.1.2.3 Osmotherapy

Osmotic agents, such as mannitol and hypertonic saline, may also have a place as they shrink cells suffering from cellular oedema, especially vascular endothelial cells, and this may enhance return of perfusion. Mannitol is also a free radical scavenger and hypertonic saline may have immunomodulatory actions.

Diuretics (e.g. furosemide) may be useful to help fluid mobilisation and redistribution, to reduce tissue and pulmonary oedema, and to help restore urine output. (Also very useful with cardiogenic shock; where vasodilators also play a role.)

26.6.1.2.4 Anti-arrhythmics

May be necessary. See Chapters 25 and 27.

26.6.1.3 Other Therapeutic Interventions
26.6.1.3.1 Acid–base Disturbance Correction

Fluid therapy and restoration of renal function go a long way to sorting out many of these problems. See Chapters 21 and 23.

26.6.1.3.2 Correct Electrolyte Disturbances

Acid–base disturbances may also influence electrolyte concentrations. Acute hyperkalaemia is probably the most life-threatening electrolyte abnormality (see Chapter 24). Correct chronic changes slowly, and acute changes in electrolyte concentrations more rapidly.

26.6.1.3.3 Tight Glycaemic Control

Endeavour to normalise blood glucose concentration. Both hypoglycaemia and hyperglycaemia have adverse consequences. Some patients may also be diabetic, and critically ill patients often have a degree of insulin resistance (type 2 diabetes mellitus), possibly requiring insulin with or without glucose infusions; monitor electrolytes (especially potassium) too. Although many 'maintenance' crystalloid fluids contain some glucose, these do not contain sufficient glucose for nutritional requirements.

26.6.1.3.4 Attend to Caloric Requirements and Provide Gastrointestinal Ulcer Prophylaxis

Provide calories (enteral/parenteral nutrition) as soon as a patient cannot eat for itself. Negative energy balance is common in critically ill patients. Small volume (pharmacological/trophic) enteral feeds help to keep the gut active and healthy, even if most calorie requirements must be met by parenteral nutrition. Oral glutamine may help aid gastrointestinal tract villus epithelial restitution, although the evidence for supplementation of conditionally essential amino acids (glutamine, arginine, cysteine, taurine), is conflicting. Other pharmaco-nutrients such as omega 3 fatty acids (anti-inflammatory effects), anti-oxidants (vitamins C and E and selenium), trace elements (e.g. zinc), and mitochondrial therapies (co-enzyme Q10) require further investigations.

Prophylaxis against GI ulcers may be important, although reducing gastric acidity may allow survival of bacteria that would otherwise be destroyed by stomach acid.

26.6.1.3.5 *Control Fever; Prevent Hypothermia*
Whilst mild hypothermia reduces O_2 requirements, beware excessive hypothermia, as shivering certainly increases O_2 requirements and can compromise ventilatory efficiency.

26.6.1.3.6 *Antibiotics*
Where infection is present, suspected, or likely to develop, broad spectrum antibiotics covering Gram positive, Gram negative, and anaerobic bacteria, are given until results of culture and sensitivity are known. Attention to cleanliness and aseptic technique are important for all indwelling intravascular cannulae, and oxygen delivery, urinary, and feeding catheters.

26.6.1.3.7 *Anti-inflammatories, Anti-endotoxins, Anti-oxidants, and Rheological Agents*
Several NSAIDs have an anti-NFκB effect as well as causing COX ($\pm$5–LOX) inhibition. Glucocorticoids inhibit phospholipase A2, and therefore reduce flux through COX and 5-LOX pathways and reduce PAF production, thereby exerting some of their anti-inflammatory effects. Corticosteroids also promote production of IκBα, thus inhibiting NFκB activation, thereby exerting further anti-inflammatory effects by further reducing cytokine, eicosanoid, and NO production. They have a permissive/facilitatory effect on the actions of catecholamines (e.g. through COMT inhibition [which delays breakdown of catecholamines, thus prolonging their effects] and up-regulation of β receptor expression); thus improving patient response to endogenous catecholamines and also positive inotropes and vasopressors, and reducing exogenous inotropic/pressor requirements. They tend to make animals feel better too (said to be euphoric). The side effects of NSAIDs and glucocorticoids may, however, preclude their usefulness, although there is some renewed interest in low dose hydrocortisone in critical illness.

Pentoxifylline is a methylxanthine derivative that inhibits phosphodiesterase enzymes, increasing cellular cAMP, which interferes with MAPK pathway activation, producing anti-inflammatory effects, and also inhibits the phosphorylation of IκB and so reduces the activation of NFκB. It is therefore a potent anti-inflammatory, especially in the face of endotoxin challenge. It may also be used as a 'rheological' agent to decrease blood viscosity and platelet aggregation, cause selective vasodilation, and help offset some of the haemodynamic consequences of endotoxaemia.

The β_2 adrenoceptor agonists, e.g. clenbuterol, have anti-inflammatory effects through regulating NFκB activation by multiple mechanisms (e.g. increased cellular cAMP increases cytosolic IκB, which prevents NFκB activation and translocation to the nucleus).

Ketamine, and possibly some of the opioids, also have anti-NFκB actions. Further research is needed before definitive advice on their use can be given.

Lidocaine, when administered intravenously, has anti-inflammatory properties and may reduce inflammatory cell adhesion to endothelium as well as causing some vasodilation. These actions have been suggested to help promote reperfusion by preventing the 'no-reflow' phenomenon. That is, even with fluid therapy, some vascular beds remain 'blocked', not always by microthrombi or cell debris, but rather possibly by vasoconstriction/vasospasm (due to high intracellular calcium concentration in vascular smooth muscle cells and/or endothelin release) or adhered inflammatory cells, or due to vascular endothelial cellular oedema, or even due to extrinsic compression by interstitial oedema. Vasodilators may occasionally be appropriate (alongside well monitored fluid therapy and haemodynamic function) in the hope that they improve tissue perfusion and oxygen delivery.

Natural antioxidants are present within cells, even inside different cell organelles, and also in the extracellular environment. Antioxidants are present in both the aqueous and lipid phases. They include: non-enzymatic molecules, which scavenge ROS, such as vitamin C, vitamin A, vitamin E, co-enzyme Q-10; proteins with sulphydryl groups (albumin, haptoglobin, caeruloplasmin); and enzymes that minimise ROS generation and activity, such as catalase, superoxide dismutase, and glutathione peroxidase, for which selenium is an important cofactor.

Theoretically, the following compounds have antioxidant properties:

- Allopurinol (inhibits xanthine oxidase)
- Superoxide dismutase (converts superoxide radicals into hydrogen peroxide, H_2O_2)
- Dimethyl sulphoxide (DMSO) (scavenges hydroxyl radicals and inhibits NFκB)
- Deferoxamine (suppresses Fe-dependent free-radical reactions)

Inclusion of some of the above during therapy may help to limit ischaemia-reperfusion/re-oxygenation injury and may improve the chances of survival, but good evidence is so far lacking.

Lazeroids (synthetic 21 aminosteroids) were at one time promoted, especially for acute CNS injuries, as potent anti-oxidants with no glucocorticoid activity. They no longer appear to be popular.

Pyruvate is a scavenger of ROS (including hydrogen peroxide), and its administration has been shown to improve organ function in models where there is oxidant-mediated cellular injury, although it is relatively unstable in aqueous solution. A more stable compound, ethyl pyruvate, has therefore been trialled in various experimental models of critical illness, and has shown some promising results; in addition to its ROS scavenging actions it appears to have other anti-inflammatory actions.

Decoy oligodeoxynucleotides, which can inhibit NFκB activity, have also been tried, but with equivocal results.

Monoclonal antibodies directed against 'O' antigens (e.g. Stegantox™) are specific to a particular bacterial strain, whereas monoclonal antibodies directed against the core antigens (e.g. hyperimmune serum) or lipid A have cross-reactivity across many Gram negative bacteria. There is some evidence to support the use of equine hyperimmune serum where endotoxin has an important role in the presenting patient's condition.

In people, intravenous human immunoglobulin has been shown to improve outcome in some cases of Gram negative sepsis and may warrant further investigations in animals.

Polymixin B, a cyclic cationic peptide antibiotic, acts like a detergent. It forms a stable 1 : 1 complex with the lipid A part of endotoxin. Its usefulness, however, is limited because of its own side effects (nephro- and neuro-toxicity).

Antibodies to, or antagonists of, CD14 and TLR4 receptors have so far proved disappointing, as have monoclonal antibodies directed against the various cytokines and their receptors. TNFα remains membrane-bound on the inflammatory cells that produce it, until it is released by the TNFα-converting enzyme 'TACE'. As free TNFα is the most 'active', TACE-inhibitors should therefore reduce the amount of 'active' TNFα. The clinical benefits of TACE-inhibitors, however, have yet to be proven.

26.6.1.3.8 *TLC (Tender Loving Care)*
Good nursing with physiotherapy to encourage patient mobilisation and stimulate interest can also help.

26.7 Take Home Message

The complex and interlinking inflammatory, coagulation, and immune pathways will likely preclude one single panacea; rather multiple interventions (the treatment bundle concept), with good supportive care, may yet provide the best outcomes. The reader is referred to the reference section for further information.

26.8 Anaphylaxis

Anaphylaxis is an acute, serious hypersensitivity reaction that is rapid in onset and may cause death. Triggers include medications such as the penicillin-type antibiotics and neuromuscular blockers, blood transfusions, and imaging contrast agents such as radiographic and MRI contrast agents. The reaction occurs without warning. *Distinction between anaphylactic and anaphylactoid reactions is no longer recommended as both the clinical picture and emergency treatment are similar, regardless of the pathophysiologic mechanism.*

Most anaphylactic episodes are of the allergic type and involve an immediate hypersensitivity reaction following allergen interaction with cell-bound immunoglobulin E (IgE). Less commonly, other mechanisms (allergic/immune or non-allergic/non-immune) are involved. Regardless of the inciting mechanism, the final common pathway involves release of histamine and other mediators from mast cells and basophils. The severity of the reaction can vary from mild anaphylaxis (e.g. urticaria/itching) to full-blown anaphylactic shock that can be fatal. Symptoms usually occur within five to 30 minutes of exposure to the trigger factor, although occasionally they do not develop for several hours. The quicker the onset, the more severe the reaction is. Anaphylaxis may be fatal within minutes, usually through cardiovascular or respiratory compromise, or both.

26.8.1 Typical Signs

- Cutaneous symptoms and signs are the most common manifestations of anaphylaxis, occurring in 90% of cases. These include generalised urticaria, erythema (flushing/redness of the skin), itching/pruritus, and angioedema (swelling of the subcutaneous tissues, especially around the head and face). Note that cutaneous signs may not be obvious until cardiovascular resuscitation has taken place.
- Respiratory signs (wheezing, dyspnoea) occur because bronchoconstriction, mucosal oedema, laryngeal, and/or pharyngeal oedema and excessive mucus production cause respiratory obstruction. Such signs occur in about 70% of cases.
  - Looks like asthma attack; wheezing, dyspnoea, excessive salivation/mucus production around mouth
- Gastro-intestinal signs (vomiting; diarrhoea, which may be haemorrhagic) occur in around 40% of cases.

- Hypotension and cardiovascular collapse (due to vasodilation and increased capillary permeability with extravasation of fluid) occurs in 10–30% of cases.
  - May see acute bradycardia ('paradoxical bradycardia' associated with the Bezold-Jarisch reflex response to acute, massive depletion of intravascular volume), which may be sustained
  - May see transient bradycardia, followed by increase in HR/tachycardia
  - May see tachycardia rapidly giving way to bradycardia
  - May see arrhythmias
  - Arterial blood pressure falls dramatically
  - $ETCO_2$ will fall due to reduced cardiac output and reduced pulmonary perfusion
- CNS signs: restlessness, inco-ordination; mental dullness; collapse; seizures or coma

26.8.1.1 Species-specific Reactions

In dogs, the major 'shock organs' are the liver and GI tract. Specifically, the hepatic portal vein constricts, causing portal hypertension and pooling of blood in the abdominal viscera, which results in hepatic and GI oedema with subsequent out-pouring of haemorrhagic effusion into the gut lumen, which can be seen as almost immediate haemorrhagic diarrhoea. Conscious dogs may also vomit. Abdominal ultrasonography usually reveals oedema/striation of the gallbladder wall (the 'halo' or 'double-rim' sign), and mild (to moderate) haemoperitoneum may also accompany anaphylaxis in dogs (beware unnecessary emergency exploratory laparotomy).

In cats, the major 'shock organ' is the lungs, with the GI tract as a secondary shock organ, so that dyspnoea, salivation, and also vomiting and diarrhoea are common signs.

26.8.2 Treatment Outline

With treatment, the clinical signs generally resolve, but in a small number of patients, signs can recur within 6–12 hours ('biphasic' reactions) despite successful initial treatment, so further treatment is required. Epinephrine (adrenaline) is widely advocated as the main treatment in those individuals experiencing anaphylaxis. The use of epinephrine in anaphylaxis is based on tradition and on evidence from fatality series (in which most individuals dying from anaphylaxis had not received prompt epinephrine treatment). Although the evidence base in support of the use of epinephrine is unclear, there is no other medication with a similar effect on the many body systems that are potentially involved in anaphylaxis. **Epinephrine appears to be life-saving when injected promptly**, however, there is no evidence from randomised controlled trials for or against the use of epinephrine in the emergency treatment of anaphylaxis.

Epinephrine is widely advocated as the initial treatment of choice for anaphylaxis either intramuscularly or by intravenous infusion, or both. It is an alpha- and beta-adrenergic receptor agonist, with bidirectional cyclic AMP-mediated pharmacologic effects on target organs and a narrow therapeutic index.

Epinephrine treatment results in:

- vasoconstriction (and therefore increased peripheral vascular resistance)
- decreased capillary permeability (and therefore decreased oedema formation)
- positive inotropic and chronotropic effects (i.e. increased force and rate of cardiac contraction, respectively)
- bronchodilation
- decreased mediator release from mast cells and basophils

The optimal dose of epinephrine to administer IM or IV has not yet been defined in humans or animals. The risk of adverse side effects (usually on the heart) following epinephrine treatment is also unquantified, but side effects tend to occur in the setting of inappropriate dosing (an overdose, an inadequately diluted intravenous dose, or an overly rapid rate of infusion). There is, however, now increased awareness that the heart itself may be a target organ in anaphylaxis and that electrocardiographic changes suggesting myocardial ischaemia, and dysrhythmias, can occur in the absence of epinephrine administration. (Excessive endogenous catecholamine release, or exogenous epinephrine administration, may result in acute, reversible, systolic dysfunction, possibly associated with adrenergic receptor desensitisation, and which has been termed Takotsubo syndrome in people.) In summary, the use of epinephrine in anaphylaxis appears to be based largely upon extrapolation from first principles, expert opinion, and tradition.

Note that **atropine should be avoided in cases of paradoxical bradycardia** (which is thought to be a physiological response that tries to preserve diastolic ventricular filling in the face of profound hypovolaemia) as it may induce cardiac arrest.

26.8.2.1 Evidence for Epinephrine Use in Dogs

In a canine model of fully developed anaphylactic shock:

- Epinephrine 0.01 mg/kg IM was ineffective
- An intravenous bolus of 0.01 mg/kg resulted in transient improvement
- Intravenous infusion at ~0.05 µg/kg/min was the only method to produce a sustained improvement, but only due to its positive inotropic effect on the heart. No increases in either systemic vascular resistance or pulmonary

arterial wedge pressure were noted. Thus, if a severe reaction develops and epinephrine is administered at the generally recommended doses for anaphylaxis (see below), it might not adequately counteract the effects of vasodilation and distributive-hypovolaemic shock on its own, even when given as an intravenous infusion.

26.8.2.2 Treatment Protocol

- Secure the airway and provide 100% oxygen (STOP the anaesthetic if severe reaction)
- Secure IV access if not already available
  - Start crystalloid fluids at shock rate
    - ○ 90 ml/kg/h, dog (or bolus in aliquots of 20 ml/kg)
    - ○ 60 ml/kg/h, cat (or bolus in aliquots of 10 ml/kg)
- For peracute *moderate* reactions, give 0.01 mg/kg epinephrine IM; repeat every 5–15 minutes until haemodynamic and respiratory status improve (maximum dose 0.3 mg/kg [<40 kg]; or 0.5 mg/kg [>40 kg])
  - Note 0.01 mg/kg = 0.01 ml/kg of epinephrine 1 : 1000
- For any *severe* reactions, give epinephrine 0.01 mg/kg IV; repeat with ½ the dose within two minutes if poor response. (Human data suggest initial epinephrine doses of 0.05–0.1 mg/kg may be indicated for the most severe reactions/in the face of cardiac arrest, but adequate IV fluid resuscitation must also be provided; and both too low and too high doses of epinephrine can be associated with adverse outcomes)
  - For IV administration, epinephrine 1 : 1000 is easier to use if diluted
    - ○ Take 1 ml of epinephrine 1 : 1000 and add 9 ml saline to make 10 ml of 1 : 10000 epinephrine
    - ○ Now 0.01 mg/kg = 0.1 ml/kg of epinephrine 1 : 10000
- If life-threatening hypotension persists
  - Consider an epinephrine infusion (start ~0.05 μg/kg/min; and titrate to effect)
    - ○ Add 2 ml (2 mg) epinephrine 1 : 1000 to a 500 ml bag of saline; start infusion at ~1 ml/kg/h (= 0.07 μg/kg/min), then titrate to effect
  - Consider phenylephrine (0.01 mg/kg SLOW IV q. 15 minutes or infusion ~0.05–3 μg/kg/min); or dopamine (5–10 μg/kg/min), as alternatives. (Vasopressin and glucagon may also be considered.)
- If respiratory distress occurs, administer terbutaline (a β2 agonist bronchodilator) at 0.01 mg/kg SC (or slow IV, but beware if already tachycardic)
- Consider antihistamines (most effective if given within the first 10 minutes); chlorphenamine
  - Dogs: 2.5–10 mg per dog SLOW IV
  - Cats: 2.5–5 mg per cat SLOW IV
- Consider corticosteroids
- Consider gastro-protectants (including H$_2$-blockers); anti-emetics; and other supportive care as required

26.8.2.3 Diagnosis

The diagnosis of anaphylaxis is based largely on history and clinical findings. Laboratory tests have proven to be disappointing in clinical practice. Plasma histamine may be elevated, but it is only reliable when measured within one hour of onset and the concentrations are not stable during routine sample handling, so it is seldom used. Serum or plasma tryptase levels greater than 15 ng/ml within 12 hours (preferably within 3 hours) of the onset of an episode is more widely used as a confirmatory test, but serial measurements may be more helpful than single measurements.

26.9 Notes

26.9.1 The Complement System

The complement cascade is activated in a number of ways. The classical pathway can be activated by contact with antigen-bound antibodies or contact with some viral and bacterial surfaces. The classical pathway starts with C1, which has three parts: C1q, C1r, C1s; and C1r and C1s have proteolytic activity when activated. The alternate pathway (starting with C3) is activated by 'activating surfaces' (e.g. bacteria, viruses, endotoxin, aggregated immunoglobulins). The third method of complement activation involves acute phase proteins called mannose-binding proteins. These bind to the mannose-containing glycoproteins of bacterial cell walls to act as opsonins, which can stimulate the alternate complement pathway. Interestingly, the mannose-binding proteins have some structural homology with C1q, and via serum proteases, may also activate the classical pathway. The terminal pathway of the complement system results in formation of the 'membrane-attack-complex', which forms a large pore that inserts itself, and 'punches holes' into, cell membranes resulting in cell death.

Regulation of the complement system is important. The natural inhibitor of the classical pathway is C1-inhibitor (or C1-inactivator). This blocks the activation of C1r and C1s. The alternate pathway has several regulatory proteins (e.g. the decay-accelerating-factor). There are also inhibitors of the formation of the membrane attack complex (e.g. protectin).

In sepsis, a reduction in active C1-inhibitor has been correlated with increased mortality; and administration of exogenous C1-inhibitor has been shown to reduce the need for vasopressors in patients with sepsis.

C1-inhibitor is also important in regulating the intrinsic coagulation system.

26.9.2 Coagulation

According to **Virchow's triad,** three things are necessary for thrombosis to occur:

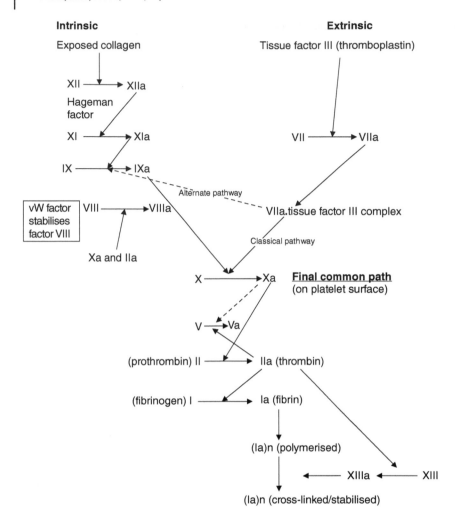

Ca^{2+} (often called factor IV) is necessary in all steps bar XII → XIIa; and XI →XIa

Figure 26.5 Brief summary of coagulation pathways.

- Hypercoagulable state
- Stasis/slow blood flow
- Vascular endothelial 'damage' (incl. hypoxic/ischaemic damage)

Figure 26.5 outlines the classic coagulation cascade, but we now only really use this to help guide results of the [one stage] prothrombin time ([OS]PT, which relates to the extrinsic pathway) and activated partial thromboplastin time ([A]PTT, which relates to the intrinsic pathway), coagulation assays because actually, the vascular endothelium, platelets, and clotting factors are all important players in coagulation *in vivo*.

The cell surface model is more representative of how coagulation actually occurs *in vivo* and consists of three overlapping stages. Calcium and phospholipid surfaces are important for the majority of the stages.

Initiation phase: Vascular damage exposes TF (thromboplastin or tissue factor III) on extravascular cells, which binds to factor VII or VIIa in a 1 : 1 complex (see Figure 26.6).

During the initiation phase, small amounts of Xa, IXa, Va, and IIa are produced. Once activated, TF : VIIa complex leaves its local environment and is rapidly inactivated by tissue factor pathway inhibitor (TFPI) or antithrombin III (AT III). If any Xa moves away from the vicinity of the cell surface where it was activated, it is slowly inactivated by TFPI or AT III, whereas IXa is not affected by TFPI and is only very slowly degraded by AT III.

Amplification phase: Occurs on platelet surfaces. The small amount of thrombin (IIa) generated in the initiation phase can diffuse away from the TF-bearing cell to help activate platelets (along with their exposure to extracellular matrix components), and certain other clotting

Figure 26.6 Summary of the initiation phase of coagulation in the cell surface model.

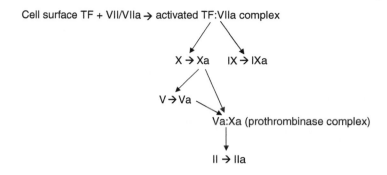

Figure 26.7 Summary of the 'thrombin burst' part of the propagation phase of coagulation in the cell surface model.

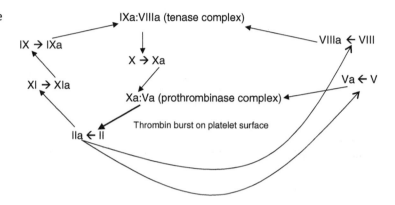

factors that have accessed the interstitium. That is, thrombin activates clotting factor V to Va, XI to X1a, and it cleaves factor VIII off von Willebrand factor, activating it in the process (VIIIa).

Propagation phase: Occurring on the surface of activated platelets, VIIIa can now bind IXa to produce the tenase complex. The tenase complex and the prothrombinase complex act in concert, alongside thrombin's ability to activate factors V, VIII, and XI, to result in a burst of thrombin production (see Figure 26.7).

Finally, thrombin cleaves fibrinogen (factor I) to form a fibrin monomer (factor Ia); which forms a loosely associated fibrin polymer, forming the initial clot. Thrombin also activates factor XIII (fibronectin), and activated factor XIIIa stabilises the fibrin clot through the formation of covalent bond cross-links.

26.9.2.1 Natural Modulators of Haemostasis

Several mechanisms prevent widespread coagulation far from the site of injury. Some of the regulators of coagulation are listed below.

- Antithrombin III (requires heparin as a cofactor; heparin is present in the endothelial surface layer); inhibits IIa (thrombin), Xa and, poorly, IXa.
- Activated protein C (i.e. Ca) (vitamin K dependent, and needs a cofactor, protein S); cleaves Va and VIIIa. (The thrombin/thrombomodulin complex activates protein C; thrombomodulin is an endothelial cell surface receptor.)
- TFPI; rapidly inactivates TF : VIIa complex (and Xa and possibly very slowly, IXa).
- Thrombin-activatable fibrinolytic inhibitor (TAFI); removes lysine residues from the fibrin clot making it less recognisable as a substrate for plasmin. TAFI is activated by thrombin/thrombomodulin complex.
- Tissue plasminogen activator (tPA): activates fibrinolysis by activating plasmin (fibrinolysin).
- Prostacyclin (PGI$_2$), produced by endothelial cells, is a potent inhibitor of platelet adhesion and aggregation.
- Fibrin degradation products also bind to platelets and reduce their reactivity, and inhibit thrombin (IIa), and fibrin (Ia).
- α1 anti-trypsin, α2 macroglobulin, α2 anti-plasmin, PAI1; all inhibit plasmin (fibrinolysin) activity.

26.9.2.2 Platelets
26.9.2.2.1 Surface Receptors
- Glycoprotein Ib (GpIb) binds to von Willebrand's factor (VWF) to mediate platelet adhesion to each other. (As vWF also binds to exposed collagen, this enables vWF-bound platelets to bind directly to collagen, see next point.)
- Glycoprotein Ia/IIa receptor complex (an integrin) helps platelets to bind to exposed subendothelial collagen.

- GpIIb–IIIa (an integrin adhesion protein) binds platelets to fibrinogen (and von Willebrand's factor). (Ideally the final common pathway of coagulation occurs on platelet surfaces.) There are three commercially available GpIIb–IIIa antagonists.

26.9.2.3 Disseminated Intravascular Coagulopathy (DIC)

Diagnosis of DIC is not easy, unless acute or fulminant DIC is present (severe bleeding from everywhere). Serial measurements may be more helpful as the clinical picture can change rapidly. Subclinical and chronic forms are harder to diagnose, but classically have been suggested to be present with **three or more of** the following:

- Reduced platelet number and platelets may be slightly dysfunctional, perhaps partly due to increased fibrin degradation (split) products (FD[S]Ps).
- Reduced fibrinogen acutely (fibrinogen may increase chronically).
- Reduced antithrombin III (but may already be low because it decreases as part of acute phase reaction in most species, bar cats).
- Reduced coagulation factors.
- Increased FD[S]Ps; particularly D-dimers, D-E fragment. (Significant liver disease can also raise FD[S]Ps due to reduced clearance.)
- Prolonged one stage prothrombin time ([OS]PT).
- Prolonged activated partial thromboplastin time ([A]PTT).
- Prolonged thrombin time (TT).
- Presence of schizocytes (schistocytes) on peripheral blood smear due to microangiopathic pathology (but this is not unique to DIC).
- Prolonged bleeding time (e.g. buccal mucosal bleeding time > 4 minutes for dogs and cats; or some say >4.2 minutes in dogs, and >2.4 minutes in cats).
- Measurement of the viscoelastic properties of clot formation and dissolution using various viscoelastometry analysers (e.g. TEG™, ROTEM, Sonoclot™ or the VCM™ [Viscoelastic Coagulation Monitor]) can help analyse the process of clot formation and dissolution, but the exact abnormalities for definitive diagnosis of DIC remain to be determined and validated at this moment.

26.9.2.3.1 Effects of DIC

Early in SIRS/shock states, with haemoconcentration (loss of plasma water [±proteins] into the interstitial space through leaky capillaries), vascular endothelial basement membrane exposure, adherence of inflammatory cells, sludging of blood flow through the capillaries (slowed circulation because of reduced cardiac output and cell/platelet adherence to swollen capillary endothelial cells causing some occlusion), and many other pro-coagulant triggers, there is an **initial hypercoagulable state**. Activation of coagulation by multiple pathways results in thrombosis outstripping thrombolysis, despite valiant attempts by antithrombin III and various other natural antithrombotic substances. The patient therefore has a tendency to clot. The formation of microthrombi in capillaries further reduces tissue perfusion, contributes to MODS/MOF, and promotes the patient's demise. Pulmonary thromboemboli may also cause trouble.

As time progresses, more pro- and anti-thrombotic agents are produced (including NO, which has antithrombotic activity), platelets and clotting factors are consumed and there is a shift in balance towards a **later hypocoagulable state**. The patient now has a tendency to bleed (and is in a dangerous situation). Petechiae and/or ecchymoses may be observed on unpigmented mucous membranes and glabrous areas of skin.

26.9.2.3.2 Treatment of DIC

The treatment for DIC depends upon if the patient is clotting excessively or bleeding excessively.

If clotting excessively, then unfractionated heparin may be favoured.

If bleeding excessively, then fresh whole blood, fresh or fresh-frozen plasma, cryoprecipitate, factor concentrates, and platelet rich plasma can be administered. It may be appropriate to administer vitamin K. Antifibrinolytics such as tranexamic acid may also be required if hyperfibrinolysis can be demonstrated. Protease inhibitors may also be considered.

If no excessive bleeding or clotting can be demonstrated, then prophylactic low molecular weight heparin may be administered. Low molecular weight heparin has a longer half-life and fewer side effects than unfractionated heparin because it only inhibits the action of factor Xa, and not IIa; its actions are more easily antagonised by protamine too.

At one time, heparin was thought necessary to add to fresh or fresh-frozen plasma in order to fully activate all the antithrombin III present, thereby making it superior for transfusion into animals with DIC. However, fresh-frozen plasma or fresh plasma, or even fresh whole blood, is probably just as good.

Activated protein C (protein Ca) has antithrombotic actions via inhibition of factors Va and VIIIa. In some human trials, when extra protein Ca was given to patients with SIRS, a strongly positive influence on outcome was seen. However, in some patients, there was an increased tendency to bleed which caused problems.

26.9.2.3.3 Protein-losing Nephropathy and Enteropathy

Thromboembolic disease is sometimes associated with protein-losing nephropathy because in addition to albumin, other small proteins such as antithrombin III, are also 'lost' in the urine. With the loss of this anticoagulant factor, the blood is more likely to clot.

Thromboembolic disease can also accompany protein-losing enteropathies, but larger proteins can also be lost with this condition and these larger proteins tend to include the pro-coagulant factors, so there is then a more balanced loss of pro- and anticoagulant factors, so sometimes no change in overall coagulability is apparent.

Further Reading

Abelson, A.L., O'Toole, T.E., Johnston, A. et al. (2013). Hypoperfusion and acute traumatic coagulopathy in severely traumatized canine patients. *Journal of Veterinary Emergency and Critical Care* 23: 395–401.

Alcott, C.J., Sponseller, B.A., Wong, D.M. et al. (2011). Clinical and immunomodulating effects of ketamine in horses with experimental endotoxemia. *Journal of Veterinary Internal Medicine* 26: 935–943.

Barton, M.H., Parviainen, A., and Norton, N. (2004). Polymixin B protects horses against induced endotoxaemia *in vivo. Equine Veterinary Journal* 36: 397–401.

Boller, A.M. and Otto, S.M. (2015). Sepsis and septic shock. In: *Small Animal Critical Care Medicine*, 2e, vol. 91 (eds. D.C. Silverstein and K. Hopper), 472–480. Missouri, USA: Elsevier Saunders.

Brianceau, P. and Divers, T.J. (2001). Acute thrombosis of limb arteries in horses with sepsis: five cases (1988-1998). *Equine Veterinary Journal* 33: 105–109.

Brown, A. (2012). Vasodilatation and vasoplegia in septic shock. Proceedings of the Multidisciplinary Systems Review in conjunction with the 18th International Veterinary Emergency and Critical Care Symposium. September 2012 San Antonio, Texas. 29–32.

Bruchim, Y. (2012). Canine heatstroke. *Israel Journal of Veterinary Medicine* 67: 92–95.

Bruchim, Y., Aroch, Y., Saragusty, J., and Waner, T. (2008). Disseminated intravascular coagulation. *Compendium on Continuing Education for the Practicing Veterinary Surgeon* 30: E1–E16.

Bruchim, Y., Horowitz, M., and Aroch, I. (2017). Pathophysiology of heatstroke in dogs – revisited. *Temperature* 4: 356–370.

Cap, A. and Hunt, B.J. (2015). The pathogenesis of traumatic coagulopathy. *Anaesthesia* 70 (Suppl. 1): 96–101.

Cassutto, B.H. and Gfeller, W.G. (2003). Use of intravenous lidocaine to prevent reperfusion injury and subsequent multiple organ dysfunction syndrome. *Journal of Veterinary Emergency and Critical Care* 13: 137–148.

Ceron, J.J., Eckersall, P.D., and Martinez-Subiela, S. (2005). Acute phase proteins in dogs and cats: current knowledge and future perspectives. *Veterinary Clinical Pathology* 34: 85–99.

Chandler, M. (2008). Nutritional support for the hospitalised small animal patient. *In Practice* 30: 442–448.

Cheng, T., Mathews, K.A., Abrams-Ogg, A.C.G., and Wood, D. (2011). The link between inflammation and coagulation: influence on the interpretation of diagnostic laboratory tests. *Compendium: Continuing Education for Veterinarians*. February 2011, https://pdfs.semanticscholar.org/d10e/569e61241f9b48dca1b73e2e73b6f48e0b42.pdf.

Cudmore, L.A., Muurlink, T., Whittem, T., and Bailey, S.R. (2013). Effects of oral clenbuterol on the clinical and inflammatory response to endotoxaemia in the horse. *Research in Veterinary Science* 94: 682–686.

De Laforcade, A. and Silverstein, D.C. (2015). Shock. In: *Small Animal Critical Care Medicine*, 2e, vol. 5 (eds. D.C. Silverstein and K. Hopper), 26–30. Missouri, USA: Elsevier Saunders.

De Laforcade, A. (2015). Systemic inflammatory response syndrome. In: *Small Animal Critical Care Medicine*, 2e, vol. 6 (eds. D.C. Silverstein and K. Hopper), 30–34. Missouri, USA: Elsevier Saunders.

Dewachter, P. and Savic, L. (2019). Perioperative anaphylaxis: pathophysiology, clinical presentation and management. *BJA Education* 19: 313–320.

Ebo, D.G., Clarke, R.C., Mertes, P.-M. et al. (2019). Molecular mechanisms and pathophysiology of perioperative hypersensitivity and anaphylaxis: a narrative review. *British Journal of Anaesthesia* 123: e38–e49.

Epstein, K.L. (2014). Coagulopathies in horses. *Veterinary Clinics of North America: Equine Practice* 30: 437–452.

Epstein, K.L., Brainard, B.M., Giguere, S. et al. (2013). Serial viscoelastic and traditional coagulation testing in horses with gastrointestinal disease. *Journal of Veterinary Emergency and Critical Care* 23: 504–516.

Feige, K., Schwarzwald, C.C., and Bombeli, T.H. (2003). Comparison of unfractionated and low molecular weight heparin for prophylaxis of coagulopathies in 52 horses with colic: a randomized double-blink clinical trial. *Equine Veterinary Journal* 35: 506–513.

Fink, M.P. (2004). Ethyl pyruvate: a novel treatment for sepsis and shock. *Minerva Anastesiologica* 70: 365–371.

Fink, M.P. (2007). Ethyl pyruvate: a novel anti-inflammatory agent. *Journal of Internal Medicine* 261: 349–362.

Flournoy, W.S., Macintire, D.K., and Wohl, J.S. (2003). Heatstroke in dogs: clinical signs, treatment, prognosis and prevention. *The Compendium on Continuing Education for the Practising Veterinarian: Small Animal/Exotics* 25: 422–431.

Fogle, J., Jacob, M., Blikslager, A. et al. (2017). Comparison of lipopolysaccharides and soluble CD14 measurement between clinically endotoxaemic and nonendotoxaemic horses. *Equine Veterinary Journal* 49: 155–159.

Gajanayake, I. and Chan, D. (2009). Nutritional support for the critical care patient. *In Practice* 31: 386–389.

Garvey, L.H., Dewachter, P., Hepner, D. et al. (2019). Management of suspected immediate perioperative allergic reactions: an international overview and consensus recommendations. *British Journal of Anaesthesia* 123: e50–e64.

Giunti, M., Troia, R., Bergamini, P.F., and Dondi, F. (2015). Prospective evaluation of the acute patient physiologic and laboratory evaluation score and an extended clinicopathological profile in dogs with systemic inflammatory response syndrome. *Journal of Veterinary Emergency and Critical Care* 25: 226–233.

Goggs, R.A.N. and Lewis, D.H. (2015). Multiple organ dysfunction syndrome. In: *Small Animal Critical Care Medicine*, 2e, vol. 7 (eds. D.C. Silverstein and K. Hopper), 35–46. Missouri, USA: Elsevier Saunders.

Goggs, R., Mastrocco, A., and Brooks, M.B. (2018). Retrospective evaluation of 4 methods for outcome prediction in overt disseminated intravascular coagulation in dogs (2004-2014): 804 cases. *Journal of Veterinary Emergency and Critical Care* 28: 541–550.

Gommeren, K., Desmas, I., Garcia, A. et al. (2019). Cardiovascular biomarkers in dogs with systemic inflammatory response syndrome. *Journal of Veterinary Emergency and Critical Care* 29: 256–263.

Gottlieb, D.L., Prittie, J., Buriko, Y., and Lamb, K.E. (2017). Evaluation of acute traumatic coagulopathy in dogs and cats following blunt force trauma. *Journal of Veterinary Emergency and Critical Care* 27: 35–43.

Hayes, G., Mathews, K., Doig, G. et al. (2010). The Acute Patient Physiologic and Laboratory Evaluation (APPLE) score: a severity of illness stratification system for hospitalized dogs. *Journal of Veterinary Internal Medicine* 24: 1034–1047.

Hollenbach, M., Hintersdorf, A., Huse, K. et al. (2008). Ethyl pyruvate and ethyl lactate down-regulate the production of pro-inflammatory cytokines and modulate expression of immune receptors. *Biochemical Pharmacology* 76: 631–644.

Hopper, K. and Bateman, S. (2005). An updated view of hemostasis: mechanisms of hemostatic dysfunction associated with sepsis. *Journal of Veterinary Emergency and Critical Care* 15: 83–91.

Iba, T., Levy, J.H., Raj, A., and Warkentin, T.E. (2019). Advance in the management of sepsis-induced coagulopathy and disseminated intravascular coagulation. *Journal of Clinical Medicine* 8: 728. https://doi.org/10.3390/jcm8050728 *(Useful graphics for coagulation and related pathways and interesting overview of how sepsis-induced coagulopathy can progress to DIC.).*

Jeffery, U., Brooks, M.B., and LeVine, D.N. (2017). Development of a fibrinolysis assay for canine plasma. *The Veterinary Journal* 229: 19–25.

Johnson, V., Gaynor, A., Chan, D.L., and Rozanski, E. (2004). Multiple organ dysfunction syndrome in humans and dogs. *Journal of Veterinary Emergency and Critical Care* 14: 158–166.

Kane, A.D., Kothmann, E., Giussani, G.A. (2020). Detection and response to acute systemic hypoxia. *BJA Education* 20: 58–64.

Kao, K.K. and Fink, M.P. (2010). The biochemical basis for the anti-inflammatory and cytoprotective actions of ethyl pyruvate and related compounds. *Biochemical Pharmacology* 80: 151–159.

Kato, D., Takahashi, M., Yonezawa, T., Ohmi, A., Takeda, S., Nakagawa, T., Hosoda, S., Kanemoto, H., Fukushima, K., Ohno, K., Matsuki, N., Tsujimoto, H. (2020). Evaluation of an automated point-of-care test system for measuring thrombin-antithrombin complex in dogs. *Journal of Veterinary Emergency and Critical Care* 30: 102–106.

Kelmer, G., Doherty, T.J., Elliott, S. et al. (2008). Evaluation of dimethyl sulphoxide effects on initial response to endotoxin in the horse. *Equine Veterinary Journal* 40: 358–363.

King, J.N. and Gerring, E.L. (1989). Antagonism of endotoxin-induced disruption of equine bowel motility by flunixin and phenylbutazone. *Equine Veterinary Journal* 21 (Supplement 7): 38–42.

Koster, L.S., Fosgate, G.T., Suchodolski, J. et al. (2019). Comparison of biomarkers adiponectin, leptin, C-reactive protein, S100A12, and the Acute Patient Physiologic and Laboratory Evaluation (APPLE) score as mortality predictors in critically ill dogs. *Journal of Veterinary Emergency and Critical Care* 29: 154–160.

Kwak, J., Yoon, H., Kim, J. et al. (2018). Ultrasonographic measurement of caudal vena cava to aortic ratios for determination of volume depletion in normal beagle dogs. *Veterinary Radiology and Ultrasound* 59: 203–211.

Lamia, B., Chemla, D., Richard, C., and Teboul, J.-L. (2005). Clinical review: interpretation of arterial pressure wave in shock states. *Critical Care* 9: 601–606.

Lang, K.M. and Kirby, R. (2008). An update on cardiovascular adrenergic receptor physiology and potential pharmacological applications in veterinary critical care. *Journal of Veterinary Emergency and Critical Care* 18: 2–25.

Levi, M. and Scully, M. (2018). How I treat disseminated intravascular coagulation. *Blood* 131: 845–854.

Lisciandro, G. and Lisciandro, S. (2019). Sonographic changes of the gallbladder associated with anaphylaxis in dogs. *Journal of Veterinary Emergency and Critical Care* 29: 214–215.

Lisowski, Z.M., Pirie, R.S., Blikslager, A.T. et al. (2018). An update on equine post-operative ileus: definitions, pathophysiology and management. *Equine Veterinary Journal* 50: 292–303.

Mackenzie, C.A., McGowan, C.M., Pinchbeck, G., and Carslake, H.B. (2018). Comparison of two blood sampling techniques for the determination of coagulation parameters in the horse: jugular venipuncture and indwelling intravenous catheter. *Equine Veterinary Journal* 50: 33–338.

Marx, G. (2003). Fluid therapy in sepsis with capillary leakage. *European Journal of Anaesthesiology* 20: 429–442.

Marx, G. and Schuerholz, T. (2010). Fluid-induced coagulopathy: does the type of fluid make a difference. *Critical Care* 14: 118–119.

McMichael, M. and Moore, R.M. (2004). Ischaemia-reperfusion injury pathophysiology, part I. *Journal of Veterinary Emergency and Critical Care* 14: 231–241.

McMichael, M. (2004). Ischaemia-reperfusion injury: assessment and treatment, part II. *Journal of Veterinary Emergency and Critical Care* 14: 242–252.

McMichael, M.A. and Smith, S.A. (2011). Viscoelastic coagulation testing: technology, applications and limitations. *Veterinary Clinical Pathology* 40 (2): 140–153.

Meneghini, C., Rabozzi, R., and Franci, P. (2016). Correlation of the ratio of caudal vena cava diameter and aorta diameter with systolic pressure variation in anaesthetized dogs. *American Journal of Veterinary Research* 77: 137–143.

Moore, J.N., Norton, N., Barton, M.H. et al. (2007). Rapid infusion of a phospholipid emulsion attenuates the effects of endotoxaemia in horses. *Equine Veterinary Journal* 39: 243–248.

Moore, J.N. and Vandenplas, M.L. (2014). Is it the systemic inflammatory response syndrome or endotoxemia in horses with colic? *Veterinary Clinics of North America: Equine Practice* 30: 337–351.

Mulier, K.E., Beilman, G.J., Conroy, M.J. et al. (2005). Ringer's ethyl pyruvate in hemorrhagic shock and resuscitation does not improve early hemodynamics or tissue energetics. *Shock* 23: 248–252.

National Institute for Health and Care Excellence (NICE) (2013). Diagnostics Assessment Programme. Viscoelastometric point-of-care testing (ROTEM, TEG and Sonoclot systems) to assist with detecting, managing and monitoring of haemostasis. Final scope (August 2013).

Piagnerelli, M., Zouaoui Boudjeltia, K., Vanhaeverbeek, M., and Vincent, J.-L. (2003). Red blood cell rheology in sepsis. *Intensive Care Medicine* 29: 1052–1061.

Rabozzi, R., Armenise, A., and Franci, P. (2013). Caudal vena cava and aortic diameter ratio (cvc/ao) as an index to predict fluid volume deficit in anaesthetized injured dogs. *Journal of Veterinary Emergency and Critical Care* 23: S24. https://doi.org/10.1111/vec.12088.

Radcliffe, R.M., Buchanan, B.R., Cook, V.L., and Divers, T.J. (2015). The clinical value of whole blood point-of-care biomarkers in large animal emergency and critical care medicine. *Journal of Veterinary Emergency and Critical Care* 25: 138–151.

Raftery, A.G. (2018). When should we measure cardiac troponin I? *Equine Veterinary Education* 30: 85–87.

Rhodes, A., Evans, L.E., Alhazzani, W. et al. (2017). Surviving sepsis campaign: international guidelines for management of sepsis and septic shock. *Intensive Care Medicine* 43: 304–377.

Roy, M.-F., Kwong, G.P.S., Lambert, J. et al. (2017). Prognostic value and development of a scoring system in horses with systemic inflammatory response syndrome. *Journal of Veterinary Internal Medicine* 31: 582–592.

Schroeder, E.L., Holcombe, S.J., Cook, V.L. et al. (2011). Preliminary safety and biological efficacy studies of ethyl pyruvate in normal mature horses. *Equine Veterinary Journal* 43: 341–347.

Scroggin, R.D. and Quandt, J. (2009). The use of vasopressin for treating vasodilatory shock and cardiopulmonary arrest. *Journal of Veterinary Emergency and Critical Care* 19: 145–157.

Segev, G., Aroch, I., Savoray, M. et al. (2015). A novel severity scoring system for dogs with heatstroke. *Journal of Veterinary Emergency and Critical Care* 25: 240–247.

Semrad, S.D., Hardee, G.E., Hardee, M.M., and Moore, J.N. (1987). Low dose flunixin meglumine: effects on eicosanoid production and clinical signs induced by experimental endotoxaemia in horses. *Equine Veterinary Journal* 19: 201–216.

Silverstein, D.C. and Hopper, K. (2015). *Small Animal Critical Care*, 2e (eds. D.C. Silverstein and K. Hopper). Missouri, USA: Elsevier Saunders.

Simmons, J.W. and Powell, M.F. (2016). Acute traumatic coagulopathy: pathophysiology and resuscitation. *British Journal of Anaesthesia* 117 (S3): iii37–iii43.

Smith, S.A. (2009). The cell-based model of coagulation. *Journal of Veterinary Emergency and Critical Care* 19: 3–10.

Thachil, J. (2016). Disseminated intravascular coagulation, a practical approach. *Anesthesiology* 125: 230–236.

Troia, R., Mascalzoni, G., Calipa, S. et al. (2019). Multiorgan dysfunction syndrome in feline sepsis: prevalence and prognostic implication. *Journal of Feline Medicine and Surgery* 21: 559–565.

Sykes, B.M. and Furr, M.O. (2005). Equine endotoxaemia: a state-of-the-art review of therapy. *Australian Veterinary Journal* 83: 45–50.

Wada, H., Matsumoto, T., and Yamashita, Y. (2014). Diagnosis and treatment of disseminated intravascular coagulation (DIC) according to four DIC guidelines. *Journal of Intensive Care* 2: 15. https://jintensivecare.biomedcentral.com/articles/10.1186/2052-0492-2-15.

Werners, A.H., Bull, S., and Fink-Gremmels, J. (2005). Endotoxaemia: a review with implications for the horse. *Equine Veterinary Journal* 37: 371–383.

Wilkins, P.A. (2018). What's in a word: the needs for SIRS and sepsis definitions in equine medicine and surgery. *Equine Veterinary Journal* 50: 7–9.

Witkowska-Pilaszewicz, O.D., Zmigrodzka, M., Winnicka, A. et al. (2019). Serum amyloid A in equine health and disease. *Equine Veterinary Journal* 51: 293–298.

Wong, D.M. and Wilkins, P.A. (2015). Defining the systemic inflammatory response syndrome in equine neonates.

Veterinary Clinics of North America: Equine Practice 31: 463–481.

Zhang, B., Li, Q., Shi, C., and Zhang, X. (2018). Drug-induced pseudoallergy: a review of the causes and mechanisms. *Pharmacology* 101: 104–110.

Note that a special issue of the *Journal of Veterinary Emergency and Critical Care* was devoted to the subject of haemostasis: Volume 19, February 2009.

Self-test Section

1 Define 'shock' and list the main types/causes.

2 What are the three main phases of coagulation as portrayed by the cell surface model?

3 True or False? In cats, antithrombin III is an acute phase protein.

27

Gastric Dilation/Volvulus (GDV)

See also Chapter 26 on shock.

27.1 The Problems

- Obstructed oesophagus (cannot swallow or vomit productively); salivary losses (and potential aspiration).
- Massively dilated stomach + fluid sequestration within stomach ('third-space' losses).
- Compromised blood supply to stomach +/− spleen.
- Abdominal distension results in 'splinting' of diaphragm (similar to bloat in cattle and tympanic colic in horses); ventilation becomes compromised leading to respiratory acidosis and hypoxaemia.
- Abdominal distension can also interfere with venous return, and therefore cardiac output (i.e. obstructive shock).
- Abdominal compartment syndrome (occurs with very high intra-abdominal pressures) can cause myriad problems for multiple organs (both within and outside the abdomen itself).
- Fluid sequestration in stomach and salivary losses lead to hypovolaemia and hypovolaemic shock.
- Compromised blood supply to stomach can lead to ischaemia (may get haemorrhagic fluid losses into stomach) and result in bacterial translocation and endotoxin absorption, and therefore distributive shock and disseminated intravascular coagulopathy (DIC).
- Fluid losses can also cause acid–base and electrolyte imbalances (these are unpredictable; see below).
- Acid–base and electrolyte disturbances may be:
  - Metabolic alkalosis (often early on, acid loss into stomach greater than salivary bicarbonate loss).
  - Metabolic acidosis (as shock develops, lactic acidosis occurs).
  - Respiratory acidosis ('splinted' diaphragm and hypoventilation).
  - Respiratory alkalosis (may develop as a compensatory response for metabolic acidosis).
  - Hypokalaemia (often accompanies alkalosis; K$^+$ lost in gastric secretions too).
  - Hyperkalaemia (often accompanies severe acidosis because of H$^+$/K$^+$ transcellular exchange); arrhythmias may occur.
  - Hypochloraemia (often accompanies early alkalosis, Cl$^-$ lost in stomach secretions).
  - Hypernatraemia (Na$^+$ not lost to any great degree in stomach secretions, but haemoconcentration occurs with developing hypovolaemia).
- Hyper- or hypo-glycaemia can occur at different stages of 'shock'.
- Low cardiac output/shock results in reduced pulmonary perfusion (adds to hypoxaemia).
- Low cardiac output/shock also results in myocardial compromise (i.e. cardiogenic shock) (worsened by electrolyte-abnormality-induced arrhythmias).
- Myocardial hypoxia results in (ventricular) arrhythmias, which, rather than occurring acutely, often develop within one to three days of the Gastric Dilation/Volvulus (GDV) occurring.
- Changes in packed cell volume (PCV)/total solids (TS) and coagulation profile. Haemoconcentration results from hypovolaemia, but haemorrhagic fluid losses into the stomach lumen are also possible. This all adds to much variation in what the haematological and electrolyte profiles can be.
- Many of these dogs are the giant deep-chested breeds (e.g. Great Danes) that are also prone to atrial fibrillation.
- Prognostic indicators may include various biomarkers, including lactate, myoglobin, and cardiac troponins.
- Ischaemia with subsequent reperfusion injury, upon initial treatment of shock and de-rotation of the stomach,

Veterinary Anaesthesia: Principles to Practice, Second Edition. Alexandra H. A. Dugdale, Georgina Beaumont, Carl Bradbrook, and Matthew Gurney.
© 2020 John Wiley & Sons Ltd. Published 2020 by John Wiley & Sons Ltd.
Companion website: www.wiley.com/go/dugdale/veterinary-anaesthesia

can fuel SIRS (systemic inflammatory response syndrome), which in turn can complicate the post-operative recovery period.

27.2 Approach

A detailed history and thorough clinical examination should be expedited and blood samples taken for evaluation of baseline haematology, biochemistry, electrolytes, and acid–base status (and potential prognostic biomarkers), if possible. Pre-anaesthetic medical/haemodynamic resuscitation/stabilisation is of paramount importance in reducing the risks associated with general anaesthesia and surgery. Pre-existing atrial fibrillation further compromises cardiac output and increases the risks: check the medical history for this and other conditions and current treatments. Cardiac arrhythmias (often secondary to myocardial ischaemia), tend to occur within the first one to three days following development of the condition and can be fatal, but often the first 6–12 hours are free of such arrhythmias (although beware electrolyte-abnormality-induced arrhythmias). Post-operative arrhythmias are common and warrant close patient monitoring.

Initially, the stomach should be decompressed if possible, whether by passing a stomach tube or by percutaneous trocarisation. Hypovolaemia and electrolyte imbalances should be addressed at this time too, although electrolyte measurement is not always available. Intravenous fluid therapy is the mainstay of stabilisation and resuscitation. Large bore cannulae are chosen and placed into more than one vein if necessary. If the patient's cardiovascular system is very compromised, a 'cut down' procedure may be required to locate a suitable vein for cannulation. The crystalloid/colloid debate continues. Large volumes of balanced crystalloids are often required, which may promote the development of interstitial oedema/fluid sequestration in many tissues. Although smaller volumes of colloids (relative to using crystalloids) usually produce adequate initial intravascular volume restoration, they eventually gain access to the interstitium, especially if increased capillary permeability (capillary 'leak') is present, and water follows, so that interstitial fluid sequestration may still occur – which may be more difficult to treat (e.g. with diuretics) than when this occurs with crystalloids. A small volume of hypertonic saline can also be used for immediate (but relatively transient) intravascular volume 'resuscitation', but must be followed by more balanced crystalloids; and furthermore, it is useful to know the pre-treatment plasma sodium and potassium concentrations, as hypertonic saline can worsen pre-existing hypernatraemia and

hypokalaemia. As with all fluid therapy, the initial aim is to restore circulating blood volume, and the patient's response (clinical, haemodynamic) to treatment is monitored as a guide to the effectiveness of this therapy.

27.3 Premedication

Some patients may struggle during attempted passage of a stomach tube, requiring sedation, whilst others may initially present with subdued mentation due to shock (prior to initial stabilisation/resuscitation), and although not needing much sedation, these patients are at even greater risk of aspiration during passage of a stomach tube. If sedation is required before initial fluid resuscitation can be completed, low doses may be sufficient. Sedation may provide premedication that itself can reduce the required doses of anaesthetic agents.

Opioids alone can provide good sedation alongside analgesia, but morphine should be avoided as it may cause vomiting, which is distressing if these animals have oesophageal obstruction and cannot vomit productively. Acepromazine causes vasodilation, which compounds the hypovolaemic shock, so tends to be avoided. The α2 agonists also cause haemodynamic changes that may be poorly tolerated in patients with shock. They can also occasionally induce vomiting which, as for morphine, is distressing. Benzodiazepines may, however, be useful adjuncts to opioids and can also be used as co-induction agents.

27.4 Anaesthetic Induction

Pre-oxygenate if possible, and if the patient tolerates it; using a mask is more effective than simply providing flow-by oxygen, although the latter is better than nothing.

If a benzodiazepine (diazepam or midazolam; the latter causes slightly more cardiorespiratory depression at the higher end of the dose range) has not been given as part of the premedication, it can be administered as a co-induction agent, followed by either propofol or alfaxalone, given slowly, to effect. Etomidate offers another possibility for anaesthetic induction as it provides excellent cardiovascular stability, but the increased muscle tone that it causes may make tracheal intubation more difficult, so it should also be used alongside a benzodiazepine. In addition, the suppression of adrenal activity it produces may be an unwanted side effect in patients with shock. Other co-induction agents include fentanyl (c. 2+µg/kg); lidocaine (c. 0.5–1mg/kg), which may also provide useful anti-arrhythmic activity; and ketamine (c. 0.5mg/kg), which can also provide useful analgesia.

Whatever agent/s are chosen, the anaesthetic induction process should not be too prolonged because a cuffed endotracheal tube should be placed as soon as possible (have a laryngoscope ready) in order to protect the airway (especially if de-rotation of the oesophagus/stomach has not been possible). Suction should be available if possible.

27.5 Anaesthetic Maintenance

- Ensure provision of adequate oxygen.
- Nitrous oxide should be avoided until the stomach is decompressed and/or de-rotated as it will increase any gaseous distension of the stomach, causing more difficulties for the patient and the surgeon. Once the stomach has been decompressed, however, N_2O can be used, although if there is any doubt over gastric motility, it may be better avoided so as to reduce the potential for re-distension.
- The patient should be turned into dorsal recumbency gently to reduce any sudden further compression of the caudal vena cava or hepatic portal vein.
- Ventilation may need to be assisted or provided (ventilation is impaired when the diaphragm is effectively splinted by the increased intra-abdominal pressure). Monitoring end tidal carbon dioxide tension and blood gases, where possible, will help to direct any necessary interventions to 'correct' any disturbances. Beware the mechanical and chemical side effects of mechanical ventilation.
- The provision of good intra-operative anti-nociception and balanced/multimodal post-operative analgesia is of paramount importance for helping to achieve as stable as possible a plane of anaesthesia during surgery and to reduce unnecessarily high sympathetic tone post-operatively.
- Maintenance of anaesthesia is usually achieved with a combination of inhalation agents (sevoflurane or isoflurane are common choices as they are minimally arrhythmogenic) and injectable agents (lidocaine, ketamine and fentanyl infusions are common choices).
- Intravenous fluid therapy is continued intra-operatively according to the patient's requirements. Crystalloids, colloids (synthetic or natural), and blood/blood products may be required.
- The patient's physiological status must be monitored closely: heart rate, pulse rate, ECG, breathing/ventilation rate, SpO_2 (by pulse oximetry), mucous membrane colour, arterial blood pressure (direct/continuous if possible), central venous pressure, end tidal CO_2 tension, blood gases, temperature (even core : periphery gradient), electrolytes, blood glucose, lactate, and urine output.

- Cardiac arrhythmias may occur, although they are more common during post-operative recovery. During splenic handling, however, ventricular premature complexes/contractions (VPCs) are very common. An intra-operative lidocaine infusion can provide useful anti-arrhythmic activity, alongside intra-operative anti-nociception and some anti-inflammatory and anti-reperfusion-injury actions.
- Beware pneumothorax as a complication of circumcostal gastropexy.

27.6 Recovery

- Fluids/blood/plasma are continued or provided as necessary. Monitoring heart rate, arterial blood pressure, urine output, and urine specific gravity may be helpful in guiding ongoing fluid therapy.
- Monitor blood gases, pH, electrolytes, and lactate if possible. Acid–base and electrolyte disturbances are treated as necessary.
- Monitor ECG and be prepared to treat arrhythmias if necessary (see below).
- Monitor breathing rate, effort, and SpO_2. Nasal oxygen supplementation may be provided (e.g. nasal prongs providing c. 200 ml/kg/min [2–10 l/min for 10–50 kg], increase inspired oxygen to about 50%).
- Monitor abdominal girth and/or ultrasound findings according to surgeon's advice.
- Monitor patient's pain scores and provide analgesia as appropriate.
- Good general nursing; continuous observation if possible.

27.7 When Is an Arrhythmia 'Malignant'?

'When the animal's haemodynamics are affected', i.e. when there is significant cardiac output reduction to result in forward cardiac failure.

- When the ventricular rate is too rapid (e.g. >180 bpm sustained for long periods).
- When any abnormal complexes are frequent (>15/min, or >15 consecutively), especially if associated with pulse deficits.
- When VPCs are multiform/polymorphic (multiple ectopic foci) because ventricular fibrillation is possible. (Check for low serum potassium and magnesium.)
- When VPCs occur very close together; the so-called 'R on T' phenomenon is a pre-fibrillatory rhythm.

Further Reading

Adamvik, K.N., Burgener, I.A., Kovacevic, A. et al. (2009). Myoglobin as a prognostic indicator for outcome in dogs with gastric dilation-volvulus. *Journal of Veterinary Emergency and Critical Care* 19: 247–253.

Buber, T., Saragusty, J., Ranen, E. et al. (2007). Evaluation of lidocaine treatment and risk factors for death associated with gastric dilation and volvulus in dogs: 112 cases (1997–2005). *Journal of the American Veterinary Medical Association* 230: 1334–1339.

Burgener, I.A., Kovacevic, A., Maulden, G.N., and Lombard, C.W. (2006). Cardiac troponins as indicators of acute myocardial damage in dogs. *Journal of Veterinary Internal Medicine* 20: 277–283.

Canyon, S.J. and Dobson, G.P. (2004). Protection against ventricular arrhythmias and cardiac death using adenosine and lidocaine during regional ischemia in the *in vivo* rat. *American Journal of Physiology, Heart and Circulatory Physiology* 287: H1286–H1295.

de Papp, E., Drobatz, K.J., and Hughes, D. (1999). Plasma lactate concentration as a predictor of gastric necrosis and survival among dogs with gastric dilation-volvulus:102 cases. *Journal of the American Veterinary Medical Association* 215: 49–52.

Muir, W.W. (1982). Gastric dilatation-volvulus in the dog, with emphasis on cardiac arrhythmias. *Journal of the American Veterinary Medical Association* 180: 739–742.

Muir, W.W. (1982). Acid–base and electrolyte disturbances in dogs with gastric dilatation-volvulus. *Journal of the American Veterinary Medical Association* 181: 229–231.

Muir, W.W. and Weisbrode, S.E. (1982). Myocardial ischemia in dogs with gastric dilatation-volvulus. *Journal of the American Veterinary Medical Association* 181: 363–366.

Nielsen, L.K. and Whelan, M. (2012). Compartment syndrome: pathophysiology, clinical presentations, treatment and prevention in human and veterinary medicine. *Journal of the Veterinary Emergency and Critical Care Society* 22: 291–302.

Schober, K.E., Cornand, C., Kirbach, B. et al. (2002). Serum cardiac troponin I and cardiac troponin T concentrations in dogs with gastric dilatation-volvulus. *Journal of the American Veterinary Medical Association* 221: 381–388.

Tivers, M. and Brockman, D. (2009). Gastric dilation-volvulus syndrome in dogs 1. Pathophysiology, diagnosis and stabilisation. *In Practice* 31: 66–69.

Tivers, M. and Brockman, D. (2009). Gastric dilation-volvulus syndrome in dogs 2. Surgical and postoperative management. *In Practice* 31: 114–121.

28

Equine Sedation and Premedication

LEARNING OBJECTIVES

- To be familiar with the main groups of drugs, their effects and side effects.
- To be able to discuss the factors affecting drug choice for sedation/standing chemical restraint and for premedication.

28.1 Introduction

Before any drugs are administered, a full and pertinent history should be obtained, including details of patient age, vaccination status, and previous and current illnesses and treatments. If the patient and time allow, as full a clinical examination as possible should be conducted, at the very least it should include the cardiovascular and respiratory systems. Several factors usually need to be considered before a final choice of agent and method can be made.

Bear in mind that horses are driven by their sympathetic nervous systems (the fight or flight response), and in the absence of more dominant animals to look to for guidance, horses will tend to want to run away from any potentially 'new' situation. Physical restraint alone, including 'twitching', may suffice for certain procedures, but is more often considered an adjunct to chemical restraint, and should never be considered sufficient as the only means of restraint where painful interventions are anticipated. Therefore, before any drug choice decisions are made, it is important to first consider:

- The patient's temperament, tractability, and degree of excitement (possibly affected by breed)
- The patient's physiological condition (concurrent illness or pregnancy)
- Available personnel, and their experience and ability to help
- Facilities and environment available

- Intensity and duration of desired effect
- Your familiarity with the drug/s
- The patient's weight

The properties of an ideal sedative/premedicant drug have been discussed in Chapter 4. No such ideal drug is available yet, although where one drug alone is insufficient, combinations of two or more may be more effective. Drug combinations may allow optimisation of desired effects, whilst simultaneously minimising undesirable side effects. Anxiolytics, sedatives, and narcotic analgesics are defined in Chapter 4. Whenever the term *muscle relaxation* is used below, it describes only the nonspecific effects of the agents considered here.

The effectiveness of any 'sedative' drug, or combination of drugs, will always be influenced by external factors, some of which will be beyond your control. For example, the state of excitement of the horse may affect the outcome, and, where possible, the patient (and possibly the owner too) should be allowed to, or encouraged to, calm down before drugs are administered. The general environment in which the drug is administered (i.e. the level of stimulation/distraction to which the horse is subjected) is important. Aim for a quiet environment, with few distractions, especially where drugs are to be administered by intramuscular or oral routes, when the onset of action is expected to be delayed; and in these circumstances, do not be impatient but allow sufficient time for the response to become apparent. The route of drug administration and volume of

Veterinary Anaesthesia: Principles to Practice, Second Edition. Alexandra H. A. Dugdale, Georgina Beaumont, Carl Bradbrook, and Matthew Gurney.
© 2020 John Wiley & Sons Ltd. Published 2020 by John Wiley & Sons Ltd.
Companion website: www.wiley.com/go/dugdale/veterinary-anaesthesia

injectate may require consideration: a small volume may be easier to inject quickly into a needle-shy animal, whereas for a slow, controlled intravenous injection, a larger volume may be easier to handle.

Try to choose the right drug/s for the effect desired. For example, the following scenarios may well require different approaches:

- Standing sedation for clipping; sweating is undesirable.
- Sedation for boxing/travelling (consider purpose of journey [e.g. is the horse being taken to a show], length of journey and return journey).
- Sedation for standing castration or wound suturing.
- Sedation for shoeing, radiography, or diagnostic nerve blocks; ataxia undesirable.
- Sedation for laryngeal endoscopy; excessive α2 agonist sedation may be undesirable.
- Premedication (also requires patient preparation; elective versus emergency surgery).

Horses, when sedated, may still be arousable and deliver well-aimed kicks and bites

The reader is referred to Chapter 4 for information regarding the pharmacological actions of the different drug groups and their mechanisms of effects and side effects.

28.2 Phenothiazines

Of these drugs, only **acepromazine** (acetylpromazine) is licenced in the EU. It is available as a yellow solution for injection (5 and 10 mg/ml formulations; not to be confused with the 2 mg/ml small animal formulation) and as a 35 mg/ml oral gel.

28.2.1 Dose

- 0.01–0.05 mg/kg IV (0.5–2.5 ml for 500 kg horse)
- 0.03–0.1 mg/kg IM
- 0.1–0.25 mg/kg PO

The sedative effects of acepromazine alone are unpredictable, but can be improved by combination with an opioid.

The onset of action of acepromazine, noted by a slight lowering of the head position, occurs around 5 minutes following IV administration, but the peak sedative effect takes 20 minutes to develop. Onset times are longer (15–20 minutes) following IM, oromucosal, or oral administration and peak effects take at least 30–40 minutes to develop. Ideally, the animal should be left undisturbed whilst the drug is taking effect, no matter what route of administration is used. If possible, the animal should also be calm before the administration of acepromazine (as with any sedative). Only about 70% of animals respond in the expected manner, and there is no way of forecasting which animals will respond. The same animal may also respond differently under different circumstances. The administration of further doses usually prolongs the degree of tranquillisation observed, without increasing its depth. However, further doses will also worsen the hypotension and its duration, and the cardiovascular effects outlast the observed sedative effects.

Obvious sedative effects tend to wane after around 2 hours, but the elimination half-life is between 6 hours and 8.5 hours (following IV or oral administration, respectively). Although the duration of observable effects is dose-dependent, some authors recommend that horses should not be ridden for 36 hours following the administration of acepromazine. Urinary metabolites may be found for at least three days post-dosing so that acepromazine is not recommended for any horse (e.g. race-horse) likely to undergo a urine test (for doping) within the following four days of dosing.

28.2.2 Effects

The **anxiolytic** effect of acepromazine may be all that is required in certain situations, e.g. for loading and transport of apprehensive horses, to help calm horses that need to be box-rested, and occasionally to enable clipping or dental attention. Acepromazine has been administered for long-term (up to six weeks) box rest without noticeable ill effects. The major problem is the unreliability of the effects, although the ease of oral administration allows owner dosing, which may be an advantage.

Where acepromazine's anxiolytic/sedative effect may be judged to be insufficient, its **combination with an opioid may improve the response**. The following opioids may be used:

- Morphine: 0.05–0.1–0.3 mg/kg IM or IV
- Methadone: 0.05–0.1–0.3 mg/kg IM or IV
- Butorphanol: 0.025–0.05–0.1 mg/kg IM or IV
- Buprenorphine: 0.005–0.01 mg/kg IM or IV

It is believed that some of the 'excitement' phenomena (e.g. increased locomotor activity) following high-dose opioid administration in horses are due to an increase in central dopamine activity, and as acepromazine has antidopaminergic actions, it may be useful to help control opioid-induced excitement. When acepromazine is chosen to help reduce the possible manifestations of opioid-induced 'excitement', it should be given first and allowed time to act (minimum 30 minutes by whichever route) before the opioid is given.

The confidential enquiry into peri-operative equine fatalities (CEPEF) studies demonstrated a reduction in mortality when acepromazine was included in the anaesthetic protocol. In addition to its **sedative effects** (which also tend to reduce the doses of other agents required and may contribute to calmer recoveries), and possible **anti-arrhythmic effects** (see Chapter 4), it has been shown to **improve cardiac output and arterial partial pressure of oxygen** (through improved ventilation-perfusion matching) in horses under α2 agonist-based sedation and dissociative anaesthesia (although the overall potential improvement in tissue oxygen delivery may be somewhat offset by a reduction in the haematocrit due to splenic sequestration of red cells due to both acepromazine [the effect can be marked, of the order of 20% reduction] and α2 agonists). A **small decrease in mean arterial blood pressure**, mainly due to **vasodilation** (causing a decrease in peripheral [systemic > pulmonary] vascular resistance) is accompanied by an improvement in cardiac output (probably due to the reduced afterload). The vasodilation (due to antagonism at α1 adrenoceptors) and improved tissue perfusion resulting from acepromazine's administration may be helpful in the treatment of both post-anaesthetic myopathy and laminitis, where acepromazine's **weak anti-inflammatory effects** may also be beneficial.

Although acepromazine has been shown to be **spasmolytic**, its use has not been associated with any increased risk of post-operative ileus (possibly because of its sympatholytic effects), although its use may predispose to the development of oesophageal choke. Although older texts suggested acepromazine as a potential treatment for 'spasmodic colics', its use is cautioned in any animals that are cardiovascularly compromised (e.g. hypovolaemic).

Acepromazine **reduces locomotor activity** and **reduces muscle tone**, although ataxia is rarely noted. Acepromazine may be used as an adjunct in the treatment of tetanus to allay anxiety, to reduce locomotor activity, and to produce some reduction in muscle tone. In mares, especially maiden mares or foster mares, it has been used to help increase milk production, and alongside oxytocin (which stimulates the milk-ejection reflex), it may encourage milk let-down through providing anxiolysis.

In male animals (especially stallions, but also reported in geldings), the retractor penis muscle becomes relaxed and penile protrusion occurs; this is usually transient (lasts for a similar duration to the sedative effect), but sometimes the retractor penis muscle becomes paralysed and prolonged penile protrusion may result in dependent congestion and/or traumatic damage of the distal penis and **paraphimosis**. Although a role for testosterone has been suggested, there should be no testosterone in gelded animals, hence this suggestion is difficult to support. Transient penile protrusion, however, does follow antagonism of the normal sympathetic (α1 adrenoceptor-mediated) retractor penis muscle tone by acepromazine's α1 antagonistic effects. A dose-related effect has been reported.

Occasionally, **priapism** (sustained erection) may also occur, which, through prolonged, persistent engorgement/tumescence, may result in paraphimosis with eventual penile paralysis. The aetiology of priapism is thought to be due to the α1 antagonistic effects of acepromazine on the sympathetically-mediated signals for penile detumescence.

Acepromazine may also cause vasodilation/relaxation of vascular/cavernous smooth muscle within the penile structure, particularly the corpus cavernosum penis, thus facilitating any engorgement and helping to maintain priapism or promoting the development of paraphimosis during penile protrusion. Paraphimosis and priapism may both ultimately require penile amputation, which is disastrous for breeding animals. Therefore, the use of acepromazine in breeding stallions is contra-indicated in the drug's data sheet. In reality, the incidence of permanent penile dysfunction (mostly following paralysis/prolonged prolapse) is less than around 1 in 10,000, and in a recent survey, it appeared that although veterinary anaesthetists were aware of the potential problems, they tended to use acepromazine in stallions where they thought there was a clinical indication to do so, albeit being extra vigilant for complications.

Should complications occur, it is important to recognise them early and intervene as soon as possible for the best possible outcome. Attempted support of the penis, e.g. by use of a sling, or, better, replacement of the prolapsed penis within the sheath and retention there by the use of purse-string sutures, appears efficacious in most cases. Diuretics and massage to reduce oedema may be warranted. In these cases, massage/Esmarch bandaging to achieve exsanguination of the penis, hydrotherapy, and mechanical support may be employed. Additionally, the administration of benzatropine mesylate, a compound with anti-cholinergic and anti-histaminic actions (dose c. 20 μg/kg IV) may facilitate detumescence in cases of priapism. Other suggested strategies have centred around the use of decongestants (α1 agonist vasopressors such as phenylephrine), either applied topically or irrigated intracavernously (through the corpus cavernosum penis) or anti-thrombotics, such as heparin, to try to maintain penile perfusion in order to avoid ischaemic damage. Aspiration of stagnant blood or clots, the creation of surgical shunts, and phallectomy are usually last-resort surgeries.

Overdosage is usually manifested as excitement, possibly increased locomotor activity, yet muscle weakness, ataxia, and tremors. Tachycardia, tachypnoea and sweating have also been reported. It is possible that all of these observed effects are reactions to a more profound hypotension, although the Parkinsonian-like (extrapyramidal) effects may well be due to over-suppression of central dopaminergic neurotransmission. There are no specific antidotes, although intravenous fluid therapy, vasopressors, amphetamines, methylxanthines, weak antimuscarinics/antihistaminics (diphenhydramine, benzatropine), and analeptics (CNS stimulants such as 4-aminopyridine or doxapram) have all been suggested.

Intracarotid injection has been associated with excitement, collapse, and seizures. Diazepam may be required to treat the seizures.

28.3 Thioxanthenes

These compounds are generally used as human antipsychotic agents and have anti-dopaminergic and anti-adrenergic actions, and depress the release of many hypothalamic and pituitary hormones. Zuclopenthixol acetate (or even decanoate) may occasionally be used to provide relatively long-acting mild sedation for wild or feral Equidae. The reader is referred to specialist texts for details regarding the chemical immobilisation of wild and feral Equidae.

28.4 Benzodiazepines

- **Diazepam** (5 mg/ml): dose 0.01–0.2 mg/kg IV only (often 0.05 mg/kg for adults, and 0.1–0.25 mg/kg for foals).
- **Midazolam** (5 mg/ml): dose 0.01–0.2 mg/kg IV or IM.
- **Zolazepam** (in combination with tiletamine) is often used for the chemical restraint of feral Equidae.

Experimentally, diazepam doses of 0.05–0.4 mg/kg (IV) in adult horses produce minimal cardiovascular and respiratory depressant effects, although doses greater than 0.2 mg/kg often result in increased muscular weakness; muscle fasciculations especially of the head, neck, and forequarter muscles, ataxia; and even recumbency. Sedation is not very obvious until doses of at least 0.2 mg/kg.

Higher doses (e.g. 0.6 mg/kg) result in some cardiorespiratory depression, whereas lower doses, although producing no obvious cardiorespiratory effects themselves, can enhance the cardiorespiratory depressant effects of other agents.

Horses were not reported to extend and lower their heads, as seen with 'sedation', although they did appear to be less aware of their surroundings, and therefore were 'tranquillised'.

Occasionally, horses showed strange behavioural reactions, such as mouthing food, or attempting to pace (which may have been a response to the centrally produced muscle relaxation). Table 28.1 outlines the results of the study.

Benzodiazepines, which act as allosteric modulators of $GABA_A$ receptors (at benzodiazepine binding sites associated with $GABA_A$ receptors) to enhance GABA (inhibitory neurotransmitter) binding and/or activity, may reduce anaesthetic dose requirements as many anaesthetic agents also act via $GABA_A$ receptors. Benzodiazepines and barbiturates additionally appear to promote each other's binding to these $GABA_A$ receptor complexes.

28.4.1 Effects

In **mature** animals, **transient ataxia/excitement and recumbency** can occur with doses that produce some (but minimal), mental 'calming', and thus benzodiazepines **tend not to be used for standing chemical restraint**. It is suggested that the feeling of muscular weakness causes horses to panic, so they try to run away, which is not easy if they are ataxic. However, due to the muscle relaxant effects produced, benzodiazepines are a **useful adjunct to ketamine anaesthesia**. Benzodiazepines, especially the longer acting diazepam, may 'enhance' the muscle relaxation produced by other centrally acting muscle relaxants (e.g. guaiphenesin), and the muscle weakness it produces may, theoretically, also compound that produced by peripherally acting neuromuscular blocking agents, although this does not appear to be clinically significant.

In **foals**, since recumbency is less of a problem (the feeling of **muscular weakness** seems to be **tolerated better**

Table 28.1 Results of diazepam administration to horses.

Duration of clinical effect (min)	Dose (mg/kg)	Head lowering	Fixed gaze	Muscle fasciculations	Ataxia	Recumbency	Other
5	0.05	No	Yes	Yes	No	No	Mouthed food, paced
20–50	0.1	No	Yes	Yes	Yes	No	Not reported
50	0.2	No	Yes	Yes	Yes	Rare (for 3 minutes)	Not reported
50–120	0.4	No	Yes	Yes	Yes	More often (for 7–21 minutes)	Not reported

by foals, which seem to accept the weak feeling and just lie down), and is less dangerous for the handlers and is even desirable, benzodiazepines are often chosen to produce sedation with minimal cardiorespiratory side effects in animals younger than six weeks old. Occasionally, however, **'disinhibition'** (paradoxical excitement) will occur.

Benzodiazepines are also useful for the **treatment of seizures;** 10–100 mg diazepam per horse is the starting dose.

Overdoses can be treated with supportive measures, e.g. support of ventilation and circulation. However, specific **benzodiazepine antagonists** (e.g. **flumazenil**) are available, although tend to have shorter half-lives than the agonists, so re-dosing may be necessary, and they are often expensive. A dose rate for horses is not recorded in the literature, but, as for dogs, a dose of 10 μg/kg is suggested, which may have to be repeated due to its relatively short-lasting effects. Compounds such as theophylline derivatives and anticholinesterases were once used in an attempt to 'reverse' benzodiazepine sedation before the introduction of flumazenil.

28.5 α2 Adrenoreceptor Agonists

These are **sedative–analgesics** with some **muscle relaxant** properties. Those licenced for use in horses include:

- **Xylazine** (injectable 100 mg/ml and 20 mg/ml solutions); a thiazine derivative. Dose: 0.25–1.1 mg/kg IV or IM.
- **Detomidine** (injectable 10 mg/ml solution and an oral transmucosal gel formulation 7.6 mg/ml); an imidazoline derivative. Dose: 0.005–0.08 mg/kg IV or IM. Also well absorbed across mucous membranes and can be administered in a relatively small volume by the sublingual, oromucosal route, at a dose of c. 40 μg/kg (i.e. 2–3 ml of the oromucosal gel for the average 500 kg horse).
- **Romifidine** (injectable 10 mg/ml solution); an imidazoline derivative (but does not contain an imidazole ring). Dose: 0.025–0.1 mg/kg IV (not licenced for IM).

Medetomidine and **dexmedetomidine**, also imidazoline derivatives, are not currently licenced for use in horses, but have gained much popularity. Doses are around 5–10 μg/kg IV for medetomidine and around half of this for dexmedetomidine.

Doses at the lower end of the range should be used for large breed and draught horses because of 'allometric' (as opposed to isometric) scaling of doses. That is, larger horses have relatively smaller surface areas, relatively slower metabolic rates, and require reduced doses, especially when these are calculated according to body weight (i.e. on a mg/kg basis). Perhaps we should dose according to body surface area, as is now suggested for dexmedetomidine in dogs.

28.5.1 Effects

Sedation is characterised by head-lowering, ptosis, drooping of the lower lip, some ataxia, and penile protrusion in males.

Muscle relaxation manifests as ataxia or limb incoordination. It may be the result of:

- Reduced vigilance and lack of concentration that accompanies the anxiolysis and sedation
- Local anaesthetic type of action on motor nerves
- Central actions on imidazoline receptors may occur (such receptors are thought to be similar to, or connected with, benzodiazepine receptors, and hence mediate 'central' muscle relaxation, perhaps via effects at glycine and GABA$_A$ receptors).

Lowering of the head may be partly a response to the muscle relaxation as well as a result of the induced sedation. Penile protrusion also occurs, but there have been no reports of problems associated with this, unlike with acepromazine. Smooth and striated muscles are affected. Beware animals with laryngeal paralysis where these drugs may obscure the diagnosis and promote respiratory obstruction.

The **analgesia** afforded by α2 agonists includes visceral and superficial somatic analgesia, although analgesia can be difficult to study because of the accompanying sedation. The sedation and analgesia provided by α2 agonists are not unlike those produced by opioids, and there are two possible reasons why this is so:

- α2 and opioid receptors are found in similar locations in the brain and spinal cord.
- These receptors share common signal transduction pathways (involving G proteins) and similar effector mechanisms (e.g. changes in ion permeabilities).

The various **endocrine effects**, including **diuresis**, are explained in more detail in Chapter 4. The reduction in release of 'stress hormones' may reduce the 'stress response' associated with anaesthesia and surgery, but whether this is of benefit or detriment to the animal is not fully understood. It may be that modulation of the 'inflammatory response to surgery', rather than of the stress response, is more important to eventual outcome, at least in healthy patients. **Sweating** is often observed, especially on recovery from sedation, and may be due to changes in autonomic nervous system (ANS) balance and regional blood flow, and to the reduction in anti-diuretic hormone (ADH) and aldosterone.

Uterine α2 receptor stimulation tends to result in **uterine contraction** (although the contractions may not be well co-ordinated), and an **increase in intra-uterine**

Table 28.2 Uterine effects of α2 agonists in non-pregnant mares.

Drug	Xylazine	Detomidine	Romifidine
Dose ('equipotent')	1.1 mg/kg	40 μg/kg	80 μg/kg
Intra-uterine P ↑	+ + + +	+ +	+
Duration of IU P ↑	+(+)	+ +	+

pressure in the **non-gravid equine uterus** that causes concern about potential ecbolic (abortifacient) effects. In the non-gravid uterus, xylazine causes the greatest increase in intra-uterine pressure, detomidine having intermediate effects and romifidine causing the least increase in intra-uterine pressure. The results of one study, using 'equipotent' sedative doses (i.e. subjectively indistinguishable degree and duration of sedation) of the three available α2 agonists in non-pregnant mares, are outlined in Table 28.2.

In **pregnant mares**, on the other hand, **detomidine** administered at 20 or 40 μg/kg IM was shown to **reduce uterine electrical activity** (and presumably, therefore reduced intra-uterine pressure), although at the higher dose of 60 μg/kg it had no effect on uterine electrical activity. This does not necessarily mean that α2 agonists can be safely used in pregnant mares because all **α2 agonists potentially cause uteroplacental vasoconstriction**, and in addition to reducing cardiac output in the dam, they cross the placenta to **depress foetal cardiovascular function**, all of which **may compromise foetal viability**, regardless of whether or not they affect uterine tone. The foetus also becomes sedated.

There is inconclusive evidence about the safety and possible teratogenic effects of α2 agonists on the developing embryo and foetus in the first trimester of pregnancy (organogenesis stage), and, overall, there still remains some fear about α2 agonist use in pregnant animals, especially in the last trimester of pregnancy (during which their use is contra-indicated in the data sheets). Two studies, which administered multiple doses of detomidine to pregnant mares either throughout pregnancy or during the last trimester, however, failed to demonstrate any adverse outcomes. The distress caused by not sedating an anxious mare might be more detrimental than a dose of α2 agonist. If multiple top-ups or an infusion of α2 agonist are required, then it is often recommended to administer clenbuterol (800 ng/kg IV at the start of the procedure and again 12 hours later) in the hope of preserving uteroplacental perfusion. Clenbuterol administration has also been recommended when pregnant mares undergo general anaesthesia, where the anaesthetic protocol includes an α2 agonist.

Overall, **gut motility is reduced** (both large and small intestine) and passage of food through the GI tract becomes slowed (i.e. gut transit time is increased). The increase in oesophageal transit time may predispose animals to the development of oesophageal 'choke', thus horses should not be fed soon after sedation. The reduction in gut motility may help to relieve the pain associated with certain forms of 'colic' (e.g. spasmodic colic), but, associated with the reduction in gut motility, there may be vasoconstriction of the mesenteric blood vessels, which may further compromise an already ischaemic gut. Reduced gastro-intestinal motility may also predispose to ileus, but so can high sympathetic tone which accompanies pain and distress.

Thermoregulation is suppressed centrally, resulting in decreased thermogenesis. The usual slight overall increased peripheral vasoconstriction may offset body heat loss to some extent. **Sweating**, however, **may also influence body temperature**. Febrile horses have been noted to become tachypnoeic after α2 agonist administration, thought to be due to an antipyretic effect,

Administration of α2 agonists **tends to reduce intra-ocular pressure** (see Chapter 4). This may, however, be **offset by the lowered head carriage** (secondary to sedation). Furthermore, the initial arterial hypertension and rise in central venous pressure following intravenous administration of α2 agonists may transiently increase intra-ocular pressure.

Decreases in both PCV and TP occur due to splenic sequestration of red cells and possibly secondary to the mild hyperglycaemia, with resultant shift of water into the intravascular space. Blood pH and blood gas tensions also remain essentially unchanged in previously healthy animals. Platelet aggregation is theoretically enhanced, but clinical problems have not been reported. Hyperglycaemia is common, but is not usually accompanied by glycosuria. Splenic size may also increase with the sequestration of red blood cells.

28.5.2 Use for Sedation

α2 agonists reliably produce predictable sedation in >80% of horses. Failure of a response may be seen in animals that are excited, in pain, or stressed or fearful, and is due to their higher sympathetic activity that 'competes' better with the drug-induced sympatholysis. In such animals, further doses may be required, or the procedure could be abandoned and attempted another day when the animal should be calmed first if possible. All animals should be left in a quiet environment after drug administration, for sedation to become apparent, before further interventions are begun. Following IV administration, the onset of sedation occurs within 3–5 minutes and peak sedation is observed within 5–15 minutes, whereas following oromucosal administration, although onset of sedation occurs within around 20–30 minutes, peak effects take about 45–60–100 minutes to develop.

A feature of the sedation produced with α2 agonists is that horses may be aroused by sudden stimuli, especially touch and noise, and can still deliver well-aimed kicks. To increase the 'reliability' of the sedation (especially in fractious animals), increase the analgesia, and reduce the responsiveness to stimuli, α2 agonists are often combined with opioids, butorphanol being the most commonly used, mainly because it is not a controlled drug and is thus readily available for ambulatory equine veterinarians.

Sedation can be difficult to assess in horses, with the degree of head lowering often being taken as an objective measurement for depth and duration of sedation. Analgesia and sedation can also be difficult to differentiate

The sedation produced by α2 agonists is dose-dependent with a ceiling effect (a dose beyond which the depth of sedation is not increased further by increasing the dose, but the duration of sedation continues to increase). Analgesia is also thought to be dose-dependent, and to persist for only about one-third to two-thirds of the duration of the observed sedation. Although xylazine and detomidine seem to obey these 'rules', there has been much debate over romifidine. The sedation (head lowering) is much less obvious following romifidine than the other agents, meaning perhaps a less deep sedation; and some authors believe that the analgesia afforded by romifidine is the least (least predictable) of all the agents. The three commonly used α2 agonists are compared in Table 28.3 at equipotent doses.

Equipotent IV sedative doses are believed to be:

$$\text{Xylazine 1 mg/kg} \equiv \text{Detomidine 15 µg/kg} \left(\text{or } 20-40 \text{ µg/kg}\right)$$
$$\equiv \text{Romifidine 80 µg/kg}$$

The ceiling doses for sedation are believed to be:

- Xylazine 1.1 mg/kg
- Detomidine 40 µg/kg
- Romifidine 80–100 µg/kg (some believe that higher doses of romifidine are associated with a reduction in, or reversal of, the observed sedation).

At these doses, the cardiopulmonary effects are similar, and after these doses it is assumed safe to ride the horse:

- 8 hours after xylazine
- 24 hours after detomidine
- Up to 48 hours after romifidine

The **addition of an opioid improves the reliability of the sedation and reduces the possibility of arousal and reaction to stimulation, but never trust a sedated-looking animal**. The addition of opioids generally does not increase the cardiovascular depression already produced by the α2 agonist, but may increase the respiratory depression and ataxia observed.

Opioids are always quoted for their ability to cause 'excitement' reactions when administered, especially intravenously, to horses (and cats), but much of this dogma results from early experiments where huge doses were given to non-painful animals. Such 'excitement' usually manifests as increased locomotor activity and restlessness, occasional head-pressing (if they walk into a corner and try to keep going), muscle tremors (especially around the face), and ataxia. It usually occurs soon after IV administration, and later gives way to sedation. These reactions are due mainly to activity at µ receptors, but κ receptor stimulation may augment locomotor activity and ataxia, and occasionally causes bizarre behaviour such as sham-drinking and yawning. When opioids are to be administered, the sedative

Table 28.3 Features of the three common α2 agonists when administered at 'equipotent' sedative doses.

α2 agonist	Xylazine	Detomidine	Romifidine
Dose (IV)	1 mg/kg	15 µg/kg	80 µg/kg
Onset of action	Within 3 minutes	Within 5 minutes	Within 5 minutes
Duration of action	Average 20 minutes	Average 80 minutes	>80 minutes
Sedation	+ + +	+ +	+(+)
Muscle relaxation	+ +	+ + +	+
Ataxia[a]	+ + +(+)	+ +(+ +)	+
Analgesia	+ + + +	(>10 µg/kg) + + + +	+(+)
Sweating		Difficult to predict	

[a] May be influenced by speed of IV injection.

agent is usually given first, and then the opioid is given once sedation has been assured. If the injections cannot be separated, be aware of the potential side effects seen with high dose opioid administration, especially in relatively pain-free animals.

Butorphanol is the most commonly used opioid by ambulatory equine practitioners. Its intravenous use has not been associated with histamine release, and the volume for injection is convenient. Its use is also not complicated by legislation requiring a written record to be made for each dose administered. As a sole agent, doses as low as 50 μg/kg IV may induce some increase in locomotor activity and mild ataxia. (Doses up to 200 μg/kg [or more] may be necessary to provide adequate analgesia in some circumstances.) Butorphanol alone causes minimal haemodynamic and respiratory effects, but can enhance the respiratory depressant effects of other agents. It tends to produce excitement effects and ataxia, especially at higher doses in non-painful animals, but these later give way to sedation, which can augment that resulting from other sedative agents.

Buprenorphine can also be given alongside α2 agonists at doses of 0.005–0.01 mg/kg, although the higher dose tends to stimulate an increase in locomotor activity, especially in non-painful animals. More recently, a sustained-release formulation of buprenorphine was reported to result in colon impaction and a prolonged increase in locomotor activity, which will likely preclude its clinical use, despite the potential for it providing antinociception/analgesia for up to 48 hours.

When used in combination with α2 agonists, butorphanol is usually administered at doses of 25–50 μg/kg; and buprenorphine at 5–10 μg/kg. The α2 agonists can then also be administered in 'lower' doses (e.g. xylazine 0.5 mg/kg; detomidine 10 μg/kg; romifidine 40 μg/kg).

α2 agonists may also be combined with acepromazine, although reduced doses of each should be used. A useful combination for intramuscular administration in fractious animals, which ensures a good quality of sedation, is given below (other opioids can be used in place of butorphanol). The addition of acepromazine seems to assure a good background anxiolysis and further reduces the animal's response to environmental and other stimuli. It also improves the haemodynamics and arterial oxygenation.

The doses commonly used (in combination) are:

Detomidine 20 μg/kg + acepromazine 30 μg/kg + butorphanol 50 μg/kg IM.

The animal must be left undisturbed for a good 30 minutes after this injection.

For a 500 kg horse this combination would mean: 10 mg detomidine (1 ml) + 15 mg acepromazine (1.5 ml, if using the 10 mg/ml formulation) + 25 mg butorphanol (2.5 ml); total volume = 5 ml.

Usually foals less than four to six weeks old can be nicely sedated with benzodiazepines, possibly including an opioid. However, for older, and more boisterous younger foals, α2 agonists may be used to facilitate handling. The following doses have been used without problems in **healthy** foals, but remember that foals tend not to resist the feeling of muscle weakness and so often become recumbent. Recumbency may facilitate the planned intervention, but also promotes the development of postural hypoxaemia (common in neonatal foals anyway), such that provision of supplemental oxygen should be considered if recumbency is prolonged. Also be aware of the foal's hydration status and its temperature. Sick foals may only require very small doses.

Doses in healthy foals:

- Xylazine 0.2–1 mg/kg IV
- Detomidine 5–40 μg/kg IV
- Romifidine 20–70 μg/kg IV
- Butorphanol can be administered alone or alongside benzodiazepines or α2 agonists at 0.05–0.2 mg/kg to enhance sedation and/or provide analgesia.
- Pethidine 3.5–5 mg/kg IM (not IV) can be given to foals to provide analgesia and some sedation, and can also be a useful adjunct to benzodiazepine or α2 agonist sedation.
- Buprenorphine can be administered to foals at 0.005–0.01 mg/kg to provide analgesia. As with other opioids, increased locomotor activity may be seen with the higher doses in non-painful animals; also sedation and tachypnoea have been reported in non-painful foals at the higher dose.

28.5.3 Use, by Continuous Infusion, for Standing Chemical Restraint

The licenced, and, as yet, unlicensed, α2 agonists have all been studied for administration by continuous infusion to provide a stable level of sedation/analgesia for standing procedures (or a stable level of background sedation/analgesia during general anaesthesia, where their provision can reduce inhalation agent requirements and improve recovery quality; see Chapter 30). Of all the α2 agonists, those with the shortest half-lives are the most suitable for administration by continuous infusion as they are the most titratable and least cumulative. These include xylazine, medetomidine, and dexmedetomidine. Romifidine can also be given by continuous infusion, but although it produces the least ataxia, it is the hardest to titrate to effect. As a general rule for the α2 agonists, half of the initial effective/loading dose is infused per hour, but the rate can be varied according to the patient's response/requirements. An algorithm has recently developed by Ghent veterinary school to assist in scoring the adequacy of standing chemical restraint, and how to alter the rate of α2 agonist infusions.

Whenever standing surgery is proposed, it is important to prepare as if the horse requires a general anaesthetic as conversion to this may become necessary. The horse's temperament is also important as some patients just do not tolerate standing procedures. An idea of the duration of the procedure is helpful, as is an idea of how invasive/noxious it is likely to be, and whether complementary systemic opioids and local/regional anaesthetic techniques could be used. Intravenous access is mandatory and be aware of horses leaning forward on the stocks and occluding their jugular veins, as this will stop any gravity-flow infusions. The aim is for a patient that remains standing, without excessive ataxia, and that is non-responsive to noxious stimuli like pain and non-responsive to external stimuli like noise. Standing chemical restraint techniques also capitalise on balanced (multi-modal) analgesic techniques.

Although many variations have been reported in the literature, a basic technique is described below and can be modified to suit any particular patient. First of all, acepromazine (0.03 mg/kg IM) may be given around 30–40 minutes before jugular venous cannulation is achieved (if there are no contraindications to its use). IV access must then be secured. An α2 agonist, preferably the one that has been chosen for infusion is then given IV and sedation is allowed to develop for at least five minutes before an opioid is administered. An NSAID can be given at this time, if appropriate. Once the patient has reached peak sedation from the initial bolus, a follow-on infusion of α2 agonist can be started. Although intermittent IV top-ups of sedatives and analgesics may be given, the peaks and troughs of sedation can make surgical progress difficult, hence continuous infusions are usually preferred because a more stable level of sedation can be achieved (the infusion rate can easily be altered according to the patient's response).

α2 agonists and opioids are the most common drugs chosen for administration by continuous infusion, although lidocaine and ketamine may also be considered (see Tables 28.4 and 28.5 below). Lidocaine (without epinephrine) can be given at a loading bolus dose of 1–2 mg/kg over 5–10 minutes, followed by a continuous infusion at 25–50 μg/kg/min. Ketamine can be administered at a loading dose of 0.2–0.5 mg/kg SC or IM, or at a dose of 0.1–0.25 mg/kg slowly IV as a 'ketamine stun' (but note that even small doses of ketamine, if given too rapidly IV, can cause agitation and even recumbency in some horses); followed by infusion at around 0.5 mg/kg/h. Once settled on the infusion/s, consider if any local/regional anaesthetic techniques would be suitable: These must be performed,

Table 28.4 Examples of drug doses for continuous infusion for standing procedures.

Drug	Loading dose (IV)	Initial infusion rate
Xylazine	1 mg/kg	c. 0.5 mg/kg/h
Detomidine	6–10–40 μg/kg	c. 5–20 μg/kg/h The lowest loading dose requires a higher initial 'maintenance' infusion rate, starting out around 35 μg/kg/h, but usually this can be reduced within the first 15 min and further reductions may subsequently be necessary
Romifidine See Table legend	50–80 μg/kg	c. 20–40 μg/kg/h
Medetomidine	5–10 μg/kg	c. 3–5 μg/kg/h
Morphine	0.1–0.2 mg/kg	0.03–0.05 mg/kg/h
Butorphanol	0.05–0.1 mg/kg	0.01 mg/kg/h
Ketamine	0.1–0.25 mg/kg (0.2–0.5 mg/kg SC)	c. 0.5 mg/kg/h
Lidocaine (without epinephrine)	1–2 mg/kg	1.5–3 mg/kg/h (25–50 μg/kg/min)

Note that although romifidine is included in this table, its pharmacokinetic profile precludes it from easy titration during standing chemical restraint. It may, however, be administered in a partial/supplemental intravenous anaesthesia protocol during general anaesthesia, where it can be diluted in a small total volume of sterile saline to be delivered by syringe driver.

and the blocks allowed to develop, before surgery is allowed to commence (see Chapter 16).

28.5.4 Use for Premedication

Predictable sedation and calming of horses prior to induction of anaesthesia greatly smooths the course of anaesthesia. If excessive ataxia is to be avoided, agents such as romifidine may be preferred, or lower doses of the other agents may be sufficient.

Residual sedation at the end of surgery also smooths the recovery period by reducing the excitement to which horses seem prone, especially if romifidine has been used, because the ataxia is minimal. Alternatively, additional doses of α2 agonists may be given at the beginning of the recovery period to serve the same purpose. The different α2 agonists produce slightly different features in recovery, e.g. with respect to suppression of swallowing (e.g. romifidine tends to delay return of swallowing, so do not always wait for

Table 28.5 Quick guide to setting up an infusion.

Drug	Quantity to add to 500 ml 0.9% saline	Infusion rate (Rates usually need to be varied according to the patient's response)	Expected volume to be infused per hour for a 500 kg horse	Drops per second (assumes standard giving set, which gives 20 drops/ml)
Xylazine	500 mg	0.5 mg/kg/h	250 ml	1.5
Detomidine	10 mg	10 µg/kg/h	250 ml	1.5
Medetomidine	3.5 mg	3.5 µg/kg/h	250 ml	1.5
Morphine	60 mg	30–50 µg/kg/h	125–210 ml	c. 1
Butorphanol	10 mg	10 µg/kg/h	250 ml	1.5
Ketamine	500 mg	0.5 mg/kg/h	250 ml	1.5
Lidocaine	1500 mg (75 ml of 2%)	50 µg/kg/h	500 ml	c. 3

swallowing to return before removing the endotracheal tube), and how long they spend in sternal recumbency before attempting to stand.

α2 agonists, when administered for premedication, greatly reduce the requirements for other anaesthetic agents, both induction and maintenance agents.

There seem to be no obvious differences among the characteristics of anaesthesia when different α2 agonists have been used for premedication. Heart rates, arterial blood pressures, and breathing rates and patterns all seem similar, all other factors being equal.

28.5.5 Problems Associated with the Use of α2 Agonists

- Bradycardia and bradyarrhythmias, especially A-V blocks. It is believed that horses exhibiting physiological A-V blocks prior to sedation are at no extra risk. Occasionally heart rates below 20 bpm have been recorded. Atropine (0.01 mg/kg IV) is an effective treatment but is not without its own side effects (severe tachycardia and hypertension, possibly arrhythmias, intestinal ileus, mydriasis and central excitement). Some prefer to use glycopyrrolate (2 µg/kg IV), which has less dramatic cardiovascular effects, is longer acting, and does not cross the blood–brain barrier, although it may have more profound GI effects. Another alternative is hyoscine butylbromide (dose c. 0.1 mg/kg), but it is only very short-acting (5–10 minutes). Anticholinergic agents may be given prior to α2 agonist administration, but their prevention of the reflex bradycardia in response to the α2-mediated initial hypertension may have adverse haemodynamic effects. Also, the tachycardia resulting from anticholinergic administration increases myocardial oxygen demand, which may cause problems if hypoxaemia already exists

(see also Chapter 4). Partial antagonism of the α2 agonist with atipamezole may be an alternative strategy, but sedation will also be antagonised.

- Respiratory obstruction can develop, due to nasal oedema (if prolonged head drooping), and relaxation of the nostrils and may cause stertorous breathing. Horses with laryngeal paralysis may suffer further inspiratory dyspnoea due to relaxation of laryngeal muscles. These agents are not a good choice for sedation for the assessment of laryngeal function.
- Diuresis and increased urination may cause problems where urethral obstruction exists.
- Sweating (+/− piloerection) may cause problems if sedation is necessary for clipping, or, e.g. for taking pinchgrafts of the skin.
- Ataxia may be problematical for shoeing or lameness examinations, and beware in Wobblers.
- Although lameness may be masked by the analgesic effects of these drugs, the shorter-acting α2 agonists have been shown to be acceptable for sedation for diagnostic nerve blocks during lameness workups.
- The use of these agents is controversial in pregnant animals, uteroplacental perfusion probably being more affected than intra-uterine pressure.
- Reduced gastrointestinal motility theoretically increases the risk of oesophageal choke, impactions, and ileus; and ischaemic gut may be further compromised by vasoconstriction. Thus be aware of these potential problems in 'colics', and perhaps use the shorter acting α2 agonists where possible.
- Subcutaneous or intramuscular administration occasionally causes localised inflammatory reactions.
- Urticarial rashes have been observed following detomidine and romifidine administration, but required no specific treatment.

- Occasional tachypnoea with antipyresis has been observed following the IV administration of xylazine and detomidine in pyrexic animals. Treatment is not usually necessary.
- Intra-arterial injections have been associated with rapid onset of disorientation, excitement, seizures, and collapse. Treatment by induction of barbiturate anaesthesia, with or without benzodiazepine anticonvulsants, and the provision of oxygen, may provide a favourable outcome. The use of IV α2 antagonists is not advised as a first line treatment because the reaction is thought to be due more to general cerebral irritation/vasoconstriction than the specific central actions of the drugs. Papaverine, a potent vasodilator, is theoretically a good choice of drug to give into that artery to offset the vasoconstriction, but access to the same artery may not be available, or indeed safe, in a seizuring animal.
- Beware use in shocky/hypovolaemic animals because the resulting bradycardia, hypotension, and reduced cardiac output may compromise the animal's ability to compensate cardiovascularly. Small doses of the shortest acting agents, xylazine (medetomidine or dexmedetomidine), are preferred if necessary (e.g. in colic cases) and can provide useful analgesia.
- Large breeds (e.g. draught horses) were believed to be more sensitive to α2 agonists, whereas smaller breeds were thought to be more resistant. This apparent differential sensitivity may be due to 'metabolic weight' differences, i.e. the allometric (as opposed to isometric) scaling of body size. That is, dosing should be related more to body surface area than to actual body weight. With these precautions in mind, smaller doses (mg/kg) should be considered for large breed horses.
- The contemporaneous administration of detomidine and intravenous trimethoprim potentiated sulphonamides has been associated with fatal cardiac arrhythmias. Although this may have been an effect of the antibiotic alone (probably the solvent or 'carrier'), precaution should be observed.
- There are reports that there may be some deterioration in the activity of xylazine in bottles that have been broached for some days.
- Beware especially with sedation for shoeing or dentistry (where you may leave the farm once the animal has been sedated), and indeed for all occasions of sedation, because you are responsible for the horse (and safety of the horse and any attending personnel) until the horse is fully recovered.
- Beware accidental owner- or self-administration (e.g. across mucous membranes) as profound cardiorespiratory depression and sedation result, necessitating respiratory and circulatory support and the use of specific antagonists.
- Xylazine is contra-indicated as a sedative prior to Somulose™ (quinalbarbital and cinchocaine) euthanasia. It seems to worsen the quality of death, possibly by altering cardiac output so that 'slow' injection is not slow enough, although the other α2 agonists do not seem to cause the same problems. Perhaps xylazine's central α1 receptor actions may be partly responsible.

28.5.6 Epidural (Extradural) Administration

Epidural administration of α2 agonists can complement standing chemical restraint for obstetrical manoeuvres and surgery involving the hindquarters and tail. Different doses and combinations (with local anaesthetic agents and opioids), have been published. The use of α2 agonists alone should negate the possibility of motor nerve blockade, ataxia and recumbency, and consequent patient panic. However, administration of α2 agonists by the epidural route still allows their systemic absorption, so sedation and some ataxia may still be observed, and their local anaesthetic type activity (especially xylazine) can also produce some motor nerve blockade, and therefore ataxia. Just a few of these combinations are listed below (see also Chapter 16).

28.5.6.1 Xylazine Alone
Xylazine has a wide dose range by this route (0.03–0.35 mg/kg), but the preferred dose seems to be 0.17–0.35 mg/kg for sacro-coccygeal or inter-coccygeal injection. The resulting volume can be diluted into about 10 ml normal saline to provide an easier volume for administration. This should produce good analgesia for three to five hours. The analgesia provided by epidural xylazine outlasts that provided by epidural detomidine, possibly because of its greater α1 agonist effects, thereby causing greater localised vasoconstriction which delays its systemic absorption, and possibly also due to its better local anaesthetic type action (which may be related to their ability to reduce the I_h repolarisation current).

28.5.6.2 Detomidine Alone
Detomidine 60 μg/kg seems to be preferred for sacro-coccygeal or inter-coccygeal injection, again diluting the final volume into 10 ml normal saline. This should provide two to three hours of analgesia.

28.5.6.3 Combinations
In combination with morphine (0.05–0.1 mg/kg), use half the above doses of α2 agonist. Note that preservative-free morphine should be used.

In combination with local anaesthetic solutions, e.g. 0.17 mg/kg xylazine can be combined with 0.22 mg/kg lidocaine.

28.5.7 Antagonism

One of the advantages of the use of α2 agonists is the potential for their specific antagonism ('reversal'). Before the availability of specific antagonists, agents such as 4-amino-pyridine and doxapram (non-specific CNS stimulants) were used. There are a number of α adrenoceptor antagonists available with differing α2 : α1 selectivity:

- Prazosin: α1 > α2
- Tolazoline: α1 = α2
- Idazoxan, yohimbine: α2 > α1
- Atipamezole: α2 >> α1

28.5.7.1 Atipamezole

Atipamezole is not licenced for use in horses, but can be used where antagonism of α2 agonist effects is warranted, e.g. adverse reactions (e.g. excessive ataxia). Remember that analgesia will also be antagonised with the antagonism of sedation, but the cardiopulmonary effects may not be entirely antagonised when sedation is obviously reversed. Some authors suggest that opioid analgesia may also be partly antagonised by α2 antagonists, just as naloxone may also antagonise α2 agonist-induced analgesia, although there is much controversy (see Chapter 3).

The dose of atipamezole has not been determined for each α2 agonist and will depend upon the dose of agonist administered and the time elapsed since that administration. However, as a guide, 50 μg/kg is a starting point, and may need to be repeated. Atipamezole should be administered by IM or slow IV injection. Rapid IV injection results in rapid displacement of agonist from peripheral α2 receptors, with a sudden hypotension and reflex tachycardia. There has been some suggestion that atipamezole may also result in a degree of sedation in horses, which has not been reported in any other species.

28.5.7.2 Vatinoxan

Previously known as MK-467, vatinoxan is a peripherally-acting α2 antagonist and its administration alongside an α2 agonist can reduce the unwanted peripheral side effects such as cardiovascular changes and reduced GI motility, similarly to how N-methylnaltrexone or alvimopan have been tried as peripherally-restricted opioid antagonists in the hope of reducing opioid side effects, particularly on gut motility. Preliminary work is promising, but it is not yet commercially available.

28.5.8 Anticholinergics

See Chapter 4 on small animal sedation and premedication. Because of the mydriasis that follows atropine and glycopyrrolate (which can cause photophobia, blurred vision, and excitement), and due to the reduction in gut motility and the possibility of this leading to impaction type colics, these drugs are not generally favoured, and therefore tend to be reserved for emergency situations.

Doses used are: atropine 0.01 mg/kg IV and glycopyrrolate 2 μg/kg IV. In one study, atropine at 0.044 mg/kg reduced GI motility for 3–12 hours in ponies; whereas 5 μg/kg glycopyrrolate reduced GI motility for only 2–6 hours.

Hyoscine butylbromide (butylscopolamine) has been administered to anaesthetised horses (0.1–0.2 mg/kg) in an attempt to increase heart rate, blood pressure, and cardiac output, but the effects were only short lasting (c. 5–10 minutes). It also acts as a GI spasmolytic, but beware when assessing colics that have received a recent dose because the heart rate will be increased for 5–10 minutes.

Further Reading

Adams, A. and Hendrickson, D.A. (2014). Standing male equine urogenital surgery. *Veterinary Clinics of North America. Equine Practice* 30: 169–190.

Amadon, R.S. and Craigie, A.H. (1935). The actions of morphine on the horse. Preliminary studies: morphine, dihydromorphine, codeine, dihydropseudocodeine, dionine and dihydromorphinone (dialudid). University of Pennsylvania Bulletin. *Veterinary Extension Quarterly* 36 (60): 3–26.

Bradbury, L.A., Dugdale, A.H.A., Knottenbelt, D.C. et al. (2008). The effects of anesthesia on laryngeal function and laryngeal/pharyngeal trauma in the horse. *Journal of Equine Veterinary Science* 28: 461–467.

Boller, M., Fuerst, A., Ringer, S. et al. (2005). Complete recovery from long-standing priapism in a stallion after propionylpromazine/xylazine sedation. *Equine Veterinary Education* 17: 305–309.

Bryant, C.E., England, G.C.W., and Clarke, K.W. (1991). Comparison of the sedative effects of medetomidine and xylazine in the horse. *Veterinary Record* 129: 421–423.

Carregaro, A.B., Luna, S.P.L., Mataqueiro, M.I., and de Queiroz-Neto, A. (2007). Effects of buprenorphine on nociception and spontaneous locomotor activity in horses. *American Journal of Veterinary Research* 68: 246–250.

Carter, S.W., Robertson, S.A., Steel, C.J., and Jourdenais, D.A. (1990). Cardiopulmonary effects of xylazine sedation in the foal. *Equine Veterinary Journal* 22: 384–388.

Combie, J., Douhgerty, J., Nugent, E., and Tobin, T. (1979). The pharmacology of narcotic analgesics in the horse IV. Dose and time response relationships for behavioral responses to morphine, meperidine, pentazocine, anileridine, methadone and hydromorphone. *Journal of Equine Medicine and Surgery* 3: 377–385.

Cooke, C.D. (2015). What can I give to calm this stallion down? *Equine Veterinary Education* 27: 496–497.

De Cozar, M.J. (2019). Can I give alpha-2 agonists for blocking and accurately assess the horse's lameness once blocked? (Critically Appraised Topic). *Equine Veterinary Education.* 31: 111–112.

Deniau, V., Depecker, M., Bizon-Mercier, C., and Courouce-Malblanc, A. (2013). Influence of detomidine and xylazine on spleen dimensions and splenic response to epinephrine infusion in healthy horses. *Veterinary Anaesthesia and Analgesia* 40: 375–381.

De Vries, A., Pakkanen, S.A.E., Raekallio, M.R. et al. (2016). Clinical effects and pharmacokinetic variables of romifidine and the peripheral alpha 2 adrenoceptor antagonist MK-467 in horses. *Veterinary Anaesthesia and Analgesia* 43: 599–610.

Driessen, B., Zarucco, L., and Bertolotti, L. (2011). Contemporary use of acepromazine in the anaesthetic management of male horses and ponies: a retrospective study and opinion poll. *Equine Veterinary Journal* 43: 88–98.

Ducharme, N.G., Hackett, R.P., Fubini, S.L., and Erb, H.N. (1991). The reliability of endoscopic examination in assessment of arytenoid cartilage movement in horses. Part II. Influence of side of examination, re-examination and sedation. *Veterinary Surgery* 20: 180–184.

England, G.C.W., Clarke, K.W., and Goossens, L. (1992). A comparison of the sedative effects of three alpha 2 adrenoceptor agonists (romifidine, detomidine and xylazine) in the horse. *Journal of Veterinary Pharmacology and Therapeutics* 15: 194–201.

England, G.C.W. and Clarke, K.W. (1996). Alpha 2 adrenoceptor agonists in the horse: a review. *British Veterinary Journal* 152: 641–657.

Fielding, C.L., Brumbaugh, G.W., Matthews, N.S. et al. (2006). Pharmacokinetics and clinical effects of a subanesthetic continuous rate infusion of ketamine in awake horses. *American Journal of Veterinary Research* 67: 1484–1490.

Gibbs, H.M. and Troedsson, M.H.T. (1995). Effect of acepromazine, detomidine and xylazine on myometrial activity in the mare. *Biology of Reproduction Monographs Series* 1: 489–493.

Gozalo-Marcilla, M., Gasthuys, F., Luna, S.P.L., and Schauvliege, S. (2018). Is there a place for dexmedetomidine in equine anaesthesia and analgesia? A systematic review (2005–2017). *Journal of Veterinary Pharmacology and Therapeutics* 41: 205–217.

Gozalo-Marcilla, M., de Oliviera, A.R., Fonseca, M.W. et al. (2019). Sedative and antinociceptive effects of different detomidine constant rate infusions, with or without methadone in standing horses. *Equine Veterinary Journal* 51: 530–536.

Grimsrud, K.N., Mama, K.R., Thomasy, S.M., and Stanley, S.D. (2009). Pharmacokinetics of detomidine and its metabolites following intravenous and intramuscular administration in horses. *Equine Veterinary Journal* 41: 361–365.

Jedruch, J. and Gajewski, Z. (1986). The effect of detomidine hydrochloride (Domosedan) on the electrical activity of the uterus in cows. *Acta Veterinaria Scandinavica. Supplement* 82: 189–192.

Jedruch, J., Gajewski, Z., and Kuussaari, J. (1989). The effect of detomidine hydrochloride on the electrical activity of the uterus in pregnant mares. *Acta Veterinaria Scandinavica* 30: 307–311.

Katila, T. and Oijala, M. (1988). The effect of detomidine (Domosedan) on the maintenance of equine pregnancy and foetal development: ten cases. *Equine Veterinary Journal* 20: 323–326.

Komaromy, A.M., Garg, C.G., Ying, G.-S., and Liu, C. (2006). Effect of head position on intraocular pressure in horses. *American Journal of Veterinary Research* 67: 1232–1235.

Kendall, A., Mosley, C., and Broejer, J. (2010). Tachypnea and antipyresis in febrile horses after sedation with alpha 2 agonists. *Journal of Veterinary Internal Medicine* 24: 1008–1011.

Knych, H.K., Seminoff, K., McKemie, D.S., and Kass, P.H. (2018). Pharmacokinetics, pharmacodynamics and metabolism of acepromazine following intravenous, oral and sublingual administration to exercised thoroughbred horses. *Journal of Veterinary Pharmacology and Therapeutics* 41: 522–535.

L'Ami, J.J., Vermunt, L.E., van JPAM, L., and Sloet van Oldruitenborgh-Oosterbaan, M.M. (2013). Sublingual administration of detomidine in horses: sedative effect, analgesia and detection time. *The Veterinary Journal* 196: 253–259.

LeBlanc, M.M., Hubbell, J.A.E., and Smith, H.C. (1984). The effects of xylazine hydrochloride on intrauterine pressure in the cow. *Theriogenology* 21: 681–690.

Lees, P. and Serrano, L. (1976). Effects of azaperone on cardiovascular and respiratory functions in the horse. *British Journal of Pharmacology* 56: 263–269.

Leonardi, F., Costa, G.L., Dubau, M., Sabbioni, A., Simonazzi, B., and Angelone, M. (2019). Effects of intravenous romifidine, detomidine, detomidine combined with butorphanol and xylazine on tear production in horses. Equine Veterinary Education. http://doi.org/10.1111/eve.13040.

Levionnois, O.L., Graubner, C., and Spadavecchia, C. (2018). Colon constipation in horses after sustained-release buprenorphine administration. *Veteirnary Anaesthesia and Analgesia* 45: 876–880.

Love, E.J., Taylor, P.M., Murrell, J., and Whay, H.R. (2012). Effects of acepromazine, butorphanol and buprenorphine on thermal and mechanical nociceptive thresholds in horses. *Equine Veterinary Journal* 44: 221–225.

Luukkanen, L., Katila, T., and Koskinen, E. (1997). Some effects of multiple administrations of detomidine during the last trimester of equine pregnancy. *Equine Veterinary Journal* 29: 400–403.

Marntell, S., Nyman, G., Funkquist, P., and Hedenstierna, G. (2005). Effects of acepromazine on pulmonary gas exchange and circulation during sedation and dissociative anaesthesia in horses. *Veterinary Anaesthesia and Analgesia* 32: 83–93.

McDonnell, S.M. (2005). Managing the paralysed penis, priapism and paraphimosis in the horse. *Equine Veterinary Journal* 17: 310–311.

Memon, M.A., Usenik, E.A., Varner, D.D., and Meyers, P.J. (1988). Penile paralysis and paraphimosis associated with reserpine administration in a stallion. *Theriogenology* 30: 411–419.

Messenger, K.M., Davis, J.L., LaFevers, D.H. et al. (2011). Intravenous and sublingual buprenorphine in horses: pharmacokinetics and influence of sampling site. *Veterinary Anaesthesia and Analgesia* 38: 374–384.

Michou, J. and Leece, E. (2012). Sedation and analgesia in the standing horse 1. Drugs used for sedation and systemic analgesia. *In Practice* 34: 524–531.

Michou, J. and Leece, E. (2012). Sedation and analgesia in the standing horse 2. Local anaesthesia and analgesia techniques. *In Practice* 34: 578–587.

Muir, W.W., Sams, R.A., Huffman, R.H., and Noonan, J.S. (1982). Pharmacodynamic and pharmacokinetic properties of diazepam in horses. *American Journal of Veterinary Research* 43: 1756–1762.

Naylor, J.M., Garven, E., and Fraser, L. (1997). A comparison of romifidine and xylazine in foals: the effects on sedation and analgesia. *Equine Veterinary Education* 9: 329–334.

Oijala, M. and Katila, T. (1988). Detomidine (Domosedan) in foals: sedative and analgesic effects. *Equine Veterinary Journal* 20: 327–330.

Pakkanen, S.A.E., Raekallio, M.R., Mykkanen, A.K. et al. (2015). Detomidine and the combination of detomidine and MK-467, a peripherally-acting alpha-2 adrenoceptor antagonist, as premedication in horses anaesthetized with isoflurane. *Veterinary Anaesthesia and Analgesia* 42: 527–536.

Parry, B.W. and Anderson, G.A. (1983). Influence of acepromazine maleate on the equine haematocrit. *Journal of Veterinary Pharmacology and Therapeutics* 6: 121–126.

Parry, B.W., Anderson, G.A., and Gay, C.G. (1982). Hypotension in the horse induced by acepromazine maleate. *Australian Veterinary Journal* 59: 148–152.

Pearson, H. and Weaver, B.M.Q. (1978). Priapism after sedation, neuroleptanalgesia and anaesthesia in the horse. *Equine Veterinary Journal* 10: 85–90.

Pimenta, E.L.M., Teixeiro Neto, F.J., Pignaton, P.A.S.A.W., and Garofalo, N.A. (2011). Comparative study between atropine and hyoscine-N-butylbromide for reversal of detomidine induced bradycardia in horses. *Equine Veterinary Journal* 43: 332–340.

Rezende, M.L., Grimsrud, K.N., Stanley, S.D. et al. (2014). Pharmacokinetics and pharmacodynamics of intravenous dexmedetomidine in the horse. *Journal of Veterinary Pharmacology and Therapeutics* 38: 15–23.

Robertson, S.A., Sanchez, L.C., Merritt, A.M., and Doherty, T.J. (2005). Effect of systemic lidocaine on visceral and somatic nociception in conscious horses. *Equine Veterinary Journal* 37: 122–127.

Santos, M., Fuente, M., Garcia-Iturralde, P. et al. (2003). Effects of alpha 2 adrenoceptor agonists during recovery from isoflurane anaesthesia in horses. *Equine Veterinary Journal* 35: 170–175.

Schatzmann, U., Josseck, H., Stauffer, J.-L., and Goossens, L. (1984). Effects of alpha 2 agonists on intrauterine pressure and sedation in horses: comparison between detomidine, romifidine and xylazine. *Journal of Veterinary Medicine A* 41: 523–529.

Schauvliege, S., Cuypers, C., Michielsen, M. et al. (2019). How to score sedation and adjust the administration rate of sedatives in horses: a literature review and introduction of the Ghent sedation algorithm. *Veterinary Anaesthesia and Analgesia* 46: 4–13.

Seabaugh, K.A. and Schumacher, J. (2014). Urogenital surgery performed with the mare standing. *Veterinary Clinics of North America. Equine Practice* 30: 191–209.

Sellon, D.C., Monroe, V.L., Roberts, M.C., and Papich, M.G. (2001). Pharmacokinetics and adverse effects of butorphanol administered by single intravenous injection or continuous intravenous infusion in horses. *American Journal of Veterinary Research* 62: 183–189.

Tapio, H., Raekallio, M.R., Mykkanen, A. et al. (2019). Effects of vatinoxan on cardiorespiratory function and gastrointestinal motility during constant-rate medetomidine infusion in standing horses. *Equine Veterinary Journal* 51: 646–652.

Taylor, P., Coumbe, K., Henson, F., and Taylor, A. (2014). Evaluation of sedation for standing clinical procedures in horses using detomidine combined with buprenorphine. *Veterinary Anaesthesia and Analgesia* 41: 14–24.

Tomasic, M., Mann, L.S., and Soma, L.R. (1997). Effects of sedation, anesthesia and endotracheal intubation on respiratory mechanics in adult horses. *American Journal of Veterinary Research* 58: 641–646.

Van Niekerk, C.H. and Morgenthal, J.C. (1982). Fetal loss and the effect of stress on plasma progestagen levels in pregnant thoroughbred mares. *Journal of Reproduction and Fertility. Supplement* 32: 453–357.

Vigani, A. and Garcia-Pereira, F.L. (2014). Anesthesia and analgesia for standing equine surgery. *Veterinary Clinics of North America. Equine Practice* 30: 1–17.

Walker, A.F. (2007). Sublingual administration of buprenorphine for long-term analgesia in the horse. *Veterinary Record* 160: 808–809.

Wong, D.M., Davis, J.L., and White, N.A. (2011). Motility of the equine gastrointestinal tract: physiology and pharmacotherapy. *Equine Veterinary Education* 23: 88–100.

Self-test Section

1 True or False? The features of co-administration of vatinoxan (MK-467) with an α2 agonist in horses include:

   A Lowered head position

   B Bradyarrhythmias

   C Reduced gut motility

   D Analgesia

2 True or False? Paraphimosis:

   A May occur after acepromazine administration in stallions

   B Never occurs after acepromazine administration in geldings

   C May occur after reserpine administration in stallions

   D May result in the need to perform distal phallectomy

29

Equine Heart Murmurs

29.1 Physiological/Functional/Flow Murmurs

Tend to become more intense after mild exercise and generally localise over the aortic and pulmonic valves. Usually systolic, grades I to II; soft and blowy sounds, although can be 'clicks'.

Haemic murmurs associated with anaemia are due to reduced blood viscosity and increased turbulence of blood flow.

In hypovolaemic states (e.g. colics), the heart is less 'full' so the valve rings become distorted, so that murmurs become more likely. The situation may also be compounded by a high heart rate, a hyperdynamic circulation, and a change in blood viscosity if packed cell volume and/or total protein increase.

29.2 Young Racehorses in Training

Tricuspid and mitral regurgitation are common systolic murmurs. The heart hypertrophies with exercise, but valve leaflets cannot grow, so the valves become leaky as the valve rings (annuli) 'stretch'. Tend to be low grade but can affect performance if severe.

29.3 Aortic Regurgitation

Middle-aged to older animals. Diastolic murmur over aortic region, but also a systolic murmur may be heard over the mitral region. The left ventricle becomes volume-overloaded (due to the aortic regurgitation), and so hypertrophies (eccentrically, so the chamber dilates), leading to secondary mitral valve regurgitation. The condition will progress, but the time course of deterioration is difficult to predict. Affected horses, however, are prone to developing arrhythmias.

Bounding pulses are a feature of aortic regurgitation. Back-flow of blood from the aorta into the left ventricle augments left ventricular volume for the next ejection phase. The leaky aortic valve, however, facilitates a rapid fall in arterial pressure. This means that the pulses are easy to feel because the pulse pressure (systolic pressure minus diastolic pressure) is larger than 'normal'.

29.4 Mitral Regurgitation

Systolic murmur over mitral valve region. May be secondary to endocardiosis-type ageing changes or to bacterial endocarditis. Ruptured chordae tendineae also result in a murmur of mitral insufficiency.

A systolic murmur may also be heard over the tricuspid valve region as tricuspid regurgitation can develop secondary to pressure-overload of the right heart. (Mitral insufficiency results in volume overload of the left ventricle, which, in turn, increases back pressure on the pulmonary circulation.)

29.5 Tricuspid Regurgitation

Systolic murmur over tricuspid valve region. If not physiologic (i.e. racehorses), may be secondary to mitral regurgitation (see above) or to other causes of pulmonary hypertension such as chronic respiratory disease. Check for atrial fibrillation as right atrial enlargement can develop secondary to volume overload and predisposes to atrial fibrillation. Differentiate from ventricular septal defects (see below).

Veterinary Anaesthesia: Principles to Practice, Second Edition. Alexandra H. A. Dugdale, Georgina Beaumont, Carl Bradbrook, and Matthew Gurney.
© 2020 John Wiley & Sons Ltd. Published 2020 by John Wiley & Sons Ltd.
Companion website: www.wiley.com/go/dugdale/veterinary-anaesthesia

29.6 Ventricular Septal Defects

Pansystolic murmur. Common congenital defect, especially small pony breeds (e.g. Welsh section A and Shetlands). Often located in the membranous portion of the interventricular septum, just beneath the tricuspid valve, so that the murmur is loudest over the tricuspid valve area on the right side. A systolic ejection murmur is also heard over the pulmonic valve, usually one grade softer than the murmur over the tricuspid valve. (Left to right shunting of blood through a ventricular septal defect causes the loudest sounds to be heard over the tricuspid valve area. The slightly softer murmur over the pulmonic valve area is due to the increased volume of blood passing through a 'normal' pulmonic valve, which represents a 'relative' pulmonic stenosis.)

Further Reading

Jago, R. and Keen, J. (2017). Identification of common equine cardiac murmurs. *In Practice* 39: 222–232.

30

Equine Anaesthesia

LEARNING OBJECTIVES

- To be able to discuss possible reasons for the relatively high risk of anaesthesia for Equidae.
- To be familiar with the available drugs and techniques.

30.1 Introduction

The risks of morbidity or mortality associated with general anaesthesia in the horse are far greater than those for dogs and cats, although not too dissimilar to those for rabbits. The peri-anaesthetic mortality rate for elective procedures in horses is most frequently published at around 1 in 100–1 in 200. The peri-operative mortality rate for compromised and emergency cases is even worse at around 1–2 in 10.

30.2 Factors Influencing Anaesthetic Risks

Factors (other than emergencies or colic) that may influence the risks associated with anaesthesia in the horse are listed below. Their consideration is important in helping us to both inform owners and also to take steps to minimise them where possible.

30.2.1 Size

Size really does matter and it is important to accurately measure or estimate the body mass of patients where possible. Size not only influences how easily the horse can be handled before, during, and after anaesthesia, but also affects the risks associated with anaesthetic recovery. A larger horse suffering from ataxia or having a bad recovery has more momentum and is more likely to injure itself. Larger horses are thought to be at more risk from post-operative myopathy/neuropathy syndrome (but this may be more related to breed; see later).

Large horses also appear more susceptible to developing hypoxaemia and large alveolar–arterial (A-a) oxygen tension differences, especially with dorsal recumbency that promotes the development of compression atelectasis. Other factors, however, including reabsorption atelectasis (from the use of high inspired oxygen concentrations), hypoventilation, and hypotension (including poor pulmonary perfusion) likely also contribute to ventilation–perfusion mismatches and the resultant hypoxaemia.

Size is obviously related to breed, but obesity, regardless of the underlying frame size, may also complicate not only the choice of drug doses, but also the course of a general anaesthetic (See Chapter 40).

30.2.2 Breed

There are certain breeds of horses and ponies that may be at greater anaesthetic risk. Draught breeds, at least when immature, appear to be at increased risk of developing spinal cord malacia; and draught types are prone to equine polysaccharide storage myopathy (EPSM), which may not become apparent until post-anaesthetic myopathy develops during recovery from anaesthesia. Quarter horses may suffer from hyperkalaemic periodic paralysis (HYPP), which may cause problems pre-, intra- and post-operatively. Welsh mountain ponies are about 20 times more likely than other breeds to suffer from congenital heart abnormalities such as ventricular septal defects (VSD) or tetralogy of Fallot, whereas large horses are more prone to developing atrial fibrillation and also laryngeal paralysis.

Within some breeds, certain types of horse may be at greater risk, e.g. the fit Thoroughbred that has fractured a

Veterinary Anaesthesia: Principles to Practice, Second Edition. Alexandra H. A. Dugdale, Georgina Beaumont, Carl Bradbrook, and Matthew Gurney.
© 2020 John Wiley & Sons Ltd. Published 2020 by John Wiley & Sons Ltd.
Companion website: www.wiley.com/go/dugdale/veterinary-anaesthesia

leg on the racecourse is probably one of the greatest challenges to the equine anaesthetist due to the temperament, fitness, and high levels of circulating catecholamines.

30.2.3 Temperament

A horse's best means of defence is to run away from any threat. This means that many horses are 'flighty' or nervous in strange circumstances and tend to have a lot of circulating catecholamines, which are not good for anaesthesia. During recovery from anaesthesia, some horses may try to stand (to run away) too soon after regaining consciousness as they may 'feel safer' on their feet. Some horses may respond to fear by barging, biting, or kicking, and can be a danger to personnel. Horses in pain may be difficult to handle too.

30.2.4 Sex

Sex is important as it not only relates to temperament (stallions, mares), but also to some specific risks associated with anaesthesia. For example, the use of acepromazine is contra-indicated in breeding stallions as there is a small risk of priapism (sustained penile erection) or paraphimosis (inability to retract the penis following paralysis of the retractor muscles). In mares, the use of α2 agonists is not recommended in the last trimester of pregnancy. (See Chapters 4 and 28.) Care is needed in anaesthetising heavily pregnant mares as the gravid uterus may impede venous return from the caudal vena cava in dorsal recumbency, and most anaesthetic agents cross the placenta (see Chapter 39).

30.2.5 Age

Young animals have an increased anaesthetic risk because of immature physiology and metabolism (see section on foal anaesthesia and Chapter 37). Old horses may suffer from concurrent medical problems such as liver disease (e.g. chronic ragwort toxicity), osteoarthritis and/or osteoporosis (which may impact induction and recovery quality), and pituitary pars intermedia dysfunction (equine Cushing's disease). How much these conditions increase the risk of anaesthesia is unclear.

30.2.6 Surgical Time

Anaesthetic durations of more than two hours are associated with a marked increase in risk of peri-operative morbidity/mortality. Every attempt should therefore be made to reduce anaesthesia time (i.e. clip surgery site before anaesthetic induction, complete surgery as swiftly as possible).

30.2.7 Time of Day of the Procedure

Due to the nature of equine veterinary work, a significant number of anaesthetics occur 'out-of-hours'. There is both veterinary and medical evidence that 'out-of-hours' anaesthesia carries more risk than at other times, even in patients that are not compromised. The reasons for this seem to centre around adverse human factors at the circadian nadir (e.g. reduced vigilance, cognitive function, and psychomotor skills), compounded by chronic sleep deprivation, circadian rhythm disturbance, and fatigue that accompany typical veterinary working hours. Furthermore, the patient is at its own circadian nadir overnight and suffers interruption of its normal circadian rhythmicity, especially with respect to the normal sleep–wake and food intake patterns.

30.2.8 Anaesthetic Agents?

In most studies on peri-operative equine fatalities, there have been no widely-used anaesthetic agents where their specific use has been significantly associated with an increased risk of anaesthesia. However, lack of premedication/sedation before anaesthesia has been associated with an increased risk, whereas premedication with acepromazine markedly decreased the risk. Possible reasons include the purported anti-arrhythmic effects of acepromazine through: blocking cardiac α1 adrenergic receptors; reducing catecholamine release (due to its sedative effects); and preventing the sensitisation of cardiomyocytes to catecholamines caused by, e.g. halothane. Acepromazine therefore reduces the chances of catecholamine-induced arrhythmias (e.g. secondary to hypercapnia or inadequate anaesthetic depth). The vasodilation that results from its use may also be protective of tissue perfusion, i.e. cardiac output is better maintained when acepromazine is co-administered with α2 agonists (specifically romifidine), despite the accompanying reduction in arterial blood pressure. Although its combination with α2 agonists (specifically romifidine) has been shown to improve PaO_2 (via improved pulmonary perfusion and better ventilation-perfusion matching), the reduction in haematocrit that it causes may offset this potential for improved tissue oxygen delivery.

30.2.9 Health Status

One of the most important influences on risk associated with general anaesthesia, and not just in horses, is the metabolic and physiological state of the patient. The ASA classification system is described in Chapter 2. Pre-anaesthetic assessment is vitally important. Following thorough history-taking, a full clinical examination should be performed, with particular focus on the cardiovascular and respiratory systems. The reproductive state of the animal may well influence choices as may the state of its musculoskeletal system.

30.3 Preparation for Anaesthesia

As stated above, all animals that undergo elective anaesthesia should be given a full pre-anaesthetic assessment. If that assessment highlights any areas for concern, then those areas should be investigated before the animal undergoes anaesthesia (e.g. blood tests, imaging etc.). (Although there is much debate about the usefulness of pre-operative blood tests for outwardly healthy animals, a minimum database [e.g. packed cell volume, total plasma protein and perhaps some other biochemistry analytes], may be useful.)

The animal's weight should also be measured (e.g. weigh-bridge) or estimated (e.g. weight-tape) as accurately as possible, and its body condition score should be assessed.

30.3.1 Assessment for Pain

A number of pain assessment tools have become available for horses, some suited more to orthopaedic pain and others to visceral pain, and several have been validated to at least some degree. As yet, no universal pain scale has been agreed although a composite of some of the behavioural changes alongside facial grimace signs might be a way forward as proposed by one equine hospital in 2016.

30.3.2 Food Restriction

Horses cannot vomit, but reflux/regurgitation of predominantly liquid gastric contents can occur (visible at the nares) where intestinal obstruction is present, and warrants special consideration before, and at the time of, anaesthetic induction and during endotracheal intubation, and later, at the time of tracheal extubation. Restriction of feeding before equine anaesthesia is, therefore, not primarily aimed at reduction of vomiting/reflux/regurgitation and the possibly consequent pulmonary aspiration. Pre-operative food withholding has, instead, been traditionally suggested to reduce diaphragmatic 'splinting' and vena caval compression by an otherwise full stomach/intestine during recumbency (particularly dorsal recumbency), with the hope of better preserving pulmonary functional residual capacity (FRC) (and alveolar ventilation), and also venous return (and therefore cardiac output). The overall hope is that alveolar ventilation-perfusion matching is better maintained to prevent hypoxaemia or at least to reduce its severity. Withholding of food for at least 18 hours is,

however, required to reduce gut fill significantly, and, even then, recumbency itself appears to have the most detrimental effect on FRC. Indeed, only minimal (and non-significant) differences were found in PaO_2 when horses were deprived of concentrates for 17 hours before anaesthesia (compared to 4 hours) or hay for 11 hours pre-anaesthesia (compared with 1 hour).

Revision of human guidelines with respect to food and liquid withholding before anaesthesia, and the importance of prehabilitation, have led to the veterinary community reconsidering its stance too. An open discussion at the Association of Veterinary Anaesthetists' meeting in March 2019 failed to reach consensus regarding the duration of pre-operative food restriction for mature animals. Questions remained about the type of food: whether forage (and then whether fresh, dry-conserved, or ensiled), and/or concentrates, are equally important to consider, and whether prior large, intermittent meals or ad-lib access to food, require different strategies. Opinions seemed to be that recent access to large quantities of concentrates or fresh forage (grass and particularly the legume Lucerne) may predispose to large intestinal tympany, and, in the case of fresh forages, also increase gut bulk. On the other hand, where horses have ad lib access to pasture, hay, or haylage, then minimal restriction before premedication may be appropriate, despite these fibre sources usually being accompanied by, or encouraging, large volumes of water intake, and therefore increased GI bulk. The type of surgery also warrants consideration, e.g. laparoscopy (whether to be performed in standing [sedated] or recumbent [anaesthetised], horses) may necessitate reduced gut fill to facilitate surgical access, for which horses may require feed restriction for two to three days.

It was agreed that the impact of pre-operative food withholding strategies upon the occurrence of post-anaesthetic colic is hard to disentangle from the effects of: pre-operative management changes (including transport to the surgery); pre-operative sedation/s for surgical planning purposes, which also include periods of food and water withhold/reduced access; the anaesthetic and surgery itself (with incurred stress response and inflammatory response); the administration of antimicrobial drugs; post-operative pain (and its management); and management practices surrounding the post-operative re-introduction of food. It was, however, acknowledged that changes in husbandry (including feeding practices) are well-known triggers of colic episodes.

It was generally agreed that **access to clean, fresh water should be allowed up until the time of premedication**. Until conclusive evidence becomes available, for elective cases, **restricting access to concentrates and large meals of forages for around four to six hours prior to**

premedication might be a prudent starting point to limit gut fill and the development of tympany so as to limit increases in intra-abdominal pressure. Ideally, non-edible bedding (e.g. shavings or shredded paper) should be used to reduce the chances of a hungry horse then eating its bedding. Although muzzles may be used, some horses struggle to drink through them and their use pre-operatively has resulted in post-anaesthetic colic, most likely secondary to large intestinal impactions because of dehydration. **For animals that are grazing or have truly ad lib access to conserved or ensiled forages, then it is hard to justify any restriction of such access.** If, however, access to food is allowed right up until the time of premedication, the mouth must be washed out thoroughly, especially if an endotracheal tube is to be placed, because 'dirty mouths' were commonly reported with this strategy. Therefore, **potentially restricting access to these kinds of feed for one to two hours prior to anaesthesia** might address this problem whilst mitigating against the detrimental effects (physiological, biochemical, endocrine, behavioural, and welfare) of restricting food intake. Again, attention should be paid to providing non-edible bedding materials.

30.3.3 Re-perform Basic Clinical Examination Immediately Prior to Surgery

If the patient was admitted to the hospital the day prior to surgery, it should be re-examined on the day of surgery (basic clinical examination including temperature, pulse rate/quality and respiratory frequency), to make sure that it has not developed any problems that may influence anaesthesia such as respiratory infection (from mild viraemia to shipping fever).

30.3.4 Vascular Access Should Be Secured

Before any horse or pony is anaesthetised, a wide-bore cannula should be placed and secured, e.g. in a jugular vein. This is usually done around the time of premedication.

30.3.5 Theatre Head Collar/Tail Bandage

A leather padded head collar is used for aiding control of the horse at anaesthetic induction.

- Leather is less likely than nylon-webbing to cause trauma, such as friction burns, if pulled tight against the horse's skin.
- The padding is to protect superficial nerves near bony prominences from the metal rings in the head collar.
- A soft cotton rope is then attached to the head collar as this is less likely to cause friction burns to the handler's skin if pulled rapidly through his or her hands.

- A tail bandage should be placed to reduce contamination of theatre and to prevent long tails tripping up the horse during recovery from anaesthesia.

30.3.6 Shoe Removal/Surgery Clip

Ideally all shoes are removed before induction of anaesthesia and any sharp hoof should be rasped smooth. This is for horse and handler safety, and to protect induction box flooring. Removing shoes before anaesthetic induction may not be possible, but shoe removal after induction increases anaesthesia time. For the same reason, it is helpful if the surgery site is clipped before anaesthetic induction, however, some horses do not tolerate clippers very well.

30.3.7 Mouth Wash

The mouth should be washed out with water using either a hose or a large dosing syringe. This is to remove as much food material that may have aggregated there as possible. Otherwise when the endotracheal (ET) tube is passed 'blindly', any remaining food material may be 'collected' by the tube and passed down into the trachea. Particular attention should be paid to the space between the cheeks and the cheek-teeth, but food can also be accumulated at the back of the mouth.

30.3.8 Personal Protective Equipment

In the light of recent reminders that equine veterinarians are amongst those most likely to suffer injuries at work, sturdy shoes, gloves, a hard hat, and perhaps even a body protector should be considered.

30.3.9 Pre-Anaesthetic Medications

In many cases, antibiotics and/or non-steroidal anti-inflammatory drugs (NSAIDs) may need to be administered before anaesthesia.

- Sodium penicillin (Crystapen™) can cause hypotension and bradyarrhythmias, and so should be administered slowly and ideally at least 20 minutes before anaesthetic induction so that any haemodynamic effects will have subsided by this time. It also tends to cause horses/ponies to pass watery-ish droppings within 10 minutes of administration; it is preferable to avoid contamination of the induction/recovery box environment with this material. Its use has also been associated with an increased incidence of post-anaesthetic colic.
- Intravenous trimethoprim-potentiated sulphonamides (TMPS) can cause fatal arrhythmias if administered around the same time as intravenous detomidine. (Some

operators are similarly cautious about the administration of other α2 agonists.)

- Many NSAIDs are not licenced for pre-operative use.

30.4 Premedication/Sedation

See Chapter 28 on equine premedication/sedation. When using α2 agonists and opioids for premedication, the α2 agonist should be given first and sedation allowed to develop (e.g. wait five minutes) before the opioid is administered. This reduces the locomotor stimulatory effects of the opioid, which is particularly noticeable with butorphanol. Some operators prefer to give the opioid after anaesthetic induction.

This author also favours the administration of acepromazine, as long as no contra-indications exist, at least 30–45 minutes before administration of α2 agonists and opioids. Acepromazine *may* also reduce the locomotor stimulation side effects of opioids.

30.5 Induction of Anaesthesia

During induction of general anaesthesia, the horse/pony must undergo the transition from a (usually) standing position to recumbency as safely as possible. A safe induction area should be sought, whether this is a field (beware steep gradients, hard or stony ground, barbed-wire fences and nearby roads, watercourses or pools), padded induction box, squeeze-gated padded induction area, or padded tilt-table. You are responsible for the safety of the horse and any people helping you.

Although the chosen anaesthetic induction agent may influence the quality of induction, the biggest influence is to have a calm, and, preferably well-sedated, patient. Handling techniques range from 'free-fall', through manual assistance, through using a swinging padded door/gate as a 'squeeze-gate', to slings and tilt-tables. The choice of technique is manly determined by familiarity and availability.

30.5.1 Induction Agents

See Chapters 5 and 8, and also the section on foals later. For adult animals, injectable anaesthetic agents are usually preferred, whereas inhalation techniques may be chosen for some foals. For standing animals, injectable agents are usually administered in boluses of estimated doses because it is not possible to titrate them IV slowly to effect, unlike the situation in small animals. Because of this, small, relative 'overdoses' are commonly administered, but are usually well tolerated. It is always advisable to have at least one spare top-up dose of the appropriate injectable agent

available, and may be an alternative agent too. At the moment, there are few licenced intravenous induction agents that may be used in horses. Most animals are premedicated before induction (see Chapter 28).

30.5.1.1 Ketamine

Ketamine is a dissociative anaesthetic agent. It has excitatory and inhibitory effects on different parts of the CNS (see Chapter 5 on induction agents and Chapter 3 on pain). The simplest way to think of it is that it 'disconnects' consciousness from sensory inputs. Although it rapidly crosses the blood–brain barrier to reach its effect site (thought to be mainly NMDA receptors), its actions at these receptors are not immediately obvious such that induction of dissociative anaesthesia can take up to two minutes.

Ketamine became a schedule 2 controlled drug on 30 Nov 2015 in UK, so a controlled drugs register detailing its acquisition, use, and disposal is a legal requirement. It must also be stored in a lockable cabinet.

Before ketamine is administered for induction of anaesthesia, adequate sedation must be achieved, otherwise the smoothness of induction will be compromised. Therefore α2 agonist-based premedication is best. To test the adequacy of sedation, some workers tap the forehead of the animal to check its response – which should be 'minimal arousal'. Aceopromazine/opioid combinations usually produce insufficient sedation for guaranteed, smooth anaesthetic induction with ketamine (at the 'usual' doses).

30.5.1.1.1 Clinical Use

Dose: 2–3 mg/kg IV is commonly quoted, **following profound sedation** (α2 agonist-based), but the injectate volume is then rounded up to the nearest whole ml or two for most animals >100 kg. Ketamine has a wide safety margin, so small overdoses are well tolerated. Adjuncts include:-

- Diazepam or midazolam (at around 0.02–0.05 mg/kg IV) is commonly included (just before or with the ketamine) to reduce the increased muscle tone associated with ketamine and to provide better conditions for tracheal intubation and surgery.
- Guaiphenesin (GG) (infusion, around 30–100 mg/kg IV) can be used as an alternative centrally-acting skeletal muscle relaxant to the benzodiazepines, just before the ketamine. Irritant to tissues if extravascular or transvascular deposition occurs. It is usually administered by infusion to effect and produces mild sedation at higher doses. Similar to the benzodiazepines, it produces minimal cardiovascular depression, but does not allow (much) reduction of ketamine induction doses because of ketamine's unique dissociative action. The ketamine dose may be able to be reduced to around 1.7 mg/kg, but most people prefer to administer 2–3 mg/kg to ensure anaesthetic induction.

When ketamine is administered as a bolus (with or without prior benzodiazepine or GG), anaesthetic induction usually follows within 60–120 seconds. Induction is usually characterised by the horse 'crumpling'/sinking to the ground gently by flexing all 4 limbs. Occasionally, however, a horse may dog-sit and off-balance itself when its head tilts up, or it may stumble forwards if the hindlimbs fail to flex. For these reasons, if holding the horse for anaesthetic induction, it is advisable to try to keep the head low/prevent it from lifting too high, and steady the shoulder once the horse starts to sink. Beware your own feet and face as these are likely to be in close proximity to moving parts of the horse.

Characteristics of ketamine-based anaesthetic inductions:

- Post-induction apnoea may follow (up to 120 seconds). Irregular and/or apneustic breathing patterns may also be observed.
- Minimal CV depression; even slight stimulation. Ketamine's direct negative inotropic and vasodilative effects are offset by the sympathetic stimulation it causes. However, hypovolaemic animals with already high sympathetic tone may not have much sympathetic reserve and so mild cardiovascular depression may occur. (Premedication drugs may also affect the haemodynamic consequences of ketamine given for anaesthetic induction.)
- Cranial nerve reflexes are maintained. If swallowing and laryngeal closure cause problematic tracheal intubation, a small dose of thiopental or further small doses of α2 agonists or benzodiazepines may be helpful.
- The duration of anaesthesia following one induction dose of ketamine is around 10–20 minutes. During this time, anaesthetic maintenance by whatever means (injectable or inhalation) should be initiated.
- May be metabolised to norketamine, which has about ¼ the activity of the parent drug (and may be responsible for some dysphoria), but can be further metabolised to inactive compounds. Otherwise, ketamine can be excreted unchanged in the urine. Multiple doses are cumulative and the effects are complicated by the production of norketamine.
- Although ketamine provides excellent somatic analgesia, multimodal analgesic strategies are encouraged.
- Can increase intracranial and intra-ocular pressure, so beware in cases where these are likely to cause problems and be aware of other factors affecting these intracompartmental pressures.

At this present time, no other licenced injectable agents are readily available in UK, although a veterinary licenced version of thiopental can be imported from Australia under a Special Treatment Certificate from the Veterinary Medicines Directorate.

A typical protocol employing ketamine for anaesthetic induction would be:

0.02 mg/kg acepromazine (IM or IV), wait 30 minutes
60–80 μg/kg romifidine IV, wait 5 minutes
0.2 mg/kg morphine IV, wait 5 minutes
c. 2.5 mg/kg ketamine ($\pm$0.05 mg/kg diazepam) IV as a bolus

30.5.1.2 Thiopental

Thiopental is an ultra-short-acting intravenous barbiturate anaesthetic agent. At body pH, because of tautomerism, it rapidly undergoes keto-enol transformation so that there is increased availability of the fat-soluble keto tautomer, which rapidly crosses the blood–brain barrier to reach its effect site (the $GABA_A$ receptor). It is very irritant to tissues if accidental extravascular deposition occurs. Therefore, pre-placement of an IV cannula is strongly advised and this should be checked to ensure it is still correctly positioned in the vein and patent.

30.5.1.2.1 Clinical Use

Dose: 3–5 mg/kg IV following profound sedation (α2 agonist-based); **up to 5–10 mg/kg** following acepromazine-based premedication; and up to 25 mg/kg if no premedication.

- Diazepam or midazolam (at around 0.05 mg/kg IV) may be administered as co-induction agents and help to reduce the required dose of thiopental a little, if minimal premedication is given.
- Guaiphenesin (infusion, around 30–100 mg/kg IV) can be used as an alternative centrally-acting muscle relaxant to the benzodiazepines. Irritant to tissues if extravascular or transvascular deposition occurs. It is usually administered by infusion to effect (just before the thiopental is given), and produces mild sedation at higher doses. Similar to the benzodiazepines, it produces minimal cardiovascular depression and allows reduction of the thiopental induction dose if minimal other premedication is given.

When thiopental is administered as a bolus (with or without prior benzodiazepine or GG), anaesthetic induction should follow within 30–60 seconds and is often preceded by a deep breath/sigh. Anaesthetic induction is usually characterised by the horse suddenly collapsing to the ground like a felled tree, following a deep sigh – rather inelegant and inco-ordinated compared to ketamine inductions. Expect the unexpected if you are the handler!

Characteristics of thiopental-based anaesthetic inductions:

- Post-induction apnoea may follow, but usually not quite as long as after ketamine (may be up to 60 seconds), although partly depends upon the dose administered.
- Cardiovascular depression is usually mild. Hypotension can be more profound in previously hypovolaemic patients. Arrhythmias may occur (thiopental sensitises

the myocardium to the arrhythmogenic effects of catecholamines). (Premedication drugs may also affect the haemodynamic consequences of thiopental given for anaesthetic induction.)

- Cranial nerve reflexes are lost. Tracheal intubation conditions should be good.
- The duration of anaesthesia following one induction dose is around 20–30 minutes (depends upon the dose given and premedication too). During this time, anaesthetic maintenance by whatever means (injectable or inhalation) should be initiated.
- Thiopental provides no analgesia.
- Slow metabolism means that redistribution is important for return of consciousness. Thin animals with poor muscling and little body fat have a reduced sink for thiopental's redistribution, so recovery is prolonged. Large doses can also 'fill' redistribution depots and also delay recovery.

Typical protocols employing thiopental for anaesthetic induction would be:

0.05 mg/kg acepromazine IM or IV, wait 30 minutes
0.2 mg/kg morphine IV, wait 5 minutes
10 mg/kg thiopental IV bolus
OR
60–80 μg/kg romifidine IV, wait 5 minutes
0.2 mg/kg morphine IV, wait 5 minutes
5 mg/kg thiopental IV bolus

30.5.1.3 Propofol

Propofol is a substituted phenol and produces unconsciousness by interaction with GABA$_A$ receptors in the CNS. It undergoes very rapid metabolism, with sites other than the liver facilitating this; it must, therefore, be given IV to be effective. It is not yet licenced for use in equidae and the large volumes required can be expensive. The quality of anaesthetic induction is not always good, especially if premedication is not provided. Recovery quality is not always as good as hoped either, but many factors influence this, with horse temperament perhaps being the biggest.

30.5.1.3.1 Clinical Use

Dose: 2–5 mg/kg following premedication (lower end of this range after α2 agonist-based premedication; higher end following acepromazine based premedication). Although it can be administered without premedication, larger doses are required and it can be expensive.

- There is one description of propofol (0.5 mg/kg) administration simultaneously with GG (100 mg/kg) in horses [following detomidine premedication], and another of 90 mg/kg GG followed by 3 mg/kg propofol.
- There are no reports of propofol administration following benzodiazepines in horses.

When propofol is administered as a bolus, anaesthetic induction should follow within 30–90 seconds.

Characteristics of propofol-based anaesthetic inductions:

- Induction quality is similar to that following thiopental.
- Post-induction apnoea is common and often lasts up to 120 seconds or longer (depends upon dose and possibly speed of injection). Marked respiratory depression can be a problem when propofol is administered by infusion for maintenance of anaesthesia.
- Cardiovascular depression is slightly more profound than following thiopental. Hypotension can be even more profound in previously hypovolaemic patients. (Premedication drugs may also affect the haemodynamic consequences of propofol used for anaesthetic induction.)
- Cranial nerve reflexes are lost. Tracheal intubation conditions should be good.
- The duration of anaesthesia following one induction dose is around 20–30 minutes (depends upon the dose administered and premedication too). During this time, anaesthetic maintenance by whatever means (injectable or inhalation) should be initiated.
- Propofol provides insignificant analgesia.
- Rapid metabolism theoretically facilitates good quality recoveries, but this is not always the case as recovery quality is determined by other factors too.

30.5.1.4 Alfaxalone

Alfaxalone is a neuroactive steroid presented in aqueous solution thanks to a novel cyclodextrin formulation, and is unique in that it is closely related to endogenous progesterone compounds (e.g. allopregnanolone), which themselves have hypnotic effects. Like thiopental, it has a dual action at GABA$_A$ receptors, being a positive allosteric modulator at low doses yet providing direct GABA$_A$ agonism at higher doses.

30.5.1.4.1 Clinical Use

Not yet licenced for use in horses, but reports have been published.

Dose c. 1 mg/kg IV, following good sedation with α2 agonists.

- Diazepam or midazolam (at around 0.02–0.05 mg/kg IV) may be included to reduce the increased muscle tone associated with alfaxalone and to provide better conditions for tracheal intubation and surgery.
- One study reported xylazine (0.5 mg/kg) and GG (35 mg/kg) premedication followed by 1 mg/kg alfaxalone induction. Induction quality was similar to xylazine/GG premedication followed by ketamine (2.2 mg/kg) induction, but more muscle tremors were seen after alfaxalone.
- One study compared anaesthetic induction with 1 mg/kg alfaxalone combined with 0.02 mg/kg diazepam against

2.2 mg/kg ketamine with 0.02 mg/kg diazepam, both after premedication with 100 µg/kg romifidine and 0.05 mg/kg butorphanol. Induction was slightly quicker after alfaxalone, but induction quality was good for both protocols. Top-up doses (0.2 mg/kg alfaxalone or 0.5 mg/kg ketamine) were administered as necessary in order to complete the castration; more horses needed alfaxalone top-ups than ketamine top-ups. Recovery quality was good in both groups, but ever so slightly less good after alfaxalone.

- A further study evaluated anaesthesia for castration with the following protocol: premedication with 100 µg/kg romifidine and 0.05 mg/kg butorphanol followed by anaesthetic induction with alfaxalone 1 mg/kg and diazepam 0.02 mg/kg, and anaesthetic maintenance with top-ups of 0.2 mg/kg alfaxalone as required. Anaesthetic time could be extended as necessary. Induction and recovery quality were good.
- One study compared 1 mg/kg with 2 mg/kg alfaxalone following premedication with 6 µg/kg medetomidine and 0.02 mg/kg midazolam. Induction and recovery qualities were good in both groups, but recovery was prolonged in the 2 mg/kg dose group, and more severe respiratory depression at the greater dose suggested that oxygen supplementation should be provided, especially when larger doses are used.
- One study evaluated anaesthetic induction with 35 mg/kg GG and 2 mg/kg alfaxalone following premedication with 0.03 mg/kg acepromazine and 7 µg/kg medetomidine. A similar study evaluated anaesthetic induction with 1 mg/kg alfaxalone following premedication with 7 µg/kg medetomidine, 0.025 mg/kg butorphanol, and 0.05 mg/kg midazolam. Both reported good induction qualities and anaesthetic was continued with infusions of alfaxalone alongside other agents (see later).
- A recent study evaluated anaesthetic induction with 35 mg/kg GG and 1 mg/kg alfaxalone following premedication with 0.03 mg/kg acepromazine and 1 mg/kg xylazine. Anaesthetic induction quality was good, and anaesthesia was continued with infusion of alfaxalone to effect (see later).

When alfaxalone is administered as a bolus (following suitable premedication and possibly after benzodiazepine or GG administration), anaesthetic induction follows within 60–90 seconds (this author's experience), although other authors report induction times of 20–35 seconds. Differing effects of premedication on haemodynamics may help to explain these differences.

Characteristics of alfaxalone-based anaesthetic inductions:

- Post-induction apnoea may follow (respiratory depression is dose-dependent).
- Mild cardiovascular depression. (Premedication drugs may also affect this.)

- Cranial nerve reflexes are abolished so tracheal intubation conditions should be good, but if muscle relaxation is poor following premedication and if benzodiazepines or GG are omitted, muscle tone, including jaw tone, may be increased, making placement of a gag prior to tracheal intubation somewhat troublesome.
- The duration of anaesthesia following one induction dose is around 10–20 minutes (but abrupt earlier recovery/movement is possible). Should anaesthetic time need to be prolonged, then anaesthetic maintenance by whatever means (injectable or inhalation) should be initiated as soon as possible after induction.
- Rapid metabolism theoretically facilitates good quality recoveries, but this is not always the case as recovery quality is determined by other factors/drugs too. In one study of field castrations, recoveries following alfaxalone were not quite as good as following ketamine.
- Not analgesic.

30.5.1.5 Guaiphenesin

Also known as guaifenesin, glyceryl guaiacolate ether (GGE), or glyceryl guaiacolate (GG); a propanediol derivative from wood tar.

- A centrally-acting skeletal muscle relaxant, inhibiting the internuncial neuronal relay in the spinal cord, brainstem, and subcortical brain areas thereby producing postural muscle weakness primarily.
- Has some sedative properties, possibly due to actions in the reticular formation.
- Minimal cardiovascular depression (mild hypotension), but irritant to tissues if deposited extravascularly and to the vein if deposited transvascularly (e.g. upon withdrawal of the IV catheter, if this is not thoroughly flushed through first). Can cause thrombosis and haemolysis – somewhat dependent upon concentration of solution and species (See Chapter 17).
- Minimal respiratory depression at therapeutic doses.
- Available as a licenced product in UK (Myorelax™, a 10% solution). Both 10% and 15% solutions have variably been available from other European countries (which can be imported to the UK under Special Import Certificates, available from the Veterinary Medicines Directorate). These higher percentage solutions can be diluted down to 5% in dextrose-saline; but use of such diluted solutions constitutes 'off-licence' use. Solutions in excess of 10–12% can cause haemolysis, but, in horses, this is most significant with concentrations greater than 15% and if 'stabilisers' are excluded from the solution.
  - Excipients of commercially available solutions often include dextrose and N-methyl pyrrolidone, which is an industrial solvent (that has been used as a paint-stripper!)

and that can be irritant. Dextrose is included as a 'stabiliser' to try to help protect erythrocytes from osmotic damage and reduce haemolysis.

- **Dose: 30–100 mg/kg IV usually administered by infusion** until the 'second wobble'/hind-quarter sway occurs, at which point the horse can no longer resist the muscular relaxation. (At the 'first wobble', the horse usually drops it head and knuckles at the fetlocks, but then usually manages to strengthen its stance for a brief period until the second wobble.) Lethal dose is around 300 mg/kg. Doses >150 mg/kg produce some cardio-respiratory depression.
- GG is metabolised by the liver and the metabolites are excreted in the urine; one metabolite catechol (or a compound with cross-reactivity to catechol) appears to be responsible for some of the effects of large (>150 mg/kg) doses, e.g. paradoxical muscular twitches/rigidity and irregular/apneustic breathing (which can sometimes be mistakenly interpreted as the animal being under-dosed and too light). Pony stallions appeared to metabolise GG more slowly than mares, but there were no differences in dose requirements for recumbency.

30.5.2 Inhalation Agents

Inhalation agents may be used for induction of anaesthesia in well-sedated or obtunded foals. Administration by mask, naso-pharyngeal or naso-tracheal insufflation is possible. Pre-oxygenation facilitates inhalation induction. Try to perform the technique in as stress-free a way as possible. The CEPEF study suggested that induction of anaesthesia with inhalation agents was associated with higher morbidity/mortality than following injectable agents. This may have reflected the fact that this technique may have been reserved for the sickest animals. Also, halothane was the inhalation agent most commonly used at that time; and halothane sensitises the myocardium to the arrhythmogenic effects of catecholamines, so if the induction process was at all stressful, arrhythmias may have resulted and contributed to the observed mortality.

Sevoflurane, being less soluble in blood than isoflurane and halothane, should produce the most rapid induction of anaesthesia. Despite not being licenced, sevoflurane may, therefore, be favoured over isoflurane for inhalation induction of anaesthesia in foals. Neither isoflurane nor sevoflurane sensitise the myocardium to the arrhythmogenic effects of catecholamines, so would normally be favoured over halothane. All the volatile agents produce dose-dependent cardio-respiratory depression, but there are slight differences. Halothane is said to be least pungent and produces least respiratory depression, whereas isoflurane is usually blamed for producing the most respiratory depression, although sevoflurane may be just as bad as isoflurane or even worse. Foals, however, seem less affected by the respiratory depressant effects of volatile agents compared with mature horses, such that isoflurane or sevoflurane are both suitable. The cardiovascular depression that accompanies halothane anaesthesia is mostly due to direct negative inotropy, whereas following isoflurane and sevoflurane, vasodilation is the biggest cause of hypotension. Nevertheless, for a similar anaesthetic depth, halothane produces the most reduction in cardiac output, whilst sevoflurane produces the least (although isoflurane is very similar). None of the inhalation agents provides significant analgesia. Halothane is no longer commonly available and at the time of writing, only isoflurane is licenced for equine use, at least in the UK. Desflurane is not licenced for equine use although a few practices use it; it has even lower blood solubility than sevoflurane, and therefore anaesthetic depth change can be very quick. Its pungency, however, precludes its use for inhalation induction (particularly in humans, although some veterinary species may tolerate it better), although the more rapid recovery may, if well controlled by judicious use of sedation, facilitate 'better quality' recovery from equine anaesthesia. Desflurane also causes dose-dependent cardiorespiratory depression, but to a slightly lesser degree than sevoflurane and isoflurane at similar anaesthetic depths. (See Chapter 8.)

30.5.3 Post-induction Patient Care

After anaesthetic induction, it is important to:

- Ensure that vital signs are still present; patient monitoring should begin as soon as possible
- Place an endotracheal tube, if one is required/thought necessary
- Move the patient into the desired position and secure it there (if applicable)
- Protect the eyes from dirt, debris, and direct sunlight
- Initiate maintenance of anaesthesia by whichever technique is desired (if applicable)

30.5.4 Analgesia

For each patient, a multimodal (balanced) analgesic approach should be adopted, wherein analgesic drugs of several different classes may be used to target the pain pathway at several different sites in order to provide the best possible intra-operative anti-nociception and prevention/treatment of pre- and post-operative pain for the fewest possible overall side effects. α2 adrenoceptor agonists, opioids, and NSAIDs form common components of such an approach (see Chapters 3, 4, 6, and 28). Local/regional anaesthetic techniques should also be employed where possible (see Chapter 16).

Multimodal/balanced anaesthetic techniques similarly involve the use of several classes of drugs to produce the most desirable features of general anaesthesia (i.e. unconsciousness/hypnosis, muscle relaxation, antinociception/analgesia, and autonomic stability), whilst minimising their unwanted side effects. (Such techniques therefore necessarily incorporate multimodal analgesic techniques.) To this end, the intra-operative provision of further drugs providing sedative, hypnotic, muscle-relaxant, and analgesic effects for anaesthetic maintenance (beyond those provided by premedication, anaesthetic induction, and single-agent anaesthetic maintenance) has become popular (see below and Further Reading).

30.5.5 Maintenance of Anaesthesia

Anaesthesia can be maintained with inhalation and/or injectable agents. Local or regional anaesthesia/analgesia should be provided where possible and such techniques are often performed after premedication or once the patient is under general anaesthesia (See Chapter 16). During the maintenance period, intravenous fluid therapy is usually provided (see Chapter 23).

30.5.5.1 Inhalational Anaesthesia
- Requires expensive equipment
- Not easy to transport for use 'in the field'
- Endotracheal tube essential
- Ensures oxygen delivery
- Can provide positive pressure ventilation either manually or by using a large animal ventilator
- Depth of anaesthesia may be easier to alter than with injectable agents

See Chapter 8 on inhalational agents and Chapter 9 on breathing systems. Inhalational anaesthesia requires an anaesthetic breathing system. A large animal circle (LAC) or 'To-and fro' are the two main types available (although a small animal circle or a non-rebreathing system with a suitably sized reservoir bag can be used for foals). Anaesthetic breathing systems need to be maintained. Both the LAC and the 'To-and-fro' require carbon dioxide absorbent, which also needs to be changed when exhausted. Oxygen flow rates for horses on the LAC are around 1 l/100 kg, with the adjustable pressure limiting (APL) valve open. For horses, 'inhalation agents' usually means only the volatile agents as nitrous oxide may partition into insoluble-gas-filled spaces within the gut, causing an increase in their volume and/or pressure, which can have adverse consequences of its own.

30.5.5.2 Total Intravenous Anaesthesia (TIVA)
- Minimal equipment required
- Easy to do 'in the field'
- Does not, itself, deliver oxygen, but some anaesthetists ensure provision of supplemental oxygen by insufflation or demand valve (via nasopharyngeal or ET tube), to TIVA-anaesthetised horses.
- Depth of anaesthesia may not be so easy to alter (especially to 'lighten') quickly; once administered, the agents cannot be taken back
- Anaesthetic depth and provision of anti-nociception are potentially able to be addressed separately
- Drugs can be expensive
- Ventilatory support may be necessary

TIVA can be achieved in two main ways, by 'top-up' bolus injections or by continuous (drip) infusions. TIVA produces a much **diminished anaesthesia stress response** compared with inhalation anaesthesia, and is therefore often regarded as a physiologically superior method of anaesthesia. The main drawbacks are highlighted above. It is usually advised to limit the duration of TIVA techniques to no longer than about 90 minutes, if possible, because of the accumulation of injected drugs that can delay recovery and reduce its quality.

30.5.5.2.1 'Top-Up' TIVA
After induction of anaesthesia (usually with intravenous agents), anaesthesia is maintained by the intermittent bolus administration of injectable (IV) agents, either when the horse shows signs of becoming 'light' or at regular time intervals.

Ketamine
For example:

Premedication with acepromazine (0.02 mg/kg), followed, after 30–40 minutes by
Xylazine (1 mg/kg) and opioid, wait until adequate sedation, then
Anaesthetic induction with c. 2.5 mg/kg ketamine ($\pm$ 0.05 mg/kg diazepam), provides 10–15 minutes surgical anaesthesia
+
If necessary, for first top-up, give 1/3–1/2 induction dose of ketamine (i.e. 0.8–1.2 mg/kg ketamine)
And similar for xylazine (i.e. 0.3–0.5 mg/kg xylazine)
+
If necessary, for second and subsequent top-ups, give about 1/4–1/3 of original induction dose of ketamine (i.e. 0.6–0.8 mg/kg)
And similar for xylazine (i.e. 0.25–0.3 mg/kg)

If detomidine or romifidine were given for premedication, instead of xylazine, then because these are longer acting, they only require top-ups about every third to fifth ketamine top-up, respectively. Should medetomidine or dexmedetomidine be used, then top-ups with each ketamine top-up would be likely required as these both have short half-lives. An alternative strategy is to give only ketamine for the majority of top-ups, but to ensure that an α2 agonist is given alongside the ketamine at the very last top-up. (Recoveries from 'ketamine alone' are often of poor quality.)

Ketamine (± α2 agonist) can also be given 'by-the-clock' about every 10 minutes. For example:

Premedication with acepromazine (0.02 mg/kg),
followed, after 30–40 minutes by
Xylazine (1 mg/kg) and opioid, wait until adequate sedation, then
Anaesthetic induction with c. 2.5 mg/kg ketamine (± 0.05 mg/kg diazepam) provides 10–15 minutes surgical anaesthesia
+
After 10 minutes, give 1/3–1/2 induction dose of ketamine (i.e. 0.8–1.2 mg/kg ketamine)
And similar for xylazine (i.e. 0.3–0.5 mg/kg xylazine)
+
After each further 10 minutes, give about 1/4–1/3 of original induction dose of ketamine (i.e. 0.6–0.8 mg/kg)
And similar for xylazine (i.e. 0.25–0.3 mg/kg)

Again, ketamine can be administered without further α2 agonist for the first few doses (2–4, respectively), if detomidine or romifidine were given in the premed because these are longer acting. Some people prefer to only re-dose with a half-dose of α2 agonist at the 'last' ketamine top-up, or as recovery starts, so that the horse does not recover from ketamine alone, which can produce more excitable recoveries.

Recently, a comparison between anaesthetic induction with ketamine 2.2 mg/kg and ketamine 5 mg/kg (both with 0.03 mg/kg diazepam) following premedication with 0.05 mg/kg acepromazine, 0.7 mg/kg xylazine and 0.025 mg/kg butorphanol, for field castration, showed slightly superior surgical conditions with the higher dose of ketamine, with reduced requirements for further top-ups (0.25 mg/kg xylazine and 0.5 mg/kg ketamine), and with only very little deterioration in recovery quality.

Alfaxalone (Not Yet Licenced)

For example:

Premedication with acepromazine (0.02 mg/kg),
followed, after 30–40 minutes by
Xylazine (1 mg/kg) and opioid, wait until adequate sedation, then
Anaesthetic induction with c. 1 mg/kg alfaxalone (± 0.05 mg/kg diazepam) provides 10–15 minutes surgical anaesthesia
+

If necessary, for first top-up, give 1/3–1/2 induction dose of alfaxalone (i.e. 0.3–0.5 mg/kg alfaxalone)
And similar for xylazine (i.e. 0.3–0.5 mg/kg xylazine)
+
If necessary, for subsequent top-ups, give about 1/4–1/3 of original induction dose of alfaxalone (i.e. 0.25–0.3 mg/kg)
And similar for xylazine (i.e. 0.25–0.3 mg/kg)

If detomidine or romifidine are used for premedication, then they do not require such frequent top-ups because they are longer-acting. Should medetomidine or dexmedetomidine be used, then top-ups with each alfaxalone top-up would be likely required.

30.5.5.2.2 *Continuous Infusion TIVA*
Ketamine-GG-α2 Agonist 'triple-drip' After induction (normally achieved with injectable agents), anaesthesia is maintained with a combination of injectable agents, which, together, provide all the components of the 'triad' of anaesthesia.

The three components of the 'triple-drip' are:

- **Ketamine** to provide the analgesia and 'anaesthesia'.
- **GG (guaiphenesin)** to provide muscle relaxation (± some sedation).
- **α2 agonist** to provide sedation (counter any excitatory effects of ketamine), some analgesia, and muscle relaxation.

See Chapter 31 on field anaesthesia for recipes. Because there is normally a limited amount of anaesthesia time available (i.e. around 90 minutes) when using 'triple-drip' infusion, cases should be selected very carefully to ensure that the surgical procedure can be completed well within this time. Packing ears with cotton wool and covering eyes may reduce auditory and visual stimuli, and increase anaesthesia depth and time.

Monitoring of horses receiving 'triple-drip' can be difficult as the horses can swallow, blink, and show some ear and other facial movements, generally appearing 'light', which can result in the infusion rate being increased more than necessary. A general increase in muscle tone and strange respiratory patterns (which appear to indicate an increased ventilatory drive) can be due to the buildup of catechol, a metabolite of GG, which causes excitatory phenomena and can lead you into thinking the animal is too light, when in fact it is too deep.

Care should be taken to ensure that excessive doses of GG are not given (aim to keep total dose <150 mg/kg) as GG is a cumulative centrally-acting muscle relaxant. Therefore, if the horse receives too much, it will be ataxic on recovery or remain recumbent for a long period. The buildup of catechol may also cause an excitable recovery.

Other disadvantages of 'triple-drip' are that the ratios of doses of the individual components are fixed so they can only be administered in that ratio; and once the solution is made up, it should be used that day. If only a small amount of a solution is used the rest is wasted, so 'triple-drips' can be expensive.

30.5.6 Alfaxalone Infusion

- One study evaluated anaesthetic induction with 35 mg/kg GG and 2 mg/kg alfaxalone following premedication with 0.03 mg/kg acepromazine and 7 μg/kg medetomidine, and then anaesthesia was maintained with separate infusions of medetomidine 5 μg/kg/h and alfaxalone 2 mg/kg/h for 45 minutes. Anaesthetic conditions were good and both induction and recovery qualities were good.
- A similar study evaluated anaesthetic induction with 1 mg/kg alfaxalone following premedication with 7 μg/kg medetomidine, 0.025 mg/kg butorphanol and 0.05 mg/kg midazolam. Anaesthesia was then maintained with infusions of 5 μg/kg/h medetomidine, 0.03 mg/kg/h butorphanol and 2 mg/kg/h alfaxalone for 60 minutes. Anaesthetic conditions were good as were induction and recovery qualities, *but* respiratory depression was noted. The inclusion of a benzodiazepine and opioid (which have mild respiratory depressant effects of their own) might compound the mild respiratory depression from alfaxalone and might necessitate the provision of supplementary oxygen and ventilatory support.
- A recent study evaluated anaesthetic induction with 35 mg/kg GG and 1 mg/kg alfaxalone following premedication with 0.03 mg/kg acepromazine and 1 mg/kg xylazine. Anaesthesia was then maintained for 180 minutes with an infusion of alfaxalone that was tailored to the individual requirements of the horses, and, after starting at 5 mg/kg/h (a rate which the authors later suggested was too high), averaged 3 mg/kg/h. Anaesthesia was characterised by the presence of brisk palpebral reflexes, intermittent nystagmus, and spontaneous swallowing that were not consistently associated with gross purposeful movements. Recoveries were good despite noise- or tactile stimulus-induced muscle twitches/tremors, rigidity, or gross paddling movements. Cardiovascular effects were minimal, *but* ventilatory support was required in the majority of horses.

30.5.6.1 Partial (or Supplementary) Intravenous Anaesthesia (PIVA or SIVA)

- Requires placement of an endotracheal tube, but enables oxygen and ventilation provision
- Requires equipment for both inhalation and injectable agent provision, but oxygen supplementation is assured and the means for supporting ventilation is also available
- A cumbersome technique for in-field use
- Depth of anaesthesia potentially more titratable, and both anaesthetic depth and provision of anti-nociception may be able to be tailored to the animal's needs separately
- Offers the best of both worlds

As all the volatile anaesthetic agents cause dose-dependent cardiorespiratory depression and promote the stress response, any techniques that can reduce the requirement for volatile agents during anaesthesia and surgery may be advantageous. Since the first edition of this book, there has been an explosion of publications regarding different drug protocols, which are impossible to do justice to here. Amongst the techniques, however, has been the increasing interest in delivering infusions of α2 agonists, intra-operatively and into the early recovery period, as it is generally agreed that provision of some sort of sedation in the recovery period *can* improve the overall recovery quality. Intra-operative infusions of other drug classes, such as opioids, lidocaine, and ketamine, are also popular. The anaesthetist must, however, be vigilant concerning the total dose of ketamine administered (large doses may reduce recovery quality, especially where only racemic ketamine is available) and remember that lidocaine can increase ataxia in early recovery, so its infusion should be stopped, where possible, around 30 minutes before the end of anaesthesia. The reader is referred to Chapter 28 on equine sedation as the recipes given there for the various drug infusion protocols can be used for horses under general anaesthesia as well as for the provision of standing chemical restraint.

30.5.7 Monitoring Horses under General Anaesthesia

This section should be read in conjunction with Chapter 18 on monitoring. The anaesthetised horse presents the anaesthetist with some extra risk because unwanted movement can be very dangerous both to the horse and to personnel. Always be aware of personnel standing in potentially dangerous positions. Below are some brief points about monitoring that specifically relate to horses.

30.5.7.1 CNS/Reflexes

- In horses (compared with dogs and cats), eye position is a relatively unreliable indicator of anaesthetic depth.
- Palpebral reflex (check both eyes if possible) is often 'just' maintained at depths of anaesthesia suitable for surgery, but becomes refractory if the stimulation is repeated too frequently.
- Perineal reflex/anal tone can be a useful index of anaesthetic depth.

Horses anaesthetised with ketamine maintain cranial nerve reflexes so they have brisk palpebral and gag reflexes; their lips and ears may twitch as well. This makes it hard to tell whether the horse is 'light' or not.

30.5.7.2 Cardiovascular System

The cardiovascular system of horses seems to be particularly susceptible to depression under anaesthesia, especially volatile anaesthesia, and cardiovascular support is often required. **Arterial hypotension** is a **common** consequence of anaesthesia, especially under inhalation agents and especially with dorsal recumbency.

Horses have a huge amount of cardiac reserve, thus in response to an increased sympathetic tone they may not increase their heart rate to achieve an increase in cardiac output; instead they just increase their stroke volume. This means that heart rate is not necessarily a good indicator of a horse becoming light, whereas arterial blood pressure can be more helpful and is one reason why we monitor arterial blood pressure in anaesthetised horses.

Peripheral arterial blood pressure should also be monitored as horses are susceptible to developing post-anaesthetic myopathies. One of the risk factors for the development of myopathies is ischaemia due to poor perfusion of muscles. The mean arterial blood pressure is usually maintained around 70 mmHg in the hope of maintaining adequate muscle perfusion during recumbency on a standard padded 'bed'. Positive inotropes and vasopressors may be required to aid maintenance of adequate arterial blood pressure (see Chapter 25). IV fluid therapy may help a little, especially in previously hypovolaemic animals.

Be aware of certain drugs (e.g. α2 agonists, hyoscine, clenbuterol) or diseases (e.g. grass sickness) that may affect the heart rate even when the horse is anaesthetised.

30.5.7.3 Respiratory System

Intra-operative **hypoxaemia and hypercapnia are common** in anaesthetised horses.

Horses also have a huge respiratory reserve and so may not increase their respiratory rate as they become 'light'. They may, however, suddenly change their respiratory pattern or take a sudden intake of breath when light.

Ketamine (and sometimes thiopental) predisposes horses to develop 'periodic breathing' patterns. This means that the horse will take several breaths in relatively quick succession before then holding its breath for a longer period of time. This can make determining respiratory rates difficult and make the anaesthetist think the horse is lighter/deeper than it actually is. Ketamine can also cause apneustic breathing, where there is an end-inspiratory pause, rather than the normal end-expiratory pause.

General anaesthesia in horses, either with volatile agents or with most injectable agents, tends to cause respiratory depression. Supplementary oxygen is usually provided to the horse, and ideally some method of monitoring blood oxygenation (at least percentage saturation of arterial blood haemoglobin with oxygen) should be used.

Intra-operative hypoxaemia has several causes:

- Low inspired oxygen percentage/oxygen supply failure
- Hypoventilation:
  - Malpositioned or obstructed endotracheal tube, preventing fresh gases from reaching the lungs.
  - Reduced ventilatory drive, even with hypercapnia and hypoxaemia, due to volatile agents.
  - Splinting of the diaphragm with recumbency, especially dorsal (Figure 30.1). This can be exacerbated by increased intra-abdominal pressure such as pregnancy, obesity, and GI distension.
  - Reduced respiratory muscle tone and inhibition of sighing/yawning under general anaesthesia (also facilitate a reduction in FRC).
- Should hypercapnia develop due to hypoventilation, the increased alveolar CO_2 tension reduces alveolar O_2 tension/availability. Furthermore, hypercapnia shifts the haemoglobin-oxygen dissociation curve to the right, thus reducing haemoglobin-oxygen carriage.
- Compression atelectasis of dependent lung areas (Figure 30.1) promotes regional intrapulmonary shunting of blood.
- Absorption/resorption/oxygen-induced atelectasis (i.e. because we commonly provide 100% inspired O_2) also promotes intrapulmonary shunting of blood.
- Hypoxic pulmonary vasoconstriction is inhibited by inhalation agents, which results in reduced opposition to the development of intrapulmonary shunting of blood.
- Reduced cardiac output results in reduced pulmonary perfusion and promotes the development of alveolar dead space regions. Reduced systemic cardiac output also results in reduced mixed venous (pulmonary arterial) oxygen tension.

Ventilation/perfusion mismatching is a common result of most of the above (Figure 30.2).

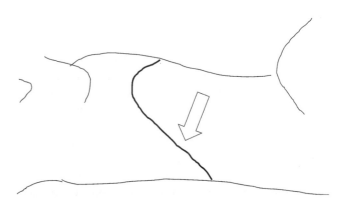

Figure 30.1 Abdominal viscera compress and 'splint' the diaphragm, especially during dorsal recumbency.

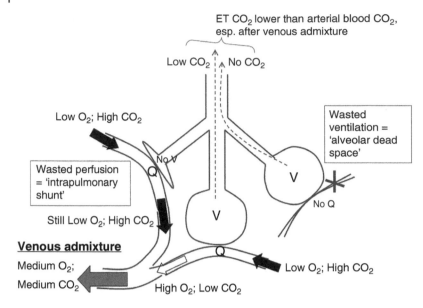

ET CO$_2$ lower than arterial blood CO$_2$, esp. after venous admixture

Low CO$_2$ · No CO$_2$

Low O$_2$; High CO$_2$

No V

Q

Wasted perfusion = 'intrapulmonary shunt'

Still Low O$_2$; High CO$_2$

V

Venous admixture

Medium O$_2$;

Medium CO$_2$

Q

High O$_2$; Low CO$_2$

V

No Q

Wasted ventilation = 'alveolar dead space'

Low O$_2$; High CO$_2$

Figure 30.2 Ventilation/perfusion mismatching is outlined in this diagram showing alveoli under normal (matched ventilation and perfusion), and two extreme conditions (no ventilation, but perfusion; no perfusion, but ventilation). Deoxygenated blood reaching alveoli in pulmonary arteries is shown by black arrows. The white arrow shows re-oxygenated blood in a pulmonary vein leaving areas of good ventilation and perfusion. The grey arrow shows how admixture of pulmonary venous blood of different oxygen saturations occurs to result in overall desaturation. The degree of desaturation depends upon, ultimately, the overall proportion of cardiac output which constitutes 'intrapulmonary shunt'. V = (alveolar) ventilation; Q = (alveolar) perfusion; ET = end tidal.

Treatment of the resultant hypoxaemia includes:

- Increasing the inspired O$_2$ percentage (although it may already be being delivered at 100%). (High [e.g. >50–60%] inspired oxygen concentrations can also exacerbate absorption atelectasis.)
- Providing mechanical ventilation in the form of positive pressure ventilation, with or without some form of alveolar recruitment manoeuvre and positive end expiratory pressure (PEEP). (Beware possible reduction in cardiac output due to both the increased intrathoracic pressures and changes in PaCO$_2$.) Optimal ventilatory support strategies (including optimal mixtures of inspired gases and optimal inspired oxygen concentration) have not yet been determined for all equine body shapes, sizes, and recumbent positions, nor their impacts on the haemodynamics of animals presenting in different physiological states. The reader is referred to the Further Reading section for more information.
- Bronchodilators (intratracheal/bronchial [e.g. salbutamol, 1–2 µg/kg administered during inspiration] seem to produce fewer side effects than intravenous [e.g. clenbuterol, 0.8 µg/kg slowly IV]), which actually work as local vasodilators and help to turn lung units at/near the 'alveolar dead space' end of the spectrum into units with better ventilation-perfusion matching. Salbutamol inhalers tend to deliver 100 µg per metered dose, so 1–2 puffs are required per 100 kg body weight. Propellants present in metered dose inhalers may not only interfere with anaesthetic agent monitoring (where infrared absorption spectroscopy is used), but may also damage the analyser.
- Maintain adequate mean arterial pressure (commonly used as a proxy measure of cardiac output).

30.6 The Recovery Period

This is perhaps the most dangerous time for a horse undergoing general anaesthesia. Not only do increased size and worse temperament of the patient increase the chances of the animal injuring itself (or others), but when equine patients are placed into the recovery box, all the monitoring and support is usually withdrawn (for safety reasons). It is not uncommon for sick colics to survive the anaesthesia period itself, but then to succumb in the recovery box.

Many techniques are used throughout the world. Recovery may be 'free stand', where the horse is not assisted to its feet at all, or may include the use of ropes on the head and/or tail to assist standing. Such rope-assisted recoveries have become more common in recent years, but cannot guarantee successful recoveries. Other techniques are sometimes used including: slinging, tilt-tables, inflatable mattresses that are deflated rapidly when the horse is ready to stand, hydropools, or rafts anchored in swimming pools. The number of techniques in use reflects the difficulty in finding one solution to the problem of recovering all patients safely. Any one technique is also probably not suitable for all patients, but neither is every technique available at all hospitals, nor are all anaesthetists necessarily familiar with every technique.

30.6.1 The Recovery Environment

- Choose a place with minimal chance for the horse to injure itself, e.g. a large flat grassy field, a loose box with bedded floor and bales stacked against the walls (make sure the bales are secure and will not fall onto the horse), or a padded recovery box. The floor should offer 'padded' support and should also provide good traction.

- Ideally, some means of supplementing oxygen should be available.
- Emptying the bladder increases general comfort and delays the animal's urge to stand. It can also reduce the soiling of bandages.
- All horses tend to develop hypothermia to some degree during anaesthesia/recovery, and one study has shown an association between the duration of recovery and the number of attempts to stand with the degree of hypothermia. It thus seems prudent, as with other species, to try to prevent hypothermia during anaesthesia and in the recovery box as this may well help to improve recovery quality. This, however, might be easier said than done.
- A quiet, calm environment is more likely to result in smoother recoveries. Sudden loud noises, especially horses trotting past or whinnying, will likely result in sudden arousal that may be detrimental to recovery quality. Ear plugs may help to reduce the noise-sensitivity of the patient, but not all ear plugs are equal with respect to their noise-reduction performance (and they require later removal). A constant level of background noise may be preferable, e.g. radio chatter or music. Whilst classical music has been shown to calm anxious racehorses, to this author's knowledge, different sorts of noise or music have not yet been tested during equine recovery and horses would probably need a period of acclimatisation beforehand.
- Dimly lit or darkened boxes (or putting a cloth over the animal's eyes) were at one time thought to reduce external stimulation and increase the chances of a smoother recovery, but this assertion was not supported in a clinical study.
- Equine appeasing pheromone (EAP) has been shown to reduce horses' reactions to novel situations, but it remains to be determined whether EAP can improve recovery quality.

30.6.2 Positioning the Horse for Recovery

Ideally, the horse should be placed in the same lateral recumbency that it endured throughout anaesthesia. Occasionally, there may be justification to put the horse into the opposite lateral recumbency for recovery, e.g. after surgery on the medial aspect of a leg. In these situations, the benefits of having an affected leg uppermost for ease of standing up must be weighed against the deleterious effects of the horse having to breathe from a congested lung. When a horse is turned over after a prolonged period (20+ min) in one lateral recumbency, then atelectasis develops in the newly dependent lung quicker (in 10–20 minutes) than it clears in the previously dependent (new uppermost) lung.

If the horse was in dorsal recumbency for surgery, then it should be placed in whichever lateral recumbency facilitates access to the jugular vein cannula or so that the limb that had undergone surgery is uppermost (although some people suggest that the affected limb may also be dependent). Although there should be a theoretical advantage of left lateral recumbency because the uppermost right lung is bigger, studies have shown no difference.

The horse should be positioned so that there is enough room in front of it to allow it to stand easily. The horse should be placed with its back nearest to the access point into the box so that it is facing away from that point.

The dependent foreleg is often protracted to fan out the triceps muscles to minimise overall pressure on the muscles to help reduce the chances of triceps myopathy developing. This action may also help protect against radial neuropathy. However, it is also an unnatural position for the dependent forelimb and may cause increased struggling to attain sternal recumbency.

All hobbles, ropes, and overshoes should be removed. The recovery floor should be as non-slippery as possible.

For 'field' recoveries, the patient's eyes should be protected from direct sunlight and also from any loose substratum (dust, long grass, etc.) in the recovery environment. Where endotracheal tubes are used, then their open, external ends must also be protected against potential aspiration of such loose material. Dark coat/skin colours readily absorb heat, and so recovery in direct sunlight on hot days should be avoided where possible; instead, shady areas should be chosen.

30.6.3 Monitoring during the Recovery Period

When the horse is first placed into the recovery box an immediate assessment should be made of anaesthetic depth as many horses respond to the stimulus of being moved.

If appropriate, an oxygen demand valve can be used to provide oxygen (via the ET tube), and even support ventilation. A nasopharyngeal tube and perhaps a nasal oxygen insufflation tube can also be placed. The purpose of the nasopharyngeal tube is to prevent the soft palate from obstructing the upper airway and to ensure some kind of nasal airway through probably oedematous nasal passages (although the nasal tube will be narrower than the nasal passages would normally be, it may still offer less resistance than oedematous nasal airways). Horses are obligate nose-breathers and often develop nasal mucosal oedema/hyperaemia/congestion during surgery (especially if in dorsal recumbency when the head is often 'below' the level of the heart and venous return from the head is compromised despite valves in the jugular veins). An alternative approach to the problem of nasal mucosal congestion is to use a topical decongestant at the end of surgery (e.g. phenylephrine). This intervention, however, has to be timed correctly because reactive hyperaemia develops as the effect of the decongestant wanes: the hope is that the horse has recovered to at least a sternal position (head now above heart) by the time the decongestant's effect has worn off, so that dependent nasal oedema is less likely to re-form with a vengeance.

For endotracheal tube removal, one school of thought advocates tracheal extubation whilst the horse is relatively deeply anaesthetised, thus incurring fewer problems with laryngospasm or stimulating the horse to try to stand too soon, but another advocates waiting until swallowing has returned (relatively lightly anaesthetised) to ensure the patient can reposition its soft palate (i.e. during swallowing) and protect its airway. If horses are sedated for the early part of the recovery period, however, the swallowing reflex may be suppressed; this seems particularly so with detomidine and romifidine, but less so after xylazine.

Removing the ET tube before the horse is too 'light' (normally around the first signs of nystagmus) is usually less of a worry with horses (which cannot vomit, and, at least when otherwise 'healthy', are unlikely to regurgitate), than with small animals (which can gag, retch, and vomit or regurgitate at light planes of anaesthesia). At very light planes, the horse may bite down on the tube (if the gag has been removed), preventing its removal and causing respiratory obstruction (especially if the ET tube cuff has not yet been deflated); it is therefore important to remember to remove the tube before the gag is removed. Some horses may displace their soft palate on removal of the ET tube, especially if at relatively deeper planes of anaesthesia, so you should always check for adequate airflow from the nostrils or nasopharyngeal tube after ET tube removal. For horses in which there may be regurgitated gut contents, blood, or other material in the throat region, then as much material as possible should be removed before the horse enters the recovery box, and then tracheal extubation is usually performed once the animal's swallowing reflex has returned (the tube's cuff may be left inflated, or at least partly inflated, during its removal). Remember to remove the gag once the ET tube has been removed. The horse should then be observed from a safe position to ensure that no respiratory obstruction occurs and that the nasopharyngeal tube, if present, remains patent. Some anaesthetists prefer to leave the ET (either oro-tracheal or naso-tracheal) tube in place during recovery until the horse has regained its feet. If this is to be done, then the tube must be secured well as tubes can sometimes be inhaled. There is also a big question surrounding whether the cuff should be deflated

or not. Leaving it inflated means that the tube's outer, open end provides the only route for air entry into the animal's respiratory tract. Should the horse then kink or otherwise obstruct this end of the tube, then total respiratory obstruction develops (see below). Should the cuff be deflated, however, then although total respiratory obstruction should be much less possible, the patient's airway is not fully protected from aspiration of any materials that may be in the throat region.

Many horses that are agitated or frightened on recovery respond to a calming voice. Making the decision to re-enter a recovery box if, e.g. the horse has got cast, depends upon the experience of the anaesthetist and the potential danger to the patient/anaesthetist. Manually-assisted recoveries should not be attempted in confined recovery boxes for anything other than small horses or foals, and only then if you have adequate help.

30.6.4 Problems Associated with Recovery from Anaesthesia

30.6.4.1 Trauma

Trauma can result in damage ranging from mild contusions and small cuts to dislocations and fractures of limbs or the neck. Whilst post-anaethetic myopathies/neuropathies may contribute to weakness/ataxia-associated injuries (see below), rubber-floored boxes are susceptible to becoming very slippery if they get very wet. It is therefore important to try to minimise possible sources of liquid by: catheterising the bladder intra-operatively (or in early recovery) to drain the urine; drying excess sweat off the horse; and putting down some form of bedding to provide grip.

30.6.4.2 Post-anaesthetic Myopathy/Neuropathy Syndrome (PAM/N)

Equidae that undergo general anaesthesia are at risk of developing myopathies and/or neuropathies. The aetiology of post-anaesthetic myopathy is complex, multi-factorial, and still not fully understood. Myopathy may be localised to one or two muscle groups or may become generalised to include multiple muscles. As muscles swell, nerves can become compressed, so neuropathies can accompany myopathies; however, neuropraxic neuropathies can also occur independently of myopathies due to poor padding over the bony prominences near which nerves run.

Some of the factors that may contribute to post-anaesthetic myopathies:

- Ischaemia/reperfusion injury (poor perfusion: hypotension, occlusion of vessels, compartmental syndrome)
- Poor positioning and inadequate padding

- Hypoxaemia
- Prolonged anaesthesia time, especially >2 hours
- Repeated anaesthetics
- EPSM (a glycogen storage/mobilisation problem), which affects especially Draught breeds
- HYPP (a sodium channel problem), which affects especially Appaloosas and Quarter horses
- Recent exercise/fit horses
- Recent feeding, which appears to go hand in hand with fit/in-work horses (i.e. high concentrate diets)

30.6.4.2.1 Diagnosis

Horses suffering from myopathy may show any or all of the following:

- Affected muscles feel firm and swollen
- Sweating (especially over affected muscles)
- Pain
- Reluctance to move or stand
- Lameness; from mild to non-weight bearing
- Myoglobinuria
- Raised aspartate aminotransferase (AST) and creatine kinase (CK); but concentrations do not always parallel the clinical severity of the condition

In cases of neuropraxic neuropathy, where only nerves are affected, the symptoms depend upon the actual nerve affected, but usually horses show no or little pain, rather they may be anxious with the dysfunctionality. Radial nerve paresis (common following poor padding over triceps muscles) results in a dropped elbow, inability to protract the forelimb, and reluctance to stand or move. Facial nerve pareses may result in, e.g. unilateral lip droop, ptosis, or ear droop. Recovery depends upon the degree of nerve damage. Ocular care (if blinking is affected), assisted feeding (if prehension of food is difficult), and musculoskeletal support (with limb neuropathies) may be necessary.

30.6.4.2.2 Treatment for Myopathy

The goals of treatment are to calm the horse, provide analgesia, increase blood flow to the affected muscles, reduce inflammation, and promote diuresis (to prevent myoglobin from blocking renal tubules and causing renal failure):

- Sedation if necessary (acepromazine can be useful as the vasodilation it causes may increase perfusion of affected muscles)
- Analgesia. Consider systemic NSAIDs (beware renal function), opioids, α2 agonists; these may also be administered by continuous infusion, as may drugs such as lidocaine and ketamine
- Fluids: intravenous fluids (extracellular fluid volume replacers) can be administered at two to three times maintenance, at least initially

- DMSO (dimethyl sulphoxide): intravenous or topically applied (may be anti-inflammatory, anti-free radical, and promotes local vasodilation)
- Physiotherapy: massage, hydrotherapy, and hot/cold compresses may help

If there has been no improvement in the horse's condition after 24–36 hours, then the prognosis is poor, especially if the horse has not stood, or in cases of generalised myopathy. Nursing of recumbent patients is logistically difficult. Although some patients may tolerate slings, these are not without their own problems.

30.6.4.2.3 Prevention

Fortunately, our greater awareness of PAM/N and some of its causal factors has reduced its frequency and severity. However, even with all the common precautionary steps (listed below), the condition can still occur.

- Maintain peripheral mean arterial blood pressure > 70 mmHg (to maintain perfusion pressure of c. 35 mmHg in the face of intracompartmental pressures of c. 35 mmHg
- Keep anaesthesia times as short as possible (e.g. remove shoes, clip surgical site before anaesthetic induction)
- Avoid unnecessary repeat anaesthetics
- Use appropriate head and limb supports and bedding (e.g. air mattresses). In lateral recumbency, the dependent forelimb should be protracted and both non-dependent limbs should be supported parallel to lower limbs; in dorsal recumbency, hindlimbs should not both be extended caudally at the same time
- EPSM: if this is suspected and surgery cannot be delayed, then three teacups of vegetable oil administered by stomach tube before anaesthesia is said to help.
- HYPP: acetazolamide treatment for several days before anaesthesia may help; otherwise, be familiar with treatments for acute hyperkalaemia.

30.6.4.3 Spinal Cord Malacia

This is also known as spinal cord myelopathy, myelomalacia, haematomyelia, and poliomyelomalacia. It is a form of ischaemic necrosis of the spinal cord and occurs sporadically. It is most often encountered in young male Draught breeds, especially after dorsal recumbency, but has also been reported in smaller breeds, mares, and also after lateral recumbency. Typically, the preceding anaesthetic is uneventful and short, although a hypertensive episode may be noted, thought to be associated with the onset of spinal pathology. The horse then fails to stand in recovery, but is seen dog-sitting with its hind limbs often extended. The condition typically affects the thoracolumbar spinal cord. There is a cranial progression, with initial loss of perineal sensation and anal tone/reflex, progressing to loss of hind limb deep pain and voluntary movement, and eventually the panniculus reflex is affected. Horses are usually not distressed. No improvement occurs with time or treatment such as corticosteroids. Indeed, deterioration may occur over time as the pathology ascends the spinal cord and intercostal muscles become affected (animals may start to become distressed).

The exact aetiology of the ischaemia is yet to be determined. It has been suggested that young horses' vertebral columns grow faster than their spinal cords, so the spinal cord is easily stretched during dorsal recumbency, which reduces its perfusion. It has also been suggested that dorsal recumbency in these large horses compresses the caudal vena cava and azygos vein, resulting in venous congestion of tissues in the caudal part of animal, including the spinal cord, so compromising its perfusion. Dorsal recumbency also tends to increase the cerebrospinal fluid pressure within and around the cord, which may compromise its perfusion. Micro-thromboemboli or fibrocartilagenous emboli may also be involved, and perhaps verminous arteritis is a predisposing factor, of either the emboli or reduced perfusion. Vitamin E and selenium deficiencies have also been proposed, such that oxidative cord damage might be involved. Some have suggested anomalous or poor vasculature in the thoracolumbar spine region in Draught horses, but this has never been proved. The prognosis is hopeless.

30.6.4.4 Post-Anaesthetic Respiratory Obstruction (PARO)

Nasal mucosal oedema/congestion/hyperaemia can be a problem, especially in horses that have been in dorsal recumbency for long periods, and its severity can be gauged by either digitally exploring the nasal passages or observing the degree of chemosis and eyelid oedema that are usually also present. It is caused by hydrostatic congestion. Nasopharyngeal tubes or topical decongestants (e.g. phenylephrine) can be used, but beware of rebound hyperaemia as the decongestant wears off. In most cases, the congestion/hyperaemia/oedema reduces significantly after a short period of time in recovery and even faster once sternal recumbency is achieved and the head is once again above heart height. Nasopharyngeal tubes can help to avert obstruction due to soft palate displacement.

Post-anaesthetic respiratory obstruction is perhaps more recognised in equidae than other species because they are obligate nose-breathers. Dyspnoea is not uncommon in the recovery period. It can range from mild snoring to complete respiratory obstruction. Whilst the cause of nasal oedema is positional, the exact cause of bilateral laryngeal paresis/paralysis is unresolved, although may include stretch-ischaemia of the recurrent laryngeal nerves by over-extended positions of the head and neck. Severe/complete respiratory obstruction can quickly become fatal and can be caused by: severe bilateral nasal oedema; dorsal displacement of the soft palate; laryngospasm; bilateral laryngeal paresis/paralysis; or unusual patient positions during recovery that result in occlusion of the open end of the ET tube (especially if the cuff is still inflated), or both nostrils. Some cases of bilateral laryngeal paralysis may not become immediately obvious after tracheal extubation, but instead become apparent some time later, usually when the horse requires increased respiratory effort, e.g. to whinny or to walk back to its loose box. Even if the cause of the obstruction is quickly rectified, negative pressure pulmonary oedema (with a component of neurogenic pulmonary oedema, due to hypoxaemia) is a common sequel to respiratory obstruction (seen as pink frothy fluid at the nostrils and possibly also lips), and unless treated aggressively, can be fatal. Treatment includes re-establishment of an airway by the quickest possible means: endotracheal intubation or tracheostomy tube (re-induction of anaesthesia may be unnecessary in a cyanotic, collapsed animal); provision of oxygen with positive pressure ventilation is recommended; suction may also be necessary to help remove copious quantities of frothy fluid; furosemide speeds resolution of the oedema. At one time, ethanol was suggested as a topical anti-foaming agent, but is no longer advised; bronchodilators such as IV clenbuterol are no longer favoured as they may have adverse effects in the wake of the hyperadrenergic state (due to the CNS hypoxic/ischaemic response), which accompanied the obstruction. Besides the neurogenic component to the pulmonary oedema, another complication following the massive sympathetic discharge that accompanies CNS hypoxia is neurogenic cardiomyopathy, which can manifest as delayed-onset (around three days later) cardiac arrhythmias. Recovery (a few weeks) from laryngeal paralysis has been documented.

Pulmonary thromboemboli are a rare cause of dyspnoea and occasionally death in recovery.

30.6.4.5 Horner's Syndrome

This sympathetic neuropathy may occasionally become apparent after anaesthesia and may be associated with jugular venepuncture complications or cervical spinal injury during induction or recovery. The clinical signs include ptosis, enophthalmos, protrusion of the third eyelid, miosis, and sweating over the face and upper neck.

30.6.4.6 CNS Ischaemia

Neurological signs (blindness, abnormal behaviour, seizures) may not be immediately apparent in recovery, but may be delayed in onset (hours to days). CNS injury is most probably secondary to intra-operative interruptions in cerebral oxygen delivery whether due to ischaemia, hypoxaemia, or embolic events, but other causes of neurological behaviour such as hepatic encephalopathy and hyperammonaemia should also be ruled out.

30.6.4.7 Jugular Cannula or 3-Way Tap Damage or Leakage

If the jugular intravenous cannula or 3-way tap is damaged or displaced so as to effectively uncap the cannula, there can often be haemorrhage from an 'up' the jugular vein catheter, especially once the patient has recovered to a position where the head is 'above' the heart. Although it may look dramatic, such haemorrhage is not usually life-threatening as clotting usually limits blood loss during the time that it takes for you to be able to safely enter the recovery box to address the problem. Blood and blood clots on the recovery box floor, however, can be quite slippery. Venous cannulae placed 'down' the jugular vein may entrain air if they become uncapped and the patient has its head 'above' its heart. Venous air emboli are potentially fatal. (See Chapter 7.)

30.6.4.8 Jugular Venous Thrombosis

May develop within the first few days of surgery (see Chapter 7).

30.6.4.9 Post-anaesthetic Colic (PAC)

May develop within the first 72 hours post-operatively. Several causes have been proposed (see Further Reading).

30.6.4.10 Horse Will Not Get Up

Most horses should regain their feet within 90 minutes of the end of anaesthesia. **A prolonged recovery is considered to be one in excess of 30 minutes for every hour of anaesthesia time**. If the horse is still recumbent after this time, the anaesthetist should start to consider the following possibilities:

- Horse exhausted or cold, e.g. (colic) after long surgery
- Osteoarthritis – especially in old horses
- Myopathy/neuropathy (see above)
- Fracture/dislocation/severe trauma
- Spinal cord malacia

30.7 Anaesthesia of Foals

See Chapter 37 on neonates. The age of the foal is very important as this reflects how developed the organ systems, metabolism, and homeostasis are. Some of the factors to consider include:

- Most foals come with their dam, and she may require sedation. She may also be in-foal again. Although α2 agonists are contra-indicated in the last trimester (because in non-pregnant mares, they increase uterine tone in the order: xylazine>detomidine>romifidine), in pregnant mares, detomidine was shown to have no effect on, or even reduced, uterine tone and intra-uterine pressure. α2 agonists, however, reduce not only maternal, but also foetal, cardiac output (due to bradycardia and increased afterload), which coupled with likely uteroplacental vasoconstriction (α2 agonism), may well reduce uteroplacental perfusion and compromise foetal well-being. The foetus possibly suffers more from the reduction in cardiac output than the dam because of being less tolerant of bradycardia. See Chapter 28 on equine sedation for further details and the possible use of clenbuterol in pregnant mares where α2 agonists are administered.

- Cardiac output is largely dependent upon heart rate in neonates (first two weeks of life), as the ventricles are less compliant; take care with drugs that depress cardiac function, especially heart rate. For the first week of life, a transitional circulation exists, in which the foetal ductus arteriosus and foramen ovale are only functionally closed. Should anything happen to cause a relative pulmonary hypertension, the pressure gradient across these channels reverses, which can cause them to re-open, therefore re-establishing a foetal-type circulation that leads to a vicious circle of progressively worsening hypoxaemia because there is no longer a placenta to provide any oxygenated blood. Causes of pulmonary hypertension include: hypovolaemia, hypothermia, hypoxaemia, acidosis, and pain.

- Liver metabolism is immature until about four weeks of age.

- Hypothermia can quickly develop due to the large surface area : volume ratio, little subcutaneous fat and no brown fat, immature control of vasomotor tone (especially peripherally), high susceptibility to hypoglycaemia (which limits immature shivering and non-shivering thermogenesis mechanisms), and an immature hypothalamic thermostat.

- Neonates are susceptible to hypoglycaemia. The neonatal liver has a limited ability to store glycogen and its ability for gluconeogenesis is poorly developed, yet the basal metabolic rate is high so there is a high demand for glucose.

- Neonates have a highly compliant chest wall, yet relatively stiff lungs, which, along with their high breathing rate, results in a high work of breathing. Minute ventilation is largely dependent upon breathing rate. The highly compliant chest wall means that the end-expiratory intrapleural pressure is close to atmospheric pressure (rather than being negative, as in the mature animal), which facilitates airway/alveolar collapse during normal tidal ventilation, especially when combined with recumbency that lowers the FRC further. The relatively low FRC and relatively high closing capacity (the lung volume at which small airways/alveoli collapse) promotes this so-called postural hypoxaemia. Their high minute ventilation means that neonates are very sensitive to drugs that depress respiratory activity.

- Neonates have a poor ability to concentrate urine or excrete a water load in the first week or two of life so are poorly tolerant of hypervolaemia/hypovolaemia. They may also struggle with acid–base balance for the first month of life until renal function is mature.
- Always check IgG levels in neonates.
- Foals are prone to gastrointestinal ulcers whose development may be influenced by poor perfusion and stress. Foals should be monitored for bruxism, salivation, and dorsal recumbency (i.e. signs of colic/ulcers). Most gastro-protectants are not licenced for neonatal foals, but sucralfate may be useful where there are fears of increasing gastric pH with subsequent increased risk of systemic invasion of harmful bacteria.
- Foals are, however, precocious, so that by about one month old, their physiology is more like that of a mature horse.
- Have you got appropriate (e.g. appropriately-sized) equipment and facilities?

30.7.1 Pharmacological Considerations

Neonates are said to be more sensitive to the effects of drugs than adults. This may result from pharmacokinetic and pharmacodynamic differences:

- Increased body water content and higher ECF : ICF ratio increases the volume of distribution of water-soluble and poorly protein-bound drugs
- Potential for hypoalbuminaemia (although not usually observed in foals compared with neonates of other species); reduced protein binding increases the concentration of free (active) drug
- Low body fat (2% c.f. 5–15% in adults), and muscle mass limit the re/distribution of drugs
- Immature hepatic and renal excretion pathways delay drug elimination
- Increased blood–brain barrier permeability, for the first month of life, increases drug access to the CNS
- Receptor differences, e.g. foetal/neonatal neuromuscular junction nicotinic receptors respond differently to neuromuscular blocking drugs than adult type receptors (neonates behave as mini-myasthenics); and perhaps neonatal adrenergic receptors have different expression/sensitivities compared to adults also (neonates are vagally-dominant).

30.7.2 Pre-anaesthetic Evaluation/Preparation

- History is important. Was the birth difficult? Passed meconium? Urinated? Suckled? IgG status?

- Clinical examination. Most foals under the age of five days will have a patent ductus arteriosus (i.e. continuous machinery murmur), heart rate 70–90 bpm, respiratory rate about 30 bpm.
- Check temperature and blood glucose concentration.
- Do not deny suckling; but if a foal has just had a large drink, it may be prudent to wait 20–30 minutes before administering drugs to give the milk time to clot in the stomach to reduce any risk of regurgitation.
- Measure the foal's weight.
- If possible and stress-free, pre-oxygenate the foal, e.g. during sedation/recumbency and before/during induction of anaesthesia.
- Secure IV access before anaesthetic induction if the foal allows.

30.7.3 General Anaesthesia

Have all the appropriate equipment ready and ensure that all personnel present are aware of the plan. If possible, ensure the environment is warm. Sedate the mare if necessary and have a safe stable available for her. It is advisable to have contingency plans too, as some foals belie their age or physiological status and become distressed and/or unhandleable and require a sudden change in plan. Below is one example protocol for a young or sick foal.

30.7.3.1 Young <4 Weeks (or Sick) Foals

- Weigh.
- Achieve restraint by gentle handling.
- Diazepam or midazolam (0.1–0.25 mg/kg IV) often provides useful sedation and the foal may even become voluntarily recumbent. (α2 agonists are avoided where possible because of the marked reduction in heart rate and cardiac output that they cause.) Recumbency prior to anaesthetic induction also helps to smooth the induction of anaesthesia in that it removes the necessity for transition from standing to recumbent.
- Consider an opioid for painful interventions: pethidine (3.5–5 mg/kg), butorphanol (0.025–0.5 mg/kg), or buprenorphine (0.005–0.01 mg/kg).
- Apply local anaesthetic cream/gel to the rostral-most part of the nasal passages, and, after a suitable delay for the local anaesthetic to take effect, then introduce either a nasopharyngeal or nasotracheal tube. Inflate the cuff (of the latter) or occlude the other nostril (if using a nasopharyngeal tube). Attach an appropriate anaesthetic breathing system (e.g. non-rebreathing system for the smallest foals or a small animal circle for larger foals) and start by administering oxygen. Then quickly increase the inspired concentration of volatile agent to ensure rapid transition through any induction excitement phase.

- Once a stable plane of anaesthesia is achieved, then a larger diameter (lower resistance) oro-tracheal tube can be placed if necessary, and anaesthesia maintained with a volatile agent in oxygen.
- Try to conserve body heat as much as possible – minimise clipping/wetting of surgical sites, use insulative blankets, heated mattresses, forced warm air devices, etc. and remember to wrap the limbs where possible as these appendages have high surface area compared to their volume and much heat can be lost from them. Use warm fluids for IV administration and surgical lavage if possible.
- Monitor as much as possible: anaesthetic depth, cardiovascular and respiratory variables (pulse rate, arterial blood pressure, oxygenation [at least by pulse oximetry if blood gas analysis is not available], end tidal carbon dioxide tension), blood glucose, and temperature. Ventilation may require support, but positive pressure ventilation is well-tolerated (and generally less detrimental to venous return) in foals (compared with adults), because of their compliant chest walls and less negative intrapleural pressures. Being more vagally-dominant, foals often tolerate lower mean arterial blood pressure (MAP) than mature animals. This author generally tries to maintain MAP ≥60 mmHg.
- The judicious administration of IV fluids may be required.
- Consider other means of providing analgesia: are local/regional anaesthetic techniques appropriate?
- For recovery, keep the foal warm and dry and continue oxygen administration until sternal recumbency can be attained. If recovery is slow, check the foal's temperature, blood glucose, and oxygenation.
- Assist to stand if smaller than 100–150 kg. Once the foal is steady on its feet, the dam can be brought to the foal. They should re-bond immediately and a good sign is that the foal suckles more or less straight away.

Older (>4 weeks), healthy foals can usually be considered as similar to mature animals in that α2 agonists can be used in the premedication and injectable agents are generally preferred for anaesthetic induction. Premedication may also result in recumbency, which is helpful in that it helps to smooth anaesthetic induction by removing the necessity for the transition between standing and recumbency.

30.7.3.1.1 *Uroperitoneum*
See Chapter 44.

30.8 Fractures

- Beware excessive ataxia after premedication, especially if the horse has a full limb-length splint. However, some patients are very agitated and very painful. Good analgesia is required.

- Slings are very useful, if tolerated. Assisted inductions, e.g. against a wall, are usually best if tilt-tables and slings are unavailable. The fractured leg is best made available to manipulation by one of the assistants so that it does not get into abnormal positions during the transition from standing to recumbent.
  - If slings are used for anaesthetic induction, lower the horse to the floor quickly and gently to relieve the cardiorespiratory compromise caused by the sling.

30.9 Head/Eye Injuries

- If raised intracranial or intra-ocular pressure are to be avoided, beware the low head carriage that follows α2 agonist sedation. Support the head in a natural/high position. α2 agonists themselves lower intra-ocular pressure through extra-ocular muscle relaxation, reduced production of aqueous humour, and an increase in its drainage; but if the head is allowed to 'drop', the intra-ocular pressure can increase. Bilateral jugular venous occlusion can also increase intra-ocular pressure should a horse lean forwards hard against the front bar of stocks.
- A recent paper investigating the effects of anaesthetic protocols on intra-ocular pressure found xylazine (0.5 mg/kg) premedication followed by head-held-neutral position before GG (~55 mg/kg) and thiopental (4 mg/kg; 10% solution) induction produced lowering of intra-ocular pressure; whereas xylazine (0.5 mg/kg), GG (~55 mg/kg), and ketamine (2 mg/kg) caused an increase in intra-ocular pressure. Ketamine appears to increase intra-ocular pressure in horses through increasing extra-ocular muscle tone.
- Various helmets are available to protect the head/eyes from trauma/further trauma during anaesthetic induction (and recovery). However, in this author's experience, the sizes available never quite fit the animal with the problem, and a badly-fitting helmet can be worse than none at all.

30.10 Colics

GI tract obstructions can be:

- **Strangulating**
- **Non-strangulating**

With non-strangulating obstructions, secretions sequester into the gut lumen (extracellular fluid loss) and promote the development of hypovolaemia. Gas may also build up following bacterial fermentation of gut contents. Increased fluid and gas within the gut lumen causes distension of gut, which is painful, and also initially causes hypermotility of the gut (also painful) to try to move the cause of the distension on downstream. If gut distension persists, eventually the gut becomes fatigued of its hypermotility and becomes hypomotile. Distended gut and displaced gut may also put traction on the mesentery, which adds to the pain. Stretch of the gut wall also compromises its perfusion so it becomes ischaemic, hypoxic, and oedematous (and eventually, even necrotic). Oedema tends to compromise its perfusion further so a vicious cycle is entered, which results in further compromise so that the mucosa becomes 'leaky' and eventually endotoxaemia (SIRS) complicates the earlier hypovolaemia.

With strangulating lesions, the mucosal barrier becomes compromised much sooner, allowing translocation of bacteria and toxins into the blood stream, so that endotoxaemia (SIRS) and hypovolaemia almost co-exist from the start. As ischaemic bowel becomes necrotic, peritonitis may also develop, which further adds to the pain.

Clinical signs of hypovolaemia/hypovolaemic shock are those of sympathetic stimulation. Initially (compensatory phase), these include tachycardia, weak peripheral pulses, cold and pale extremities (peripheral vasoconstriction tries to 'centralise' the remaining blood volume for vital organ perfusion), and tachypnoea. (Pain itself is rarely the sole cause of tachycardia in colicky horses.) Stimulation of chemoreceptors by hypoperfusion and by acidaemia (anaerobic metabolism with the production of lactic acid, accompanies tissue hypoperfusion during hypovolaemia), and stimulation of baroreceptors (due to hypotension) that can also result in stimulation of the respiratory centre, both contribute to the tachypnoea. The tachypnoea helps to produce a respiratory alkalosis to offset/compensate for the metabolic acidosis that commonly develops.

Eventually, when the animal can no longer compensate, and the periphery demands more perfusion, massive peripheral vasodilation occurs, dropping the blood pressure dramatically and loading the blood with acidic metabolites. Decompensation thus occurs, and the animal rapidly deteriorates clinically.

Endotoxaemic (SIRS/sepsis) horses tend to be much sicker (dull and depressed, but this may be masked if painful). Endotoxins play havoc with vascular integrity/permeability and tone (via stimulation of inflammatory cells to produce inflammatory mediators, and via interactions with endothelial cells, the endothelial glycocalyx, platelets, and clotting factors), resulting in vasodilation, capillary leakiness, and disseminated intravascular coagulopathy (DIC) (petechiae, ecchymoses). Horses tend to have congested (vasodilated) mucous membranes (± petechiae), with sluggish perfusion (prolonged capillary refill time; CRT).

30.10.1 Problems

- Pain. Visceral pain from distended/ischaemic gut and mesenteric traction causes the 'typical' colic signs of pawing, Flehmen sign (upper lip curled up), flank-watching, rolling, kicking at the belly. Parietal pain can be more predominant with peritonitis; the animal will 'board' its abdomen and be unwilling to move rather than typically show the more overt and violent signs of pain. Animals may show signs of both.
- Hypovolaemia (+ increased packed cell volume [PCV]). Compromised circulation (due to fluid loss, increased blood viscosity, and abdominal distension).
- Endotoxaemia (SIRS). Compromised circulation and pulmonary gas exchange (pulmonary capillaries are also affected by endotoxaemia).
- Compromised ventilation due to abdominal distension and possible 'splinting' of the diaphragm (especially with large colon torsions).

30.10.1.1 Why Is There Pain?

- Due to distension of gut with fluid and gas
- Due to mesenteric stretch or traction
- Due to hypermotility that is unsuccessful in relieving the local distension
- Due to early ischaemia of the gut wall (once necrotic, the gut is no longer painful)
- Due to inflamed gut
- Due to peritoneal inflammation if peritonitis present

30.10.2 Clinical Examination and Preparation

A quick but thorough clinical examination should take place. Initial concerns centre around the provision of analgesia, and also the safety of handlers and attending personnel.

Listed below are the main factors that are useful in determining a suitable approach to anaesthesia of each case.

- Assess whether the horse is in pain and safe to approach. It may need analgesia/sedation in order to make it safe to examine. Anyone who has witnessed a horse with severe pain from colic will appreciate how distressed and uncontrollable the animal can be. Furthermore, these painful episodes can appear suddenly with no warning. Thus, administration of analgesics relieves pain and facilitates examination and supportive therapy to be administered with a higher degree of safety for both horse and personnel.
- Assess how long it has been since the horse was last normal.

- Determine its cardiovascular and respiratory status:
  - Assess pulse rate, rhythm, and pulse pressure.
  - Assess respiratory rate: may indicate metabolic acidosis.
  - Auscultate heart and lungs.
  - Check mucous membrane colour and CRT.
  - Measure PCV and total solids (TS). Splenic contraction (increased sympathetic tone) can increase PCV markedly.
  - Measure blood and peritoneal fluid lactate (and possibly also glucose) concentration.
- Check stomach for accumulation of fluid. This can be done by passing a nasogastric tube and establishing a syphon. Ultrasound can also be used to detect dilation of the duodenum, which, in the horse, is abnormal and may indicate gastric distension. Some authors advocate leaving a stomach tube secured in place during anaesthetic induction to reduce the chances of stomach rupture. However, a stomach tube (if placed with its distal tip through the cardia) may encourage fluid passage out of the stomach not only through its lumen, but also around the outside of the tube as well, which can increase the risk of inhalation/aspiration before a cuffed endotracheal tube can be placed. It may be better to make a concerted effort to relieve as much gastric distension as possible by stomach tube, and then either reverse the tube slightly so that its internal tip lies within the oesophagus (it can be re-advanced into the stomach once the airway has been protected), or remove it completely before induction of anaesthesia.
- Caecal or colonic trocarisation is occasionally required to decompress the abdomen. Although this risks gut laceration, it can be life-saving in tympanic colics with severe cardiorespiratory compromise.
- Abdominocentesis: test fluid for cellularity, protein, and lactate.
- Findings upon rectal examination and transabdominal ultrasound may help to determine the site of the lesion.

30.10.2.1 Considerations for Anaesthesia

- Emergency
- Horse may be in (sometimes severe) pain; can be dangerous to handle
- No control of previous drugs administered by referring vet
- Shock (hypovolaemia ± endotoxaemia/SIRS)
- Abdominal distension ('splints' the diaphragm to compromise ventilation and may also compromise venous return due to compression of abdominal vena cava, and therefore reduces cardiac output). Abdominal compartment syndrome may occur with severe intra-abdominal hypertension

- Risk of regurgitation and aspiration
- Acid–base and possible electrolyte abnormalities
- Often unsociable hours; tired personnel

30.10.3 Approach to Anaesthesia

- Analgesia (± sedation), including gut decompression where appropriate.
- Fluids; possibly pre-operatively (possibly hypertonic saline or colloids), also intra-operatively and post-operatively.
- Acid–base and electrolyte disturbances may require attention.
- Use of drugs with minimal cardio-respiratory depressant effects.
- Drugs with anti-endotoxic effects (some NSAIDs, polymixin B, etc.). Beware hypovolaemia & renal toxicity.
- Avoid N_2O (at least until the gut is decompressed) as it partitions into 'low-solubility-gas'-filled spaces (e.g. gas pockets entrapped in gut) and worsens the problems of increased intra-abdominal pressure for the surgeon and the anaesthetist alike. Some anaesthetists avoid N_2O in all horse anaesthetics as it *may* increase gut distension and predispose to post-operative colic.
- Ventilatory support may be required, especially if massive abdominal distension is present. (Note: positive pressure ventilation, especially in hypovolaemic animals, may significantly reduce thoracic vena caval blood flow and venous return to the heart, thereby reducing cardiac output and blood pressure, etc.)
- Dorsal recumbency further compromises venous return and cardiac output (because the great vessels [vena cava and aorta; although veins are the most easily compressible] get squashed), especially in hypovolaemic animals, and may cause an animal to decompensate acutely and die between anaesthetic induction and the operating table (e.g. when hoisted up by its legs). Body position changes should be performed relatively slowly and gently.
- Beware of reperfusion/re-oxygenation injury, e.g. re-establishment of blood flow to previously compromised gut (with subsequent entry of anaerobic metabolism products into the main circulation), and production of reactive oxygen species in previously ischaemic/damaged tissue. Animals can 'crash' shortly after affected gut is un-twisted. (DMSO and lidocaine were, at one time, advocated due to their free radical scavenging abilities.)

30.10.3.1 Analgesics

This section is specifically aimed at the immediate pre- and peri-operative period. Remember that decompression (e.g. gastric) can afford pain relief too.

Sometimes a dose of hyoscine butylbromide will provide sufficient spasmolytic effect on the gut to enable safe patient examination. If the pain is more severe and relentless, then xylazine is often administered as it produces good visceral analgesia, partly through depressing gut motility and it also produces sedation. Relatively small doses (especially if cardiovascularly compromised) should be given intravenously, to effect, beginning with doses as low as 0.2 mg/kg. Opioids may also be administered. Different anaesthetists have different preferences for these drugs, and each has their advantages and disadvantages (see Chapter 3). This author has favoured morphine (0.3 mg/kg IV) once the decision for surgery has been made. If there are concerns over masking pain, then shorter-acting drugs such as butorphanol (0.1 mg/kg IV) or pethidine (5 mg/kg IM) are suitable. This author has also given fentanyl (2 μg/kg IV), which produced excellent analgesia for around 12 minutes.

Once the decision for surgery has been made, an NSAID is usually administered (providing the horse has not previously received one), despite concerns over their use in hypovolaemic states. Flunixin is often preferred (despite its potential adverse effects on gut mucosal restitution and permeability) due to its apparently superior analgesic properties over several other available NSAIDs, although more recently, a COX-2 selective (COX-1 sparing) NSAID, firocoxib, has been demonstrated to provide a similar level of analgesia. Other NSAIDs such as carprofen, meloxicam, ketoprofen, and phenylbutazone may, however, have already been given. Flunixin reduces the degree of cardiovascular dysfunction associated with endotoxaemia more than phenylbutazone, whereas phenylbutazone appears to oppose the reduction in GI motility associated with endotoxaemia more than flunixin. Flunixin, meloxicam, and carprofen have also been shown to inhibit the activation of nuclear transcription factor κB-dependent genes, with a subsequent anti-inflammatory effect that is additional to their COX inhibiting effects. (Endotoxin causes activation of NFκB, amongst other pathways, with the consequent production of pro-inflammatory mediators.)

Lidocaine and ketamine infusions may also have a place. Lidocaine infusion is also often advocated for its purported prokinetic effect on 'compromised' gastrointestinal tract, possibly through analgesic, anti-inflammatory, and anti-reperfusion injury mechanisms, although direct effects on myenteric plexi and gut smooth muscle have also been demonstrated. α2 agonists are currently less popular (at least outwith the anaesthetic period) because they may reduce GI motility and also gut perfusion. Nevertheless, pain itself, through increasing sympathetic tone, is a powerful inhibitor of gut motility and also perfusion.

Local/regional anaesthetic techniques are currently being explored, and it may be that some forms of truncal block could provide useful additional analgesia.

30.10.3.2 Fluid Therapy

In colic cases, there may be any or all of the following: hypovolaemia, dehydration, endotoxaemia (SIRS), electrolyte imbalances, and acid–base abnormalities. On presentation, it is important to assess the status of the cardiovascular system (see above). Whilst clues can be gained (or deductions made) about likely acid–base/electrolyte status at this time, it is often not until blood samples are analysed that a clearer picture is gained.

For horses that are in shock (i.e. PCV >45%, heart rate > 80 beats per minute, cool extremities, poor pulse pressure, CRT >3–4 seconds etc.), either 4–5 ml/kg hypertonic (7.2 or 7.5%) saline over ~10 minutes or 4–5 ml/kg of a synthetic colloid (pentastarch or tetrastarch used to be favoured) over ~10 minutes, can be administered to improve the intravascular volume before anaesthetic induction and early maintenance of anaesthesia. (At least most horses will then survive the relative physiological insult of anaesthetic induction.) Both these treatments should be followed by isotonic crystalloids.

It is important not to administer isotonic 'extracellular fluid volume replacers' (Hartmann's solution, 0.9% saline) at too high a rate until any compromised gut is isolated, otherwise fluid may sequester from the circulation into the gut wall and lumen, further exacerbating distension and possibly compromising anastomosis sites. Indeed, crystalloid fluid overload is associated with oedema of many organs.

Many horses with colic have acid–base abnormalities. Although there is no one consistent acid–base abnormality at the time of admission, most horses with any degree of hypovolaemia will have a mild metabolic acidosis (lactic acidosis) due to increased anaerobic metabolism where tissue perfusion is compromised. More severe metabolic acidosis may develop where there is gut strangulation because of the additional production of lactic acid in the ischaemic gut. During fluid therapy and rehydration, improvements in the peripheral circulation can 'wash' previously sequestered products of anaerobic metabolism into the general systemic circulation so the situation may appear to worsen, initially. A subsequent reduction in lactate is usually a good prognostic sign.

Alkalotic horses are normally only encountered as a result of over-treatment with bicarbonate or when magnesium salts have been administered by the referring veterinary surgeon.

Horses which hypoventilate under anaesthesia can develop respiratory acidosis, and this may compound a previously existing metabolic acidosis causing a very low blood pH.

In colic cases, it is impossible to over-emphasise the benefit derived from serial blood gas and acid–base measurements over the course of treatment. Venous blood is adequate if one is interested only in the degree of metabolic acidosis or alkalosis. Arterial samples provide extra information on the adequacy of ventilation and oxygenation. In the conscious horse, the sites from which to draw arterial blood include the transverse facial artery and the carotid artery directly 'behind/beneath' the jugular vein, about 10 cm above the point where the pectoral muscle crosses the jugular groove (in an average 500 kg horse). (The jugular vein should be digitally displaced to one side to enable an uncontaminated arterial stick.) After any arterial blood sample is obtained by needle puncture, digital pressure over the arterial puncture site is required for a good five minutes to prevent haematoma formation.

Many horses anaesthetised for colic surgery are hypotensive, so the use of vasopressors and positive inotropes is often necessary (+ IV fluids) to support peripheral arterial blood pressure (see Chapter 25).

Norepinephrine (40 μg/ml), or phenylephrine solution (100 μg/ml), administered IV to effect can be useful when diastolic pressure is low (<40 mmHg) such that coronary perfusion is compromised, and tachycardia accompanies hypovolaemia. Vasoconstrictor therapy can then, hopefully, be withdrawn as fluid resuscitation progresses.

Dobutamine solution (250 μg/ml) can also be administered to effect if/once the heart rate is nearer the normal range. Dobutamine is not this author's first choice where tachycardia is present in conjunction with low arterial blood pressure and low diastolic pressure (see Chapter 25).

30.10.3.3 Anaesthetic Protocols

Once the decision has been made to take a colic horse to surgery, if time and the patient allow, try to get an accurate weight and remove shoes.

There is a lot of debate about what the best anaesthetic protocol is for horses with colic, but there are many types of colic and no one protocol is perfect for all the possibilities. Although some protocols may carry some theoretical advantages, familiarity is often safer. Below are some general points:

- Acepromazine is often contraindicated as it exacerbates hypotension.
- In sick cases, start with low doses of α2 agonists.
- Be careful not to overdose the horse with NSAIDs.
- Inhalational anaesthesia tends to be more commonly practiced for anaesthetic maintenance as surgeries tend to be long, but PIVA/SIVA techniques with agents such as lidocaine, ketamine, and opioids help to reduce the volatile agent requirement, which may improve cardiovascular status. Loading doses are usually given before infusions are begun; if not, then it takes longer to reach a 'steady state' plasma concentration.

For cases that are not showing signs of hypovolaemic or endotoxaemic shock, then a standard induction protocol may be used. Some anaesthetists prefer to use xylazine instead of detomidine or romifidine in the premedication.

The justification for this is that any deleterious cardiovascular and GI effects will not last as long.

Xylazine 0.1–0.75 mg/kg IV, wait 2–3 minutes
Morphine 0.2–0.3 mg/kg IV, wait 5 minutes
Ketamine 2.2 mg/kg (± 0.05 mg/kg diazepam or midazolam) IV
Isoflurane or sevoflurane in oxygen
Consider lidocaine infusion/ketamine infusion

For animals that are severely hypovolaemic, if the use of α2 agonists is more limited, and the operator is more wary of ketamine-based anaesthetic inductions, an alternative strategy could be as follows.

No sedation
Morphine 0.2–0.3 mg/kg IV
5, 10 or 15% GG solution infused IV to effect (30–50 mg/kg) followed by 5 mg/kg thiopental IV
Isoflurane or sevoflurane in oxygen
Consider lidocaine infusion/ketamine infusion

GG/thiopental inductions often produce a more dramatic onset of unconsciousness where the horse literally falls to the floor, so unless it is assisted into recumbency (by the aid of an induction 'squeeze' gate or similar), distended stomach or intestine may rupture on impact.

After induction, it is important to place a cuffed ET tube and inflate the cuff as soon as possible to protect the airway from potential refluxed/regurgitated material.

30.10.3.4 Monitoring

Colic cases require careful monitoring and the use of multiparameter monitoring equipment is almost essential. Sudden changes in physiological status can occur, e.g. when endotoxins/inflammatory mediators are released into the general circulation when strangulated portions of intestine are untwisted, or when a large mesenteric artery is torn.

30.10.3.5 Recovery

As stated earlier, the recovery period is a dangerous time for any horse. Some colic horses will be exhausted and have very prolonged recoveries.

30.10.3.6 Post-operative Care

It is important that all cases are carefully monitored and supported in the first few days after surgery. Analgesia is paramount, as is judicious fluid therapy. Acid–base and electrolyte status may require interventions. Nutritional support is also vital and 'pharmacological' enteral nutrition likely has an important role. The reader is referred elsewhere for further details regarding enteral and parenteral nutrition. Post-operative ileus is a common complication.

Further Reading

Aarnes, T.K., Bednarski, R.M., Bertone, A.L. et al. (2014). Recovery from desflurane anesthesia in horses with and without post-anaesthetic xylazine. *The Canadian Journal of Veterinary Research* 78: 103–109.

Abass, M., Picek, S., Garzon, J.F.G. et al. (2018). Local mepivacaine before castration of horses under medetomidine isoflurane balanced anaesthesia is effective to reduce perioperative nociception and cytokine release. *Equine Veterinary Journal* 50: 733–738.

Ambrosio, A.M., Ida, K.K., Souto, M.T.M.R. et al. (2013). Effects of positive end-expiratory pressure titration on gas exchange, respiratory mechanics and haemodynamics in anaesthetized horses. *Veterinary Anaesthesia and Analgesia* 40: 564–572.

Auckburally, A. and Flaherty, D. (2009). Recovery from anaesthesia in horses. Part 1: what can go wrong? *In Practice* 31: 340–347.

Auckburally, A. and Flaherty, D. (2009). Recovery from anaesthesia in horses. Part 2: avoiding complications. *In Practice* 31: 362–369.

Auckburally, A. and Nyman, G. (2017). Review of hypoxaemia in the anaesthetised horse: predisposing factors, consequences and management. *Veterinary Anaesthesia and Analgesia* 44: 397–408.

Auer, U., Schramel, J.P., Moens, Y.P. et al. (2019). Monitoring changes in distribution of pulmonary ventilation by functional electrical impedance tomography in anaesthetized ponies. *Veterinary Anaesthesia and Analgesia* 46: 200–208.

Bardell, D. (2017). Managing orthopaedic pain in horses. *In Practice* 39: 40–427.

Bettschart-Wolfensberger, R., Bowen, M.I., Freeman, S.L. et al. (2001). Cardiopulmonary effects of prolonged anaesthesia via propofol-medetomidine infusion in ponies. *American Journal of Veterinary Research* 62: 1428–1435.

Bettschart–Wolfensberger, R., Kalchofner, K., Neges, K. et al. (2005). Total intravenous anaesthesia in horses using medetomidine and propofol. *Veterinary Anaesthesia and Analgesia* 32: 348–354.

Bettschart-Wolfensberger, R. and Larenza, P. (2007). Balanced anesthesia in the equine. *Current Techniques in Equine Practice* 6: 104–110.

Bidwell, L.A. (2013). Anesthesia for dystocia and anesthesia of the equine neonate. *The Veterinary Clinics of North America. Equine Practice* 29: 215–222.

Boscan, P., Van Hoogmoed, L.M., Pypendop, B.H. et al. (2006). Pharmacokinetics of the opioid antagonist N-methylnaltrexone and evaluation of its effects on gastrointestinal tract function in horses treated or not treated with morphine. *American Journal of Veterinary Research* 67: 998–1004.

Bradbury, L.A., Dugdale, A.H.A., Knottenbelt, D.C. et al. (2008). The effects of anesthesia on laryngeal function and laryngeal/pharyngeal trauma in the horse. *Journal of Equine Veterinary Science* 28: 461–467.

Briganti, A., Portela, D.A., Grasso, S. et al. (2015). Accuracy of different oxygenation indices in estimating intrapulmonary shunting at increasing infusion rates of dobutamine in horses under general anaesthesia. *The Veterinary Journal* 204: 351–356.

Brosnahan, M.M., Holbrook, T.C., Gilliam, L.L. et al. (2009). Intra-abdominal hypertension in two adult horses. *Journal of Veterinary Emergency and Critical Care* 19: 174–180.

Casoni, D., Spadavecchia, C., and Adami, C. (2014). Cardiovascular changes after administration of aerosolized salbutamol in horses: 5 cases. *Acta Veterinaria Scandinavica* 56: 49. http://www.actavetscand.com/content/56/1/49.

Casoni, A., Spadavecchia, C., Wampfler, B. et al. (2015). Clinical and pharmacokinetic evaluation of S-ketamine for intravenous general anaesthesia in horses undergoing field castration. *Acta Veterinaria Scandinavica* 57: 21. https://doi.org/10.1186/s13028-015-0112-4.

Chesnel, M.A. and Clutton, R.E. (2013). A comparison of two morphine doses on the quality of recovery from general anaesthesia in horses. *Research in Veterinary Science* 95: 1195–1200.

Clark-Price, S.C. (2013). Recovery of horses from anesthesia. *The Veterinary Clinics of North America. Equine Practice* 29: 233–242.

Clark-Price, S.C., Posner, L.P., and Gleed, R.D. (2008). Recovery of horses from general anaesthesia in a darkened or illuminated recovery stall. *Veterinary Anaesthesia and Analgesia* 35: 473–479.

Clutton, R.E. (2010). Opioid analgesia in the horse. *The Veterinary Clinics of North America. Equine Practice* 26: 493–514.

Cook, V.L. and Blikslager, A.T. (2008). Use of systemically administered lidocaine in horses with gastrointestinal tract disease. *Journal of the American Veterinary Medical Association* 232: 1144–1148.

Cook, V.L. and Blikslager, A.T. (2015). The use of nonsteroidal anti-inflammatory drugs in critically ill horses. *Journal of Veterinary Emergency and Critical Care* 25: 76–88.

Corletto, F., Raisis, A., and Brearley, J.C. (2005). Comparison of morphine and butorphanol as pre-anaesthetic agents in combination with romifidine for field castration in ponies. *Veterinary Anaesthesia and Analgesia* 32: 16–22.

Cowles, C.E. Jr. and Culp, W.C. Jr. (2019). Prevention and response to surgical fires. *BJE Education* 19: 261–266.

Crumley, M.N., McMurphy, R.M., Hodgson, D.S., and Kreider, S.E. (2013). Effects of inspired oxygen concentration on ventilation, ventilatory rhythm, and gas exchange in isoflurane-anesthetized horses. *American Journal of Veterinary Research* 74: 183–190.

Day, T.K., Gaynor, J.S., Muir, W.W. et al. (1995). Blood gas values during intermittent positive pressure ventilation and spontaneous ventilation in 160 anesthetized horses positioned in lateral or dorsal recumbency. *Veterinary Surgery* 24: 266–276.

Del Barrio, M.C.N., David, F., Hughes, J.M.L. et al. (2018). A retrospective report (2003-2013) of the complications associated with the use of a one-man (head and tail) rope recovery system in horses following general anaesthesia. *Irish Veterinary Journal* 71: 6.

Dobromylskyi, P., Taylor, P.M., Brealey, J.C. et al. (1996). Effects of pre-operative starvation on intra-operative arterial oxygen tension in horses. *Journal of Veterinary Anaesthesia* 23: 75–77.

Driessen, B. (2005). Assisted recovery in horses awakening from general anaesthesia. In: *Recent advances in anesthetic management of large domestic animals* (ed. E.P. Steffey), International Veterinary Information Service. www.ivis.org.

Dugdale, A. (2013). How to prevent and manage post-anaesthetic neuropathies and myopathies. Proceedings of the British Equine Veterinary Association Congress, Manchester, UK. (September 2013): 181–182.

Dugdale, A. (2015). Nutrition of the surgical colic patient: what's the evidence? Proceedings of British Equine Veterinary Association Congress, Liverpool, UK. (September 2015): 132–133.

Dugdale, A.H.A., Obhrai, J., and Cripps, P.J. (2015). Twenty years later: a single-Centre, repeat retrospective analysis of equine perioperative mortality and investigation of recovery quality. *Veterinary Anaesthesia and Analgesia* 43: 171–178.

Dugdale, A.H.A. and Taylor, P.M. (2016). Equine anaesthesia-associated mortality: where are we now? *Veterinary Anaesthesia and Analgesia* 43: 242–255.

Elmas, C.R., Cruz, A.M., and Kerr, C.L. (2007). Tilt table recovery of horses after orthopedic surgery: fifty-four cases (1994-2005). *Veterinary Surgery* 36: 252–258.

Ferreira, T.H., Brosnan, R.J., Shilo-Benjamini, Y. et al. (2013). Effects of ketamine, propofol or thiopental administration on intraocular pressure and qualities of induction and recovery from anesthesia in horses. *American Journal of Veterinary Research* 74: 1070–1077.

Fischer, B. and Clark-Price, C. (2015). Anesthesia of the equine neonate in health and disease. *The Veterinary Clinics of North America. Equine Practice* 31: 567–585.

Gleerup, K.B. and Lindegaard, C. (2016). Recognition and quantification of pain in horses: a tutorial review. *Equine Veterinary Education* 28: 47–57.

Gozalo-Marcilla, M., Gasthuys, F., Luna, S.P.L., and Schauvliege, S. (2018). Is there a place for dexmedetomidine in equine anaesthesia and analgesia? A systematic review (2005-2017). *Journal of Veterinary Pharmacology and Therapeutics* 41: 205–217.

Gozalo-Marcilla, M., Gasthuys, F., and Schauvliege, S. (2014). Partial intravenous anaesthesia in the horse: a review of intravenous agents used to supplement equine inhalation anaesthesia. Part 1: lidocaine and ketamine. *Veterinary Anaesthesia and Analgesia* 41: 335–345.

Gozalo-Marcilla, M., Gasthuys, F., and Schauvliege, S. (2014). Partial intravenous anaesthesia in the horse: a review of intravenous agents used to supplement equine inhalation anaesthesia. Part 2: opioids and alpha 2 adrenoceptor agonists. *Veterinary Anaesthesia and Analgesia* 42: 1–16.

Grint, N., Gorvy, D., and Dugdale, A. (2007). Hyperthermia and delayed-onset myopathy after recovery from general anesthesia in a horse. *Journal of Equine Veterinary Science* 27: 221–227.

Grosenbaugh, D.A. and Muir, W.W. (1998). Cardiorespiratory effects of sevoflurane, isoflurane and halothane anesthesia in horses. *American Journal of Veterinary Research* 59: 101–106.

Haga, H.A., Lykkjen, S., Revold, T., and Ranheim, B. (2006). Effect of intratesticular injection of lidocaine on cardiovascular responses to castration in isoflurane-anesthetized stallions. *American Journal of Veterinary Research* 67: 403–408.

Hubbell, J.A.E., Aarnes, T.K., Bednarski, R.M. et al. (2011). Effect of 50% and maximal inspired oxygen concentrations on respiratory variables in isoflurane-anesthetized horses. *BMC Veterinary Research* 7: 23. http://www.biomedcentral.com/1746-6148/7/23.

Hubbell, J.A.E. and Muir, W.W. (2015). Oxygenation, oxygen delivery and anaesthesia in the horse. *Equine Veterinary Journal* 47: 25–35.

Hudson, N.P.H. and Pirie, R.S. (2015). Equine post-operative ileus: a review of current thinking on pathophysiology and management. *Equine Veterinary Education* 27: 39–47.

Ida, K.K., Fantoni, D.T., Ibiapina, B.T. et al. (2013). Effects of postoperative xylazine administration on cardiopulmonary function and recovery quality after isoflurane anesthesia in horses. *Veterinary Surgery* 42: 877–884.

Ida, K.K., Fantoni, D.T., Souto, M.T.M.R. et al. (2013). Effect of pressure support ventilation during weaning on ventilation and oxygenation indices in healthy horses recovering from general anaesthesia. *Veterinary Anaesthesia and Analgesia* 40: 339–350.

Jago, R.C., Corletto, F., and Wright, I.M. (2015). Peri-anaesthetic complications in an equine referral hospital: risk factors for post-anaesthetic colic. *Equine Veterinary Journal* 47: 635–640.

Johnson, C.B. (1993). Positioning the anaesthetised horse. *Equine Veterinary Education* 5: 57–60.

Johnston, G.M., Eastment, J.K., Wood, J.L.N., and Taylor, P.M. (2002). The confidential enquiry into perioperative equine fatalities (CEPEF): mortality results of phases 1 and 2. *Veterinary Anaesthesia and Analgesia* 29: 159–170.

Johnston, G.M., Eastment, J.K., Taylor, P.M., and Wood, J.L.N. (2004). Is isoflurane safer than halothane in equine anaesthesia? Results from a prospective multicentre randomised controlled trial. *Equine Veterinary Journal* 36: 64–71.

Johnston, G.M., Taylor, P.M., Holmes, M.A., and Wood, J.L.N. (1995). Confidential enquiry of perioperative equine fatalities (CEPEF-1): preliminary results. *Equine Veterinary Journal* 27: 193–200.

Kelmer, G., Doherty, T.J., Elliott, S. et al. (2008). Evaluation of dimethyl sulphoxide effects on initial response to endotoxin in the horse. *Equine Veterinary Journal* 40: 358–363.

Langdon Fielding, C., Brumbaugh, G.W., Matthews, N.S. et al. (2006). Pharmacokinetics and clinical effects of a subanesthetic continuous rate infusion of ketamine in awake horses. *American Journal of Veterinary Research* 67: 1484–1490.

Leece, E.A., Corletto, F., and Brearley, J.C. (2008). A comparison of recovery times and characteristics with sevoflurane and isoflurane anaesthesia in horses undergoing magnetic resonance imaging. *Veterinary Anaesthesia and Analgesia* 35: 383–391.

Leece, E.A., Girard, N.M., and Maddern, K. (2009). Alfaxalone in cyclodextrin for induction and maintenance of anaesthesia in ponies undergoing field castration. *Veterinary Anaesthesia and Analgesia* 36: 480–484.

Lin, H.C., Passler, T., Wilborn, R.R. et al. (2015). A review of the general pharmacology of ketamine and its clinical use for injectable anaesthesia in horses. *Equine Veterinary Education* 27: 146–155.

Lisowski, Z.M., Pirie, R.S., Blikslager, A.T. et al. (2018). An update on equine post-operative ileus: definitions, pathophysiology and management. *Equine Veterinary Journal* 50: 292–303.

Love, E.J., Taylor, P.M., Clark, C. et al. (2009). Analgesic effect of butorphanol in ponies following castration. *Equine Veterinary Journal* 41: 552–556.

Love, E.J., Taylor, P.M., Whay, H.R., and Murrell, J. (2013). Postcastration analgesia in ponies undergoing castration. *Veterinary Record* https://doi.org/10.1136/vr.101440.

Lukasik, V.M., Gleed, R.D., Scarlett, J.M. et al. (1997). Intranasal phenylephrine reduces post-anaesthetic upper airway obstruction in horses. *Equine Veterinary Journal* 29: 236–238.

MacFarlane, P.D., Mosing, M., and Burford, J. (2010). Preliminary investigation into the effects of earplugs on sound transmission in the equine ear. *Pferdeheilkunde* 26: 199–203.

Mackenzie, C. (2017). Do opioids cause colic? *Equine Veterinary Education* 29: 401–402.

Malone, E., Ensink, J., Turner, T. et al. (2006). Intravenous continuous infusion of lidocaine for treatment of equine ileus. *Veterinary Surgery* 35: 60–66.

Marntell, S., Nyman, G., Funkquist, P., and Hedenstierna, G. (2005). Effects of acepromazine on pulmonary gas exchange and circulation during sedation and dissociative anaesthesia in horses. *Veterinary Anaesthesia and Analgesia* 32: 83–93.

Marntell, S., Nyman, G., and Hedenstierna, G. (2005). High inspired oxygen concentrations increase intrapulmonary shunt in anaesthetized horses. *Veterinary Anaesthesia and Analgesia* 32: 338–347.

Martin, D., McKenna, H., and Galley, H. (2018). Rhythm and cues: role of chronobiology in perioperative medicine. *British Journal of Anaesthesia* 121: 345–349.

Mayerhofer, I., Scherzer, S., Gabler, C., and van den Hoven, R. (2005). Hypothermia in horses induced by general anaesthesia and limiting measures. *Equine Veterinary Education* 17: 53–56.

McCoy, A.M., Hackett, E.S., Wagner, A.E. et al. (2011). Pulmonary gas exchange and plasma lactate in horses with gastrointestinal disease undergoing emergency exploratory laparotomy: a comparison with an elective surgery horse population. *Veterinary Surgery* 40: 601–609.

McFadzean, W. and Love, E. (2017). How to do equine anaesthesia in the field. *In Practice* 39: 452–461.

McKay, J.S., Forest, T.W., Senior, M. et al. (2002). Postanaesthetic cerebral necrosis in five horses. *Veterinary Record* 150: 70–74.

Menzies, P.L., Ringer, S.R., Conrot, A. et al. (2016). Cardiopulmonary effects and anaesthesia recovery quality in horses anaesthetized with isoflurane and low-dose S-ketamine or medetomidine infusions. *Veterinary Anaesthesia and Analgesia* 43: 623–634.

Milligan, M., Beard, W., Kukanich, B. et al. (2007). The effect of lidocaine on postoperative jejunal motility in normal horses. *Veterinary Surgery* 36: 214–220.

Moens, Y. (2013). Mechanical ventilation and respiratory mechanics during equine anesthesia. *The Veterinary Clinics of North America. Equine Practice* 29: 51–67.

Moens, Y. and Bohm, S. (2011). Ventilating horses: moving away from old paradigms. *Veterinary Anaesthesia and Analgesia* 38: 165–168.

Monticelli, P. and Adami, C. (2019). Aspiration pneumonitis (Mendelson's syndrome) as perianaesthetic complication occurring in two horses: a case report. *Equine Veterinary Education* 31: 183–187.

Mosing, M., Auer, U., MacFarlane, P. et al. (2018). Regional ventilation distribution and dead psace in anaesthetized horses treated with and without continuous positive airway pressure: novel insights by electrical impedance tomography and volumetric capnography. *Veterinary Anaesthesia and Analgesia* 45: 31–40.

Mosing, M., MacFarlane, P., Bardell, D. et al. (2016). Continuous positive airway pressure (CPAP) decreases pulmonary shunt in anaesthetized horses. *Veterinary Anaesthesia and Analgesia* 43: 611–622.

Mosing, M., Rysnik, M., Cripps, P.J., and MacFarlane, P. (2013). Use of continuous positive airway pressure (CPAP) to optimize oxygenation in anaesthetized horses – a clinical study. *Equine Veterinary Journal* 45: 414–418.

Moudgil, R., Michelakis, E.D., and Archer, S.L. (2005). Hypoxic pulmonary vasoconstriction. *Journal of Applied Physiology* 98: 300–403.

Muir, W.W., Lerche, P., and Erichson, D. (2009). Anaesthetic and cardiorespiratory effects of propofol at 10% for induction and 1% for maintenance of anaesthesia in horses. *Equine Veterinary Journal* 41: 578–585.

Nelson, B.B., Lordan, E.E., and Hassel, D.M. (2013). Risk factors associated with gastrointestinal dysfunction in horses undergoing elective procedures under general anaesthesia. *Equine Veterinary Journal* 45 (Suppl 45): 8–14.

Nyman, G. and Hedenstierna, G. (1989). Ventilation-perfusion relationships in the anaethetised horse. *Equine Veterinary Journal* 21: 274–281.

Pakkanen, S.A.E., Raekallio, M.R., Mykkanen, A.K. et al. (2015). Detomidine and the combination of detomidine and MK-467, a peripherally-acting alpha-2 adrenoceptor antagonist, as premedication in horses anaesthetized with isoflurane. *Veterinary Anaesthesia and Analgesia* 42: 527–536.

Parviainen, A.K.J. and Trim, C.M. (2000). Complications associated with anaesthesia for ocular surgery: a retrospective study 1989-1996. *Equine Veterinary Journal* 32: 555–559.

Patschova, M., Kabes, R., and Krisova, S. (2010). The effects of inhalation salbutamol administration on systemic and pulmonary hemodynamics, pulmonary mechanics and oxygen balance during general anaesthesia in the horse. *Veterinární Medicína* 55: 445–456.

Portier, K.G., Jaillardon, L., Leece, E.A., and Walsh, C.M. (2009). Castration of horses under total intravenous anaesthesia: analgesic effects of lidocaine. *Veterinary Anaesthesia and Analgesia* 36: 173–179.

Portier, K.G., Sena, A., Senior, M., and Clutton, R.E. (2010). A study of the correlation between objective and subjective indices of recovery quality after inhalation anaesthesia in equids. *Veterinary Anaesthesia and Analgesia* 37: 329–336.

Pratt, S., Cunneen, A., Perkins, N. et al. (2019). Total intravenous anaesthesia with ketamine, medetomidine and guaifenesin compared with ketamine, medetomidine and midazolam in young horses anaesthetised for computerised tomography. *Equine Veterinary Journal* 51: 510–516.

Proudman, C.J., Dugdale, A.H.A., Senior, J.M. et al. (2006). Pre-operative and anaesthesia-related risk factors for mortality in equine colic cases. *The Veterinary Journal* 171: 89–97.

Radcliffe, R.M., Buchanan, B.R., Cook, V.L., and Divers, T.J. (2015). The clinical value of whole blood point-of-care biomarkers in large animal emergency and critical care medicine. *Journal of Veterinary Emergency and Critical Care* 25: 138–151.

Ragle, C., Baetje, C., Yiannikouris, S. et al. (2011). Development of equine post anesthetic myelopathy: 30 cases (1979–2010). *Equine Veterinary Education* 23: 630–635.

Raisis, A.L. (2005). Skeletal muscle blood flow in anaesthetized horses. Part I: measurement techniques. *Veterinary Anaesthesia and Analgesia* 32: 324–330.

Raisis, A.L. (2005). Skeletal muscle blood flow in anaesthetized horses. Part II: effects of anaesthetics and vasoactive agents. *Veterinary Anaesthesia and Analgesia* 32: 331–337.

Raisis, A.L., Blissitt, K.J., Henley, W. et al. (2005). The effects of halothane and isoflurane on cardiovascular function in laterally recumbent horses. *British Journal of Anaesthesia* 95: 317–325.

Rigotti, C., De Vries, A., and Taylor, P.M. (2014). Buprenorphine provides better anaesthetic conditions than butorphanol for field castration in ponies: results of a randomized clinical trial. *Veterinary Record* https://doi.org/10.1136/vr.102729.

Rioja, E., Cemicchiaro, N., Costa, M.C., and Valverde, A. (2012). Perioperative risk factors for mortality and length of hospitalization in mares with dystocia undergoing general anesthesia: a retrospective study. *Canadian Veterinary Journal* 53: 502–510.

Robertson, S.A. and Bailey, J.R. (2002). Aerosolized salbutamol (albuterol) improves PaO2 in hypoxaemic anaesthetized horses – a prospective clinical trial in 81 horses. *Veterinary Anaesthesia and Analgesia* 29: 212–218.

Robertson, S.A. and Sanchez, L.C. (2010). Treatment of visceral pain in horses. *The Veterinary Clinics of North America. Equine Practice* 26: 603–617.

Robertson, S.A., Sanchez, L.C., Merritt, A.M., and Doherty, T.J. (2005). Effect of systemic lidocaine on visceral and somatic nociception in conscious horses. *Equine Veterinary Journal* 37: 122–127.

Russold, E., Ambrisko, T.D., Schramel, J.P. et al. (2013). Measurement of tidal volume using respiratory ultrasonic plethysmography in anaesthetized, mechanically ventilated horses. *Veterinary Anaesthesia and Analgesia* 40: 48–54.

Santos, M., Fuente, M., Garcia-Iturralde, P. et al. (2003). Effects of alpha 2 adrenoceptor agonists during recovery from isoflurane anaesthesia in horses. *Equine Veterinary Journal* 35: 170–175.

Scarabelli, S. and Rioja, E. (2018). Retrospective evaluation of correlation and agreement between two recovery scoring systems in horses. *Veterinary Record* https://doi.org/10.1136/vr.104546.

Schauvliege, S., Cuypers, C., Michielsen, A. et al. (2019). How to score sedation and adjust the administration rate of sedatives in horses: a literature review and introduction of the Ghent Sedation Algorithm. *Veterinary Anaesthesia and Analgesia* 46: 4–13.

Schauvliege, S. and Gasthuys, F. (2013). Drugs for cardiovascular support in anesthetized horses. *The Veterinary Clinics of North America. Equine Practice* 29: 19–49.

Schoster, A., Mosing, M., Jalali, M. et al. (2016). Effects of transport, fasting and anaesthesia on the faecal microbiota of healthy adult horses. *Equine Veterinary Journal* 48: 595–602.

Schramel, J.P., Wmmer, K., Ambrisko, T.D., and Moens, Y.P. (2014). A novel flow partition device for spirometry during large animal anaesthesia. *Veterinary Anaesthesia and Analgesia* 41: 191–195.

Seddighi, R. and Doherty, T.J. (2012). Anesthesia of the geriatric equine. *Veterinary Medicine: Research and Reports* 3: 53–64.

Senior, J.M., Pinchbeck, G.L., Allister, R. et al. (2006). Post anaesthetic colic in horses: a preventable complication? *Equine Veterinary Journal* 38: 479–484.

Senior, J.M., Pinchbeck, G.L., Allister, R. et al. (2007). Reported morbidities following 861 anaesthetics given at four equine hospitals. *Veterinary Record* 160: 407–408.

Senior, M. (2005). Post-anaesthetic pulmonary oedema in horses: a review. *Veterinary Anaesthesia and Analgesia* 32: 193–200.

Shelly, M.P., Robinson, A.A., Hesford, J.W., and Park, G.R. (1987). Haemodynamic effects following surgical release of increased intra–abdominal pressure. *British Journal of Anaesthesia* 59: 800–805.

Staffieri, F., Bauquier, S.H., Moate, P.J., and Driessen, B. (2009). Pulmonary gas exchange in anaesthetised horses mechanically ventilated with oxygen or a helium/oxygen mixture. *Equine Veterinary Journal* 41: 747–752.

Thibault, C.J., Wilson, D.V., Robertson, S.A. et al. (2019). A retrospective study of fecal output and postprocedure colic in 246 horses undergoing standing sedation with detomidine, or general anaesthesia with or without detomidine. *Veterinary Anaesthesia and Analgesia* 46: 458–465.

Thompson, K.R. and Bardell, D. (2016). The effect of two different intra-operative end tidal carbon dioxide tensions on apneic duration in the recovery period. *Veterinary Anaesthesia and Analgesia* 43: 163–170.

Tzelos, T., Blissit, K.J., and Clutton, R.E. (2015). Electrocardiographic indicators of excitability in horses for predicting recovery quality after general anaesthesia. *Veterinary Anaesthesia and Analgesia* 42: 269–279.

Valente, A.C.S., Brosnan, R.J., and Guedes, A.G.P. (2015). Desflurane and sevoflurane elimination kinetics and recovery quality in horses. *American Journal of Veterinary Research* 76: 201–207.

Valverde, A. and Gunkel, C.I. (2005). Pain management in horses and farm animals. *Journal of Veterinary Emergency and Critical Care* 15: 295–307.

Valverde, A., Gunkel, C., Doherty, T.J. et al. (2005). Effect of a constant rate infusion of lidocaine on the quality of recovery from sevoflurane or isoflurane general anaesthesia in horses. *Equine Veterinary Journal* 37: 559–564.

Van Loon, J.P.A.M., de Grauw, J.C., and Van Oostrom, H. (2018). Comparison of different methods to calculate venous admixture in anaesthetized horses. *Veterinary Anaesthesia and Analgesia* 45: 640–647.

Van Oostrom, H., Schaap, M.W.H., and van Loon, J.P.A.M. (2017). Oxygen supplementation before induction of anaesthesia in horses. *Equine Veterinary Journal* 49: 130–132.

Voulgaris, D.A. and Hofmeister, E.H. (2009). Multivariate analysis of factors associated with post-anesthetic times to standing in isoflurane-anesthetized horses: 381 cases. *Veterinary Anaesthesia and Analgesia* 6: 414–420.

Wagner, A.E. (2009). Complications in equine anesthesia. *The Veterinary Clinics of North America. Equine Practice* 24: 735–752.

Wettstein, D., Moens, Y., Jaeggin-Schmucker, N. et al. (2006). Effects of an alveolar recruitment maneuver on cardiovascular and respiratory parameters during total intravenous anesthesia in ponies. *American Journal of Veterinary Research* 67: 152–159.

White, K. (2015). Total and partial intravenous anaesthesia of horses. *In Practice* 37: 189–198.

Wiese, A.J., Brosnan, R.J., and Barter, L.B. (2014). Effects of acetylcholinesterase inhibition on quality of recovery from isoflurane-induced anesthesia in horses. *American Journal of Veterinary Research* 75: 223–230.

Wilderjans, H. (2005). Advances in assisted recovery from anaesthesia. In: *Proceedings of the British Equine Veterinary Association Congress*, Harrogate, UK (September 2005): 36–38.

Wilderjans, H. (2011). The 1 man rope assisted recovery from anaesthesia in horses. Proceedings of the 12th International Congress of the World Equine Veterinary Association, Hyderabad, India. (November 2011), reprinted by IVIS (www.ivis.org).

Wolff, K. and Moens, Y. (2010). Gas exchange during inhalation anaesthesia of horses: a comparison of between immediate versus delayed start of intermittent positive pressure ventilation – a clinical study. *Pferdeheilkunde* 26: 706–711.

Wong, D.M., Davis, J.L., and White, N.A. (2011). Motility of the equine gastrointestinal tract: physiology and pharmacotherapy. *Equine Veterinary Education* 23: 88–100.

Woodhouse, K.J., Brosnan, R.J., Nguyen, K.Q. et al. (2013). Effects of postanesthetic sedation with romifidine or xylazine on quality of recovery from isoflurane anesthesia in horses. *Journal of the American Veterinary Medical Association* 242: 533–539.

Wylie, C.E., Foote, A.K., Rasotto, R. et al. (2015). Tracheal necrosis as a fatal complication of endotracheal intubation. *Equine Veterinary Education* 27: 170–175.

Young, S.S. and Taylor, P.M. (1993). Factors influencing the outcome of equine anaesthesia: a review of 1,314 cases. *Equine Veterinary Journal* 25: 147–151.

Ziegler, A.L., Freeman, C.K., Fogle, C.A. et al. (2019). Multicentre, blinded, randomized clinical trial comparing the use of flunixin meglumine with firocoxib in horses with small intestinal strangulating obstruction. *Equine Veterinary Journal* 51: 329–335.

Self-test Section

1 True or False? Tracheal extubation (if performed at return of deglutition), may be delayed until after first movement in recovery, if romifidine (but not detomidine or xylazine) is chosen for sedation in early recovery, following inhalation anaesthesia.

2 True or False? Post-anaesthetic spinal cord malacia has been associated with the following:
   - Young draught breeds
   - Males
   - Females
   - Dorsal recumbency
   - Lateral recumbency
   - Hypotension
   - Prolonged anaesthesia time

31

Equine Intravenous Anaesthesia in the Field and Standing Chemical Restraint

31.1 Field Anaesthesia

- First of all, consider if general anaesthesia is really necessary. Can you achieve the same investigation/surgery with sedation with or without a local or regional block?
- If possible, take some experienced help with you; another veterinary surgeon or a nurse.
- Check out the local environment. Soft ground is best, e.g. a well-grassed paddock, and definitely not stony ground. A flat field or one with a gentle gradient is best. Ensure there are no barbed wire fences, ponds, lakes, water courses, or busy roads in the vicinity of where anaesthesia or surgery is proposed.
- Take a good history and perform a clinical examination as you would for an in-hospital case.
- Check tetanus vaccination status.
- After explaining the associated risks to the owner or agent, a consent form should be signed.
- The horse's weight should be estimated; weigh-tapes or formulae based on various morphometric measures can be used (it is unlikely that a weighbridge will be available).
- Minimum anaesthesia equipment should include: intravenous cannulae, extension sets, injection bungs and flush; sufficient sedative, anaesthetic, and analgesia drugs; padded head collars of different sizes; soft ropes; small towels (for covering and protecting eyes).
- Some people like to take a small oxygen cylinder and some means of delivering it to the patient (by insufflation or by demand valve, via naso- or oro-tracheal or nasopharyngeal tube).
- Clippers, surgical scrub, swabs, instruments, and suture material as necessary for the particular surgery will also be required. The complexity of surgery attempted in the field will dictate the degree to which the hospital is exported to the field, but only simple procedures should be attempted away from the 'relative safety' of a well-equipped and well-staffed hospital.

31.1.1 Sedation/Premedication

- Phenothiazines: Acepromazine (acetylpromazine) may be useful as a 'pre-premed', but sufficient time should be allowed for it to work (30–40 minutes undisturbed). It provides useful background anxiolysis; may provide an anti-arrhythmic effect, and, in combination with α2 agonists, improves haemodynamics.
- α2 agonists provide more reliable sedation.
  - Xylazine (1.1 mg/kg IV) provides 10–20 minutes sedation, analgesia, some muscle relaxation, slight ataxia.
  - Detomidine (10–20 μg/kg IV) gives up to 80 minutes sedation, analgesia, some ataxia.
  - Romifidine (60–100 μg/kg IV) gives minimum 80 minutes sedation, some analgesia, minimal ataxia.

31.1.2 Analgesia

- Pre-empt surgical/inflammatory pain with NSAIDs where possible.
- Local anaesthetic blocks can provide a useful part of balanced analgesia.
- Opioids provide good analgesia and increase sedation (synergy with sedatives).
  - Butorphanol (0.05–0.2 mg/kg IV) provides around 60–90 minutes analgesia.
  - Morphine (0.12–0.25 mg/kg IM or slow IV) provides two to four hours analgesia.
  - Methadone (0.1–0.25 mg/kg IV) provides two to four hours analgesia.
  - Pethidine (3.5–5 mg/kg IM) provides 30–40 minutes analgesia.
- Buprenorphine (0.006–0.01 mg/kg IM) provides up to 12 hours analgesia (onset 30–45 minutes).

Veterinary Anaesthesia: Principles to Practice, Second Edition. Alexandra H. A. Dugdale, Georgina Beaumont, Carl Bradbrook, and Matthew Gurney.
© 2020 John Wiley & Sons Ltd. Published 2020 by John Wiley & Sons Ltd.
Companion website: www.wiley.com/go/dugdale/veterinary-anaesthesia

31.1.3 Induction of Anaesthesia

In the field, anaesthetic induction can be hard to control, so guaiphenesin (GG), which can cause ataxia during induction, may be avoided at this stage. By avoiding GG for anaesthetic induction, however, more is available for its use during anaesthetic maintenance (see below). Whatever drug (± adjuncts) are chosen for anaesthetic induction, be sure to always have at least one top-up dose available.

Anaesthesia may be induced with, e.g.:

- Ketamine (2.5–5 mg/kg) after effective α2 agonist premedication.
- Ketamine (2.5–5 mg/kg) with benzodiazepine (0.05 mg/kg diazepam OR midazolam) after effective α2 agonist premedication.
- Alfaxalone (1–2 mg/kg) after effective α2 agonist premedication.
- Thiopental:

  - 5–8 mg/kg (± 0.05 mg/kg benzodiazepine) after effective α2 agonist premedication.
  - 10–15 mg/kg (± 0.05 mg/kg benzodiazepine) after only acepromazine (± opioid) premedication.
  - Try not to far exceed 15 mg/kg (25 mg/kg maximum) total thiopental dose, or recovery may be prolonged. The use of thiopental for anaesthetic induction therefore also limits the number of top-ups you can give.

31.1.4 Maintenance of Anaesthesia

- Try to keep anaesthesia time to ≤2 hours.
- Ensure careful limb positioning.
- Protect eyes from dirt, dust, debris, grass, etc., and direct sunlight.
- Minimise environmental stimulation as much as possible to improve and increase anaesthetic time; cotton wool can be placed in the ears and a blanket over the eyes (lubricant should be put into the eyes).
- **Incremental top-up IV bolus doses of:**

  - Ketamine ± α2 agonist. If top-up doses are to be given only as necessary, then try to pre-empt the requirement a little because these extra doses take time to produce their effect. Otherwise, top-up doses can be given every 10 minutes by the clock.
    - If xylazine was administered as the premedicant, xylazine, and ketamine can be administered (e.g. every 10 minutes) at 1/3–1/2 the original premedication and induction doses, respectively, for at least the first top-up. As ketamine is slightly cumulative and has a partially active metabolite (norketamine) in some horses, and as xylazine can also be slightly cumulative (and at large doses, some α1 agonist

activity [stimulatory effects] may develop), their subsequent doses should be decreased a little (e.g. 1/4–1/3 of original induction doses) and/or the dosing interval may be able to be increased.
    - If detomidine was administered for premedication, only ketamine need be included for the first two top-ups. A half-dose of detomidine need only be administered about every 30 minutes (i.e. with every third ketamine top-up).
    - If romifidine was administered for premedication, then a further dose of romifidine (1/3–1/2 the original dose) need only be administered after about 1 hour of anaesthesia.
  - Alfaxalone 0.2+ mg/kg ± α2 agonist (as above).
  - Thiopental 1 mg/kg (range 0.5–2.5 mg/kg). (Keep a track of the total dose administered.) Thiopental produces a much quicker effect than ketamine, so is useful if the horse moves suddenly.
  - A benzodiazepine *may* be administered alongside either ketamine or thiopental top-ups. Doses of diazepam or midazolam (around 0.025 mg/kg) can be administered every 20–30 minutes, *but* after three such doses (especially of diazepam), the time interval between top-ups should be increased to 60 minutes or else recovery quality may be affected by the increased risk of muscle weakness.

Ketamine (0.25–1 mg/kg) can be administered after a thiopental induction.

Thiopental (0.5–1+ mg/kg) can be administered after a ketamine induction.

- **Continuous intravenous infusions**, based on combinations of GG, ketamine, and an α2 agonist. Several different combinations have been reported:
  - **GG 5% (50 mg/ml) + xylazine (0.5 mg/ml) + ketamine (1 mg/ml).**
    - To a 500 ml bottle of 5% GG, add 250 mg xylazine and 500 mg ketamine.
  - **GG 10% (100 mg/ml) + xylazine (1 mg/ml) + ketamine (2 mg/ml).**
    - To a 500 ml bottle of 10% GG, add 500 mg xylazine and 1000 mg ketamine.
  - **GG 15% (150 mg/ml) + xylazine (1.5 mg/ml) + ketamine (3 mg/ml).**
    - To a 500 ml bottle of 15% GG, add 750 mg xylazine and 1500 mg ketamine.
  - **GG 10% (100 mg/ml) + detomidine (0.02 mg/ml) + ketamine (2 mg/ml).**
    - To a 500 ml bottle of 10% GG, add 10 mg detomidine and 1000 mg ketamine.
  - **GG 15% (150 mg/ml) + detomidine (0.03 mg/ml) + ketamine (3 mg/ml).**

o To a 500 ml bottle of 15% GG, add 15 mg detomidine and 1500 mg ketamine.
- **GG 10% (100 mg/ml) + romifidine (0.05 mg/ml) + ketamine (2 mg/ml).**
  o To a 500 ml bottle of 10% GG, add 25 mg romifidine and 1000 mg ketamine.
- **GG 15% (150 mg/ml) + romifidine (0.06–0.075 mg/ml) + ketamine (3 mg/ml).**
  o To a 500 ml bottle of 10% GG, add 30–37.5 mg romifidine and 1500 mg ketamine.

For all of these, the combination is infused 'to effect', but remember that horses will 'look light' (i.e. they tend to have spontaneous palpebral reflexes, may swallow or have occasional ear movements), so beware of overdosing and producing deep anaesthesia. As a rough guide the infusion rate is around 1 ml/kg/hour for all the above mixtures, but often the infusion rate can be reduced over time. Try not to exceed 150 mg/kg GG, or signs of toxicity may develop: arrhythmias, muscle spasms, and prolonged and ataxic recoveries. When using a standard 20 drops/ml giving set, then for a 500 kg horse, the initial administration rate will be nearly 3 drops/second. The rate is adjusted pro-rata for other body weights. The infusion should be started as soon as possible after the induction of anaesthesia.

- **Continuous intravenous infusions**, based on alfaxalone and α2 agonists. The most common infusion rate for alfaxalone has been around 2 mg/kg/hour, and horses under alfaxalone anaesthetic maintenance may 'look light', but the reader is warned that many of the published studies reported respiratory depression that may require oxygen supplementation and ventilatory support. The reader is referred to Chapter 30, in which more details on published protocols can be found.

31.2 Prolonged Sedation for Procedures on the Standing Patient

Although top-ups of sedative agents can be given, infusions of sedatives (and also opioids and perhaps even low dose ketamine etc.) may offer advantages (see below and Chapter 28 on equine sedation). Some authors talk of CRIs – which are usually defined as either *constant rate infusions* or *continuous rate infusions*. This author finds such terminology confusing as the whole point of infusions is that their rates should be able to be varied according to patient needs, and *continuous* implies *infusion* and so is a tautology. This author therefore proposes the term VRI (variable rate infusion) for the remainder of this chapter.

Potential uses for VRIs are for prolonged standing procedures, such as dental extractions, frontal bone trephination, thoracoscopy, or laparoscopy for ovariectomy or orchiectomy. For further details and recipes, please see Chapter 28 on equine sedation.

31.2.1 Advantages of VRIs

- No need for repeated top-ups.
- Aims to maintain an even plane of sedation.
- Can anticipate changes in level of sedation.
- IV cannula already in place should emergencies arise and IV access be required.

31.2.2 Disadvantages of VRIs

- Time taken to set up.
- IV cannula is a pre-requisite.
- Cost.
- Possibility of profound sedation if not observant.

31.2.3 Xylazine Infusion

- Acepromazine 0.02 mg/kg IV or IM can be given some 20–40 minutes beforehand.
- The horse is then sedated with 1 mg/kg xylazine IV (allow 2–5 minutes for full effect).
- Morphine 0.12–0.25+ mg/kg IM or slow IV can be administered once sedation has developed.
- Prepare the infusion: add 500 mg xylazine to 500 ml of normal saline (=1 mg/ml).
- For a 500 kg horse, the initial drip rate is around 2 drops/second (about 12 μg/kg/minute) (adjust for other body weights).
- When adequate sedation is achieved, the infusion rate should be reduced to 1-2 drops/second.
- After the end of the procedure, the horse should be able to be led back to its loose box about 10–15 minutes after stopping the infusion.

31.2.4 Detomidine Infusion

- Acepromazine 0.02 mg/kg IV or IM can be given some 20–40 minutes beforehand.
- The horse is first sedated with 6–7.5 μg/kg detomidine IV (allow 5 minutes to achieve full effect).
- An opioid is also usually administered once sedation has developed, e.g. butorphanol 0.05–0.1 mg/kg IV or morphine 0.12–0.25+ mg/kg IM or slow IV.
- Prepare the detomidine infusion: add 12 mg of detomidine to 500 ml of normal saline (=24 μg/ml).

- For a 500 kg horse, the initial drip rate is around 4 drops/second (about 0.6 µg/kg/minute); this initial rate should be adjusted pro-rata for other body weights.
- When adequate sedation is achieved, the infusion rate is reduced to around 1–2 drops/second.
- After the end of the procedure, the horse should be able to be led back to its loose box around 15–20 minutes after stopping the infusion.

Note that for this protocol, the initial loading dose of detomidine may seem quite low and the initial infusion rate is therefore relatively fast. This is to try to avoid greater initial ataxia and might enable a smoother overall level of sedation to be achieved by titration of the infusion compared with alternative protocols that start with a greater loading dose and slower infusion rate where a smoother plane of sedation might actually be more difficult to achieve in the earlier stages.

31.2.5 Medetomidine Infusion (Not Licenced in the UK)

- Acepromazine 0.02 mg/kg IM or IV can be given 20–40 minutes beforehand.
- Prepare the infusion: add 3.5 mg medetomidine to 500 ml normal saline (=7 µg/ml).
- Loading dose 5 µg/kg IV, then immediately start infusion at 3.5–5 µg/kg/hour; or loading dose 7 µg/kg IV, then wait 5 minutes, and then start infusion at 3.5 µg/kg/hour
- For the 7 µg/ml solution, around 1.5 drops/second for a 500 kg horse gives 3.5 µg/kg/hour.
- An opioid can be administered once sedation becomes apparent.
- The diuresis due to α2 agonists seems to be much more obvious with medetomidine infusions than with xylazine, detomidine, and romifidine.

Recently, an algorithm has been published that should help to optimise adjustment of infusion rates during standing procedures, but also warns that conversion to general anaesthesia may be necessary and should always be planned for.

31.3 Difficult-to-handle Horses

For 'difficult' horses, the following combination usually works well (often dubbed 'magic mixture'):

Acepromazine (0.03 mg/kg) + **detomidine** (0.02 mg/kg) + **butorphanol** (0.05 mg/kg) **all in one syringe, administered IM.**

Xylazine (1.1 mg/kg) can be used instead of detomidine, but the effect is shorter lasting. Morphine (0.2–0.3 mg/kg) can also be used in place of detomidine. Allow a good 30 minutes, undisturbed, for it to take effect.

Some people use romifidine (100 µg/kg) instead of detomidine, but romifidine is not licenced for IM use, and when mixed with acepromazine in the same syringe, the mixture will go cloudy ('banana milkshake'). If left, however, the mixture will clear again, and there are anecdotal reports of this cleared mixture being administered IM to good clinical effect.

For wild/feral Equidae, try:

Acepromazine (0.05 mg/kg) + **detomidine** (0.08 mg/kg) + **morphine** (0.5 mg/kg) IM.

For clipper-shy, box-shy, or needle-shy horses, try:

Acepromazine oral gel (35 mg/l): c. 0.15 mg/kg, which is around 2–2.5 ml for a 500 kg horse. The transparent yellow/orange gel should be administered into the cheek pouch, but can also be mixed with food if the horse is head-shy. (It can be difficult to dose animals <200 kg accurately because of problems with the delivery of such small volumes.) Allow at least 40 minutes for the effect to develop, during which time the horse should be left quiet.

Detomidine oromucosal gel (7.6 mg/ml): c. 40 µg/kg, which is around 2.5 ml for a 500 kg horse. The translucent blue gel should be administered sublingually. The horse should be left quiet for a good 30–40 minutes to allow sedation to develop. Detomidine oromucosal gel can also be given at least 40 minutes after acepromazine gel to deepen the sedation.

The role of **reserpine** to 'calm' equidae requires further investigation.

32

Donkeys

LEARNING OBJECTIVES

- To appreciate that donkeys are not just small horses.
- To be aware of the potential difficulties with regard to tracheal intubation and jugular venous cannulation.
- To be aware of the anatomical differences for epidural/extradural injections.
- To be familiar with the differing pharmacokinetics of some NSAIDs.

32.1 Introduction

Donkeys come in three sizes: miniature, standard, and mammoth.

Mule = jack × mare.
Hinny = jenny × stallion.

32.1.1 Normals

- Heart rate 35–55 bpm; respiratory rate 20–35 breaths/minute.
- Horse and pony weigh tapes are not accurate. If appropriate weigh scales are not available, a weight estimator fact sheet can be downloaded from the Donkey Sanctuary website (see Further Reading).
- A five-point body condition scoring system tends to be favoured (see Further Reading).

32.1.2 Key Anatomical and Physiological Variations from Horses

- Donkeys have **relatively thick skin** over the jugular groove, so nicking the skin prior to jugular venous cannula insertion may be required (appropriate cannula sizes would be 14 or 16 g). The well-developed longus colli muscle sometimes obscures the jugular groove.
- Donkeys **have relatively large heads** compared to their bodies, so there is a tendency to over-estimate endotracheal (ET) tube size. However, donkeys also tend to have

disproportionately small tracheas for their size, so it is important to have small ET tubes available.

- The angle of opening of the glottis from the pharynx is more acute than in horses, but the epiglottis is softer and easier to displace (and possibly easier to retrovert, which can obstruct passage of the tube into the trachea). They also have a relatively deep pharyngeal recess and the ET tube tip may get stuck here during attempts to advance it. If difficulty occurs when attempting to pass an orotracheal tube, the nasotracheal route could be tried as an alternative, but the ventral nasal meatus is relatively narrow (compared to that in horses), so, once again, relatively small tubes tend to be more appropriate.
- Donkeys have a larger intracellular fluid compartment: extracellular fluid compartment ratio than horses, which means that, being **desert-adapted**, their packed cell volume (PCV) tends to increase only once dehydration has reached 12–15%.
- Donkeys tend to have faster hepatic (oxidative) metabolism than horses, so the half-lives of many drugs are shorter.
- Donkeys are **prone to hyperlipaemia** if starved or off food, especially for >3 days.
- Auricular arteries are generally preferred for cannulation as they are bigger than mandibular and transverse facial arteries.
- The spinal cord terminates at vertebra Sa2, but the dural meningeal sheath extends to Co1–2. To perform an epidural/extradural injection, you may need to employ a

Veterinary Anaesthesia: Principles to Practice, Second Edition. Alexandra H. A. Dugdale, Georgina Beaumont, Carl Bradbrook, and Matthew Gurney.
© 2020 John Wiley & Sons Ltd. Published 2020 by John Wiley & Sons Ltd.
Companion website: www.wiley.com/go/dugdale/veterinary-anaesthesia

slightly different angle than in horses and you may occasionally, accidentally, puncture the dura to discover cerebrospinal fluid.

32.1.3 Drug Responses

- Some of the literature suggests that donkeys may be more resistant to the effects of anaesthetic agents than horses. This may, however, be due to allometric scaling whereby, because of their relatively larger body surface area compared to body size and weight, they require seemingly higher doses.
- Donkeys are, on the whole, more stoical than horses, and are also prepared to argue the toss as to whether they will do what you require of them or not. That is, they seem more prepared to 'fight' rather than to take the 'fright and flight' option.
- They are less inclined than horses to suffer emergence excitement upon recovery from general anaesthesia, or indeed excitement upon induction of anaesthesia. When they do stand, they get up more like cows (hind end first). (Mules tend to recover more like horses.)
- If the animal is not tame, then it may require a larger dose of sedative, especially regarding the α2 agonists. However, tame donkeys require similar doses of α2 agonists as horses, and the level of sedation produced appears to be dose-dependent.
- The half-life of ketamine is shorter in donkeys than in horses, so if using top-up doses, be prepared to re-dose more frequently.

- The MAC of inhalation agents is similar in donkeys and horses.
- The eyes are 'quieter' under anaesthesia than in horses, and definitely not a reliable indicator of anaesthetic depth.
- Arterial blood pressure seems better maintained in donkeys than in anaesthetised horses and can be used as an indicator of anaesthetic depth.
- Noxious stimuli may result in breath-holding at lighter planes of anaesthesia.
- Non-steroidal anti-inflammatory drugs (NSAIDs): there is much debate about their effectiveness. Meloxicam has a very short half-life. Flunixin and phenylbutazone are metabolised and cleared more rapidly than in horses; however, carprofen is cleared more slowly.

32.1.4 Pain and Pain Recognition

Donkeys demonstrate a greater cerebral cortical response to a noxious stimulus than ponies. Their behavioural expression of pain, however, is subtle and they exhibit a different repertoire of pain behaviours compared to horses, often leading to inadequate analgesia provision through difficulty in pain recognition. Pain-related behaviours that have been identified as very important by veterinary surgeons and owners were: dullness for colic-associated pain; keeping the foot lifted and lameness for foot and limb pain; and inability to chew properly for head and dental pain. Preliminary investigations have also been made into the facial changes associated with pain in donkeys.

Further Reading

Burden, F. (2012). Practical feeding and condition scoring for donkeys and mules. *Equine Veterinary Education* 24: 589–596. **(Includes guide to body condition scoring and equations to estimate body weight.)**.

Burden, F.A., Hazell-Smith, E., Mulugeta, G. et al. (2016). Reference intervals for biochemical and haematological parameters in mature domestic donkeys (Equus asinus) in the UK. *Equine Veterinary Education* 28: 134–139.

Burnham, S.L. (2002). Anatomical differences of the donkey and mule. *Proceedings of the American Association of Equine Practitioners annual convention* 48: 102–109.

Grint, N.J., Johnson, C.B., Clutton, R.E. et al. (2015). Spontaneous electroencephalographic changes in a castration model as an indicator of nociception: a comparison between donkeys and ponies. *Equine Veterinary Journal* 47: 36–42.

Grint, N.J., Whay, H.R., and Murrell, J.C. (2015). Investigating the opinions of donkey owners and veterinary surgeons towards pain and analgesia in donkeys. *Equine Veterinary Education* 27: 365–371.

Hagag, U. and Tawfiek, M.G. (2018). Blind versus ultrasound-guided maxillary nerve block in donkeys. *Veterinary Anaesthesia and Analgesia* 45: 103–110.

Lizarraga, I. and Beths, T. (2012). A comparative study of xylazine induced mechanical hypoalgesia in donkeys and horses. *Veterinary Anaesthesia and Analgesia* 39: 533–538.

Lizarraga, I., Castillo-Alcala, F., Varner, K.M., and Robinson, L.S. (2015). Sedation and mechanical nociception after intravenous administration of detomidine in donkeys: a dose-effect study. *Veterinary Record* 176: 202. https://doi.org/10.1136/vr.102569.

Lucas Castillo, J.A., Gozalo-Marcilla, M., Werneck Fonseca, M. et al. (2018). Sedative and cardiorespiratory effects of low doses of xylazine with and without acepromazine in Nordestino donkeys. *Equine Veterinary Journal* 50: 831–835.

Maloiy, G.M.O. and Boarer, C.D.H. (1971). Response of the Somali donkey to dehydration: hematological changes. *American Journal of Physiology* 221: 37–41.

Matthews, N.S., Peck, K.E., Mealey, K.L. et al. (1997). Pharmacokinetics and cardiopulmonary effects of guaiphenesin in donkeys. *Journal of Veterinary Pharmacology and Therapeutics* 20: 442–446.

Matthews, N. and van Loon, J.P.A.M. (2013). Anaesthesia and analgesia of the donkey and mule. *Equine Veterinary Education* 25: 47–51.

National Equine Welfare Council (NEWC) (2009). *Equine Industry Welfare Guidelines Compendium for Horses, Ponies and Donkeys*, 3rd Edition. *(Includes body condition scoring systems for Equidae.)*

Perez-Ecija, A. and Mendoza, F.J. (2017). Characterisation of clotting factors, anticoagulant protein activities and viscoelastic analysis in healthy donkeys. *Equine Veterinary Journal* 49: 734–738.

Reghan (nee Ashley), F.H., Hockenhull, J., Pritchard, J.C. et al. (2016). Identifying behavioural differences in working donkeys in response to analgesic administration. *Equine Veterinary Journal* 48: 33–38.

Sprayson, T. and Thiemann, A. (2007). Clinical approach to castration in the donkey. *In Practice* 29: 526–531.

VanDierendonck, M.C., Burden, F.A., Rickards, K., and van Loon, J.P.A.M. (2018). Objective pain assessment in donkeys: scale construction. Abstract. *Equine Veterinary Journal* 50 (Suppl. 52): 9.

Yousef, M.K., Dill, D.B., and Mayes, M.G. (1970). Shifts in body fluids during dehydration in the burro, Equus asinus. *Journal of Applied Physiology* 29: 345–349. www.thedonkeysanctuary.org.uk/sites/uk/files/2018-10/donkey-weight-estimator-chart.pdf.

Self-test Section

1 Describe the differences between horses and donkeys that affect endotracheal intubation?

2 True or False? The half-life of ketamine is shorter in donkeys than in horses.

3 True or False? The half-life of carprofen is shorter in donkeys than in horses.

33

Ruminants

Local and General Anaesthesia

LEARNING OBJECTIVES

- To be familiar with the risks of general anaesthesia in ruminants (e.g. regurgitation, aspiration, bloat), and therefore why local/regional anaesthetic techniques +/− sedation tend to be preferred.
- To be able to describe the precautions necessary when having to perform general anaesthesia in ruminants.
- To be able to discuss drug and technique choices.
- To be able to recognise the options for providing analgesia: both systemic and local techniques.

33.1 General Anaesthesia

General anaesthesia in ruminants is associated with several factors that complicate the course of anaesthesia and may even endanger the animal's life. These are due to the effects of both recumbency and anaesthesia itself and include:

- Restraint and handling risks.
- Body weight is often unknown and may be inaccurately estimated.
- Ruminal tympany (bloat).
- Regurgitation of reticuloruminal contents.
- Aspiration of regurgitated material or saliva, leading to aspiration pneumonia.
- Hypoventilation with subsequent hypercapnia and possibly hypoxaemia.
- Hypotension.
- Neuropathy (myopathy is uncommon, especially in the more bony dairy cattle breeds).
- Fluid and electrolyte imbalances (loss of bicarbonate and phosphate in saliva).
- Limited number of licenced drugs.

33.1.1 Reducing the Risks

33.1.1.1 Considerations for Preventing Ruminal Tympany, Regurgitation, and Aspiration
33.1.1.1.1 Pre-operative Starvation
Withholding food from ruminating animals for 18–24 hours reduces the rate of fermentation and the subsequent development of bloat, although the quantity and quality of ingesta also influence the fermentation rate. Starvation for longer than 24 hours may result in ketoacidosis in high production animals, but, alternatively, it can result in alkalosis in less metabolically stressed animals, possibly due to changes in volatile fatty acid production and an increased pH of rumen contents. Body temperature has been shown to decrease in animals starved for over 24 hours, and this is accompanied by a reduction in metabolic rate and changes in pH status. Starvation for longer than 24 hours also results in increased fluidity of rumen contents and increases the likelihood of regurgitation. Furthermore, food withholding in small ruminants (sheep and goats) tends to result in increased water intake and increased fluidity of reticuloruminal contents.

So, is there an ideal duration of food (and water?) withhold? How does this vary with age, species, production-level, and

Veterinary Anaesthesia: Principles to Practice, Second Edition. Alexandra H. A. Dugdale, Georgina Beaumont, Carl Bradbrook, and Matthew Gurney.
© 2020 John Wiley & Sons Ltd. Published 2020 by John Wiley & Sons Ltd.
Companion website: www.wiley.com/go/dugdale/veterinary-anaesthesia

intended surgical intervention? And should it differ for milk-, forage-, and concentrate-based foodstuffs? Ruminants presenting for emergency procedures and for which it has not been possible to deny ad lib access to conserved forage (hay in particular), appear to be less likely to regurgitate under anaesthesia (author's observations), whilst those that have recently eaten a large meal of concentrates are at increased risk of bloating, and those that have had access to copious amounts of fresh forage (particularly spring grass or alfalfa) may be predisposed to regurgitation due to the increased water content of these feedstuffs.

Depending upon the intended surgery, there may be little advantage in denying access to ad lib conserved forage, although the risks of tympany and regurgitation cannot be completely ignored so that a few hours (perhaps 6–12 hours) of food withhold would be appropriate. As for concentrates and large quantities of fresh 'rich' or ensiled, 'wet' forages, until more evidence is gathered, these should possibly be withheld for at least 6–12 hours. For young (pre-ruminating) milk-fed calves, lambs, and kids, milk should not be withheld at all, and creep feeds should probably not be withheld for more than one to two hours. Procedures on the gastrointestinal (GI) tract, however, may require longer pre-operative food (and water?) withholding.

Although it used to be recommended to deny access to water for 12–18 hours in order to reduce reticuloruminal bulk and fermentation rate, dehydration can ensue (packed red cell volume increases). It is now generally recommended that access to clean, fresh water should be available at all times for all ages.

Induction of anaesthesia should, where possible, be swift ('rapid sequence induction') followed by rapid endotracheal (ET) intubation with a cuffed ET tube in order to 'secure the airway' to guard against aspiration. As tympany worsens with increased duration of recumbency/anaesthesia, vigilance is required, especially for longer procedures, but moderate to severe bloat may need relieving at any time during a procedure. Recumbency itself can increase the risk of bloating because the cardia may become 'submerged'. Although left lateral recumbency helps to keep the cardia 'above' the liquid level in the reticulorumen, it prevents access to the left flank to trocarise the rumen if ruminal intubation (by naso- or oro-gastric tube) is unsuccessful in relieving gaseous distension.

33.1.1.1.2 Use of Cuffed ET Tubes

Cuffed ET tubes should always be used because aspiration of saliva or regurgitated reticuloruminal contents is one of the greatest hazards of ruminant anaesthesia and can result in aspiration pneumonitis/pneumonia (known as Mendelson's syndrome in people). **Regurgitation** can be **active** or **passive**. Active regurgitation occurs during light planes of anaesthesia,

whereas passive regurgitation occurs during deeper anaesthesia. Active regurgitation may occur during attempts to intubate the trachea, making intubation a critical occasion during general anaesthesia. To reduce the risk of regurgitated fluid entering the airway during tracheal intubation attempts, it has been suggested to try to maintain the animal in sternal recumbency, with its head held up. This, however, may not always be possible, so if the animal is laterally recumbent, a sand bag or similar can be placed under its head so as to raise its poll, so that the glottis is 'uphill' and hopefully 'above' any saliva or regurgitated liquor that pools under the influence of gravity. Because regurgitation may occur before the airway is secured, the risk of aspiration can be reduced by the following (if it is impossible to lower the animal's head below the level of its body to encourage drainage by gravity):

- Apply 'cricoid pressure' by pushing hard against the larynx in order to squash closed the oesophagus that lies behind it (akin to Sellick's manoeuvre in people). Although this may prevent further regurgitated material from reaching the pharynx, it will not help prevent aspiration of any already regurgitated material which may be near the glottis.
- Place a cuffed ET tube into the oesophagus, inflate the cuff and try to duct any refluxed material away from the pharynx. (It is not easy to achieve correct cuff inflation, however, and regurgitated material tends to stream around the outside of the tube too.) Another cuffed ET tube is then required to intubate the trachea and the space available within the mouth can be limiting for the placement of this.

If, after all these precautions, regurgitated material still enters the airway, drainage under gravity or the use of suction can help to clear it away, but cannot usually guarantee total removal of all the material. There remains debate about whether withholding artificial (manual or mechanical) ventilation, usually in the form of positive pressure ventilation, and therefore relying on the animal's spontaneous breathing efforts, reduces the severity of any subsequent aspiration pneumonia, but this must be weighed against the risks of hypoventilation itself.

33.1.1.1.3 Use of Anticholinergics as 'Drying Agents' (Antisialogogues)

Saliva production is copious: cows produce 50–150 l/day, whereas sheep produce around 10 l/day, depending upon their diet; and **saliva production tends to continue under anaesthesia**. Not only can this be another source of material for aspiration and obstruction of the respiratory tract, but it also represents a substantial fluid loss, and within that fluid, many electrolytes and especially buffers such as bicarbonate and phosphate are lost (so the animal may become acidotic; see below). Although atropine, butylscopolamine (hyoscine butylbromide), and glycopyrrolate will reduce the volume of saliva produced, this is by reducing the watery part of the secretions, so the saliva that is produced is then much more viscous and more difficult to clear from either the animal's throat or indeed its airway if aspiration occurs. Furthermore, these agents reduce mucociliary function, and therefore reduce the clearance of pre-existing mucus/infectious agents from the respiratory tract and also of any aspirated material, which may increase the chances of subclinical infections 'taking hold' and/or of aspiration pneumonitis/pneumonia developing. For these reasons, and their effects on the GI tract (see below), anti-muscarinic-anti-cholinergics are therefore no longer commonly favoured as part of any premedication.

33.1.1.2 Considerations Regarding Hypoventilation

Ruminants **tend to hypoventilate** under general anaesthesia as evidenced by shallow breaths, which are not fully compensated for by the increase in breathing rate that usually occurs. It is therefore common to provide artificial (usually positive pressure) ventilation of their lungs under general anaesthesia (muscle relaxants are not necessary to do this). Tidal volumes of around 10 ml/kg (i.e. 1 l/100 kg body weight), and rates of around 10 breaths per minute make a good starting point, providing that the peak inspiratory pressure does not exceed ~25 cmH$_2$O. Ruminant lungs contain less fibrous connective tissue than horse lungs, so they are more prone to alveolar rupture and pneumothorax if inadvertently high peak airway pressures are delivered during positive pressure ventilation. If end tidal CO$_2$ tension can be monitored, it reflects (but may be lower than) the systemic arterial carbon dioxide partial pressure, and can be used as a guide to the adequacy of ventilation.

Recumbency itself allows the large heavy GI tract to 'press on' the diaphragm, resulting in some 'splinting' of diaphragmatic movements, and thus hypoventilation. (One proposed benefit of pre-operative food/water withhold is to reduce GI bulk in order to minimise this, but because of the effects of recumbency alone, very prolonged starvation may be required to produce noticeable benefits.) General anaesthesia also causes a degree of respiratory depression via, not only a reduction in thoracic and diaphragmatic breathing movements (due to 'muscular relaxation'), but also a reduction in ventilatory drive (because of depression of chemoreceptors, which normally respond to blood CO$_2$ tension and pH). (The hypoxic drive to ventilation is also depressed until or unless moderate-to-severe hypoxaemia occurs.)

Lung volume and functional residual capacity (FRC) are also reduced: by compression of the thoracic cavity by abdominal contents pushing on the diaphragm (during recumbency); by smaller tidal breaths; and by the abolishment of normal sighing and yawning. (FRC is that volume of air remaining in the lungs after a normal tidal exhalation and its presence allows gaseous exchange to continue throughout the end-expiratory pause.) When FRC is reduced, the 'gas reserve' in the lung alveoli is reduced, alveoli and small airways may start to collapse (atelectasis), and ventilation-perfusion mismatches start to develop. Atelectasis is promoted during recumbency and anaesthesia by both compression (recumbency- and muscle relaxation-related), and reabsorption (especially when gas mixtures of high oxygen percentage and excluding highly insoluble gases [e.g. nitrogen] are used). Hypoxic pulmonary vasoconstriction is also blunted by many anaesthetic agents, which further promotes the development of ventilation-perfusion mismatching (see Chapter 8).

33.1.1.3 Considerations Regarding Hypotension

Hypotension is less commonly observed in anaesthetised cattle (compared to anaesthetised horses), except under very deep planes of anaesthesia (usually with inhalation agents). Large doses of xylazine, or inclusion of acepromazine in the premedication can, however, contribute to the development of hypotension. When in dorsal recumbency, the weight of the viscera, particularly the reticulorumen, can compress especially the caudal vena cava, reducing venous return and compromising cardiac output and arterial blood pressure. (Historically, another reason for prolonged pre-operative food/water withholding was to try to reduce this effect, but even very prolonged starvation cannot fully empty the reticulorumen to prevent this.) Why healthy cattle generally maintain better arterial blood pressure than similarly large horses under anaesthesia remains a mystery, but several ideas have been proposed:

- Because cattle hypoventilate under general anaesthesia, hypercapnia develops and this stimulates the sympathetic nervous system, so that overall there is gentle cardiovascular stimulation. This sounds good, but when artificial ventilation is instituted to maintain normocapnia, cattle can still maintain near 'normal' blood pressures (even despite the often-detrimental cardiovascular effects of the positive pressure ventilation). Furthermore, variation in P$_a$CO$_2$ has complex and variable effects on blood pressure.
- Vagal activity appears to predominate in conscious cattle and is actually further enhanced by starvation (i.e. slower heart rates are observed in starved [especially >48 hours] cattle), whereas general anaesthesia may change the autonomic balance so that sympathetic activity predominates. (This suggestion has not yet been proven or disproven.)

Should hypotension develop (definitions differ, but commonly a mean arterial pressure less than 70 mmHg), then attention to the depth of anaesthesia, reduction of the peak inspiratory pressure created by positive pressure ventilation, intravenous fluid therapy, and the use of positive inotropes and vasopressors can be considered, similar to other species. Vasopressors and positive inotropes, however, are not yet licenced for use in any veterinary species, so they can only be administered to food producing animals under the 'cascade' in the UK.

33.1.1.4 Considerations Regarding Patient Positioning

Post-anaesthetic myopathy is not common in cattle, especially the more bony dairy type breeds. Prolonged postoperative recumbency, however, may be associated with hypocalcaemia, especially in peri-parturient cattle. Neuropathies are more common than myopathies, especially in the more bony milking breeds, and occur if the animal is poorly positioned, insufficient padding is used over bony prominences, and/or recumbency is prolonged. Careful padding and positioning are therefore important as in horses. It is also important to protect the patient from heat and cold, especially if outdoors, and also to protect the eyes from dust, debris, and direct sunlight.

33.1.1.5 Considerations Regarding Fluid and Electrolyte Losses

Saliva (which is rich in buffers) continues to be produced during anaesthesia, but cannot be swallowed, so tends to flow from the mouth and is lost. Regurgitation of reticuloruminal contents may also occur, exacerbating fluid and electrolyte losses during anaesthesia.

Intravenous crystalloids, usually Hartmann's solution, are commonly administered at around 3–5 ml/kg/h, but if surgery is unduly prolonged, then electrolytes and pH should be monitored, and any derangements treated as necessary, paying particular attention to calcium, magnesium, and bicarbonate (and possibly phosphate). Saliva and any regurgitated material can be collected in a bucket placed beneath the animal's head (which is lowered/tilted slightly downwards) and can be returned to the animal by stomach tube at the end of the procedure.

33.2 Sedation/Premedication

For all the drugs mentioned in this chapter, it is important to be familiar with which products are licenced for use in food-producing farm animals in your country of practice.

Ruminants tend to be much more docile than horses and may be amenable to standing surgery under local/regional anaesthesia without sedation. Sedation, however, may reduce the stress response to surgery, and systemic analgesia should be provided for standing surgical techniques. Sedation and/or analgesia may also be required to increase both patient and operator safety.

Similarly, whilst premedication may be thought unnecessary in docile animals, it can reduce the dosage requirements of both anaesthetic induction and maintenance agents and provide systemic analgesia. Although ruminants do not tend to suffer from emergence excitement during recovery from anaesthesia, the residual effects of premedication after short-ish anaesthetics may help to smooth the recovery process, or further sedation and analgesia can be administered if required.

33.2.1 Xylazine

Xylazine is an $\alpha2$ adrenoreceptor agonist, and as such is a sedative-analgesic with muscle relaxant properties. It is licenced for cattle in the UK. It may be administered intramuscularly, intravenously, or subcutaneously (but different manufacturers' recommendations may vary), and its effects are dose-dependent, although they can be a little unpredictable, especially in previously 'excited' animals. Ruminants are more 'sensitive' to xylazine than horses (possibly because long-acting active metabolites are produced, and also due to differences in post-receptor signalling between species), so the 2% solution is preferred over the 10% solution for more accurate dosing volumes. Xylazine should be used with care in pregnant ruminants because of its potential to increase uterine tone and possibly compromise uteroplacental perfusion, with the worry that it might cause abortion in the last trimester (see below). Its safety during embryogenesis in the first trimester has not yet been proven.

In cattle, the dose range is 0.05–0.3 mg/kg IM or 0.03–0.1 mg/kg IV. The degree of sedation is dose-dependent such that once the dose increases above 0.1 mg/kg IM, recumbency (sternal to lateral), usually occurs. Generally, about one-third of the IM dose will produce the same effect if administered IV.

In sheep and goats, which may be more difficult to dose accurately (or perhaps are even more 'sensitive'), doses range between 0.05 mg/kg to 0.1 mg/kg IM, or not more than 0.05 mg/kg IV. If patients become recumbent, attempts should be made to elevate the poll to encourage saliva to drain away from the pharynx/larynx.

33.2.2 Detomidine

Detomidine is another $\alpha2$ agonist, but is more $\alpha2$-selective than xylazine. It is licenced for use in cattle in the UK at doses of 10–40 μg/kg IM or IV: the degree of sedation is dose-dependent, but recumbency cannot always be guaranteed at the higher doses. Manufacturers caution against its use in the last trimester of pregnancy for similar reasons to xylazine (see above, but also below).

33.2.3 Effects of α2 Agonists

- Xylazine and high dose (40–60 μg/kg) detomidine, but not low dose (20 μg/kg) detomidine, increase uterine tone (and intra-uterine pressure) in both non-pregnant and pregnant cattle and sheep, but without causing synchronised uterine contractions. However, they may also vasoconstrict the utero-placental blood vessels, and reduce both maternal and foetal cardiac output, thereby possibly compromising uteroplacental perfusion and foetal viability. Their oxytocin-like ecbolic actions have been suggested to increase the risk of abortion, so manufacturers warn to avoid their use, if possible, in the last trimester of pregnancy. That said, low dose detomidine has no effect on (or even reduces) intra-uterine pressure in pregnant cattle, so may be preferable to xylazine if sedation is absolutely required. Acepromazine, although not licenced, has been suggested as an alternative sedative for pregnant cattle.
- Reduce reticuloruminal activity and increase the chance of tympany because they reduce eructation. (Interestingly, diarrhoea may be observed 12–24 hours after sedation.)
- May (controversial) reduce cardiac sphincter tone, so may increase the likelihood of regurgitation.
- Reduce swallowing, leading to pharyngeal accumulation of saliva and regurgitated material that increases the risk of aspiration. Animals tend to drool saliva because swallowing is reduced, not because saliva production is increased (in fact, saliva production is somewhat reduced by these drugs).
- Reduce laryngeal activity, which increases the risk of aspiration.
- Cause diuresis. Interestingly, glycosuria is a more common feature in cattle than, e.g. in horses, so a component of the diuresis is due to an osmotic diuresis, in addition to reduced antidiuretic hormone secretion and activity (see Chapters 4 and 28).
- Reduce gastrointestinal motility by reducing acetylcholine release from the presynaptic terminals of post-ganglionic parasympathetic fibres in the gut wall. There are presynaptic α2 receptors on these cholinergic nerve endings, and presynaptic α2 receptor activity is enhanced by α2 agonists, which results in a reduction of transmitter release (in this case, acetylcholine).
- Increase airway resistance (due to bronchoconstriction) and may cause pulmonary hypertension, especially in small ruminants (sheep and goats). This may result in the development of pulmonary oedema, which can be

one of the many causes of hypoxaemia under general anaesthesia. This can be severe enough to be fatal. Low doses are therefore advised in sheep and goats, and also in animals that have, or have had, respiratory infections. If any signs of pulmonary oedema develop, antagonism (e.g. with atipamezole) is recommended as soon as possible, as it appears to become refractory to treatment after about 10 minutes.
- Hypertension is rarely detected following the IM administration of α2 agonists, but bradycardia and hypotension (especially with repeated or higher doses) can be observed.
- Repeated doses of xylazine over several days are accompanied by the development of tolerance to the drug. This could be due to α2 receptor down-regulation/desensitisation, or to the induction of hepatic microsomal enzymes for its metabolism. Repeated doses of xylazine given over minutes-hours may not deepen the level of sedation and may even result in increased excitatory effects, thought to be due to increasing α1 agonist activity, which can overcome the sedative effects of α2 agonism.
- Effects on thermoregulation have been variously described, with both increases and decreases in rectal temperature observed for several hours following xylazine administration.

33.2.4 Atipamezole

Although atipamezole is not licenced for use in ruminants, it is useful to antagonise sedation and shorten post-operative recumbency following α2 agonists. Doses of 20–50 μg/kg IM (or slow IV) are usually suggested.

33.2.5 Acepromazine

Not licenced for use in ruminants. Reduces cardiac sphincter tone, so increases the likelihood of regurgitation.

33.2.6 Atropine, Hyoscine Butylbromide, and Glycopyrrolate

Neither atropine nor glycopyrrolate is licenced for use in ruminants although, according to European Union (EU) regulations (EU Commission Regulation No.37/2010), atropine and butylscopolamine (hyoscine butylbromide) may be used in all food producing species and no MRL is required. These drugs all reduce both the upper and lower oesophageal sphincter tone and may facilitate reflux and regurgitation, but they also reduce overall gut motility and thereby possibly encourage the development of bloat. The ruminant dose for atropine is variously quoted as 0.02–0.1 mg/kg IV. The ruminant dose for glycopyrrolate is suggested to be c. 2–5 μg/kg IV.

33.2.7 Benzodiazepines

There are no licenced benzodiazepines for use in food producing animals. Diazepam and midazolam, however, are the most commonly available and cause minimal cardiovascular and respiratory depression. They can be very useful when administered alone for the sedation of young and small ruminants and produce dose-dependent central nervous system (CNS) depression from anxiolysis to sedation. They also produce muscle relaxation due to a central action in the spinal cord (and brainstem), where they inhibit the reflex spinal relay that normally helps to maintain postural muscle strength. Ruminants tend not to panic at the feeling of muscular weakness, but rather give in to it and become recumbent if high enough doses are given. Occasionally, however, animals may become 'excited' due to disinhibition. Appetite may also be stimulated (as sometimes is seen in small animals).

Quoted dose rates vary widely, from 0.02–0.25 mg/kg IV and even up to 0.5 mg/kg IV. Lower doses are favoured in mature cattle, possibly because diazepam has been blamed for increased salivation and ruminal atony. However, as the oesophagus of ruminants (and dogs) is all striated muscle, and, at least in dogs, diazepam increases lower oesophageal sphincter tone and may reduce the incidence of reflux/regurgitation, this is a potential advantage in ruminants also.

The higher dose rates can be used alone for sedation of calves, sheep, and goats for non-painful procedures such as radiography; e.g. 0.25–0.5 mg/kg diazepam or midazolam IV gives recumbent sedation in sheep, goats, and calves.

Diazepam has poor bioavailability if administered IM, but midazolam can be administered by this route. Although midazolam is said to be twice as potent as diazepam and shorter acting, the two are often difficult to distinguish clinically, so similar doses are used.

Benzodiazepines, at 0.05–0.1 mg/kg IV, are a useful adjunct to ketamine anaesthesia to provide some skeletal muscular relaxation to counteract the increased muscular tone associated with ketamine. (Similarly, guaiphenesin, also known as glyceryl guaiacolate ether [GGE] or glyceryl guaiacolate [GG], may be used alongside ketamine; see later.)

Benzodiazepines are also useful anticonvulsants.

33.2.8 Opioids

Opioids enhance the sedative effects of benzodiazepines, and the sedative and analgesic effects of $\alpha2$ agonists. Opioids tend to slow gut motility (by reducing propulsive peristalsis) and may reduce lower oesophageal sphincter tone. (See later under epidural analgesia.) None is licenced for use in farm animal species in the UK, but, of all the opioids available, butorphanol is the most commonly administered under the 'cascade' to provide analgesia and sedation in addition to that provided by $\alpha2$ agonists.

- Butorphanol is a useful adjunct to $\alpha2$ agonists or benzodiazepines, providing sedation and analgesia (especially at the higher doses). Dose 0.02–0.05 (to 0.1) mg/kg IV; or up to 0.2 mg/kg IM.
- Buprenorphine 0.006–0.03 mg/kg IV or IM (N.B. buprenorphine has a relatively short duration of action in sheep and goats, but work on a slow-release formulation has shown promise).
- Morphine 0.1–0.3 mg/kg IM (care with the IV route because of a small risk of histamine release).
- Methadone 0.25 mg/kg IM or IV.
- Pethidine 3.5–5 mg/kg IM (avoid IV injection because of the risk of histamine release).

33.3 Intravenous Access

If possible, intravenous access should be secured by placing an IV cannula prior to anaesthetic induction with injectable agents. Premedication/sedation may facilitate this. Bovine skin is often very thick and very mobile, so long cannulae are preferred to try to ensure that at least the tip remains in the vein should the animal move freely. In cows, the jugular vein, or occasionally the 'milk vein' (cranial superficial epigastric vein) are useful sites for IV access. In bulls, it is often very difficult to find jugular veins through the thick, mobile neck skin and subcutaneous tissues, so that a 'cut-down' approach may be required. However, locating the jugular vein may also be dangerous to personnel if the animal is restrained in a neck-yoke, but maintains the ability to slide its neck forwards and backwards and/or up and down through the yoke. The auricular veins may offer a useful alternative site for venous access, after first ensuring that the animal is adequately sedated and/or its head is secured through a neck-yoke and then restrained gently to one side, facilitating access to the opposite ear. Once a venous cannula is in place, an extension set can be useful to reduce its dislodgement potential should the patient fidget excessively during subsequent drug administration.

33.4 Anaesthetic Induction

Anaesthesia can be induced with injectable drugs, administered by either the intravenous or intramuscular route, or by inhalational techniques. (See also chapters 5 and 8.)

33.4.1 Ketamine

Ketamine, an arylcyclohexylamine, is a dissociative anaesthetic, analgesic, and anti-hyperalgesic due to its non-competitive antagonism at NMDA receptors (amongst other actions). It is now licenced for use in cattle, sheep, goats, and pigs in the UK and can be administered either IV or IM. Following IV administration, ketamine usually results in induction of anaesthesia within 1–2 minutes, whereas 5–10 minutes must be allowed if the IM route is used.

The dose required for induction of anaesthesia is 2–5 mg/kg by either route. After α2 agonist premedication, the lower end of the dose range (2–2.5 mg/kg) is usually sufficient, whereas if no premedication is given, or poor sedation is achieved after premedication, doses of 4.5–5+ mg/kg may be required. When larger doses are given, the duration of effect is longer before a top-up may be required. Ketamine is analgesic at sub-anaesthetic doses, e.g. 0.1–0.5 mg/kg IM or SC. (Occasionally transient excitement or even recumbency can be seen with these relatively small doses if given rapidly IV.)

Although ketamine preserves, and even enhances, cranial nerve reflexes (e.g. gag and swallowing), it will not guarantee a protected airway, especially if an α2 agonist was included in the premedication (i.e. the trachea should be intubated with a cuffed ET tube to ensure a protected airway). Sometimes the increased muscle tone that ketamine causes will make ET intubation difficult, hence α2 agonists, benzodiazepines, or GG (which provide a degree of muscular relaxation) are useful adjuncts. Although ketamine itself tends not to alter lower oesophageal sphincter tone, the other agents used alongside it often reduce cardiac sphincter tone and increase the risk of reflux/regurgitation. Ketamine does, however, tend to increase salivation.

Ketamine can be administered in combination with other drugs, e.g. GG and an α2 agonist, as an IV infusion for maintenance of general anaesthesia. Care is required if xylazine is chosen for such a combination, with doses around 1/10th those suggested for horses (see Chapter 31) because of the increased sensitivity of cattle to xylazine compared with horses.

Although ketamine tends to produce minimal cardiovascular depression in healthy animals, it does cause direct myocardial depression (negative inotropy) and vasodilation, but this is not usually noticeable because it also stimulates the sympathetic nervous system. However, in animals where the sympathetic nervous system is already working hard, or is even exhausted, e.g. in very excited or shocky animals, ketamine's administration may well result in some hypotension and reduced cardiac output because of the reduced sympathetic reserve.

Ketamine produces minimal respiratory depression, but will cause post-induction apnoea after rapid IV bolus injection; and occasionally irregular breathing patterns or apneustic breathing (end-inspiratory pauses) may be observed.

33.4.2 Guaiphenesin

Guaiphenesin, also known as glyceryl guaiacolate (GG) or glyceryl guaiacolate ether (alternatively, guaiacol glyceryl ether) (GGE), like the benzodiazepines, is a centrally acting skeletal muscle relaxant, with some sedative, but no analgesic, properties. (It is referred to as GG from here on.) Central muscle relaxation (of postural, skeletal muscles) is due to blockade of internuncial neurotransmission in the spinal cord, brainstem, and sub-cortical areas of the brain. The formulations of GG currently available for horses (10 and 15% solutions) can be diluted in 5% dextrose or dextrose-saline solutions, but are not licenced for use in food producing animals.

GG must be administered IV and preferably via a pre-placed IV cannula, which must be flushed before removal because GG is extremely irritant if extravascular or transvascular deposition occurs. It can also cause haemolysis, the haemolytic threshold in solutions without 'stabilisers' (glucose or fructose) being around 8–10% in cattle. Therefore, solutions of 5% should be used for cattle and administered to effect.

Usual doses are 30–100 mg/kg. It is cumulative, and high doses can cause problems (see below), so a maximum dose of 100–150 mg/kg should not be exceeded in any 24 hour period. If doses in excess of 150 mg/kg are given, recoveries can be prolonged and cardiac arrhythmias, CNS 'excitement reactions' (seizure-like activity/opisthotonos/paradoxical muscle rigidity), and apneustic breathing patterns (end-inspiratory pause rather than the normal end-expiratory pause) can all occur. 'Excitement' may be due to one of its metabolites, catechol, or at least a compound with cross-reactivity to catechol (reminiscent of catecholamines). It can be administered along with either thiopental or ketamine for induction and/or maintenance of anaesthesia (up to 1[–2] hours' duration), or can be administered during anaesthesia to improve muscular relaxation, e.g. for relocation of dislocated hips or shoulders.

33.4.3 Barbiturates

Thiopental sodium, an ultra-short acting barbiturate, is the sodium salt of thiobarbituric acid, which, because of keto-enol tautomerism is only soluble in aqueous solution at very alkaline pH (around 10.5). It is therefore very irritant if extravascular deposition occurs, necessitating placement of an IV cannula that must be flushed before removal. Sodium thiopental exists as a racemic mixture of two unstable structural isomers (the keto and enol forms), called tautomers, with a predominance of the enol (water soluble) form at pH 10.5 (in solution in the bottle). With a pKa of 7.6, however, once injected into the body (blood pH around 7.4), the two isomers become present in more or less equal quantities: the keto form being more lipid-soluble, whereas the enol form is more water-soluble. This increased availability of the lipid-soluble keto isomer, which can rapidly cross the blood brain barrier to reach its effect site within the CNS (it is a dose-dependent positive allosteric modulator and direct agonist of $GABA_A$ receptors), means that anaesthetic induction is rapid (within about 30–50 seconds) and it is relatively easy to judge the adequacy of dosing.

Thiopental is not currently available under veterinary licence in the UK, but a veterinary product in Australia (which is licenced for dogs, cats, horses, cattle, sheep, and pigs) may be imported under a Special Treatment Certificate from the Veterinary Medicines Directorate. In the EU, thiopental can be used in all food producing animals and no MRL is required.

If a total dose much in excess of 15–25 mg/kg is administered, then recovery will be prolonged, but, without premedication, doses up to 15 mg/kg may be required: therefore, premedication is advised where possible in order to reduce the required dose to 5–10 mg/kg. Thiopental can also be combined with, or used after, GG to reduce the dose of thiopental necessary. Because initial recovery depends upon redistribution into muscles and fat (metabolism is slow), high doses are best avoided in young or debilitated animals (with relatively little body fat and poor muscling).

Thiopental causes mild cardiovascular and respiratory depression. The cardiovascular depression results in hypotension, which is partly compensated for by a reflex (albeit somewhat damped) tachycardia. Occasional arrhythmias may be seen (thiopental sensitises the myocardium to the arrhythmogenic effects of catecholamines).

33.4.4 Propofol

Propofol, a positive allosteric modulator of $GABA_A$ receptors, is a substituted phenol, and, being insoluble in water, is most commonly presented as a macro-emulsion in Intralipid™. Although not irritant if deposited extravascularly, it must be administered IV (preferably via an IV cannula) in order to induce anaesthesia, because its rapid metabolism prevents a sufficiently rapid increase in effect-site concentration to induce anaesthesia following absorption after non-IV (e.g. IM) administration. Not currently licenced for use in food producing animals in the UK, it can, however, be used according to the 'cascade'. The dose required for induction of anaesthesia is 2–6 mg/kg, but can be reduced by premedication. Administration relatively

slowly and 'to effect' (i.e. over one to two minutes, if circumstances allow safe administration this slowly) can further reduce the required dose compared with a fast bolus technique (i.e. over ~5 seconds). Such dose reduction also reduces the side effects of mild-to-moderate hypotension due to vasodilation and negative inotropy (usually without any reflex tachycardia), and post-induction apnoea (which can last for several minutes). However, the required injection volumes are expensive for large patients, and they are also unwieldy and impractical. That said, it can be a useful drug in smaller patients, although death has been reported following its use in some breeds of goat.

33.4.5 Alfaxalone (Alfaxan™)

This neuro-active steroid, which is also a dose-dependent positive allosteric modulator and agonist of $GABA_A$ receptors, is not yet licenced for use in farm animals in the UK, and, currently, animals that have been given alfaxalone must never be intended for human consumption. Alfaxalone is, however, an excellent short-acting injectable anaesthetic agent that can be administered IV (and also IM in smaller patients), and has undergone extensive research in sheep and goats with promising results for both anaesthetic induction and maintenance. Should it become licenced, it will offer an excellent alternative to propofol for, e.g. anaesthetising goat kids to enable disbudding. (Preliminary data suggest doses of 3–5 mg/kg, but analgesia must also be provided as alfaxalone has no inherent analgesic activity.)

33.5 Anaesthetic Induction Using Inhalation Agents

This is possible most commonly in smaller ruminants via either face-mask or via nasopharyngeal insufflation after passage of a nasopharyngeal tube. Oro- or naso-tracheal intubation may also be possible after sedation or premedication, thus facilitating administration of inhalation agents with minimal environmental pollution.

Volatile agents can be administered, usually in oxygen, by mask to anaesthetise goat kids for disbudding, but beware of the high oxygen concentration in the presence of a hot disbudding iron. Precautions must therefore be taken to make an effective seal around the mask (e.g. wet cotton wool if a rubber diaphragm is not available to help seal the mask around the muzzle), and clip away or dampen down the hair around the horn buds to reduce the risk of ignition of the hair should oxygen leakage occur. Alternatively, the mask can be removed briefly for the moments of actual disbudding to reduce the risk of setting fire to the hair. Injectable techniques may, however, be preferable.

33.5.1 Halogenated Anaesthetic Agents

None of these agents is licenced for use in food producing farm animals in Europe, although isoflurane can be used under the 'cascade'. Isoflurane is a halogenated ether derivative of relatively low blood and fat solubility: these properties enabling relatively rapid change of anaesthetic depth (including induction and recovery). It is minimally metabolised (~0.2%) by the liver such that recovery from anaesthesia is mainly dependent upon its exhalation. It causes dose-dependent cardiorespiratory depression, with hypotension being mainly due to vasodilation as it causes minimal negative inotropic effects on the heart. It does not sensitise the heart to the arrhythmogenic effects of catecholamines. Hypoventilation may require ventilatory support. The MAC of isoflurane is 1.25% in mature cattle. For further information, see Chapter 8.

33.5.2 Nitrous Oxide

Beware the use of nitrous oxide in mature ruminants for long procedures as it will partition into 'low-solubility-gas'-filled spaces to increase their volume or pressure. It may therefore encourage the formation of ruminal tympany because the rumen contains methane and hydrogen (both of which are less soluble in the blood than N_2O), so N_2O enters the rumen quicker than either of these two gases can leave. High intra-abdominal pressure can compromise both venous return (and therefore cardiac output), and diaphragmatic movements through 'diaphragmatic splinting' (resulting in hypoventilation).

33.6 Breathing Systems

For small lambs and kids (<10 kg), a T-piece or mini-Lack may be appropriate, although modern circle systems (with their smaller diameter and smooth-bore tubing, small absorber canisters, low-resistance one-way valves, and small rebreathing bags) can offer a very suitable alternative. For animals between 10 and 135 kg, standard small animal circles can be used, but the capacity of the rebreathing bag should be appropriate for the size of patient (it should have a volume of at least twice the animal's normal, resting tidal volume), and the absorber canister should also have a capacity of at least twice the animal's normal tidal volume. For animals >135 kg, a large animal circle (or To and Fro) is more appropriate, again paying attention to the capacity of rebreathing bag (the largest available have capacities of around 20–50 l). Ensure that there is an appropriately sized ET tube connector available to connect the ET tube to the circle's Y-piece.

33.7 ET Intubation

Deep sedation with muscle relaxation after α2 agonists (and possibly after benzodiazepines) may be sufficient to allow ET intubation. Usually, however, administration of an anaesthetic induction agent is required.

To facilitate ET intubation of calves, goats, and sheep, the patient may be kept in sternal recumbency with the head raised by assistants. The head/neck angle is then straightened, and a gag is placed in the mouth, or tapes are used, to open the jaw. A laryngoscope with a long straight blade is useful to help visualise the larynx. The labial fissure is small, as is the degree of mouth opening, so a laryngoscope is highly recommended. Although not a strictly correct way of using the laryngoscope, the tip of the blade *may* be used to gently depress the tip of the epiglottis in order to improve visualisation of the glottis. An ET tube introducer/bougie/stylette is often helpful. (See below regarding use of topical laryngeal local anaesthetic in sheep and goats.)

An alternative technique is that of 'blind intubation'. For this, the animal of often in lateral recumbency with the head and neck extended. Straight ET tubes are often easier to use than curved tubes. The ET tube is passed through the mouth to the pharynx, then the larynx is 'held' externally with one hand, whilst the other hand attempts to advance the tube; thus the tube can be manoeuvred into and through the larynx whilst simultaneously manipulating the larynx over the tube. A final technique for tracheal intubation in these smaller ruminants is to restrain them on a table in dorsal recumbency with the head hanging over the edge of the table. This position enables the head and neck to be easily extended and also allows any regurgitated material to drain away from the glottis, but operator eye/face protection should be worn to protect them against drooled saliva and regurgitated material.

Sheep and goats have more sensitive larynges than cattle, so application of a little short-acting topical local anaesthetic (by spray or deposition of a small volume of solution down the ET tube after its tip is located just at the larynx) is necessary to facilitate tracheal intubation. If the surgical procedure is short and the larynx has been desensitised with topical local anaesthetic, be vigilant during the recovery from anaesthesia because the laryngeal reflexes may still be numbed, so laryngeal protection may be poor. However, as tracheal extubation is not usually performed until the animal is actively swallowing and chewing at the very least (and the actual trachea itself should still be sensitive to foreign material so the cough reflex should be minimally impaired), use of topical local anaesthetic on the larynx should not create any great problems.

ET intubation in mature cattle can be attempted either in sternal recumbency with the head held up (to try to mini-mise the risk of aspiration should regurgitation occur), or, as is often more practical, in lateral recumbency (where the risk of aspiration of regurgitated material before the airway can be 'secured' is greater). In either position, the ET intuba-tion itself is usually achieved by digital (per-oral) palpation of the larynx and manually-guided passage of the ET tube into the trachea. One or two Drinkwater gag/s can be placed to reduce the chance of bite-injury from sharp cheek teeth, and also to help preserve the integrity of the ET tube and its cuff. Room to manoeuvre an arm and the ET tube inside the mouth is often limited because of the relatively narrow labial fissure and lingual torus. Cattle seem much less prone to laryngospasm than other species, such that gentle palpation of the epiglottis seems only to elicit wiggling of the tongue-tip, and a lubricated ET tube can usually be easily advanced through the larynx and into the trachea. As soon as the ET tube is in place, the cuff should be inflated.

Another way of facilitating ET intubation is to first advance a stomach tube (smaller diameter than the intended ET tube) via the mouth into the trachea (often easier if the head–neck axis is kept straight). The stomach tube's position in the airway is then verified (you may see condensation forming inside the tube with each exhaled breath, or feel air movements through the tube with breath-ing, or check with capnography). Then the ET tube is advanced ('railroaded') 'over' the stomach tube, using the stomach tube as a guide. Once the ET tube is in place, the cuff should be inflated and the stomach tube withdrawn.

Whenever tracheal intubation is undertaken, it is impor-tant to be aware of the risks of regurgitation (both passive and active) and subsequent aspiration. Laryngeal spasm/ obstruction may occasionally be provoked by intubation attempts, but is usually recognised and can be promptly remedied (by deepening the plane of anaesthesia, applying topical local anaesthetic, using a smaller ET tube with introducer, or providing an emergency airway if necessary etc.). Less noticeable (unless heart rate and blood pressure are monitored during this time period), is the autonomic response to laryngeal stimulation that can either be that of sympathetic stimulation (not normally too much of a prob-lem, as it is usually transient) or that of a parasympathetic (vagal) response, which can be profound enough to result in bradycardia to the point of asystole.

33.8 Positioning

Positioning is often dictated by surgery. If lateral recum-bency is required, elevation of the poll, to encourage drainage of saliva and refluxed material away from the

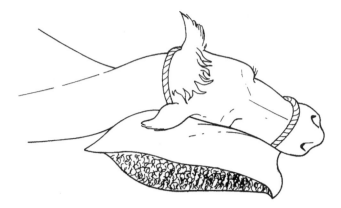

Figure 33.1 Cow's head inclined over a support to allow saliva and regurgitated material to freely drain out of the mouth. *Source:* Reproduced from Hall et al. (2001) with permission from Elsevier.

pharynx, is recommended (Figure 33.1), or perhaps a gentle head-down tilt. The upper limbs should also be supported so that they are parallel with those on the table or ground. If general anaesthesia is performed in the 'field', it is important to protect the eyes from direct sun-light, dirt, and trauma; and remember that animals, espe-cially black-coated, can get heatstroke if left for hours in full sun.

33.9 Maintenance of Anaesthesia

Anaesthesia may be maintained by injectable agents, given IV either as intermittent boluses or by infusion tech-niques (e.g. GG/ketamine/xylazine or GG/thiopental type combinations), but be aware of the total doses given because recovery may be prolonged and its quality com-promised by large cumulative doses. If anaesthesia is to be maintained by injectable agents, the airway must still be protected, and the provision of supplemental oxygen should be considered.

If anaesthesia is to be maintained by injectable agents, ketamine top-ups or infusion (in combination with xyla-zine) are the most common techniques. Ketamine top-up boluses can be given either every 10 minutes by the clock or when the patient is deemed to require another dose. Top-up doses are usually of the order of 1/4–1/2 the original induction dose, with the first top-up dose being nearer 1/2 the original induction dose, and subse-quent top-up doses being reduced in order to minimise drug accumulation that tends to impact on recovery quality.

If a GG/ketamine/xylazine combination is permitted for maintenance of anaesthesia, then to 500 ml of 5% GG, add 500 mg ketamine and 25 mg xylazine. This results in a solution of 50 mg/ml GG, 1 mg/ml ketamine, and 0.05 mg/ml xylazine. It is infused 'to effect', with a rough starting guide being 1 ml/kg/hour. For a 500 kg animal and a giving set that delivers 20 drops/ml, this is roughly 3 drops/second.

If GG is omitted, then to a 500 ml bag of normal saline, add 500 mg ketamine and 25 mg xylazine. Again, this results in a solution containing 1 mg/ml ketamine and 0.05 mg/ml xylazine. The starting infusion rate is also around 1 ml/kg/hour, i.e. about 3 drops/second.

Anaesthesia may also be maintained by inhalational techniques with one of the halogenated agents being supplied in oxygen-enriched carrier gas/es. None is licenced for farm animals in the UK, although isoflurane can be used according to the 'cascade' as it is licenced for use in horses. A combination of inhalation and injectable agents may also be used, similar to the partial (or supplemental) intravenous anaesthesia techniques used in horses and small animals. Choosing minimally cumulative injectable agents and inhalation agents with low blood (and preferably also low fat) solubility can help to avoid unduly prolonged recoveries.

33.10 Monitoring the Anaesthetised Patient

See Chapter 18. Eyeball position is an excellent indicator of anaesthetic depth in cattle, but is less reliable in sheep and goats. The eyeball rotates ventrally between the animal being awake and being lightly anaesthetised. As anaesthesia deepens, it rotates back centrally, but palpebral and pupillary reflexes are absent and lacrimation is reduced. As anaesthesia is lightened, the changes occur in the reverse order, i.e. from deep to lighter anaesthesia, the eyeball moves from central to ventrally rotated; and from light anaesthesia to awake, it moves from the downwards rotated position to central again. Lacrimation increases and palpebral reflexes become more active as the depth of anaesthesia decreases.

Other monitoring is as for small animals (see Chapter 18), e.g. heart rate, pulse rate (auricular, radial, femoral, or metatarsal arteries), breathing rate (although artificial ventilation is often required), mucous membrane colour, and capillary refill time and temperature (especially for young and small patients) should form part of basic monitoring. Pulse oximetry, capnography, electrocardiography, arterial blood pressure, and blood gases and electrolytes can also be monitored if the equipment is available. Neonates should be monitored closely for the development of hypoglycaemia and hypothermia.

33.11 Recovery

Recoveries are usually smooth due to the placid temperament of these animals. The head should be positioned so that drainage of fluid etc. from the mouth is possible (i.e. elevate the poll above the nose/mouth during lateral recumbency, Figure 33.1). Aim to get the patient into sternal recumbency as soon as possible because whilst in lateral recumbency, there is risk of regurgitation and also of the development of bloat. Usually left lateral is considered better than right lateral to discourage bloat (i.e. encourage eructation) because the cardia is less likely to be submerged by reticuloruminal liquor. Left lateral recumbency, however, denies access to the rumen for trocarisation (using a needle or trocar) should this be required (e.g. if passing a stomach tube does not help to relieve ruminal tympany).

The ET tube is usually left in place and with the cuff inflated for as long as the animal tolerates it, and until the pharyngeal/laryngeal reflexes have returned. The ET tube may then be either fully withdrawn with the cuff still inflated, or, if the inflated cuff gets stuck at the larynx, partial, or full cuff deflation may be required to facilitate tracheal extubation.

33.12 Analgesia

Several surveys from the early 2000s highlighted the under-provision of analgesia for farm animals following a wide variety of surgeries. Reasons for this appeared to include: the difficulty in assessing pain in farm animals, which, as prey species, tend not to display overt signs of pain; concerns regarding the side effects of analgesic drugs; and financial constraints. Increased education, supported by veterinary anaesthesia colleges and associations, and continuing research have, however, begun to turn this tide. Furthermore, validated pain scores are now available for cattle and sheep and a sheep grimace scale has also recently been published, all of which should improve the objectivity of pain assessment and enable evaluation of efficacy of the chosen analgesic treatment/s.

In the UK in 2017, a joint consensus statement between the British Cattle Veterinary Association and the British Veterinary Association recommended administration of a non-steroidal anti-inflammatory drug (NSAID), in addition to the use of local anaesthesia, to all calves undergoing disbudding or castration. Most NSAIDs, however, are not safety tested for use in young animals (i.e. most likely to be undergoing such husbandry procedures), and care must be taken to ensure that they are healthy and unlikely to be or become dehydrated. It is also now widely recognised that parturition, mastitis, lameness, and many other illnesses and infectious conditions can be associated with significant pain.

Wherever possible, 'balanced analgesia' should be practised, that is, the use of several analgesic drugs with different, but complementary, mechanisms of action that produce an overall optimum effect, whilst possibly allowing reduced doses of each drug (because of synergism) and therefore reduced side effects. Consider opioids, local anaesthetics, NSAIDs, α2 agonists, and ketamine.

The following NSAIDs are licenced for cattle in the UK, but *not* for sheep or goats (although meloxicam appears in Table 1 [Allowed substances] in the Annex of the EU Commission Regulation No. 37/2010 where its use is permitted in goats):

- Carprofen: 1.4 mg/kg IV or SC once; can be given to lactating animals.
- Flunixin: 2–2.2 mg/kg IV or IM once daily, for up to five consecutive days; can be given to lactating animals. Also available as a transdermal pour-on solution for single application of 3.33 mg/kg.
- Ketoprofen: 3 mg/kg IV or deep IM, for up to three consecutive days; can be given to lactating animals.
- Meloxicam: 0.5 mg/kg IV or SC, once; can be given to lactating animals. Data sheets suggest to avoid in calves <1 week old; and in older calves to ensure against dehydration.
- Metamizole (dipyrone): 40–50 mg/kg, in combination with butylscopolamine (hyoscine butylbromide) 0.32–0.4 mg/kg IV or IM, up to twice daily for three days; not permitted for use in lactating cattle.
- Tolfenamic acid: 4 mg/kg IV (or SC in young cattle) once, but may be repeated after 48 hours; can be given to lactating animals.
- Sodium salicylate: 40 mg/kg once daily PO (can be divided between drinks/meals), in drinking water or milk replacer, for one to three days. Not in calves <2 weeks old. Must not be administered to animals producing milk for human consumption.

33.13 Local Anaesthesia

Local/regional anaesthetic techniques are often favoured in ruminants because of the afore-mentioned problems associated with general anaesthesia. Furthermore, these techniques require less expensive drugs and equipment, and can easily be performed on the farm. Ruminants, and especially cattle, tend to be very amenable to local/regional anaesthetic techniques because they are generally docile, although sedation may be warranted (see above).

33.13.1 Local Anaesthetic Agents Licenced for Use in Ruminants

According to the EU Commission Regulation No. 37/2010, benzocaine and tetracaine may be used in all food producing species and these agents require no MRL. That said, no licenced products containing either of these local anaesthetics are currently available in the UK.

Procaine 5% with adrenaline (epinephrine) is currently the only licenced local anaesthetic for cattle in the UK and has a 'zero days' withholding period for both meat and milk. (In 2016, a marketing authorization was granted for a 4% solution of procaine with epinephrine for cattle, horses, pigs, and sheep to be marketed in Spain; no MRL is required.) Procaine's indications include field blocks and perineural infiltration, including cornual blocks, but it is contraindicated for epidural administration, intravenous administration (and therefore intravenous regional anaesthesia [IVRA]), and intra-articular analgesia, probably more due to the epinephrine and preservatives (chlorocresol and sodium metabisulphite) that it contains than the procaine itself, although higher concentrations of local anaesthetics are associated with greater degrees of neurotoxicity and chondrotoxicity. As an ester-linked local anaesthetic, procaine is a benzoic acid derivative and one of its metabolites is para amino benzoic acid (pABA). pABA itself can cause hypersensitivity reactions and can also antagonise the antibacterial effects of sulphonamides (which are structural analogues of pABA), and therefore also trimethoprim-potentiated sulphonamides.

Lidocaine (1 or 2%) may be licenced for use in cattle and other farm species in different countries, and is a popular choice, offering better tissue penetration and longer duration of action than procaine. Its licence, however, was withdrawn in the UK due to concerns over one of its metabolites (2, 6-xylidine), which is produced extensively in cattle and pigs and has potential genotoxic/carcinogenic effects in laboratory rodents.

Lidocaine is first metabolised to MEGX (mono-ethyl glycine xylidide), which is then metabolised to GX (glycine xylidide). Both MEGX and GX are subsequently metabolised to 2, 6-xylidine (also known as 2, 6-dimethyl aniline, DMA) in cattle and pigs. The 2, 6-xylidine itself and especially its hydroxylated metabolites (DMAP and DMHA) can damage DNA both directly and also via enhancing the production of reactive oxygen species and other reactive intermediates.

In 2001, the European Medicines Agency (EMeA) considered that an MRL was not required for lidocaine, but restricted its use to local/regional anaesthesia in Equidae (because they do not produce 2, 6-xylidine). However, because lidocaine was listed, with 'No MRL required', in

Table 1 of the Annex of Commission Regulation (EU) No. 37/2010, it may be used in farm species according to the so-called 'cascade', especially where procaine is not advised (e.g. for epidural anaesthesia), or where veterinary surgeons feel that lidocaine would provide superior local anaesthesia to procaine. When used under these circumstances, the suggested withholding periods are, however, 15 days (rather than the more usual 7) for milk and 28 days for meat.

All the techniques described below can be performed with 2% lidocaine (either with or without epinephrine; and when epinephrine should be excluded will be highlighted) or similar volumes of procaine 5% (with epinephrine). Many of the techniques described below are with mature cattle in mind, although the techniques are applicable to other ruminants, but the doses must be reduced pro-rata for smaller ruminants. For young lambs and kids, the local anaesthetic solution can be diluted in sterile saline to reduce the risk of toxicity. The maximum safe dose of lidocaine is about 3 (plain) to 7 (with epinephrine) mg/kg, and perhaps nearer 1–2 mg/kg for young lambs and kids. Procaine is generally considered to be less toxic than lidocaine; the maximum safe dose being in the region of 4 mg/kg (plain) to 8 mg/kg (with epinephrine). For young lambs and kids, maximum doses of around 3–4 mg/kg (with epinephrine) might be more prudent.

33.13.2 Local Anaesthetic Techniques for Facial and Cornual Procedures (Based on Cattle)

Figure 33.2 shows the locations of perineural nerve blocks around the head.

33.13.2.1 Infraorbital Nerve Block

This desensitises the ipsilateral nose/muzzle, upper lip and face rostral to the infraorbital foramen. The infraorbital foramen can be difficult to palpate through tough thick skin in large cattle, but should lie just rostral to the facial tuberosity, roughly midway along a line between the second upper cheek tooth and the nasomaxillary notch (Figure 33.2; see C). This block may be useful for suturing wounds to the nose or rostral part of the upper lip, and, when performed bilaterally, for inserting rings into bulls' noses. Good restraint of the head is essential for safety whilst performing the injection. For mature cattle, an 18 g needle would be appropriate for injection of 5–10 ml local anaesthetic (after aspiration to ensure intravascular injection is avoided), where the infraorbital nerve leaves the foramen (fan out the injection volume over a small arc just rostral to the foramen).

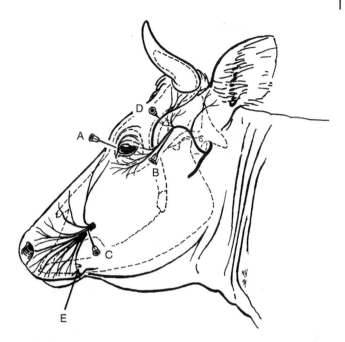

Figure 33.2 Local anaesthetic techniques used for bovine heads. *Source:* Modified from Tranquilli et al. (2007) with permission of Blackwell Publishing Ltd. A = local infiltration of eyelids. B = auriculopalpebral nerve block. C = infraorbital nerve block. D = cornual nerve block. E = mental nerve block.

33.13.2.2 Mental Nerve Block

This block desensitises the lower lip on the ipsilateral side, but not any teeth, unless the needle is inserted a few cm into the foramen (which risks nerve damage and often produces an aversive patient reaction, even if sedated) (Figure 33.2; see E). The mental foramen tends to be found in the rostral 1/3rd of the diastema, on the lateral aspect of the mandible, and is usually approached transcutaneously. For mature cattle, 5–10 ml local anaesthetic is injected where the mental nerve leaves the foramen, after initial aspiration to check for inadvertent intravascular injection.

33.13.2.3 Cornual Nerve Block

The main cornual nerve is a branch of the lacrimal nerve (also called zygomaticotemporal), which is a branch of the ophthalmic division of the trigeminal nerve. Each cornual nerve lies beneath the bony temporal ridge which is palpable extending caudally from the lateral canthus of the eye to the ipsilateral horn base.

In young calves, 2–5 ml of local anaesthetic is best injected into each temporal fossa (the depression beneath the temporal ridge, just caudal to the lateral bony orbital rim), but not too deep (5/8–1″ needle), and extending the needle caudally just beneath the temporal ridge, for about half its length (see Figure 33.2, D). Aspirate before injection to avoid inadvertent injection into the artery or vein that also accompany the nerve. Ptosis and/or drooping of the ear may be seen, indicating inadvertent block of the auriculo-palpebral nerve (a branch of the facial nerve, which carries only motor fibres), which lies in close proximity to the cornual nerve (See Figure 33.2, B and D). Whilst ptosis often accompanies a good block of the cornual nerve, its absence does not necessarily mean that the cornual nerve block has not been successful.

In older cattle, where the horns have developed to some degree and acquired a more substantial innervation, in addition to the cornual nerve block (either as above, or by performing two separate injections – the first into the temporal fossa and the second just beneath the temporal ridge, roughly halfway along its length), extra infiltration of local anaesthetic into the subcutaneous tissues in an arc around the caudal base of the horn is necessary in order to desensitise the cutaneous branches of the second (and sometimes also the first) cervical nerve. Injection into the dense, fibrous subcutaneous fascia, however, can be difficult. Depending upon the size of the patient, 5–10 ml of local anaesthetic may be required at each of the three injection sites, and sufficient time (5–10 minutes) must be allowed for the block to develop. A stout 1″ needle is required.

Occasionally, the horn may remain sensitive because of other sources of innervation. The medial aspect of the more well-developed horn is innervated by the cornual branch of the infratrochlear nerve (also a branch of the ophthalmic division of the trigeminal nerve). This can be desensitised either where the nerve emerges from a small notch in the upper bony orbital rim, just dorsolateral to the medial canthus, or roughly halfway along a line between the medial canthus and medial horn base. Alternatively, the arc block around the caudal aspect of the horn base can be extended medially to block the innervation from the infratrochlear nerve. Indeed, performing a more complete ring-block around the entire horn base would help to ensure block of both cornual nerves in addition to any innervation arising from the second, and sometimes also the first, cervical segmental nerves.

Any further residual sensation may be due to the frontal (supra-orbital) nerve. The frontal (supra-orbital) nerve supplies innervation to the frontal sinus, which becomes integral with the horn (and which is broached) in older cattle with more well-developed horns. This nerve can be blocked roughly half-way along the upper bony orbital rim. Depending upon breed and individual maturation rate, the horn bud and frontal bone 'fuse' at around eight weeks of age; and by around eight to nine months, pneumatisation of the horn begins, after which there is increased risk of broaching the frontal sinus, and therefore requirement for blockade of the frontal nerve during dehorning.

Whilst it has been common practice for farm vets to add some α2 agonist (commonly xylazine) to the local anaesthetic to be injected, this not only has the advantage of resulting in systemic uptake, and therefore sedation and analgesia, but α2 agonists may enhance perineural blocks through their own suppression of nerve conduction by blocking the hyperpolarisation-activated cation (I_h) current. Typically, 1–5 ml of xylazine (20 mg/ml) is added to 100 ml local anaesthetic, resulting in a final concentration of 0.2–1 mg/ml xylazine. Now, if say 5 ml is used for each cornual block for a young calf of around 50 kg, then 10 ml of the mixture is used in total, which would deliver between 2 and 10 mg, which would mean a xylazine dose of 0.04–0.2 mg/kg, which is within the intramuscular dose range of 0.05–0.3 mg/kg.

Goat horns are supplied by the cornual branches of both the lacrimal and infratrochlear nerves (Figure 33.3). To desensitise the cornual branch of the lacrimal nerve, local anaesthetic can be infiltrated halfway along a line between the lateral canthus of the eye and the lateral horn base. To desensitise the cornual branch of the infratrochlear nerve, local anaesthetic can be infiltrated halfway along a line between the medial canthus of the eye and the medial horn base. The dose for mature animals is 2–3 ml local anaesthetic at each site.

The application of topical local anaesthetic onto the surgical site after disbudding has been shown to improve the

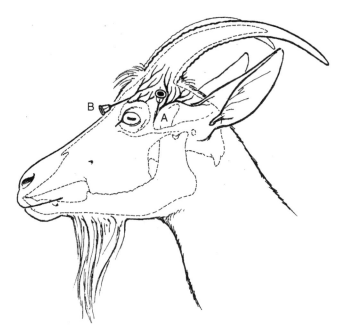

Figure 33.3 Nerve blocks for dehorning goats. *Source:* Reproduced from Tranquilli et al. (2007) with permission of Blackwell Publishing Ltd. A = cornual branch of lacrimal nerve (ophthalmic V). B = cornual branch of infratrochlear nerve (ophthalmic V).

analgesia after a cornual block alone, but no studies have been performed to explore whether topical local anaesthetics interact with other topically applied agents such as antibacterial agents. Furthermore, for young goat kids, care must be taken to avoid local anaesthetic toxicity, as some local anaesthetic agents designed for topical application are supplied in concentrated solutions and can be rapidly absorbed.

Research supports the administration of systemic analgesics, especially NSAIDs, in all situations where there are no contra-indications.

33.13.3 Local Anaesthetic Techniques for Ocular and Peri-ocular Structures

The literature can be confusing as several different versions of similar techniques exist.

33.13.3.1 Retrobulbar Block

See Figure 33.4. This block aims to desensitise cranial nerves II (optic), III (oculomotor), IV (trochlear), VI (abducens), and the ophthalmic and maxillary branches of V (trigeminal); and therefore all the extra-ocular muscles, the entire globe, and conjunctivae. Complete motor block of the eyelids (i.e. block of the orbicularis oculi muscle) will, however, require an additional palpebral block (see below). Evidence of successful retrobulbar block is by loss of corneal sensation, reduced lacrimation, exophthalmos, and mydriasis (although some of these signs may not be recognisable in

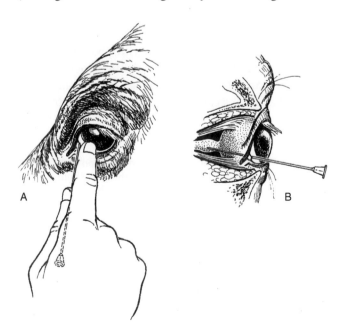

Figure 33.4 Retrobulbar block. With needle placement through the medial canthus (A), see how the needle tip reaches the orbital apex (B). *Source:* Reproduced from Tranquilli et al. (2007) with permission of Blackwell Publishing Ltd.

diseased eyes, and the deposition of local anaesthetic behind the globe can itself result in proptosis).

Retrobulbar block is most commonly achieved by either a one-point technique or a four-point technique (or variations of these). Needles can be inserted either percutaneously through the eyelids, or through the conjunctival fornix and even through the base of the third eyelid. For trans-conjunctival approaches, topical local anaesthetic agent (e.g. tetracaine) can be instilled into the conjunctival sac first.

The one-point technique uses either: a long, curved needle, inserted just dorsomedial to the lateral canthus and curved around the globe so as to penetrate the extra-ocular muscle cone (conus ocularis) somewhere near its apex; or a straight needle, inserted just ventrolateral to the medial canthus and along the floor of the orbit towards the apex of the extra-ocular muscle cone, again aiming to deposit local anaesthetic within the conus ocularis. This latter technique not only usually requires placement of the needle through the base of the third eyelid (and therefore should be avoided if this structure is affected by infection or neoplasia), but also carries a greater risk of injection into the cerebrospinal fluid (CSF) within the meningeal sheath surrounding the optic nerve, as the needle tip is more likely to lie in very close proximity to the optic nerve (which although good for blocking the nerve, risks penetration of the meningeal sheath around it; see below).

The four-point technique involves making injections laterally, medially, dorsally, and ventrally around the orbit. If straight or only slightly curved needles are used, the needle tips are unlikely to reach beyond the equator of the globe and if the needle tip remains outside the conus ocularis during injection of local anaesthetic, then this technique is more correctly a peribulbar (extraconal) block rather than a retrobulbar (intraconal) block. Because larger volumes of local anaesthetic tend to be used with the four-point peribulbar technique and because the local anaesthetic is deposited outwith the conus ocularis, it spreads more easily to block the palpebral nerve, thus often negating the requirement for an additional palpebral block.

Long (10–15 cm) needles are required, and a total of 10–20 ml local anaesthetic is deposited, after careful aspiration to try to avoid inadvertent intravascular or intrathecal injection.

Complications include:

- Puncture of the globe.
- Increased intra-ocular pressure because of proptosis/exophthalmos and the volume of local anaesthetic solution deposited behind the globe. This may encourage globe rupture where deep ulcerations or lacerations are present. This is less of a worry where enucleation is intended, unless there is a risk of infection or tumour spread.
- Retrobulbar haemorrhage, if blood vessels are damaged.

- Optic nerve damage.
- Injection of local anaesthetic into the cerebrospinal fluid which is present in the meningeal sheath which surrounds the optic nerve, with resultant acute CNS toxicity (seizures, collapse). The 1-point, curved-needle, 'dorso-medial to lateral canthus' approach carries a slightly lower risk of penetrating the optic nerve/meningeal sheath, than the one-point, straight-needle, 'ventrolateral to medial canthus' approach, as the optic nerve enters the globe more medioventrally.
- Occasionally the deposition of a large-ish volume of local anaesthetic solution behind the globe will stimulate the oculo-cardiac reflex; although once the block has developed, this reflex should be prevented.
- Possible seeding of tumour, or infection, to peri-ocular tissues along the track of needle insertion/s.

33.13.3.2 Peterson's Block

Anaesthesia of the globe and orbit is provided by the Peterson block (Figure 33.5; see A), whilst total akinesia of the eyelids requires the additional (auriculo)palpebral block (Figure 33.5; see B), of which only the palpebral part is really necessary. Although this block is technically more difficult to perform than the retrobulbar block, it is preferred if tumours of the globe and its adnexa are present (e.g. squamous cell carcinomata) because it avoids needle insertion through potentially affected tissues. Complications are as for those of the aforementioned retrobulbar techniques.

- When combined with a palpebral block, this technique *can* produce almost complete anaesthesia of the side of the head/face, i.e. it blocks all three branches of cranial nerve V (whilst the ophthalmic and maxillary branches exit the cranial vault via the foramen orbitorotundum, the mandibular branch exits the cranial vault via the nearby foramen ovale)

- cranial nerve II (exits cranium via optic foramen)
- cranial nerves III, IV, and VI (which exit the cranium via the foramen orbitorotundum)
- the palpebral branch of the facial nerve, VII (which provides only motor supply to the orbicularis oculi muscle)

In order to perform the block, firstly locate the depression where the caudal rim of the orbit meets the zygomatic arch; rostral to the coronoid process of the mandible and inject a bleb of local anaesthetic subcutaneously. Then, insert a straight (or slightly curved needle) (10–15 cm long) into the depression through the subcutaneous local anaesthetic bleb and aim rostroventrally towards the foramen orbitorotundum, adjacent to the apex of the conus ocularis (optic foramen) in the pterygopalatine fossa (Figure 33.5; see A). Aspirate before injection of 10–20 ml of local anaesthetic to reduce the risk of inadvertent intravascular injection (the ventral maxillary artery is nearby). The needle is then partly withdrawn until its tip lies just subcutaneously, then it can be re-directed caudally for about 2–3 cm, and a further 5 ml local anaesthetic is deposited at the dorsal rim of the highest point of the zygomatic arch to block the palpebral nerve. The block will reduce blinking, so the eye becomes vulnerable to dust entry or trauma, although this is not a post-operative concern if the block is performed before enucleation.

33.13.4 Local/Regional Anaesthetic Techniques for Limbs, Digits, Tail, and Perineum

33.13.4.1 Perineural Infiltration

Perineural infiltration is possible with good anatomical knowledge. The skin, however, is tightly adhered to the distal limbs and the fascia is dense, which can sometimes make such injections difficult. If cellulitis is present,

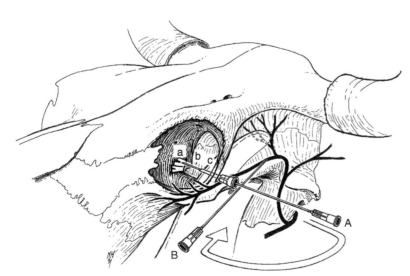

Figure 33.5 Peterson eye block (A), with (auriculo) palpebral block (B). *Source:* Reproduced from Tranquilli et al. (2007) with permission of Blackwell Publishing Ltd. a = foramen orbitorotundum; b = pterygoid crest; c = coronoid process.

perineural injections may be contra-indicated, not only because the local anatomy becomes unrecognisable, but also because injections should not be made into potentially infected tissues.

33.13.4.2 'Proximal' Lower Limb Nerve Blocks

For desensitisation of the hock and limb distal to the hock, the following nerves must be blocked (Figure 33.6): A, the common peroneal nerve (branch of sciatic nerve); and B, the tibial nerve (branch of sciatic nerve).

The common peroneal nerve passes caudal to the lateral collateral ligament of the stifle. It can be blocked at a point just behind the caudal most edge of the lateral tibial plateau, just proximal to where the nerve passes between peroneus longus and the lateral digital extensor. A 5 cm, 18–20 g needle and 10–20 ml local anaesthetic will be required.

The tibial nerve can be blocked about 10 cm proximal to the point of the hock, between the common calcaneal and deep digital flexor tendons, on the medial aspect of the limb. A 5 cm, 18–20 g needle and 10–20 ml local anaesthetic will be required. Cattle usually cope well with a desensitised lower limb and will usually remain standing.

For desensitisation distal to the carpus, the following nerves must be blocked (see Figure 33.7): the medial and dorsal antebrachial nerves that are branches of the musculocutaneous (A) and radial (A') nerves; the ulnar nerve (B); and the median nerve (C). To block A and A', 10–20 ml local anaesthetic is injected in a line across the dorsal aspect of the distal radius. To block B, about 5 ml of local anaesthetic is injected approximately 10 cm proximal to the accessory carpal bone, on the caudolateral surface of the radius between flexor carpi ulnaris and ulnaris lateralis (the nerve may be palpable here). To block C, around 20 ml local anaesthetic can be injected at a site about 5 cm distal to the elbow on the medial aspect of the limb, along the caudomedial radius. Cattle usually cope well with a desensitised lower limb and should remain standing.

33.13.4.3 'Distal' Lower Limb Nerve Blocks

To desensitise the interdigital cleft, 5–10 ml local anaesthetic can be injected at sites D (axial digital nerves) as depicted in Figures 33.7 and 33.8.

To desensitise both medial and lateral forelimb digits, local anaesthetic must be injected at A, B, C, D and E in Figure 33.8. If only the lateral digit is to be desensitised, then injections at B, C, D and E are required, whereas for the medial digit, injections at A, D, and E are required. The reader is referred to anatomy and other anaesthesia texts for more details on these blocks.

For desensitisation of the hindlimb digits (Figure 33.9), the superficial peroneal nerve (at A), the deep peroneal

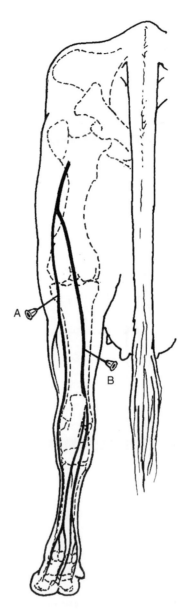

Figure 33.6 Hindlimb 'proximal' nerve blocks. *Source:* Reproduced from Tranquilli et al. (2007) with permission of Blackwell Publishing Ltd. A = common peroneal nerve; B = tibial nerve.

nerve (at B), and the medial and lateral plantar metatarsal nerves (at C: medially and laterally) must be blocked. Again, the reader is referred to anatomical and other anaesthetic texts for more details on these nerve blocks.

33.13.4.4 Ring Block

Normally, local anaesthetic solution without epinephrine is used for these blocks so as not to compromise the blood supply to the distal limb and to allow greater spread of the local anaesthetic in the tissues for a better block. This block can be performed proximal to regions of cellulitis, but injections should not be made into inflamed and potentially infected tissues.

33.13.4.5 Intravenous Regional Anaesthesia (IVRA) or Bier's Block

This is usually easiest to perform if the cow is cast into lateral recumbency (e.g. by Reuff's method), or occasionally is possible when cows are restrained in a crush, but adequate precautions must be taken to ensure safety of personnel and the patient. A suitable superficial vein must first be identified; cellulitis may preclude this. A tourniquet is then applied proximal to the area to be blocked (Figures 33.10 and 33.11); common sites are just above or below the carpus or tarsus. If above the hock, then bandage rolls (or similar) are used so as to 'fill' the bilateral depressions between the Achilles tendon and the tibia, to reduce damage to the tendons and to increase the efficacy of the tourniquet. The superficial vein distal to the tourniquet is then re-located and the skin at the injection site is clipped and prepared as aseptically as possible. For mature cattle, 20–35 ml local anaesthetic is injected, usually against the direction of blood flow in the vein (i.e. towards the foot), and as rapidly as possible (the rapidity of injection is suggested to help the spread of

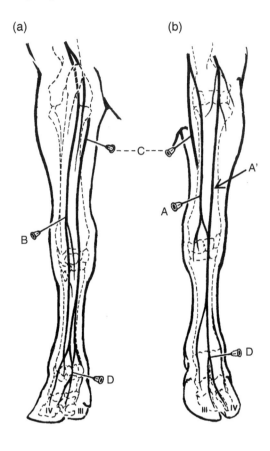

Figure 33.7 Forelimb 'proximal' nerve blocks. *Source:* Modified from Tranquilli et al. (2007) with permission of Blackwell Publishing Ltd. A = musculocutaneous nerve; A' = radial nerve; B = ulnar nerve; C = median nerve; D = axial digital nerves.

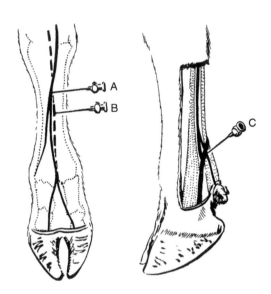

Figure 33.9 Nerve blocks of the distal hindlimb. *Source:* Reproduced from Hall et al. (2001) with permission from Elsevier.

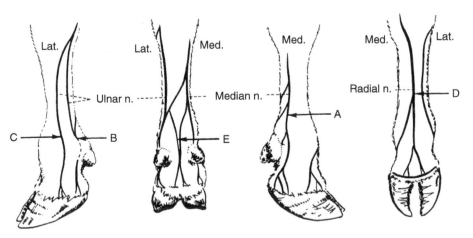

Figure 33.8 Nerve blocks of the lower forelimb. *Source:* Reproduced from Hall et al. (2001) with permission from Elsevier.

the local anaesthetic). Lidocaine without epinephrine is usually preferred; the absence of epinephrine facilitates maximum spread of local anaesthetic into the tissues and the short duration of action of lidocaine ensures that safe release of the tourniquet can performed after around 20 minutes. Volumes towards the lower end of the range are more suitable when the tourniquet is placed distal to the hock or carpus; larger volumes are indicated when the tourniquet is placed proximal to the hock or carpus. For a mature sheep (50–70 kg), 5–10 ml local anaesthetic (again, lidocaine without epinephrine) is usually sufficient; the volume also depending upon the position of the tourniquet. Some operators have suggested that a more certain block is achieved if the limb is first exsanguinated before tourniquet application (by raising the limb above the heart for a few minutes, or, better, by applying an Esmarch bandage, but this may be contra-indicated in a very inflamed leg). It can be helpful to ensure that a vein is cannulated before the limb is exsanguinated, but it is also easy to dislodge the pre-placed cannula whilst applying, and then unwrapping, an Esmarch bandage. See also Chapter 14.

Once the local anaesthetic has been injected, allow a good 10–20 minutes for full desensitisation to occur. Test for anaesthesia of the digit/limb by needle-pricking. As the interdigital fossa is the last site to become desensitised, this is a useful test site to assess if the block has worked. It should be noted that if the tourniquet is not tight enough, this site will not block completely.

The toxic dose of lidocaine varies a little between species, but is probably >3 mg/kg (without epinephrine). As 30 ml of 2% lidocaine only contains 600 mg lidocaine (30 times 20), then this would be 1 mg/kg for a 600 kg cow, which is well below the toxic dose. Therefore, should the tourniquet be or become loose 'too soon' (it is usually recommended not to release them for at least 15–20 minutes), and this lidocaine enters the systemic circulation, it is highly unlikely to have serious consequences. If, however, large volumes of local anaesthetic that include epinephrine (usually at around 0.01 mg/ml) are inadvertently injected intravascularly, there may be some cardiovascular effects, but these are usually transient as the overall dose is relatively small.

There is debate regarding how long tourniquets can safely be left in place without causing extensive ischaemic tissue damage to distal limb structures or risking serious reperfusion injury after their release. In horses and cattle, because they have relatively more tendons and less muscle mass in the distal limbs than humans, tourniquets can be left on safely for 2–2.5 hours, and they have even been left in place for 3 hours without obvious problems. A useful 'side effect' of tourniquet application for IVRA is haemostasis in the surgical field that can be helpful for digit amputations. Although ischaemic anaesthesia (reversible conduction block in both motor and sensory fibres) occurs in the distal limb around 15–45 minutes after tourniquet application, it must not be relied upon to provide surgical anaesthesia. Initial application of the tourniquet is itself a noxious stimulus (probably

Figure 33.10 Forelimb IVRA: superficial veins. *Source:* Reproduced from Tranquilli et al. (2007) with permission of Blackwell Publishing Ltd. a = common dorsal metacarpal vein; b = lateral palmar digital vein (more commonly the medial palmar digital vein, a branch of the radial vein, is used; on the medial aspect of the limb); c = lateral palmar metacarpal vein; the medial palmar metacarpal vein can also be used.

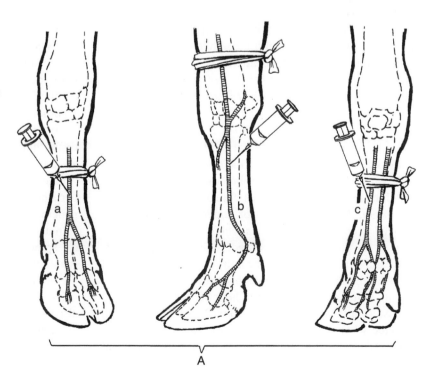

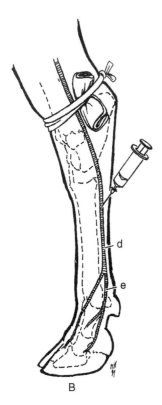

B

Figure 33.11 Hindlimb IVRA: superficial veins. *Source:* Reproduced from Tranquilli et al. (2007) with permission from Blackwell Publishing Ltd. d = lateral saphenous vein (lateral aspect); e = lateral plantar digital vein.

due to mechanical compression), and pain at the site of the tourniquet can persist whilst it is in place. This tourniquet pain probably contributes to the 'tourniquet effect' (increase in arterial blood pressure and possibly also heart rate that occurs upon tourniquet application).

33.13.4.6 Epidural (also known as Extradural) Block
33.13.4.6.1 *Terminology*
Caudal, low (low-dose), or *posterior* are terms applied to epidural anaesthesia where only the most caudal part of the body is desensitised (i.e. tail, perineum, part of the escutcheon, caudal pelvic structures), but the animal retains its hindlimb motor activity, and therefore remains able to stand.

Cranial, high (high-dose), or *anterior* are the terms applied to epidural anaesthesia where more of the caudal part of the patient is desensitised, including its hind legs and caudal trunk, such that the animal loses motor control of its hindlimbs and is not able to stand.

The difference between *caudal* and *cranial* epidural anaesthesia therefore depends upon the quantity of drug injected when the injection site is the same. Both can be achieved from the sacro-coccygeal or inter-coccygeal injection site.

Segmental 'belts' of anaesthesia, however, can also be produced by lumbar or thoracic injection at specific sites.

Epidural catheters can be advanced cranially up the vertebral canal, by a premeasured length (from a more caudal insertion site), and then injection of drugs at the tip of the catheter results in a belt of analgesia/anaesthesia in the proximity of the catheter's tip. Catheters can also be left in situ (if asepsis is preserved) to enable longer term analgesia by administering top-up doses. The reader is referred to other anaesthesia texts for more information regarding the placement and use of epidural catheters.

Injections are usually made into the epidural space between the last sacral and first coccygeal vertebrae (Sa5–Co1), or, between the first two coccygeal vertebrae (Co1–Co2) as there may be fusion between the sacrum and the first coccygeal vertebra (Figure 33.12). As the spinal cord terminates at vertebrae Lu6/Sa1 in cows, and the meningeal sac continues only to Sa2–Sa3, there should be no danger of entering the intrathecal space (and injecting into cerebrospinal fluid), with sacro-coccygeal or inter-coccygeal injections. The situation is somewhat similar for sheep and goats, but sacro-coccygeal (Sa5–Co1) or inter-coccygeal (Co1–Co2) epidural injections may be associated with increased risk of performing inadvertent intrathecal injections as the dural sac may extend further caudally.

Lumbo-sacral injection is more rarely performed, and there is an increased chance of performing an intrathecal injection. However, this site is sometimes used in sheep and calves, see below.

33.13.4.6.2 *Sacro-coccygeal or Inter-coccygeal and 'Caudal' Epidural Technique*
The Sa5–Co1 or Co1–Co2 space is located by pumping the tail-head up and down to feel for the intervertebral space with the most movement. The site should be prepared aseptically.

Although hypodermic needles can be used, stylleted spinal needles with a short bevel (and therefore said to be relatively 'blunt') can enhance the feeling as the needle is advanced into the epidural space. Needles of 3–5 cm are usually used for mature cattle. As the needle is inserted, perpendicularly to the skin in both orthogonal planes, it penetrates, in order: the skin, subcutaneous tissue, supraspinous ligament (between the dorsal tips of adjacent dorsal spinous processes), inter-spinous ligament (between the shafts of adjacent dorsal spinous processes), and finally, the inter-arcuate ligament (between the dorsal surfaces of adjacent vertebral bodies). The inter-arcuate ligament is also called the yellow ligament or ligamentum flavum and is tougher than the other ligaments, so on penetration of this ligament, a 'popping' sensation can be felt, especially when a spinal needle (relatively blunt) is used. Sometimes

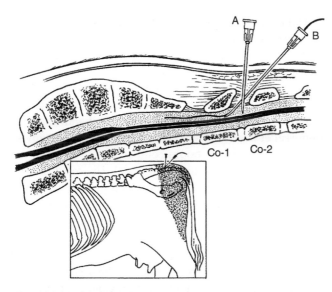

Figure 33.12 Epidural (extradural) injection into inter-coccygeal space Co1–Co2. *Source:* Reproduced from Tranquilli et al. (2007) with permission of Blackwell Publishing Ltd. A = normal needle placement; B = needle placement for insertion of an epidural catheter.

the needle advances so easily that its tip may hit the ventral floor of the vertebral canal before you can halt its progression. If this happens, you may need to withdraw it slightly, as otherwise injection may be difficult if the needle tip is hard against the floor of the canal. Always gently aspirate to ensure subsequent injections are not intravascular. Injection is usually made with the bevel of the needle pointing cranially. Ideally, injections should be made relatively slowly (over one to two minutes), especially for larger volumes, and injectate should be warmed to reduce the chance of Durrans' sign (tachypnoea and hyperpnoea).

The shaded area in Figure 33.12 shows the region of perineal desensitisation after injection of about 5 ml of local anaesthetic in an average 500 kg cow. The tail should be desensitised too. (Larger injectate volumes increasingly risk hindlimb motor block and recumbency such that caution is advised with volumes of ≥10 ml for 500 kg cattle.) For similar effects in mature sheep and goats, 1–2 ml local anaesthetic is administered.

Sometimes epidural injections result in quite patchy or unilateral effects. It may be that uneven epidural fat deposits or fibrous tissue within the epidural space interferes with the even spread of the injectate.

33.13.4.6.3 Sacro-coccygeal or Inter-coccygeal and 'Cranial' Epidural Technique

If recumbency is intended and hindlimb, udder, or flank anaesthesia is required, then volumes of 10–15 (−25) ml local anaesthetic /100 kg have been reported for such 'cranial' epidural anaesthetic techniques. Doses of nearer 25 ml/100 kg have been reported to provide anaesthesia as

far cranially as the diaphragm. When using cranial epidural techniques, care should be taken to prevent the animal from 'doing the splits' whilst losing (or regaining) motor and proprioceptive function of its hindlimbs (e.g. hobbles can be pre-placed). Incomplete, patchy, or unilateral blocks may also occur with the 'cranial' epidural technique. Hypotension (hindquarter vasodilation) usually accompanies this technique; see below.

33.13.4.6.4 To Help Check that the Needle is in the Correct Place

- Loss of, and/or lack of, resistance to injection. In addition to a popping sensation being felt as the needle is advanced through the ligamentum flavum (inter-arcuate ligament), there should be minimal resistance to injection. Using a 5 ml syringe, into which is drawn 3 ml sterile saline and 1 ml air, repeated/continual injection attempts can be made as the needle is advanced. Upon entry of the needle tip into the epidural space, a sudden loss of resistance to injection occurs; the saline injects easily (and there is sometimes the impression that it is being sucked in), and the 'cushion' of air (which sits on top of the saline when the syringe is connected to the needle hub) is not compressed.
- The hanging drop technique. Once the needle tip is beneath the skin, the stylette is removed and a bleb of sterile saline is placed into its hub before it is then advanced slowly. Upon entry of the needle tip into the epidural space, the saline is sucked into the needle because there is normally a slight negative pressure at this region of the epidural 'space'. In cattle with increased intra-abdominal pressure (e.g. bloat), there may not be negative pressure in this caudal region of the epidural space. Note that the needle may become blocked by a core of tissue (after the stylette is removed), so a negative result does not always mean that the needle placement was incorrect.
- The whoosh or swoosh tests. Once it is felt that the needle is in the correct location, air or saline (or a mixture) is injected rapidly, whilst listening to the area cranial to the needle with a stethoscope, and a whooshing (following air injection) or swooshing (following liquid injection or mixtures of air and liquid) sound should be heard.

In the absence of convincing results from the above tests, but where local anaesthetic has nevertheless been injected, the tail should become flaccid and anal tone should be lost within 5–10 minutes.

33.13.4.6.5 What to Inject?

Local anaesthetics, opioids, and α2 agonists can be administered into the epidural (extradural) space, although the exact drugs that can be administered by this route in food-producing animals will depend upon licencing in different countries.

All drugs intended for epidural injection, especially if the injection is to be repeated, are best if preservative-free.

Local Anaesthetics

Local anaesthetic agents can cause motor as well as sensory block, so hindlimb ataxia and recumbency can be unintended potential complications. The hindlimbs of mature cattle can be hobbled to prevent them doing the splits, which may happen if they become ataxic and go down or, if having gone down, they struggle to stand whilst ataxic. Hindlimb ataxia and recumbency are usually less risky for smaller ruminants that can be more easily manually-assisted.

Lidocaine is a common choice for short surgical procedures. Epinephrine may be included and may provide some local anaesthetic action of its own as well as prolonging the block (through vasoconstriction, reducing systemic absorption). By localising the injectate volume near the injection site, epinephrine may also reduce cranial spread of the injected drug (although there is the theoretical potential for local ischaemia following vasoconstriction). In the UK, lidocaine may be used according to the cascade, especially as the licenced procaine formulations (which include epinephrine) carry a contra-indication for use by the epidural route because of their high concentration (5%), acidic pH, and the included epinephrine and preservatives, all of which may increase the risk of toxicity (neural/vascular) when administered neuraxially.

Local anaesthetics administered for caudal epidural anaesthesia can be useful for tail, perineal, anal, and vulval surgery and can help to reduce the abdominal straining during/after parturition, or during/after replacement of rectal, vaginal, or uterine prolapses. Whilst caudal epidural anaesthesia can reduce the abdominal straining associated with the pelvic reflex during assisted calvings, it does not always totally abolish all straining because it can be difficult to desensitise the whole birth canal without also producing motor block of the hindlimbs. Epidural anaesthesia also has little impact on the Ferguson reflex (uterine contraction associated with oxytocin release), so *uterine* contractions *can* persist even without much abdominal straining. With cranial epidural anaesthesia, the pelvic reflex, and therefore abdominal straining, should be totally abolished, and, depending upon the dose of local anaesthetic injected, the flank may also be desensitised, such that calving attempts can be easily converted into surgical Caesarean section without much delay. The major side effect of cranial epidural anaesthesia, however, is hypotension because the sympathetic supply to the hind end of the animal is also blocked so that massive vasodilation occurs. This can result in significant heat loss as well as hypotension, so beware in animals that are hypovolaemic and/or likely to become hypothermic. Animals are usually hobbled to prevent them doing the splits, both as they become recumbent and also as they recover to standing.

α2 Agonists

Most reports have used xylazine. Whilst α2 agonists can be used alone, the onset of action is slower than after lidocaine (i.e. 20 minutes for xylazine compared with about 5 minutes after lidocaine), although the duration of action is longer (i.e. three to six hours compared with one to two hours), probably because of the local vasoconstriction caused. Xylazine also has some local anaesthetic properties (which may be associated with the ability of α2 agonists to reduce the repolarisation (I_h) current), which along with the sedation (from systemic absorption), increases the risk of ataxia and recumbency.

Alone, xylazine (for mature cattle) can be used at around 0.05–0.07 mg/kg, usually made up to a volume of around 5–7 ml in total for injection. Alternatively, it can be combined with lidocaine, i.e. 0.03 mg/kg xylazine plus c. 0.22 mg/kg lidocaine 2%.

For mature sheep (50–70 kg body mass), a useful combination is 1.75 ml lidocaine 2% plus 0.25 ml xylazine 2%.

Opioids

None are licenced, but morphine at 0.1–0.2 mg/kg provides analgesia, at least up to the last rib, and even up to the thoracic limbs. Analgesia may be slow to onset (1–4 hours), but can last up to 24 hours. The final volume of injectate (as well as the dose) influences the rostral spread of analgesia, and may need adjusting by addition of sterile saline or sterile water (but dilution may also result in poorer/more patchy block). Epidural opioid analgesia is usually insufficient for surgical/incisional (epicritic) pain, so must be combined with a local anaesthetic (or possibly an α2 agonist) if surgery is being contemplated. If a combination of drugs is to be injected at the sacro-/inter-coccygeal site, rather than mix the two agents, it has been suggested to administer the opioid first and the local anaesthetic last to possibly enable better analgesia provision by the opioid, but to prevent too much cranial spread of the local anaesthetic block. Neuraxially-administered morphine is poorly absorbed into the systemic circulation, and therefore produces fewer systemic side effects such that reduced gut motility (which may result in tympany) is less of a risk.

33.13.4.6.6 *Contra-indications to Epidural Blocks*

Obesity (rarely a problem for dairy breeds), local skin infection, perhaps distant foci of infection too, distorted pelvic/tailhead anatomy, coagulopathies, pre-existing neuropathies.

33.13.4.6.7 *Risks Associated with Epidural Injections*

Nerve damage, hypotension, hypothermia, systemic toxicity (inadvertent IV injection), introduction of infection with resultant meningitis, osteomyelitis etc. Intrathecal (subarachnoid) injection should not occur, at least in cattle, at the Sa–Co1 or Co1–Co2 sites, as only coccygeal nerves are present. Ataxia/recumbency can be a nuisance, but also increases the risk of fractures or dislocations if animals do the splits.

33.13.4.6.8 *Lumbo-sacral Epidural Technique*

Lumbo-sacral epidural block can be performed in calves, sheep, and goats (Figure 33.13), for procedures such as vasectomy and occasionally Caesarean section (although the ewe may remain recumbent/unable to stand for one to two hours after surgery, which may delay suckling by the lambs). Injection of local anaesthetic at this site produces anaesthesia somewhat cranial to as well as caudal to the injection site. A recent study in dogs has shown similar cranial spread (up the vertebral canal) following injection of the same volume (albeit of contrast agent), whether injection was performed at the lumbo-sacral or sacro-coccygeal site. Whether the same will be true for other species remains to be determined.

The injection site is located similarly to its location in dogs (see Chapter 14). Injection of 1 ml local anaesthetic per 4.5 kg body weight (11–15 ml per 50–70 kg mature sheep) is usually required to ensure sufficient anaesthesia. This will result in hindlimb motor block and recumbency. Xylazine (0.05–0.2 mg/kg) can be used in combination with a local anaesthetic (now reduced to 1 ml per 10 kg body weight). Occasionally, insertion of the needle at this site will result in penetration of the dura mater, and therefore CSF will either flow from the needle hub or be easily aspirated. If this occurs, even if the needle is withdrawn slightly, any drugs injected may now have direct access to the CSF. It is therefore advisable to either abandon this block or reduce the dose/s injected to perform a true spinal (intrathecal) block; normally, only about a quarter of the intended epidural dose is administered intrathecally, and preferably, only using agents that do not contain epinephrine and preservatives.

33.13.4.7 True Spinal/Subarachnoid/Intrathecal Block

True spinal (subarachnoid or intrathecal) injections are performed more rarely in cattle, but may be accidental or intentional during injection at the lumbo-sacral site in sheep (e.g. for vasectomy). This block will result in hindlimb paresis and recumbency: the dose of local anaesthetic used should be about 1/4 of that for epidural injection at this site (see above). Local anaesthetic without epinephrine should be used, and preferably, also without preservatives. Lower concentrations of local anaesthetics are generally less directly neurotoxic, but the acidic pH of commercial solutions has also been implicated in neurotoxicity. See Chapter 14 for comparison between epidural and intrathecal blocks.

33.13.5 Local/Regional Anaesthetic Techniques for Udder and Teats

33.13.5.1 Udder

- Paravertebral (PV, Lu1, Lu2), and caudal epidural or pudendal block may provide partial desensitisation.
- Cranial epidural should provide more complete desensitisation (recumbency is likely).

The cranial portion of the udder receives its nerve supply from branches of the first two lumbar segmental nerves, which also supply the flank (Figure 33.14). The bulk of the udder receives its innervation from branches of the third and fourth lumbar segmental nerves (which also supply the hindlimbs). The caudal most area and escutcheon is innervated by branches of the perineal and other nerves from the second, third, and fourth sacral nerves (which also supply the hindlimbs).

33.13.5.2 Teats

- Ring block around the base of the teat. Use local anaesthetic without epinephrine so as not to compromise teat blood supply (A in Figure 33.15).
- IVRA if you can find a tiny local superficial teat vein; a tourniquet (stretchy bandage) is placed proximally, around the base of the teat, up against the udder (D in Figure 33.15).
- Infusion of local anaesthetic into the teat cistern after milk is stripped out. (A tourniquet is placed around the teat base before milk is stripped out and local anaesthetic instilled to localise the local anaesthetic solution to the teat cistern.) This will desensitise the mucosal lining of teat cistern (C in Figure 33.15).
- Inverted 'V' block proximal to the wound (B in Figure 33.15).

33.13.6 Local/Regional Anaesthetic Techniques for Genitalia

33.13.6.1 Epidural Block

Epidural injection of local anaesthetics can be used, but in order to ensure adequate anaesthesia in male animals, a more cranial epidural technique is required, and so recumbency is usually inevitable.

33.13.6.2 Pudendal Nerve Block

The block was originally described by Larson and is useful for penile examination or surgery in males, and to reduce straining after vaginal or cervical trauma in females. The pudendal nerve comprises a main branch from the third and fourth sacral segmental nerves and a communicating

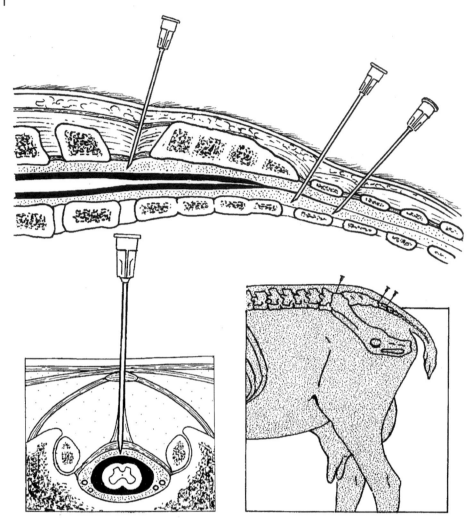

Figure 33.13 Goats and sheep: sites for epidural injection. *Source:* Reproduced from Tranquilli et al. (2007) with permission of Blackwell Publishing Ltd.

branch from the sciatic nerve (Lu6/Sa1/2) (Figure 33.16). The pudendal nerve is sensory to the whole penis, but motor to only the distal two-thirds of the retractor penis muscle. The caudal rectal nerve (early branch off the pudendal nerve) is motor to the proximal one-third of the retractor penis muscle. The deep and superficial perineal nerves (later branches of the pudendal nerve) are sensory to the perineum, prepuce (external lamina), and scrotum (not testicles) of males, and the escutcheon and caudal udder of females.

33.13.6.2.1 Technique

The following must be performed bilaterally. During per rectum examination, the cranial part of the lesser sciatic foramen is identified along the ventrolateral pelvic wall, dorsolaterally to the obturator foramen which lies on the floor of the pelvis. The caudal part of the lesser sciatic foramen is obscured by the coccygeus muscle. Also ventrolaterally within the pelvic

canal lies the internal iliac artery, which continues as the internal pudendal artery as it traverses (but does not exit), the lesser sciatic foramen, from where it continues along the pelvic floor towards the ischial arch. Once the internal iliac / pudendal artery can be felt pulsating, about a finger's width dorsally lies the main bulk of the pudendal nerve (which is composed of several interconnecting branches), and which, along with the internal pudendal artery, can be followed caudally, traversing the lesser sciatic foramen. A tiny communicating branch from the sciatic nerve joins the pudendal nerve, ventrally, as it traverses the lesser sciatic foramen. The caudal rectal nerve is an early branch off the pudendal nerve, coursing dorsally relative to the main pudendal nerve.

The usual approach for blocking, bilaterally, the pudendal nerves, the caudal rectal nerves, and the communicating branches from the sciatic nerves is via the ischiorectal fossae (Figure 33.17). Each ischiorectal fossa is located between the ischial tuberosity ventrally, the sacrosciatic

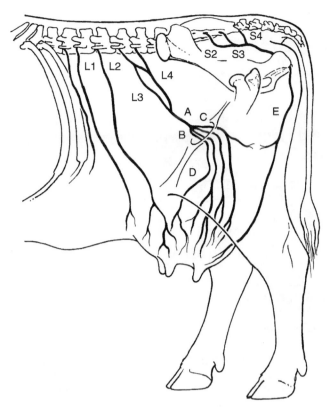

Figure 33.14 Udder innervation. *Source:* Reproduced from Tranquilli et al. (2007) with permission of Blackwell Publishing Ltd. A, B, C, and D = inguinal nerves; E = perineal nerve.

ligament dorsolaterally, and the rectal wall medially. After aseptic preparation and subcutaneous local anaesthetic bleb deposition, a long (10–15 cm) needle is inserted into each ischiorectal fossa, in turn, and the needle tip is guided to near the pudendal nerve with help from the hand that is within the rectum. Around 20–25 ml local anaesthetic is injected just cranial to the most cranial/soft part of the lesser sciatic foramen, and massaged around (using the hand within the rectum) to ensure that the main branches (schematically A and B in Figure 33.16) of the pudendal nerve are blocked. Then the needle tip is re-directed more caudo-dorsally (after slight withdrawal) before a further 10–15 ml local anaesthetic is injected to block the caudal rectal nerve (C in Figure 33.16). Finally, the needle tip is re-directed slightly more ventrally than the initial position, just distal to where the communicating branch from the sciatic nerve (D in Figure 33.16) joins the pudendal nerve, and a further 10–15 ml local anaesthetic is injected. A good 30 minutes should be allowed for the block to take full effect, and, in males, penile protrusion may slightly precede complete loss of sensation.

The ischiorectal fossae lie either side of the tailhead and are easily visible in bony cattle as the depressions on either side of the tailhead, just proximal (dorsomedial) to the pin-bones (ischial tuberosities). However, in beef breeds or fatter dairy animals, the fossae may be obscured by fat or muscle.

Figure 33.15 Local anaesthetic techniques for teats. *Source:* Reproduced from Tranquilli et al. (2007) with permission of Blackwell Publishing Ltd.

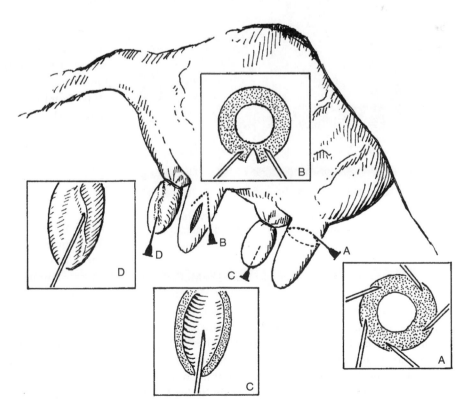

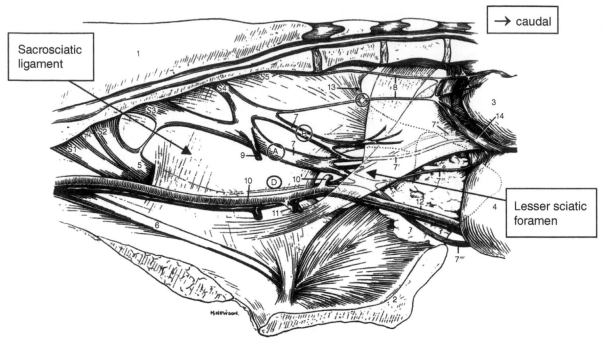

Figure 33.16 Nerves and vessels on medial surface of bovine pelvic wall. *Source:* Modified from Dyce et al. (2002) with permission from Elsevier. Internal pudendal (pudic) nerve = A and B. Caudal rectal nerve = C. Communicating branch of sciatic nerve to pudendal nerve = D. Sciatic nerve = 5. Internal iliac artery = 10; becomes the internal pudendal artery = 12. Obturator nerve = 6. Sacrum = 1. Pubic symphysis = 2.

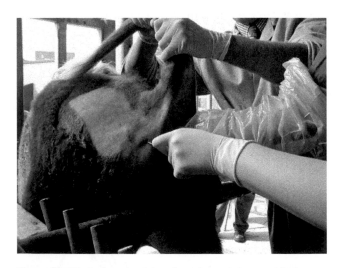

Figure 33.17 Left pudendal and caudal rectal nerve block performed from left ischiorectal fossa in a young bullock.

An alternative, lateral, approach (developed by McFarlane) (Figure 33.18) is to insert the needle cranio-medially through each sheet-like sacrosciatic ligament; again using the 'internal' hand to direct the needle tip to near the nerves to be blocked, just cranial to the 'soft' part (most cranial aspect) of each lesser sciatic foramen. To locate the lateral injection site, with a thumb on the cranial ischial tuberosity, place the tip of the index finger on the sacral end of the sacrotuberous ligament, then using this 'length of the sacrotuberous ligament' as a 'radius', swing the index fingertip ventrally until the thumb-to-fingertip line is parallel with the dorsal midline, and then the fingertip marks the injection site. There is a potentially slightly greater risk of penetrating the rectal wall with this approach if the needle entry angle is too steep.

If performing penile surgery, at the end of the procedure, the penis should be replaced into the sheath and a piece of bandage tied around the distal sheath to protect the penis from trauma until the block has worn off (duration of lidocaine block around one to two hours), at which time the bandage must be removed.

33.13.6.3 Intratesticular Block

After prior aspiration to guard against inadvertent intravascular injection, a single injection of 3–5 ml (or up to 10 ml for larger animals) local anaesthetic into the body of each testicle provides sufficient anaesthesia for castration within around three minutes, but rapid uptake of the local anaesthetic into testicular lymphatics and the pampiniform plexus means that anaesthesia wanes after 10 minutes, giving a short window of surgical anaesthesia for castration. Rapid spread of the local anaesthetic agent occurs from the testicular body to the spermatic cord; the only tissues not

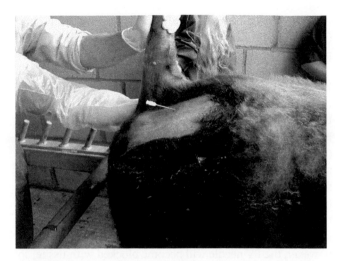

Figure 33.18 Right pudendal and caudal rectal nerve block performed from the lateral approach.

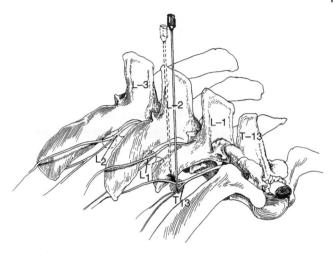

Figure 33.19 Paravertebral block. *Source:* Reproduced, with kind permission, from Skarda (1987).

blocked are the cremaster muscle and the skin at the incision site. A small bleb of local anaesthetic can be deposited subcutaneously at the skin incision site.

Where possible, the injection/s should be performed under aseptic technique, especially where bloodless castration is to be performed.

Local anaesthetic with epinephrine is preferred to slow the rate of systemic absorption.

33.13.7 Local/Regional Anaesthetic Techniques for Laparotomies

33.13.7.1 Epidural Block

A 'cranial' epidural block is required, so recumbency is more likely (with local anaesthetics). Other techniques are therefore preferred.

33.13.7.2 Paravertebral (PV) Block

This is commonly performed to desensitise the flank for surgical incisions at the sublumbar (paralumbar) fossae, which requires that the thirteenth thoracic and first two lumbar segmental nerves must be blocked at paravertebral sites close to where these segmental nerves leave their intervertebral foramina. The very caudal part of the sublumbar fossa is also innervated by branches of the third and fourth lumbar segmental nerves, but if these are blocked, there may be some hind leg weakness because these nerves also supply some motor fibres to the hindlimb muscles. Therefore, local infiltration may be preferable to extend the field of anaesthesia in order to complete surgery at this site.

The aim of the PV block is to desensitise the segmental nerves shortly after they leave the intervertebral foramina, before they have had much time to branch (Figure 33.19).

By keeping the injected local anaesthetic distant to the site of surgery, there is less distortion of the surgical site and some believe that wound closure and therefore healing is improved.

Several techniques have been described, broadly categorised into proximal and distal techniques. Proximal techniques aim to block the nerves as proximally as possible, whereas distal techniques block the nerves a little farther away from where they leave the intervertebral foramina. Once the nerves have emerged from their foramina, they divide into dorsal and ventral branches. The ventral branches then course beneath the lumbar transverse processes, diagonally-caudally. The dorsal branches also course diagonally and caudally, and supply cutaneous branches that innervate a long way down the flank. Both dorsal and ventral branches supply muscle, and the ventral branches also significantly contribute to skin innervation, especially ventrally, but also extending dorsally quite considerably. The ventral branches also supply the peritoneum and carry sympathetic nerves (some of which carry 'pain' information from the viscera). Thus, both dorsal and ventral branches must be blocked to anaesthetise the flank fully (and provide some visceral analgesia, but bilateral blocks are required to fully produce visceral analgesia). Block of the sympathetic nerves also results in vasodilation.

The proximal technique was first described by Farquharson and was modified by anaesthetists at Liverpool and Cambridge veterinary schools (Figure 33.19). The lumbar transverse processes are initially palpated. Normally the transverse process of the fifth lumbar vertebra is the first lumbar transverse process palpable cranial to the 'hook bone' (tuber coxae). From here, the other transverse processes can be counted cranially, but the transverse process of the first lumbar vertebra is shorter and narrower than the others and is often obscured behind the last rib. Using your fingers like callipers, having gauged the distance between say the second and third lumbar transverse processes, the location of the transverse process of the first lumbar vertebra can now be determined in relation to the second.

The sites to prepare for injection are: just cranial to the transverse process of the first lumbar vertebra; over and between the transverse processes of the first and second lumbar vertebrae; and between the transverse processes of the second and third lumbar vertebrae; and for each of these sites, about halfway between the dorsal spinous processes and the lateral tips of the transverse processes. After aseptic preparation of the injection sites, subcutaneous (and slightly deeper into the epaxial muscles) blebs of local anaesthetic are injected at the sites where the larger PV needles will later be inserted. This helps to reduce spasm of longissimus dorsi muscles when a PV needle is subsequently inserted.

33.13.7.2.1 The Liverpool Technique

The PV needle can then be inserted at right angles to the skin, about half-way along the length of the transverse process, starting at the site between the second and third lumbar vertebrae. The needle tip is aimed to just hit the caudal edge of the transverse process of the second lumbar vertebra from where it can be 'walked off' the caudal edge of the process. As the needle slides off the caudal edge of the transverse process, it should 'pop' through the inter-transverse ligament, and the ventral branch of the second lumbar segmental nerve lies under here. For a mature cow, 20–30 ml of local anaesthetic is injected, whilst gently moving the needle around to redirect it a little (and aspirating before each injection to guard against inadvertent intravascular or intraruminal injection), to facilitate adequate spread of the local anaesthetic solution. As the needle is withdrawn, once its tip is deemed 'above' the intertransverse ligament, another 5–10 ml of local anaesthetic is injected to block the dorsal branch of the second lumbar nerve. This whole process is repeated by next aiming for the caudal edge of the transverse process of the first lumbar vertebra to block the ventral and dorsal branches of the first lumbar segmental nerve. Finally, before the needle is removed totally, it is aimed at the cranial border of the transverse process of the first lumbar vertebra, slightly nearer the dorsal midline of the animal, to block the thirteenth thoracic segmental nerve below and above the intertransverse ligament in a similar manner. (For mature sheep, the doses required are around 5 ml of local anaesthetic for the ventral branch and 3–5 ml for the dorsal branch of each segmental nerve.)

PV needles with short bevels are akin to spinal needles in that they are said to be relatively blunt, which enables a better appreciation of the sensation of passing through the intertransverse ligament. Once the PV needle's tip is inserted beneath the skin, and after its stylette is removed (if applicable), if a little local anaesthetic or sterile saline is placed into its hub, then should accidental penetration of the dorsal part of the abdominal cavity occur, the liquid will be sucked in, due to the usual negative pressure at this location. The needle should be withdrawn slightly, until no further negative pressure is appreciated, before injection of local anaesthetic is performed. However, in recumbent (especially gravid) animals, there is less likely to be appreciable negative pressure in the dorsal peritoneal cavity. Should the rumen be inadvertently penetrated, ruminal contents (gas and liquid) will usually egress the needle rapidly. In this situation, it is better to withdraw the needle completely and start over with another sterile needle. (Sometimes, however, the PV needle will become blocked with tissue, so that the use of these tests to confirm or refute penetration of the peritoneal cavity or rumen, will rendered useless.)

33.13.7.2.2 The Cambridge Technique

The PV needle is inserted slightly nearer the dorsal midline of the animal than in the Liverpool technique (about 1 cm closer to the dorsal spinous processes), and is directed at the cranial borders of the lumbar transverse processes instead. Therefore, the second lumbar segmental nerve is blocked at the cranial edge of the transverse process of the third lumbar vertebra; the first lumbar segmental nerve is blocked at the cranial border of the transverse process of the second lumbar vertebra; and the thirteenth thoracic segmental nerve is blocked at the cranial edge of the transverse process of the first lumbar vertebra. Local anaesthetic doses are as above.

33.13.7.2.3 The Cornell Technique

Magda and Cakala described this distal PV technique that results in less scoliosis than the proximal techniques as the epaxial and hypaxial muscles tend to be spared (see below). The segmental nerves are approached from the distal tips of the lumbar transverse processes, advancing the needles parallel with the long axes of the transverse processes, and depositing local anaesthetic above and below them. The thirteenth thoracic segmental nerve is therefore blocked just above and below the distal tip of the transverse process of the first lumbar vertebra; the first lumbar segmental nerve is blocked just above and below the distal tip of the transverse process of the second lumbar vertebra, but the third lumbar segmental nerve courses closer to the tip of the transverse process of the fourth lumbar vertebra than that of the third, and so it is blocked just above and below the distal tip of the fourth lumbar transverse process. Each injection is made in a fan shape, with the needle being moved around gently to increase the success of the block. This approach is more difficult in well-muscled or fat animals, as the tips of the transverse processes may be very difficult to find. That said, the proximal techniques are also more tricky in fatter or well-muscled animals, and may require longer needles and larger doses of local anaesthetic.

33.13.7.2.4   How Can You Tell If the Block Has Worked?

The flank becomes warm (local vasodilation), and with proximal unilateral blocks, because of unilateral flank and back muscle relaxation, the flank bows out on the side of the block so that the spine tends to curve, with the convexity to the side of the block (Figure 33.20). If bilateral blocks are performed, a mild kyphosis may be observed because of bilateral relaxation of the longissimus dorsi muscles. Because of vasodilation, oozing haemorrhage may be increased, which can be a nuisance for surgery. The muscle relaxation usually helps surgery, although the bowing of the flank may make approximation of muscles and skin (at the end of surgery) more difficult without some tension.

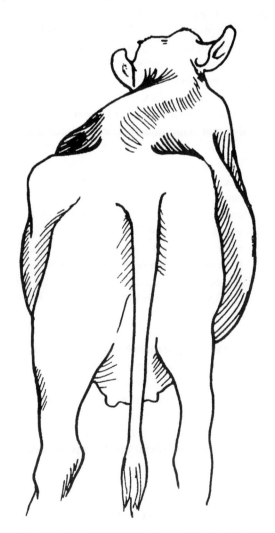

Figure 33.20   When the paravertebral block has worked, the spine bows out on the blocked side. *Source:* Reproduced from Hall et al. (2001) with permission from Elsevier.

33.13.7.3   Inverse 'L' (or Reverse 7) Block

The flank is infiltrated along the lines of black dots illustrated in Figure 33.21a; hence the name 'inverted L' (or 'reversed 7') block when operating on the left flank. (When operating on the right side, the block would be a 'rotated L' or a 'standard 7' block.) The open circle depicts the occasional caudal extent of the block required.

About 100 ml local anaesthetic is needed for a mature cow and an 18–20 g, 3.5 cm needle; or around 25 ml for a mature sheep (the local anaesthetic solution can be diluted to facilitate the block whilst reducing the risk of toxicity).

Starting from one initial desensitised site (superficial tissues, then deeper muscles and finally the peritoneum), the block can be advanced by placing the next needle at the edge of the previously desensitised area, so that the animal does not react to all the subsequent needle insertions. Local anaesthetic is infiltrated 'down' the flank along the caudal border of the last rib, and then along a 'horizontal' line extending caudally from the last rib, just ventral to the transverse processes of the lumber vertebrae, and extending as far caudally as the transverse process of lumbar vertebra four (or perhaps more caudally if required).

One advantage of this block is that it does not require detailed anatomical knowledge. It gives decent muscle relaxation, but can be time-consuming to perform and requires a relatively large volume of local anaesthetic. The toxic dose of lidocaine is in the region of/greater than about 4 (plain) to 8 (with epinephrine) mg/kg, so for a 500 kg cow, this could be between 2,000 and 4,000 mg, which is equivalent to 100 ml of 2% lidocaine plain, or 200 ml of 2% lidocaine solution with epinephrine (note: 2% solution = 20 mg/ml). If such volumes are required, or even exceeded, then observe the animal closely: if the cow looks slightly sleepy, and she was not sedated, the sedation may well be due to systemic absorption of the lidocaine.

33.13.7.4   Line Block (Infiltration Along Proposed Incision Site)

Again, not much anatomical knowledge is required. Local anaesthetic solution is infiltrated along the intended incision line (e.g. Figure 33.21b). For a mature cow, around 100 ml local anaesthetic will be required.

For a mature (50–70 kg) sheep, for a flank 'line' block for Caesarean section, 10–25 ml local anaesthetic should be sufficient. It can also be diluted to a larger volume to facilitate performing the block whilst reducing the risk of toxicity.

Problems include:

- Lack of muscle relaxation.
- Potential formation of haematomas and presence of 'pockets' of local anaesthetic along the incision line (which makes surgery harder as this can distort the local anatomy).

(a)

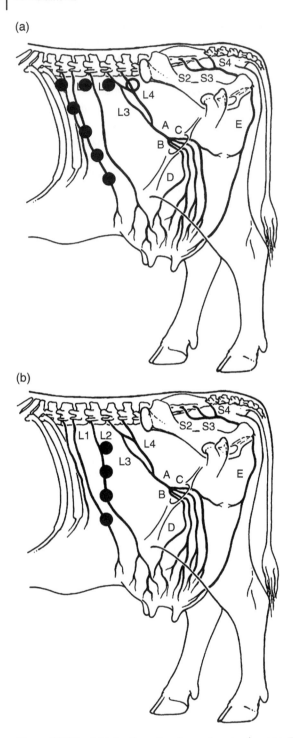

(b)

Figure 33.21 (a) Injection sites for performing 'reverse 7' block. (b) Line block of the flank. *Source:* Reproduced from Tranquilli et al. (2007) with permission of Blackwell Publishing Ltd.

- Possible interference with wound healing; beware especially if epinephrine is included with the local anaesthetic and if environmental temperatures are also low, as both encourage vasoconstriction.
- Systemic toxicity if large doses of local anaesthetic are used.

33.13.7.5 Local/Regional Anaesthetic Techniques for Lower Abdominal Wall or Ventral Abdominal Surgery

For umbilical herniorrhaphy, a cranial epidural from the sacro-/inter-coccygeal site or a lumbo-sacral epidural could be performed, both producing recumbency and risking hypotension and hypothermia. Bilateral PV blocks may offer an alternative strategy, but require excellent technique to guarantee good anaesthesia of the ventral midline. Although a 'ring block' around the hernial sac is easy to perform, it may distort the local anatomy at the surgical site. Therefore, interest in alternative techniques for truncal blocks has grown, although none of these 'compartment blocks' has been completely evaluated and proven clinically at the time of writing.

33.13.7.5.1 Quadratus Lumborum Block

Not yet described for clinical use in cattle, but has been studied in canine cadavers following its description in people. Ultrasound-guided injection of local anaesthetic is made, bilaterally, into the plane between the fascia of the quadratus lumborum (one of the lumbar hypaxial muscles) and that of the psoas major and minor muscles, usually at the level of the first or second lumbar vertebrae in order to block the ventral branches of the lumbar nerves with their sympathetic component. The extent of anaesthesia of the ventral abdomen (in the cranial to mid abdominal section) depends upon the volume of local anaesthetic injected and how well it spreads in the inter-fascial plane to block the lumbar segmental nerves. More recently, the human literature has described this technique as a type of indirect PV block (PV by proxy) for producing truncal anaesthesia, which almost brings us back full-circle to considering bilateral PV blocks.

33.13.7.5.2 Transversus Abdominis Plane (TAP) Block

The TAP block anaesthetises the nerves of the lateral abdominal wall, extending towards the ventral midline, but not always including it. The lateral abdominal musculature is composed of three muscle layers, from superficial to deep: external abdominal oblique (EAO), internal abdominal oblique (IAO), and transversus abdominis (TA). The last several thoracic and first few lumbar segmental nerves and the cranial and caudal iliohypogastric and ilioinguinal nerves run in the fascial plane in between the TA and the IAO muscles. In humans, several approaches to this block have been described, and although some use only anatomical landmarks, the concomitant use of ultrasound guidance is recommended.

In calves, as in dogs, the block can be performed, with ultrasound guidance, by injecting local anaesthetic at either a single injection site or at several injection sites on each flank. As yet, the optimal injection site/s and local anaesthetic volume/s have not been determined. For the single injection site, a needle is inserted midway between the last rib and the iliac crest, in-plane with the ultrasound transducer: when the three muscle layers have been identified, needle insertion is 'observed' by ultrasound, and local anaesthetic solution deposition can be witnessed as 'hydrodissection' in the fascial plane between the IAO and TA muscles. The block should be performed bilaterally to effect anaesthesia of the abdominal wall for surgery. However, this block may only provide somatic analgesia (i.e. blockade of sympathetic/visceral innervation is not always achieved); the extent of the block is highly dependent upon interfascial spread of injected local anaesthetic, and it cannot always guarantee desensitisation of the ventral midline. Therefore, for umbilical hernia repair, a complementary (or even totally alternative) block, may be the rectus sheath block (see below). A true PV block technique is thought to be the only technique to guarantee visceral analgesia alongside somatic analgesia (see Chapter 16 for further discussion of this).

33.13.7.5.3 *Rectus Sheath Block*

The external and internal sheaths of the rectus abdominis muscles are composed of the aponeuroses of the rectus abdominis muscles with, variously (depending upon the actual cranial-to-caudal anatomical location), those of the EAO, IAO, and TA. The rectus sheaths completely enclose the rectus abdominis muscles over their cranial-most three-quarters, but cover only the external aspect of the rectus abdominis muscles over their caudal-most quarters. For the caudal-most quarter of each rectus abdominis muscle, there is no internal rectus sheath as such, rather the rectus abdominis muscle is in direct contact with the transversalis fascia. Injection of local anaesthetic solution 'within' the rectus sheath, either beneath/inside the internal sheath (or beneath/inside the transversalis fascia if far caudally), or beneath/inside the external sheath, can produce anaesthesia of the ventral midline and nearby ventral abdominal wall. Furthermore, this anaesthesia can extend cranial and caudal to the umbilicus, depending upon the site/s of the injections and the volumes of local anaesthetic injected.

Ultrasound-guided injection of local anaesthetic solution 'within' the rectus abdominis sheath has been described in people. This technique can be used to complement the TAP block, but has also been used as a standalone technique in people to provide sufficient analgesia for umbilical herniorrhaphy. The most common injection site is adjacent, but craniolateral to, the umbilicus, bilaterally. For very large umbilical hernias or where infection is suspected, and the surgical site is somewhat distant to the ventral midline, the TAP block may be preferable, which somewhat distances the injection sites from the hernial contents.

References

Dyce, K.M., Sack, W.O., and CJG, W. (eds.) (2002). The pelvis and reproductive organs of female ruminants. In: *Textbook of Veterinary Anatomy*, 3e, 691–712. Elsevier.

Hall, L.W., Clarke, K.W., and Trim, C.M. (eds.) (2001). Anaesthesia of cattle. In: *Veterinary Anaesthesia*, 10e, 315–339. Elsevier.

Skarda, R.T. (1987). Local and regional analgesia. In: *Principles and Practice of Veterinary Anesthesia* (ed. C.E. Short), 91–133. Baltimore, MD, USA: Williams and Wilkins.

Tranquilli, W.J., Thurmon, J.C., and Grimm, K.A. (eds.) (2007). *Lumb and Jones' Veterinary Anesthesia and Analgesia*, 4e. Blackwell Publishing Ltd.

Further Reading

Abrahamsen, E.J. (2008). Ruminant field anesthesia. *Veterinary Clinics of North America: Farm Animal Practice* 24: 429–444.

Adams, J. (2017). Assessment and management of pain in small ruminants. *Livestock* 22: 324–328.

Bell, N. and Mahendran, S. (2017). Local anaesthesia and analgesia guidance for surgical treatment of cows with necrotic hoof lesions. *Livestock* 22: 298–304.

Caulkett, N.A., MacDonald, D.G., Janzen, E.D. et al. (1993). Xylazine hydrochloride epidural analgesia: a method for providing sedation and analgesia to facilitate castration of mature bulls. *The Compendium on Continuing Education for the Practising Veterinarian: Food Animal Practice* 15: 1155–1159.

Clutton, R.E. (2018). A review of factors affecting analgesic selection in large animals undergoing translational research. *The Veterinary Journal* 236: 12–22.

De Oliveira, F.A., Luna, S.P.L., do Amaral, J.B. et al. (2014). Validation of the UNESP-Botucatu unidimensional composite pain scale for assessing postoperative pain in cattle. *BMC Veterinary Research* 10: 20.

Edmondson, M.A. (2008). Local and regional anaesthesia in cattle. *Veterinary Clinics of North America: Farm Animal Practice* 24: 211–226.

Garcia-Villar, R., Toutain, P.L., Alvinerie, M., and Ruckebusch, Y. (1981). The pharmacokinetics of xylazine hydrochloride: an interspecific study. *Journal of Veterinary Pharmacology and Therapeutics* 4: 87–92.

Habel, R.E. (1956). A source of error in the bovine pudendal nerve block. *Journal of the American Veterinary Medical Association* 128: 16–17.

Hager, C., Biernot, S., Buettner, M. et al. (2017). The sheep grimace scale as an indicator of post-operative distress and pain in laboratory sheep. *PLoS One* 12 (4): e0175839.

Hendrickx, M.-O. (2015). Lidocaine use in pigs, cattle and horses. *Veterinary Record* 176: 630.

Hodgkinson, O. and Dawson, L. (2007). Practical anaesthesia and analgesia in sheep, goats and calves. *In Practice* 29: 596–603.

Jedruch, J. and Gajewski, Z. (1986). The effect of detomidine hydrochloride (Domosedan) on the electrical activity of the uterus in cows. *Acta Veterinaria Scandinavica Supplementum* 82: 189–192.

Kaestner, S.B.R. (2006). Alpha 2 agonists in sheep: a review. *Veterinary Anaesthesia and Analgesia* 33: 79–96.

Larson, L.L. (1953). The internal pudendal (pudic) nerve block for anesthesia of the penis and relaxation of the retractor penis muscle. *Journal of the American Veterinary Medical Association* 123: 18–27.

Laven, R. (2018). Managing pain in lame cattle. *Livestock* 23: 161–167.

LeBlanc, M.M., Hubbell, J.A.E., and Smith, H.C. (1984). The effects of xylazine hydrochloride on intrauterine pressure in the cow. *Theriogenology* 21 (5): 681–690.

Lin, H.C. (2015). Comparative anaesthesia and analgesia of ruminants and swine. In: *Veterinary Anaesthesia and Analgesia*, the fifth edition of Lumb and Jones (eds. K.A. Grimm, L.A. Lamont, W.J. Tranquilli, et al.), 743–753. Iowa, USA: Wiley Blackwell.

Lomax, S., Witenden, E., Windsor, P., and White, P. (2017). Effect of topical vapocoolant spray on perioperative pain response of unweaned calves to ear tagging and ear notching. *Veterinary Anaesthesia and Analgesia* 44: 163–172.

McFarlane, I.S. (1963). The lateral approach to the pudendal nerve block in the bovine and ovine. *Journal of the South African Veterinary Medical Association* 34: 73–76.

McLennan, K.M., Rebelo, C.J.B., Corke, M.J. et al. (2016). Development of a facial expression scale using footrot and mastitis as models of pain in sheep. *Applied Animal Behaviour Science* 176: 19–16.

Peterson, D.R. (1951). Nerve block of the eye and associated structures. *Journal of the American Veterinary Medical Association* 118: 145–148.

Plummer, P.J. and Schleining, J.A. (2013). Assessment and management of pain in small ruminants and camelids. *Veterinary Clinics of North American: Farm Animal Practice* 29: 185–208.

Potter, T.J., Hallowell, G.D., and Aldridge, B. (2012). Head and ocular surgery in farm animals. *In Practice* 34: 518–522.

Remnant, J.G., Tremlett, A., Huxley, J.N., and Hudson, C.D. (2017). Clinician attitudes to pain and use of analgesia in cattle: where are we 10 years on? *Veterinary Record* https://doi.org/10.1136//vr.104428.

Rizk, A., Herdtweck, S., Offinger, J. et al. (2012). The use of xylazine hydrochloride in an analgesic protocol for claw treatment of lame dairy cows in lateral recumbency on a surgical tipping table. *The Veterinary Journal* 192: 193–198.

Sakamoto, H., Kirihara, H., Fujiki, M. et al. (1997). The effects of medetomidine on maternal and fetal cardiovascular and pulmonary function, intrauterine pressure and uterine blood flow in pregnant goats. *Experimental Animals* 46: 67–73.

Schulz, K. (2008). Field surgery of the eye and para-orbital tissue. *Veterinary Clinics of North America: Farm Animal Practice* 24: 527–534.

Siva, T., Taffarel, M., Oliveira, R., and Denadai, L. (2019). Validation of the UNESP-Botucatu composite pain scale for assessing postoperative pain in sheep. Proceedings of the spring meeting of the Association of Veterinary Anaesthetists, Bristol, UK. 47.

Torneke, K., Bergstrom, U., and Neil, A. (2003). Interactions of xylazine and detomidine with alpha 2 adrenoceptors in brain tissues from cattle, swine and rats. *Journal of Veterinary Pharmacology and Therapeutics* 26: 205–211.

Valverde, A. and Sinclair, M. (2015). Ruminant and swine local anesthetic and analgesic techniques. In: *Veterinary Anaesthesia and Analgesia*, fifth edition of Lumb and Jones (eds. K.A. Grimm, L.A. Lamont, W.J. Tranquilli, et al.), 941–959. Iowa, USA: Wiley Blackwell.

Waldvogel, D. and Bleul, U. (2014). Effect of xylazine, isoxuprine and lidocaine on Doppler sonographic uterine and umbilical blood flow measurements in cows during the last month of pregnancy. *Theriogenology* 81: 993–1003.

Walkowiak, K.J. and Graham, M.L. (2015). Pharmacokinetics and antinociceptive activity of sustained-release buprenorphine in sheep. *Journal of the American Association for Laboratory Animal Science* 54: 763–768.

Wessels, M.E., Scholes, S.F.E., Kemp, R., and Hodgkinson, O. (2007). Hindlimb paralysis following epidural anaesthesia in a ram. *Letter: Veterinary Record* 161: 459.

Zaugg, J.L. and Nussbaum, M. (1990). Epidural injection of xylazine: a new option for surgical analgesia of the bovine abdomen and udder. *Veterinary Medicine* 85: 1043–1045.

Zoff, A., Dugdale, A., Coates, A.N., and Rioja, E. (2017). Transversus abdominis plane block in two calves undergoing umbilical herniorrhaphy. *Veterinary Record Case Reports* 5: e000447, 1–5. Doi: https://doi.org/10.1136/vetreccr-2017-000447.

Self-test Section

1 True or False? The following may be complications of prolonged starvation in ruminants:

   A Increased fluidity of reticuloruminal contents

   B Ketoacidosis in high production animals

   C Increased heart rate

   D Decreased body temperature

2 Which cranial nerves exit the cranium via the foramen orbitorotundum in cattle?

   A II, III, IV, V (ophthalmic, maxillary), VI

   B II, III, IV, V (ophthalmic, maxillary, and mandibular), VI

   C III, IV, V (ophthalmic, maxillary), VI

   D III, IV, V (ophthalmic, maxillary, and mandibular), VI

34

Lamoids (South American Camelids)

LEARNING OBJECTIVES

- To be familiar with the ruminant-like and horse-like characteristics of lamoids (South American Camelids) and the associated risks of general anaesthesia.
- To be able to recognise the potential problems with respect to venous cannulation and endotracheal intubation.
- To be able to devise a protocol for sedation and general anaesthesia; recognising the need to provide analgesia

---

34.1 Introduction

Llamas and alpacas have been domesticated from (and are therefore descendants of) their wild relatives, the guanacos and vicugnas, respectively. Llamas are used as pack animals and/or for their fleece, whereas alpacas are kept mainly for their fleece. The two types of alpaca are distinguishable by their fleece: the more common Huacaya alpacas have shorter more crimpy, spongy fibres (similar to sheep), whereas Suri alpacas have longer straight fibres with no crimp. Young lamoids are called crias. Parturition is referred to as *unpacking* or *criation*. Llamas and alpacas can cross-breed with their offspring being called huarizo.

Shearing, toe-clipping, ear-tagging, and diagnostic procedures (such as radiography, ultrasonography) may be possible with only sedation and/or analgesia. Where sedation with local/regional anaesthesia is inappropriate or the patient is not amenable, general anaesthesia will be necessary, e.g. for fracture fixation, enucleation, castration, Caesarean section and colic surgery (e.g. uterine torsion is common in late gestation).

Lamoids can be temperamental and occasionally **aggressive**, especially the males; beware spits, bites, kicks, and strikes.

Male llamas weigh 150–250 kg; female llamas weigh 100–200 kg. Male alpacas weigh 60–90 kg; female alpacas weigh 50–60 kg. It can be **hard to estimate their weight** because of their thick hair coat.

Jugular veins can be difficult to cannulate. There are **no well-defined jugular furrows**, lots of jugular venous **valves**, and males have **thick tough skin**, and **cervical vertebral transverse processes** (especially Ce 5 and Ce 6) can 'cover' (fold over) the vein. The best sites for venous cannulation are high up the neck, towards the vein's bifurcation at the angle of the mandible or low down the neck near the thoracic inlet. If one imaginary line is drawn along the ventral border of the horizontal ramus of the mandible, and another from the base of the ear along the caudal aspect of the vertical ramus of the mandible, the jugular vein should be located where these two lines intersect. For adult animals, 16 g cannulae are commonly used and a scalpel blade may be used to make a small skin nick to facilitate passage of the cannula through the skin without damaging it. Cannulating the right jugular vein avoids the risk of causing oesophageal trauma. Cephalic and auricular veins may sometimes be used too; 18 or 20 g cannulae, respectively, would be appropriate. **Venous blood often looks more 'red' than you would expect** in our more usual lower altitude species because of the lower P_{50} (17.5–22 mmHg) of lamoid haemoglobin, which therefore remains well saturated at the venous

Veterinary Anaesthesia: Principles to Practice, Second Edition. Alexandra H. A. Dugdale, Georgina Beaumont, Carl Bradbrook, and Matthew Gurney.
© 2020 John Wiley & Sons Ltd. Published 2020 by John Wiley & Sons Ltd.
Companion website: www.wiley.com/go/dugdale/veterinary-anaesthesia

partial pressures of oxygen commonly measured at lower altitudes (see Further Reading).

The **trachea can be difficult to intubate**. Desensitising the larynx with topical local anaesthetic may help. A laryngoscope with long blade and an endotracheal (ET) tube intubating stylette or bougie will help. With the head and neck held extended (aim for a 180° head-on-neck angle), the jaws are then parted as wide as possible using tapes to 'distract' them (the labial fissure is narrow). Gentle traction is applied to the tongue. Like ruminants, there is a lingual 'torus' to negotiate. If orotracheal intubation fails, try the nasotracheal route with tubes 1–2 sizes smaller than the orotracheal ET tube, but lamoids are prone to epistaxis on nasotracheal (and nasopharyngeal) intubation and extubation, and beware the nasopharyngeal diverticulum (see star mark in Figure 34.1).

Lamoids are also prone to airway obstruction, both on intubation, and especially after tracheal extubation; possibly due to laryngospasm/laryngeal oedema. It is advisable to have the necessary drugs and equipment available for performing emergency ET intubation or even tracheostomy.

Nasal oedema may develop during anaesthesia, as in horses, and can cause upper respiratory tract obstruction in recovery, but nasopharyngeal tubes can be used as for horses (beware epistaxis).

Lamoids are similar to ruminants in many respects, but are said to be obligate nose-breathers like horses. They can, however, mouth-breathe, but find it distressing to have to do so.

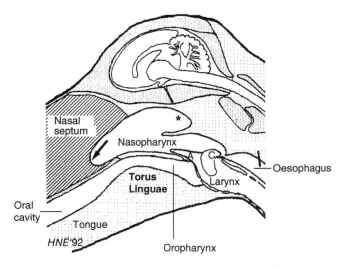

Figure 34.1 Sagittal section through lamoid head. The nasopharyngeal diverticulum is marked with a star. *Source:* Reproduced from Riebold et al. (1994) with kind permission of the American Veterinary Medical Association.

They have a stoic nature, so often do not require sedation pre-induction or pre-recovery. Premedication can, however, reduce the required doses of anaesthetic induction and maintenance agents, and can reduce any aggressive behavioural responses provoked by the anxiety of the novel situation with novel handlers, etc.

Lamoids are modified ruminants and have a three-compartment 'stomach'. They ruminate and under anaesthesia are **prone to continued salivation, drooling, regurgitation, and aspiration**. They appear to be less prone to the development of ruminal tympany than true ruminants. Food (and water) withholding prior to general anaesthesia can reduce bulk and fermentation rate in the first two stomach compartments (C1/C2), and may help to reduce the risk of regurgitation and tympany, but does not reduce the chance of the animal spitting (spitters are said to be more prone to regurgitation). Any reduction in C1/C2 bulk may also reduce cardiovascular and respiratory compromise during recumbency (especially dorsal). That said, the optimal time for food withholding and which type of foods are most important to withhold are unknown; recent suggestions for ruminants are that water should be available at all times and perhaps ad libitum access to conserved forage (e.g. hay, rather than the wetter ensiled variants), until about 6 (−12) hours before general anaesthesia, may be preferred.

Regurgitation may occur during very light or very deep planes of anaesthesia. In particular, active regurgitation can be provoked during tracheal intubation attempts under light anaesthesia, where it poses risks for aspiration. Furthermore, at light planes of anaesthesia, lamoids are said to respond, not only to tracheal intubation, but also to surgical stimuli, with vagal (rather than sympathetic) responses, so may require anticholinergics: either atropine 0.02 mg/kg IV (or 0.04 mg/kg IM), or glycopyrrolate 5–10 µg/kg IV. Anticholinergics, however, reduce gut motility, enhance oesophageal reflux (by reducing cardiac sphincter tone), reduce the watery parts of respiratory secretions and saliva (which become more viscous and harder to clear), reduce respiratory mucociliary activity, and result in bronchodilation (which increases dead space and enhances rebreathing). Therefore, these drugs tend not to be administered routinely as a part of the premedication, but must be available in case of emergency.

Although stomach tubes can be placed into the oesophagus to direct any regurgitated material away from the pharynx/larynx, they tend to increase the amount of fluid regurgitated and even provoke regurgitation, which can pour down the outside of the tube too. In order to prevent the glottis from being submerged by fluids in the pharyngeal/laryngeal region, the poll should be raised above the stomach and nose levels with a sand bag under the throat region, much as for cattle; or the head should be lowered so that material can drain away from the throat. Cuffed ET tubes should be used.

Lamoids are **prone to stress-related third stomach compartment ulcers**. Minimise stress if possible, keep hospital stay as short as possible, and perhaps bring a companion animal from the herd. When non-steroidal anti-inflammatory drugs (NSAIDs) form part of the analgesic protocol, anti-ulcer medications should probably be included in the treatment plan (see below).

Adaptations to high altitude and arid environments include relatively small, flat elliptoid red blood cells with relatively high haemoglobin content. These erythrocytes are flexible yet highly resistant to osmotic lysis. Normal PCV is 27–40%.

Prophylaxis against third compartment (C3) ulcers has not been absolutely proven, but the following may help:

- Cimetidine, an H2 antagonist, 5 mg/kg q.i.d. IV only changes C3 pH for two hours after each dose, so some people advocate 3.3 mg/kg every two hours.
- Ranitidine, an H2 antagonist, 1.5 mg/kg IV produces minimal and transient (<1 hour), reduction in C3 acidity.
- Omeprazole, an irreversible proton pump inhibitor, produces only short duration reduction in C3 acidity. In mature, ruminating animals, it has very low bioavailability by the oral route, but may help increase C3 pH at 1.4 mg/kg t.i.d. PO in pre-ruminant crias. In ruminating animals, 0.4–0.8 mg/kg IV can suppress C3 acid production, but re-dosing is required every two hours.
- Pantoprazole, an irreversible proton pump inhibitor, 1–1.5 mg/kg once daily IV or SC appears to produce clinically useful suppression of C3 acid production.
- Misoprostol, a PGE1 analogue, 10 µg/kg once daily, slowly IV, may be effective, but adverse reactions may be commonly

observed such as collapse, recumbency, disorientation, and regurgitation. Avoid in pregnant animals.
- Sucralfate, a basic aluminium complex of sulphated sucrose which is an ulcer cytoprotective agent, 20–40 mg/kg q.i.d. PO may be useful should C3 ulcers already exist.
- Non-specific antacids: empirical dose.

34.2 Drugs and Details for Anaesthesia

Try to maintain a calm environment and handle these animals gently. Provide a soft, non-slippery floor as South American Camelids tend to cush (assume sternal recumbency) once sedated.

34.2.1 Premedication

- Allays fear and anxiety that facilitates handling and venous cannulation.
- Can provide analgesia.
- Generally smooths anaesthetic induction and reduces the doses of anaesthetic induction and maintenance agents required.

34.2.1.1 Phenothiazines

Acepromazine is rarely used as it produces a poorly predictable response, and it promotes vasodilation with consequent hypotension and hypothermia. It also reduces lower oesophageal sphincter tone and may increase the risk of regurgitation. It is not analgesic.

34.2.1.2 Benzodiazepines

Useful in immature and sick animals as they produce minimal cardiorespiratory depressant effects. Not analgesic, but can be combined with opioids. (See Table 34.1.)

Table 34.1 Benzodiazepine-based sedation.

Drug/s	Dose/route	Effects
Diazepam or midazolam	0.1 mg/kg IV	Co-operation/possibly recumbency, in neonates, geriatrics, pregnant, or sick patients Duration about 15 min
Diazepam or midazolam	0.3 + mg/kg IV	Possibly recumbent sedation Duration about 30 min
Diazepam or midazolam + Butorphanol	0.1 mg/kg IV 0.1 mg/kg IV	Recumbent sedation for up to 30 min

34.2.1.3 α2 Agonists

Produce predictable, dose-dependent sedation, analgesia, and muscle relaxation, but have profound cardiovascular side effects (care in young or sick animals), and cause diuresis (care if urethral obstruction). Xylazine has been the most commonly used agent, so there is less information about detomidine and romifidine; and no information, as yet, about oral transmucosal delivery of detomidine. Medetomidine, however, is becoming more popular as an alternative to xylazine. Beware in pregnant animals, although not known to cause abortion. Combination with opioids enhances the sedation and analgesia. Atipamezole can be used as an antagonist if required. (See Table 34.2.)

Low (sub-anaesthetic) dose ketamine (sometimes called a ketamine stun) can be added to xylazine and butorphanol to produce an even deeper sedation, with recumbency, which may be useful for procedures such as radiography, cast placement, or even joint flush. A useful combination, producing 20–30 minutes sedation (with recumbency for at least the first 10–15 minutes of this) is:

$$\text{Xylazine}\left(0.3\,\text{mg/kg}\right) + \text{butorphanol}\left(0.1\,\text{mg/kg}\right) \\ + \text{ketamine}\left(0.3\,\text{mg/kg}\right) \text{given IV}$$

The IV route of administration produces more reliable results than if the drug combination is administered IM. Sedation/recumbency can be prolonged by further doses of 0.15 mg/kg ketamine IV.

34.2.1.4 Opioids

Provide analgesia and some sedation. Produce minimal cardiorespiratory side effects at commonly used doses, but can reduce gut motility. (See Table 34.3.)

34.2.2 Anaesthetic Induction

A calm environment with a soft, non-slippery floor is important. Premedication helps to smooth anaesthetic induction, whether induction is achieved by injectable or inhalation agents. Injectable techniques are usually favoured in larger/mature animals, with IV administration of induction agents favoured over IM. Intravenous access should be secured beforehand, where possible, no matter by what route the induction agent is administered. Inhalation induction of anaesthesia may be preferred in young or sick crias; inhalation agents can be administered either by a facemask or by nasopharyngeal tube insufflation. Mask inductions can become quite messy because

Table 34.2 α2 agonist-based sedation.

Drug/s	Dose/route	Effects
Xylazine	0.1–0.15 mg/kg IV 0.2–0.3 mg/kg IM	Standing sedation for around 15 min
Xylazine	0.3–0.5 mg/kg IV 0.6–1.0 mg/kg IM	Recumbent sedation for around 20–30 minutes
Xylazine + Butorphanol	0.1–0.25 mg/kg IV + 0.05–0.2 mg/kg IV (Double these doses for IM)	Standing to recumbent sedation for up to 30–40 min (dose-dependent)
Medetomidine	0.01–0.03 mg/kg IV 0.05–0.15 mg/kg IM	Recumbency with higher doses Duration 30–90 min (dose-dependent)
Atipamezole	0.05–0.25 mg/kg IM (IV in emergency)	Should be effective within 5 min of administration

Table 34.3 Opioid doses.

Drug	Dose/route	Duration
Butorphanol	0.02–0.2 + mg/kg IV, IM, SC	30–60 min (dose-dependent)
Buprenorphine	0.002–0.01 mg/kg IV, IM	6–8 + h
Morphine	0.05–0.25 mg/kg IM, IV	2–4 h
Pethidine	3.5–5 mg/kg IM	1 h

saliva production continues under anaesthesia and can accumulate in the mask; clear masks enable better visualisation than black rubber masks.

34.2.2.1 Inhalation Agents

Both isoflurane and sevoflurane are usually well tolerated for inhalation induction. Sevoflurane is slightly less soluble in blood than isoflurane, which enables a very slightly faster induction. Sevoflurane is also suggested to be a little less pungent than isoflurane, so may offer a slightly smoother induction, with less breath-holding.

34.2.2.2 Injectable Agents
34.2.2.2.1 Ketamine

Ketamine is a dissociative anaesthetic agent, and, even at sub-anaesthetic doses, it is analgesic and anti-hyperalgesic. It has a high therapeutic index and can be administered IV, IM, or even oral-transmucosal. It produces minimal cardiorespiratory side effects in healthy patients. When administered alone, it can cause an unwanted increase in muscle tone such that it is usually used following, or in combination with, $\alpha2$ agonists, benzodiazepines, or guaiphenesin to reduce the muscle rigidity and improve tracheal intubation conditions.

Ketamine 2–5 mg/kg IV (5–10 mg/kg IM) may be given in combination with diazepam or midazolam 0.05–0.2 mg/kg IV to improve muscle relaxation (if benzodiazepines have not already been given as part of the premedication).

34.2.2.2.2 Guaiphenesin

Guaiphenesin is also known as glyceryl guaiacolate ether (GGE) or glyceryl guaiacolate (GG). It is a centrally acting muscle relaxant with some sedative properties and minimal cardiorespiratory side effects at commonly used doses. Must be administered IV, preferably via an IV cannula (which must be flushed adequately at the end of the injection/infusion), as it is very irritant if deposited extravascularly or transvascularly. Can cause haemolysis in concentrations of 10% or greater, but higher concentrations can be diluted in 5% dextrose or dextrose-saline solutions. Although it can be administered alone at around 15–25 mg/kg IV to produce sedation, it is more commonly given in doses of around 50–100 mg/kg IV, alongside ketamine, to reduce the increased muscle tone associated with ketamine.

34.2.2.2.3 Propofol

A substituted phenol, presented most commonly as a macro-emulsion in Intralipid™. It must be administered IV to be effective because following IM administration, its rapid metabolism, following absorption, prevents it ever reaching a high enough concentration in the brain to cause unconsciousness. Propofol causes moderate cardiorespiratory depression and is not analgesic. It is best administered relatively slowly IV, 'to effect'. Large doses and/or rapid IV injection tend to produce more profound respiratory depression, possibly requiring ventilatory support. Doses of around 2–6 mg/kg IV are required for anaesthetic induction: prior premedication tends to reduce the required induction dose to the lower end of this dose range.

Propofol and ketamine combinations have also been researched for induction of anaesthesia and enable reduced doses of each agent, but post-induction apnoea may still necessitate tracheal intubation and provision of artificial ventilation.

34.2.2.2.4 Alfaxalone

This neuroactive steroid, solubilised in aqueous solution by complexing it with large sugar molecules, called hydroxypropyl beta cyclodextrin, can be administered IV or IM, and produces only mild cardiorespiratory effects. Large doses and/or rapid IV administration can, however, produce more profound respiratory depression, possibly requiring ventilatory support. Alfaxalone can also cause muscle stiffness or tonic/clonic movements at induction and/or recovery, especially if administered without prior sedation/premedication. It does not provide any analgesia. There is currently limited information regarding the use of alfaxalone in lamoids, but preliminary investigations with 2 mg/kg alfaxalone suggest that ventilatory support may be required and that sedation/premedication may be important to offset unwanted muscular activity.

34.2.3 Tracheal Intubation

See above for further details. For orotracheal intubation, long, cuffed ET tubes of about 12 mm internal diameter are required for adult llamas; and down to 8–9 mm internal diameter, for alpacas. Crias will need smaller tubes of around 5 mm internal diameter. If nasotracheal intubation is preferred, tubes of 1 or 2 sizes smaller are used and good lubrication, including local anaesthetic and decongestant, is necessary to help reduce trauma and epistaxis.

34.2.4 Maintenance of Anaesthesia

The method of maintaining anaesthesia depends upon location (field versus hospital) and the availability of the necessary equipment and drugs. Injectable techniques (see above) employ either intermittent boluses or the provision of intravenous infusions. Inhalational techniques, however, are more flexible regarding extension of general anaesthesia time because inhalants are much less cumulative. They also ensure supplemental oxygen provision.

Examples of injectable anaesthetic protocols that can be used in the field are given in Table 34.4. Tracheal intubation is not always necessary, as positioning the head carefully by elevating the poll (as for cattle) can encourage saliva and any regurgitated material to drain away from the larynx, reducing the chance of aspiration.

Isoflurane or sevoflurane may be used, and both offer relatively rapid recoveries. Nitrous oxide, although analgesic, is less favoured as it partitions into spaces where gases of low solubility occur (e.g. methane in the gastrointestinal tract and air [nitrogen] in the ET tube cuff), and increases the volume of and/or pressure in these spaces. Some degree of cardiorespiratory compromise can occur should the gut volume and/or intra-abdominal pressure increase massively because of compression of the caudal vena cava and 'splinting' of the diaphragm.

Attention should be paid to ensure careful positioning on a well-padded bed, especially at pressure points, as neuropathies seems to be more of a risk than myopathies. The long flexible neck should also be carefully supported to avoid airway or jugular occlusion and attempts should be made to keep the throat clear of saliva and/or regurgitated material accumulation. If a head-down position is used, nasal congestion/oedema may develop that can cause upper respiratory obstruction after tracheal extubation.

Lamoids have prominent eyes that are prone to injury and must be protected from dust and direct sunlight (if outdoors), and saliva, regurgitated material, surgical scrub, and direct trauma (in all situations).

34.2.5 Anaesthetic Breathing Systems

The anaesthetic breathing system chosen will depend upon the patient's size. For alpacas (50–90 kg), a small animal circle is suitable. For llamas up to around 135–150 kg, a small animal circle is suitable, whereas a large animal circle will be required for animals larger than this. For crias <10 kg, a T-piece or mini-Lack may be used, but also some circle systems are now available that are suitable for such small patients.

As a rough guide, when using circle systems, the absorber canister should have a volume of at least twice the normal, resting tidal volume (i.e. $\geq 2 \times 10$ ml/kg); and the rebreathing bag should also have a capacity of at least twice the resting tidal volume (i.e. $\geq 2 \times 10$ ml/kg). Therefore, for alpacas, an absorber canister of 2–4 l and a rebreathing bag of 2–5 l capacity would be appropriate; whereas for llamas, an absorber canister of 4–10 l and a rebreathing bag of 5–10–15 l capacity would be more appropriate.

34.2.6 Monitoring

The physiological status and anaesthetic depth of the patient should be monitored as for other species. In lamoids, eyeball position and reflexes, as a guide to anaesthetic depth, are quite variable (they are more like horses than cattle). End tidal anaesthetic agent monitoring (if volatile agents are used for anaesthetic maintenance) can help guide anaesthetic depth.

Table 34.4 Injectable combinations for field anaesthesia.

Premedication/Induction	Opioid	Duration of effect
Xylazine 0.3 mg/kg IV Either with, or followed by, after 3 minutes: Ketamine 3 mg/kg IV	Butorphanol 0.05–0.1 mg/kg IV or IM Or Morphine 0.05–0.1 mg/kg IV or IM	Around 15 min recumbent anaesthesia. Can top up with 1/3–1/2 doses of xylazine and ketamine to extend recumbency by 5–10 min
Diazepam 0.2 mg/kg IV Either just before, or mixed with: Ketamine 4 mg/kg IV	Butorphanol 0.05–0.1 mg/kg IV or IM Or Morphine 0.05–0.1 mg/kg IV or IM	Around 15–20 min recumbent anaesthesia. Can top up with 1/3–1/2 original doses to extend duration by 5–10 min
5% GG infused to effect IV (~50–100 mg/kg) Followed by: Ketamine 2 mg/kg IV	Butorphanol 0.05–0.1 mg/kg IV or IM Or Morphine 0.05–0.1 mg/kg IV or IM	Around 15–20 min recumbent anaesthesia. Beware topping up GG as max dose ~150 mg/kg. Can give 1/3–1/2 original ketamine dose to extend time by 5–10 min

Cardiorespiratory monitoring should include: pulse rate, breathing rate, mucous membrane colour and capillary refill time (CRT), capnography, pulse oximetry (but due to the low P_{50} of lamoid haemoglobin, SpO_2 values may remain high in the face of quite severe hypoxaemia), arterial blood pressure, ECG, temperature, blood gases, and electrolytes. Cannulation of auricular arteries enables direct arterial blood pressure monitoring, which can help anaesthetic depth evaluation and also allows sampling of blood for arterial blood gas analysis. For crias, temperature and blood glucose monitoring are especially important. All reasonable attempts to prevent undue heat loss should be made, especially in crias: warm operating environment, insulation, use of rebreathing systems if possible (or coaxial non-rebreathing systems), use of heat and moisture exchangers, warmed IV and lavage fluids, heated mattresses, forced warm air 'blankets', etc.

34.2.7   Intra-operative Support

Lamoids may hypoventilate under general anaesthesia, especially in dorsal recumbency, so be prepared to provide artificial (manual or mechanical) ventilation, usually in the form of positive pressure ventilation. Respiratory depression may also worsen as the duration of anaesthesia increases.

Hypotension may occur under deeper planes of inhalation anaesthesia. Required interventions may include: lightening of anaesthesia, attention to intravascular volume status and ventilator settings, and possibly the use of positive inotropes and vasopressors. Bradycardia, which may be accompanied by hypotension, may result from a vagal/vasovagal response to visceral traction or noxious stimuli, especially at relatively light planes of anaesthesia, but may also accompany the administration of α2 agonists. Required interventions may include: brief suspension of surgery, antagonism of α2 agonists, administration of anticholinergics, administration of ephedrine, administration of analgesics, and deepening the plane of anaesthesia.

34.2.8   Fluids

Although fluid therapy is important for compromised/hypovolaemic patients, Hartmann's solution is often administered at around 3–5 ml/kg/h to help to replace losses from regurgitation, continued saliva production, evaporation from the respiratory tract and the surgical site, and any pre-operative withholding deficits. Fluid administration also helps ensure an 'open vein', as any problems with the IV access hopefully become quickly apparent and can be rectified so that if IV access is needed in an emergency, it should be available. For neonates, glucose may

need to be supplemented. Blood electrolytes and pH may warrant monitoring during long procedures, and abnormalities should be addressed as necessary.

34.2.9   Analgesic Options

34.2.9.1   Opioids
See above.

34.2.9.2   NSAIDs
NSAIDs are acidic compounds, and if given orally, absorption can be slow or erratic as the pH in the first two stomach compartments can be near neutral, which reduces the unionised fraction available for absorption. Beware third compartment stomach ulcers (see above).

- Flunixin 0.5–1 mg/kg once daily IV, PO.
- Phenylbutazone 2–5 mg/kg every 24–48 hours IV (possibly PO).
- Ketoprofen 1–2 mg/kg once-twice daily IV (possibly PO).
- Meloxicam 0.5 mg/kg IV once; or 1 mg/kg PO (possibly every 72 hours).
- Carprofen, currently no dose information is available.

34.2.9.3   Local Anaesthetic Techniques
Local/regional anaesthetic techniques should be used where possible as part of an overall balanced analgesic technique (see below). Toxic doses of local anaesthetic drugs are unknown in South American Camelids, but maximum doses should probably be around 3 mg/kg for plain lidocaine (4–7 mg/kg for lidocaine with epinephrine), 1.5–3 mg/kg for ropivacaine, and 1–2 mg/kg for bupivacaine. The available solutions can be diluted with sterile saline if necessary. For all the techniques described, aseptic preparation of injection sites is important, and aspiration should always be performed before injection so as to reduce the risk of inadvertent intravascular injection.

Local anaesthetic agents can be used for:

- Topical/surface application (e.g. conjunctival, laryngeal [for tracheal intubation], intra-articular)
- Non-specific infiltration (e.g. ring block, field block, intratesticular)
- Local/regional blocks (e.g. specific perineural blocks, regional nerve blocks [e.g. brachial plexus block], neuraxial anaesthesia)
- Intravenous regional anaesthesia (IVRA)
- Intravenous infusion (systemic analgesia)

34.2.9.3.1   Techniques for Facial, Dental, and Ocular Interventions
Infraorbital Nerve Block   Injection of 1–2 ml local anaesthetic where the infraorbital nerve exits the infraorbital

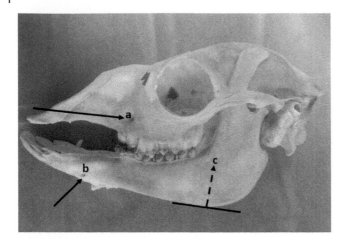

Figure 34.2 Alpaca skull showing infra-orbital foramen (a), mental foramen (b), and location of position of mandibular foramen (c) on medial aspect of mandible.

foramen (Figure 34.2a) desensitises the ipsilateral facial soft tissue structures (upper lip, nose) rostral to the foramen. The infraorbital foramen is usually located 1–3 cm dorsal to the upper premolars on a line between the first premolar and the medial canthus.

Mental Nerve Block

Injection of 1–2 ml local anaesthetic where the mental nerve exits the mental foramen (Figure 34.2b) desensitises the ipsilateral soft tissue structures of the lower lip and chin rostral to the foramen. The mental foramen is located on the lateral aspect of the rostral mandible, around 2–3 cm caudal to the lower incisors and roughly at the midpoint of the diastema (in the rostro-caudal direction), but nearer to its ventral border (in the dorso-ventral direction).

Mandibular Foramen Block

Injection of 3–5 ml local anaesthetic at the mandibular foramen (Figure 34.2c) desensitises all the ipsilateral intra-oral and extra-oral soft tissues and teeth rostral to the foramen. The mandibular foramen lies on the medial aspect of the mandible 2–4 cm 'up' a line drawn perpendicularly to the ventral border of the mandible, just where the upslope of the vertical ramus begins to curve away from the horizontal ramus.

Retrobulbar (Intraconal) Techniques

Local anaesthetic (5–10 ml) can be deposited 'behind' the globe, near the apex of the extra-ocular muscle cone by several different techniques. An additional palpebral block may be required to improve eyelid akinesis. Precautions and complications are as described for small animals and ruminants (see Chapters 13 and 33).

- Trans-orbital approach: A curved needle can be introduced under the orbital rim, dorso-medially to the lateral canthus (in the 2 o'clock position if looking at the left eye, or the 10 o'clock position if looking at the right eye), and advanced around and behind the globe towards the apex of the conus ocularis.
- Dorsal approach: A straight needle can be inserted into the supra-orbital fossa and advanced ventrally; when the globe is seen to rotate dorsally, the needle tip has penetrated the conus ocularis and local anaesthetic can now be injected.
- Lateral approach, reminiscent of the Peterson's block: a straight (or slightly curved) needle is placed into the angle formed where the caudal rim of the orbit meets the zygomatic arch, and advanced into the pterygopalatine fossa, rostral to the coronoid process of the mandible.

34.2.9.3.2 Techniques for Distal Limb and Foot Procedures

- IVRA: a tourniquet can be placed above or below the hock or carpus (for up to two hours), and 1 ml lidocaine 2% (without epinephrine) per 15 kg body weight is injected into an accessible vein distal to the tourniquet (and injecting toe-wards).
- Digital nerve blocks: in order to block the axial and abaxial branches of the digital nerves for both digits, the 6 injection sites are: subcutaneously, at the level of the distal fetlock (medio-dorsally and latero-dorsally as well as medio-palmarly/plantarly and latero-palmarly/plantarly), and into the interdigital cleft (on both the dorsal and plantar/palmar aspects). At each injection site, 1–2 ml of local anaesthetic is deposited, after aspiration to guard against inadvertent intravascular injection.

34.2.9.3.3 Techniques for Flank Anaesthesia

Similar techniques to those used for cattle and small ruminants are also suitable for lamoids. For further details, see Chapter 33.

- Line block
- Inverted 'L' (reverse 7) block
- Paravertebral block: block of the twelfth thoracic spinal segmental nerve and the first two lumbar segmental nerves is required for most flank approaches to abdominal surgery, with occasionally a little extra local infiltration to block any contribution from the third lumbar segmental nerve. (Note that paravertebral block of the third lumbar segmental nerve may cause ipsilateral hindlimb weakness). Note also that lamoids have 12 thoracic vertebrae and 7 lumbar vertebrae.
- Neuraxial (epidural, spinal) anaesthesia.

34.2.9.3.4 Neuraxial Techniques

Epidural (Extradural) Injection at the Sacro- or Inter-coccygeal Site   This can be useful for surgical procedures of the tail, perineum, pelvic structures, hindlimbs and caudal abdomen. For details regarding technique and contra-indications, see Chapter 33. The injection site is found, as for small animals and ruminants, in the midline at the most moveable articulation at the tailhead when the tail is pumped up and down.

- 'Caudal' epidural: for procedures on only the tail or perineum, 0.5 mg/kg lidocaine is usually sufficient.
- 'Cranial' epidural: for procedures on the tail, perineum, pelvic structures, hindlimbs, or caudal abdomen, 2–3 mg/kg lidocaine is required, but sometimes the block can be a bit patchy or lateralised to only one side. Note that this 'cranial' technique produces recumbency because of hindlimb motor block.

Epidural (Extradural) Injection at the Lumbo-sacral Site

The injection site is found, as for small animals and small ruminants, in the 'dip' caudal to the dorsal spinous process of the seventh lumbar vertebra, in the dorsal midline, between the two tuber coxae. Injections can be made in standing animals or those that are 'cushed' (in sternal recumbency).

For procedures on the tail, perineum, pelvic structures, hindlimbs, or caudal abdomen, 1–2 mg/kg lidocaine or 1 mg/kg ropivacaine should be sufficient. Note that this technique will also produce recumbency due to hindlimb motor block.

Intrathecal/Subarachnoid (True Spinal) Injection at the Lumbo-sacral Site

For procedures on the tail, perineum, pelvic structures, hindlimbs, or caudal abdomen, doses of around ¼–½ of those used for extradural techniques should be sufficient, e.g. 0.5–1 mg/kg lidocaine or 0.25–0.5 mg/kg ropivacaine. Preservative-free preparations should be used, preferably also of low concentration and without epinephrine. This technique will produce recumbency due to hindlimb motor block.

34.2.9.3.5 Techniques for Castration

Although 'cranial' epidural or intrathecal neuraxial techniques will produce sufficient anaesthesia for castration, hindlimb motor block may be a nuisance. Intratesticular injection of local anaesthetic is, therefore, preferred, along with infiltration of a bleb of local anaesthetic subcutaneously at the proposed skin incision site. The total dose (for both testicles) should be kept to a maximum of 3 mg/kg plain lidocaine (or c. 5 mg/kg lidocaine with epinephrine).

34.2.10   Recovery from General Anaesthesia

Lamoids, similarly to true ruminants, tend not to suffer emergence excitement during recovery, so stay relatively calm. In the early stages of recovery, when still in lateral recumbency, it is important to keep the poll raised (relative to the nose and cardia) to ensure drainage of material away from the larynx. Following the attainment of sternal recumbency, which should be encouraged as soon as possible, the head may be raised, whilst keeping the nose pointing down. This helps to stop newly regurgitated material from reaching the throat, yet enables previously regurgitated material, or any saliva, to drain or continue to drain from the mouth. Raising the head also helps any nasal congestion to resolve before tracheal extubation (see below regarding placing nasopharyngeal tubes and/or using nasal decongestants). Try to continue to protect against heat loss and/or provide rewarming as necessary, but also beware of the development of hyperthermia in animals with heavy coats in warm environments. If recumbency is unduly prolonged, but vital signs, body temperature, blood glucose, pH, and electrolytes are normal, consider administering antagonists (e.g. atipamezole to antagonise α2 agonists).

Supplementary oxygen can be provided through the ET tube until tracheal extubation (and subsequently via the nasopharyngeal tube, if placed). Tracheal extubation can either be performed whilst anaesthesia is relatively deep (so that regurgitation and laryngospasm are not provoked; but this risks aspiration), or, more usually, tracheal extubation is recommended only when the animal is awake enough to be actively chewing and swallowing (so that it can guard its own airway), although this may stimulate laryngospasm. The ET tube may be removed with the cuff either inflated or partially inflated, in order to try to avoid leaving any regurgitated material/saliva within the trachea. Mouth-breathing and dyspnoea after tracheal extubation may be due to nasal oedema. This complication can be treated, or, even better, pre-empted, by placing a well-lubricated nasopharyngeal tube or applying topical decongestant (e.g. phenylephrine solution) into the nasal passages as soon as problems arise, or, better still, prior to tracheal extubation.

Maintain patient observation throughout recovery as respiratory obstruction may occur sometime after tracheal extubation. If the upper airways are obstructed (by nasal congestion/oedema or laryngeal spasm), immense negative intrathoracic pressures can be generated during inspiratory attempts. Such upper respiratory tract obstruction, if severe enough, can result in non-cardiogenic pulmonary oedema (partly due to the negative pressure and partly due to a neurogenic component [i.e. the high sympathetic tone that accompanies hypoxaemia]). Such pulmonary oedema is seen as pinky-white froth from the nose and mouth. If this happens, try to re-establish an airway however possible (re-intubate the trachea, emergency tracheostomy), supply oxygen preferably by positive pressure ventilation, suction may be required (to remove froth from the airways), and furosemide c. 1 mg/kg IV may be beneficial.

Reference

Riebold, T.W., Engel, H.N., Grubb, T.L. et al. (1994). Orotracheal and nasotracheal intubation in llamas. *Journal of the American Veterinary Medical Association* 204 (5): 779–783.

Further Reading

Amsel, S.I., Kainer, R.A., and Johnson, L.W. (1987). Choosing the best site to perform venipuncture in a llama. *Veterinary Medicine* 82: 535–536.

Bradbury, L. (2008). Field anaesthesia in camelids. *In Practice* 30: 460–463.

Cebra, C.K., Tornquist, S.J., Van Suan, R.J., and Smith, B.B. (2001). Glucose tolerance testing in llamas and alpacas. *American Journal of Veterinary Research* 62: 682–686.

Christensen, J.M., Limsakun, T., Smith, B.B. et al. (2001). Pharmacokinetics and pharmacodynamics of antiulcer agents in llama. *Journal of Veterinary Pharmacology and Therapeutics* 24: 23–33.

Del Alamo, A.M., Mandsager, R.E., Riebold, T.W., and Payton, M.E. (2015). Evaluation of intravenous administration of alfaxalone, propofol and ketamine-diazepam for anaesthesia in alpacas. *Veterinary Anaesthesia and Analgesia* 42: 72–82.

Grint, N. and Dugdale, A. (2009). Brightness of venous blood in South American camelids: implications for jugular catheterisation. *Veterinary Anaesthesia and Analgesia* 36: 63–66.

Navarre, C.B., Ravis, W.R., Campbell, J. et al. (2001a). Stereoselective pharmacokinetics of ketoprofen in llamas following intravenous administration. *Journal of Veterinary Pharmacology and Therapeutics* 24: 223–226.

Navarre, C.B., Ravis, W.R., Nagilla, R. et al. (2001b). Pharmacokinetics of phenylbutazone in llamas following single intravenous and oral doses. *Journal of Veterinary Pharmacology and Therapeutics* 24: 227–231.

Navarre, C.B., Ravis, W.R., Nagilla, R. et al. (2001c). Pharmacokinetics of flunixin meglumine in llamas following a single intravenous dose. *Journal of Veterinary Pharmacology and Therapeutics* 24: 361–364.

Plummer, P.J. and Schleining, J.A. (2013). Assessment and management of pain in small ruminants and camelids. *Veterinary Clinics of North America: Food Animal Practice* 29: 185–208.

Poulsen, K.P., Smith, G., Davis, J., and Papich, M.G. (2006). Pharmacokinetics of oral omeprazole in llamas. *Journal of Veterinary Pharmacology and Therapeutics* 28: 539–543.

Smith, G., Davis, J., Smith, S.M. et al. (2010). Efficacy and pharmacokinetics of pantoprazole in alpacas. *Journal of Veterinary Internal Medicine* 24: 949–955.

Taylor, S.D., Baird, A.N., Weil, A.B., and Ruple, A. (2017). Evaluation of three intravenous injectable anaesthesia protocols in healthy adult male alpacas. *Veterinary Record* https://doi.org/10.1136/vr.104085.

Self-test Section

1 Roughly what is the P_{50} of lamoid haemoglobin?

35

Pigs

Sedation and Anaesthesia

35.1 Special Considerations

Pigs may be presented for veterinary attention under a wide variety of circumstances: as pet pigs, commercial farm pigs, or research pigs; each with different economic implications. Procedures may have to be performed 'on farm' or veterinary hospital facilities may be available.

35.1.1 Weight

Pigs come in a huge range of sizes, from 0.5 kg piglets to boars weighing over 350 kg; and if weigh-scales/weigh-bridges are not available, their weight must be estimated, which has implications for calculating drug doses. Pigs have a propensity to become obese such that some form of body condition scoring may alert the anaesthetist to be mindful of the effects of obesity on drug doses and the physiological consequences of recumbency and anaesthesia.

Patient size and physique (i.e. emaciated/lean/fat) may influence the choice of anaesthetic technique and equipment. Patient size also has implications for heat loss.

35.1.2 Age and Physiological Status

Piglets or pigs of any age and physiological status, including reproductive status, may require sedation or anaesthesia. Whilst age/maturity also influences weight, it has its own pharmacological and physiological implications.

Attempts should also be made to grade each patient's physiological status according to the American Society of Anesthesiologists (ASA) system, perhaps even including 'G' ('gravid') for pregnant animals as has been proposed for the human grading system.

35.1.3 Breed

Some breeds are prone to **malignant hyperthermia** (see later).

35.1.4 Plentiful Subcutaneous Fat

Mature pigs tend to have a substantial depth of subcutaneous fat over much of their bodies, which makes it difficult to deliver intramuscular injections accurately. If a poor response is observed following the supposed intramuscular delivery of a drug or combination of drugs, it can be difficult to know if the dose/s given was/were insufficient, or whether the injectate was just delivered into fat.

35.1.5 Little Hair But Plentiful Subcutaneous Fat

The lack of a dense, insulative hair coat, yet the thick layer of subcutaneous fat can affect thermoregulation. Skin colour can also affect thermoregulation: black-skinned pigs more rapidly become hyperthermic than pink-skinned

Veterinary Anaesthesia: Principles to Practice, Second Edition. Alexandra H. A. Dugdale, Georgina Beaumont, Carl Bradbrook, and Matthew Gurney.
© 2020 John Wiley & Sons Ltd. Published 2020 by John Wiley & Sons Ltd.
Companion website: www.wiley.com/go/dugdale/veterinary-anaesthesia

animals if left in direct sunlight on hot sunny summer days. Pink-skinned pigs, however, are prone to sunburn.

35.1.6 Paucity of Easily Accessible Superficial Veins

Thick skin and the often substantial layer of subcutaneous fat make locating suitable veins for venous access challenging. Auricular vessels are usually the most accessible, but are not easy to locate in animals with small ears (e.g. neonates) or animals that have had aural haematomas with subsequent scarring. Furthermore, awake subjects are not usually amenable to venous cannulation without good physical or chemical restraint. Jugular veins often require cut-down techniques to assist cannulation, with or without ultrasound-guidance, and require good patient restraint (usually chemical). Cephalic veins can be difficult to locate, especially in awake animals. The cranial superficial epigastric vein (which anastomoses with the caudal superficial epigastric vein) forms the subcutaneous abdominal vein (also known as the 'milk vein' in females), lying just dorsolateral to the mammary chain. Pressure on this vein just caudal to the elbow results in visible filling, enabling venepuncture or cannulation.

35.1.7 Problems of Handling

Pigs have evolved to move about through dense undergrowth and thus have a 'slippery' surface with short appendages that do not make good 'handles'. Pigs resent restraint by squealing loudly and they will struggle for freedom. Larger pigs can be restrained by using a snare around the snout (upper jaw, with the snare loop located behind the canines), when they will usually pull back, sit down, and squeal. Smaller pigs can be held in lateral or dorsal recumbency by holding their legs. Although pigs can squeal deafeningly, this is not always associated with a massive stress response. Ear defenders are, however, recommended for the operators.

Malignant hyperthermia appears to be related to the porcine stress syndrome, such that careful handling and minimising exertion or excitement when handling pigs before sedation or anaesthesia is also important (see later).

35.1.8 Temperament

This can vary enormously. Pigs are very intelligent and can be trained easily, but can learn bad habits too. Pet pigs have a tendency to get too fat, and for Vietnamese pot-bellied pigs, this can exacerbate their problems of entropion. Pigs with sore eyes that cannot see very well may become very grumpy and aggressive when approached around the head. Temperament may also be related to age and sex, with older boars being potentially more aggressive, but gilts and sows can guard their litters aggressively too.

Where pigs, which are normally housed in groups, require sedation or anaesthesia, they should not be returned to the group until fully recovered because of attack/cannibalism by other group members.

35.1.9 Pain Recognition

Currently there is no validated pain assessment tool for pigs, although a recent report using facial recognition technologies shows promise for the evaluation of the 'emotional' states of pigs, perhaps eventually enabling us to identify distress and pain.

35.1.10 Tracheal Intubation Is Difficult

Pigs are prone to respiratory obstruction, especially if brachycephalic, so endotracheal (ET) intubation is advised. Laryngospasm is common and stimulation of the larynx during attempted tracheal intubation can stimulate either a sympathetic response or, less commonly, a vagal response that can cause profound bradycardia, even to the point of asystole. Topical local anaesthetic applied to the larynx can help prevent laryngospasm and reduce the severity of autonomic reflexes.

Pigs: have a relatively narrow glottis and trachea compared to their body size; a long soft palate; often 'excessive' cheeks/jowls/pharyngeal tissue and a relatively large tongue (like brachycephalic dogs); cannot open their mouths very wide; have sharp teeth; and have interesting laryngeal anatomy. They have: chunky arytenoids and bipartite vocal cords (longitudinally), which may impede ET tube passage; a long downwards-sloping thyroid cartilage; a long thyrocricoid ligament on the floor of the larynx (which may act as a blind end to tube passage through the glottis); and the trachea then slopes upwards away from the larynx. The larynx therefore presents a 'U' bend between the glottic opening and the trachea. They also have a pharyngeal recess just above the larynx and a laryngeal recess between the base of the epiglottis and the thyroid cartilage in the midline on the ventral floor of the larynx, both of which can hinder ET tube passage (Figure 35.1). Their relatively short neck, and therefore trachea, and presence of an eparterial (tracheal) bronchus means that care must be taken to ensure that ET tubes are not so long as to bypass, block, or even enter this bronchus. The carina is also reported to be prone to puncture if sharp intubating stylettes are used.

Figure 35.1 Pig larynx in sagittal section.

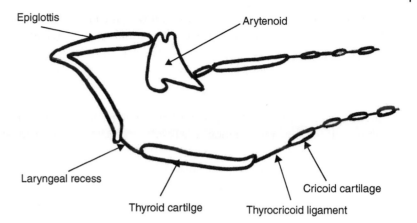

Epiglottis

Arytenoid

Laryngeal recess

Thyroid cartilge

Thyrocricoid ligament

Cricoid cartilage

35.2 Approach to Chemical Restraint: Sedation and General Anaesthesia

- Regarding withholding food before sedation or anaesthesia, it is important to note that if food is withheld, then bedding should also be removed as hungry pigs will eat whatever they can find. Whilst occasional reports in the literature have raised concerns regarding vomiting, this does not appear to be a common problem. At the 2019 Association of Veterinary Anaesthetists' Congress, the following suggestions were offered:
  - Pre-weaning – do not restrict suckling or access to creep feed
  - Post-weaning – other than for minipigs and micropigs (which should not have food restricted as they may become hypoglycaemic), perhaps restrict access to food for 0–1 hour before premedication/the procedure (pigs normally have a rapid gastric emptying time). If, however, it is felt that the act of actually removing food will disturb the pig/s and cause distress, it may be better not to.
  - If abdominal surgery is contemplated, then food withhold times may need to be longer, but this may depend upon the actual surgical procedure and liquid diets may be preferred instead. If food is to be withheld for more than one hour, then bedding should also be removed.
- Access to water should be allowed up until the time of premedication or the procedure.
- Aim to minimise the stress of the procedure, especially for those prone to malignant hyperthermia, e.g. Landrace and Pietrain pigs; and in malignant hyperthermia-prone breeds, consider avoiding exposure to inhalation agents.
- For intramuscular injections, use needles that are 'long enough'; up to 7 cm long may sometimes be required.

Intramuscular injection sites include the neck muscles (epaxially or laterally behind the ear), triceps, epaxial lumbar muscles, gluteals, and quadriceps. The choice of site may be determined by the intended 'use' of the pig, i.e. avoid the gluteals and quadriceps if the pig is intended for meat production for human consumption. Injections into neck muscles are generally best tolerated. Distance injection techniques may facilitate successful IM injections in wriggling or moving animals: inserting an extension line (Luer-locked at either end) between the syringe and needle enables the injection to be continued (and hopefully completed) even if the animal moves. (The dead space in the extension set must be accounted for, by either including extra injectate volume in the syringe, or by including sufficient air in the syringe to 'chase' all the injectate volume through the extension set and into the animal.)

Pig boards or snares may be necessary to restrain larger animals; smaller animals can usually be restrained manually.

- Be prepared to intubate the trachea. A gag (or, e.g. strips of bandage or tape to distract the jaws), laryngoscope, topical local anaesthetic to desensitise the larynx, and ET tubes of several sizes should be available.
- Check the environmental temperature; if possible, avoid very cold or very hot conditions. Black pigs can get heatstroke on hot sunny days; pink pigs are prone to sunburn. Pigs can easily become hypothermic on cold days.
- Prepare for positioning and padding the patient.
- Protect the eyes from dust, debris (e.g. tusk fragments, surgical scrub), and direct sunlight.
- Respiratory obstruction may occur even under sedation, especially in brachycephalic pigs, just as with brachycephalic dogs. It is therefore advisable to have a number of ET tubes of various sizes to hand, an ET tube introducer/stylette/bougie, a laryngoscope with a long (straight)

blade, some bandage to use to hold the jaws apart for intubation, some lidocaine spray for the larynx, and some means of inducing anaesthesia to reduce the gag reflex. Although not always possible in the field, it is reassuring to have oxygen and some means of artificial ventilation available. In the field, emergency ventilation can be provided by mouth-to-tube (or mask; see below), or better, by using a self-inflating resuscitation type bag.

In research settings, short-acting muscle relaxants (e.g. succinylcholine [suxamethonium] chloride, a depolarising neuromuscular blocker) may be administered IV to facilitate tracheal intubation instead of topical lidocaine spray for the larynx. Neuromuscular blockers will, however, cause respiratory muscle paralysis, and so require that ventilation can be supported. Suxamethonium can also trigger malignant hyperthermia (see later).

Given that pigs, especially brachycephalic breeds, are prone to respiratory obstruction, heightened vigilance is required during their sedation, and equipment and drugs should be available to establish an airway (e.g. to perform emergency tracheal intubation/needle or tube tracheostomy), should this become necessary.

For pigs undergoing general anaesthesia, tracheal intubation would appear to be the best option for ensuring a patent airway, but it may not always be necessary and is certainly not without its complications. Tracheal intubation itself may be difficult to achieve and pigs are also prone to suffering laryngospasm: not just at tracheal intubation but also after tracheal extubation. In anaesthetised pigs, where ET intubation has not been performed, or, has not been possible to perform, increased vigilance for airway obstruction is required, and the necessary drugs and equipment for establishing an airway, should an emergency arise, must be available. Supraglottic airway devices (such as laryngeal mask airways) have been advocated for pigs as an alternative technique to tracheal intubation for 'securing' an airway, and may provide a tight enough seal around the larynx to facilitate the provision of artificial (manual or mechanical) ventilation. These devices, however, are not without their own complications and may actually cause laryngeal obstruction when their insertion can retrovert the epiglottis (this may happen when the relatively large epiglottic tip is located dorsal to the soft palate prior to insertion of the supraglottic airway device). Bougie-assisted insertion of these devices has been described to overcome this problem.

If low-grade upper respiratory tract obstruction occurs, sternal recumbency, with the head extended slightly forwards (and the tongue pulled forwards if possible), may help to reduce airway obstruction. However, if the head is extended too far forwards, the potential for laryngeal obstruction increases because of the anatomy of the throat region. Interestingly, turning a pig into dorsal recumbency may improve air flow because all the excessive soft tissues in the pharyngeal region flop away from the glottis. Artificial ventilation by a well-fitting facemask is most efficient in pigs in dorsal recumbency; ideally, the tongue should be pulled forwards and out of mouth, and 'forward' pressure should be put behind the vertical ramus of the mandible to increase the space available in the pharynx. This position also results in less stomach inflation (meteorism) than if mask-ventilation is attempted in sternal or lateral recumbency.

35.2.1 Sedation and Premedication

35.2.1.1 Butyrophenones

Butyrophenones tend to cause excitement before sedation finally occurs. They are said to cause less cardiorespiratory depression and interference with thermoregulation than phenothiazines, but are more potent anti-emetics. Sedation, which is said to occur in the absence of anxiolysis, is due to a combination of anti-dopaminergic, anti-noradrenergic, and GABA-mimetic activity in the reticular activating system in the CNS.

35.2.1.1.1 Azaperone

- Cheap, effective, and licenced for pigs as a 40 mg/ml solution.
- Azaperone can be used to control fighting amongst pigs, e.g. when weanlings are mixed, and can decrease maternal aggression/rejection of piglets.
- Dose range 1–2 mg/kg deep IM, with the lower dose advised in larger animals due to allometric scaling (whereby dosing is related to metabolic body weight [which itself is related more to body surface area, than to actual body mass]).
- Doses >1 mg/kg are best avoided in boars, as they have been associated with penile prolapse with secondary trauma.
- If the first dose does not appear to produce the desired effect, the data sheets caution against administering further doses on the same day because slow release of the initial dose from subcutaneous fat could lead to eventual overdosage.
- After injection, pigs are best left undisturbed for at least 20 minutes. Excitement reactions can still occur during the onset of sedation, but are more likely if the pig is disturbed before the sedative effects have peaked.
- Azaperone sometimes causes increased salivation and panting, especially after larger doses.
- Azaperone does cause some peripheral vasodilation (α1 adrenoreceptor blockade), and hence some degree of

hypotension and an increase in heat loss should be expected. Data sheets suggest that azaperone should be avoided in very cold conditions because of the possibility of cardiovascular collapse secondary to peripheral vasodilation and hypothermia. Vasodilation of the ear veins may, however, make them easier to locate and cannulate.

- Can be used in pregnant and lactating animals.

Azaperone can be administered in various drug combinations to produce 'deeper' sedation:

- Azaperone 1–2 mg/kg and midazolam 0.3 mg/kg together deep IM.
- Azaperone 1 mg/kg and ketamine 5 mg/kg together deep IM.
- Azaperone 1 mg/kg, midazolam 0.1 mg/kg and ketamine c.5 mg/kg all together deep IM.
- Azaperone 1–2 mg/kg, ± butorphanol 0.1–0.2 mg/kg, and ketamine c.5 mg/kg all together deep IM.

35.2.1.2 Phenothiazines

Not commonly used as azaperone tends to be preferred (see above).

35.2.1.2.1 Acepromazine

- Not licenced for use in pigs intended for human consumption in the UK.
- Although the effects of this drug can be very unpredictable, it has been used at doses of 0.03–0.1 mg/kg deep IM.
- Sufficient time (20–40 minutes) must be allowed for the effect to become apparent and reach its peak; and it is important that the pig should be left undisturbed during this time.
- Acepromazine, through antagonism of adrenergic α1 receptors, causes peripheral vasodilation, hypotension, and increases heat loss.
- It may be used in combination with other drugs, e.g. acepromazine 0.03–0.05 mg/kg and ketamine c. 5+ mg/kg together deep IM.

35.2.1.3 Benzodiazepines

Not commonly used in practice, especially as the sole agent, but may be combined with other agents; may be useful for young piglets.

35.2.1.3.1 Diazepam and Midazolam

- Not licenced for use in pigs intended for human consumption in the UK.
- When used alone, benzodiazepines do not tend to produce very reliable sedation in adult animals.
- Doses vary from 0.1 mg/kg up to 1(–2) mg/kg.

- Best administered by deep IM injection, but as the bioavailability of diazepam after IM injection is poor, midazolam is a better choice for IM administration.
- Young piglets have been successfully sedated by intranasal and even rectal midazolam.
- Benzodiazepines can be used in combinations, e.g. midazolam 0.2++ mg/kg and ketamine c. 5+ mg/kg both together deep IM, or as described above (see under Azaperone).

35.2.1.4 α2 Agonists

None is licenced for use in pigs intended for human consumption in the UK.

35.2.1.4.1 Xylazine

- Xylazine is said to be much less potent in pigs than in cattle or horses (potency: pig < horse < cow), although intra-fat administration may be the cause of some of the reported sedation failures.
- It is not often administered alone.
- Occasionally it can induce vomiting in pigs, as in small animals.
- It is most often used in combination with ketamine, after which a good 10–20 minutes should be allowed for the effect to develop, e.g. xylazine 1–3 mg/kg, ± butorphanol 0.1–0.2 mg/kg and ketamine c. 5 mg/kg, all together deep IM.

35.2.1.4.2 Detomidine

Like xylazine, this is most often used in combination with ketamine, e.g. detomidine 0.1 mg/kg, butorphanol 0.1–0.2 mg/kg and ketamine c. 5 mg/kg all together deep IM.

35.2.1.4.3 Medetomidine and Dexmedetomidine

These are most often used in combinations, e.g. medetomidine 30–80 μg/kg, butorphanol 0.1–0.2 mg/kg and ketamine c. 5 mg/kg combination by deep IM. This particular combination is reported to produce 'field anaesthesia' rather than just sedation. For only sedation, it is suggested to omit the butorphanol.

35.2.1.4.4 Romifidine

Also most commonly used in combinations, e.g. romifidine 120 μg/kg, butorphanol 0.1 mg/kg and ketamine 5–8 mg/kg all together by deep IM injection.

Azaperone (c. 1 mg/kg) may be administered IM 20 minutes before the above α2 agonist-based combinations for more profound chemical restraint.

35.2.2 Induction and Maintenance of Anaesthesia

The sedation provided by some of the above combinations may be of sufficient depth to allow tracheal intubation, and then anaesthesia can be maintained, e.g. with an inhalation agent (in oxygen ± nitrous oxide or medical air, if these are available). Alternatively, sedation should allow venous cannulation (if this was not possible beforehand), so that drugs may be administered intravenously for anaesthetic induction (± maintenance). Failing these, inhalation agents may be administered by facemask once the animal is at least sedated to some degree, or further drug doses of injectable agents may need to be administered by the deep IM route to deepen or prolong sedation or anaesthesia.

35.2.2.1 Injectable Drugs

35.2.2.1.1 Arylcyclohexylamines

35.2.2.1.1.1 Ketamine Ketamine can be used in food-producing pigs in the EU; no MRL is required. A licenced product is available in the UK for induction of anaesthesia (following azaperone premedication) at doses of 15–20 mg/kg IM. Ketamine at such high doses can cause a marked increase in skeletal muscle tone. Ketamine can, however, be administered at lower doses (more commonly 5–10 mg/kg IM), where an increase in muscle tone is less likely, and especially if it is administered in combination with other agents with muscle-relaxing properties (α2 agonists or benzodiazepines).

Ketamine produces minimal cardiovascular depression in healthy animals and even causes gentle stimulation. It provides excellent analgesia (especially somatic). Although ketamine is supposed to maintain (or even enhance) laryngeal reflexes, this should never be relied upon for the maintenance of a patent airway because ketamine sometimes causes hypersalivation, and the other drugs administered may compromise airway protection through their sedative and muscle-relaxant effects.

When ketamine is administered as part of a sedative combination [see above] (at doses of c. 5 mg/kg IM), sedation may be deepened and/or its duration extended by the administration of further doses of c. 5 mg/kg ketamine IM or IV. Further doses of benzodiazepines or α2 agonists may also be required.

If ketamine has been administered as part of a sedative combination [see above] (at doses of c. 5 mg/kg IM), for premedication purposes, then anaesthesia can be induced by administration of further doses of c. 5+ mg/kg ketamine IV (± diazepam or midazolam at 0.1 mg/kg IV), which should be sufficient to allow tracheal intubation. If IV access is impossible to establish, further doses of c. 5+ mg/kg ketamine may alternatively be given by deep IM injection.

35.2.2.1.2 Carboxylated Imidazoles: Metomidate and Etomidate

35.2.2.1.2.1 Metomidate Metomidate is no longer available as a licenced product in the UK. Following azaperone sedation, metomidate administered IV produced anaesthesia for about 30 minutes with minimal cardiovascular depression and only transient apnoea after rapid IV administration. It was non-cumulative because of rapid plasma esterase hydrolysis and hepatic metabolism. It occasionally caused pain on injection, probably because of the propylene glycol solvent, which was also blamed for occasional haemolysis. The disadvantages were that it did not provide any analgesia and the quality of muscle relaxation was poor.

35.2.2.1.2.2 Etomidate Etomidate (not licenced) is sometimes used in experimental pigs. Dose 0.2 mg/kg IV, and often with midazolam (or diazepam) at 0.1 mg/kg IV to improve muscular relaxation. Salivation may sometimes occur.

35.2.2.1.3 Barbiturates

35.2.2.1.3.1 Thiopental Thiopental can be used in food-producing pigs in the EU and requires no MRL. Licenced products are still available, but not currently in the UK or EU. They may, however, be imported into the UK under a Special Treatment Certificate obtained from the Veterinary Medicines Directorate (VMD). Thiopental produces mild cardiorespiratory depression and can sensitise the heart to the arrhythmogenic effects of catecholamines, such that premedication is advised and keeping a calm and stress-free environment is important.

Thiopental is irritant to tissues if accidental extravascular deposition occurs, and therefore it must be administered intravenously, preferably via a pre-placed (position- and patency-checked) intravenous cannula.

The dose required depends upon the depth of prior sedation/premedication, but for healthy animals, generally lies between 5 and 15 mg/kg IV. Hepatic metabolism is slow such that recovery is highly dependent upon redistribution into muscle and fat (which are plentiful in most adult pigs), but large total doses will still prolong the recovery period, so top-ups should be given with the total cumulative dose in mind.

35.2.2.1.4 Neuro-active Steroids

35.2.2.1.4.1 Alfaxalone Not yet licenced for use in food-producing animals in the UK. Early reports, however, suggest that, following azaperone premedication at 1–2 mg/kg, alfaxalone administered at 2–3 mg/kg IV produces acceptable tracheal intubating conditions and anaesthesia for around 15 minutes. Another report has described deeper sedation and superior quality of subsequent inhalation anaesthetic induction following dexmedetomidine (0.01 mg/kg) plus alfaxalone (5 mg/kg) IM, compared with dexmedetomidine (0.01 mg/kg) plus ketamine (10 mg/kg) IM.

Alfaxalone causes only mild cardiorespiratory depression although it may cause more moderate hypoventilation/transient apnoea following rapid IV injection. Muscular twitches may occasionally occur after induction and/or during recovery, such that premedication is advised. Top-ups or infusions (IV) may be given without unduly prolonging recovery as alfaxalone undergoes relatively rapid hepatic metabolism; ventilatory support may, however, be required under these circumstances. Alfaxalone is also effective following IM administration, although the large injectate volume required for large pigs may be cumbersome. Alfaxalone is not irritant if inadvertent extravascular deposition occurs.

One study has reported that a combination of lidocaine (2 mg/kg) and alfaxalone (6 mg/kg), given intratesticularly, produced deep sedation and adequate testicular anaesthesia in neonatal pigs undergoing castration.

35.2.2.1.5 Substituted Phenols

35.2.2.1.5.1 Propofol
Propofol undergoes rapid hepatic and extrahepatic metabolism; therefore, to be effective, it must be administered IV, necessitating prior venous cannulation. The required dose is up to 6–8 mg/kg in unpremedicated animals, but is usually less following sedation/premedication. Propofol causes moderate cardiovascular and respiratory depression, although it can cause transient/prolonged apnoea following rapid bolus IV injection. Propofol is minimally cumulative, so top-up doses or infusions can be administered, although this might be expensive in larger pigs and artificial ventilation is often required. Propofol therefore tends to be reserved for research animals. One study comparing propofol and alfaxalone for anaesthetic maintenance reported slightly better maintained cardiovascular variables with alfaxalone, but slightly improved recovery quality with propofol. Propofol has also been combined with ketamine for anaesthetic maintenance.

35.2.2.2 Inhalation Agents
The volatile halogenated anaesthetic agents should be avoided in malignant hyperthermia-prone animals.

Volatile anaesthetic agents can be administered by facemask or via an ET tube or supraglottic airway device. They can be employed for induction and/or maintenance of anaesthesia and may be useful for anaesthetic maintenance for procedures likely to take longer than 40–60 minutes, where, otherwise, extra doses or infusions of injectable agents would be required, most of which are cumulative. Halothane is no longer available, but none of the halogenated agents is licenced for use in pigs intended for human consumption in the UK, although isoflurane can be used according to the cascade. For research work, isoflurane, sevoflurane, or desflurane may be used. The choice between the inhalation agents is as for other species (see Chapter 8). Isoflurane and desflurane are considered to be the most pungent of the agents, and therefore not the first choice for mask induction. Although sevoflurane might then be considered the best choice for inhalation induction, isoflurane has also been used successfully.

Nitrous oxide can be included to provide a little analgesia, but has similar contra-indications for all species (see Chapter 8).

The anaesthetic breathing system must be chosen to suit the patient size. For pigs between 0.5 kg and around 10 kg, a T-piece or mini Lack, or circle suitable for such small patients would be appropriate. For patients between about 10 kg and up to about 135–150 kg, a standard small animal circle system would be appropriate. For pigs larger than 135–150 kg, a large animal circle or large animal To-and-Fro is required. When using circle systems, it is important to ensure that the rebreathing bag is of an appropriate size (at least twice the normal, resting tidal volume) and the carbon dioxide absorber canister also has suitable capacity (also at least twice the normal, resting tidal volume). It is also important that there is an appropriately sized ET tube connector available to connect the required ET tube to the chosen anaesthetic breathing system.

35.2.2.2.1 Endotracheal Intubation
A laryngoscope is required (long straight blades are often preferred), and it is advisable to have a large range of ET tube sizes to hand. An ET tube introducer/stylette/bougie is also useful. Because pigs are prone to laryngospasm, the larynx should be desensitised with topical local anaesthetic (usually lidocaine) before intubation is attempted. After topical application of lidocaine, however, at least 30 seconds should be allowed before intubation attempts begin. (Alternatively, short-acting neuromuscular blocking agents, usually succinylcholine, can be administered, but the necessary equipment and facilities must be available to ensure intubation and artificial ventilation can be provided.)

Pigs have an eparterial (tracheal) bronchus (as do ruminants), but because pigs have a relatively short neck, it is easy to bypass or block this bronchial root with a long ET tube (or its inflated cuff), which results in compromised ventilation of the right apical lung lobe (hypoxaemia [often noted by falling SpO_2 values] and hypercapnia will develop). (It may also be possible to insert a relatively small tube into this bronchus, thus bypassing the substantial remaining lung volume, such that hypoxaemia and hypercapnia will develop very quickly.) Therefore, consider the length of the ET tubes that you are using, and try to ensure that the tip (or at least the inflated cuff) lies proximal to the root of the tracheal bronchus. ET tube introducers/bougies

(a)

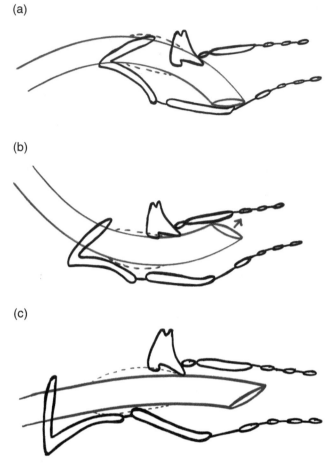

(b)

(c)

Figure 35.2 Insertion of a curved ET tube without the assistance of a bougie.

should be used gently to avoid causing trauma to the airway.

Tracheal intubation in pigs can be performed when they are held in sternal recumbency, lateral recumbency, or dorsal recumbency. As well as operator experience and preference, the choice may also depend upon the size of the pig and the help available.

If a flexible bougie is used as a guide for the ET tube, then this can first be directed into the trachea, being careful to guide it through the 'U' bend (see above), and the ET tube can then be 'railroaded' over it. Without using an ET tube introducer, tracheal intubation can be a little more challenging (see Figure 35.2).

For curved ET tubes, and with the pig in sternal recumbency, start off with the tube tip pointing downwards. The tube tip is then advanced just through the glottis, but resistance will be found if attempts are made to further insert the tube because its tip will abut the thyroid cartilage or thyrocricoid ligament (along the floor of the larynx) (Figure 35.2a). Occasionally, the tube tip may also get stuck at the laryngeal recess. Therefore, at this point, the tube

should be turned through 180° about its long axis to free its tip so that it can now be gently advanced (Figure 35.2b). It should start to enter the trachea, which continues on from the larynx in an upward sloping direction. Having advanced the tube a little, it is often necessary to turn it back through 180° again to enable easy passage on down the trachea (Figure 35.2c).

35.2.2.2.2 *Malignant Hyperthermia*

Known affected breeds are: Landrace, Pietrain, Duroc, and Poland China. Malignant hyperthermia (MH) is triggered by stress, succinylcholine, and all volatile halogenated anaesthetic agents (halothane is the most potent trigger); the 'size' of the trigger determines the 'size' of the response. Nitrous oxide and ketamine were once thought to be weak triggers, but are now pretty much regarded not to be triggers.

MH is caused by a dysfunction (due to genetic mutation) of the **ryanodine-sensitive calcium channel** in the sarcoplasmic reticulum, which results in a failure of regulation of the intracellular ionised calcium concentration. The condition is a hereditary autosomal recessive disorder in pigs; only homozygotes express the condition, and it is usually fulminant and often fatal. It can be tested for by the halothane/caffeine muscle contracture test, but fresh skeletal muscle tissue is required. DNA tests may replace the need for muscle biopsies in time, but more than one genetic mutation may be responsible.

35.2.3 Clinical Signs

The speed of onset of clinical signs depends upon the severity of the trigger.

- Muscle rigidity (due to sustained muscle contraction) causes the toes to splay or 'separate' and the eyeballs become retracted deep into the orbits so the third eyelids look obvious.
- Increased carbon dioxide and heat production, resulting from hypermetabolism and sustained muscle contraction.
- The skin becomes very hot and pink/red (in pink-skinned pig), and the mucous membranes also become very pink.
- Tachypnoea, tachycardia, and an increased core temperature develop.
- If monitoring includes capnography, then an increase in the end tidal CO_2 (ETCO$_2$) tension *may* be one of the first indicators of trouble, reflecting accelerated muscle metabolism. However, this early marked increase in ETCO$_2$ tension is most commonly reported for animals under neuromuscular blockade (and therefore where the patient's lungs are being ventilated at a constant pre-set rate); whereas in spontaneously breathing animals, a marked increase in respiratory rate and effort is usually

observed first (before ETCO$_2$ values increase). Respiratory muscles can, however, spasm, reducing spontaneous ventilation efficiency (see below).

- Mixed metabolic and respiratory acidosis (accelerated metabolism often outstrips oxygen supply such that anaerobic respiration supervenes; respiratory muscles may spasm, reducing ventilatory efficiency in eliminating carbon dioxide).
- Rhabdomyolysis (due to: increased turnover of membrane phospholipids due to calcium-induced activation of phospholipases; and eventually, to energy supply failure), can result in hyperkalaemia and myoglobinaemia/myoglobinuria, which, in turn, can cause cardiac arrhythmias and acute renal failure, respectively.
- Rhabdomyolyis and hyperthermia can also result in disseminated intravascular coagulopathy.

35.2.4 Treatment

MH is difficult to treat once clinically obvious.

Volatile anaesthetic agent administration must be stopped immediately; the breathing system should ideally be changed to a new one that is not contaminated by volatile agent (although the pig's exhaled breath will still contain volatile agent and will therefore contaminate a new system). It used to be thought that non-rebreathing systems were best but, for large patients, it may not be possible to increase the fresh gas flow sufficiently to eliminate the increased carbon dioxide load (and to ensure no re-breathing of volatile agent from the patient's anatomical dead space gases). Therefore, a new circle system may be used, but activated charcoal filters must be inserted on both the inspiratory and expiratory limbs to adsorb the exhaled volatile agent, and, in-so-doing, to reduce contamination of the plastic/rubber components of the breathing system and also to reduce harbouring of exhaled volatile agent in the new carbon dioxide absorbent. If activated charcoal filters are not available, the rebreathing bag should be 'dumped' frequently to reduce buildup of exhaled volatile agent within the new breathing system and high fresh gas flows should be used.

Cool/cold fluids should be administered IV, and consider cold fluids for bladder lavage, colon lavage, and even gastric lavage to enhance core cooling. Application of cold water or alcohol to the skin can help cooling, which can be assisted by the use of a fan. Ice packs may also be applied to the skin, but must first be covered by a thin layer of material to prevent direct ice-burns. Submergence in cold running water is often not practically possible mid-surgery.

Pigs can develop metabolic acidosis (due to hypermetabolism) and respiratory acidosis (because respiratory muscles can spasm, thereby reducing ventilatory efficiency), therefore ventilatory and circulatory support will probably be required; ventilatory support at least whilst still anaesthetised. Intravenous fluids are also necessary to protect the kidneys from myoglobin released from damaged muscles. If possible, monitor for hyperkalaemia that can occur secondary to potassium release from dying muscle cells.

Dantrolene at 2–10 mg/kg IV may help, but is better given prophylactically. Dantrolene doses should be repeated until a response is observed. Dantrolene is very expensive and has a short shelf-life, so often none is available. Dantrolene, however, is not without its own side effects, such as arrhythmias, ataxia, and hepatopathy.

Dantrolene sodium is a postsynaptic muscle relaxant that reduces excitation-contraction coupling in muscle cells. It achieves this by inhibiting Ca^{2+} ion release from sarcoplasmic reticulum stores by antagonising the calcium-induced calcium release when ryanodine-sensitive calcium channels are activated. It is the primary drug used for the treatment and prevention of MH. It is also used in the management of neuroleptic malignant syndrome and serotonin syndrome. Dantrolene vials contain 20 mg, solubilised in mannitol, which itself may also help the treatment of MH through its free radical scavenging and osmotic/osmotic diuretic effects.

If initial treatment is successful, vigilance is important as the clinical signs of MH can recur up to several hours after their initial resolution.

35.3 Analgesia

35.3.1 NSAIDs

Licenced drugs include:

- Flunixin: 2 mg/kg once daily by deep IM injection, can repeat for up to 3 consecutive days.
- Ketoprofen: 3 mg/kg once by deep IM injection; can repeat every 24 hours for up to three injections if required.
- Meloxicam: 0.4 mg/kg once by deep IM injection or PO (in food or water); can repeat after 24 hours if required. Can be administered to pregnant or lactating animals.
- Metamizole (dipyrone): 50 mg/kg with butylscopolamine (hyoscine butylbromide) 0.4 mg/kg once by deep IM injection.
- Sodium salicylate: 25 mg/kg per day PO (in drinking water) for three to five days. Not in piglets <4 weeks old.
- Tolfenamic acid: 2 mg/kg once only by deep IM injection.

35.3.2 Paracetamol

Licenced; 30 mg/kg daily (divided between two meals) PO, for up to five days. Can be administered to pregnant and lactating animals.

35.3.3 Opioids

None is licenced for use in pigs, but opioids can be used at similar doses to those used for dogs (although pigs may often require higher doses or shorter dosing intervals).

- Morphine 0.1–0.5 mg/kg IM.
- Methadone 0.25 + mg/kg IM.
- Pethidine 3.5–5 mg/kg IM.
- Butorphanol 0.1–0.5 mg/kg IM.
- Buprenorphine 0.006–0.02 mg/kg IM.

35.3.4 α2 Agonists

None is licenced for use in pigs in the UK, but they are commonly used for research or pet pigs. These drugs provide analgesia alongside sedation and muscle relaxation, but all these effects are antagonised by atipamezole.

35.3.5 Local/Regional Anaesthetic Techniques

Local/regional anaesthetic techniques can be used as an adjunct to sedation or general anaesthesia.

Local blocks can provide excellent analgesia, but often they are impractical to 'top up', so other forms of analgesia should also be provided. According to EU Commission Regulation No. 37/2010, benzocaine, tetracaine, and procaine can be used in food-producing pigs; no MRL is required for these agents. Currently, there is no commercially available licenced product containing procaine for pigs in the UK, but such a product does exist in Spain and may be imported under a Special Import Certificate available from the VMD. Although lidocaine is not licenced for use in food-producing pigs in the UK, it may be used according to the 'cascade', but pigs, like cattle, produce 2,6-xylidine as a major metabolite of lidocaine, which is potentially carcinogenic (see Chapter 33).

35.3.5.1 Lumbosacral Epidural (Extradural)

Epidural anaesthesia may be provided for castration, obstetrical, and perineal surgeries. It is easier to perform if the pig is first sedated.

The landmarks are the same as those used for dogs (just caudal to a transverse line joining the iliac crests), but can be hard to locate easily in very large or fat pigs. Therefore, it is suggested to draw an imaginary vertical line up from

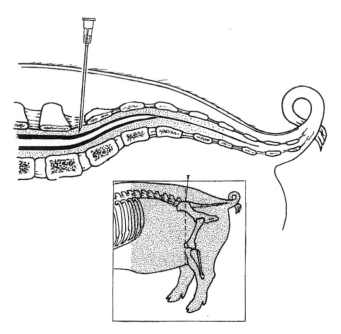

Figure 35.3 Porcine epidural injection site and the extent of block possible. *Source:* Reproduced from Tranquilli et al. (2007) with permission of Blackwell Publishing Ltd.

the patellae, and then the lumbosacral space should be 2–3 cm caudal to where this line crosses the spine (Figure 35.3).

An intradermal bleb of local anaesthetic is placed prior to insertion of the epidural needle, which may need to be 5–10 cm long, depending upon the size of pig. Aspiration prior to injection is important to avoid inadvertent intravascular or intrathecal injection. Pigs have five or six lumbar vertebrae; the spinal cord terminates between the last two lumbar vertebrae, but the meningeal sac continues to mid sacral level, so occasionally the dura will be penetrated and cerebrospinal fluid will be obtained.

For pigs of around 50 kg, 10 ml lidocaine 2% will usually result in recumbency because of motor as well as sensory block to the hind end. The duration of block is one to two hours.

Xylazine/lidocaine combinations can also be used. For example, 1 mg/kg xylazine made up to a total volume of 10 ml with lidocaine 2% provides analgesia for up to six hours.

Opioids may be used alone or in combination with local anaesthetic agents and/or α2 agonists. The reader is referred to the literature for doses.

35.3.5.2 Intratesticular Local Anaesthetic for Castration

This can be suitable in young pigs, possibly up to about six months old. Older animals are often better castrated under general anaesthesia, but analgesia can still be augmented with local anaesthetic.

Depending upon the size of the pig, 2–15 ml lidocaine 2% is required per testicle, with most of the volume being injected into the body of the testicle (perhaps with some into the spermatic cord), and 1–2 ml deposited subcutaneously beneath the scrotal skin (at the proposed incision site) as the needle is withdrawn. Around three to five minutes should be allowed to elapse for the block to take effect before surgery is performed. Local anaesthetic, however, is quickly absorbed from the testicle into the systemic circulation, such that surgery should be completed within 10 minutes where possible.

35.3.5.3 Local Infiltration
Local infiltration into the flank is possible to aid Caesarean section or other laparotomies.

35.3.5.4 Intravenous Regional Anaesthesia
This has also been described. It is an excellent technique as long as a suitable superficial vein can be located.

35.3.5.4.1 Monitoring Several physiological variables should be monitored in addition to indicators of anaesthetic depth such as jaw tone, general muscle tone, and ocular position/reflexes. The physiological variables monitored should include heart rate (stethoscopy), pulse rate (it may be difficult to palpate pulses because of the thick skin and subcutaneous fat), breathing rate, mucous membrane colour, rectal temperature, and skin temperature (subjective assessment is often good enough to tell if malignant hyperthermia is developing). Pulse oximetry, capnography, ECG, and arterial blood pressure monitoring can also be helpful. Blood pressure can be monitored non-invasively with a Doppler flow probe or an oscillometric device. Superficial arteries, for direct blood pressure monitoring, can be difficult to locate/cannulate. As with all monitoring, trends can be very useful. See Chapter 18.

35.3.5.4.2 Intra-operative Fluid Therapy If intravenous access has been secured, then, at least in healthy animals, Hartmann's solution at 3–5 ml/kg/h is often administered. However, more specific fluid therapy should be directed to the individual patient's requirements.

35.3.5.4.3 Recovery Close observation is important, especially after tracheal extubation, because pigs can develop laryngeal spasm/obstruction much in the same way as cats, and such respiratory obstructions during recovery are often 'silent'. Once the righting reflex has been regained and a sternal position can be maintained, monitoring can become a little more 'hands off'.

A warm environment is important, especially for small pigs and young piglets. Blankets and heat lamps may be required. If a pig should be slow to recover, its temperature should be checked as hypothermia can delay recovery. Pigs should not be recovered amongst 'awake' pigs because their pen-mates may attack them whist they are still groggy. Only once fully recovered should a pig be returned to its pen-mates.

If slow recovery is thought to be due to the prolonged effects of some of the premedication drugs, antagonists may be given, but none is licenced for use in food-producing pigs, at least in the UK.

Atipamezole can be administered to antagonise the effects of α2 agonists. Recommended doses are 20–50 μg/kg IV or IM, although doses up to 250 μg/kg may be necessary. Generally, a small dose is administered first and can be repeated every 5–10 minutes if necessary. Atipamezole has a relatively short duration of action compared to the α2 agonists.

Flumazenil can be given to antagonise the effects of benzodiazepines. Doses are unknown, but 1 mg flumazenil for every 13 mg benzodiazepine given has been suggested, which is around 10 μg/kg. Additional doses may be required as flumazenil has a relatively short duration of action.

Reference

Tranquilli, W.J., Thurmon, J.C., and Grimm, K.A. (eds.) (2007). *Lumb and Jones' Veterinary Anesthesia and Analgesia*, 4e. Blackwell Publishing Ltd.

Further Reading

Baumgartner, C.M., Brandl, J.K., Pfeiffer, N.E. et al. (2015). A comparison of the hemodynamic effects of alfaxalone and propofol in pigs. *Symbiosis Online Journal, Anesthesiology and pain management* 2: 1–8.

Bradbury, A.G., Eddleston, M., and Clutton, R.E. (2016). Pain management in pigs undergoing experimental surgery: a literature review (2012-2014). *British Journal of Anaesthesia* 116: 37–45.

Bradbury, A.G. and Clutton, R.E. (2016). Review of practices reported for preoperative food and water restriction of laboratory pigs (*Sus scrofa*). *Journal of the American Association for Laboratory Animal Science* 55: 35–40.

Brederlau, J., Muellenbach, R., Kredel, M. et al. (2008). Comparison of arterial and central venous cannulations using ultrasound guidance in pigs. *Veterinary Anaesthesia and Analgesia* 35: 161–165.

Clutton, R.E. (2018). A review of factors affecting analgesic selection in large animals undergoing translational research. *The Veterinary Journal* 236: 12–22.

Haga, H.A. and Ranheim, B. (2005). Castration of piglets: the analgesic effects of intratesticular and intrafunicular lidocaine injection. *Veterinary Anaesthesia and Analgesia* 32: 1–9.

Hancock, T.M., Caulkett, N.A., Pajor, E.A., and Grenwich, L. (2018). An investigation of the effects of intratesticular alfaxalone and lidocaine during castration in piglets. *Veterinary Anaesthesia and Analgesia* 45: 858–864.

Hodgkinson, O. (2007). Practical sedation and anaesthesia in pigs. *In Practice* 29: 34–39.

Keates, H. (2003). Induction of anaesthesia in pigs using a new alphaxalone formulation. *Veterinary Record* 153: 627–628.

Lervik, A., Raszplewicz, J., Ranheim, B. et al. (2018). Dexmedetomidine or fentanyl? Cardiovascular stability and analgesia during propofol-ketamine total intravenous anaesthesia in experimental pigs. *Veterinary Anaesthesia and Analgesia* 45: 295–308.

Lin, H.C. (2015). Comparative anesthesia and analgesia of ruminants and swine. In: *Veterinary Anesthesia and Analgesia, the Fifth Edition of Lumb and Jones* (eds. K.A. Grimm, L.A. Lamont, W.J. Tranquilli, et al.). Chapter 38, 743–753. Iowa, USA: Wiley-Blackwell.

Morath, U., Skogmo, H.K., Ranheim, B., and Levionnois, O.L. (2014). The use of bougie-guided insertion of a laryngeal mask airway device in neonatal pigs after unexpected complications. *Veterinary Record Case Reports* 2: e000040. https://doi.org/10.1136/vetreccr-2013-000040.

Santos, M., Bertran de Lis, B.T., and Tendillo, F.J. (2016). Effect of intramuscular dexmedetomidine in combination with ketamine or alfaxalone in swine. *Veterinary Anaesthesia and Analgesia* 43: 81–85.

Schoos, A., Devreese, M., and Maes, D.G.D. (2019). Use of non-steroidal anti-inflammatory drugs in procine health management. *Veterinary Record* 185: 172. https://doi.org/10.1136/vr.105170.

Snook, C.S. (2001). Use of the subcutaneous abdominal vein for blood sampling and intravenous catheterization in potbellied pigs. *Journal of the American Veterinary Medical Association* 219: 809–810, 764.

Trim, C.M. and Braun, C. (2011). Anesthetic agents and complications in Vietnamese potbellied pigs: 27 cases (1999-2006). *Journal of the American Veterinary Medical Association* 239: 114–121.

Valverde, A. and Sinclair, M. (2015). Ruminant and swine local anesthetic and analgesic techniques. In: *Veterinary Anesthesia and Analgesia, Fifth Edition of Lumb and Jones* (eds. K.A. Grimm, L.A. Lamont, W.J. Tranquilli, et al.). Chapter 51, 941–959. Iowa, USA: Wiley-Blackwell.

Self-test Section

1 Describe the anatomical structures of the porcine head and larynx that can make tracheal intubation difficult in this species.

2 What compound is also present in dantrolene sodium, and which might also be helpful in the treatment of malignant hyperthermia?

36

Rabbit Anaesthesia

36.1 Risk of Peri-anaesthetic Morbidity

Rabbits are famed for being high-risk candidates for anaesthesia; the morbidity rate was recently determined as 1 in 72. Some of the reasons for the higher risk of peri-anaesthetic morbidity compared to other species are given below.

36.1.1 Underlying Disease

- Malnourishment (common in rabbits requiring dental treatment), and dehydration. A thorough history might help to determine if hyporexia/anorexia/decreased faecal output pre-exists.
- Obesity is prevalent in rabbits and increases the incidence of post-anaesthetic gastrointestinal (GI) complications and the risk of peri-anaesthetic hypoxaemia.
- Many rabbits are effectively geriatric when presenting for conditions other than neutering.
- Sub-clinical respiratory disease (e.g. Pasteurellosis) can affect the rabbit's oxygenation during anaesthesia, and may progress to a clinical infection post-operatively.
- Uterine carcinomas may complicate ovariohysterectomy by placing pressure on the great vessels and the thorax during dorsal recumbency, affecting ventilation and blood pressure.

36.1.2 Lack of Familiarity and Expertise

Anaesthetic dose requirements for pet rabbits will often be much lower than those published from experimental studies, where healthier (specific pathogen free) rabbits had been used (Table 36.1).

36.1.3 Size

- Ranges from dwarfs to giant French lops.
- Beware hypothermia (relatively large surface area: body mass).
- Intravenous cannulation and endotracheal intubation require appropriately sized equipment, but can also be technically challenging. Beware excessive resistance and dead space within the anaesthetic breathing system.

36.1.4 Endotracheal Intubation

Challenging due to a narrow gape, long incisors, and a fleshy tongue, all of which can make visualisation of the larynx difficult. The glottis is also relatively small. Laryngospasm can occur during endotracheal intubation and may be influenced by the choice of anaesthetic protocol (see Further Reading). Gentle endotracheal intubation is advised to avoid excessive laryngeal trauma.

36.1.5 Pain

Rabbits are a prey species and so will be unwilling to show signs of pain, especially when housed near cats and dogs. Vets tend to be less familiar with pain recognition in this species than with that in dogs and cats. Behavioural changes include a reduction in appetite (and thus faecal output and body weight), and spending less time on exploring their surroundings and moving around. Grimace scales have been developed for use in rabbits using changes in facial expression (namely, orbital tightening, cheek flattening, nose shape, whisker position, and ear position) to quantify pain. The difficulties associated with pain assessment in this species should not prevent analgesia provision.

Veterinary Anaesthesia: Principles to Practice, Second Edition. Alexandra H. A. Dugdale, Georgina Beaumont, Carl Bradbrook, and Matthew Gurney.
© 2020 John Wiley & Sons Ltd. Published 2020 by John Wiley & Sons Ltd.
Companion website: www.wiley.com/go/dugdale/veterinary-anaesthesia

Table 36.1 Pre-anaesthetic medication and induction doses taken from studies on pet rabbit populations.

Pre-anaesthetic medication	Induction of anaesthesia	References
	Ketamine 15 mg/kg + midazolam 3 mg/kg IM	Grint and Murison (2008)
	Ketamine 15 mg/kg + medetomidine 0.25 mg/kg IM or SC	Grint and Murison (2008) Orr et al. (2005)
	Ketamine 15 mg/kg + medetomidine 0.5 mg/kg SC	Orr et al. (2005)
Fentanyl/fluanisone 0.1 ml/kg IM	Propofol IV to effect (mean dose 2.2 mg/kg)	Martinez et al. (2009)
Fentanyl/fluanisone 0.1 ml/kg IM	Midazolam IV to effect (mean dose 0.7 mg/kg)	Martinez et al. (2009)
Fentanyl/fluanisone 0.2 ml/kg IM	Midazolam 0.2 mg/kg IV	Benato et al. (2013)
Buprenorphine 0.03 mg/kg IM	Alfaxalone 2–3 mg/kg IV	Grint et al. (2009)

36.1.6 Gastrointestinal System

- Rabbits are caeco-colic fermenters.
- Post-operative ileus is common even in the face of prokinetics. Predisposing factors include pain, starvation, stress, and alteration of diet.
- Gastrointestinal tract tympany due to gut stasis can promote cardiovascular and respiratory embarrassment under anaesthesia due to diaphragmatic splinting and occlusion of the abdominal great vessels.
- Prokinetics can be administered in an attempt to prevent ileus: ranitidine seems to be favoured and some operators suggest to administer a dose of 4 mg/kg per os at the same time that local anaesthetic cream is applied to the IV access site. Metoclopramide can also be used.

36.2 Approach to Rabbit Anaesthesia

36.2.1 Pre-anaesthetic Preparation

- Stabilise condition before anaesthesia.
- Allow food up to the point of premedication to: help maintain blood glucose concentration, sustain body heat production, and prevent gut stasis.

36.2.2 Pre-anaesthetic Medication

- Rabbits are easily stressed. Struggling before anaesthesia can result in: fractured vertebrae; catecholamine induced arrhythmias. Stress also promotes gut stasis.
- The provision of pre-anaesthetic medication will have all the same benefits as for other species (see Chapter 4).

- Drugs include acepromazine, benzodiazepines, α2 adrenergic agonists, and opioids. A neuroleptanalgesic combination of fentanyl and fluanisone, (Hypnorm™) is licenced for use in rabbits in the UK. The administration of buprenorphine after this combination is sometimes practised ('sequential analgesia') so that there is lessening of fentanyl's respiratory depression, but the continued provision of analgesia.

36.2.3 Intravenous Access

Facilitates accurate and 'to effect' dosing of intravenous induction agents and administration of fluid therapy and emergency drugs. Cannulae (usually 22 or 24 g) can be placed in the marginal ear vein (see Figure 36.1 and Chapter 7) or cephalic vein. Cannulation is facilitated by topical local anaesthetic cream (e.g. EMLA™ applied to a clipped area of the insertion site and covered with an occlusive dressing for 30–40 minutes); or gel (Ametop™ [amethocaine, also known as tetracaine], which works in 5–10 minutes after application) before catheter placement.

36.2.4 Pre-oxygenation

As sub-clinical respiratory infections are common in pet rabbits (which may affect their gas exchange), and endotracheal intubation may not be as swift in this species as in others, pre-oxygenation before induction of anaesthesia is a useful technique (if stress-free), usually by face mask (Figure 36.2); flow-by oxygen provides lower levels of inspired oxygen. Any pre-oxygenation achieved by placing a rabbit in an 'oxygen tent' is soon lost when the rabbit is lifted out for induction.

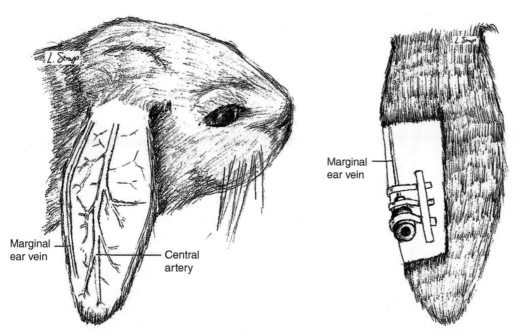

Figure 36.1 Showing marginal ear vein and central auricular artery. *Source:* Image courtesy of Dr. Lee Strapp BVetMed MRCVS.

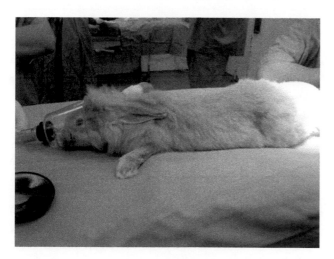

Figure 36.2 A mask can be used to pre-oxygenate a rabbit before endotracheal intubation is attempted.

36.2.5 Induction of Anaesthesia

Can be achieved by intravenous, intramuscular or inhalational administration of various drugs, all of which have relative advantages and disadvantages (see Table 36.1 and Chapters 5 and 8).

Alfaxalone is now licenced in the UK for anaesthetic induction in pet rabbits. It produces minimal cardiorespiratory depression, slightly less than propofol, yet also offers fairly rapid metabolism and recovery. It can be administered IM as well as IV (where 'slowly to effect' via a cannula is best).

Inhalation induction is possible via face mask or chamber. The rabbit should be adequately sedated before volatile agent is administered. Sevoflurane is often preferred for a fast induction, which appears to be well tolerated; isoflurane is more pungent and less well tolerated. Neither of these volatile agents sensitise the myocardium to the arrhythmogenic effects of catecholamines should the rabbit become stressed. With inhalation induction by both techniques (mask or chamber), oxygen alone should be delivered initially before slowly increasing the delivery of volatile agent; sudden large increases in volatile agent delivery may cause breath-holding.

36.2.6 Endotracheal Intubation

Recommended for all except the shortest procedures where a mask may be sufficient. A paediatric laryngoscope (especially one with a slimmed down blade-tip, the Flecknell small animal laryngoscope™), or otoscope can be used to visualise the larynx, then a stylette or bougie (or a urinary catheter [with the Luer adapter removed if using an otoscope]) can be introduced into the trachea, and finally the endotracheal tube can be 'railroaded' over this. An alternative technique is the 'blind' method, where the rabbit's head position is 'key' (it must be held so the nose is pointing to the sky and the hard palate is perpendicular to the table, Figure 36.3); then the anaesthetist relies on hearing breath sounds (or using your eye to 'feel' breaths) coming through the endotracheal tube as the tube is advanced. If the breath sounds disappear, then endo-oesophageal intubation is

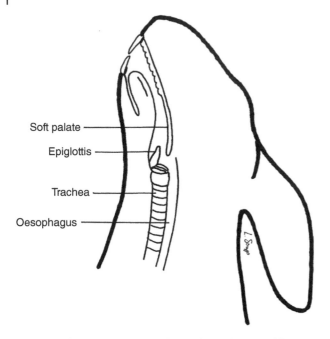

Soft palate

Epiglottis

Trachea

Oesophagus

Figure 36.3 Optimal positioning of the rabbit's head for endotracheal intubation. *Source:* Image courtesy of Dr Lee Strapp BVetMed MRCVS.

suspected; the tube should be withdrawn and redirected. When endotracheal intubation is successful, breath sounds will become louder and the rabbit may cough. Capnography can also be used to guide and/or verify endotracheal tube placement. Topical lidocaine onto the larynx may prevent laryngospasm during endotracheal intubation attempts. Do not pull the tongue too hard or vagal stimulation can result in profound bradycardia; this can also happen upon laryngeal stimulation. Supra-glottic airway devices (SGADs), such as laryngeal mask airways (LMAs) and rabbit v-gels™, have also been used to maintain airways in rabbits with the advantages of being an easier technique and requiring less induction agent for placement. Careful positioning of LMAs, however, has been advised in order to avoid lingual vascular compression, which can result in cyanosis of the tongue.

36.2.7 Maintenance of Anaesthesia

- Some induction protocols may produce anaesthesia of sufficient duration for short procedures, although oxygen should always be supplemented.
- For delivery of volatile agents, a non-rebreathing system (e.g. Jackson Rees modification of the Ayre's T-piece) should be used in all but the largest rabbits. Fresh gas flow calculations should be based on a higher minute ventilation rate compared with dogs and cats, approximately 250 ml/kg/min.
- Nitrous oxide may be used, although will limit the fraction of inspired oxygen, so monitoring of pulse oximetry

(SpO_2) is recommended. Nitrous oxide may accumulate in the gas-filled gastrointestinal tract of the rabbit (similar to the horse, see Chapter 8), so monitoring for tympany during the anaesthetic is advised.
- Ocular lubricant should be applied and care taken to avoid ocular damage. Ocular reflexes are not usually helpful to judge anaesthetic depth.
- Forelimb withdrawal reflexes are said to be more reliable than hindlimb reflexes to help monitor anaesthetic depth. (Jaw tone is very difficult to assess.)

36.2.8 Fluid Therapy

The intravenous route is preferred. Subcutaneous or intra-peritoneal routes are alternatives, although glucose-containing fluids are not recommended via these routes. The type of fluids and rates of infusion will be determined by the likely imbalances present (see Chapter 23). Rabbit blood volume is around 50 ml/kg, and maintenance requirements have been estimated to be around 100 ml/kg/day due to their high metabolic rate.

36.2.9 Monitoring during Anaesthesia

- Minimum: breathing rate, heart rate, pulse rate (see below), and temperature. Steps should be taken to maintain body temperature (see Chapter 20).
- Pulse oximetry, capnography, and the ECG may be monitored. Some monitors, especially pulse oximeters that have been designed for humans, may not be able to display the relatively high pulse rates that occur in these small animals. Paediatric capnograph connectors should be chosen to minimise breathing apparatus dead space.
- The auricular artery (runs down the middle of the ear) can be palpated, and can be cannulated for direct blood pressure measurement. Due to the small size of some rabbits, oscillometric blood pressure measurement may be difficult, but blood pressure can be measured using the Doppler technique (see Chapter 18).

36.2.10 Analgesia

Multi-modal analgesia should be considered. Medetomidine, ketamine, and fentanyl/fluanisone, commonly used in premedication/induction protocols, are inherently analgesic. Buprenorphine is a popular choice of opioid due to its relatively long duration of action. Non-steroidal anti-inflammatory drugs (NSAIDs) such as meloxicam and carprofen will also provide longer term analgesia. Local anaesthetic techniques can be used, although accurate calculation of doses is critical to avoid overdose. Retrobulbar block used to be relatively contraindicated, as the rabbit has a large venous plexus behind the globe that is easily penetrated, however, an ultrasound-guided technique for a periconal block has recently been published with few complications recorded to date (See Further Reading).

36.2.11 Recovery from Anaesthesia

- Ensure a warm, calm (minimal stress) environment away from predators.
- Continue monitoring.

- Short-acting anaesthetic drugs promote shorter and more 'complete' recoveries, which allow a rapid return of appetite and thermoregulation. Antagonists may be considered, where appropriate.
- Offer food as soon as the rabbit is sufficiently recovered to prevent ileus and provide a source of glucose. Syringe-feeding with high-fibre gruels/mashes may be necessary in some cases.
- Continue analgesia. (Pain can also promote ileus.)

Further Reading

Benato, L., Chesnel, M., Eatwell, K., and Meredith, A. (2013). Arterial blood gas parameters in pet rabbits anaesthetised using a combination of fentanyl-fluanisone-midazolam-isoflurane. *Journal of Small Animal Practice* 54: 343–346.

Benato, L., Rooney, N.J., and Murrell, J. (2019). Pain and analgesia in pet rabbits. *Veterinary Anaesthesia and Analgesia* 46: 151–162.

Beswick, A., Dewey, C., Johnson, R. et al. (2016). Survey of Ontario veterinarians' knowledge and attitudes on pain in dogs and cats in 2012. *The Canadian Veterinary Journal* 57: 1274–1280.

Brodbelt, D.C., Blissitt, K.J., Hammond, R.A. et al. (2008). The risk of death: the confidential enquiry into perioperative small animal fatalities. *Veterinary Anaesthesia and Analgesia* 35: 365–373.

Clarke, K.W. and Hall, L.W. (1990). A survey of anaesthesia in small animal practice. AVA/BSAVA report. *Journal of Veterinary Anaesthesia* 17: 4–10.

Cruz, M.I., Sacchi, T., Luna, S.P. et al. (2001). Use of a laryngeal mask for airway maintenance during inhalation anaesthesia in rabbits. *Veterinary Anaesthesia and Analgesia* 27: 112–116.

Farnworth, M.J., Walker, J.K., Schweizer, K.A. et al. (2011). Potential behavioural indicators of post-operative pain in male laboratory rabbits following abdominal surgery. *Animal Welfare* 20: 225–237.

Grint, N.J. and Murison, P.J. (2008). A comparison of ketamine-midazolam and ketamine-medetomidine combinations for induction of anaesthesia in rabbits. *Veterinary Anaesthesia and Analgesia* 35: 113–121.

Grint, N.J., Smith, H.E., and Senior, J.M. (2009). Clinical evaluation of alfaxalone in cyclodextrin for the induction of anaesthesia in rabbits. *Veterinary Record* 163: 395–396.

Kazakos, G., Anagnostou, T.L., Savvas, I., and Kazakou, I.M. (2007). Use of the laryngeal mask airway in rabbits: placement and efficacy. *Lab Animal* 36: 29–34.

Keating, S.C.J., Thomas, A.A., Flecknell, P.A., and Leach, M.C. (2012). Evaluation of EMLA cream for preventing pain during tattooing of rabbits: changes in physiological, behavioural and facial expression responses. *PLoS One* 7: 11.

Keown, A.J., Farnworth, M.J., and Adams, N.J. (2011). Attitudes towards perception and management of pain in rabbits and Guinea pigs by a sample of veterinarians in New Zealand. *New Zealand Veterinary Journal* 59: 305–310.

Lee, H.W., Machin, H., and Adami, C. (2018). Peri-anaesthetic mortality and non-fatal gastrointestinal complications in pet rabbits: a retrospective study in 210 rabbits. *Veterinary Anaesthesia and Analgesia* 45: 520–528.

Lee, L.Y., Lee, D., Ryu, H. et al. (2019). Capnography-guided endotracheal intubation as an alternative to existing intubation methods in rabbits. *Journal of the American Association of Laboratory Animal Science* 58: 240–245.

Martinez, M.A., Murison, P.J., and Love, E. (2009). Induction of anaesthesia with either midazolam or propofol in rabbits premedicated with fentanyl/fluanisone. *Veterinary Record* 164: 803–806.

Najman, I.E., Ferreira, J.Z., Abimussi, C.J.X. et al. (2015). Ultrasound-assisted periconal ocular blockade in rabbits. *Veterinary Anaesthesia and Analgesia* 42: 433–441.

Orr, H.E., Roughan, J.V., and Flecknell, P.A. (2005). Assessment of ketamine and medetomidine anaesthesia in the domestic rabbit. *Veterinary Anaesthesia and Analgesia* 32: 271–279.

Weaver, L.A., Blaze, C.A., Linder, D.E. et al. (2010). A model for clinical evaluation of perioperative analgesia in rabbits (Oryctolagus cuniculus). *Journal of the American Association of Laboratory Animal Science* 49: 845–851.

Self-test Section

1 List five factors that contribute to the high risk of rabbit anaesthesia.

2 What strategies can help to prevent post-operative ileus?

37

Neonates/Paediatrics

LEARNING OBJECTIVES

- To be able to discuss the physiological and pharmacological differences from adults.
- To be able to discuss options for chemical restraint.

37.1 Definitions

- **Neonates = up to four weeks old** (pups, kittens) **or up to two weeks old** (more precocious: foals and farm species).
- **Infants = two to six weeks old.**
- **Juveniles = six weeks to three to six months old.**
- Infants and juveniles are also **paediatric** patients.

37.2 Physiological Differences

37.2.1 Central Nervous System

Increased blood–brain barrier permeability to drugs.

37.2.2 Autonomic Nervous System

Parasympathetic system is mature at birth; sympathetic system is not: vagal dominance.

37.2.3 Cardiovascular System

At birth, the right ventricle is equivalent in size to the left or slightly larger. The ductus arteriosus can remain slightly patent for up to five days: machinery murmur audible.

Pulmonary vasculature is very muscular and responsive/sensitive to changes in blood gases, pH, and temperature. In the first few days of life, any increase in pulmonary vascular resistance (pulmonary hypertension) can cause re-opening of the foetal ducts (foramen ovale and ductus arteriosus), which 'closed' at birth (at least, functionally and physiologically [by constriction], respectively), and reversion to right-to-left shunting of blood. This recreates a foetal-like circulation, and results in systemic hypoxaemia because now there is no placenta to rely on for gaseous exchange. (Acidosis, hypoxaemia, and hypothermia during the first week of life can therefore pose a threat to the neonate when the circulation is 'transitional'.) (Anatomical closure of the foetal ducts can take months to years.)

The neonatal heart is poorly compliant, but resistant to hypoxia. This 'stiffness' limits its ability to increase stroke volume, so **cardiac output** is mainly **heart rate dependent**.

Limited stroke volume and vagal dominance provide limited cardiovascular reserves, and a poor ability to respond to sudden and/or large changes in blood volume/pressure (i.e. **poor haemodynamic stability).**

37.2.4 Respiratory System

High basal metabolic rate means high O_2 demand, which requires **high minute ventilation**.

Neonatal chest wall is very compliant, yet lungs are relatively stiff: these factors limit the achievable tidal volume, so **minute ventilation** is **breathing rate dependent. High breathing rate means high work of breathing;** therefore, **prone to respiratory fatigue.** Dead space forms a greater proportion of tidal volume than in the adult.

Intrapleural pressure is less negative (compliant chest wall) than adults, so alveoli can close easily between breaths.

Veterinary Anaesthesia: Principles to Practice, Second Edition. Alexandra H. A. Dugdale, Georgina Beaumont, Carl Bradbrook, and Matthew Gurney.
© 2020 John Wiley & Sons Ltd. Published 2020 by John Wiley & Sons Ltd.
Companion website: www.wiley.com/go/dugdale/veterinary-anaesthesia

Low functional residual capacity (due to immature alveolar number, compliant chest wall, and stiff lungs), and relatively high closing capacity compared to adults, makes neonatal lungs prone to atelectasis. During recumbency, **postural hypoxaemia** is quite commonly seen in foals (See chapter 30). Response to hypoxia is biphasic (i.e. initial response is unsustained):

- Transient increase in respiratory rate (respiratory muscle fatigue is also a factor in this transient response).
- Decreased respiratory rate, even to apnoea.

The overall foetal response to hypoxia is to 'shut down' (i.e. reduced muscle activity, bradycardia, bradypnoea, etc.), which is thought to be protective in the short term.

37.2.5 Haematology

Small size means small total blood volume (although c. 10–12% body mass compared with about 8–9% for adult [dog/horse]).

Dogs, and to some extent, horses, do not have a distinct foetal type of haemoglobin, but have less red cell 2,3, diphosphoglycerate (2,3-DPG). After birth, new red cells are made with increasing amounts of 2,3-DPG. Coagulation cascades and their control loops are immature with an increased tendency for coagulopathies.

37.2.6 Kidneys

Post-natal glomerular filtration matures over two to three weeks in dogs, compared to one week in horses and calves.

Renal tubular (especially secretory) function develops over four to eight weeks in dogs, compared to four to six weeks in horses.

A higher proportion of extracellular water in neonates means a higher daily water requirement (Figures 37.1 and 37.2). A higher rate of water turnover and immature kidneys increase the susceptibility to dehydration and overhydration. Immature renal function means:

- Poor ability to concentrate urine.
- Poor ability to excrete a water load.
- Poor acid–base regulation.

37.2.7 Liver

The immature liver has poor gluconeogenic ability and limited glycogen stores; these in combination with a high metabolic rate (and demand for glucose) make neonates **very susceptible to hypoglycaemia.** Within the first month of life, hepatic function matures rapidly.

37.2.8 Thermoregulation

Thermoregulatory control is immature. Neonates are prone to hypothermia despite their high metabolic rate and brown fat metabolism (although brown fat has not been found in piglets and foals), because:

- Large body surface area: body mass ratio.
- Little insulating subcutaneous fat (white adipose tissue).

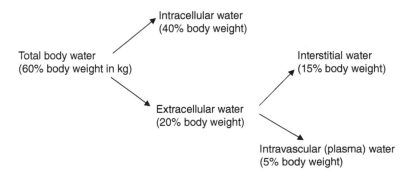

Figure 37.1 Water distribution in the adult (dog/horse). Daily water requirement is c. 40–60 ml/kg/day. Urine output is c. 1.5 ml/kg/h.

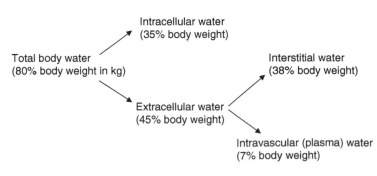

Figure 37.2 Water distribution in the neonate. Daily water requirement is c. 80–120 ml/kg/day. Urine output is c. 6 ml/kg/h.

- Poorly matured mechanisms for shivering thermogenesis (includes low muscle mass).
- Limited ability for non-shivering thermogenesis (limited liver glycogen reserves; brown fat is not always present).
- Susceptibility to hypoglycaemia.
- Immature control of vasomotor tone.

Hypothermia itself has detrimental effects (see Chapter 20).

37.2.9 Neuromuscular Junctions

Neonates are 'mini-myasthenics' (see Chapter 17).

37.3 Pharmacological Considerations

- Higher body water content and higher extracellular:intracellular fluid ratio means increased volume of distribution for water soluble/poorly protein bound drugs.
- Relative hypoalbuminaemia (not seen commonly in foals) leads to increased 'free' (active) concentration of protein-bound drugs. (Acidic drugs bind albumin, whereas basic drugs prefer to bind to α1-acid glycoprotein.)
- Low body fat (and relatively poor muscling) limits drug redistribution.
- Immature renal and hepatic metabolism/excretion pathways delay drug elimination.
- Increased blood–brain barrier permeability (especially for the first month of life), increases drug access to the central nervous system (CNS) (which helps to reduce the MAC of inhalation anaesthetic agents).
- Receptor differences: 'mini-myasthenics'; adrenoceptors (may respond poorly to endogenous and exogenous agonists, e.g. potentially poor response to vasopressors, inotropes, and possibly also anticholinergics).

37.4 Considerations for Chemical Restraint (Sedation/Anaesthesia)

- **No (or minimal) starvation** pre-operatively, **monitor blood glucose regularly.**
- **Weigh accurately.**
- **Temperature conservation**. Try to minimise heat loss (Chapter 20).
- **Premedication should be carefully considered and dosed appropriately.** Try to **use drugs that require minimal metabolism.** Try to **avoid drugs that reduce heart rate. Pethidine used to be favoured** amongst the opioids due to its ability to maintain heart rate (rather than reduce it), but now appears to be less commonly used. **Low dose methadone** may also be used. **Benzodiazepines provide useful sedative effects in neonatal/paediatric patients.**

- **Anaesthetic induction**. Secure **IV access** (small veins). **Pre-oxygenate** if possible without stressing the patient. Choose **drugs that require minimal metabolism** and allow **rapid recovery. Inhalation agents** like isoflurane or sevoflurane may be used and can be delivered by chamber, mask, or nasopharyngeal insufflation in as stress-free a manner as possible (the chosen method depending upon patient species, size and co-operativity). Inhalation anaesthetic agent MAC is reduced in neonates. Intravenous anaesthetic agents (propofol or alfaxalone [which can be diluted in saline to 1 mg/ml, off-licence]) should be given slowly and to effect.
- **Maintenance. Oxygen**. Medical air or N_2O maybe included if patient oxygenation sufficient. (N_2O role in pulmonary hypertension equivocal.) Monitoring of SpO_2 is advised to help determine sufficiency of oxygen provision. Inhalation anaesthetic agents preferred over injectables because they can be more easily titrated to effect and recovery only requires ventilation (although the various agents can also be metabolised to different degrees).
- **Anaesthetic breathing system**. Choice depends upon patient size, e.g. from Jackson-Rees modified Ayre's T-piece to small animal circle. Heat and moisture exchangers may help prevent hypothermia, but beware the additional apparatus dead space (although neonatal sizes are available). Try to **minimise apparatus dead space**.
- **Endotracheal tubes or mask?** The airway should be secured with an endotracheal tube, ideally cuffed and with careful assessment for any leak present. (Over-inflation of the cuff may result in tracheal damage.) Face masks are not recommended for use for maintenance of anaesthesia. Caution should be exercised with the use of red rubber tubes due to their cuff design, risk of obstruction if bent, and inability to visualise any material that may lead to an internal obstruction. Beware over-long tubes (excess dead space if the tube extends 'externally' too far beyond the 'incisor arcade'; or risk of endobronchial intubation if the tube extends too far 'internally'). Tubes should be measured against the patient prior to use (nose to thoracic inlet).
- **Ventilatory assistance** (artificial ventilation in the form of positive pressure mechanical or manual ventilation) is often required. **Be gentle**. Positive pressure ventilation is usually well tolerated by the cardiovascular system because of the compliant chest wall and lack of normal negative intrapleural end-expiratory pressure.
- **Monitoring**. See Chapter 18.

- **Fluids**. Beware over- and under-hydration. The relatively stiff myocardium means that the heart is not as responsive to fluid loading (in terms of Starling's law and increased inotropy) as in adults, and over-hydration and pulmonary oedema can be a consequence of excess IV fluids. Fluid (usually Hartmann's solution or normal saline, ± 5% glucose) rates of around 10 ml/kg/h are probably OK short term, if the patient was not previously hypovolaemic. IV access can be challenging: intra-osseous access represents an alternative. Burette-type or paediatric fluid giving sets, each with micro-droppers which deliver 60 drops/ml, can be useful, especially if infusion pumps are not available.
- Check **blood glucose** regularly.
- **Analgesia** Provide balanced analgesia where possible, but few agents are licenced. Beware local anaesthetic overdose toxicity (dilute solutions with sterile saline if necessary). See Chapters 12–16.

Further Reading

Dugdale, A. (2004). Sedation and anesthesia of foals. In: *Equine Neonatology: Medicine and Surgery* (eds. D.C. Knottenbelt, N. Holdstock and J.E. Madigan), 441–453. Saunders, London, UK.

Grubb, T.L., Perez Jimenez, T.E., and Pettifer, G.R. (2015). Neonatal and pediatric patients. In: *Veterinary Anesthesia and Analgesia, the Fifth Edition of Lumb and Jones* (eds. K.A. Grimm, L.A. Lamont, W.J. Tranquilli, et al.), 983–987. Iowa, USA: Wiley Blackwell.

Ousey, J.C. (1990). Heat production and its clinical implications in neonates. *Equine Veterinary Journal* 22 (2): 69–72.

Rigotti, C.F. and Brearley, J.C. (2016). Anaesthesia for paediatric and geriatric patients. In: *BSAVA Manual of Canine and Feline Anaesthesia and Analgesia* (eds. T. Duke-Novakovski, M. de Vries and C. Seymour), 418–427. Gloucester, UK: BSAVA.

Self-test Section

1 Define the closing capacity and its relation to the functional residual capacity in neonates.

2 Why was pethidine once favoured for neonatal opioid-analgesia and why might it be less favoured nowadays?

3 In which of the following has brown adipose tissue not been found?
   A Puppies
   B Kittens
   C Foals
   D Calves

4 What are your five main considerations for anaesthesia of the neonate?

38

Senescent/Geriatric Patients

38.1 Ageing Changes

Ageing changes are gradual, progressive, and generally irreversible, and centre around reduced organ function/capacity. Lifespans vary, but an individual is **considered geriatric when it has completed 75–80% of its expected natural lifespan. Medium-sized dogs > 8 years (small dogs > 12 years; giant breeds > 6 years), cats > 12 years and horses > 15 years** are often considered geriatric, although can be considered 'senior' for about the three years preceding geriatricity (see Further Reading).

Consider the chronological and physiological ages of an animal because factors other than its breed and genetics, such as nutrition and work, can influence senescence. Watch out for animals that look 'old for their years'. With advancing age, chronic diseases may be superimposed on ageing changes.

38.1.1 Central Nervous System/Peripheral Nervous System

- Progressive central nervous system (CNS) neuronal atrophy and decreased neurotransmitter release lead to **senility** (which can decrease the minimum alveolar concentration [MAC] of inhalation anaesthetic agents, making overdose more likely).
- Increased blood–brain barrier permeability (drugs reach CNS easily, also increasing likelihood of overdose).
- Decreased thermoregulatory ability.
- Decreased reflex activity (baroreceptor and chemoreceptor).

- Decreased visual and auditory acuity: patients are **more anxious** in strange places; **approach these patients quietly and carefully so as not to startle them, and consider the use of anxiolytic medications where appropriate.**
- Decreased conduction velocity in peripheral nerves may lead to some incoordination.
- Decreased number of nicotinic acetylcholine receptors at neuromuscular junctions causes increased sensitivity to non-depolarising neuromuscular blocking agents.

38.1.2 Cardiovascular System
Decreased cardiovascular reserves:

- Decreased **cardiac output**; decreased **blood pressure due to:**
  - **Increased vagal tone**.
  - Decreased baro- and chemoreceptor sensitivity.
  - Decreased responsiveness to catecholamines (β1 receptors appear to be down-regulated with age).
- **Slightly** decreased **blood volume**.
- **Cardiac output becomes preload-dependent.**

Cardiac degenerative changes (endocardiosis, valvular insufficiencies, cardiomyopathies, etc.) can predispose to **arrhythmias (ECG monitoring recommended)**. Hypertension, however, may be a consequence of conditions such as chronic renal disease. Atherosclerosis can occur in dogs, secondary to hyperlipaemia, which is most commonly associated with hypothyroidism. Where possible, (systolic) arterial blood pressure should be assessed prior to

Veterinary Anaesthesia: Principles to Practice, Second Edition. Alexandra H. A. Dugdale, Georgina Beaumont, Carl Bradbrook, and Matthew Gurney.
© 2020 John Wiley & Sons Ltd. Published 2020 by John Wiley & Sons Ltd.
Companion website: www.wiley.com/go/dugdale/veterinary-anaesthesia

premedication so that 'normal for that patient' can be documented, but many patients are very anxious, which precludes obtaining true values.

38.1.3 Respiratory System

Decreased ventilatory reserves (decreased functional residual capacity [FRC]; increased closing capacity; increased work of breathing), therefore increased risk of atelectasis and hypoxaemia, especially in the immediate recovery period (careful patient monitoring is advised):

- Decreased chest wall compliance (calcification of costochondral junctions and muscular atrophy).
- Decreased lung elasticity (calcification and fibrosis).
- Increased airway dead space.
- Decreased 'diffusing capacity' of alveolar/capillary gas diffusion 'membrane'.
- Decreased chemoreceptor and protective reflexes (e.g. coughing).

Diseases (e.g. chronic bronchitis, neoplasia, laryngeal paresis) may also reduce ventilatory reserves.

Obesity can increase peri- and intrathoracic fat that may restrict chest wall excursion, lung inflation, and also cardiac function (Pickwickian syndrome).

38.1.4 Kidneys

Reduced overall glomerular filtration rate (GFR). Decreased number of functional nephrons. Decreased cardiac output. Overall:

- May be azotaemic.
- May be isosthenuric (polydipsic/polyuric).
- Decreased excretory ability.

There may also be chronic renal disease.

38.1.5 Liver

- Decreased hepatic blood flow (decreased cardiac output); can delay drug metabolism.
- Decreased hepatocyte number and function:
  - Decreased albumin production (increased 'free'/active drug concentrations).
  - Decreased clotting factor production leading to coagulopathies.
  - Decreased metabolic functions (decreased basal metabolic rate [BMR]; decreased drug/toxin detoxification).
- Diseases (lipidosis; cirrhosis; neoplasia).

38.1.6 Endocrine

- Decreased stress responses.
- Endocrine disorders common, e.g. hypothyroidism.

38.1.7 Gastrointestinal Tract

- Decreased lower oesophageal sphincter tone (**increased risk of reflux/regurgitation**).
- Increased gastric acidity (**increased risk of reflux oesophagitis**).
- In **horses**, dental problems reduce food intake and the subsequent decreased fibre digestion in the large intestine significantly decreases heat production.

38.1.8 Thermoregulation

Geriatrics are prone to hypothermia, but laryngeal paresis and impaired panting (dogs) can lead to hyperthermia. Factors contributing to hypothermia include:

- Decreased muscle mass (less effective shivering).
- Decreased BMR.
- Decreased temperature homeostasis (CNS changes).
- Higher vagal tone reduces control of peripheral vasoconstriction abilities.
- Lack of brown fat (usually).
- Adiposity (white adipose tissue) variable (variable insulation).
- Possible hormonal alopecia.
- Reduced fibre digestion in equine large intestine.

38.1.9 Musculoskeletal

- Decreased muscle mass (sarcopenia) and increased fat mass (even in non-obese animals, sarcopaenic obesity is common with increased fat: lean ratio): alters the compartments for drug redistribution. Lack of soft tissue over bony skeletal structures may make positioning during anaesthesia painful in itself, even during diagnostic, non-invasive procedures. Drug administration by the IM route may be complicated by the reduced muscle mass, and may result in less predictable effects.
- Osteoarthritis/spondylosis: requires gentle positioning during anaesthesia and for restraint during, e.g. IV cannula placement, and can 'distort' local anatomy for, e.g. epidural injections. Also, care should be taken with neck movement during endotracheal tube placement.
- Obesity may obscure anatomical landmarks for local blocks. Obesity also decreases epidural dose requirements due to increased adipose tissue presence in the epidural 'space' and the effects of increased intra-abdominal pressure.
- Narrowed intervertebral foramina (fibrosis/ossification): epidural dose requirements are reduced.

38.2 Approach to Anaesthesia

- Time permitting, **determine any existing organ dysfunction and stabilise before general anaesthesia** to optimise anaesthetic management.
- Routine pre-anaesthetic blood testing is often advised in dogs over 8 years of age and cats over 10–12 years, even if they appear 'healthy' on physical examination and after taking a thorough history.
- **Handle gently**. Offer plenty of tender loving care (TLC) in the peri-operative period. Geriatrics suffer more 'emergence delirium' than any other patients, possibly due to senile changes, increased blood–brain barrier permeability, and increased anxiety. Thoughtful and appropriate opioid dosing, according to pain assessment/scoring, may aid in reducing opioid-related dysphoria.
- **Premedication**. **Small doses** (elimination prolonged). Drugs with minimal cardiovascular and respiratory side effects. Opioids are commonly chosen. Sedatives can be administered if necessary: low doses of acepromazine (c. 0.005–0.01 mg/kg); α2-adrenoreceptor agonists (medetomidine 1–3 μg/kg, dexmedetomidine 0.5–1 μg/kg) or benzodiazepines (e.g. midazolam 0.1–0.2 mg/kg), but some animals suffer 'disinhibition-excitement' with benzodiazepines, therefore not advised to be used as a sole agent in the 'healthy' geriatric.
- **Pre-oxygenate** if possible without stress.
- **Secure IV access**.
- **Anaesthetic induction**. Injectable anaesthetic induction agents should be given IV slowly (where possible) 'to effect'. Injectable agents are generally preferred for anaesthetic induction; inhalation induction must be stress-free and beware the reduced MAC of inhalation anaesthetic agents in older patients.
- **Maintenance of anaesthesia**. Supply O₂. Consider **balanced anaesthetic techniques**. The MAC of inhalation agents is reduced in old age, therefore, if used for (or as part of) anaesthetic maintenance, the depth of anaesthesia should be carefully and frequently assessed. **Ventilatory support** may be required no matter what drug/s are used for anaesthetic maintenance. Intravenous **fluids** (preferably Hartmann's solution) are usually administered at c. 5 ml/kg/h if not previously hypovolaemic.
- **Analgesia**. Multimodal approach. Check renal/hepatic function. May also facilitate non-invasive/diagnostic procedures due to reduction of pain associated with musculoskeletal disease, such as osteoarthritis.
- **Monitoring** see Chapter 18.

Recovery. Ensure **continued analgesia** and **good nursing**. Geriatric animals are **prone to emergence delirium**: TLC often works wonders. Quick return to the owners can be beneficial. Careful use of low doses of sedatives/anxiolytics may be warranted if delirium occurs. Check temperature if recovery appears delayed. Possibly continue IV fluids until oral intake resumes. Ensure empty bladder (improves comfort in recovery). Older animals are often reluctant to defecate or urinate in a strange place; and arthritic, stiff, or sore animals may be reluctant to stand and posture to urinate and defecate; good analgesia is essential in this period.

Further Reading

Brosnahan, M.M. and Paradis, M.R. (2003). Demographic and clinical characteristics of geriatric horses: 467 cases: 1989–1999. *Journal of the American Veterinary Medical Association* 223: 93–98.

Burns PM (2015) Top 5 considerations for anesthesia of a geriatric patient. Clinician's Brief June 2015, 71–75.

Carpenter, R.E., Pettifer, G.R., and Tranquilli, W.J. (2005). Anesthesia for geriatric patients. *Veterinary Clinics of North America: Small Animal Practice* 35: 571–580.

Coupland, S. and Reynolds, H. (2018). Do dog owners recognise behavioural indicators of canine cognitive dysfunction and can environmental enrichment techniques slow its progression? *The Veterinary Nurse* 9: 118–123.

Davies, M. (2012). Geriatric screening in first opinion practice – results from 45 dogs. *Journal of Small Animal Practice* 53: 507–513.

Davies, M. (2016). Focusing on geriatric pets. *In Practice* 38: 39–42.

Fortney, W.D. (2012). Implementing a successful senior/geriatric health care program for veterinarians, veterinary technicians and office managers. *Veterinary Clinics of North America: Small Animal Practice* 42: 823–834.

Grubb, T.L., Perez Jimenez, T.E., and Pettifer, G.R. (2015). Senior and geriatric patients. In: *Veterinary Anesthesia and Analgesia, The Fifth Edition of Lumb and Jones* (eds. K.A. Grimm, L.A. Lamont, W.J. Tranquilli, et al.), 988–992. Iowa, USA: Wiley Blackwell.

Malik, A. and Gregerson, S. (2019). Managing pain in common end-of-life conditions. *The Veterinary Nurse* 10: 173–181.

Matthews, N.S. (2002). Anesthetic considerations of the older equine. *Veterinary Clinics of North America: Equine Practice* 18: 403–409.

Rigotti, C.F. and Brearley, J.C. (2016). Anaesthesia for paediatric and geriatric patients. In: *BSAVA Manual of Canine and Feline Anaesthesia and Analgesia* (eds. T. Duke-Novakovski, M. de Vries and C. Seymour), 418–427. Gloucester, UK: BSAVA.

Seddighi, R. and Doherty, T.J. (2012). Anesthesia of the geriatric equine. *Veterinary Medicine: Research and Reports* 3: 53–64.

Willems, A., Paepe, D., Marynissen, S. et al. (2017). Results of screening of apparently healthy senior and geriatric dogs. *Journal of Veterinary Internal Medicine* 31: 81–92.

Self-test Section

1 True or False? Geriatric animals are prone to anxiety and post-anaesthetic emergence delirium.

2 True or False? Drug doses for epidural injection should be reduced in elderly patients.

3 What do you understand by the term 'sarcopaenic obesity'?

39

Pregnancy and Caesarean Sections

LEARNING OBJECTIVES

- To be able to discuss the physiological changes occurring during pregnancy and their influences on anaesthesia.
- To be able to devise an anaesthetic plan.

39.1 Physiological Changes during Pregnancy

39.1.1 Cardiovascular System

Increased cardiac output (by up to approx. 40%), increased myocardial work:

- Increased heart rate.
- Increased stroke volume.
- Decreased systemic vascular resistance (progesterone effect).
- Decreased responsiveness to vasoactive medications, including vasopressors, positive inotropes, and anticholinergics. (Progesterone reduces [whereas oestrogen increases] sensitivity to catecholamines by affecting adrenoceptor expression.)

39.1.2 Blood

Physiological anaemia and decreased blood viscosity:

- Increased plasma volume.
- Slightly increased red cell mass.
- Slightly decreased total protein.
- Platelet count may increase near term.

Hypercoagulable state: increased clotting factors and increased risk of thromboemboli (see hepatic effects below).

39.1.3 Respiratory System

- Increased minute ventilation as a result of an increased O_2 demand, increased basal metabolic rate (BMR), and progesterone's effect on CO_2 sensitivity:
  - Increased breathing rate; overcomes decreased tidal volume with advancing gestation.
  - Progesterone increases central chemoreceptor sensitivity to CO_2. P_aCO_2 reduces to produce a slight respiratory alkalosis (e.g. 40 mmHg [5.3 kPa] → c. 35 mmHg [4.7] kPa). Blood pH remains normal, however, due to a compensatory, offsetting metabolic acidosis (due to increased renal excretion of bicarbonate).
- Decreased functional residual capacity (FRC) (as intra-abdominal pressure increases), decreases 'gas reserves' in the lungs and increases potential for hypoxaemia (e.g. during post-induction apnoea), although alveolar gas composition can change more quickly in the smaller FRC during inhalational anaesthesia (and therefore anaesthetic depth can change more rapidly). Closing capacity 'approaches' the FRC during late pregnancy leading to an increased risk of atelectasis.
- Airway dilation (progesterone effect) reduces resistance, but increases dead space.
- Decreased P_aCO_2 theoretically shifts the Hb/O_2 dissociation curve to the left, but increased 2,3- diphosphoglycerate (2,3-DPG) offsets this.

Veterinary Anaesthesia: Principles to Practice, Second Edition. Alexandra H. A. Dugdale, Georgina Beaumont,
Carl Bradbrook, and Matthew Gurney.
© 2020 John Wiley & Sons Ltd. Published 2020 by John Wiley & Sons Ltd.
Companion website: www.wiley.com/go/dugdale/veterinary-anaesthesia

39.1.4 Uterus

Perfusion (proportional to placental and foetal size):

- Depends upon the arterio-venous blood pressure difference. Maintaining adequate maternal blood pressure during anaesthesia is essential.
- Is inversely proportional to uterine tone and vascular resistance.
  – Uterine contractions may decrease perfusion.
- Uterine blood flow is sensitive to P_aCO_2 (increased CO_2 leads to vasodilation; decreased CO_2 leads to vasoconstriction).

39.2 Aorto-caval Compression Syndrome/Supine Hypotensive Syndrome

During dorsal recumbency (if heavily pregnant), the weight of the gravid uterus squashes the large blood vessels that run close to the spine, including the caudal vena cava (most compressible major vessel) and descending aorta. Vena caval compression reduces venous return to the right side of the heart, subsequently reducing cardiac output and may lead to reduction in arterial blood pressure. Reflex tachycardia usually occurs in response to the hypotension, but sudden severe reduction in venous return (e.g. if animal turned into dorsal recumbency quickly), especially if superimposed on pre-existing hypovolaemia (absolute or relative [e.g. sympathetic block accompanying epidural anaesthesia]), can also stimulate the Bezold-Jarisch reflex, which results in inappropriate vasodilation and bradycardia (and can result in vaso-vagal syncope). Compression of the abdominal aorta also risks reducing uteroplacental perfusion. Gentle, slow changes in patient position are recommended and rolling slightly (a 15° tilt is suggested for people), to the left side of dorsal (away from the vena cava), reduces pressure on the vena cava.

39.2.1 Gastrointestinal Tract

- Cranial displacement of the stomach increases the risk of gastric reflux and also 'splints' the diaphragm leading to decreased ventilatory reserves.
- Delayed gastric emptying and decreased cardiac sphincter tone (both due to progesterone which relaxes smooth muscle) lead to increased intragastric pressure and increased risk of reflux/regurgitation. (Raised intra-abdominal pressure, due to the gravid uterus, also increases intragastric pressure and the risk of reflux/regurgitation).
- Increased gastric acid secretion (effect of prolactin and foetal/placental gastrin), increases the acidity of any regurgitated material, which is potentially more harmful if aspirated.

39.2.2 Renal

Increased frequency of micturition:

- Increased urine output (increased cardiac output).
- Bladder squashed by increased intra-abdominal pressure.

39.2.3 Hepatic

- Decreased serum proteins, including plasma cholinesterase.
- Increased clotting factors, increased fibrinogen and plasminogen inhibitor, decreased antithrombin III and plasminogen activator, leading to hypercoagulability.

39.2.4 Other

- Increased blood–brain barrier permeability and central nervous system (CNS) depressant effects (both due to progesterone/its metabolites), increase sensitivity to drugs. Sedatives and injectable anaesthetic agents should be given in reduced doses and the MAC of volatile anaesthetic agents is reduced. (Endogenous opioid release around the time of parturition may also help to reduce MAC further.) Progesterone (especially its 3-alpha-hydroxy steroid metabolites) also sedates the foetus/es. Therefore, titrate injectable and inhaled anaesthetic drug administration to effect to reduce the risk of overdose.
- Engorged epidural (extradural) veins reduce epidural 'space' and decrease epidural dose requirements. Progesterone also increases sensitivity to local anaesthetics.
- Insulin resistance (physiological) may develop in the face of increased progesterone (and other hormone) concentrations.

39.3 Placental Transfer of Drugs

In general, placental exchange can occur via bulk flow (water), active transport, pinocytosis (immunoglobulins and other large molecules), direct mixing (in haemochorial placentae of humans, apes, rabbits, and rodents), and diffusion. The placental transfer of respiratory gases and most anaesthetic drugs occurs via diffusion, which is dependent upon their physicochemical properties and the concentration gradient between maternal and foetal circulations.

39.3.1 Physicochemical Properties

- Molecular size (smaller molecules can potentially diffuse more rapidly).
- Molecular shape (isomerism).
- Molecular charge (ionisation; pKa) (non-ionised molecules cross membranes more readily).

- Lipophilicity (fat solubility)/hydrophilicity (aqueous solubility) (e.g. partition coefficient).
- Protein binding (blood and tissue proteins).
- Stability (chemical and/or enzymatic degradation).

39.3.2 Factors Affecting Concentration Gradient between Maternal and Foetal Circulations

- Maternal drug dose.
- Maternal pharmacokinetics and pharmacodynamics ([re]distribution/elimination).
- Placental blood flow.
- Placental thickness and 'surface area' for exchange.
- The pH gradient between dam and foetus. Foetus usually more acidic leading to ion-trapping of basic drugs.
- Placental drug metabolism.
- Foetal pharmacokinetics and pharmacodynamics ([re] distribution/elimination).

39.4 Caesarean Sections (C-sections)

The mother's life is usually the priority. Orphan neonates have decreased survival. **For viable young**, you must **avoid foetal hypoxia**.

Causes of foetal hypoxia, at the time of C-section, include:

- Premature placental separation.
- Impaired maternal ventilation (drug- or position-induced respiratory depression).
- Drug- or position-induced maternal hypotension.
- Drug-induced foetal depression (foetal cardiovascular depression; neonatal cardio-respiratory depression).

Most anaesthetic agents (bar the highly ionised muscle relaxants) will readily cross the placenta, so **an anaesthetised mother means anaesthetised foetus/es as well**.

39.4.1 Options

39.4.1.1 Sedation + Local Anaesthetic Technique

Extra physical restraint often necessary. Sedative drugs given to the dam will affect the foetus/es. Local anaesthetics can cross placenta (bupivacaine least as highly protein-bound); placental transfer is dependent upon pKa of the drug, maternal and foetal pH, and the degree of protein binding. The quantity of local anaesthetic in the foetal circulation increases during foetal acidosis (ion-trapping). Local anaesthetic epidurals in the dam lead to caudal sympathetic block, which can decrease arterial blood pressure and placental perfusion; so ensure IV access, and aggressive fluid therapy etc. may be required.

In foaling horses an EXIT (ex-utero, intrapartum therapy/treatment) procedure may be considered, where oxygen is administered to the foal (via a naso-tracheal tube, if its head can be reached within the birth canal), during foetal manipulation (and before placental separation), for attempted controlled vaginal deliveries, or during C-section (usually under general anaesthesia) if this is subsequently required.

39.4.1.2 General Anaesthesia

General anaesthesia is often the most practical technique, but **most drugs cross the placenta** to also affect the young. The technique should be aimed at maintaining maternal oxygenation and blood pressure (placental perfusion and oxygen delivery to the foetus).

Decreased placental perfusion → decreased foetal oxygen supply → foetal bradycardia and acidosis.

Ketamine, opioids, and local anaesthetics are weak bases. If the foetus becomes very acidotic, **ion trapping** of these drugs is promoted.

39.4.1.2.1 Approach to General Anaesthesia

- History and clinical examination: **emergency** (recent meal?) **or elective?**
- **Minimal, but effective, premed.** Often **opioid-based** (pethidine), at least until foetus/es delivered. Anticholinergics? (see below). Debate concerning α2 agonists is further explored in Chapter 28 (equine sedation) and in Further Reading.
- Consider **local anaesthesia**, including epidural techniques (lumbo-sacral or sacro-/inter-coccygeal) and local infiltration along the linea alba/midline/incision site.
- Ensure **IV access**; exhausted dams may require pre-operative stabilisation.
- **Pre-oxygenate** without stress if possible (to increase the dam's oxygen reserves).
- Try to **pre-clip** the belly if possible (saves time).

39.4.2 Anaesthetic Induction

Injectable anaesthetic agents are administered IV to effect, but, do not unduly delay anaesthetic induction due to the risk of regurgitation (increased intra-abdominal pressure secondary to gravid uterus and reduced lower oesophageal sphincter pressure), and aspiration. Propofol or alfaxalone are common choices for small animals and ketamine-based techniques for horses, but familiarity with the agent/protocol is also important. In one study, alfaxalone use was associated with better neonatal vitality during the first hour of life compared with propofol, although overall survival was similar between agents.

For small animals, induction of anaesthesia with **inhalation** agents can be achieved by mask or chamber, following pre-oxygenation, as long as the dam remains unstressed. Inhalation induction tends to be relatively quick because of the high minute ventilation and reduced FRC (despite the higher cardiac output), but patients can still experience 'stage II, involuntary excitement', where they appear to struggle/writhe, so be prepared for this (these techniques tend to be less favoured than injectable techniques). Isoflurane and sevoflurane should result in fewer cardiac arrhythmias during a stressful (high catecholamine) induction than halothane. A relatively rapid induction is important, to enable rapid control of the airway, due to the risk of regurgitation and aspiration.

39.4.3 Tracheal Intubation

Cuffed ET tube as soon as possible. Keep head elevated until the ET tube is secured and the cuff inflated to reduce the risk of regurgitation and aspiration.

39.4.3.1 Anaesthetic Maintenance

- Inhalation agents usually preferred (less potential for prolonged recoveries of dam and neonates). The MAC of volatile agents is reduced due to CNS depressant (GABA$_A$) effects of progesterone and/or its metabolites.
- Always supplement oxygen.
- N$_2$O controversial (theoretical possibility of diffusion hypoxia in the delivered young).
- **Careful positioning**: 'dorsal, with a slight tilt to the left'. **Changes of position should be done slowly and gently**.
- Artificial ventilation (i.e. manual or mechanical ventilation), and usually in the form of positive pressure ventilation may be required: **beware over-ventilation** because excessive reduction of end tidal CO$_2$ (ETCO$_2$) tension (and therefore P$_a$CO$_2$) will shift the Hb/O$_2$ dissociation curve further to the left, and reduce O$_2$ transfer to the foetus; and hypocapnia results in vasoconstriction of uterine vessels, with possible compromise of foetal oxygenation. (Positive pressure ventilation can also promote hypotension through mechanical and chemical [P$_a$CO$_2$] effects.)
- **Muscle relaxants may be considered**. Neuromuscular blocking agents are highly ionised and **do not cross the placenta**. (If used, the patient will require artificial ventilation and careful monitoring of anaesthetic depth as well as the degree of neuromuscular blockade and its reversal.) See Chapter 17.
- **Epidural** local anaesthetic can afford excellent analgesia, but performing the technique may increase anaesthetic time. Reduce epidural doses and beware the side effect of hypotension if local anaesthetics are used. Epidural

opioids do not produce hypotension in the dam and also do not cause temporary paraplegia that can complicate nursing. Epidural opioids alone, however, do not provide good 'incisional' analgesia/anti-nociception.

- **Loco-regional anaesthesia** may be more appropriate depending upon the species, including paravertebral nerve block (ruminants), or local infiltration techniques, including the linea alba/midline ± intraperitoneal 'splash' (companion animals), or line/'inverted L' block of the flank (ruminants).
- **Analgesia**. Systemic **opioids** can be given to the dam **after foetal delivery**; they do cross the placenta and also enter milk to a small degree, and so can make the offspring sleepy (both the foetus and milk are slightly acidic, so basic drugs like opioids can ion-trap there). **NSAIDs** readily cross the placenta, although, being acidic, do not ion-trap in the usually more acidic foetus. NSAIDs therefore can be given as soon as the young are delivered, but most people prefer to wait until the dam has 'recovered' from the anaesthetic (as hypotension may occur during anaesthesia). Due to their high protein binding and acidic nature, NSAIDs tend to be only minimally transferred to milk. Even so, some people consider gastro-protectant administration in the delivered young (e.g. sucralfate). Currently, there are no NSAIDs licenced in the UK for use in pregnant or lactating companion animals. (Administration of NSAIDs to a near-term dam might theoretically delay parturition, although this has not been documented as a problem. NSAIDs may also cause premature closure of the foetal ductus arteriosus by reducing PGE$_2$ production, one of the factors responsible for maintaining its patency. The relevance is debatable for one-off NSAID exposure, but chronic exposure to NSAIDs during human pregnancy has revealed an association with persistent pulmonary hypertension of the newborn.) The recommended 'withdrawal period' for milk and meat in large and production animals varies among products; it is essential that this information is communicated to owners before administration. For dogs, **paracetamol** is an alternative, or indeed adjunct, to conventional NSAIDs, but also readily crosses the placenta and a small amount will get into the milk.
- Intravenous **fluids** (Hartmann's solution often chosen) should be considered peri-operatively, and at c. 3–5 ml/kg/h intra-operatively, although be prepared to increase the rate when the gravid uterus is lifted, manipulated, or exteriorised or the foetus delivered (the sudden reduction in intra-abdominal pressure can result in hypotension).
- **Uterine traction** occasionally results in vagal (rather than sympathetic) reflexes such that **anticholinergics may be indicated**: **glycopyrrolate** is often preferred

because it **does not cross the placenta**, although it is slightly slower in onset than atropine.

- **Monitor** pulse rate, ECG, breathing rate, SpO_2, $ETCO_2$ tension, arterial blood pressure if possible, temperature, and arterial blood gases if possible (horses).
- Should **gastric reflux/regurgitation** occur, gently lavage the oesophagus with warm water (ensure ET tube cuff inflated), retrograde-flush the nasal passages, and ensure a clear pharynx before tracheal extubation.
- **Oxytocin** is often administered to aid uterine involution.

39.4.4   Recovery

Beware vomition/aspiration by the dam (especially small animals). If rapidly eliminated anaesthetic drugs were administered, then recovery should be quick, and the young should be allowed to **suckle and bond as soon as possible**. If not given already, **NSAIDs** may now be given to the dam.

39.4.5   Neonatal Resuscitation

- You will need **help**; the more pairs of hands the better, especially for large litters and foals.
- Assess heartbeat, muscle 'tonus', respiratory and reflex activity, mucous membrane colour, vocalisation, and suckling reflex. Neonate vigour/vitality/viability has been assessed using a modified APGAR score. This system was first used to assess human neonatal physical condition one minute after birth/delivery: A (appearance/skin colour), P (pulse), G (grimace/reflex irritability), A (activity/muscle tone), R (respiration); see Further Reading. The acronym 'APGAR' was coined some ten years after the original scoring system was reported by Virginia Apgar, and is therefore sometimes referred to as a 'backronym'.

- Ensure the airway is clear and that membranes and mucus are removed from nose and mouth. Gentle **suction** (catheter attached to syringe may suffice) may be required to clear mucus from the throat. Holding the head-down may help to clear the airways.
- Umbilical cords are usually clamped.
- Lots of **warm dry towels** to **rub (gently)**, especially over the ribs, to stimulate breathing.
- Stimulation of the nasal philtrum (**acupuncture point GV26**), with a towel or something sharper (straw/needle for calves/foals), may help to initiate breathing.
- **Naloxone** and **atipamezole** can be considered if neonatal respiratory depression is thought to be related to the dam's analgesia or sedation.
- If necessary, flow-by oxygen can be supplied.
- **Tracheal intubation** with a small ET tube or cannula may also be attempted, followed by gentle **insufflation with air** (which usually suffices), exhaled breath, or O_2.
- Keep neonate/s warm with **warm insulative blankets**, radiant heat lamp (beware burns though), forced warm air 'blanket', or heat pad (young pups and kittens often not heavy enough to feel the warmth though).
- **Re-unite neonate/s with dam as soon as possible** for suckling and bonding.

Previously used but currently unavailable medications include:

- **Doxapram** drops administered sublingually were once commonly used. However, doxapram may be detrimental in the presence of hypoxaemia as it increases myocardial and cerebral O_2 demand, which is not good in hypoxic neonates.
- **Etamiphylline** gel (stimulates respiratory activity by increasing sensitivity to CO_2, and enhances diaphragmatic activity), administered sublingually, was often favoured in farm species for neonatal resuscitation.

Further Reading

Claude, A. and Meyer, R.E. (2016). Anaesthesia for caesarean section and for the pregnant patient. In: *BSAVA Manual of Canine and Feline Anaesthesia and Analgesia*, 3e (eds. T. Duke-Novakovski, M. de Vries and C. Seymour), 366–375. Gloucester, UK: British Small Animal Veterinary Association.

Corley, K.T. and Furr, M.O. (2000). Cardiopulmonary resuscitation in newborn foals. *Compendium on Continuing Education for the Practising Veterinarian* 22: 957–966.

De Kramer, K.G.M., Joubert, K.E., and Nothling, J.O. (2017). Puppy survival and vigor associated with the use of low dose medetomidine premedication, propofol induction and maintenance of anesthesia using sevoflurane

gas-inhalation for caesarean section in the bitch. *Theriogenology* 96: 10–15.

Doebeli, A., Michel, E., Bettschart, R. et al. (2013). Apgar score after induction of anesthesia for canine cesarean section with alfaxalone versus propofol. *Theriogenology* 80: 850–854.

Griffiths, S.K. and Campbell, J.P. (2015). Placental structure, function and drug transfer. *Continuing Education in Anaesthesia, Critical Care and Pain* 15: 84–89.

Johnston, G.M. (1992). Perioperative care of mares subjected to Caesarean section. Part 1: anaesthesia. *Equine Veterinary Education* 4: 26–30.

Johnston, G.M. (1992). Perioperative care of mares subjected to Caesarean section. Part 2: perioperative support of the mare and foal. *Equine Veterinary Education* 4: 78–83.

Kinsella, S.M. and Tuckey, J.P. (2001). Perioperative bradycardia and asystole: relationship to vasovagal syncope and the Bezold-Jarisch reflex. *British Journal of Anaesthesia* 86: 859–868.

Luna, S.P.L., Cassu, R.N., Castro, G.B. et al. (2004). Effects of four anaesthetic protocols on the neurological and cardiorespiratory variables of puppies born by Caesarean section. *Veterinary Record* 154: 387–389.

Moon, P.F., Erb, H.N., Ludders, J.W. et al. (2000). Perioperative risk factors for puppies delivered by cesarean section in the United States and Canada. *Journal of the American Animal Hospital Association* 36: 359–368.

Moon-Massat, P.F. and Erb, H.N. (2002). Perioperative factors associated with puppy vigor after delivery by cesarean section. *Journal of the American Animal Hospital Association* 38: 90–96.

Perez, R., Sepulveda, L., and SantaMaria, A. (1991). Xylazine administration to pregnant sheep: Effects on maternal and fetal cardiovascular function, pH, and blood gases. *Acta Veterinaria Scandinavica Supplement* 87: 181–183.

Raffe, M.R. (2015). Anesthetic considerations during pregnancy and for the newborn. In: *Veterinary Anesthesia and Analgesia: The Fifth Edition of Lumb and Jones* (eds. K.A. Grimm, L.A. Lamont, W.J. Tranquilli, et al.), 708–719. Ames, Iowa, USA: Wiley Blackwell.

Rioja, E., Cernicchiaro, N., Costa, M.C., and Valverde, A. (2012). Perioperative risk factors for mortality and length of hospitalization in mares with dystocia undergoing general anaesthesia: a retrospective study. *Canadian Veterinary Journal* 53: 502–510.

Robertson, S. (2016). Anaesthetic management for caesarean sections in dogs and cats. *In Practice* 38: 327–339.

Romagnoli, M., Barbarossa, A., Cunto, M. et al. (2019). Evaluation of methadone concentrations in bitches and in umbilical cords after epidural or systemic administration for Caesarean section: a randomised trial. *Veterinary Anaesthesia and Analgesia* 46: 375–383.

Sakamoto, H., Kirihara, H., Fujiki, M. et al. (1997). The effects of medetomidine on maternal and fetal cardiovascular and pulmonary function, intrauterine pressure and uterine blood flow in pregnant goats. *Experimental Animals* 46: 67–73.

Self, I. (2019). Anaesthesia for canine Caesarean section. *Companion Animal* 24: 84–90.

Self-test Section

1 True or False? Progesterone increases sensitivity to catecholamines.

2 Which of the following statements is correct?
  A NSAIDs readily cross the placenta, ion-trapping in the more acidic foetus; and also ion-trap in the milk.
  B NSAIDs readily cross the placenta, ion-trapping in the more acidic foetus; but do not ion-trap in the milk.
  C NSAIDs readily cross the placenta, but do not ion-trap in the more acidic foetus; although they do ion-trap in the milk.
  D NSAIDs readily cross the placenta, but do not ion-trap in the more acidic foetus; and they do not ion-trap in the milk.

40

Obesity

LEARNING OBJECTIVES

- To outline the physiological and metabolic/endocrinologic consequences of obesity and how they impact anaesthesia and the peri-operative period.
- To be familiar with the pharmacokinetic consequences of obesity with respect to anaesthetic and adjunctive agents.

40.1   Introduction

Companion animal obesity is increasing in parallel with that of human obesity in Western societies such that some 20–40% of companion animal populations (dogs, cats, rabbits, and Equidae) are now overweight or obese. *Obesity* is defined as 'excessive body fat content sufficient to cause impairment to health or bodily function' and it is associated with increased morbidity and mortality. The reduction of life expectancy that accompanies obesity is likely due to its medical sequelae that include type 2 (insulin-resistant) diabetes mellitus, altered circulating lipid profiles, cardiovascular and respiratory disease, musculoskeletal disease, skin disease, infertility, and neoplasia. Obesity, however, may also be the consequence of other conditions, most notably endocrine disease. In addition, advancing age tends to reduce metabolic rate and physical activity, which can increase the risk of the development of sarcopaenic obesity whether other medical conditions are present or not.

40.2   General and Pharmacokinetic Complications of Obesity

- Clinical examination may be hindered; the chest more difficult to auscultate (and apex beat may be more difficult to palpate), and the abdomen may be more difficult to palpate.
- Increased subcutaneous fat may result in poor drug delivery after intended intramuscular administration.
- The low perfusion of adipose tissue may delay absorption of subcutaneously administered drugs.
- Veins and arteries may be more difficult to identify when large amounts of subcutaneous fat are present. Pulses may be more difficult to palpate.
- Anatomical landmarks may be obscured, thus rendering local/regional anaesthetic/analgesic techniques more challenging. If epidural anaesthesia is to be performed, then doses should be reduced by about ¼ because of the smaller epidural 'space' due to fatty tissue deposition and often engorged epidural blood vessels (because of increased intra-abdominal pressure).
- Endotracheal intubation may be complicated by the presence of excessive fatty tissues in the oropharyngeal region and tongue.
- Surgical access is often more difficult, thus prolonging anaesthetic time, which increases risk and potentially lengthens recovery time.
- Increased body fat is accompanied by a reduction in total body water (on a ml/kg basis). The volume of distribution of water-soluble drugs is therefore reduced. For water-soluble drugs, e.g. the peripherally-acting non-depolarising neuromuscular blocking agents, initial loading doses should therefore be calculated according to the patient's ideal body weight. Subsequent doses must be tailored to the patient's requirements.
- For lipid-soluble drugs, e.g. sedative and anaesthetic agents, not only is the volume of distribution increased, but their clearance is potentially delayed because they enter a larger mass of adipose tissue whose perfusion is relatively slow. For some of the anaesthetic adjuncts,

Veterinary Anaesthesia: Principles to Practice, Second Edition. Alexandra H. A. Dugdale, Georgina Beaumont, Carl Bradbrook, and Matthew Gurney.
© 2020 John Wiley & Sons Ltd. Published 2020 by John Wiley & Sons Ltd.
Companion website: www.wiley.com/go/dugdale/veterinary-anaesthesia

such as opioids, and especially if administered intra-muscularly, it may be preferable to dose according to the patient's actual (total) bodyweight, so that, after redistribution into fat, an effective plasma/effect site concentration is achieved and maintained. If administered intravenously, however, a more profound effect (and side effects) may be observed initially with doses based on actual weight. For rapid-acting injectable anaesthetic induction agents, intravenously-administered induction doses scaled according to lean/ideal body mass may be preferable because it is the rapid increase in brain concentration that produces the initial effect, the size of the fat sink only acting later to delay elimination. Anaesthetic induction doses based on actual body weight risk overdosing (although in most circumstances, such drugs are titrated, slowly, to effect). Lean tissue mass tends to increase slightly as adipose tissue mass increases and some people prefer to dose according to an adjusted body weight to account for this (see below). Maintenance doses/infusions of injectable anaesthetics, however, may scale more according to total body weight. During prolonged administration of inhalation agents, which may easily occur in obese patients when surgery is often relatively complicated, the blood-solubility of the agents becomes less important than their fat-solubility for influencing recovery from anaesthesia. Halothane is most fat-soluble; sevoflurane is slightly more fat-soluble than isoflurane; and desflurane (and nitrous oxide) are least fat-soluble. The potential for prolonged recoveries is therefore greatest with halothane, but is also a possible nuisance with sevoflurane and even isoflurane.

- Increased circulating free fatty acids, triglycerides, and cholesterol may compete with acidic anaesthetic agents for protein-binding with albumin, thus increasing 'free/active' drug concentrations. In contrast, the increased α1-acid glycoprotein concentration found in obese states can increase the binding of basic drugs (ketamine, opioids, local anaesthetics), thus reducing their 'free/active' concentrations.

- Obesity is considered to confer an inflammatory state upon the patient. Despite this, patients are generally considered to be at increased risk of wound infection/breakdown, although this may be partly a consequence of increased surgical time.

- Fatty infiltration of the liver *may* accompany obesity, but is also associated with endocrine disorders. Hepatomegaly can increase the diaphragmatic splinting and hypoventilation that accompany obesity. Hepatic function is not normally reduced in uncomplicated obesity, but where other diseases are present and hepatic function is impaired, drug elimination may be delayed.

- Renal function is not normally impaired in uncomplicated obesity and renal clearance may even be increased because of slightly increased renal blood flow (secondary to increased cardiac output), and glomerular filtration rate.

- An increased risk of gastro-oesophageal reflux/regurgitation may accompany the increased intra-abdominal pressure with increased intra-abdominal fat. Aspiration risk is therefore potentially increased.

- Cerebral blood flow is usually unaltered because of cerebrovascular autoregulation, unless profound cardiovascular impairment is present.

- Increased fat mass may provide thermal insulation and predispose patients to heat-stress.

40.2.1 Respiratory Complications Due to Obesity

- Increased fat mass within the oropharyngeal soft tissues (and tongue) may increase the risk of airway obstruction and may complicate endotracheal intubation.

- Increased fat mass both outside and within the chest cavity can reduce lung and chest wall compliance, total lung capacity and functional residual capacity (FRC) (whilst leaving residual volume within normal limits), increase airway resistance, and increase the work of breathing. Internal fat within the thoracic and abdominal cavities can also 'splint' the diaphragm, exacerbating these effects. FRC reduction results in reduced oxygen reserves so that patients are less tolerant of periods of apnoea, but it also means that the depth of inhalation anaesthesia can change more quickly. Pre-oxygenation should increase the oxygen reserve and protect against desaturation during short periods of apnoea after anaesthetic induction, but often increases resorption atelectasis (especially if performed with F_IO_2 greater than around 60%). FRC may also decrease below the closing capacity (the lung volume at which small airways begin to collapse) so that atelectasis may occur even during resting tidal breathing (so some degree of hypoxaemia is common), and is therefore even more likely under sedation and anaesthesia (i.e. with respiratory depression). Blood gas disturbances are therefore common and may persist into the recovery period too.

- Oxygen consumption and carbon dioxide production are increased in obese patients because of the increased amount of tissues that require metabolic support, although normocapnia is usually maintained in the awake animal by increased minute ventilation. The ventilatory reserve is, however, reduced. Most patients, whilst awake, are said to retain their normal response to hypercapnia and hypoxaemia. In morbidly obese people, however, the Pickwickian syndrome has been described, whereby the chemoreceptors become progressively desensitised to hypercapnia such that hypoxaemia becomes the most important driver of ventilation. Relative leptin insensitivity (common in obese individuals) can worsen the reduced ventilatory response to high CO_2. The provision of high inspired oxygen concentrations can then promote hypoventilation and worsening hypercapnia because of removal of the hypoxaemic ventilatory drive.

40.2.2 Cardiovascular Complications Due to Obesity

- Blood volume is increased in absolute terms, but on a ml/kg basis, is reduced.
- Venous and arterial access may be hindered.
- Increased risk of thromboembolic disease.
- The increased fat mass demands perfusion, albeit slow, which necessitates an increase in blood volume and cardiac output that tend to reduce cardiovascular reserves.
- Myocardial oxygen requirements are increased *(an increased body mass warrants overall increased metabolic demands)*, potentially in the face of hypoxaemia. Eventually obesity-induced cardiomyopathy may result.
- Polycythaemia may accompany chronic hypoxaemia, and the increased blood viscosity increases myocardial work and may predispose to cardiac dysrhythmias and promote the development of thromboemboli. Fluid loading, in an attempt to reduce the blood viscosity, may be poorly tolerated and precipitate acute congestive cardiac failure.

40.3 Approach to the Obese Patient

- Although pre-operative weight reduction may help to reduce some of the risks and complications associated with anaesthesia and surgery, this is not possible for emergency cases, and should be done under expert direction. A crash diet over the few days before anaesthesia is not recommended.
- Many obese patients will have a degree of insulin resistance that may be exacerbated by pre-operative food withholding. At present, however, the optimum duration of pre-operative food withholding and indeed the optimal nutritional composition of any pre-anaesthetic meal are unknown (See Chapter 2). Water should, however, be freely available until the time of premedication.

- A thorough history and pre-operative evaluation of the patient are important and may direct further workup and/or treatment, time permitting.
- Intramuscular and subcutaneous drug delivery for premedication may be followed by poor absorption. Longer needles can be used to try to ensure intramuscular drug delivery. Alternatively, intravenous administration may be preferred. Premedication should aim to provide 'light' sedation (to minimise further respiratory depression), because of the increased risk of respiratory embarrassment. If possible, after premedication, the patient should be closely observed for signs of respiratory compromise. Premedication drugs, especially opioid analgesics, may be dosed according to actual body mass for IM administration, or consider dosing according to lean body mass for IV administration.
- Pre-oxygenation is usually advised and requires a fairly close-fitting face mask and oxygen delivery (200–500 ml/kg/min) for up to five minutes. If premedication was 'light', the patient may not tolerate pre-oxygenation by mask without becoming stressed; flow-by oxygen delivery is an alternative strategy, but is usually less effective.
- Induction of anaesthesia may be by intravenous or inhalation agents, although it may be preferable to ensure rapid control of the airway (orotracheal intubation), because of the possible increased risk of gastro-oesophageal reflux/regurgitation. Intravenous access may be difficult, but venous cannulation is desirable before anaesthetic induction; ultrasound guidance or cut-down is sometimes required.
- It is usually suggested to titrate injectable anaesthetic agents slowly to effect, but if a rapid anaesthetic induction is required, some idea of the dose needed would be helpful. There is debate about which derivative of the patient's body mass should be used for such a calculation: whether the lean body mass, the ideal body mass, (or the normalised versions of these, i.e. using correction factors for patient 'frame size'), or the adjusted body mass (see below). Furthermore, calculation of lean body mass and ideal body mass require certain assumptions and are not without their own problems. It is therefore likely that no single dosing scalar will be suitable for calculating loading doses of the various anaesthetic and adjunctive agents for all veterinary species. Until more information becomes available, or patient-side assessment of total fat mass, lean mass, and ideal body mass becomes easily possible, induction agent dosing according to an estimated lean, ideal, or adjusted body mass would be appropriate. The adjusted body mass, which lies somewhere between the actual body mass and what the veterinarian considers ideal, caters for the increase in lean tissue mass that occurs as adipose tissue mass

increases; e.g. the formula given below has been suggested for use in morbidly obese people. (Note that although a correction factor of 1/3 has been shown here, the value lies between 0.2 and 0.4 in people.) **Royal Canin™ has published a table for estimating Ideal Body Mass, assuming that for each body condition score value above 5 (5/9 being 'ideal'), the animal is overweight by an extra 10%. Therefore, if BCS is 7/9, then being 20% overweight, the ideal body mass is the actual mass divided by 1.2.**

$$\text{Adjusted Body Weight} = \text{Ideal Body Weight} + 1/3$$
$$\left(\text{Actual Body Weight} - \text{Ideal Body Weight}\right)$$

- It is important to have a variety of endotracheal tube sizes available, a bougie and a laryngoscope. Cuffed endotracheal tubes are normally preferred to provide adequate airway protection and to enable provision of artificial (positive pressure) ventilation.
- Anaesthetic breathing systems should be chosen according to the animal's lean body mass.
- During maintenance of anaesthesia, it may be preferable to provide positive pressure ventilation with or without positive end-expiratory pressure (PEEP), or, alternatively, continuous positive airway pressure (CPAP) if the patient is breathing spontaneously, although the cardiovascular impact (mechanical and chemical) of these strategies should not be forgotten. Tidal volumes for artificial ventilation should be based on lean body weight to avoid over-inflation of the lungs and possible damage (although peak inspiratory pressure may need to be relatively high because of reduced thoracic/lung compliance). For anaesthetic maintenance, inhalation agents, particularly isoflurane, tend to be favoured over injectable agents as the latter have uncertain pharmacokinetics in obese patients. Nitrous oxide may be able to be used as an adjunct, but if patient oxygenation is of concern, then the requirement for high inspired oxygen concentrations limits the usefulness of nitrous oxide. If the animal is to be positioned in dorsal recumbency, the increased mass of fat within the abdomen may increase pressure on the great vessels (resulting in aorto-caval compression) and potentially reduce venous return and cardiac output. Changes in body position should therefore be done slowly, and the patient may benefit from a slightly head-up tilt.
- Balanced (multimodal) analgesia should be provided where possible, however there may be contra-indications to the use of NSAIDs if concomitant hepatic, renal, gastro-intestinal, or some types of endocrine disease is present. (Patients may already be receiving NSAIDs as orthopaedic disease is a frequent complication of obesity. These drugs also compete for protein-binding.) Local/regional anaesthetic techniques may be more challenging because of obscured landmarks, however, the use of nerve-locators and/or ultrasound may help to overcome some of these problems. Epidural doses should be reduced by around ¼ (see above).
- In view of the cardiovascular complications, it seems that intra-operative dysrhythmias may be more likely in obese patients and perhaps precipitated by anaesthetic agents (which promote cardiorespiratory depression). Intra-operative monitoring should include heart (pulse) rate, ECG, breathing rate, SpO_2, temperature, blood glucose, end tidal CO_2 tension, and arterial blood pressure where possible. Blood gas and electrolyte monitoring may also be warranted. Direct arterial blood pressure may be difficult to monitor as access to superficial arteries may be complicated by overlying fat. Indirect arterial blood pressure monitoring may also be problematic because of excessive fat surrounding the various appendages that would be used, especially for oscillometric devices reliant on pressure-sensing cuffs. Doppler blood flow probes may be easier to use alongside a manually-operated sphygmomanometer.
- Intra-operative fluid therapy will depend upon the presentation of each case and should be tailored to individual patient requirements. Electrolyte disturbances may also require addressing. (See Chapters 23 and 24.) Basing calculations on ideal body weight would seem a sensible approach.
- Neuromuscular blocking agents may be used and are usually dosed according to ideal body weight rather than actual body weight. (If the depolarising agent succinylcholine [suxamethonium] chloride is used, because plasma cholinesterase concentration tends to increase with obesity, its effect may be shortened.) Artificial ventilation must be available if neuromuscular blocking agents are to be administered. Monitoring of the degree of neuromuscular blockade is highly advised, and adequate reversal of the block must be ensured before anaesthetic administration is discontinued. See chapter 17.
- Patient monitoring should be continued well into the post-operative recovery period and even for some time after tracheal extubation to ensure that the patient is ventilating adequately and maintaining good oxygenation. Antagonists may be administered for sedative agents if necessary, but beware injections inadvertently administered into subcutaneous fat.
- Alimentation should be resumed as soon as possible. (Sudden starvation may precipitate hepatic lipidosis, particularly in obese cats and equidae.)

Further Reading

Boveri, S., Brearley, J.C., and Dugdale, A.H.A. (2013). The effect of body condition on propofol induction requirement in dogs. *Veterinary Anaesthesia and Analgesia* 40: 449–454.

Clutton, R.E. (1988). The medical implications of canine obesity and their relevance to anaesthesia. *British Veterinary Journal* 144: 21–28.

Eleveld, D.J., Proost, J.H., Absalom, A.R., and Struys, M.M.R.F. (2011). Obesity and allometric scaling of pharmacokinetics. *Clinical Pharmacokinetics* 50: 751–753.

German, A.J. (2006). The growing problem of obesity in dogs and cats. *The Journal of Nutrition* 136: 1940S–1946S.

Green, B. and McLeay, S.C. (2011). Anesthetizing the obese. *Anesthesia and Analgesia* 113: 1–3.

Ingrande, J. and Lemmens, H.J.M. (2010). Dose adjustments of anaesthetics in the morbidly obese. *British Journal of Anaesthesia* 105 (S1): i16–i23.

Kopelman, P.G. (2000). Obesity as a medical problem. *Nature* 404: 635–643.

Lotia, S. and Bellamy, M.C. (2008). Anaesthesia and morbid obesity. *Continuing Education in Anaesthesia, Critical Care and Pain* 8: 151–156.

Love, L. and Cline, M.G. (2015). Perioperative physiology and pharmacology in the obese small animal patient. *Veterinary Anaesthesia and Analgesia* 42: 119–132.

Mosing, M., German, A.J., Holden, S.J. et al. (2013). Oxygenation and ventilation characteristics in obese sedated dogs before and after weight loss. *The Veterinary Journal* 198: 367–371.

National Institutes of Health (1985). Health implications of obesity. National Institutes of Health Consensus Development Conference Statement. *Annals of Internal Medicine* 103: 1073–1077.

Nightingale, C.E., Margarson, M.P., Shearer, E. et al. (2015). Peri-operative management of the obese surgical patient 2015 Guidelines (AAGBI and Society for Obesity and Bariatric Anaesthesia). *Anaesthesia* 70: 859–876.

Pelosi, P. and Gregoretti, C. (2010). Perioperative management of obese patients. *Best Practice & Research Clinical Anaesthesiology* 24: 211–225.

Trayhurn, P. and Wood, S. (2004). Adipokines: inflammation and the pleiotropic role of white adipose tissue. *British Journal of Nutrition* 92: 347–355.

Self-test Section

1 True or False? If premedication is to be delivered IM, doses should be based on actual body mass.

2 Estimate the ideal body weight for a 40 kg Labrador with Body Condition Score 9/9.

41

Dental and Oral Considerations

LEARNING OBJECTIVES

- To understand how to apply analgesic techniques in dental and oral surgery cases.
- To be familiar with potential complications and how to manage them.

41.1 Analgesia

Dental pain is under-recognised and a preventative approach to such cases should be practised. Consider the use of non-steroidal anti-inflammatory drugs (NSAIDs) prior to the procedure wherever there is evidence of periodontitis, gingivo-stomatitis, or osteomyelitis. Oral pain associated with neoplasia can be significant and should be proactively managed multimodally with opioids, local anaesthetics, NSAIDs, and adjuncts (see Chapter 3).

41.2 Nerve Blocks

For dental and oral surgery, the two nerves that require blocking are the maxillary nerve for the upper dental arcade and the inferior alveolar nerve (branch of the mandibular nerve) for the lower arcade. These nerves can be blocked at different sites. The reader is referred to Chapters 12 and 13 for specific local anaesthetic techniques. Points relevant to dental and oral surgery will be highlighted here.

Direct nerve trauma is a concern when performing any nerve block, although specifically with dental blocks, there is an increased risk of nerve trauma if needles are inserted into foramina. This is not recommended. Provided this practice is avoided, there is no greater risk with local anaesthetic techniques for dental procedures than with any other nerve block. In human dentistry, the most common nerve trauma is to the lingual nerve (66% of reports), occurring during anaesthesia of the inferior alveolar nerve. Nerve damage is possible by mechanical (direct needle-trauma), ischaemic (e.g. intraneural deposition of local anaesthetic [especially if vasoconstrictors are included], or haematoma formation), and chemical (neurotoxicity from the anaesthetic agent itself or preservatives) mechanisms. Reported rates of occurrence for lingual nerve damage vary from 1 : 26,000–1 : 160,000 and so are highly unlikely.

41.2.1 Evidence for the Use of Nerve Blocks

Evidence clearly demonstrates a reduction in post-operative pain scores and more stable intra-operative physiological variables in cats receiving nerve blocks (maxillary and inferior alveolar) prior to dental treatment. In dogs, an infraorbital nerve block with mepivacaine was documented to reduce the MAC of isoflurane by 23%. Nerve blocks are recommended whenever a dental extraction or oral surgery is to be performed.

41.2.2 Mixtures of Local Anaesthetics

The above-mentioned study evaluating nerve blocks in cats undergoing dental procedures used a combination of lidocaine 0.25 mg/kg and bupivacaine 0.25 mg/kg, and documented a positive benefit of this combination. (See Chapter 12.)

41.2.3 Onset and Duration of Action

In dental studies from the human literature using bupivacaine for inferior alveolar nerve blocks, onset times ranging from 6 to 12 minutes were documented. Occasionally,

---

Veterinary Anaesthesia: Principles to Practice, Second Edition. Alexandra H. A. Dugdale, Georgina Beaumont, Carl Bradbrook, and Matthew Gurney.
© 2020 John Wiley & Sons Ltd. Published 2020 by John Wiley & Sons Ltd.
Companion website: www.wiley.com/go/dugdale-veterinary-anaesthesia

attempts to block the inferior alveolar nerve will also successfully block the lingual nerve that provides sensory innervation to the rostral two thirds of the tongue, and this may result in self-trauma in the recovery period. Bilateral inferior alveolar nerve blocks should only be undertaken with caution and use of shorter-acting local anaesthetic agents (lidocaine) is advised.

41.3 Supra-periosteal Local Anaesthesia

Opinion varies regarding the efficacy of this technique in dogs and cats, although it is widely practised in humans. The needle is inserted into the muco-buccal fold 'above' or 'below' the roots of the target tooth and is advanced until bone is touched, after which local anaesthetic is injected and diffuses through the adjacent cancellous bone to produce anaesthesia of the pulpal nerve. This is a commonly used technique in human paediatric patients for maxillary teeth because the maxilla is more porous in young patients and is more porous than the mandible. Its efficacy in veterinary species remains to be investigated. Alternatives to this are the maxillary (and inferior alveolar) blocks. Intrapulpal injection is not recommended.

41.4 Other Supplementary Techniques

These are commonly used in people and are sometimes applied to animals:

- **Periodontal ligament (intraligamentary) injection**: using a Waites' dental syringe, local anaesthetic can be deposited into the periodontal ligament (via the gingival sulcus [or through the adjacent gingiva, aiming at the crest of the alveolar bone]) at several sites around the tooth to effect anaesthesia of the pulpal nerve (diffusion of local anaesthetic is thought to be more via adjacent cancellous bone that through the periodontal ligament to the root apex). These injections can, however, be technically challenging to achieve because they require very high pressure and are uncomfortable for the awake patient. Gingivitis may also preclude injection through inflamed/infected tissues. Deposition of local anaesthetic deep into the gingival sulcus may, however, produce some effect.
- **Intrapapillary infiltration anaesthesia**: using very short needles, injections of small volumes of local anaesthetic are made into the fleshy interdental gingival papillae, aiming a few mm below the papillary tips. Local

anaesthetics containing epinephrine will cause almost instantaneous blanching of the gum, which can help with haemostasis during periodontal surgery.
- **Intraseptal injection** is a hybrid between the intrapapillary and intraligamentary techniques: needle insertion is as for intrapapillary injection, but the needle is inserted until bone is touched and advanced just into the bone if possible.

41.5 Airway Access and Protection

Ensuring the airway (endotracheal tube, ET) is, and remains, correctly positioned and patent (beware kinks), and the breathing system remains connected (and is re-connected after temporary disconnection when changing patient position), are of paramount importance. Close attention should be paid to careful inflation and monitoring of the ET tube cuff (especially in cats). Always ensure the patient is disconnected from the breathing system prior to turning to avoid tracheal damage (tracheal tears can easily occur, especially in cats, usually involving the dorsal tracheal ligament).

A pharyngeal pack can be used to ensure fluid/debris does not accumulate around the ET tube cuff. (The pack must be removed prior to recovery.) Suction of the trachea proximal to the ET tube cuff is advised prior to tracheal extubation if lots of debris or lavage fluid is suspected.

Tracheal intubation may be challenging with oral neoplasia; a range of ET tube sizes, a reliable laryngoscope/light source, and careful positioning can be helpful. The use of a bougie or intubating stylette can also assist tracheal intubation. Pre-oxygenation is also recommended. Capnography is useful for confirming tracheal intubation and endoscopy may be necessary in some cases.

For facial and jaw fractures, orotracheal intubation may not be possible. In these circumstances, tracheal intubation by pharyngotomy (Figure 41.1) or transmylohyoid incision may be indicated, and ideally performed with an armoured (reinforced) ET tube to prevent kinking. Alternatively, if examination of occlusal alignment is required following jaw repair, rather than tracheal extubation, a short orotracheal tube can be used from which the adaptor can be temporarily removed during assessment, then replaced.

41.6 Haemorrhage

With oral tumour surgery, haemorrhage is a significant risk. Total blood volume should be calculated, and the volume of blood lost, evaluated. A plan should be made for

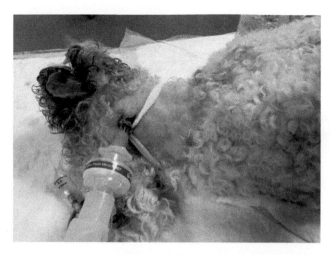

Figure 41.1 Armoured tube placed via pharyngotomy incision.

replacement of lost blood (see Chapter 23). For dental work in Greyhounds, the prophylactic use of tranexamic acid should be considered for its anti-fibrinolytic effect.

41.7 Hypothermia

With prolonged procedures and the use of copious lavage solutions, care must be paid that the patient does not become hypothermic. (Also, ensure protection of the airway during/after oral lavages.)

41.8 Mouth Gags and Post-anaesthetic Blindness

Spring-loaded gags have been shown to cause cortical blindness in cats due to occlusion of the maxillary artery (cats have poor collateral supply to the circle of Willis), and

should not be used. Prolonged opening of the jaw should be avoided in both dogs and cats.

41.9 Air Drills

Water-cooling should be ensured to guard against thermal injury and may also help to submerge the drilling site to reduce entrainment of air and the risk of venous air embolism. (Ensure protection of the airway.)

41.10 Nutrition

Hyporexia is a concern in patients with oral or dental disease, and consideration should be given to the use of feeding tubes. Attention to analgesia is also important.

41.11 Post-anaesthetic Deafness

Cases of deafness following dental and ear cleaning procedures have been reported in dogs and cats. No specific aetiology was identified, although older patients appeared more susceptible.

41.12 Pain Scoring

Although dental disease is recognised as a contributor to chronic pain states, no specific pain scoring systems are developed for dental or oral pain. Nevertheless, consideration should be given to general behavioural changes associated with pain as currently validated pain scoring systems have been used successfully in the acute setting to document improvements in pain with nerve blocks in cats.

Further Reading

Aguiar, J., Chebroux, A., Martinez-Taboada, F., and Leece, E.A. (2015). Analgesic effects of maxillary and inferior alveolar nerve blocks in cats undergoing dental extractions. *Journal of Feline Medicine and Surgery* 17: 110–116.

Barton-Lamb, A.L., Martin-Flores, M., Scrivani, P.V. et al. (2013). Evaluation of maxillary arterial blood flow in anesthetized cats with the mouth closed and open. *The Veterinary Journal* 196: 325–331.

Bell, A., Helm, J., and Reid, J. (2014). Veterinarians' attitudes to chronic pain in dogs. *Veterinary Record* 175: 428.

De Miguel Garcia, C., Whiting, M., and Alibhai, H. (2012). Cerebral hypoxia in a cat following pharyngoscopy

involving use of a mouth gag. *Veterinary Anaesthesia and Analgesia* 40: 106–108.

Diez Bernal, S. and Iff, I. (2019). Airway management by transmylohyoid endotracheal intubation in two cats with mandibular trauma. *Veterinary Anaesthesia and Analgesia* 46: 405–406.

Gunew, M., Marshall, R., Lui, M., and Astley, C. (2008). Fatal venous air embolus in a cat undergoing dental extractions. *Journal of Small Animal Practice* 49: 601–604.

Hartsfield, S.M., Gendreau, C.L., Smith, C.W. et al. (1977). Endotracheal intubation by pharyngotomy. *Journal of the American Animal Hospital Association* 13: 71–74.

Jurk, I.R., Thibodeau, M.S., Whitney, K. et al. (2001). Acute vision loss after general anaesthesia in a cat. *Veterinary Ophthalmology* 4: 155–158.

Martin-Flores, M., Scrivani, P.V., Loew, E. et al. (2014). Maximal and submaximal mouth-opening with mouth gags in cats: implications for maxillary artery blood flow. *The Veterinary Journal* 200: 60–64.

Milella, L. and Gurney, M.A. (2016). Dental and oral surgery. In: *BSAVA Manual of Canine and Feline Anaesthesia and Analgesia*, 3e (eds. T. Duke–Novakovski, M. de Vries and C. Seymour), 272–282. Gloucester, UK: BSAVA Publications.

Reiter, R.M. (2014). Open wide: blindness in cats after the use of mouth gags. *The Veterinary Journal* 201: 5–6.

Snyder, C.J. and Snyder, L.B.C. (2013). Effect of mepivacaine in an infraorbital nerve block on minimum alveolar concentration of isoflurane in clinically normal anesthetized dogs undergoing a modified form of dental dolorimetry. *Journal of the American Veterinary Medical Association* 242: 199–204.

Stevens-Sparks, C.K. and Strain, G.M. (2010). Post-anaesthesia deafness in dogs and cats following dental and ear cleaning procedures. *Veterinary Anaesthesia and Analgesia* 37: 347–351.

Stiles, J., Weil, A.B., Packer, R.A., and Lantz, G.C. (2012). Post-anesthetic cortical blindness in cats: twenty cases. *Veterinary Journal* 193: 367–373.

Self-test Section

1   Which nerve block would be used prior to removing a canine tooth on the upper arcade (104)?

   A Maxillary

   B Inferior alveolar

   C Mental

   D Infraorbital

2   List your considerations for anaesthesia for dental extractions in a cat.

42

Ocular Surgery Considerations

42.1 Introduction

Normal intra-ocular pressure (IOP) is about 15–20 mmHg and is determined by a balance between aqueous humour production and absorption, and other factors such as pupil size, corneoscleral rigidity, extra-ocular muscle tone, vascularity of the globe (itself affected by blood pressure, especially central venous pressure [CVP], and blood gas tensions), and any retrobulbar or intracranial space-occupying lesions.

Aqueous humour is produced by the ciliary processes of the ciliary body from where it flows into the anterior chamber of the eye and is absorbed into the venous system mostly via the canal of Schlemm (through the trabecular meshwork of the pectinate ligament at the 'drainage angle' of the eye). There is some absorption of aqueous humour through uveoscleral pathways, which is the most important route of drainage in horses.

42.2 Changes in IOP

42.2.1 Increase in IOP

Increased IOP is brought about by:

- Increased CVP (causes increased episcleral/choroidal venous pressure).
- Increased jugular venous pressure, e.g. jugular vein occlusion or head-down position (sedated horses); impedes venous return from head (also increases episcleral/choroidal venous pressure).
- Increased arterial blood pressure (>80 mmHg) has minimal effect.
- Increased P_aCO_2 (and decreased blood pH) (cause vasodilation and increase choroidal blood volume).
- Decreased P_aO_2 (through vasodilation).
- Increased aqueous humour production.
- Decreased aqueous humour drainage, e.g. mydriasis (especially if closed angle glaucoma tendencies).
- Increased extra-ocular muscle tone, e.g. succinylcholine (transient), ketamine in some species (man and horse).
- Increased intra-cranial pressure (ICP).
- Increased retrobulbar pressure.

42.2.2 Decrease in IOP

Decreased IOP is brought about by:

- Decreased CVP.
- Relief of any jugular vein occlusion.
- Mean arterial pressure < 80 mmHg.
- Decreased P_aCO_2 (and increased blood pH) (cause vasoconstriction and decrease choroidal blood volume).
- Increased P_aO_2.
- Increased aqueous humour drainage, e.g. miosis, osmotic diuretics.
- Decreased aqueous humour production, e.g. carbonic anhydrase inhibitors, β blockers, α2 agonists.
- Decreased extra-ocular muscle tone (allows increased aqueous drainage), e.g. most sedatives and general anaesthetics (not ketamine) and non-depolarising muscle relaxants.

Veterinary Anaesthesia: Principles to Practice, Second Edition. Alexandra H. A. Dugdale, Georgina Beaumont, Carl Bradbrook, and Matthew Gurney.
© 2020 John Wiley & Sons Ltd. Published 2020 by John Wiley & Sons Ltd.
Companion website: www.wiley.com/go/dugdale/veterinary-anaesthesia

42.3 Factors Altering CVP (and Jugular Venous Pressure)

Factors that can increase these pressures:

- Coughing
- Gagging/retching (tracheal intubation/extubation)
- Vomiting
- Straining
- Positive pressure ventilation/positive end-expiratory pressure (PEEP)
- Pneumothorax
- Pericardial tamponade
- Congestive heart failure
- Pulmonary thromboemboli
- Compression of the neck (jugular occlusion: blood sampling, poor positioning, e.g. extreme neck ventroflexion)

Factors that can decrease these pressures:

- Head up position
- Hypovolaemia/hypotension (systemic β blockers)

42.4 Changes in Pupil Size

42.4.1 Mydriasis

This is dilation of the pupil and is caused by:

- Sympathomimetics: phenylephrine, adrenaline, α2 agonists.
- Parasympatholytics/anticholinergics: atropine, hyoscine, glycopyrrolate, tropicamide, ipratropium, propantheline.
- Opioids in horses and cats.
- Ketamine.

42.4.2 Miosis

This is constriction of the pupil and is caused by:

- Sympatholytics: β blockers: timoptol, timolol.
- Parasympathomimetics/cholinergics, e.g. pilocarpine, bethanecol; or anticholinesterases, e.g. demecarium bromide, ecothiophate.
- Most general anaesthetic agents (stage III anaesthesia), but ketamine and some opioids (in cats and horses) can cause mydriasis.

42.5 Oculocardiac Reflex (Trigemino-vagal Reflex, Aschner's Reflex)

- Afferent limb: long and short ciliary nerves of ophthalmic branch of trigeminal nerve (V)
- Efferent limb: vagus nerve (X)
- Caused by: traction or pressure on eyeball
- Results in: bradycardia, asystole, A-V block, other dysrhythmias
- More a problem in animals with high resting vagal tone:
  - Very young
  - Very old
  - Horses
  - Respiratory diseases and disorders (e.g. brachycephalics)
  - Opioids and α2 agonists

The reflex usually fatigues quickly upon cessation of stimulus. May require emergency treatment with anticholinergics (atropine works fastest), or you may wish to administer anticholinergics prophylactically (glycopyrrolate and atropine similarly effective).

Retrobulbar block should abolish the reflex (although the actual injecting of local anaesthetic may cause it), whereas neuromuscular blockers may only reduce its occurrence by reducing the need to pull and push so vigorously on the globe.

42.6 Anaesthetic Agents and IOP

- **Opioids** can increase IOP (they depress the ventilatory response to CO_2; increased P_aCO2 leads to increased IOP), although the vagomimetic and miotic effects of opioids (in dogs) pretty much offset this. Opioid-induced vomiting can lead to transiently increased IOP, although cough-suppression is a useful side effect.
- **α2 agonists** decrease IOP (by reducing ADH [which helps reduce aqueous production] and increasing aqueous outflow) despite causing mydriasis. Beware low-head carriage in sedated horses though.
- **Benzodiazepines** decrease IOP.
- **Acepromazine** has minimal effects on IOP.
- **Volatile (halogenated) anaesthetic agents** cause a dose-dependent decrease of IOP (by decreasing extra-ocular muscle tone, improving aqueous drainage, and causing miosis at surgical planes of anaesthesia).
- **N_2O** causes little effect unless the eye has been 'open' and contains bubbles of air, as these will expand with N_2O to increase IOP.
- **Etomidate, propofol, alfaxalone, thiopental** all reduce IOP (similar to volatile agent anaesthesia).
- **Ketamine** can increase IOP (due to increased extra-ocular muscle tone and increased arterial blood pressure), but this is equivocal and possibly species-dependent. Its effects can be reduced by prior administration of benzodiazepines, guaiphenesin, or α2 agonists (beware low head carriage in horses).

- **Non-depolarising neuromuscular blockers** decrease IOP (due to decreased extra-ocular muscle tone).

42.7 Positive Pressure Ventilation and IOP

- The positive intrathoracic pressure may dam-back venous return and increase CVP leading to increased IOP
- Hyperventilation can reduce P_aCO_2, which decreases IOP

42.8 Requirements for Eye Surgery

- Central eye and akinetic/'still' eye, i.e. no nystagmus or blinking, good muscle relaxation
- A 'soft' eye, if globe penetration is required or perforation already exists
- Good provision of analgesia, e.g. use of local anaesthetic techniques (see Chapter 13)
- Quiet, gentle recovery to reduce trauma to eye (analgesia also important)

42.8.1 Consider

- Age
- Temperament
- Other diseases (cataract surgeries are common for diabetics)
- Elective versus emergency procedure

42.8.2 Drugs Affecting Pupil Size

Drugs affecting pupil size (e.g. topical atropine pre-operatively to ensure mydriasis) will preclude use of pupillary size for monitoring. For dog cataract surgery, topical atropine drops must be applied before premedication is given because once other drugs (especially opioids) have had their effects on pupil size, they can be hard to reverse. Pupil dilation is often insufficient during surgery, and therefore intra-ocular (intra-cameral) epinephrine (adrenaline) is used (also offers some haemostasis). Intra-ocular epinephrine may, however, cause transient cardiac arrhythmias, e.g. tachyarrythmias.

42.8.3 Anaesthetic Options

42.8.3.1 Premedication
Effective premedication leads to decreased struggling on induction, which prevents increased IOP. Antitussive effects of opioids are useful, but emetic effects are not, although the replacement of morphine with methadone in small animals has largely eliminated this concern.

42.8.3.2 Induction
Should be as **stress free** as possible. Gentle restraint important. IV induction of anaesthesia recommended.

42.8.3.3 Tracheal Intubation
Aim for **tracheal intubation** with **no gagging**: fairly deep anaesthesia or IV or topical (laryngeal) local anaesthetic (but spray application to the larynx may provoke coughing). Lidocaine IV (dog: 2 mg/kg, but not 1 mg/kg) prior to induction/tracheal intubation has been shown to reduce coughing with laryngoscopy and subsequent tracheal intubation.

42.8.3.4 Maintenance
Position the patient so as to **avoid jugular vein compression**. Some people even use a 10° head-up tilt. Consider if a local anaesthetic technique is appropriate. Newer techniques such as a sub-Tenon block (see Chapter 13) may be considered for corneal and intra-ocular surgery, particularly if muscle paralysis cannot be facilitated. Paralysis of the extra-ocular muscles may be required (see Chapter 17). Vigilant **monitoring** is important. Intravenous **fluid therapy** should be provided, as required (Chapter 23). **Analgesia** is important; consider a **multimodal approach** (Chapter 3).

42.8.3.5 Recovery
Ensure adequate reversal of neuromuscular block: respiratory depression leads to increased IOP (due to hypercapnia and hypoxaemia). Recovery should be **smooth**: patient comfort (e.g. empty bladder) and analgesia must be adequate. Tracheal extubation should be gentle (with minimal gagging), and therefore early, unless contraindicated; useful antitussive effects of opioids. If emergence delirium occurs, ensure adequate analgesia and empty bladder, then try tender loving care (TLC), and, if necessary, also consider sedation (benzodiazepines, acepromazine, or very low doses of α2 agonists). Reduce self-trauma to eyes: good analgesia, bandage paws, soft collars (preferred to hard Elizabethan collars).

42.8.3.6 Note
Birds and **reptiles** have striated iris muscles, so topical neuromuscular blockers produce mydriasis for surgery.

Further Reading

Carslake, H.B. (2019). Should I place a subpalpebral lavage system in the upper or lower eyelid? *Equine Veterinary Education* 31: 335–336.

Collins, B.K., Gross, M.E., Moore, C.P., and Branson, K.R. (1995). Physiologic, pharmacologic and practical considerations for anesthesia of domestic animals with eye disease. *Journal of the American Veterinary Medical Association* 207: 220–230.

Gross, M.E. and Pablo, L.S. (2015). Ophthalmic patients. In: *Veterinary Anesthesia and Analgesia, the Fifth Edition of Lumb and Jones* (eds. K.A. Grimm, L.A. Lamont, W.J. Tranquilli, et al.), 963–982. Iowa, USA: Wiley Blackwell.

Henriksen, M.d. and Brooks, D.E. (2014). Standing ophthalmic surgeries in horses. *Veterinary Clinics of North America: Equine Practice* 30: 91–110.

Hilton, H.G., Magdesian, K.G., Groth, A.D. et al. (2011). Distribution of flunixin meglumine and firocixib into aqueous humor of horses. *Journal of Veterinary Internal Medicine* 25: 1127–1133.

Jurk, I.R., Thibodeau, M.S., Whitney, K. et al. (2001). Acute vision loss after general anesthesia in a cat. *Veterinary Ophthalmology* 4: 155–158.

Komaromy, A.M., Garg, C.D., Ying, G.-S., and Liu, C. (2006). Effect of head position on intraocular pressure in horses. *American Joural of Veteirnary Research* 67: 1232–1235.

Marly, C., Bettschart-Wolfensberger, R., Nussbaumer, P. et al. (2014). Evaluation of a romifidine constant rate infusion protocol with or without butorphanol for dentistry and ophthalmologic procedures in standing horses. *Veterinary Anaesthesia and Analgesia* 41: 491–497.

Murgatroyd, H. and Bembridge, J. (2008). Intraocular pressure. *Continuing Education in Anaesthesia, Critical Care and Pain* 8: 100–103.

Palte, H.D., Gayer, S., Arrieta, E. et al. (2012). Are ultrasound-guided ophthalmic blocks injurious to the eye? A comparative rabbit model study of two ultrasound devices evaluating intraorbital thermal and structural changes. *Anesthesia and Analgesia* 115: 194–201.

Parviainen, A.K.J. and Trim, C.M. (2000). Complications associated with anaesthesia for ocular surgery: a retrospective study 1989-1996. *Equine Veterinary Journal* 32: 555–559.

Raw, D. and Mostafa, S.M. (2001). Drugs and the eye. *British Journal of Anaesthesia CEPD Reviews* 1: 161–165.

Roth, S. and Barach, P. (2001). Postoperative visual loss – still no answers, yet. Editorial. *Anesthesiology* 95: 575–577.

Shilo-Benjamini, Y. (2019). A review of ophthalmic local and regional anesthesia in dogs and cats. *Veterinary Anaesthesia and Analgesia* 46: 14–27.

Thomson, S.M., Oliver, J., Gould, D.J. et al. (2013). Preliminary investigations into the analgesic effects of topical ocular 1% morphine solution in dogs and cats. *Veterinary Anaesthesia and Analgesia* 40: 632–640.

Vukoja, E. (2019). Anaesthetic management of a patient undergoing unilateral phacoemulsification with concurrent diabetes mellitus. *The Veterinary Nurse* 10: 270–275.

Self-test Section

1 The afferent limb of the oculocardiac reflex is in which cranial nerve?

2 Intraocular pressure (IOP) can be increased by which of the following factors?
   A Increased CVP, increased $PaCO_2$ and increased PO_2
   B Increased CVP, decreased $PaCO_2$ and decreased PO_2
   C Increased CVP, increased $PaCO_2$ and decreased PO_2
   D Increased CVP, decreased $PaCO_2$ and increased PO_2

3 How would you approach the management of a dog with a superficial corneal ulcer requiring anaesthesia for debridement?

43

Orthopaedic and Neurosurgery Considerations

LEARNING OBJECTIVES

- To be able to devise suitable analgesic plans.
- To be familiar with the different forms of embolism, its recognition and treatment.

43.1 Analgesic Considerations for Orthopaedics

Evidence clearly demonstrates a reduction in post-operative pain scores and a decrease in the stress response where local anaesthetic techniques have been incorporated for orthopaedic surgery. Include local anaesthesia, opioids, and non-steroidal anti-inflammatory drugs (NSAIDs) where possible. Osteoarthritis produces central modulation of nociceptive input. In hip OA, total hip replacement has been shown to decrease indicators of central sensitisation in dogs. With all bone fractures, fracture-site stabilisation assists in reducing discomfort. Thoracotomies, especially sternotomies, are amongst the most painful of bony surgeries. See Chapters 12, 14, 15, and 47.

Pain after amputation may be immediate post-operative, chronic stump pain, or phantom limb pain. These may also occur in veterinary species, although particularly the last two (which are 2 components of phantom complex) can be difficult to recognise. Both limb and tail amputations can result in this phenomenon. How best to manage such patients is not clear, although pain can be greatly reduced by adhering to preventive analgesia strategies. Ensuring conduction blockade in the peripheral nerves to be transected, before actual surgical sectioning, is paramount: regional techniques (e.g. brachial plexus, neuraxial), combined with visualised individual perineural blocks just prior to nerve transection, should be used; and the American Society of Anesthesiologists recommends the use of wound catheters for continued infusion of local anaesthetic agents post-operatively.

43.2 Spinal Surgery Considerations

During spinal surgery, epidural/spinal analgesia may be contemplated but may complicate post-operative neurological assessment, especially if performed with long-acting local anaesthetics. If the epidural space and the dura mater are going to be opened at surgery, then neuraxially administered analgesic drugs may be less efficacious anyway. Topical morphine 0.1 mg/kg, however, has been shown to reduce methadone administration, based upon pain scoring, following thoracolumbar spinal surgery. The analgesic effect was enhanced when systemic opioids were administered concurrently.

Anaesthetic variables have been evaluated in dogs undergoing spinal surgery and revealed a high incidence of bradycardia and hypotension. Anaesthetic protocols should take these into account and it is recommended to incorporate analgesic infusions to reduce dependence upon volatile agents (see Chapter 6).

With spinal surgeries, there is a worry of increased gastrointestinal (GI) (and large intestine as much as stomach/small intestine) perforation with NSAIDs. (Solely *gastro*protectant drugs are therefore not always effective.) Is this because NSAIDs are commonly administered alongside corticosteroids, although corticosteroids are now clearly contraindicated for spinal injury? Or is it that with acute disc herniations, spinal cord bruising leads to a form of spinal shock with autonomic imbalance? (This is reminiscent of neurogenic shock, which basically means a massive reduction in sympathetic tone, and thus hypotension.

Veterinary Anaesthesia: Principles to Practice, Second Edition. Alexandra H. A. Dugdale, Georgina Beaumont, Carl Bradbrook, and Matthew Gurney.
© 2020 John Wiley & Sons Ltd. Published 2020 by John Wiley & Sons Ltd.
Companion website: www.wiley.com/go/dugdale/veterinary-anaesthesia

Hypotension can certainly compromise splanchnic [renal and GI] perfusion and is common under anaesthesia in these cases.)

It is also recognised that Dachshunds tend to become more bradycardic under anaesthesia than other breeds and bradycardia itself can exacerbate hypotension. Most disc herniations occur in small dogs, and the peripheral vasodilation accompanying spinal shock-induced hypotension would facilitate heat loss: hypothermia is another common problem, especially reported in small breeds like Dachshunds, and may be partly responsible for their tendency to develop bradycardia under anaesthesia. Hindquarter paresis also reduces shivering thermogenesis, and therefore promotes hypothermia (although shivering is also prevented under anaesthesia).

Factors that may have an association (no definitive association yet proven) with outcome to ambulation following decompressive spinal surgery include: primarily the grade of spinal injury at presentation; but also the duration of anaesthesia/surgery; the duration of intra-operative bradycardia and hypotension; the mean body temperature; and the mean end tidal carbon dioxide tension.

43.3 Emboli

A rare, but life-threatening risk.

43.3.1 Fat/Marrow

Marrow fragments can be seeded into the circulation during or after the fracture of long bones and possibly also during their repair. Usually 'silent', but severe embolism may result in:

- Severe respiratory compromise.
- Cerebral compromise.
- Cardiovascular compromise/collapse/shock.
- Skin/mucosal petechiation; retinal haemorrhages.
- Renal compromise; may detect fat in urine.

Intramedullary pressure may reach peaks of 1,400 mmHg during bone instrumentation (e.g. reaming). Bone marrow microemboli become surrounded by thrombocytic aggregates to form macroemboli. Wherever they lodge, they can interfere with organ perfusion and can trigger an inflammatory response, even sparking the systemic inflammatory response (SIRS), which can lead to multiple organ failure.

43.3.2 Bone Cement

Hypotension and cardiac arrest can occur (rarely) during insertion of prostheses with bone cement, or vertebroplasty with bone cement. These 'reactions' may occur when free methylmethacrylate monomer is forced into the circulation during insertion of cement, but may also be due to fat, air, thrombus, and marrow embolisation. Bone cement was reported to aggregate around the tip of a central venous catheter in one case report.

43.3.3 Thrombi

Esmarch bandaging of limbs to 'exsanguinate' them prior to surgery can dislodge venous thromboses secondary to the previous trauma, such that gravitational exsanguination is often preferred. (Trauma-associated coagulopathy may be an influencing factor.).

43.3.4 Air Emboli

Studies in dogs using volumetric capnography were able to demonstrate the occurrence of air emboli without apparent clinical effect during anaesthesia, but effects are volume-, rate-, and gas-dependent (see also Chapter 7).

Facilitated by:

- Use of air drills.
- Surgical site located 'above' heart level and when large veins or marrow cavities (including skull diploe) are exposed (e.g. spinal or cranial surgery).
- Where 'down the vein' jugular vein catheters become uncapped (e.g. in a standing horse).
- During contrast cystography where air is forced into the bladder under pressure.
- During laparoscopic surgery where the abdomen is inflated with gases. (Usually CO_2, which is the safest gas because it is highly soluble in blood, so any bubbles are quickly 'dissolved'.)
- Sometimes where positive pressure (mechanical or manual) ventilation is overzealous.

Clinical signs of pulmonary emboli are: those of a low cardiac output state, with reflex tachycardia and peripheral vasoconstriction; tachypnoea/hyperpnoea with hypoxaemia/cyanosis; and increased jugular distension. Under anaesthesia, an acute reduction in end tidal carbon dioxide tension may be seen, although the patient's arterial carbon dioxide tension is increased, such that, eventually, the end tidal carbon dioxide tension will also increase. If the patient is awake, the condition can be painful/distressing with dyspnoea and orthopnoea.

43.3.4.1 Treatment for Venous Air Emboli
- Reduce further air entry:
  - Flood or submerge the surgical site with saline.
  - Prompt haemostasis (i.e. occlude 'open' veins, which may not be easy to identify as venous bleeding may not

be obvious, especially if air is being entrained rather than blood exiting the damaged vessel).
- Lower the operating site to below the heart.
- For head/neck surgery, compress both jugular veins (increases venous back-pressure).
- Rapid IV fluids (to increase central venous pressure [CVP]).
- Stop N_2O administration.
- Provide positive pressure ventilation if possible with 100% O_2 as hypoxaemia is likely. Apply positive end-expiratory pressure (PEEP) during positive pressure ventilation, or continuous positive airway pressure (CPAP) during spontaneous breathing, to increase CVP.

- Positive inotropic and/or vasopressor support may be required if hypotensive.
- Cardiocentesis (ultrasound guided) may be considered in order to remove large air bubbles.

43.3.4.2 Treatment for Marrow/Fat/Thrombo-emboli

Anticoagulants (heparin), thrombolytics (streptokinase/urokinase), or mechanical fragmentation could be attempted if the necessary drugs and expertise are available. Respiratory and cardiovascular support are important; control of the systemic inflammatory response, which may develop into SIRS, is more tricky.

Further Reading

Abdul-Jalil, Y., Bartels, J., Alberti, O., and Becker, R. (2007). Delayed presentation of pulmonary polymethylmethacrylate emboli after percutaneous vertebroplasty. *Spine* 32: E589–E593.

Donaldson, A.J., Thomson, H.E., Harper, N.J., and Kenny, N.W. (2009). Bone cement implantation syndrome. *British Journal of Anaesthesia* 102: 12–22.

Fenn, J., Laber, E., Williams, K. et al. (2017). Associations between anesthetic variables and functional outcomes in dogs with thoracolumbar intervertebral disk extrusion undergoing decompressive hemilaminectomy. *Journal of Veterinary Internal Medicine* 31: 814–824.

Gupta, A. and Reilly, C.S. (2007). Fat embolism. *Continuing Education in Anaesthesia, Critical Care and Pain* 7: 148–151.

Harrison, R.L., Clark, L., and Corletto, F. (2012). Comparison of mean heart rate in anaesthetised dachshunds and other breeds of dog undergoing spinal magnetic resonance imaging. *Veterinary Anaesthesia and Analgesia* 39: 230–235.

Pederson, T., Viby-Mogensen, J., and Ringsted, C. (1992). Anaesthetic practice and postoperative pulmonary complications. *Acta Anaesthesiologica Scandinavica* 36: 812–818.

Romano, M., Portela, D.A., Breghi, G., and Otero, P.E. (2015). Stress-related biomarkers in dogs administered regional anaesthesia or fentanyl for analgesia during stifle surgery. *Veterinary Anaesthesia and Analgesia* 43: 44–54.

Selcer, B.A., Buttrick, M., Barstad, R., and Riedesel, D. (1987). The incidence of thoracic trauma in dogs with skeletal injury. *Journal of Small Animal Practice* 28: 21–27.

Tomas, A., Marcellin-Little, D.J., Roe, S.C. et al. (2014). Relationship between mechanical thresholds and limb use in dogs with coxofemoral joint OA-associated pain and the modulating effects of pain alleviation from total hip replacement on mechanical thresholds. *American Journal of Veterinary Research* 66: 1616–1622.

Self-test Section

1   What analgesic techniques might be considered for a lateral thoracotomy?

2   What are the initial actions for a suspected venous air embolus (VAE)?

44

Renal Considerations

LEARNING OBJECTIVES

- To be familiar with the normal kidney functions.
- To be able to devise suitable anaesthetic protocols to preserve renal function.

44.1 Normals

44.1.1 Normal Kidney Functions

- Regulation of water balance (blood volume, osmolarity [Na^+ concentration], and blood pressure).
- Regulation of electrolyte balance (some species variations); sodium, potassium, calcium, and phosphate.
- Regulation of blood pH (acid [H^+] excretion; bicarbonate 'reabsorption').
- Gluconeogenesis and other metabolic functions (e.g. reabsorption/conservation of amino acids).
- Assistance with red blood cell production (erythropoietin).
- Excretion of waste products (especially nitrogenous).
- Elimination of drugs (by filtration/secretion into urine).

44.1.2 Endocrine Functions

These include the production of:

- Erythropoietin (erythrogenin in the kidney [juxtaglomerular cells] converts erythropoietinogen [from the liver] to erythropoietin).
- Renin.
- 1, 25-dihydroxycholecalciferol; the active form of vitamin D. (Note that 25-hydroxycholecalciferol [produced in the liver by hydroxylation of vitamin D2 (ergocalciferol) and D3 (cholecalciferol)] is further hydroxylated in the kidney to the active hormone.)

44.2 Useful Values

- Renal blood flow is c. 20% of cardiac output.
- Glomerular filtration rate (GFR) is c. 125 ml/kg/h.
- Normal urine production rate is about 1% of GFR, of the order of 1–1.5 (some say 1–2) ml/kg/h. (Part of this is the minimum mandatory/obligatory urine loss in order to excrete the solute load.)
  - Anuria is defined as urine output (UO) <0.5 ml/kg/h; oliguria as UO = 0.5–1 ml/kg/h; and polyuria as UO >2 ml/kg/h.
  - Urine specific gravity (SG) can vary greatly, from 1.001 to >1.075 (dogs) and from 1.001 to >1.085 (cats). In normal, healthy, euhydrated animals, however, SG values are expected to be in the range of: 1.015–1.045 (dogs) and 1.020–1.060 (cats, although some say 1.035–1.060). Isosthenuric range of SG is 1.008–1.012 (some say up to 1.015 for cats).
- When renal failure occurs, nitrogenous waste products start to accumulate in the blood.

Azotaemia refers to an increase in one or more nitrogen-containing substances in the blood, predominantly urea and creatinine, above normal baseline values; the presence of azotaemia does not always result in clinical signs or illness in the patient. Uraemia (or 'uraemic syndrome') is the clinical manifestation of azotaemia and is most commonly associated with significant elevations in

Veterinary Anaesthesia: Principles to Practice, Second Edition. Alexandra H. A. Dugdale, Georgina Beaumont, Carl Bradbrook, and Matthew Gurney.
© 2020 John Wiley & Sons Ltd. Published 2020 by John Wiley & Sons Ltd.
Companion website: www.wiley.com/go/dugdale/veterinary-anaesthesia

urea and creatinine. Uraemia may be characterised by azotaemia, polyuria/polydipsia (PU/PD), vomiting, weight loss, depression and alterations in electrolytes, and acid–base status. A 75% loss of functional nephrons is required for isosthenuria and azotaemia. Urine concentrating ability may be lost before azotaemia appears in dogs, but cats may retain some urine concentrating ability in the presence of azotaemia.

44.3 Chronic Renal Failure

In dogs and cats, a grading system for chronic kidney disease (in addition to a system for grading acute kidney disease), has been developed by the International Renal Interest Society (IRIS), which may be used to help quantify anaesthetic risk. The IRIS grading system is based upon blood creatinine concentrations, but also considers SDMA (symmetric dimethyl arginine), proteinuria (urine protein/creatinine ratio), and hypertension.

44.4 Clinical Problems Associated with Renal Disease

- PU/PD (isosthenuric urine), which may contribute to hypovolaemia and hypokalaemia. PU/PD is sometimes noticed as nocturia, inappropriate micturition, or volume-related incontinence.
- Non-regenerative anaemia.
- Hypertension (more common in cats), which may lead to blindness (hypertensive retinopathy).
- Protein losing nephropathy (nephrotic syndrome) leads to hypercoagulability (loss of antithrombin III), hypoalbuminaemia (reduces drug-binding and promotes oedema formation), and weight loss.
- Uraemic syndrome can develop with both acute and chronic renal failure. Associated clinical signs include uraemic stomatitis/gingivitis (anorexia, halitosis, oral ulcers, petechiated/bleeding gums), uraemic gastritis (vomiting, haematemesis, melaena), uraemic pneumonitis (dypsnoea), and uraemic encephalopathy (seizures).

44.4.1 Pathophysiology of Uraemia

- High urea and creatinine
  - Uraemia interferes with platelet function, so bleeding gums and stomach lesions are more likely. The presence of blood in the stomach can also cause emesis.
  - Uraemia enhances capillary permeability and so promotes petechiation, haemorrhagic gingivitis/stomatitis/gastritis, and uraemic pneumonitis.
  - Uraemia may also cause haemolysis and bone marrow suppression, which compound the anaemia from blood loss.
- High parathyroid hormone (PTH) and high phosphates
  - Both may enhance the feeling of nausea.
  - High PTH is thought to be nephrotoxic so that the disease process is self-perpetuating.
- Enhanced permeability of the blood–brain barrier (adds to uraemic encephalopathy).
- Increased urinary protein loss and bleeding diatheses result in greater protein catabolism (weight loss).

Renal disease *can* therefore result in perturbations in many bodily functions. The presence of anaemia, disturbances in blood volume and pressure, electrolyte abnormalities, and blood pH derangements are most likely to cause concern. However, metabolism and excretion of drugs may also be altered; therefore, we must consider:

- How the renal disease affects anaesthetic choices.
- How the anaesthetic affects the underlying renal disease.

Patients should be 'stabilised' and renal function optimised before anaesthesia where possible; consider addressing hypovolaemia, azotaemia/uraemia, clinically significant anaemia, acid–base and electrolyte disturbances, especially of potassium, before induction of anaesthesia.

44.4.2 Approach

- Diurese pre-anaesthesia, correct dehydration and address electrolyte imbalances if needed. Use a balanced crystalloid solution, e.g. Hartmann's solution, but check electrolytes before starting; continue fluids intra- and postoperatively (until sufficient voluntary intake resumes).
- Beware the use of nephrotoxic drugs, e.g. antibiotics and radiographic/computed tomography (CT) and magnetic resonance imaging (MRI) contrast media. Diuresis may be indicated for several hours following the administration of contrast media if they are thought to be absolutely necessary to reach a diagnosis.
- Balanced anaesthetic protocol aimed at minimising reduction in arterial blood pressure (and renal perfusion).
- Analgesia: beware non-steroidal anti-inflammatory drugs (NSAIDs) and possibly give them only once the animal is awakening in recovery.
- UO may be measured; bladder should be emptied before recovery to improve patient comfort.

44.5 Ruptured Bladder Foals (Uroperitoneum)

44.5.1 Problems

- Hypovolaemia (decreased circulating volume, although 'third space loss' of urine into the abdomen increases the extracellular fluid compartment volume).
- Hyponatraemia.
- Hypochloraemia.
- **Hyperkalaemia** (cardiac arrhythmias if $K^+ >$ 6.2–7 mmol/l).
- Metabolic acidosis (usually due to a combination of: lactic acidosis due to hypovolaemia; reduced renal H^+ secretion; and K^+/H^+ transcellular exchange).
- Azotaemia (usually urea > creatinine).
- Occasionally ventilation is impaired (diaphragm 'splinted' by increased intra-abdominal pressure $\pm$ pleural effusion).
- Urine cannot be voided and contacts the peritoneum; beware active metabolites or drugs excreted unchanged into urine (ketamine). Increased intra-abdominal pressure adds to cardiovascular compromise.

44.5.2 Approach

Foals are neonates too (see Chapter 37).

- Stabilise pre-anaesthesia (aim for $K^+ <$ 6 mmol/l):
  - IV fluids: In a model of feline urethral obstruction, Hartmann's solution corrected the metabolic acidosis faster than normal saline (which, despite having no potassium content, and therefore being quite an appealing choice for hyperkalaemia, is quite an acidifying solution; and acidosis can promote hyperkalaemia through ion exchange mechanisms). Furthermore, whilst both solutions corrected the hyperkalaemia over a similar time-frame, better correction of overall electrolyte disturbances was seen with Hartmann's solution.
  - Possibly deny suckling (milk has high potassium content).
  - If hyperkalaemic arrhythmias are present (ECG important to aid diagnosis): consider IV calcium; IV glucose (dextrose) solutions ($\pm$ soluble insulin); possibly sodium bicarbonate (see Chapter 24). Once bladder drainage is re-established and fluid therapy underway, furosemide increases potassium excretion.
  - Drain belly SLOWLY (rapid release of previously raised intra-abdominal pressure can result in massive splanchnic vasodilation, hypotension, and syncope). Consider peritoneal dialysis/lavage with normal saline.

- Balanced anaesthesia/analgesia. Beware hypoventilation (respiratory acidosis) that may exacerbate acidaemia and promote hyperkalaemia. Ultrasonographic evaluation of the pleural space prior to anaesthesia will help determine the presence and extent of any pleural effusion (see Further Reading); drainage prior to anaesthesia/recumbency may be warranted.

44.6 'Blocked' Cats

Urethral obstructions present similar problems to those above. The approach includes stabilisation through bladder drainage and correction of fluid and electrolyte abnormalities. Bladder drainage, by cystocentesis or via urethral catheterisation, may require general anaesthesia, although benzodiazepine/opioid combinations provide useful sedation and may help to relax the urethra. α2 agonists are generally avoided in patients with cardiovascular instability; additionally, they induce diuresis and suppress insulin secretion (resulting in hyperglycaemia), which can interfere with any subsequent administration of exogenous glucose in the hope of stimulating insulin secretion in order to treat hyperkalaemia. Low doses of acepromazine may, however, help to reduce urethral spasm, due to its α1 adrenoreceptor blocking effects, and in addition, may also help to provide some anxiolysis (but be aware of the patient's cardiovascular status as acepromazine promotes hypotension). (It is important to try to minimise stress for these cats.) Prazosin, another α1 receptor antagonist, may also be useful. Sacro-coccygeal epidural anaesthesia or bilateral pudendal block can also facilitate urethral catheterisation.

Ureteral obstructions may be uni- or bilateral, and cats may present with acute oliguric/anuric renal failure and considerable renal pain. Whereas partial obstructions may be managed medically (i.e. attempts are often made to induce a diuresis to dilate the ureters in order to aid passage of the ureterolith/s), complete obstructions require urgent decompression of the dilated renal pelvis in order to preserve as much renal function as possible. Minimally invasive emergency procedures include placement of ureteral stents, subcutaneous ureteral bypass (SUB) catheters, or percutaneous nephrostomy tube placement. Patients may remain extremely painful post-operatively and can be difficult to manage. Whilst opioids may form the mainstay of peri-operative analgesia, NSAIDs are usually avoided to reduce the risks of further renal injury. Ketamine infusions and the gabapentinoids may be useful adjuncts. Lidocaine infusions have profound cardiovascular side effects in cats, with neurotoxicity also a risk, and may also cause salivation/nausea, so are rarely used for more than a few hours (e.g. one to four hours), if at all.

Post-obstructive diuresis may develop following relief of ureteral or urethral obstruction that has been relatively long-standing. Several mechanisms have been proposed, including: nephron damage leading to reduced expression of sodium transporters and reduced response to antidiuretic hormone (ADH); loss of the renal medullary concentration gradient during obstructive states; and adaptations in remaining functional nephrons that result in increased individual nephron glomerular filtration rate, reduced tubular reabsorption, and increased tubular secretion (i.e. the 'intact nephron hypothesis'). Whatever, the cause, fluid 'ins' and 'outs' and blood electrolyte concentrations should be monitored closely for the first few days following relief of obstruction, and fluid therapy may have to be greatly increased to keep up with the losses.

Further Reading

Billings, F.T. IV, Chen, S.W.C., Kim, M. et al. (2008). Alpha 2 adrenergic agonists protect against radiocontrast-induced nephropathy in mice. *American Journal of Physiology: Renal Physiology* 295: F741–F748.

Clark-Price, S.C. and Grauer, G.F. (2015). Physiology, pathophysiology and anesthetic management of patients with renal disease. In: *Veterinary Anesthesia and Analgesia, the Fifth Edition of Lumb and Jones* (eds. K.A. Grimm, L.A. Lamont, W.J. Tranquilli, et al.), 681–697. Ames, Iowa, USA: Wiley Blackwell.

Cooper, E.S. (2015). Controversies in the management of feline urethral obstruction. *Journal of Veterinary Emergency and Critical Care* 25: 130–137.

Cunha, M.G.M.C.M., Freitas, G.C., Carregaro, A.B. et al. (2010). Renal and cardiorespiratory effects of treatment with lactated Ringer's solution or physiologic saline (0.9% NaCl) solution in cats with experimentally-induced urethral obstruction. *American Journal of Veterinary Research* 71: 840–846.

Dickinson, M.C. and Kam, P.C.A. (2008). Intravascular iodinated contrast media and the anaesthetist. *Anaesthesia* 63: 626–634.

Garcia, E.R. (2018). Urogenital disease. In: *BSAVA Manual of Canine and Feline Anaesthesia and Analgesia*, 3e (eds. T. Duke-Novakovski, M. de Vries and C. Seymour), 356–365. Gloucester, UK: British Small Animal Veterinary Association.

Goic, J.B., Koenigshof, A.M., McGuire, L.D. et al. (2016). A retrospective evaluation of contrast-induced kidney injury in dogs (2006–2012). *Journal of Veterinary Emergency and Critical Care* 26: 713–719.

Hasebroock, J.M. and Serkova, N.J. (2009). Toxicity of MRI and CT contrast agents. *Expert Opinion on Drug Metabolism and Toxicology* 5: 403–416.

International Renal Interest Society (2017). IRIS Staging of CKD. http://www.iris-kidney.com/guidelines/staging.html (accessed June 2019).

Paltrinieri, S., Giraldi, M., Prolo, A. et al. (2018). Serum symmetric dimethylarginine and creatinine in Birman cats compared with cats of other breeds. *Journal of Feline Medicine and Surgery* 20: 905–912.

Shelley, M.P., Robinson, A.A., Hesford, J.W., and Park, G.R. (1987). Haemodynamic effects following surgical release of increased intra-abdominal pressure. *British Journal of Anaesthesia* 59: 800–805.

Valle, E., Prola, L., Vergnano, D. et al. (2019). Investigation of hallmarks of carbonyl stress and formation of end products in feline chronic kidney disease as markers of uraemic toxins. *Journal of Feline Medicine and Surgery* 21: 465–474.

Webb, S.T. and Allen, J.S.D. (2008). Perioperative renal protection. *Continuing Education in Anaesthesia, Critical Care and Pain* 8 (5): 176–180.

Wilkins, P.A. (2004). Respiratory distress in foals with uroperitoneum: possible mechanisms. *Equine Veterinary Education.* 16: 293–295.

Self-test Section

1 What percentage of cardiac output do the kidneys normally receive?
   A 40%
   B 30%
   C 20%
   D 10%

2 *Oliguria* is defined as urine output of?
   A <0.5 ml/kg/h
   B 0.5–1 ml/kg/h
   C 1–2 ml/kg/h
   D >2 ml/kg/h

45

Hepatic Considerations

LEARNING OBJECTIVES

- To be able to list the functions of the liver.
- To be able to discuss how hepatic dysfunction affects anaesthesia.

45.1 Normals

45.1.1 Normal Liver Functions

- Metabolism of carbohydrates, fats, and proteins. Gluconeogenesis is an important source of blood glucose. Hepatic metabolic activity is an important source of heat.
- Stores glycogen, some fat and fat-soluble vitamins, and some minerals, including iron and copper.
- Produces blood proteins: albumin, globulins (including acute phase proteins), and most clotting factors (e.g. fibrinogen, prothrombin (II), V, VII, IX, X, XIII, antithrombin, plasminogen, α2 anti-plasmin (or α2 plasmin inhibitor), and proteins C, S, and Z; vitamin K is required for the production of factors II, VII, IX, X and C, S, and Z).
- Biotransformation of drugs, including oxidation/reduction/hydrolysis (Phase I) and conjugation (Phase II).
- Produces angiotensinogen; metabolises renin.
- Produces erythropoietinogen and some erythropoietin (15% of total; kidneys produce 85%).
- Converts vitamins D2/D3 into 25-hydroxycholecalciferol (important, after conversion to 1,25-dihydroxycholecalciferol in kidneys, for calcium absorption).
- Produces bile: salts and pigments.
- Filters bacteria from portal blood (Kupffer cells important).
- Filters toxins and GABA-mimetic compounds from portal blood.
- Converts ammonia (in portal blood) to urea.

45.1.2 Useful Facts

- The normal liver receives 25% of cardiac output.
- Portal venous blood contributes 70% of total blood flow (cf. 30% from hepatic artery), and 50–60% of oxygen.
- The portal venous system has little smooth muscle, and is not as responsive to sympathetic tone as the hepatic artery.
  - The hepatic arterial buffer response enables some intrinsic regulation of hepatic blood flow, i.e. hepatic arterial flow changes so as to buffer changes in hepatic portal vein flow, tending to regulate total hepatic flow at a constant level.
- Autoregulation at the microvascular level is poorly developed in the liver, but the hepatocytes are better extractors of oxygen than cells in any other tissue.
- 80% functional liver mass must be lost for homeostasis of blood glucose to be impaired.

45.2 Hepatic Dysfunction

Hepatic dysfunction can be associated with:

- Ascites/oedema/pulmonary oedema (especially with crystalloid fluid overload) due to:
  - Hypoproteinaemia/hypoalbuminaemia
  - Decreased hepatic destruction of renin; and/or increased sensitivity to aldosterone; and/or circulatory causes of renin/angiotensin/aldosterone system activation – all leading to increased sodium and water retention
  - Portal hypertension (cirrhosis)

Veterinary Anaesthesia: Principles to Practice, Second Edition. Alexandra H. A. Dugdale, Georgina Beaumont, Carl Bradbrook, and Matthew Gurney.
© 2020 John Wiley & Sons Ltd. Published 2020 by John Wiley & Sons Ltd.
Companion website: www.wiley.com/go/dugdale/veterinary-anaesthesia

- Polyuria (± compensatory polydipsia) due to decreased urea synthesis and decreased renal medullary concentration gradient; hypovolaemia/hypotension are possible sequelae
- Anaemia
- Hypocalcaemia (low total and also possibly low ionised calcium); may be partly secondary to decreased albumin (i.e. decreased albumin-bound calcium); and partly due to decreased vitamin D conversion)
- Hypoglycaemia
- Tendency to hypothermia
- Reduced blood clotting
- Raised blood ammonia, yet low blood urea
- Raised bile acids
- Acid–base and electrolyte abnormalities
- Urinary bi-urate crystals
- Increased bacteraemias (increased risk of infections)
- Jaundice (especially increased unconjugated bilirubin)
- Hepatic encephalopathy (increased ammonia; change in ratio of branched chain to aromatic amino acids; increased absorption of false neurotransmitters/toxic metabolites [e.g. mercaptans] from gut; increased blood–brain barrier permeability)
- Chronic hepatic disease tends to be associated with autonomic dysfunction (e.g. depressed sympathetic activity; laryngeal paresis), but the exact mechanisms are not yet understood. (May contribute to hypotension).

If total protein < 3.5 g/dl; or albumin < 1.5–2 g/dl, then you can expect oedema/ascites (interstitial/third space fluid accumulation).

45.3 How Does Liver Disease Affect Our Choice of Drugs and Technique?

- Increased fluid retention leads to increased volume of distribution for water-soluble drugs.
- Decreased plasma protein leads to increased 'free' drug concentrations, especially for drugs that are normally highly protein-bound (e.g. non-steroidal anti-inflammatory drugs [NSAIDs]).
- Decreased drug metabolism slows drug elimination; a few drugs are unaffected as they do not rely on hepatic metabolism (remifentanil, atracurium).
- Decreased plasma cholinesterase (pseudo-cholinesterase or butyrylcholinesterase) leads to prolonged action of succinylcholine (suxamethonium), mivacurium, and ester-linked local anaesthetics.

- Ascites and pleural effusion can compromise cardiovascular and respiratory function; possibly drain, slowly, and restore plasma oncotic pressure.
  - The SAAG; serum-ascites albumin gap (or gradient), calculated from samples taken simultaneously, as (serum albumin concentration minus ascitic fluid albumin concentration) can be used to help determine the likely cause of abdominal fluid accumulation. Values <1.1 g/dl are normal; raised (≥1.1 g/dl) SAAG values can accompany portal hypertension (which may, or not, be liver-related), or ruptured bladder.
  - SAAG values can also be interpreted in light of the total protein content of the ascitic fluid (ascTP). Where SAAG is <1.1 g/dl but ascTP is >2.5 g/dl, then chylous effusion, pancreatitis, or neoplastic conditions may be present; where SAAG is ≥1.1 g/dl and ascTP is >2.5 g/dl, then right heart failure may be present, or some form of veno-occlusive disease; where SAAG is <1.1 g/dl and ascTP is <2.5 g/dl, then some form of protein losing condition may be present; where SAAG is ≥1.1 g/dl and ascTP is <2.5 g/dl, then hepatic dysfunction may be present.
- Risk of oedema exacerbation with IV fluid therapy.
- The lactate in Hartmann's solution etc. is *unlikely* to cause a problem in patients with hepatic dysfunction. Balanced electrolyte solutions are generally preferable to saline solutions.
- If **coagulopathy** exists, be careful with deep IM injections and IV cannulation and avoid epidurals. Surgery will also be tricky, and wound healing may be impaired. Fresh blood transfusion may be warranted. Assessment of coagulation can include:
  - Buccal mucosal bleeding time (BMBT): >4 minutes (dogs and cats) is abnormal, [some say >2.4 minutes is abnormal for cats], and may reflect a primary clotting disorder (e.g. thrombocytopaenia, thrombocytopathia [decreased platelet function, including von Willebrand's disease], or vascular wall abnormalities). Note that BMBTs can be affected by several factors including patient restraint, and which exact device is used.
  - Prothrombin time (PT) and Activated Partial Thromboplastin time (APTT; assess secondary haemostasis (involving clotting factors).
  - Viscoelastometric analyses of coagulation: can give graphical and numerical information on *in vitro* clot formation, clot strength, and subsequent clot dissolution.
- If hyperammonaemia is present, beware hyperventilation, as alkalaemia favours NH_3 formation over NH_4^+, and ammonia crosses cell membranes, and the blood–brain barrier, more easily than ammonium.

45.3.1 Portosystemic Shunts (PSS)

Commonly found in young animals, so precautions associated with neonates/paediatric patients may also apply (see Chapter 37).

45.3.1.1 Strategy

- **Stabilise** medically first (treat hepatic encephalopathy and seizures).
- **Minimal premedication.** Short-acting opioids (e.g. butorphanol/pethidine/methadone depending upon intended procedure). **Pethidine good choice for neonates** as minimal lowering of heart rate and short duration of action, **but only IM** as it can cause severe histamine release/anaphylaxis if given intravenously.
- **Anaesthetic induction.** Injectable anaesthetic agents may be preferred (propofol or alfaxalone), and should be given slowly, to effect; ensure prior venous access. Induction with inhalation agents can also be considered, especially if venous access cannot be established before anaesthetic induction.
- **Anaesthetic maintenance.** Supply **oxygen**. Volatile anaesthetic agents are usually preferred as they do not rely on hepatic metabolism. Isoflurane or sevoflurane are common choices, although isoflurane is less metabolised by the liver and also improves hepatic oxygenation whilst preserving total hepatic blood flow (by altering the ratio of hepatic portal venous flow to hepatic arterial flow).
- Continue **analgesia** provision. **Local anaesthetic techniques** may be appropriate. **Epidural/spinal opioids** may be useful for prolonged post-operative analgesia, but **beware coagulopathies**. Beware NSAIDs in the face of hypoproteinaemia and coagulopathies (some people give half the normal dose and double the normal dosing interval, but each case will likely be different and there is an increased risk of side effects). Caution is also advised with paracetamol in dogs with hepatic disease/insufficiency (and must never be given to cats).
- Maintain **body temperature**: use active and passive warming from the time of premedication until fully recovered. Intravenous fluid therapy using a balanced electrolyte solution (e.g. Hartmann's solution) is recommended. Monitoring should include **blood glucose** (every 30–60 minutes), and supplementation if required. Central venous pressure (CVP) may help guide **fluid therapy**, but beware positional effects especially in patients with large peritoneal and pleural fluid accumulations. **Arterial hypotension** can be difficult to manage when plasma oncotic pressure is low. Consider **muscle relaxation** if indicated and if it can be appropriately managed and monitored as part of a **balanced anaesthetic technique**.
- Recovery period. Recovery may be prolonged due to slowed drug elimination, hypothermia, and/or hypoglycaemia. **Post-ligation neurological syndrome** (PLNS) may develop with a spectrum of clinical signs varying from ataxia to status epilepticus. This most commonly occurs one to three days after surgical attenuation of PSS, but can still follow more gradual shunt attenuation after the placement of cellophane bands, ameroid constrictors, or intravascular coils. **Seizures** can be difficult to control with benzodiazepines; management may include correcting underlying metabolic derangements (e.g. hypoglycaemia, elevated ammonia) and use of levetiracetam, phenobarbital (possibly as a prophylactic; although it may not prevent PLNS, it appears to reduce its severity), propofol, or even low doses of medetomidine or dexmedetomidine. Ketamine may also be considered if seizures become refractory to all these other treatments. **Portal hypertension**, **intestinal ischaemia**, and increased absorption of **endotoxins** from the gut may manifest as abdominal pain and distension, vomiting, diarrhoea, increased ascites, and cardiovascular collapse.
- Continue analgesia (beware NSAID toxicity; and also beware paracetamol in dogs with reduced liver function).
  - **N.B. Gastrointestinal ulceration and/or gastritis has been reported in a high proportion of large-breed dogs with intrahepatic PSS, with pathology still being present years after surgical occlusion of the shunt itself. Therefore, some authors suggest life-long gastro-protectants (e.g. proton-pump inhibitors) for these patients, and also for <u>any</u> patients receiving NSAIDs after PSS surgery.**

45.3.1.2 Portal Venous Pressure and CVP

In some PSS surgeries, the surgeons measure portal venous pressure during their attempts to ligate the shunt vessels. Nowadays, cellophane banding, ameroid constrictors, or minimally-invasive intravascular coil placement tend to be favoured, which result in a slower shunt occlusion so the cardiovascular system has more time to adjust.

Normal portal venous pressure is about 7–10 mmHg. With PSS, this pressure is lower because blood bypasses the liver en route to the caudal vena cava.

During intra-operative shunt ligation, surgeons do not like the portal venous pressure increasing above 15 mmHg.

CVP is normally 0–10 cmH$_2$O. With shunt ligation, the CVP decreases, as the caudal vena cava is denied of some blood, as more blood is now being forced to traverse the liver. CVP should not be more than $1\,cmH_2O$ below the pre-ligation value after three minutes post-ligation, otherwise there is a risk of portal hypertension.

45.3.2 Analgesic Options for Dogs with Chronic Hepatic Disease

In the acute peri-operative setting, a combination of systemic opioids and local/regional anaesthetic techniques tends to be the mainstay for analgesia provision. The administration of NSAIDs remains controversial because of the increased risk of side effects (due to altered protein-binding and delayed drug metabolism), which are likely to differ on a case-by-case basis. In dogs, paracetamol has been suggested as an alternative, but its chronic administration may induce further liver damage (in UK, it is licenced for administration for only five days). For the treatment of more chronic pain, however, a balance must be struck between quality and quantity of life. For example, for dogs with concurrent osteoarthritis, careful attention to NSAID dose and dose-interval (i.e. using the lowest 'effective' dose at the longest 'effective' inter-dose interval) may enable improved analgesia without overt side effects. Other drugs and strategies may also be considered, e.g. from gabapentinoids to cannabinoids to alternative therapies (see Chapter 3).

Further Reading

Aronson, L.R., Gacad, R.C., Kaminsky-Russ, K. et al. (1997). Endogenous benzodiazepine activity in the peripheral and portal blood of dogs with congenital portosystemic shunts. *Veterinary Surgery* 26: 189–194.

De Brito Galvao, J.F. and Center, S.A. (2012). Fluid, electrolyte and acid–base disturbances in liver disease. In: Fluid, Electrolyte and Acid–Base Disorders in Small Animal Practice, 4e (ed. S.P. DiBartola), 456–499. Missouri, USA: Elsevier Saunders. **(*Useful information on pathophysiology of ascites formation; and tabulation of putative 'toxins' in hepatic encephalopathy.*).**

Fryer, K.J., Levine, J.M., Peycke, L.E. et al. (2011). Incidence of postoperative seizures with and without levetiracetam pretreatment in dogs undergoing portosystemic shunt attenuation. *Journal of Veterinary Internal Medicine* 25: 1379–1384.

Garcia-Pereira, F. (2015). Physiology, pathophysiology and anesthetic management of patients with hepatic disease. In: Veterinary Anesthesia and Analgesia, the Fifth Edition of Lumb and Jones (eds. K.A. Grimm, L.A. Lamont, W.J. Tranquilli, et al.), 627–937. Iowa, USA: Wiley Blackwell.

Perrin, M. and Fletcher, A. (2004). Laparoscopic abdominal surgery. *Continuing Education in Anaesthesia, Critical Care and Pain* 4: 107–110.

Self, I. (2018). Gastrointestinal, laparoscopic and liver procedures. In: BSAVA Manual of Canine and Feline Anaesthesia and Analgesia, 3e (eds. T. Duke-Novakovski, M. de Vries and C. Seymour), 343–355. Gloucester, UK: British small animal veterinary association.

Strachan, A., Abeysundara, L., and Mallett, S.V. (2018). A concise summary of coagulation in liver disease. *Journal of Anesthesia and Intensive Care Medicine* 6 (1) https://doi.org/10.19080/JAICM.2018.06.555679.

Tisdall, P.L., Hunt, G.B., Youmans, K.R., and Malik, R. (2000). Neurologic dysfunction in dogs following attenuation of congenital extrahepatic portosystemic shunts. *Journal of Small Animal Practice* 41: 539–546.

Ziser, A. and Plevak, D.J. (2001). Morbidity and morality in cirrhotic patients undergoing anesthesia and surgery. *Current Opinion in Anaesthesiology* 14: 707–711.

Self-test Section

1   The liver receives what proportion of its oxygenation from the hepatic artery?
   A 20–30%
   B 30–40%
   C 40–50%
   D 50–60%

2   The liver produces which vitamin K-dependent clotting factors?
   A II, V, VII, X
   B II, VII, IX, X
   C II, V, IX, X
   D II, VII, X, XIII

46

Endocrine Considerations

LEARNING OBJECTIVE

- To be familiar with some of the challenges of endocrine diseases.

46.1   Diabetes Mellitus

- Type 1 (absolute insulin deficiency) is more common in dogs, whereas type 2 (insulin resistance) is more common in cats, especially with the rise in obesity. The discussion below will focus on those patients that require exogenous insulin.
- Stabilise before anaesthesia, especially if ketoacidotic. (Ketonaemia can be present without demonstrable ketonuria.)
- Schedule surgery for early morning or early afternoon to ensure recovery in time to minimise disruption of the normal insulin/feeding schedule.

  Although tight glycaemic control (6–10 mmol/l) has generally been advised for human diabetics undergoing anaesthesia and surgery, there is an increased risk of hypoglycaemia, such that slightly less tight control might reduce peri-operative morbidity. One veterinary study in diabetic dogs undergoing cataract surgery evaluated whether administration of a quarter of, or the full, morning insulin dose improved the ability to maintain blood glucose within the very tight range of 3.9–6.7 mmol/l; neither protocol achieved this, and although slightly improved control was seen with the higher dose, some of these patients developed hypoglycaemia (glucose concentrations <3 mmol/l) post-operatively. The study, however, highlighted the importance of individualised monitoring and appropriate insulin/glucose therapy. The response to insulin therapy is difficult to predict, so it is important to monitor glucose regularly from before premedication, throughout anaesthesia,

and into recovery. As a very general guide to pre-operative glucose control:
  - If pre-operative glucose <4.5 mmol/l (after food has been withheld): give no insulin yet
  - If glucose 4.5–8 mmol/l: give quarter of the morning's insulin dose
  - If glucose >8–15 mmol/l, give half of the morning's insulin dose
  - If glucose >15 mmol/l, give the whole morning's insulin dose.
- Avoid withholding insulin therapy unless documented to be hypoglycaemic.
- Remember that stress can increase blood glucose (up to 15 mmol/l), especially in cats; and that the stress response to anaesthesia/surgery can often raise glucose concentrations to >20 mmol/l.
- Consider admitting the animal for overnight IV fluid therapy prior to anaesthesia to help to correct any disturbances in fluid balance and electrolyte status.
- **Intra-operative considerations;** hyperglycaemia (hypoglycaemia usually not a problem), hypotension. Blood glucose concentration should be monitored every 30–45 minutes.

46.1.1   Premedication

Not too 'heavy' to allow return to feeding as soon as possible post-operatively. α2 agonists, although able to promote hyperglycaemia in non-diabetic patients, may not have such profound anti-insulin effects in insulin-dependent diabetics. Opioids may be administered, but be aware of

Veterinary Anaesthesia: Principles to Practice, Second Edition. Alexandra H. A. Dugdale, Georgina Beaumont, Carl Bradbrook, and Matthew Gurney.
© 2020 John Wiley & Sons Ltd. Published 2020 by John Wiley & Sons Ltd.
Companion website: www.wiley.com/go/dugdale/veterinary-anaesthesia

their effects on pupil size if intra-ocular surgery is planned, and ensure that topical mydriatics are given in advance (see Chapter 42).

46.1.2 Induction

Injectable (IV) anaesthetic induction agents are generally recommended, administered slowly IV, to effect.

46.1.3 Maintenance

Choose drugs that allow rapid and hangover-free recovery. Neuromuscular blockers may be required (e.g. cataract surgery). Balanced analgesic approach; include local/regional anaesthetic techniques if possible. Dextrose-based IV fluids are often preferred, but monitor blood glucose q. 30–45 minutes. The stress response to anaesthesia and surgery can make blood glucose control very tricky.

Hypoglycaemia: once blood glucose <4.5 mmol/l, and especially if <3.5 mmol/l, treatment should be provided with a glucose bolus (administered relatively slowly) IV, dose 0.25-0.5-1 g/kg; and/or infusion of 2.5 or 5% glucose, e.g. in Hartmann's solution or 0.9% saline.

Hyperglycaemia: once blood glucose exceeds 15–20 mmol/l, and especially once >30 mmol/l, treatment may be warranted with soluble insulin (0.05–0.1 U/kg IM or SQ; or 0.05–0.1 U/kg IV, possibly followed by infusion 0.01–0.1 U/kg/h IV). Any fluids administered should be devoid of glucose.

Overall, intra-operatively:

- If blood glucose is <4 mmol/l, a slow IV bolus of glucose may be required, followed by infusion of balanced crystalloid fluids containing 5% dextrose
- If blood glucose concentration measures 4–8 mmol/l, balanced crystalloid fluids with 5% dextrose should be sufficient
- If blood glucose is >8 mmol/l, balanced crystalloid fluids with 2.5% dextrose may be appropriate
- If blood glucose exceeds 15 mmol/l, balanced crystalloid fluids without glucose may be most appropriate.

The fluid rate is usually started at around 5 ml/kg/h for dogs and 3 ml/kg/h for cats. Management of hypotension may involve use of fluid therapy ± positive inotropes and vasopressors. (Beware giving large/rapid boluses of fluids containing 5% glucose.)

46.1.4 Recovery

Monitor blood and urine glucose (and ketones, if indicated), and patient food and water intake. Further insulin is usually given with the evening meal, when ideally the patient should be returned to its normal routine. Prepare the owner for hypoglycaemic and hyperglycaemic problems (Tables 46.1 and 46.2) over the following few days, but this is likely to settle down.

46.2 Insulinoma

- Clinical signs are associated with **hypoglycaemia** and possibly with **high sympathetic tone** (catecholamines are counter-regulatory to insulin), and so include the increased possibility of arrhythmias.
  - Two presentations of hypoglycaemia can occur: the acute form, characterised by an increase in sympathetic tone, and the chronic (central nervous system, CNS) form, characterised by mental obtundation ± seizures.
  - The clinical signs of hypoglycaemia, proven by low measured blood glucose and improved by administration of glucose, constitute **Whipple's triad**.
- If fasting overnight pre-surgery, monitor blood glucose regularly and administer a glucose-containing infusion.
- Pre-operative workup should be thorough. **Check** blood electrolytes, especially **potassium**. (Medical management with diazoxide may help to alleviate hypoglycaemia.)
- **Premedication:** An opioid, e.g. methadone; and consider a low dose of an α2 agonist, as this may aid by suppressing insulin secretion. (Although one study using low dose [5 μg/kg medetomidine] improved glycaemic control in dogs with insulinomas, it is possible that not all insulinomas may respond like normal islet cells.)
- **Induction:** There are some concerns that even a single dose of propofol may trigger pancreatitis, so other agents may have a theoretical advantage.
- **Maintenance:** A balanced anaesthetic technique is recommended, with attention to analgesia (anti-nociception) provision. Multimodal analgesia may include local/regional techniques such as: epidural/extradural opioid ± local anaesthetic; intraperitoneal local anaesthetic deposition; truncal blocks. Monitor blood glucose and electrolytes regularly (q. 30–60 minutes), and address imbalances with appropriate glucose therapy as required. Glucagon is sometimes used to treat hypoglycaemic crises.
- **Recovery:** Risk of **post-operative pancreatitis and diabetes mellitus**. Pethidine has been suggested as the best choice of opioid, although methadone and buprenorphine are commonly used. Pethidine does not increase the tone of, whereas buprenorphine has minimal effect on, and methadone theoretically increases the tone of, the sphincter of Oddi (present in cats, but probably not in dogs); but poor pain management increases the

Table 46.1 Causes, signs, and treatment of glucose disturbances.

Disturbance	Causes	Clinical signs	Treatment
Hyperglycaemia (Glucose >6.5, but especially >8–10 mmol/l)	Stress, exercise, excitement (up to 15 mmol/l) Diabetes mellitus Hyperadrenocorticism (Cushing's) or glucocorticoid therapy (both mild, 7–8 mmol/l)	Polyuria/polydipsia Altered protein and fat metabolism Weight loss Glycosuria Lactic acidosis Depressed mentation Coma	Treatment aimed at underlying pathology Insulin may be appropriate
Hypoglycaemia (Glucose <3.5 mmol/l)	Starvation or anorexia Insulin overdose Insulinoma Idiopathic in toy breeds Physiological (insufficient production in neonates/juveniles esp. in toy breeds; or excessive utilisation, e.g. exercise-induced in hunting/working dogs) May accompany hypothyroidism, Addison's disease, or deficiency of catecholamines (i.e. lack of counter-regulatory hormones to insulin)	Weakness Lethargy Collapse	2 g/kg orally or 0.25–0.5–1 g/kg **slow bolus** IV Glucose can be added to maintenance fluids (e.g. 2.5 or 5% glucose in Hartmann's solution)

Table 46.2 Differentiation of hypo- and hyper-glycaemia.

	Hypoglycaemia	Hyperglycaemia
Onset	Sudden, often restless beforehand, weakness and trembling, seizures, may become comatose	Slow insidious onset, dull and depressed, may vomit, may become comatose
Drinking	No noticeable change	Increased
Urine output	No noticeable change	Increased
Urine glucose	Negative	Positive
Urine ketones[a]	Negative	Positive (depends somewhat upon dipsticks used)
Breath	Smells normal	Smells sweet (acetone)
Breathing rate	Normal	Increased rate and depth
Mucous membranes	Normal	Tacky/dry (dehydration)
Skin turgor	Normal	Skin pinch may 'tent' (dehydration)

[a] Most urine dipsticks measure only acetoacetate and not β hydroxybutyrate (usually the most abundant ketone), so false negative test results may occur.

likelihood of post-operative ileus (e.g. high catecholamines reduce gastrointestinal motility) and inappetence (which further promotes ileus), that can also be detrimental to exocrine pancreatic function. Consider epidural/extradural morphine analgesia. Pancreatitis may develop following surgical manipulation of the pancreas; there have been occasional reports of pancreatitis following propofol anaesthesia in humans (see above). Diabetes mellitus may also develop if severe pancreatitis occurs. Monitor blood glucose (and potassium) regularly post-operatively.

46.3 Addison's Disease (Hypoadrenocorticism)

Caused by a deficiency of aldosterone with or without glucocorticoid deficiency, and derangements include:

- Hyponatraemia.
- Hyperkalaemia and cardiac arrhythmias (especially bradyarrhythmias; but some protection, as often slightly hypercalcaemic).
- Hypovolaemia and hypotension.

- Pre-renal or renal failure (azotaemia/uraemia).
- Lethargy, fatigue.
- Nausea, vomiting.
- Poor tolerance to stress.

Stabilise pre-anaesthesia and normalise potassium if possible (IV fluids; glucocorticoids/mineralocorticoids).

46.4 Cushing's Disease (Hyperadrenocorticism)

- Weak muscles, including respiratory muscles; patients may require ventilatory support under anaesthesia.
- Coagulation abnormalities common; patients prone to thromboembolic episodes such as pulmonary thromboembolism.
- Tend to have expanded intravascular volume (despite polyuria/polydipsia [PU/PD]), leading to altered drug pharmacokinetics. Patients may also be hypertensive: try to measure baseline blood pressure and aim to maintain intra-operative blood pressure around this value to help autoregulation. (Ideally, and especially if renal or cardiac co-morbidities exist, it may be worth controlling the hypertension before surgery).
- Wound healing may be a problem: increased risk of infections.

46.5 Canine Hypothyroidism

- Reduced metabolic rate: prolonged drug actions and delayed recovery.
- Often obese, with reduced exercise tolerance.
- May be anaemic.
- May have peripheral neuropathies (e.g. laryngeal paresis: beware respiratory obstruction, especially in recovery; also increased risk of aspiration pneumonitis).
- Prone to hypothermia (unless laryngeal paralysis prevents effective panting; then prone to hyperthermia too).
- May present with bradycardias/arrhythmias and hypotension.
- Prone to coagulopathies.

46.6 Feline Hyperthyroidism

- Often in older cats (see Chapter 38).
- Weight loss is common and has pharmacokinetic implications (decreased tissues for redistribution of drugs; increased relative total body water content).
- Polyuria/polydipsia common; but beware 'contracted' extracellular fluid (ECF) volume.
- Cats often hyperactive and difficult to handle.
- Cardiac problems include:

  – Tachycardia ± gallop sound ± arrhythmias. (Right bundle branch block/left anterior fascicular block, common.)
  – Cardiac murmurs; often indicative of cardiomyopathy (usually hypertrophic, but occasionally dilated). Echocardiography prior to anaesthesia may be useful.
  – Cats may present with thromboembolic disease or even congestive cardiac failure.
  – Hypertension, alongside tachycardia, may eventually lead to reduced cardiac output because of increased afterload in the face of possible reduced preload (reduced ventricular filling at high heart rates, contracted ECF).
- Hyperdynamic circulation (with increased renal blood flow) may mask early renal failure, so beware unmasking chronic renal failure with your treatment.
- Thyroid hormones (T4/T3) promote expression and sensitivity of β adrenergic receptors, so potentiate catecholamine actions. (Avoid ketamine and nitrous oxide where possible as these can both increase sympathetic tone.)
- Palpable thyroid tissue may be found in the throat region. The effective 'mass' in the neck may:
  – Press on the trachea and compromise the airway (there may be coughing/dyspnoea); and cause problems for tracheal intubation.
  – Press on the oesophagus and cause dysphagia.
  – Cause laryngeal nerve dysfunction.
  – Result in Horner's syndrome.

46.6.1 Surgical and Post-operative Problems

- Tumours are often very vascular; beware haemorrhage (blood typing and blood transfusion may be required).
- Tumour resection may result in disruption of vagosympathetic trunk/s and consequent laryngeal paralysis.
- Tumour resection may result in disruption of blood supply to parathyroid glands (or inadvertent removal of parathyroid glands), leading to risk of post-operative hypocalcaemia (monitor for up to one week post-operatively for signs of lethargy, muscle weakness, or twitches [often see tetany progressing to paresis], anorexia, convulsions).
- Tumour removal may result in poor thyroid function post-operatively.
- Trachea may suffer tracheomalacia and collapse, especially after tumour removal.
- Post-operative tissue swelling may result in pressure on airway and oesophagus; beware respiratory obstruction and dysphagia.

46.6.2 Thyroid Storm/Crisis

This can occur intra-operatively if tumour handling results in release of a lot of thyroid hormones (T4/T3), which potentiate catecholamine effects, to result in massive tachycardia and arrhythmias, hypertension, hyperthermia, and possibly progressing to 'shock' (massive O_2 demand outstrips supply etc.). Have esmolol (or labetalol) available, but aim to stabilise pre-operatively (anti-thyroid medications).

46.6.3 Chronic Renal Failure

Underlying chronic renal failure may become apparent as the hyperthyroidism is treated. Monitor urine output, creatinine, urea and arterial blood pressure post-operatively. (For further information, see the International Renal Interest Society [IRIS] guidelines for staging and sub-staging of chronic kidney disease [CKD]). Use non-steroidal anti-inflammatory drugs (NSAIDs) cautiously.

46.6.4 Approach to Anaesthesia

Stabilise pre-operatively with anti-thyroid and cardiac medications where possible.

Avoid negative inotropes and large changes in heart rate; maintain preload and afterload.

Premedication facilitates handling. Opioid and benzodiazepine combinations are popular, but alfaxalone can also be administered IM. Small doses of acepromazine may be anti-arrhythmic, but may lead to hypotension and reflex tachycardia; beware beta blocker therapy that prevents tachycardia and promotes hypotension. $\alpha2$ agonists are often avoided as they reduce cardiac output and heart rate, although they may provide some cardioprotection, and, in cases of septal hypertrophy may actually improve stroke volume and cardiac output because the increased afterload relieves the dynamic outflow obstruction during systole.

46.7 Phaeochromocytoma

These tumours are not always easy to recognise or diagnose: release of hormones is not constant. Epinephrine (adrenaline) and norepinephrine (noradrenaline) production by the tumour result in 'sympathetic' effects:

- Hypertension, yet postural hypotension, because there is a relative hypovolaemia (blood volume 'shrinks' into the 'contracted' vasculature under the high sympathetic tone).
- Sustained high heart rate can result in cardiomyopathy, so beware arrhythmias.
- High O_2 and glucose demand (high metabolic rate).

46.7.1 Stabilise Pre-operatively

Encourage an increase in blood volume, i.e. gentle treatment with $\alpha1$ antagonists (phenoxybenzamine [there is evidence to support that pre-anaesthesia stabilisation improves surgical outcome], or even acepromazine), and perhaps even β blockers to reduce heart rate if very tachycardic (see below). Phenoxybenzamine causes irreversible pre- and post-synaptic α adrenoceptor block, resulting in what is sometimes called 'chemical sympathectomy'. An alternative would be phentolamine, a competitive α ($\alpha1 > \alpha2$) adrenoceptor antagonist.

It is important to **ensure α receptor block before β blockade is considered** because the use of β blockers alone can result in unopposed vasoconstriction and a hypertensive crisis.

Magnesium is sometimes used in human medicine as it reduces catecholamine release and has hypotensive effects.

46.7.2 Premedication

Should be aimed at anxiolysis, and a little vagomimetic activity is good (but you cannot always override the high sympathetic tone). Acepromazine with an opioid is a common choice. Avoid anticholinergics.

46.7.3 Induction

Should be smooth. Pre-oxygenate where possible. Injectable agents given IV, slowly to effect, are generally preferred, to avoid the potential stress and catecholamine release associated with inhalation inductions. Intravenous agents: avoid ketamine (increases sympathetic tone), and thiopental (arrhythmogenic). Etomidate can depress normal adrenal activity for several hours even following one dose, which may complicate post-operative care. Propofol tends to obtund the baroreceptor reflex-mediated tachycardic response to hypotension, which may, or not, be useful.

46.7.4 Maintenance

Supply $O_2 \pm$ medical air. Avoid N_2O (sympathetic stimulation). Use balanced anaesthetic and analgesic techniques. Avoid neuromuscular blocking agents with ganglionic effects where possible, and reversal of neuromuscular blockade normally requires anticholinergics, which may result in adverse side effects. Epidural/extradural local anaesthetics can cause profound hypotension (through splanchnic and caudal body vasodilation), whereas epidural opioids do not, and can provide good post-operative analgesia. NSAIDs may be administered once blood volume and arterial blood pressure are stabilised and adequate. Monitor cardiovascular variables.

Tumour handling may result in massive catecholamine release, such that a vasodilator (e.g. sodium nitroprusside, nicardipine) may be required. Tumours may invade local vasculature (including vena cava), the transient clamping-off of which (to resect tumour thrombi) can reduce venous return and cardiac output, and may cause tachycardic reflexes or occasionally bradycardia through the Bezold-Jarisch (vaso-vagal) reflex.

46.7.5 Recovery

Continue to monitor cardiovascular variables; also urine output. Post-operative circulatory support with fluids, positive inotropes, and vasopressors may be required.

46.8 Paraneoplastic Syndrome Hypercalcaemia (Pseudo-hyperparathyroidism)

Often associated with lymphoid type tumours, peri-anal adenomas/adenosarcomas, some bone tumours, and multiple myelomas.

Clinical signs of hypercalcaemia

- Bradyarrhythmias.
- Muscle weakness/twitches.
- Lethargy.
- Increased thirst (PU/PD).
- Urolithiasis.
- Metastatic calcification.
- Seizures.

Treat the hypercalcaemia first

- Rehydration, dilution/diuresis (calcium-free fluids), and calciuretics, e.g. furosemide. (Corticosteroids are also calciuretic.)
- Calcitonin reduces calcium mobilisation.
- Chelate the excess calcium: tetracyclines, trisodium edetate.
- In an emergency, sodium bicarbonate may be given to induce a mild metabolic alkalosis, as this can reduce the ionised calcium concentration, at least transiently.

- Bisphosphonate compounds: bind to bone mineral, inhibit osteoclast activity and enhance osteoblast activity.
- Mithramycin (plicamycin), a chemotherapeutic drug/antibiotic: inhibits osteoclast activity (many side effects).

Bone tumours, including metastatic bone tumours, can be painful, and bisphosphonates may have analgesic actions via NMDA receptor antagonism, in addition to inhibiting osteoclast activity.

46.9 Diabetes Insipidus

- Insufficient antidiuretic hormone (ADH) release or activity.
- Animals present with polydipsia/polyuria (renal medullary washout prevents urine concentration, so urine tends to be hyposthenuric), and polycythaemia.
- Animals are relatively vasodilated (Note: ADH = arginine vasopressin); so these animals tend to be absolutely and relatively hypovolaemic, and therefore hypotensive.
- Manage medically pre-anaesthesia where possible. Desmpresson (dDAVP™) is often used. Thiazide diuretics paradoxically can reduce urine output, but can also worsen hypovolaemia and cause severe electrolyte depletions: beware hyponatraemia, hypokalaemia, and hypochloraemia.
- Under anaesthesia, especially if not stabilised on medical treatment, careful fluid and electrolyte management is warranted.

46.10 Hyperaldosteronism (Conn's Syndrome)

Tends to present with hypernatraemia, hypokalaemia, metabolic alkalosis (and possible signs of hypocalcaemia, e.g. muscle cramps or weakness), an expanded ECF volume with systemic hypertension (retinal haemorrhage) and PU/PD. If electrolyte changes have occurred slowly, it is best to correct them slowly.

Further Reading

Association of Anaesthetists of Great Britain and Ireland (2015). Guidelines: Peri-operative management of the surgical patient with diabetes 2015. *Anaesthesia* 70: 1427–1440.

Evans, R.D. and Niu, Y. (2008). Hypolipidaemic effects of high-dose insulin therapy. Editorial. *British Journal of Anaesthesia* 100: 429–433.

Guedes, A.G. and Rude, E.P. (2013). Effects of pre-operative administration of medetomidine on plasma insulin and glucose concentrations in healthy dogs and dogs with insulinoma. *Veterinary Anaesthesia and Analgesia* 40: 472–481.

Herrera, M.A., Mehl, M.L., Kass, P.H. et al. (2008). Predictive factors and the effect of phenoxybenzamine on outcome in dogs undergoing adrenalectomy for pheochromocytoma. *Journal of Veterinary Internal Medicine* 22: 1333–1339.

Idowu, O. and Heading, K. (2018). Hypoglycemia in dogs: causes, management and diagnosis. *Canadian Veterinary Journal* 59: 642–649.

Kronen, P.W.M., Moon-Massat, P.F., Ludders, J.W. et al. (2001). Comparison of two insulin protocols for diabetic dogs undergoing cataract surgery. *Veterinary Anaesthesia and Analgesia* 28: 146–155.

Morgan, R.K., Cortes, Y., and Murphy, L. (2018). Pathophysiolgy and aetiology of hypoglycaemic crises. *Journal of Small Animal Practice* 59: 659–669.

Oliver, J.A., Clark, L., Corletto, F., and Gould, D.J. (2010). A comparison of anesthetic complications between diabetic and nondiabetic dogs undergoing phacoemulsification cataract surgery: a retrospective study. *Veterinary Ophthalmology* 13: 244–250.

Simpson, A.K., Levy, N., and Hall, G.M. (2008). Perioperative i/v fluids in diabetic patients – don't forget the salt. *Anaesthesia* 63: 1043–1045.

Steiner, J.M. and Bruvette, D.S. (1996). Canine Insulinoma. *The Compendium on Continuing Education for the Practising Veterinarian* 18: 13–23.

Stubbs, D.J., Levy, N., and Dhatariya, K. (2017). The rationale and strategies to achieve perioperative glycaemic control. *BJA Education* 17: 185–193.

Turina, M., Christ-Crain, M., and Polk, H.C. Jr. (2006). Diabetes and hyperglycemia; strict glycemic control. *Critical Care Medicine* 34 (Suppl 9): s291–s300. **(*Discusses the problems of hypoglycaemia with tight glycaemic control.*)**

Van den Bergh, G. (2004). How does blood glucose control with insulin save lives in intensive care? *The Journal of Clinical Investigation* 114: 1187–1195. **(*A good review of the side effects of hyperglycaemia and also hyperinsulinaemia.*)**

Veres-Nyeki, K.O. (2016). Endocrine diseases. In: *BSAVA Manual of Canine and Feline Anaesthesia and Analgesia*, 3e (eds. T. Duke-Novakovski, M. de Vries and C. Seymour), 376–391. Gloucester, UK: British Small Animal Veterinary Association.

Vukoja, E. (2019). Anaesthetic management of a patient undergoing unilateral phacoemulsification with concurrent diabetes mellitus. *The Veterinary Nurse* 10: 270–275.

Self-test Section

1 List at least five problems associated with thyroid surgery in hyperthyroid cats.

2 What are the anaesthetic considerations for a patient with diabetes mellitus and how would you manage the two most important?

3 What complications may be associated with anaesthesia for a patient with hyperadrenocorticism (Cushing's disease)?

47

Background to Neuroanaesthesia for the Brain

LEARNING OBJECTIVES

- To be familiar with the Monro-Kellie doctrine.
- To be able to list factors that influence intracranial pressure (ICP).
- To be aware of the strategies available to 'shrink' the brain in order to reduce or prevent further increases in ICP.
- To be familiar with how the various anaesthetic agents can affect ICP.
- To be able to use the modified Glasgow coma scale.

47.1 Introduction

Brain neurosurgery and neuroanaesthesia are very specialist fields requiring specialist facilities for preparation (advanced imaging modalities), surgery, and post-operative intensive aftercare. The notes here will only overview factors influencing anaesthesia for 'brain' reasons; spinal surgery considerations are discussed in Chapter 43.

47.2 The Monro–Kellie Doctrine

The skull is a non-compliant 'closed' bony box, such that the volume of its contents is somewhat fixed. The intracranial volume consists of:

- Brain parenchyma (84%).
- Blood perfusing the brain (4%).
- Cerebrospinal fluid (CSF) (12%).

An increase in the volume of one component may be compensated for (potentially incompletely) only by a decrease in one or both of the others:

- The brain parenchyma cannot alter its volume easily.
- The intracranial blood volume can alter a little.
- The intracranial CSF volume can alter a little.

For example, any change in intracranial blood or parenchymal volume is accompanied by an opposite change in CSF volume, if ICP is to be maintained constant. Once the intracranial volume compensation mechanisms have been exhausted, however, then further increases in intracranial volume lead to a rapid rise in ICP (Figure 47.1).

47.3 The Cerebral Circulation

Cerebrovascular autoregulation is the maintenance of a fairly constant cerebral blood flow (CBF) over a wide range of arterial blood pressures (mean arterial pressure [MAP] of around 60–70 to 150–160 mmHg). Cerebral blood vessels are also normally 'responsive' to blood gases (Figure 47.2). Abnormal vascular reactivity, however, may interfere with CBF autoregulation in 'diseased' brain.

The vessels usually alter their tone:

- With changes in arterial blood pressure.
- With changes in $PaCO_2$ (i.e. changes in $[H^+]$):
  - Dilate with increased $PaCO_2$ (up to 80 mmHg/10.7 kPa).
  - Constrict with decreased $PaCO_2$ (down to 20 mmHg/2.7 kPa).
- With changes in PaO_2:
  - Dilate if $PaO_2 < 50$ mmHg (<6.7 kPa).
  - Constrict if $PaO_2 > 300$ mmHg (>40 kPa).
- With changes in temperature.

Veterinary Anaesthesia: Principles to Practice, Second Edition. Alexandra H. A. Dugdale, Georgina Beaumont, Carl Bradbrook, and Matthew Gurney.
© 2020 John Wiley & Sons Ltd. Published 2020 by John Wiley & Sons Ltd.
Companion website: www.wiley.com/go/dugdale/veterinary-anaesthesia

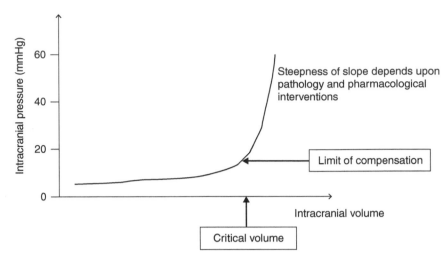

Figure 47.1 Intracranial compliance curve, illustrating how changes in intracranial volume affect intracranial pressure. Note that once the volume has reached the critical volume (limit of compensation), ICP increases dramatically.

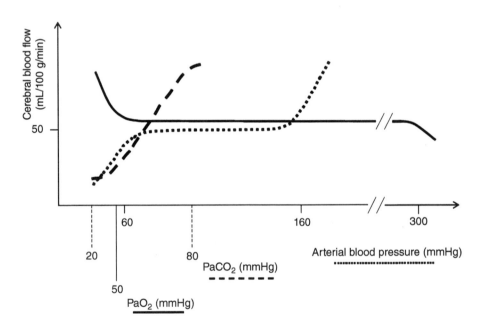

Figure 47.2 Cerebral blood flow regulation by arterial blood pressure and blood gases.

47.3.1 Coupling of CBF and Cerebral Metabolic Rate

As in many other tissues, CBF is influenced by cerebral metabolism (products of metabolism affect vessel tone), and regional variations occur:

- CBF in grey matter is c. 110 ml/100 g/min.
- CBF in white matter is c. 52 ml/100 g/min.

CBF also depends upon activity state (awake, asleep, anaesthetised).

47.3.2 Cerebral Perfusion Pressure (CPP)

$$CPP = \text{Mean arterial pressure } (MAP) - \text{Intracranial pressure } (ICP)$$

CPP and CVR (cerebral vascular resistance), determine CBF:

$$\left.\begin{array}{l} CBF = CPP/CVR \\ CBF = (MAP - ICP/CVR) \end{array}\right\} \begin{array}{l}\text{Vascular responsiveness} \\ \text{is important}\end{array}$$

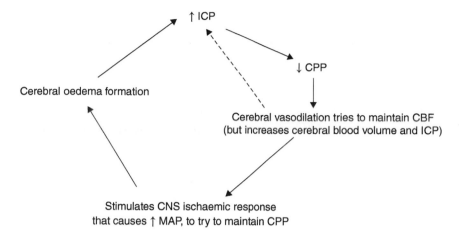

Figure 47.3 Vicious circle of raised intracranial pressure.

And:

$$ICP = MAP - CPP$$

47.3.2.1 Raised Intracranial Pressure

Normal ICP is 5–15 mmHg. With intracranial pathology, there may be:

- Alteration of neural function because of the primary pathological process itself.
- Impairment of function of the surrounding neural tissue because of oedema formation ± the development of raised intracranial pressure (with or without impaired CSF drainage).

47.3.2.1.1 Causes of Raised Intracranial Pressure

- Increased volume of brain parenchyma:
  - Cerebral oedema (4 types are recognised: vasogenic (leaky BBB), cytotoxic (hypoxia/ischaemia; impaired cellular metabolism); osmotic (hyponatraemia, hyperosmolar states); interstitial (leaky CSF:brain barrier so CSF [normally very low protein] permeates brain parenchyma)
  - Haemorrhage
  - Inflammation
  - Space occupying lesions (tumour/abscess)
- Increased volume of CSF (hydrocephalus):
  - Increased production of CSF (choroid plexus tumours)
  - Decreased drainage of CSF (brain 'swelling', space occupying lesions)
- Increased intravascular volume in cerebral vessels:
  - Head down position
  - Jugular occlusion
  - Valsalva-like manoeuvres that increase intrathoracic pressure, e.g. coughing, sneezing, retching, gagging, vomiting
  - Positive pressure ventilation (increases jugular/central venous pressure)

  - Abdominal compartment syndrome (increases jugular/central venous pressure)
  - Poor cerebral autoregulation (central nervous system [CNS] disease; anaesthetic effects; extreme hypertension)
  - Greatly increased $PaCO_2$; greatly decreased PaO_2
- Extraparenchymal:
  - Space occupying lesion
  - Haemorrhage (epidural/subdural/subarachnoid)

Once ICP increases, a vicious circle may be entered (Figure 47.3).

47.3.2.1.2 Clinical Signs of Raised Intracranial Pressure

- Decreased level of consciousness or mentation (depressed, stuporous, or comatose); changes in behaviour
- Seizures
- Cranial nerve deficits:
  - Changes in pupil size (may be different between left and right = anisocoria, or pin-point pupils)
  - Abnormal pupillary light response (PLR)
  - Reduced to absent oculo-cephalic and oculo-vestibular reflexes
  - Nystagmus and/or strabismus
  - Papilloedema (oedema/swelling of the optic discs as seen with an ophthalmoscope)
  - Blindness
  - Deafness
  - Dysphagia
  - Dysphonia
  - Dyspnoea
- Other neurological deficits (e.g. head tilt, circling, gait changes)
- Nausea and vomiting
- Circulatory and respiratory changes (**Cushing's triad,** cardiac arrhythmias, neurogenic pulmonary oedema)
  - Abnormal respiratory pattern

- Risk of brain herniation (cerebellar herniation ['coning'] is only one of many types of brain herniation)
- Decerebrate or decerebellate posture

Cushing's Triad

- Systemic hypertension.
- Bradycardia (partly reflex, due to the hypertension, and may also be partly due to compression of the vasomotor centre). BUT bradycardia is often a very late occurrence, so tachycardia may also be seen.
- Altered breathing patterns (usually due to compression of the respiratory centre).

The CNS response to rising ICP results in the 'CNS hypoxic/ischaemic response'; in which there is a massive sympathetic discharge, hence systemic hypertension (and possibly early tachycardia, with later reflex bradycardia). This massive increase in sympathetic tone may be responsible for neurogenic pulmonary oedema and cardiac arrhythmias (neurogenic cardiomyopathy).

47.4 Aims of Anaesthetic Management

- Reduce ICP (or prevent further increase in ICP).
- Promote cerebral autoregulation.
- Control seizure activity.
- Control blood glucose and beware wide swings in body temperature.
- Provide 'neuroprotection' during potential ischaemic and reperfusion episodes.

Pre-anaesthetic 'stabilisation' is important.

47.4.1 Strategies to Alleviate Raised Intracranial Pressure

- Try to shrink the brain tissue ('brain relaxation strategies').
- Reduce the CSF volume.
- Reduce the volume of blood within the CNS.
- Increase the volume allowance of the skull.

47.4.1.1 Nursing Strategies that Also Apply to Anaesthesia

Various strategies are available, many of which are aimed at reducing ICP and/or minimising further increases in ICP, and include:

- Raising the head by 30° (any more can compromise cerebral perfusion).
  - Avoid flexion, extension, and twisting of the neck, all of which might occlude the jugular veins and increase ICP.

- Minimising jugular vein pressure/occlusion; NO jugular blood samples.
- Reducing coughing, retching, and straining (Valsalva-like manoeuvres increase CVP and therefore ICP).
  - Consider bladder catheterisation and assisted bowel evacuation.
- Judicious IV fluid therapy; maintain MAP in the autoregulatory range (from 60 to 70 mmHg up to around 150–160 mmHg), although autoregulation may be impaired so that CPP becomes passively dependent upon MAP. It might, therefore, be prudent to maintain MAP between 80 and 120 mmHg, avoiding hypotension and therefore reduced cerebral perfusion with potential cerebral ischaemia, on the one hand, and also avoiding hypertension with increased CPP that increases ICP, on the other.
- Control pain and anxiety; but large doses of sedatives and opioids can obtund ventilation, with resultant hypercapnia that can further increase ICP.
- Control seizures. Seizures increase cerebral metabolic demands, so tend to promote CBF. They also promote hyperthermia and hypoglycaemia and can result in hypercapnia and hypoxaemia if ventilation is compromised. Controlling seizures also reduces the risk of cerebral damage and inflammation, which promotes further increases in ICP. Drugs, including benzodiazepines, barbiturates (e.g. phenobarbital), levetiracetam, propofol, dexmedetomidine, and ketamine may be useful in managing seizure activity. (Note that airway protection and artificial ventilation may also be required).
- Control pyrexia; ideally maintain rectal temperature between 37 and 38.5 °C. Although moderate hypothermia can be neuroprotective, it has cardiovascular, respiratory, metabolic, and rheological effects, and should only be induced with careful monitoring. Large, rapid swings in temperature should be avoided where possible.
- Monitor blood glucose and aim to keep it within normal range (normal is c. 4–6 mmol/l).
- Monitor electrolytes (especially where osmotherapy/diuresis is employed).
- Oxygen therapy may be considered/indicated, but beware with nasal prongs as they may provoke sneezing which raises ICP.
- Monitor blood gases where appropriate and aim for normoxia and normocapnia.
  - Should artificial ventilation be required, normocapnia should be targeted *unless* ICP is so high that there is imminent danger of herniation. In these cases, hyperventilation may be instituted (until other measures to reduce ICP can be instigated), but only to end tidal CO_2 (or, preferably, $PaCO_2$) tensions of around 30 mmHg. Lower values, especially once $PaCO_2$ reaches ~20 mmHg, risk cerebral ischaemia due to cerebral vasoconstriction.

Table 47.1 Modified Glasgow Coma Scale.

MODIFIED GLASGOW COMA SCALE		Score
MOTOR ACTIVITY	Normal gait, normal spinal reflexes	6
	Hemiparesis, tetraparesis, or decerebrate rigidity	5
	Recumbent, intermittent extensor rigidity	4
	Recumbent, constant extensor rigidity	3
	Recumbent, constant extensor rigidity with opisthotonos	2
	Recumbent, hypotonia of muscles, depressed, or absent spinal reflexes	1
BRAINSTEM REFLEXES	Normal PLR and oculocephalic reflexes	6
	Slow PLR and normal to reduced oculocephalic (Doll's head) reflexes	5
	Bilateral, unresponsive miosis with normal to reduced oculocephalic reflexes	4
	Pinpoint pupils with reduced to absent oculocephalic reflexes	3
	Unilateral, unresponsive mydriasis with reduced to absent oculocephalic reflexes	2
	Bilateral, unresponsive mydriasis with reduced to absent oculocephalic reflexes	1
LEVEL OF CONSCIOUSNESS	Occasional periods of alertness and responsiveness to environment	6
	Depression or delirium, capable of responding, but response may be inappropriate	5
	Semi-comatose, responsive to visual stimuli	4
	Semi-comatose, responsive to auditory stimuli	3
	Semi-comatose, responsive to repeated noxious stimuli	2
	Comatose, unresponsive to repeated noxious stimuli	1

Hyperventilation is only a transient strategy because after four to six or so hours, the brain re-sets its autoregulatory limits so that it becomes tolerant to hypocapnia-induced cerebral vasoconstriction (by a reduction in CSF and extracellular fluid bicarbonate concentration and correction of CSF/extracellular pH). If hyperventilation is now stopped abruptly, cerebral reactive hyperaemia occurs, increasing ICP dramatically. The mechanical effects of positive pressure ventilation can also increase ICP, secondary to increasing the intrathoracic pressure and thereby increasing the CVP.

- Monitor cardiorespiratory function. Note that following raised ICP, the CNS ischaemic response, with its huge increase in sympathetic tone, may result in neurogenic cardiomyopathy (arrhythmias are possible) and neurogenic pulmonary oedema (often blood-tinged).
- Monitor neurological status (modified Glasgow Coma Scale score; see Tables 47.1 and 47.2).
- Consider osmotherapy and diuresis (see below).
- Consider drugs that may reduce CSF production (see below).

47.4.1.2 Osmotherapy and Diuresis

Be aware of the patient's hydration and intravascular volume status.

Table 47.2 Interpretation of modified Glasgow Coma Scale scores.

MGCS score	Prognosis
3–8	Grave
9–14	Guarded
15–18	Good

47.4.1.2.1 Mannitol

Both 10% (100 mg/ml) and 20% (200 mg/ml) solutions are commonly used. They may require gentle warming before administration as mannitol can crystallise at lower temperatures. Both can be administered by peripheral veins, but intravenous cannulae are recommended and must be flushed well after infusion to protect against phlebitis.

- Reduces blood viscosity (shrinks red blood cells and promotes haemodilution through osmotic effects) and shrinks brain parenchyma, and also vascular endothelial cells, so may improve tissue perfusion and O_2 delivery. Improved cerebral O_2 delivery can result in cerebral vasoconstriction and reduced ICP.
- Scavenges free radicals, so possibly helps versus reperfusion injury.

- A transient increase in ICP can occur as water is drawn into the intravascular compartment before diuresis gets underway (and the direct effect of high osmolarity on blood vessels may cause some vasodilation, although this effect may be offset by the vasoconstriction which follows a decrease in blood viscosity). For this reason, **IV administration over 15–30 minutes** is recommended; some texts also advocate a dose of **furosemide pre-mannitol** in cases of severely raised ICP (see below).
- About 45 minutes after mannitol is given, an osmotic diuresis occurs (aided and abetted by its effects to increase ANP release, but inhibit ADH release), which can result in profound hypotension (which may reduce CPP and compromise cerebral perfusion). Careful monitoring of systemic blood pressure is warranted. Electrolytes should also be monitored as the diuresis can result in hypokalaemia, hypomagnesaemia, and hypophosphataemia. Loss of bicarbonate also occurs, so vigilance about blood pH is wise.
- Avoid multiple doses: rebound increased ICP may occur as mannitol can get inside brain cells and water follows.
- **Beware intracranial haemorrhage and increased blood–brain barrier permeability**: wherever blood goes, mannitol goes, and water follows.
- Dose c. 0.25–1 g/kg (this may be administered as 'split' doses totalling 1 g/kg).

47.4.1.2.2 Hypertonic Saline

- Commonly a 7.2% solution is used, but technically any saline solution stronger than 0.9% is hypertonic compared with normal plasma. Solutions over 3% are, however, best administered by a central vein (and via a cannula) to reduce the likelihood of phlebitis.
- A huge increase in intravascular volume follows its infusion, accompanied by massive intracellular and interstitial dehydration. Unlike mannitol, there is not such a profound diuresis, but rather a relatively prolonged increase in blood volume, which subsides (over about an hour), leaving the cells relatively dehydrated, but the extracellular compartments slightly hypertonic/hypernatraemic.
- Can cause hypernatraemia and hyperchloraemic metabolic acidosis; monitor electrolytes and pH.
- May be useful to reduce cerebral oedema (cytotoxic/cellular oedema) without the risk of rebound oedema formation.
- Also useful for circulatory resuscitation in trauma cases, but beware its use in cases with intracranial haemorrhage (because re-bleeding or further bleeding is promoted). In cases of traumatic brain injury, where ongoing intracranial bleeding can be ruled out, it appears to help restore neuronal membrane potential and endothelial Na^+/glutamate pump activity (which helps protect against the excito-toxic effects of excess glutamate release) and helps maintain blood–brain-barrier integrity.
- Maximum dose of 4 ml/kg of 7.2% NaCl is recommended to reduce risk of significant hypernatraemia, which can be administered incrementally in smaller doses/volumes. Monitor sodium; wide swings in sodium can result in central pontine demyelination (myelinolysis).

47.4.1.2.3 Furosemide

- Potent diuretic (also natriuretic, kaliuretic, calciuretic and magnesiuretic, so consider monitoring electrolytes).
- Resultant whole body hypovolaemia reduces cerebral blood volume and ICP.
- Decreases CSF production too.
- Potentiates effects of mannitol to improve overall 'brain relaxation'.
- Doses range from 0.5–2 mg/kg as a single IV bolus to 1 mg/kg/h as a continuous infusion.

47.4.1.2.4 Oncodiuretic Therapy

Combination of diuretic and colloid to attempt to create normovolaemic dehydration. Requires careful monitoring.

47.4.1.3 Glucocorticosteroids

Useful in reducing ICP in some cases, including certain inflammatory brain conditions, and in reducing oedema associated with tumours. Use is contraindicated in cases of head trauma. Multiple actions including:

- Diuresis.
- 'Membrane stabilisation' and anti-inflammatory activity: help to limit cellular damage following ischaemia.
- Reduction in vasogenic inflammatory or tumour-associated cerebral oedema.
- Possible modulation of neurotransmitter release.
- Dexamethasone c. 0.1–0.5 mg/kg IV.
- Methylprednisolone sodium succinate c. 30 mg/kg.
- For some cases (usually tumours), best if given for several hours (preferably days) before general anaesthesia for maximal effect.

47.4.1.4 Reduce CSF Production

Furosemide and acetazolamide are diuretics that also reduce CSF formation. Furthermore, omeprazole given IV reduces CSF production by around one quarter (in dogs), and is often administered alongside glucocorticoids (which also reduce CSF production), as a gastro-protectant.

47.4.1.5 Cerebrospinal Fluid Drainage

Occasionally done as an emergency procedure, e.g. CSF is aspirated from the cerebral ventricles (to extend the

Table 47.3 Effects of anaesthetic agents on intracranial pressure.

Drug	CBF	CMRO$_2$	CBF: CMRO$_2$ coupling	ICP
Halothane	↑↑↑	↓	Uncoupled (favourably?)	↑↑
Isoflurane Sevoflurane	↑	↓↓	Uncoupled (favourably)	↑
N$_2$O	↑	↑	?	↑
Barbiturates	↓↓↓	↓↓↓	Maintained	↓↓
Propofol	↓↓	↓↓	Maintained	↓↓
Alfaxalone	↓↓	↓↓	Maintained	↓↓
Ketamine	↑↑	↑	All but maintained	↑
Etomidate	↓↓↓	↓↓	All but maintained	↓
Benzodiazepines	↓↓	↓↓	Maintained	↓↓
Opioids	↑/↓	↓ (?)	?	↑/↓

CMRO$_2$ = cerebral metabolic rate for oxygen.

time before surgical intervention [e.g. ventriculo-peritoneal shunt placement] can be made), in cases of hydrocephalus.

47.4.1.6 Craniotomy and Durotomy
Requires surgery and therefore anaesthesia.

47.4.2 Anaesthetic Protocols for Patients with Raised ICP

See above for helpful strategies to manage ICP. The reader is referred to specialist texts. Table 47.3 outlines the effects of the common anaesthetic drugs on ICP. Many anaesthetic agents, both inhalant and injectable, also have neuroprotective properties.

Further Reading

Bradshaw, K. and Smith, M. (2008). Disorders of sodium balance after brain injury. *Continuing Education and Anaesthesia, Critical Care and Pain* 8: 129–133. (***Explains the cerebral salt wasting syndrome and brain-related causes of the syndrome of inappropriate ADH secretion.***)

Brian, J.E. Jr. (1998). Carbon dioxide and the cerebral circulation. *Anesthesiology* 88: 1365–1386.

Freeman, N. and Welbourne, J. (2018). Osmotherapy: science and evidence-based practice. *BJA Education* 18: 284–290. (***See correction in volume 19 (2019), page 34.***)

Gregory, T. and Smith, M. (2012). Cardiovascular complications of brain injury. *Continuing Education in Anaesthesia, Critical Care and Pain* 12: 67–71.

King, J.M., Roth, L., and Haschek, W.M. (1982). Myocardial necrosis secondary to neural lesions in domestic animals. *Journal of the American Veterinary Medical Association* 180: 144–148.

Lawther, B.K., Kumar, S., and Krovvidi, H. (2011). Blood–brain barrier. *Continuing Education in Anaesthesia, Critical Care and Pain* 11: 128–132.

Leece, E.A. (2016). Neurological disease. In: *BSAVA Manual of Canine and Feline Anaesthesia and Analgesia*, 3e

(eds. T. Duke-Novakovski, M. de Vries and C. Seymour), 392–408. Gloucester, UK: British Small Animal Veterinary Association.

Leonard, S.E. and Kirby, R. (2002). The role of glutamate, calcium and magnesium in secondary brain injury. *Journal of Veterinary Emergency and Critical Care* 12: 17–32.

Menon, D.K. and Summors, A.C. (1998). Neuroprotection (including hypothermia). *Current Opinion in Anaesthesiology* 11: 485–496.

Mishra, L.D., Rajkumar, N., and Hancock, S.M. (2006). Current controversies in neuroanaesthesia, head injury management and neuro critical care. *Continuing Education in Anaesthesia, Critical Care and Pain* 6: 79–82.

Moss, E. (2001). The cerebral circulation. *British Journal of Anaesthesia CEPD Reviews* 1: 67–71.

Nishiyama, T., Matsukawa, T., Yokoyama, T. Hanaoka, K. (1999). Cerebrovascular carbon dioxide reactivity during general anaesthesia: a comparison between sevoflurane and isoflurane. *Anesthesia and Analgesia* 89: 1437–1441.

Reddy, U., White, M.J., and Wilson, S.R. (2012). Anaesthesia for magnetic resonance imaging. *Continuing Education in Anaesthesia, Critical Care and Pain* 12: 140–144.

Sankhynan, N., Vykunta Raju, K.N., Sharma, S., and Gulati, S. (2010). Management of raised intracranial pressure. *Indian Journal of Paediatrics* 77: 1409–1466.

Shawkat, H., Westwood, M.-M., and Mortimer, A. (2012). Mannitol: a review of its clinical uses. *Continuing Education in Anaesthesia, Critical Care and Pain* 12: 82–85.

Tameem, A. and Krovvidi, H. (2013). Cerebral physiology. *Continuing Education in Anaesthesia, Critical Care and Pain* 13: 113–118.

White, H., Cook, D., and Venkatesh, B. (2006). The use of hypertonic saline for treating intracranial hypertension after traumatic brain injury. *Anesthesia and Analgesia* 102: 1836–1846.

Self-test Section

1 True or False? A dog with a modified Glasgow coma scale score of 16 probably has a better prognosis than one with a MGCS score of 12.

2 Which of the following agents reduces CBF?
   A Isoflurane
   B Alfaxalone
   C Ketamine
   D Nitrous oxide

48

Cardiac Considerations

LEARNING OBJECTIVE

- To be able to outline the strategies for different cardiac problems.

48.1 General Anaesthetic Aims

With cardiac compromise, the general aims during anaesthesia are:

- Maintain cardiac output.
- Avoid hypotension or hypertension.
- Avoid excessive tachycardia or bradycardia.
- Avoid increasing myocardial workload (myocardial O_2 demand).
- Avoid things that cause direct myocardial depression (negative inotropy).
- Avoid arrhythmogens.
- Maintain good ventilation, with adequate oxygenation (and avoid large changes in pH and PCO_2).
- Avoid fluid under- and over-load.

A good cardiac workup before general anaesthesia is invaluable: echocardiography, blood pressure measurement, and ECG are recommended, if indicated from the clinical examination. History of syncope or collapse is important. For dogs, **exercise tolerance is a good indicator of cardiorespiratory reserves**, but not always easy to determine if patients have painful orthopaedic disease. Increased resting heart rate (with lack of respiratory sinus arrhythmia) and increased resting breathing rate can be good indicators of underlying cardiac disease. Attempt to resolve clinical signs of congestive heart failure and arrhythmias before general anaesthesia (see also Chapter 25).

48.2 Some Particular Problems

48.2.1 A-V Valvular Insufficiencies, Especially Mitral Insufficiency

Common in older animals. Mitral insufficiency results in:

- Gradual increase in pulmonary venous pressure that causes pulmonary congestion and finally pulmonary oedema (cats often develop pleural and pericardial fluid accumulation too), leading to decreased pulmonary compliance.
- Increased left atrial pressure and left ventricular volume overload.
- Increased right ventricular work (increased afterload due to pulmonary hypertension) may result in cor pulmonale (right-sided heart failure) eventually.

48.2.1.1 Anaesthetic Considerations
- Pre-oxygenate (stress-free).
- Minimise inotropic changes (positive inotropes may actually increase the regurgitant fraction and increase myocardial work).
- Aim to maintain heart rate near 'normal'; a slight increase is better than a marked decrease, as slower heart rates increase ventricular filling time and can increase regurgitation.
- A small decrease in afterload (systemic vascular resistance) may facilitate improved cardiac output (by encouraging

Veterinary Anaesthesia: Principles to Practice, Second Edition. Alexandra H. A. Dugdale, Georgina Beaumont, Carl Bradbrook, and Matthew Gurney.
© 2020 John Wiley & Sons Ltd. Published 2020 by John Wiley & Sons Ltd.
Companion website: www.wiley.com/go/dugdale/veterinary-anaesthesia

'forwards' flow, and reducing the regurgitant fraction), but if forwards blood velocity increases, turbulence, and regurgitation may increase. Possibly avoid high doses of ketamine and N$_2$O (increase sympathetic tone and may increase systemic vascular resistance, thereby increasing the regurgitant fraction and reducing cardiac output). A slight decrease in pulmonary vascular resistance may also be beneficial as many patients develop pulmonary hypertension in later stages of the disease.

- Maintain central venous pressure (preload). (See Table 48.1.)
- Artificial ventilation (manual or mechanical ventilation, usually in the form of positive pressure ventilation) may be helpful. In the face of pulmonary congestion and oedema, positive pressure ventilation can displace some of the pulmonary blood volume back to the systemic circulation, but care with peak inspiratory pressure so as not to decrease venous return too much.

48.2.2 Cardiomyopathies

The inotropic state of the heart is compromised in both hypertrophic and dilated forms. Reduced myocardial compliance means cardiac output becomes dependent upon heart rate, so avoid large changes in heart rate; and try to maintain preload/venous return/central venous pressure (CVP). See also notes on hyperthyroidism in Chapter 46.

48.2.3 Pericardial Effusions

Rate and volume of fluid accumulation in pericardial sac determines if **cardiac tamponade** ensues.

48.2.3.1 Causes

- Idiopathic (Golden retrievers).
- Neoplastic: haemangiosarcoma (primary or secondary), heart base tumour/chemodectoma. (Abdominal ultrasonography may detect other tumours in liver and/or spleen.)
- Traumatic.

- Cardiac rupture, e.g. left atrial tears from jet lesions due to A-V valve incompetence.
- Iatrogenic (e.g. from intracardiac or attempted intracardiac injection during CPCR, or during attempted pericardiocentesis, where damage to coronary vessels or laceration of the heart itself may occur).
- Anticoagulant toxicity.

48.2.3.2 Clinical Signs

- **Beck's triad**: Increased jugular vein distension (increased CVP), muffled heart sounds (and reduced intensity of apex beat), systemic hypotension (reduced pulse pressure).
- **Ascites (hepatosplenomegaly)**, **pleural effusion**, **pulmonary oedema.**
- **Tachycardia.**
- Possible positive '**hepatojugular reflux**'. If you gently squeeze ('hug') the abdomen over the liver region, you increase the filling of the venae cavae, which increases jugular distension. Sometimes called **Kussmaul's sign**. Not to be confused with Kussmaul's respiration (see Chapter 50).
- **Pulsus paradoxus**. On inspiration, the negative intrathoracic pressure and lung expansion tend to draw blood into the lungs, so reducing venous return to the left atrium, leading to reduced left ventricular filling, which reduces left ventricular stroke volume output, which therefore reduces pulse pressure. Negative intrathoracic pressure also 'sucks' blood towards the right atrium from the venae cavae, but the high pericardial pressure precludes much of this venous return from entering the right atrium. However, any extra right ventricular filling also reduces left ventricular filling (ventricular interdependence), so worsening the noted **fall in pulse pressure during inspiration**. The paradox is that this exaggerated reduction in pulse pressure (and perhaps absence of detectable peripheral pulse) occurs when a heartbeat can be auscultated.
- **Electrical alternans** on ECG.

Table 48.1 Cardiovascular effects of common anaesthetic induction agents. Note that ketamine's effects depend upon sympathetic stimulation; therefore, in 'shocky' patients (with already high sympathetic tone or sympathetic exhaustion), its negative inotropic and direct vasodilative effects may become apparent and hypotension may occur.

Injectable anaesthetic agent	Heart rate	Arterial blood pressure	Contractility	Systemic vascular resistance	Cardiac output
Propofol	↔	↓	↓	↓	↓
Alfaxalone	↑	↔↓	↔	↔↓	↔↑
Ketamine	↑	↑	↔↑	↔↑	↑
Etomidate	↔	↔	↔	↔	↔

48.2.3.3 Sedation/Anaesthetic Considerations

Pre-operatively, drainage of even a small quantity of pericardial fluid can greatly improve the patient's condition. Drainage can be performed under sedation/local anaesthesia. Low dose acepromazine with an opioid (butorphanol or methadone) and use of infiltration local anaesthesia is a common choice. (Note that morphine causes pulmonary vasodilation that can help relieve the discomfort of dyspnoea, but if given in place of methadone, beware its emetic effect, although this can be reduced by giving acepromazine 15 minutes earlier.)

Avoid reduction in heart rate. Opioids can reduce heart rate in the order: fentanyl > methadone, morphine > butorphanol, and buprenorphine > pethidine (theoretically, at least). (In combination with acepromazine, opioid-dependent lowering of the heart rate can be somewhat moderated by the slight tachycardic response to hypotension.) Avoid reduction in CVP (venous return): IV fluids are indicated, often as a bolus pre-operatively, but beware exacerbating oedema. Have positive inotropes, vasopressors, and anticholinergics on stand-by. If positive pressure ventilation is required, deliver small tidal volumes (low peak inspiratory pressure), at a relatively fast rate, for minimal reduction of venous return/cardiac output.

48.2.4 Patent Ductus Arteriosus

- Left to right shunting of blood (until shunt reverses).
- Pulmonary blood volume is augmented leading to pulmonary hypertension/congestion.
- Systemic blood volume is diminished leading to systemic hypotension that causes increased sympathetic tone, increased renin, angiotensin, aldosterone, and antidiuretic hormone (ADH) production, which result in increased fluid retention in an attempt to increase venous return and cardiac output.
- Augmented pulmonary blood volume increases venous return to the left atrium and ventricle, leading to volume overload and eccentric hypertrophy (and A-V valve incompetence).
- Slightly increased right ventricular 'afterload' causes slight pressure overload of the right ventricle and possible concentric hypertrophy.

If pulmonary vascular resistance is greater than systemic vascular resistance, then the shunt reverses (becomes right to left [Eisenmenger's syndrome]). The 'admixture' of pulmonary arterial ('mixed venous') and systemic arterial blood results in systemic hypoxaemia; cranial mucous membranes are pink, but caudal mucous membranes are cyanosed (the ductus enters between ascending and descending parts of the aorta). Prognosis is now poor, and surgery contra-indicated because the ductus represents a pressure relief valve. Attempted closure would result in acute right heart failure and death.

48.2.4.1 Anaesthetic Considerations

- Treat signs of congestive heart failure first.
- Patients often young, but not usually truly 'neonatal': prevent hypothermia.
- Try to avoid things that increase the degree of left-to-right shunting (e.g. hypoxaemia, hypercapnia, acidosis, stress (sympathetic activation), ketamine, and N_2O [sympathetic activation]), but at the same time, you do not want to encourage reversal of flow either (e.g. marked systemic hypotension). Some people favour a slight decrease in peripheral vascular resistance, and may use a low dose of acepromazine to this end. (Acepromazine, however, may promote a reduction in systemic vascular resistance whilst leaving pulmonary vascular resistance unchanged, so *may* promote shunt reversal. *But* the systemic vasodilation also allows redistribution of blood volume away from the lungs to the systemic circulation, which can also help keep systemic pressure up.)
- Aim to use drugs with minimal C-V depressant effects as there is reduced cardiovascular reserve.
- Pre-oxygenate (in as stress-free a manner as possible).
- For thoracotomies, neuromuscular blockade and positive pressure ventilation are usually required. Positive pressure ventilation is actually very well tolerated because of the augmented pulmonary blood volume (and the open chest). Balanced analgesia can include local/regional techniques. Consider non-steroidal anti-inflammatory drugs (NSAIDs) as part of a balanced analgesia regimen too. Interestingly, NSAIDs have been used in neonates to try to encourage closure of the ductus arteriosus by reducing prostaglandin production. If the shunt is to be ligated, beware the **Branham reflex**: anticholinergics may be necessary. The **Branham reflex/sign** is the sudden reduction in heart rate at shunt ligation. Possibly due to massive left ventricular back-pressure/stretch; or due to sudden increase in systemic arterial pressure which initiates a baroreceptor reflex response. Amplatzer devices occlude more slowly, over 15 minutes, so less dramatic heart rate changes occur. Monitor cardiorespiratory variables closely. Following thoracotomy, the chest drain will need attention post-operatively.

48.2.5 Atrial and Ventricular Septal Defects

Left-to-right shunts again. Keep the shunt direction left-to-right; therefore use a similar approach to patent ductus arteriosus.

48.2.6 Pulmonic and Aortic/subaortic Stenoses

Pre-operative workup is again important. Aim to maintain pressure drop across the stenosis. Ensure adequate preload (CVP) is maintained: fluids/vasopressors. Aim for minimal myocardial depression (minimal negative inotropy). Provide supplemental oxygen. If balloon bougienage is to be performed, beware 'suicidal right ventricle' in cases of severe pulmonic stenosis, where sudden reduction in afterload results in dynamic 'collapse' of the right ventricular outflow tract (IV fluids, vasopressors and beta blockers may be required), and in all cases closely monitor the ECG intra-operatively and for 24+ hours post-operatively.

48.2.7 Pacemaker Implantation

Does the animal have any myocardial disease or just a disorder of contraction rate? It is always reassuring to have external pacing electrodes available as severe bradycardia/asystole, e.g. upon induction of anaesthesia, is the biggest risk.

48.2.8 Atrial Fibrillation in Horses

Atrial fibrillation (AF) is a relatively common arrhythmia in larger breed horses. To determine its impact on cardiovascular function, measure the pulse rate (ventricular response rate). If ventricular rate is normal (<45 bpm), then the horse is unlikely to be in heart failure (but horses have a huge cardiovascular reserve). Auscultate for additional murmurs. If in doubt, echocardiography is indicated. The diagnosis of AF may alter the decision for surgery.

If no other cardiac disease is present, then AF alone is not a contra-indication to anaesthesia, nor does it mean that normal sinus rhythm **must** be established before anaesthesia as there are risks associated with converting to normal sinus rhythm, and many sedatives, analgesics, and anaesthetic agents have vagomimetic properties and so tend to 'encourage' AF to recur. If possible, vagolytic (e.g. atropine) and sympathomimetic (e.g. dobutamine) drugs should be avoided as these can increase the ventricular rate. Otherwise, the commonly used sedative and anaesthetic agents can be used. Close monitoring, especially of pulse rate, ECG, and blood pressure are important.

Further Reading

Cross, M. and Plunkett, E. (2014). Cardiovascular physiology. In: *Physics, Pharmacology and Physiology for Anaesthetists. Key Concepts for the FRCA*, 2e, 239–280. Cambridge, UK: Cambridge University Press.

Gurney, M. and Bradbrook, C. (2016). Common ECG abnormalities in the perioperative period. *In Practice* 38: 219–228.

Humm, K.R., Senior, J.M., Dugdale, A.H., and Summerfield, N.J. (2007). Use of sodium nitroprusside in the anaesthetic protocol of a patent ductus arteriosus ligation in a dog. *The Veterinary Journal* 173: 194–196.

James, R.A. (2007). Use of pacemakers in dogs. *In Practice* 29: 503–511.

Robinson, R. and Borgeat, K. (2016). Cardiovascular disease. In: *BSAVA Manual of Canine and Feline Anaesthesia and Analgesia*, 3e (eds. T. Duke-Novakovski, M. de Vries and C. Seymour), 283–313. Gloucester, UK: British Small Animal Veterinary Association.

Scarabelli, S. and Bradbrook, C. (2016). Anaesthesia of the patient with cardiovascular disease part 1: risk assessment. *Companion Animal* 21: 280–284.

Scarabelli, S. and Bradbrook, C. (2016). Anaesthesia of the patient with cardiovascular disease part 2: anaesthesia for specific disorders. *Companion Animal* 21: 337–344.

Self-test Section

1 What is Beck's triad?
   A The three requirements for coagulation
   B The three common signs associated with raised intracranial pressure
   C The clinical signs associated with pericardial effusions/cardiac compression (tamponade)
   D The three classically described causes of hypoxia
   E The three confirmatory tests commonly used in hypoglycaemia (insulinoma) cases

2 What would be your anaesthetic considerations for a patient with mitral valve degenerative disease? List the most important five factors.

49

Respiratory Considerations

49.1 Brachycephalic Obstructive Airway Syndrome (BOAS)

BOAS is also known as brachycephalic airway obstruction syndrome (BAOS) or brachycephalic upper airway syndrome (BUAS). Breeds affected are (most to least affected): Bulldogs (English, French*), Pugs*, Boston Terriers, Pekingese, Boxers, Persian cats. (*Most frequently presented.) Components of the syndrome:

- Stenotic nares.
- Excessive, redundant pharyngeal tissue.
- Over-long ± thickened soft palate.
- Hypoplastic trachea.
- Aberrant nasal turbinates/conchae (contorted, foreshortened nasal passages).
- Relatively large and fleshy tongue (macroglossia)

Chronic upper airway obstruction makes inspiration hard work and high negative airway and intrathoracic pressures are generated:

- Pharyngeal soft tissues are sucked inwards, exacerbating the obstruction.
- Laryngeal saccule eversion leads to eventual 'laryngeal collapse'.

Chronic alveolar hypoxia causes sustained hypoxic pulmonary vasoconstriction that eventually leads to pulmonary hypertension and 'cor pulmonale' (right-sided heart failure). Animals try to compensate with postural adaptations (standing or sternal recumbency), and mouth-breathing, which help to minimise resistance to airflow. If you try to restrain the animal in lateral recumbency, you immediately destroy some of its compensatory efforts. Excitement or exercise also increase the respiratory demands and can result in decompensation. Animals may develop non-cardiogenic (negative pressure/neurogenic) pulmonary oedema with high degrees of respiratory obstruction.

Signs of chronic hypoxaemia include:

- History of syncope.
- Cyanosis.
- Poor exercise tolerance (can the animal nose-breathe at rest?).
- Polycythaemia.
- Tachycardia and tachypnoea at rest.
- Animals are prone to hyperthermia as panting is difficult and ineffective.

These animals are also affected by gastrointestinal disease, in particular, gastric reflux and regurgitation, oesophagitis, gastritis (all of which may be associated with hiatal hernia). Aspiration of gastric contents is a significant risk when the airway is unprotected, especially prior to tracheal intubation (i.e. from premedication to just after induction of anaesthesia) and, following tracheal extubation in the recovery period. Chest radiographs may be warranted at the outset of anaesthesia to detect pre-existing subclinical aspiration pneumonia. Many brachycephalics also have prominent eyes, so care must be paid to guard against inadvertent ocular trauma during handling. Severely affected cases may also be hypercoagulable.

49.1.1 Anaesthetic Considerations

Highest risks are associated with:

- Time between premedication and tracheal intubation.
- Tracheal extubation and recovery after extubation.

Veterinary Anaesthesia: Principles to Practice, Second Edition. Alexandra H. A. Dugdale, Georgina Beaumont, Carl Bradbrook, and Matthew Gurney.
© 2020 John Wiley & Sons Ltd. Published 2020 by John Wiley & Sons Ltd.
Companion website: www.wiley.com/go/dugdale/veterinary-anaesthesia

49.1.1.1 Premedication

Aim for **sedation without marked respiratory depression.** Try to **avoid drugs that can induce regurgitation and vomiting,** as this adds stress and the possibility of aspiration to the situation. Continuous observation after premedication is advised. The antitussive effect of opioids is useful and can allow relatively 'late' tracheal extubation. Brachycephalics have high resting vagal tone, so acepromazine can occasionally cause syncope. (Some people consider anticholinergics.) Consideration for their gastrointestinal disease should be included as part of the anaesthesia protocol. Use of gastroprotectants and pro-motility medications are recommended.

Pre-oxygenation (as long as it is not stressful) increases oxygen reserves if you later struggle with tracheal intubation. Ensure **intravenous access.**

49.1.1.2 Induction

- Induction should be rapid to allow **rapid tracheal intubation.** Choose drugs that also allow rapid and 'complete' recovery without hangover.
- Rapid tracheal intubation is required to rapidly gain control of the airway: be as gentle as possible. Have a **range of sizes of endotracheal (ET) tubes** on hand and also a **laryngoscope,** an ET tube introducer/stylette/**bougie,** and **suction.** Have **tracheostomy tubes on standby.** A complicating factor for rapidly gaining control of the airway, however, is that surgical assessment of palate length and laryngeal saccules may be required prior to endotracheal intubation attempts; pre-oxygenation is important, as is vigilance in case of regurgitation/aspiration. Therefore, injectable agents given more slowly and to effect may also be appropriate as long as the patient is oxygenating well enough.
- Consider **peri-operative corticosteroids** (beware concurrent non-steroidal anti-inflammatory drugs [NSAIDs]).

49.1.1.3 Maintenance

Choose drugs that require minimal metabolism for elimination, and drugs that are rapidly eliminated **so recovery will be quick and complete** (e.g. propofol, alfaxalone, isoflurane, sevoflurane). Practise **balanced anaesthesia** and ensure good analgesia. Use of N_2O is debatable as there have been concerns that it may increase pulmonary vascular resistance, and possibly more so with pre-existing pulmonary hypertension (See Chapter 8).

49.1.1.4 Recovery

Continue oxygen provision. Leave IV catheter in place until fully recovered. Ensure quiet surroundings and continuous patient observation. In hot weather, consider environmental temperature; fans or air conditioning may be required to reduce attempts to pant for thermoregulatory purposes. **Leave ET tube in place until you really have to remove it.** Most patients are happy to wake up and be able to breathe more easily than ever before so that they tolerate an ET tube remarkably well. If possible, prop the animal in a **sternal** position, as this mimics their own postural adaptations. Have **equipment and drugs available for re-intubation should it be necessary.** If problems recur, consider corticosteroids if not already given (beware if NSAIDs already given), and tracheostomy. A small dose of lidocaine (2 mg/kg IV in dogs) might help to reduce the coughing reflex upon tube manipulation during tracheal extubation. **Minor degrees of post-extubation obstruction can be remedied by keeping the animal in sternal, extending the head and neck forwards, and pulling the tongue out as far as possible, along with the use of a bite-block or gag** (e.g. roll of tape or bandage to keep the mouth open) **or a maxillary sling** (bandage used to support the maxilla so the mouth can 'hang open'). This helps to minimise airway resistance. Pain (especially thoracic or abdominal) can cause ventilatory embarrassment too, so ensure adequate **analgesia.** Consider the use of a **nasal decongestant agent** (e.g. xylometazoline hydrochloride [Otrivine™]) to reduce nasal oedema, and/or **nebulisation** with epinephrine (adrenaline) in the recovery period prior to and following extubation. Using nasal prongs to supplement oxygen can help in some patients (if they tolerate the nasal prongs). Some practices may have high-flow oxygen therapy (HFOT) wide-bore nasal prongs/cannulae available (see Chapter 50).

49.2 Bronchoscopy (and Bronchoalveolar Lavage [BAL])

It is important to note the degree of respiratory compromise that exists pre-anaesthesia.

Stress-free pre-oxygenation is advised.

For bronchoscopy, whilst a Cobb connector can allow bronchoscopy via the ET tube with minimal enviromental pollution, in small patients (<10 kg), some bronchoscopes will not fit down small ET tubes, or if they do, they block a good proportion of oxygen and anaesthetic vapour from reaching the patient's lungs. Therefore, it will often be necessary to remove the ET tube. This requires:

- Another plan to maintain anaesthesia. (Use of an IV agent; intermittent bolusing or a continuous infusion, e.g. propofol or alfaxalone.)
- Another plan to ensure an oxygen supply to the patient. One way to do this is to pass a dog urinary catheter down the airway so the tip lies at the carina. Connect the proximal end to a size 3 or 3.5 mm internal diameter ET tube connector, and thence to the anaesthetic breathing system

for oxygen delivery. You can also attach the catheter to a manually controlled jet ventilator (e.g. the Manujet™). Just one note of caution though: If the bronchoscope and catheter form a 'tight fit' down the trachea, you may block off any escape route for all the oxygen you are supplying, so beware that you do not over-inflate the lungs.

If the SpO_2 falls below 90% (and you may detect a tachycardia, or even bradycardia, with the hypoxaemia), then remove the endoscope. You may need to re-insert an ET tube, supply a decent flow of O_2, and possibly provide the odd manual breath to restore the saturation before you allow the operator to trespass down the airways again.

During BAL, instillation of relatively large volumes of saline and especially if it is cold, can stimulate vagal or vaso-vagal reflexes (sudden, profound bradycardia and hypotension), so monitoring the pulse rate and ECG is vital during this procedure. Some clinicians request terbutaline, or other β2 agonist bronchodilators, to be administered prior to bronchoscopy/BAL to enhance sample yield (especially in cats); this, however, will cause transient tachycardia. After BAL, any remaining saline is rapidly absorbed. Gentle chest coupage can help promote coughing and expectoration once recovery is progressing.

49.3 Laryngeal Paresis/Paralysis

- May be congenital or acquired. Most common in Bouviers, Bull Terriers, and older dogs of large and giant breeds.
- May accompany hypothyroidism.
- Breathing difficulty is exacerbated by hot weather and exercise: ineffective panting can lead to hyperthermia. May develop negative pressure/neurogenic pulmonary oedema with high degrees of respiratory obstruction. Similar considerations apply as to BOAS/BAOS.
- Minimise stress when handling. Light sedation helps (e.g. low dose acepromazine ± butorphanol). Oxygen supplementation methods must not increase stress: flow-by oxygen or nasal prongs are often preferred to face masks or nasopharyngeal tubes. Oxygen hoods and makeshift oxygen cages can increase heat-stress because of the build-up of humidity (and increase ventilatory drive if carbon dioxide builds up too), so are best avoided in hyperthermic patients. If patients are hyperthermic, instigate cooling methods.
- These animals cannot guard their airways very well, and even less so after laryngeal tie-backs. They may, therefore, suffer from aspiration pneumonia (both pre- and post-operatively), so avoid drugs which induce vomition.
- Antitussives are often advocated after laryngeal surgery, although some people worry that they may increase the risk of aspiration.
- Surgeons often wish to assess laryngeal function just before endotracheal intubation, so beware of premedicant drugs that reduce laryngeal motion (especially α2 agonists). Pre-oxygenate the patient where possible in a stress-free manner. Assess the larynx under 'light' anaesthesia (see Further Reading). You may need to be patient as some post-induction apnoea is common, although there appears to be a trend to using doxapram after induction to stimulate breathing.

49.4 Tracheal Collapse

- Most common in small terriers.
- Extrathoracic and/or intrathoracic portions of the trachea can be affected, which will affect clinical presentation (see Chapter 50).
- The peri-anaesthetic danger times are again around premedication and in recovery, but intrathoracic tracheal collapse can also be a problem during the maintenance phase if the ET tube does not extend through the area of collapse.

49.5 Thoracotomies

- Open chest:
  - Positive pressure ventilation is necessary.
  - Promotes heat loss.
  - Large surface area exposed from which inhalant anaesthetic agents can also 'escape' and pollute the immediate surgical environment; consider total intravenous techniques for anaesthetic maintenance.
  - Chest drain required post-operatively (see chapter 50).
- For cases with pre-existing pleural space disease, try to drain at least some fluid, gas, or air pre-anaesthesia, if possible, to increase the respiratory reserve. If a tension pneumothorax is present, avoid N_2O until the tension in the pleural cavity has been relieved.
- Ensure good analgesia: local/regional techniques form a common component of balanced analgesia. Coughing is painful, but cough suppression may not always be indicated.

49.6 Diaphragmatic Ruptures

Debate exists over how soon to repair these. Cardiac contusions can lead to arrhythmias within the first 72 hours of injury, but waiting longer increases the risks of adhesions. Pulmonary contusions may also be present, but may not become clinically apparent for one to two days.

- Positive pressure artificial ventilation is well tolerated because the negative intrapleural pressure has been lost.
- Avoid N_2O until the stomach position can be verified/corrected (torsion/dilation can occur if within chest).

- Good preparation is key; ensure the patient is pre-clipped prior to induction of anaesthesia (if possible), and the surgeon is scrubbed and ready to start surgery following tracheal intubation.
- Placing the patient on a gentle head-up slope may be helpful; patients must not be tilted head-down (until surgical correction is completed).

49.7 Equine Asthma

Equine asthma was previously known as recurrent airway obstruction (RAO), and before that, as chronic obstructive pulmonary disease (COPD). Most cases presenting with a heave line and chronic cough have only slightly increased anaesthetic risk. Horses presenting with respiratory distress and copious mucopurulent airway secretions are at greater risk. Although α2 agonists may cause some degree of bronchoconstriction, ketamine, and the halogenated inhalation agents tend to alleviate this. Additionally, α2 agonists may actually alleviate pre-existing bronchoconstriction.

If artificial ventilation (usually provided in the form of positive pressure ventilation) is required, slower lung inflation may allow time for less compliant lung areas to inflate, but be mindful of the cardiovascular effects of prolonged inspiratory times, and be sure to allow sufficient expiratory time to avoid breath-stacking. Positive pressure ventilation also risks causing air-trapping and possible alveolar rupture and pneumothorax.

Further Reading

Armitage-Chan, E. (2007). Anaesthesia for surgeries of the upper respiratory tract. *Equine Veterinary Education* 19: 197–199.

Blazquez, I.A. and Vettorato, E. (2018). How to anaesthetise the brachycephalic dog. *BSAVA Companion*, March 2018: 16–21.

Cross, M. and Plunkett, E. (2014). Cardiovascular physiology. In: *Physics, Pharmacology and Physiology for Anaesthetists. Key Concepts for the FRCA*, 2e, 239–280. Cambridge, UK: Cambridge University Press.

Downing, F. and Gibson, S. (2018). Anaesthesia of brachycephalic dogs. *Journal of Small Animal Practice* 59: 725–733.

Jackson, A.M., Tobias, K., Long, C. et al. (2004). Effects of various anaesthetic agents on laryngeal motion during laryngoscopy in normal dogs. *Veterinary Surgery* 33: 102–106.

Labuscagne, S., Zeiler, G.E., and Dzikiti, B.T. (2019). Effects of chemical and mechanical stimulation on laryngeal motion during alfaxalone, thiopentone or propofol anaesthesia in healthy dogs. *Veterinary Anaesthesia and Analgesia* 46: 435–442.

Mills, G.H. (2001). Respiratory physiology and anaesthesia. *British Journal of Anaesthesia: CEPD Reviews* 1: 35–39.

Norgate, D., Haar, G.T., Kulendra, N., and Veres-Nyeki, K.O. (2018). A comparison of the effect of propofol and alfaxalone on laryngeal motion in nonbrachycephalic and brachycephalic dogs. *Veterinary Anaesthesia and Analgesia* 45: 729–736.

Pirie, R.S., Couteil, L.L., Robinson, N.E., and Lavoie, J.-P. (2016). Equine asthma: an appropriate, translational and comprehendible terminology? *Equine Veterinary Journal* 48: 403–405.

Riggs, J., Liu, N.C., Sutton, D.R. et al. (2019). Validation of exercise testing and laryngeal auscultation for grading brachycephalic obstructive airway syndrome in pugs, French bulldogs and English bulldogs by using whole-body barometric plethysmography. *Veterinary Surgery* 48: 488–496.

Robertson, S.A. and Bailey, J.E. (2002). Aerosolized salbutamol (albuterol) improves PaO_2 in hypoxaemic anaesthetized horses: a prospective clinical trial in 81 horses. *Veterinary Anaesthesia and Analgesia* 29: 212–218.

Smalle, T.M., Hartman, M.J., Bester, L. et al. (2017). Effects of thiopentone, propofol and alfaxalone on laryngeal motion during oral laryngoscopy in healthy dogs. *Veterinary Anaesthesia and Analgesia* 44: 427–434.

Thompson, K.R. and Rioja, E. (2016). Effects of intravenous and topical laryngeal lidocaine on heart rate, mean arterial pressure and cough response to endotracheal intubation in dogs. *Veterinary Anaesthesia and Analgesia* 43: 371–378.

Woodlands, C. (2018). Perioperative care of the brachycephalic patient and surgical management of brachycephalic obstructive airway syndrome. *The Veterinary Nurse* 9: 532–538.

Self-test Section

1 Explain the pathophysiology associated with the 'brachycephalic airway obstruction syndrome'.

2 What precautions would you take when anaesthetising a French Bulldog with signs of BOAS/BAOS?

50

Respiratory Emergencies

LEARNING OBJECTIVES

- To be able to discuss the reasons for respiratory insufficiency.
- To be familiar with the methods available for supplemental oxygen administration, and importance of humidification for long-term therapy.
- To be familiar with the techniques for chest drainage and tracheostomy.

Glossary of Terms

Eupnoea	normal quiet breathing.
Tachypnoea	increased respiratory rate.
Hyperpnoea	increased rate and/or depth of breathing (usually indicating hyperventilation).
Polypnoea	rapid, shallow, panting type of breathing.
Bradypnoea	slow regular breathing.
Hypopnoea	slow and/or shallow breathing (usually indicating hypoventilation).
Apnoea	transient (or prolonged) cessation of breathing.
Orthopnoea	difficulty in breathing when in any other position than standing (e.g. increased breathing difficulty when lying down).
Trepopnoea	difficulty breathing when in one laterally recumbent position but not the other.
Platypnoea	difficulty breathing in the upright position.
Dyspnoea	laboured or distressed breathing.
Stertor	snoring sound.
Stridor	harsh, often wheezy, respiratory sound.

50.1   Respiratory Insufficiency

Respiratory insufficiency may arise because of problems at any of the following levels:

- Upper respiratory tract.
- Lower airways (lower respiratory tract).
- Lung parenchyma (lower respiratory tract).
- Pleural space.
- 'Thoracic cage', including chest wall and diaphragm.

These can also be thought of as:

- Extrapulmonary or intrapulmonary conditions affecting the process of **ventilation**, e.g. central nervous system (CNS) disorders affecting the control of breathing; neuromuscular or chest wall disorders affecting the mechanical processes of breathing; airway problems or abnormal pleural space or mediastinal filling affecting movement of air into and out of the lungs.
- Intrapulmonary conditions affecting the process of **gaseous exchange** across the alveolar-capillary barrier, e.g. pulmonary parenchymal conditions such as pneumonia or pulmonary oedema. In addition, cardiovascular conditions may affect pulmonary perfusion so as to compromise the efficacy of gaseous exchange, e.g. pulmonary emboli (air or thrombi), intrapulmonary shunting, or low cardiac output conditions such as cardiac failure or shock.

An alternative approach to differentiating the causes of respiratory insufficiency is to think of them as:

- Obstructive: of the airways or pulmonary vasculature
- Restrictive: of the pleural space or pulmonary parenchyma

Veterinary Anaesthesia: Principles to Practice, Second Edition. Alexandra H. A. Dugdale, Georgina Beaumont, Carl Bradbrook, and Matthew Gurney.
© 2020 John Wiley & Sons Ltd. Published 2020 by John Wiley & Sons Ltd.
Companion website: www.wiley.com/go/dugdale/veterinary-anaesthesia

50.1.1 Clinical Signs

As the degree of respiratory compromise increases, the clinical signs (including exercise intolerance) displayed by the animal generally progress, usually through the following stages:

- **Increased respiratory rate.**
- **Changed breathing pattern** (see below), may accompany increased rate.
- **Increased work of breathing.** Cats recruit their abdominal muscles early because their intercostal muscles are relatively weak, whereas this happens much later in dogs.
- **Postural changes.** Animals become reluctant to lie down and so become orthopnoeic (see glossary). They may stand with their back arched and their elbows abducted.
- Animals adopt the **air hunger stance**, an exaggerated form of the postural changes above, with the head and neck extended and open-mouthed breathing. Cats usually prefer to 'crouch', appearing to be in a sternal position, and open-mouthed breathing is a sign of very serious respiratory compromise. Once breathing becomes laboured to the point of being distressing to the animal, we talk of dyspnoea.
- **Cyanotic mucous membranes** (cats often appear more 'grey' than 'blue'). **Cyanosis is defined as > 5 g/dl deoxyhaemoglobin in the blood**, so its appearance depends upon the animal's initial haemoglobin concentration (i.e. very anaemic animals cannot be cyanotic because there simply is not enough haemoglobin in the first place; they look more 'white'), and also on the state of perfusion of the vascular bed (e.g. gums) being observed, and the ambient lighting. Although variable, cyanosis may be present at arterial haemoglobin oxygen saturations of <70%, or arterial oxygen tensions (PaO_2) of <50 mmHg.

Once the air hunger stance with open-mouthed breathing is adopted, it can be assumed that 75% of respiratory function has been lost.

Respiratory failure can be **defined by dyspnoea with cyanosis at rest, and PaO_2 < 60 mmHg [8 kPa]** (normal 95–105 mmHg), **and $PaCO_2$ > 46 mmHg [6.1 kPa]** (normal 35–45 mmHg) **in dogs and horses, or > c. 40 mmHg [5.3 kPa] in cats** (normal c. 31 mmHg), **whilst breathing room air** (inspired oxygen 21%).

Other **clinical signs** include:

- **Tachycardia** (response to hypoxaemia).
- **Decreased exercise tolerance** +/− **syncope.**
- **Coughing** (different 'types' are recognised: dry/hacking; soft/moist; paroxysmal; associated with exercise/excitement or eating/drinking; honking cough characteristic of tracheal collapse).
- **Change in voice** (laryngeal paresis).
- **Prone to hyperthermia** with exercise or hot weather if panting becomes inefficient (e.g. brachycephalic obstructive airway syndrome [BOAS] and laryngeal paresis).

50.1.2 Clinical Examination of the Respiratory System

- **Observe** the patient from a distance and note its breathing pattern (see below).
- **Listen** from a distance first of all. Can you hear any abnormal respiratory noises without the aid of a stethoscope? Are they inspiratory or expiratory?
- **Palpate and observe the chest wall** for respiratory excursions, and note **any asymmetry** in left and right chest wall movements. Palpate the larynx and trachea along its extrathoracic course. Is the anterior chest wall compressible in cats? Can you feel the cardiac apex beat? Is it in its normal position? And can you feel any precordial thrills?
- **Percuss** the left and right chest walls (+/− simultaneous auscultation) to help detect and define areas of hyper-resonance or abnormal dullness. (Very difficult to perform in cats, and fat or thick-coated animals, and in dyspnoeic animals.)
- **Auscultate** lung fields and over larynx and trachea. (Again, can be difficult in fat or hairy animals and in dyspnoeic animals.)

50.1.3 Breathing Sounds and Patterns

During **normal inhalation**, both the **chest and the abdomen 'expand'** because of contraction of the intercostal muscles and the diaphragm (the latter pushes the abdominal contents caudally). The opposite movements occur during exhalation. Different breathing patterns may help you to determine the site of pathology.

50.1.3.1 Inspiratory Stertor
This is associated with upper respiratory tract obstructions (nares, nasal passages, nasopharynx, soft palate problems, e.g. BOAS).

50.1.3.2 Inspiratory Stridor
This associated with laryngeal and extrathoracic tracheal obstructions (e.g. laryngeal paresis, extrathoracic tracheal collapse).

To differentiate between inspiratory stertor and stridor: Does the animal breathe quietly with its mouth open, yet noisily with its mouth closed? If so, the problem is between the nares and larynx.

50.1.3.3 Expiratory Stridor

This is associated with intrathoracic airway obstruction (e.g. intrathoracic tracheal collapse). Often accompanied by increased expiratory efforts.

50.1.3.4 Inspiratory and Expiratory Stridor

This is associated with combined extrathoracic and intrathoracic airway obstructions.

50.1.3.5 Increased Expiratory Efforts

These often occur with an abdominal push, and prolonged expiratory phase: associated with intrathoracic airway obstructions, especially small airway disease (e.g. feline asthma).

50.1.3.6 Rapid and Shallow Breathing, but with a Smooth Motion and Where the Chest Wall and Abdomen Work Together

This is associated with lung parenchymal disease (e.g. pneumonia, pulmonary oedema). In cats, cupula motion may be accentuated. The cupulae are the cranial apical portions of the left and right pleural sacs where they extend through the thoracic inlet, the left is usually larger than the right. When respiratory efforts are exaggerated, i.e. with larger than normal negative intrapleural pressures generated by exaggerated inspiratory efforts, the cupulae are 'sucked in' more than normal.

50.1.3.7 Paradoxical Abdominal Movement

- Rapid breathing, but with greatly increased work of breathing (usually seen as a rippling effect along the ribs, *and* the chest and abdomen move in a dys-synchronous fashion), is generally associated with pleural space disease (e.g. pneumothorax, haemothorax, pyothorax, pleural effusions, chylothorax, diaphragmatic hernias/ ruptures). Breathing pattern is more 'choppy' than the smooth pattern seen with lung parenchymal disorders.
- Paradoxical abdominal movement can also be seen in cases of diaphragmatic paralysis (because of the lack of normal diaphragmatic contribution to breathing), and also with upper respiratory tract obstruction because huge negative intrathoracic pressures are created in an attempt to suck air into the lungs, so the diaphragm and abdominal contents tend to be sucked towards the chest cavity, thus giving the appearance of inward abdominal movements accompanying outward chest movements during

attempted inhalation. The opposite occurs during exhalation, i.e. the chest wall relaxes (moves 'inwards') and the abdominal contents can now move caudally so the abdomen appears to expand. Note that any condition that significantly increases the work of breathing can result in fatigue of the respiratory muscles, and consequently loss of synchronous movement of chest and abdominal walls, with outward movement of the chest wall but inward movement of the abdomen on inspiration (and the opposite on expiration). Normal lung expansion can be compromised with this type of breathing pattern and it often signifies impending respiratory failure.

50.1.3.8 Flail Segments of Chest Wall

These move paradoxically (i.e. suck in on inspiration and bow out on expiration).

50.1.3.9 Paradoxical Breathing

Inward movement of the chest wall, with outward bulging of the abdomen on inspiration is often seen in anaesthetised animals at deep planes of anaesthesia, where the intercostal muscles are so 'relaxed' that inspiration becomes diaphragmatic, and appears to be abdominal. During expiration, the opposite occurs, with cranial excursion of the diaphragm tending to make the chest bulge out. This type of respiratory pattern is quite often seen in **normal cats** even in much lighter planes of anaesthesia because of their relatively weak intercostal muscles.

50.1.3.10 Apneustic Breathing

This occurs when there is an end-inspiratory pause or breath-hold, and is common under ketamine anaesthesia. (Normal awake patients have an end-expiratory pause.)

50.1.3.11 Kussmaul's Breathing

This describes regular deep and rapid breathing without much in the way of an expiratory pause. It is often seen in ketoacidotic diabetic patients that are attempting to achieve a secondary respiratory alkalosis (by blowing off CO_2) in order to try to compensate for a primary metabolic acidosis.

50.1.3.12 Cheyne–Stokes Breathing

This is characterised by waxing and waning breaths and often accompanies CNS disorders, congestive heart failure or uraemia, but has been noted in normal sleeping horses and also in 'normal' anaesthetised horses.

50.1.3.13 Biot's Breathing

This is characterised by runs of normal breaths interspersed by periods of apnoea. It is usually a sign of CNS disease (affecting the medullary respiratory centre), although is sometimes seen in anaesthetised animals, e.g. horses.

Note that horses normally have biphasic inspiration and expiration: each with an active and passive component. They are said to breathe 'around' their functional residual capacity.

50.2 Diagnostic Workup

Some form of stabilisation or resuscitation is often required: some useful techniques are considered later. Chemical restraint may be necessary.

Procedures include:

- Thoracic radiography. (Not the V/D view if the patient presents with much respiratory embarrassment.)
- Thoracic ultrasonography, including echocardiography.
- Thoracocentesis, and laboratory evaluation of any fluid removed.
- Airway endoscopy, tracheal wash, broncho-alveolar lavage.
- Haematology, including coagulation tests.
- Biochemistry.
- Blood gas analysis (arterial +/− venous).
- Lung biopsies (endoscopically guided; percutaneous needle biopsies).

50.3 Oxygen Supplementation

By oxygen supplementation (oxygen therapy), we mean any method of increasing the inspired oxygen concentration (above that of 21% in normal atmospheric air) in order to try to improve hypoxaemia.

Hypoxaemia is poor oxygenation of the blood; usually defined in terms of an abnormally low partial pressure of oxygen in the arterial blood, PaO_2 (Table 50.1). The inspired oxygen concentration and atmospheric pressure also influence the achievable PaO_2, as does the cardiorespiratory function of the patient. The oxygen content of the blood itself then depends not only upon the tiny amount of dissolved oxygen (directly measured as the PaO_2), but also (and mainly ~98%) upon the amount of haemoglobin present and its saturation with oxygen (indirectly determined from the oxygen–haemoglobin dissociation curve).

Hypoxia is poor oxygenation of tissues.

The causes of tissue hypoxia were first classified by Barcroft as follows:

- Anoxic or hypoxaemic: due to low partial pressure of oxygen in the blood.
- Anaemic: due to reduced functional haemoglobin in the blood (i.e. anaemia or haemoglobinopathies).
- Stagnant or ischaemic: due to insufficient supply of blood to the tissues.

Peters and van Slyke later added:

- Histotoxic or cytotoxic: problems with cellular oxidative processes, whereby the cells cannot utilise oxygen even if sufficient is delivered by the blood, such as happens with endotoxaemia.

50.3.1 Oxygen Humidification

Oxygen from cylinders is 'cold' (room temperature at best; but cools on expanding as it is released from the higher pressure cylinder), and 'dry'. If it is to be breathed for prolonged periods of time (more than a few [two to six] hours), especially if the upper respiratory tract (nasal passages that normally warm and moisten inspired gases) is bypassed, desiccation of respiratory mucus and compromise of the mucociliary escalator function occurs. The simplest way to achieve humidification is by bubbling the oxygen through a chamber containing water, ideally sterile (Figure 50.1).

50.3.2 Techniques of Oxygen Supplementation

50.3.2.1 Face Mask

Oxygen (from a cylinder or oxygen concentrator) is delivered through tubing or an anaesthetic breathing system to a face mask that is 'snugly' applied over the animal's nose and mouth. Oxygen flows around 5–15 l/min (determined by patient size) can increase inspired oxygen percentage greatly, depending upon the snugness of fit of the mask and entrainment of ambient air. Excessive dead-space within the mask promotes re-breathing of carbon dioxide. Be aware of condensation/humidity and heating within the face mask.

50.3.2.2 Flow-by Oxygen

Oxygen is delivered through tubing or an anaesthetic breathing system to near the animal's nose and mouth. Useful if the animal resents a face mask. Oxygen flows of 5–15 l/min are commonly used (determined by patient size) and can increase the inspired oxygen percentage to around 50%.

Table 50.1 Grades of hypoxaemia.

PaO_2 (arterial blood oxygen partial pressure) (F_iO_2 = 0.21 [room air])	Level of hypoxaemia
80–90 mmHg (10.7–12 kPa)	Mild
60–80 mmHg (8–10.7 kPa)	Moderate
<60 mmHg (<8 kPa)	Severe

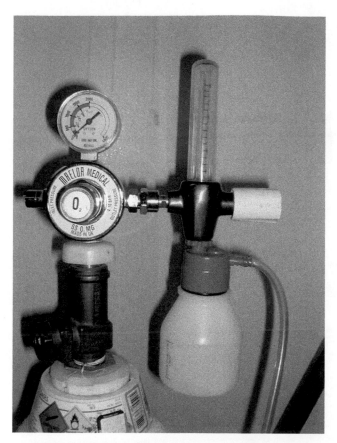

Figure 50.1 Bubble humidifier and flowmeter attached to oxygen regulator.

50.3.2.3 Oxygen Hood

Requires an Elizabethan collar (or an Oxyhood™ [Kruuse]), and then oxygen is delivered by tubing: ideally to enter the collar below the animal's chin so the oxygen flushes 'forwards' past the animal's nose and mouth to displace exhaled breath/CO_2. Transparent film may be placed over the 'open rim' of the Elizabethan collar to form a 'lid' and turn the whole assembly into a kind of oxygen tent over the animal's head, but such a 'lid' can be omitted in an emergency, as high oxygen flows delivered near the animal's nose and mouth will still increase the inspired oxygen 'within' the collar environment to above that of room air. If a 'lid' is fitted, there is usually enough inherent 'leak' in the system not to have to worry about creating an escape hole in the hood for the large/excess volume of oxygen that you are delivering; however, to improve the exit of exhaled CO_2 and to reduce the build-up of heat and humidity/condensation within the collar (which may be distressing for the patient), a small segment of the 'lid' can be left 'open'.

50.3.2.4 Oxygen Cage

Incubators are usually capable of providing an oxygen-enriched environment, although some may only deliver oxygen up to a maximum of 40%. A makeshift oxygen cage can be created by placing a cat/small dog wire mesh carrying basket inside a plastic bag into which a high flow of oxygen is delivered. Black plastic bags are most robust and easily available but are opaque, so cut a window into them and sellotape a clear plastic piece in place so that you can observe the patient. Two 'holes' in the bag/tent are required: one for oxygen entry and one for escape of excess gases. Plastic (transparent) sheeting can similarly be taped over larger kennel doors to try to make the kennel airspace into an area of oxygen enriched atmosphere. Shor-Line™ makes special kennel doors that are pretty airtight for this purpose (Figure 50.2). With all these types of oxygen cage, **increasing CO_2 and humidity inside the cage can increase respiratory demand and distress, and opening the door will immediately reduce the oxygen concentration within the kennel back towards that of room air**.

50.3.2.5 Veterinary-specific, Climate-controlled Oxygen Cages

Specially designed to control the percentage of oxygen within the cage (although opening the cage door will temporarily alter that). Most also have temperature and humidity control (many patients also require humidified oxygen) and all have carbon dioxide absorber trays (Figure 50.3).

50.3.2.6 Nasal Prongs

Commercially available for humans (Figure 50.4), therefore only suitable for patients with inter-nostril distance similar to humans (i.e. dogs, but they do not fit brachycephalics very well). Two sizes are available. They are not always well tolerated, especially at higher oxygen flows. Local anaesthetic eye drops into the conjunctival sacs will drain down the nasolacrimal tear ducts to help desensitise the nose, which might improve patient tolerance.

More recently, the use of high flow oxygen therapy (HFOT), which delivers warmed and humidified oxygen via wide-bore (snug-fitting) nasal prongs/cannulae, may offer a viable alternative to support oxygenation, and reduce the work of breathing, in patients where conventional (invasive) artificial ventilation is not available or feasible. The high flows required are of the order of 0.5-1-2 l/kg/min, which provide higher inspired oxygen concentrations than conventional nasal oxygen flows, and also provide a degree of positive end-expiratory pressure, even continuous positive airway pressure (but this depends upon whether patients attempt to mouth-breathe). Furthermore, HFOT is usually well-tolerated and improves airway secretion clearance. Mild hypercapnia may, however, develop. HFOT may also be useful in brachycephalic airway obstruction syndrome cases.

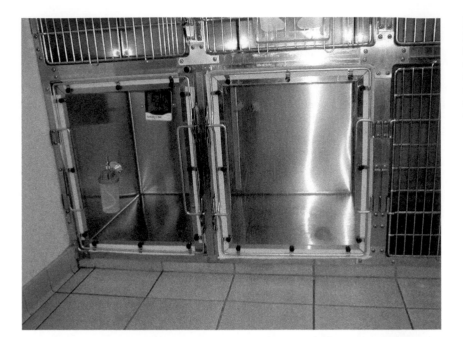

Figure 50.2 Oxygen therapy kennel doors with humidifier and thermometer/hygrometer. An ice-box/water bath (which surrounds the humidifier) is also available to deliver cooled or warmed humidified gases.

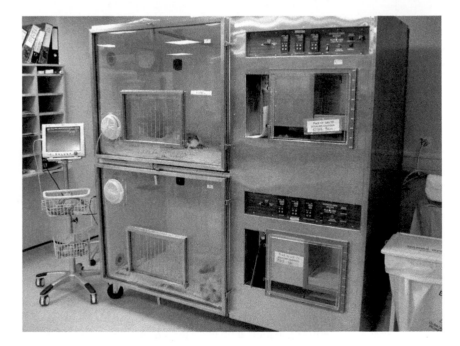

Figure 50.3 ICS-DT oxygen cages in use at Royal Veterinary College. Source: Courtesy of Robert Goggs.

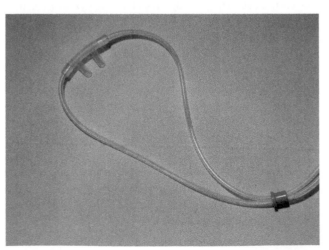

Figure 50.4 Nasal oxygen prongs (child: size 1).

(a)
(b)

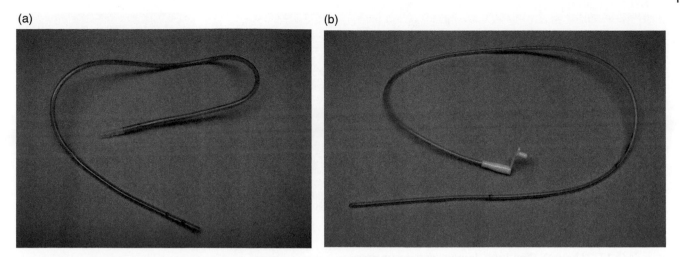

Figure 50.5 (a) Nasal oxygen catheter and (b) softer naso-oesophageal feeding tube.

50.3.2.7 Nasopharyngeal Catheters

Nasopharyngeal oxygen insufflation at 100 ml/kg/min oxygen can increase the inspired oxygen percentage to around 35%; at 200 ml/kg/min, to almost 50%; and at 500 ml/kg/min to around 80%. The exact inspired oxygen concentration will depend upon the size of tube used, the oxygen flow achieved, the position of the tube tip within the nasopharynx, and the breathing pattern of the animal. High airflow oxygen enrichment (HAFOE) venturi devices are also available to help determine more accurate inspired oxygen concentrations. Soft feeding (naso-oesophageal) tubes are often preferred (3–8 Fr) to the somewhat stiffer oxygen catheters, and are placed, with the aid of local anaesthetic, into the ventral nasal meatus, so that the tip lies in the nasopharynx (Figure 50.5a and b). The tube is pre-measured against the animal's face; the length to be inserted is noted as the distance between the nostril and the lateral canthus of the eye. (Some people use 'nares to medial canthus', but the tip of the catheter then does not always reach into the nasopharynx. Measuring to the lateral canthus gives the extra few millimetres that allow optimum positioning of the catheter tip in the nasopharynx, at least for mesaticephalic breeds.) With the animal facing you, gently push the nasal planum upwards (make the animal 'snooty-nosed') to bring the ventral nasal meatus (where the tube should go) into a straighter line with the nostril (Figure 50.6). The tube can then be inserted, advanced, and secured in place with superglue or sutures (especially with 'butterfly' tapes) to the side of the nose (just behind/beside the nasal planum), up over the bridge of the nose, and on the top of the animal's head. Elizabethan collars may be required. Tolerated better by dogs than by cats; least by brachycephalic breeds.

50.3.2.8 Trans-tracheal Oxygen Delivery

Oxygen delivery via needle tracheotomy. The bore of the needle or catheter limits the oxygen flow possible: try for

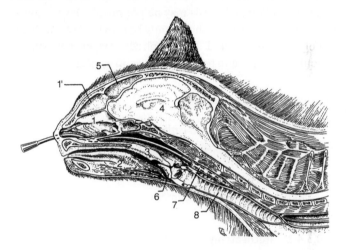

Figure 50.6 Paramedian section through cat's head. Although a naso-oesophageal feeding tube is shown in place, the route from nostril to nasopharynx is the same for a nasopharyngeal oxygen catheter. Note how the path from ventral nasal meatus to nasopharynx is not straight just caudal to the nasal planum: pushing the nasal planum 'up' helps to smooth out this course and facilitates tube passage. Source: Reproduced from Dyce, Sack, and Wensing (2002) with permission from Elsevier.

200 ml/kg/min although a maximum of only 2 l/min flow is common. Oxygen inflow may also be limited by the availability of escape routes for the extra gas volume administered, e.g. if the trachea is blocked above the site of needle entry, then care must be taken not to over-inflate the lungs. A second needle may need to be inserted to allow escape of gases so as to prevent such an over-pressure situation.

50.3.2.9 Endotracheal Oxygen Delivery

Oxygen delivery via tracheo[s]tomy tubes or endotracheal (ET) tubes. Inspired oxygen can be delivered at up to 100% by these means. Mini-tracheotomy tube kits are also available (Figure 50.7).

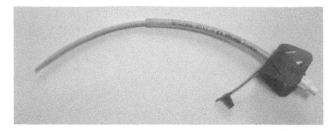

Figure 50.7 Mini-tracheotomy tube and introducer.

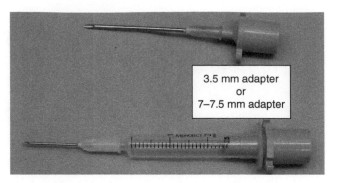

3.5 mm adapter
or
7–7.5 mm adapter

Figure 50.8 Needles can be attached to ET tube adapters for connection to an oxygen source.

50.3.3 Oxygen Toxicity

If oxygen percentages >60% are breathed for prolonged periods (>12–24 hours), then lung damage can occur (free radical generation with subsequent damage of the alveoli); and absorption atelectasis may be promoted. Oxygen therapy with >60% oxygen should only be provided when absolutely necessary; and the inspired oxygen percentage should be reduced to below 60% as soon as possible.

50.3.4 Useful Techniques

- Placing nasopharyngeal catheters
- Tracheotomy
- Thoracocentesis
- Tube thoracostomy
- Stabilising a flail chest segment

50.3.4.1 Tracheotomy

As '-ostomy' usually pertains to making a permanent 'hole' (ostium), the term *tracheostomy* should be confined to permanent surgical tracheostomies. Therefore, even when tubes are employed for several days, the correct term appears to be *tube tracheotomy*.

50.3.4.1.1 Needle Tracheotomy

In an emergency, transtracheal oxygen delivery can be achieved through a needle or catheter placed through the tracheal wall. A wide bore needle or catheter is inserted, often without local anaesthesia (in an emergency), in the midline between any two tracheal rings: distal to the site of obstruction. The hub of the needle can be connected to either a 3–3.5 mm ET tube adapter, or to a 2 ml syringe barrel that is then connected to a 7 mm or 7.5 mm ET tube connector, and then the ET tube connector is attached to an anaesthetic breathing system for oxygen delivery (Figure 50.8). The delivered oxygen flow is limited by the size of needle and degree of obstruction of the upper airway.

50.3.4.1.2 Tube Tracheotomy

Can be performed under local anaesthesia with the patient either standing (large animals) or sitting (larger dogs), and offered oxygen supplementation (e.g. flow-by or mask), although it is often easier (especially for small animals) to perform under general anaesthesia, in which case, try to pre-oxygenate the animal before inducing anaesthesia (and place an endotracheal tube if possible). Clip and aseptically prepare the ventral neck. Make a longitudinal incision along the ventral midline from the caudal border of the cricoid cartilage extending caudally some 2–3 cm (depends upon patient size and also on site of obstruction). Separate and retract the paired sternohyoideus muscles.

Identify the trachea, elevate it (a modified approach using a Penrose drain has recently been described), and then incise through the annular ligament between two adjacent tracheal rings: usually in the region of the third or fourth rings, and extend the incision circumferentially, but not further than 40% of the circumference of the trachea. (Beware the vagosympathetic trunks lying either side of the trachea.) Place stay sutures around the rings on either side of the incision, to facilitate both immediate placing of the tube and later changing of it for cleaning. Choose a suitably sized tube (usually around half the tracheal diameter), and insert it gently. Most tubes are of human design and are really a bit too angled for animal tracheas, so beware not to insert the tube so that the tip rubs tightly against the tracheal wall, or even gets occluded by abutting the tracheal wall (Figure 50.9). If you cannot find a suitable tracheotomy tube, you can cut down an ET tube (you can use some of the excess length of the tube to peel down flaps [like peeling a banana skin down] so that you can use these flaps later to help secure the tube in place). If using a cuffed tube, be careful not to overinflate the cuff. Secure in place with neck ties and/or sutures. Ensure that nothing in the

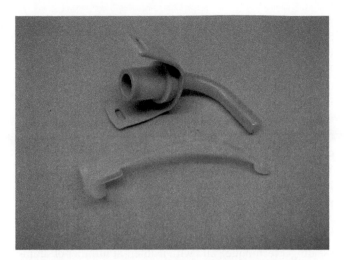

Figure 50.9 Non-cuffed 'single' tracheotomy tube with its obturator.

immediate vicinity of the animal is liable to be inhaled through the tube (care with bedding, feed, and water). Some dog breeds with excessive skin folds on the ventral neck, make bad candidates for tracheo[s]tomy procedures.

Aftercare Suction may be required every 20 minutes initially to ensure the tube is patent. Before every suction episode, the animal should be pre-oxygenated (if not already on supplementary oxygen). A small volume of sterile saline may be instilled through the tube lumen prior to suctioning and cleaning to help loosen/free-up any secretions (and it also may promote coughing that also helps to move secretions). Tubes need to be removed (briefly) for cleaning or replacing with clean tubes (initially this may be required up to twice daily, thereafter once daily may suffice); for which the stay sutures are really helpful. Have at least two spare tubes (one of the same size and one a size smaller) readily available **before** removing the tube that is in-situ.

'Double' tracheotomy tubes (for larger patients) have a removable inner tube which facilitates the cleaning process.

Complications These include: obstruction or displacement (continuous patient monitoring is therefore required); air leakage (with development of subcutaneous emphysema); coughing; respiratory infections (the upper respiratory tract with its air-filtering, warming, and humidification roles is bypassed so that mucociliary stasis occurs); tracheal stenosis/stricture. Heat and moisture exchangers incorporating filters (HMEF) are, however, available for attachment to tracheotomy tubes and may help conserve humidification of the respiratory tract, at least where the

volume of secretions is minimal, as otherwise, the HMEF may itself become blocked, causing recurrence of respiratory obstruction.

Removal The tube can be removed when the patient's condition allows. This can be assessed by temporary occlusion of the tube (e.g. with the obturator). For cuffed tubes, ensure the cuff is deflated before the tube is occluded to allow airflow into and out of the lungs. Once the tube is occluded, the patient must be monitored carefully for the return of respiratory distress. If the patient copes well, then the tube can be removed. After the tube is finally removed, the wound is cleansed and allowed to heal by second intention/granulation. (No swimming for a while!)

50.3.4.2 Thoracentesis
50.3.4.2.1 Needle Thora[co]centesis
Is therapeutic as well as diagnostic.

Site Seventh or eighth intercostal space (mid to caudal intercostal space because of the neurovascular bundle closely associated with the caudal border of each rib), halfway up chest wall (or, if the patient is in sternal recumbency, slightly higher for air, and slightly lower for fluid); and can be performed bilaterally.

Technique Hypodermic needles or butterfly needles are often preferred to catheters because catheters tend to kink or collapse. The animal may be conscious and standing, sitting, or sternal. Infiltrating the intended site of needle puncture with a bleb of local anaesthetic solution is helpful if time permits (or consider intercostal nerve blocks if time allows), but cyanotic moribund animals often will not protest in an emergency. A syringe can be attached to the needle (often via a short extension set and stopcock) to facilitate gentle aspiration as the needle is advanced, or a drop of sterile saline placed in the needle hub (before its insertion) can act as an indicator for entry into the pleural space because this drop should do one of the following:

- Be sucked in because of negative pressure in the space (intrapleural pressure is normally negative).
- Squirt out because of positive pressure in the space (e.g. with any degree of abnormal 'filling' of the space, i.e. pneumothorax, haemothorax, pyothorax). This response is more usual because, normally, a build-up of positive pressure within the pleural cavity is the reason for proceeding with chest drainage.

Once in the pleural space, the needle should be advanced more parallel to the chest wall so as to cause least possible laceration to the lungs during breathing movements. The needle should be attached to some sort of one-way valve system. Such a system can be made easily as follows: the last 20 cm of a giving set (with Luer connector) will attach to the needle hub, and the other end usually fits onto a three-way tap. You can now drain the pleural space (Figure 50.10). Fluid samples may require laboratory assessments.

Vast improvement in patient condition often follows even only partial drainage.

50.3.4.2.2 Tube Thoracostomy

This is a surgical procedure involving entry of a body cavity, and aseptic technique is therefore crucial.

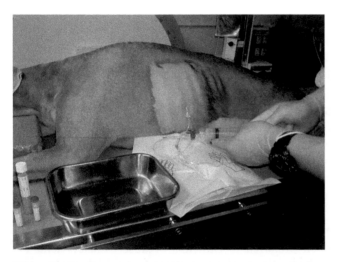

Figure 50.10 Needle thoracentesis and removal of purulent fluid from the pleural space. Five intercostal nerves were blocked (two either side of the point of drainage), evidenced by the superficial bleeding.

50.3.4.2.3 Site

Seventh or eighth intercostal space, and about half-way up the chest wall (slightly higher for air, slightly lower for fluid). Place the drain in the side that is most severely affected, as determined by clinical, radiographic or ultrasonographic investigation, or that which was most productive on needle thoracocentesis. The mediastinal pleura is often fenestrated, and is also very fragile, so that, usually, both sides of the chest are affected, but can be drained from one side. However, occasionally, especially with pyothorax, there will be 'pocketing' of the effusion, so that more than one site and possibly both sides of the chest may need to be tapped.

Different types of tubes are available (Figures 50.11 and 50.12): with or without trocars; or inserted using a wire-guide (Seldinger technique); and with a different number of drainage holes (the best have at least three side holes and an end hole). Further holes can be created, but must not be greater than a quarter of the tube's circumference or else the tube will kink easily. Some tubes have a radio-opaque marker strip. This may be combined with a 'sentinel eye': an end to, or interruption of, the marker strip at the position of the most proximal ('outermost' when the tube is in situ) hole. All holes must lie within the chest cavity after placement (confirmed by chest radiographs).

Tube size is denoted by 'French gauge' (related to outer circumference, i.e. external diameter [in mm] multiplied by 3 gives the Fr gauge, Table 50.2). Note that each 0.33 mm of external diameter therefore equates with 1 Fr. A suitable size can be guesstimated by taking the width of the mainstem bronchus (or 1/2–2/3 of the proposed intercostal space) as the largest required external tube diameter. Whereas smaller diameter tubes generally suffice for the removal of air, larger diameter tubes are better for fluid drainage, especially for thick and tenacious effusions.

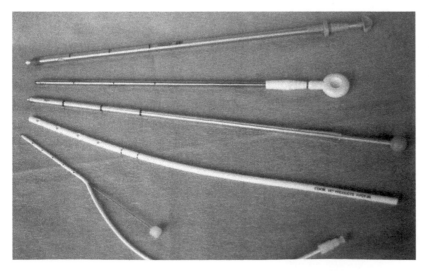

Figure 50.11 Different types of chest tubes. *Source:* Reproduced from Dugdale (2000) with permission from BVA Publications.

(a)

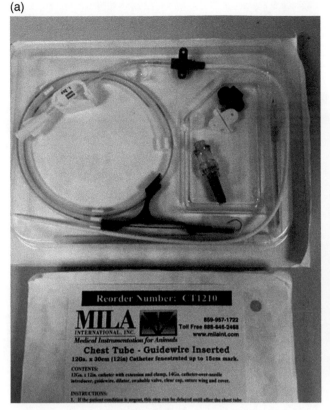

(b)

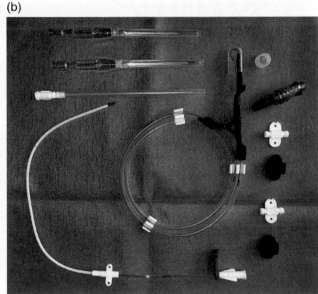

Figure 50.12 MILA™ guidewire-insertion type chest drains showing the kit in its original packaging (a), and arranged ready for use (b).

The length of tube should be such that its tip is located cranioventrally in the chest, but not further cranially than rib 2, or else the tube tends to become hindered by the pleural reflection and tissues of the thoracic inlet (Figure 50.13). Figure 50.14 shows a chest drain in situ in a horse with a pleural effusion.

50.3.4.2.4 Technique

The animal may be sitting, sternal, or laterally recumbent. The procedure is easier to perform under general anaesthesia, but local anaesthetic techniques are still helpful. ECG and pulse monitoring are useful during tube placement as arrhythmias may occur (see below).

Clip, aseptically prepare and drape the chest wall. Local anaesthetic infiltration and/or intercostal blocks are performed to desensitise the sites of tube insertion through both the skin and the chest wall. Pre-measure the length of tube to be inserted by holding it against the chest wall. Then do one of the following:

- Make a small skin incision at the tenth intercostal space; insert the tip of the tube/trocar through the incision and tunnel the whole assembly cranially, through the subcutaneous tissues, until the tip lies over the seventh or eighth intercostal space (Figure 50.15).

Table 50.2 A guide to which chest tube size to use in small animals.

Animal weight	Tube size (Fr) (mm internal diameter)
<7 kg	14–16 Fr (4 mm)
7–15 kg	16–20 Fr (5 mm)
16–30 kg	20–26 Fr (6 mm)
>30 kg	26–32 Fr (7 mm)

- An assistant pulls the skin of the lateral chest wall cranially, by about two rib spaces, so the tube can be placed directly through the skin which is now lying over the seventh or eighth intercostal space. Subsequent release of the skin automatically creates a tunnel.

Once the tube tip is positioned at the seventh or eighth intercostal space, the tube and trocar assembly are then held almost perpendicular to the body wall, aiming to slide off the cranial border of the rib concerned (eighth or ninth). A short sharp blow to the trocar 'handle' with the heel of your hand may be necessary so the trocar tip and tube tip penetrate the chest cavity; or push and twist firmly if a shorter stylette is present (Figure 50.16).

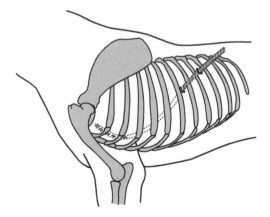

Figure 50.13 Typical position of chest tube in situ.

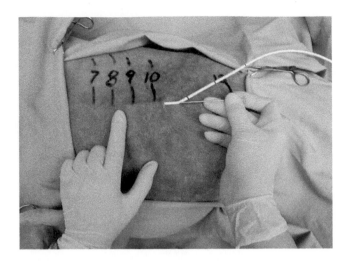

Figure 50.15 Tunnelling of chest drain beneath skin.

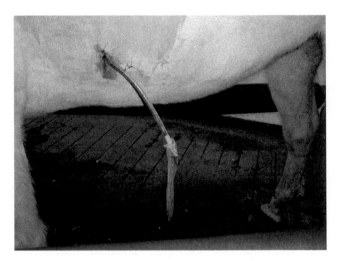

Figure 50.14 Chest drain in situ in a horse. A condom has been placed over the end of the drain to act as a one-way valve for drainage. Site for insertion is also seventh to eighth intercostal space, usually just dorsal to costochondral junctions, especially for fluid drainage.

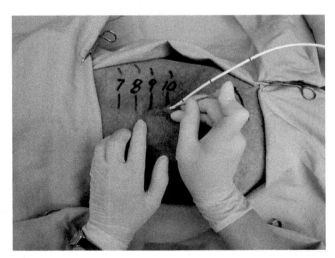

Figure 50.16 Insertion of chest drain into thoracic cavity at eighth intercostal space.

Once the tip of the trocar and tube assembly is within the chest cavity, angle it to lie more parallel with the internal chest wall and slide the tube over the trocar by about 2 cm, to 'cover' the sharp tip. The whole tube/trocar assembly can then be advanced cranially into the chest cavity, whilst keeping it more parallel with the internal chest wall so as to avoid damaging the structures within the chest. Once the tube has been inserted up to the pre-measured depth, withdraw the trocar whilst keeping a firm hold of the tube, and be ready to clamp or kink off the tube as soon as the trocar is fully withdrawn. 'Cap' the tube securely.

Newer 'Seldinger technique' type drains are available that do not require a trocar, and therefore are less traumatic.

They are available in various sizes and are placed in a similar manner as to a central venous (jugular) catheter. They are most commonly placed in dogs and cats; and necessarily being of smaller internal diameter, are most useful for the drainage of air (Figure 50.12).

Secure the tube in place using sutures (Figure 50.17):

- At the site of tube entry into the skin, place a suture through deep fascia, even adjacent rib periosteum, so as to ensure a firm anchoring for the tube. Tie several (e.g. six) knots to make a short stalk as a 'stand-off' before completing a Chinese finger trap suture around the tube. The 'stand-off' allows access to the skin to clean and inspect the wound.
- Place a suture (but not too tightly) through the skin and around the tube within its subcutaneous tunnel, about half-way along the tunnel, for extra security against air leaks.

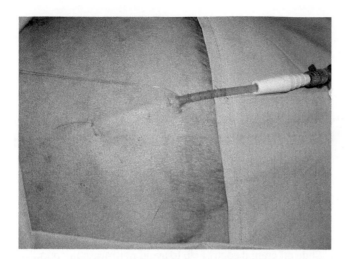

Figure 50.17 Chest drain secured in place with sutures.

- Some people like to place a suture circumferentially around the skin incision site surrounding the tube to reduce the chance of air ingress. Such sutures are like purse string sutures, but must not be over-tightened or else the skin blood supply will be compromised and necrosis may occur.
- Some people also pre-place a loose purse string suture in the skin around the tube entry site, so that at tube removal, the suture can be tightened **gently** to close the skin wound.

All connections of the tube, e.g. to the three-way tap, must be secure. Ligatures and/or superglue are often used. The tube's position should be verified with a chest radiograph.

Adequate analgesia must be provided, and may include intercostal nerve blocks, and interpleural instillation of local anaesthetic down the tube (after initial drainage) (see Chapter 15). Chest bandages, Elizabethan collars, and neck braces help to reduce interference with the tube by the patient.

Aspiration from the tube can be intermittent or continuous. Ideally, patients with chest drains should never be left unattended. If intermittent drainage is performed, gate clamps, even placed over a 'folded' section of tube, can help to ensure that the tube remains 'closed' between drainage sessions. The frequency of intermittent drainage will depend upon the rate of fluid or gas accumulation. A large syringe and three-way tap may suffice and allows measurement of the volume removed, but be careful not to apply excessive suction. For continuous drainage, a Heimlich valve or underwater seal can be used: air and/or fluid are expelled during exhalation.

Heimlich valves were at one time best suited to animals >15 kg, and for draining air (fluid tends to clog them). They consist of a one-way rubber flutter valve enclosed within a clear plastic tube, and must be securely connected to the chest drain (Figure 50.18). Smaller rigid Heimlich valves, and also 'pillow style' valves, are available for smaller patients.

An **underwater seal** consists of a sterile glass or plastic bottle, with a capacity of between 500 and 2–3,000 ml, containing sterile water or saline to a depth of a few cm (Figure 50.19). The cap has two stiff tubes placed through it; the lower tip of one is submerged about 2 cm below the level of the fluid, whilst the lower end of the other tube must remain above the fluid level. The outer end of the submerged tube is connected to the chest drain. Fluid in the submerged capillary tube imposes a back pressure on the pleural cavity, and seals it from the atmosphere. The level that the fluid attains in the tube, once connected to a chest drain, reflects the animal's intrapleural pressure. Bottles should be wide so that the level of fluid in the bottle does not fluctuate too much during breathing.

Intrapleural pressure is normally negative so that the fluid in the tube is 'sucked up' by a few (around 5) cm. During

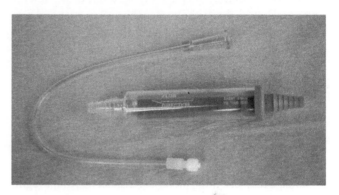

Figure 50.18 Standard size Heimlich valve. Actual size: about 16 cm long (in total) by about 2.5 cm diameter.

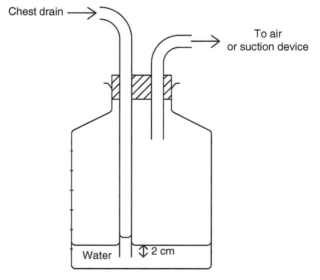

Figure 50.19 Underwater seal. The tube is normally submerged about 2 cm below the surface of the water in the bottle.

inspiration the intrapleural pressure becomes more negative, so the fluid level in the tube rises, and during expiration the pressure becomes less negative, so that the fluid level falls again (i.e. the fluid level swings slightly with breathing). With abnormal 'filling' of the pleural space (e.g. by fluid or air), the normally negative pressure becomes less negative, or even positive, so the fluid level in the tube does not rise as far or is even pushed down. If it is pushed down far enough (>2cm), then the contents of the tube can 'empty' into the bottle, and the 'excess' contents of the pleural space empty during successive expirations without the need to apply suction.

Animals should be positioned above the level of the bottle to reduce the chance of fluid syphoning back into the chest from the bottle. 'Trap' bottles can be placed between the animal's chest drain and the underwater seal bottle to reduce this risk. Trap bottles also allow measurement of drained fluid, and, by keeping any fluid out of the underwater seal bottle, the water level in the underwater seal bottle (important for its function) will not rise, so continued chest drainage is not compromised. A third bottle may also be included to act as a vacuum regulator when suction is to be applied (Figure 50.20). Should suction be necessary, 10–20 cmH$_2$O is usually sufficient. (Convenient, single-use only three-bottle systems are commercially available, e.g. Thora-seal™, Pleur-evac™, Thorametrix™).

50.3.4.2.5 Complications

- Damage to heart, lung, blood vessels, nerves, diaphragm, or liver during placement.
- Arrhythmias (heart or pericardium irritation/trauma).

- Phrenic nerve irritation with possible resultant diaphragm hemiparesis.
- Damage to vagosympathetic trunk (Horner's syndrome has been described).
- Leakage of air around or through the tube, leading to iatrogenic subcutaneous emphysema or pneumothorax.
- Infection.
- Stimulation of pleural effusion.
- Poor drainage/tube blockage (try different patient positions and/or aspiration/flushing; may be less of a problem with continuous drainage).

50.3.4.3 Reducing the Risks

- Careful aseptic technique.
- Slide off cranial edge of rib to avoid neurovascular bundle.
- Choose seventh or eighth intercostal space (further cranial or caudal risks damaging heart, diaphragm, liver).
- Create a subcutaneous tunnel between the sites of tube penetration of the body wall skin and of the chest cavity to provide some protection against air leaks.
- Pre-measure the tube length required and ensure all holes will lie within the chest cavity.
- Secure the tube in place as firmly as possible.
- Ensure all connections/tube caps are secured.
- Ensure patency and correct position of the tube.
- Use chest bandages and other devices to prevent patient interference.
- Ensure adequate analgesia.
- Ensure adequate patient observation.

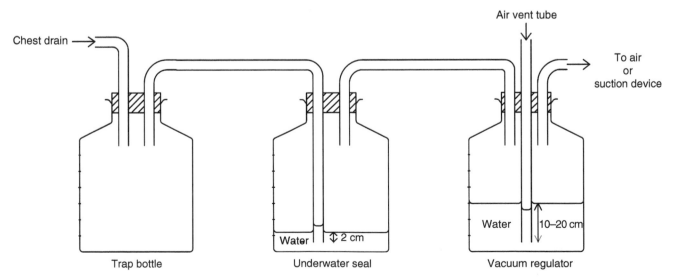

Figure 50.20 Three-bottle system. A trap or collection bottle can be interposed between the underwater seal and the patient's chest. Finally, a third bottle, the vacuum regulator, can be added: the air vent tube is usually submerged by 10–20 cm below the water surface to limit the vacuum applied to the chest to 10–20 cmH$_2$O.

50.3.4.3.1 Tube Removal Remove as soon as possible because tube presence within the pleural cavity stimulates the production of a serosanguinous pleural effusion, which can be of the order of 0.5–2 ml/kg/day. As a rough guide, tubes should be removed when no air has been aspirated for 12–24 hours or when <2 ml/kg/day fluid has been drained. The tube could be clamped off for a trial period of say 24 hours, during which time the animal is monitored closely and chest radiographs can be taken to assess progress.

50.3.4.3.2 Technique for Removal To provide some analgesia (tube removal can be quite painful), instil local anaesthetic down the tube about 30 minutes beforehand. The animal should be breathing quietly. Cut the tethering suture/s, and ensure placement of a purse-string suture (under local anaesthetic) if required and if not already pre-placed. Gently rotate the tube about its long axis to free it up from any adhesions. One person pulls out the capped tube in one quick smooth manoeuvre, whilst a second operator gets ready to gently tighten the purse string suture once the tube is out. Cleanse the wound and apply a sterile dressing and light chest bandage for 24 hours.

50.3.4.4 Flail Chest Wall Segments

Flail segments of the chest wall occur when ribs are fractured at two sites so that the mid-rib section becomes 'free' and cannot therefore move in unison with the rest of the chest wall during breathing movements. Normally during inspiration, the chest wall moves outwards, but flail segments are 'sucked in' by the increased negative intrathoracic pressure, thus moving 'paradoxically'. During expiration, the opposite occurs, i.e. the normal chest wall moves inwards, but the flail segment moves outwards. Stabilisation of flail segments greatly improves the efficacy of ventilation (reduces the air-pendulum effect) and greatly improves the animal's comfort. The reader is referred to surgical texts for approaches to flail chest stabilisation.

References

Dugdale, A. (2000). Chest drains and drainage techniques. *In Practice* 22: 2–15.

Dyce, K.M., Sack, W.O., and Wensing, C.J.G. (eds.) (2002). The head and ventral neck of the carnivores. In: *Textbook of Veterinary Anatomy*, 3e, 367–392. Elsevier.

Further Reading

Bird, F.G., Vallefuoco, R., Dupre, G., and Brissot, H. (2018). A modified temporary tracheostomy in dogs: outcome and complications in 21 dogs. *Journal of Small Animal Practice* 59: 769–776.

Dixon, D., Little, C.J.L., Harris, J., and Rishniw, M. (2018). Rapid assessment with physical examination in dyspnoeic cats: the RAPID CAT study. *Journal of Small Animal Practice* 59: 75–84.

Goggs, R. and Dugdale, A. (2006). Preliminary investigation of two oxygen therapy devices. Abstract. Proceedings of 50th Annual BSAVA Congress, Birmingham, UK. 467–468.

Hyndman, P. and Bray, J. (2017). Temporary tracheostomy: a practical approach to the placement and management of a tracheostomy tube. *Companion Animal* 22: 471–479.

Jagodich, T.A., Bersenas, A.M.E., Bateman, S.W., and Kerr, C.L. (2019). Comparison of high flow nasal cannula oxygen administration to traditional nasal cannula oxygen therapy in healthy dogs. *Journal of Veterinary Emergency and Critical Care* 29: 246–255.

Keir, I., Daly, J., Haggerty, J., and Guenther, C. (2016). Retrospective evaluation of the effect of high flow oxygen therapy delivered by nasal cannula on PaO2 in dogs with moderate-to-severe hypoxemia. *Journal of Veterinary Emergency and Critical Care* 26: 598–602.

Koterba, A.M., Kosch, P.C., Beech, J., and Whitlock, T. (1988). Breathing strategy of the adult horse (Equus caballus) at rest. *Journal of Applied Physiology* 64: 337–346.

Lilja-Maula, L., Lappalainen, A.K., Hyytiainen, H.K. et al. (2017). Comparison of submaximal exercise test results and severity of brachycephalic obstructive airway syndrome in English bulldogs. *The Veterinary Journal* 219: 22–26.

Lumb, A.B. and Thomas, C.R. (2019). High-flow nasal therapy – modelling the mechanism. *Anaesthesia* 74: 420–423.

Maltman, M. (2017). Self-assessment: dyspnea in a cat. *Companion Animal* 22: 480–485. **(Describes a case of pyothorax.)**.

Murphy, K. and Papasouliotis, K. (2011). Pleural effusions in dogs and cats 2. Placement of tubes and treatment. *In Practice* 33: 526–530.

Nicholson, I. and Baines, S. (2010). Indications, placement and management of tracheostomy tubes. *In Practice* 32: 104–113.

Pouzot-Nevoret, C., Hocine, L., Negre, J. et al. (2019). Prospective pilot study for evaluation of high-flow oxygen therapy in dyspnoeic dogs: the HOT-DOG study. *Journal of Small Animal Practice* 60: 656–662.

Riggs, J., Liu, N.C., Sutton, D.R. et al. (2019). Validation of exercise testing and laryngeal auscultation for grading brachycephalic obstructive airway syndrome in pugs, French bulldogs, and English bulldogs by using whole-body barometric plethysmography. *Veterinary Surgery* 48: 488–496.

Ryan, A., Borland, K., and Bradbrook, C. (2019). Anaesthesia in thoracic trauma. *Companion Animal* 24: 364–369.

Smith, C. and Witchell, H. (2016). Planning, managing and equipping an intensive care unit within a veterinary facility. *In Practice* 38: 2–5.

Vassilev, E. and McMichael, M. (2004). An overview of positive pressure ventilation. *Journal of Veterinary Emergency and Critical Care* 14: 15–21.

Self-test Section

1 True or False? A neurovascular bundle is associated with the caudal border of each rib.

2 How would you define *hypoxaemia* and *hypoxia*?

3 What techniques are available to provide oxygen-enriched "air" for a patient?

51

Cardiopulmonary Cerebral Resuscitation (CPCR)

LEARNING OBJECTIVES

- To be aware of different types of arrests.
- To be able to discuss Basic Life Support (now C, A, B) strategies, and for differing sizes/chest shapes of animal.
- To be familiar with Advanced Life Support (D, E, F) strategies.
- To be familiar with the drugs commonly used and the newer approaches.
- To be aware of post-resuscitation problems.

51.1 Introduction

The immediate goals of resuscitation during cardiopulmonary arrest (CPA) are to re-establish myocardial and cerebral perfusion and oxygenation, hence **cerebral** is included.

This chapter will deal with small animal CPA. For more information about horses, see Further Reading. The information in this chapter is based on the guidance provided following the RECOVER (REassessment Campaign On VEterinary Resuscitation) initiative (see Further Reading).

51.2 Types of Arrest

51.2.1 Respiratory, Cardiac or Both

Respiratory and cardiac arrest may occur almost simultaneously, or one may precede the other, e.g. one of the following can occur:

- Respiratory arrest → hypoxaemia → hypoxic myocardium → cardiac arrhythmia/arrest
- Cardiac arrest → reduced tissue perfusion/oxygenation → hypoxic medullary respiratory centre → agonal gasping → respiratory arrest.

Whatever the initiating cause, a **vicious circle** is entered, and eventually arrest of both systems occurs (CPA).

51.2.2 Acute or Chronic

Acute arrests are those that are not at all expected, e.g. the healthy bitch spay that has got a bit too deeply anaesthetised and stops breathing, or alternately, is too lightly anaesthetised and the release of catecholamines after surgical incision results in cardiac arrhythmia. Prognosis for resuscitation is excellent as long as arrest is recognised and treated early.

Chronic arrests are multifactorial, e.g. the old dog with a degree of renal failure and valvular endocardiosis perhaps now gets a little too deeply anaesthetised, respiration slows (respiratory acidosis now develops on top of pre-existing metabolic acidosis); the dog also gets a little cold under general anaesthesia and perhaps bleeds excessively so hypovolaemia is also now superimposed until a point is reached where the myocardium has just had enough; arrhythmias may be undetected until the heart finally stops. Prognosis is poor, as the 'internal milieu' is far from normal and cannot be fixed easily and quickly.

51.3 Prevention Is Better Than Cure

51.3.1 Why Do 'Arrests' Happen?

- Hypoxia/hypoxaemia.
- Hypercapnia (= hypercarbia).
- Electrolyte imbalances (especially hyperkalaemia).

Veterinary Anaesthesia: Principles to Practice, Second Edition. Alexandra H. A. Dugdale, Georgina Beaumont, Carl Bradbrook, and Matthew Gurney.
© 2020 John Wiley & Sons Ltd. Published 2020 by John Wiley & Sons Ltd.
Companion website: www.wiley.com/go/dugdale/veterinary-anaesthesia

- Acid/base abnormalities (pH changes can also affect electrolytes [especially K^+ and ionised Ca^{2+}]).
- Acute hypotension/hypovolaemia.
- Hypoglycaemia.
- Hypothermia.
- Autonomic nervous system imbalance (massive changes in either sympathetic or parasympathetic tone, often via 'reflexes').
- Pre-existing disease (cardiac, respiratory, renal, or urogenital, hepatobiliary, gastrointestinal, neurological, endocrine, haematological, immunological, neoplasia, intoxication).
- Anaesthetic overdose.

Thus, it is important to try to normalise as many of these as possible before attempting general anaesthesia and avoid their occurrence during anaesthesia.

51.3.2 Recognising that a Cardiac Arrest Has Occurred

- Unconscious patient.
- Respiratory arrest or agonal gasping ('tracheal tugs' describe the neck-flexing breathing efforts when the medullary respiratory centre is trying incredibly hard to recruit the accessory respiratory muscles [neck, and also abdominal], so breathing efforts look exaggerated).
- No heartbeat, no pulse, no haemorrhage at surgical site and the blood looks dark. (Pulse palpation is very insensitive.)
- Grey, cyanosed, or pale mucous membranes (may help indicate the initiating cause), but a fairly normal capillary refill time (CRT) may be obtained for several minutes after death.
- Central eye, unresponsive dilated pupils.
- No lacrimation (dry cornea), or salivation (dry mouth).
- No palpebral or corneal reflexes.
- Flaccid limbs, no reflexes.
- Absent capnograph trace, and minimal reading even with artificial ventilation because no circulation.

51.4 What Can We Do?

T Note the Time
H Call for Help
E follow the Emergency procedure...

C Circulation
A Airway — **Basic Life Support**
B Breathing

D Drugs (and fluids)
E Electrical defibrillation
F Follow up (and fluids) — **Advanced Life Support**
G Go home!
H Have a drink!

For humans, electrical defibrillation is now included under basic life support (BLS) because ventricular fibrillation, following myocardial infarction, is the commonest cause of out-of-hospital cardiac arrest.

51.5 Basic Life Support

Although the order of BLS used to be A, B, C; prioritisation of C has followed human evidence (in the absence of veterinary evidence to the contrary). A and B, however, may still be important, as not many animals suffer CPA because of atherosclerosis-related myocardial infarctions, but starting C as early as possible makes physiological sense.

51.5.1 C (Circulation)

External chest compressions should be commenced as soon as possible following CPA, or even *suspected CPA*. The likelihood of causing serious or lasting harm if the heart has not actually stopped beating is very low (<2%). Early C is associated with an increased chance of sustained return of spontaneous circulation (ROSC), and a higher survival rate.

- Place the patient onto a **hard, flat surface** and in a suitable position: usually lateral recumbency (see below).
- Start **compressions** at **100–120/minute** in **cycles of 2 minutes** (see below). (Even faster rates may be better, but are harder to sustain. Similarly, cycles longer than two minutes may be better, but it is very hard to maintain good technique for longer times.)
- **Compress the chest by 1/3–1/2 of its width**, taking care to **allow sufficient recoil** between compressions.
- **Cats and young animals**: compress the chest over the precordial area (two-handed technique), or circumferentially compress the anterior chest between finger and thumb (with one hand wrapped around the precordial sternum), to recruit the 'cardiac pump' with the patient positioned in **lateral recumbency**.
- **Dogs under 15 kg**, especially if **narrow-chested (keel-chested)**: compress the chest over the precordial area with compressions likely to recruit the 'cardiac pump'. **Lateral recumbency** (right lateral may be more suited to allow conversion to internal cardiopulmonary cerebral resuscitation [CPCR] if necessary), with a wedge placed under the chest, is the preferred position.
- **Round-chested or keel-chested dogs over 15 kg**: external CPCR is also performed with the patient in

lateral recumbency, but now chest compressions are recommended over the widest part of the chest to recruit the 'thoracic pump'.

- **Barrel-chested dogs** of **all sizes**: **dorsal recumbency** may be preferred (although it is not always easy to keep the patient stable in this position), with sterno-vertebral compressions (i.e. over the sternum towards the spine), in the hope of recruiting the 'cardiac pump', and possibly also the 'thoracic pump'. External chest compressions in barrel-chested dogs, no matter what their size, are not particularly effective such that some people advocate converting to internal cardiac massage sooner in these 'shapes' of dogs.

51.5.1.1 Cardiac Pump versus Thoracic Pump?

The **cardiac pump** is supposedly recruited by chest compressions centred over the heart (i.e. in the precordial region, ventrally over the third to sixth ribs). It is not usually very effective except in very small (<15 kg), and young animals with compliant chests; and may incur rib or other damage. As the chest is alternately compressed and released, the heart is supposedly also squeezed and released, establishing forwards flow through its chambers (as long as there are no leaky one-way valves).

The **thoracic pump** is the mechanism whereby most blood flow is established during external CPCR attempts in animals >15 kg. Compressions should be performed over the widest part of the chest (i.e. sixth to seventh ribs), midway down the chest wall, with the patient in lateral recumbency. The aim is not to physically compress the heart chambers, but, through evoking pressure changes within the chest (swings from positive pressure [during chest compression] to more negative pressure [during release/chest wall recoil]), to thereby facilitate alternating cardiac output and venous return. Works best when adequate 'relaxation' periods are allowed between compressions and 'normal' intrathoracic conditions exist (i.e. no pleural/pericardial effusions etc.). One-way blood flow is thus hopefully established, aided by the presence of one-way heart valves (hopefully not incompetent) and valves in the jugular veins.

51.5.2 A (Airway)

Whilst taking care not to interrupt the two-minute cycles of chest compressions, establish an **airway**: endotracheal (ET) tube, urinary catheter, tracheotomy. This may be difficult to do *during* chest compressions, but may be easier in the small interval (< 10 seconds) *between chest compression cycles*, when the animal's airway may be more accessible. (Always try not to suspend chest compressions during establishment of an airway.) **Suction** and a **laryngoscope**

may be necessary to help visualise the larynx; laryngoscopy is recommended to minimise laryngeal stimulation that may result in vagal or sympathetic reflexes. If the animal's trachea is already intubated, ensure the tube is in the correct place (capnography is useful here) and is patent. Ensure the distal tip of the ET tube lies outside the thoracic inlet, or else if the tube, or especially its cuff, lie 'within' the thoracic inlet, they may occlude the carotid arteries and compromise flow of blood towards the brain.

Turn off any halogenated anaesthetic agents and/or nitrous oxide. For rebreathing systems: increase the oxygen flow, flush with oxygen and 'dump' the bag at least twice. Ideally, aim to **deliver 100% oxygen**, although room air is also acceptable.

51.5.3 B (Breathing)

- Institute intermittent manual ventilation at a rate of **10 breaths/minute.** (Excessive rates raise the mean intrathoracic pressure for a large proportion of each minute of attempted resuscitation, which reduces venous return and cardiac output, increases intracranial pressure ([ICP], and can be detrimental. Additionally, high ventilation rates can reduce blood carbon dioxide content, which promotes cerebral vasoconstriction, potentially compromising cerebral oxygenation.)
- Aim to **inflate** the lungs **over one second with a tidal volume of 10 ml/kg**; the **chest wall should be seen to rise** (although this is not always easy to observe during rapid chest compressions).
- Try **not to exceed 15–20 cmH₂O inflation pressure.** (There may not be a manometer within the breathing system or resuscitation bag, but developing a 'feel' for such pressures when providing manual breaths for anaesthetised animals under non-urgent conditions, and where manometers are present to guide that 'feel', can provide invaluable experience.)
- **Allow the chest to deflate fully between breaths**, or 'breath-stacking' (lung hyperinflation) will hinder venous return, and hence any cardiac output you may establish.

If endotracheal intubation is impossible, as long as oxygen is supplied by **insufflation**, via a long catheter if possible (the nearer the carina the tip of the catheter, the better), then the act of chest compressions will help to move gases into and out of the lungs. The use of mouth to snout ventilation has also been documented.

For patients suffering from only respiratory arrest, you could try stimulating the Jen Chung (GV26) **acupuncture point** at the base of nasal philtrum: insert 25 g needle until it hits bone, then twist gently (or use a hen-pecking action).

Doxapram, an analeptic (central nervous system [CNS] stimulant and respiratory stimulant thought to increase the sensitivity of peripheral and central chemoreceptors to carbon dioxide and oxygen), increases cerebral and myocardial oxygen demand and can be detrimental when a patient is already hypoxaemic. Hence, it is **no longer recommended**.

51.5.4 Techniques that Have Been Tried to Help Increase the Effectiveness of External CPCR

- **Tilting the animal slightly head down** (to increase blood flow to the head) is **no longer recommended** (as it reduces venous return from the head, increasing ICP, and thereby decreases cerebral perfusion).
- **Simultaneous ventilation and compression** (SVC). Aimed to coincide occasional chest compressions with peak lung inflations to increase the 'forwards' flow of blood. **No longer recommended** because high intrathoracic pressures may dam back venous return, compromising cardiac output and also increasing central venous pressure (CVP) and ICP.
- **Raising the hindlimbs and/or hindlimb and abdominal binding** can increase initial venous return from the hind end of the animal to increase the blood volume available for vital organ perfusion. It also directs any cardiac output generated to the head end of the animal. Binding should be performed from the hind toe tips, cranially. If resuscitation is successful, binding should be released slowly, from cranially to caudally, but **beware reactive hyperaemia** of the hind end of the animal, systemic hypotension, and **reperfusion injury**.
- **Abdominal counter-pulsations (interposed abdominal compressions)**. By compressing the abdomen during chest 'relaxation', blood is encouraged to flow towards the vessels in the chest. Then, by maintaining some abdominal pressure during chest compression, blood is discouraged from returning to vessels in the abdomen, thus helping to maintain the 'head-wards' flow. Can be **difficult to co-ordinate** without training.
- **Active compression/decompression**. Theoretically, by decreasing intrathoracic pressure during chest decompression, venous return is increased. This **requires special devices** that 'attach' to the chest wall.
- **Impedance threshold devices/valves**. These attach to the airway to limit air/oxygen entering the lungs during chest recoil, thereby generating greater negative intrathoracic pressures, which increase the volume of blood returning to intrathoracic vessels (i.e. they can augment venous return). They are **not useful for patients < 10 kg**

because of the limited negative pressures generated by chest recoil in these small patients in the first place.
- **Circumferential chest compression**. This *may* **result in increased cardiac output in smaller patients**.

51.5.5 How Effective Are Your Efforts?

Within 30–60 seconds of starting CPCR, and at least every 30 seconds thereafter, and certainly during the short pauses (< 10 seconds) between compression cycles, someone should check for:

- Improvement in mucous membrane colour.
- Pupil constriction and return of pupillary light reflexes.
- Ventromedial relocation of eyes and return of corneal and palpebral reflexes.
- Return of lacrimation.
- **ECG** rhythm and any changes (beware movement artefacts).
- Increased limb tone and other reflexes.
- Return of spontaneous ventilatory efforts.
- End tidal CO_2 value increasing (capnography/capnometry). **Capnography is very useful**: You do not have to suspend your resuscitation efforts to monitor changes. (Beware overzealous ventilation.)
- A Doppler blood flow probe may be used to detect retinal blood flow, but movement artefacts can occur (practically, not very informative).
- Pulses are incredibly hard to detect during CPCR attempts, and femoral venous pulsations are commonly mistaken for arterial pulses. Therefore, check for:
  - Audible heart sounds, i.e. ROSC.
  - ECG pattern.

There is good evidence for the use of ECG and capnography:

- ECG evaluation should be performed in a rapid manner during the <10 seconds inter-cycle pauses in chest compressions (when there is no motion artefact), and can be used to inform drug choices for advanced life support (ALS).
- If $ETCO_2$ values are lower than 15 mmHg, this may signal poor compressions, such that a poor cardiac output is being generated, e.g. fatigue in the compressor or poor compression technique. When manual ventilation is first commenced, $ETCO_2$ values are likely to be high for the first breath or two, so beware not to take this as a signal of ROSC, unless the values remain high or increase. There is some evidence that higher $ETCO_2$ values (>15 mmHg [dogs] and > 20 mmHg [cats]) may be associated with an increased rate of ROSC as they generally indicate the generation of a greater cardiac output.

If no success within two minutes, try resuscitative drugs (see below). If no response within 2–5+ minutes, and especially if no ECG available, consider internal technique (you can then 'see' what the heart is doing, which may help to direct your choice of drugs).

Cease resuscitative efforts after 15–20 minutes of no response. Although the brain can normally only survive for about two minutes after its glucose and oxygen supply has ceased, animals under anaesthesia, especially if a little hypothermic, should have longer than this as the brain's energy requirements are reduced and some of the anaesthetic agents have neuroprotective properties.

51.6 Advanced Life Support (ALS)

During the performance of BLS, if not already present, **establish IV access**. Central venous access (jugular vein) is best for the 'quickest' delivery of drugs to the heart, but may not be possible in an emergency, so a peripheral venous catheter will suffice. Try not to suspend chest compression activity during venous catheterisation. Venous cut-down may be required because of the collapsed circulation. Consider intra-osseous access, especially in young animals. If intravenous access proves impossible, drugs may be administered via the trachea (see below).

Any **monitoring equipment** available should also be **attached** (e.g. ECG, capnograph) if this has not already been done during BLS.

D, E, and F can now be done more or less simultaneously and are guided by, particularly, the ECG findings. Some drugs and fluids, however, may be chosen according to any known pre-existing condition/s, e.g. if anaesthetic overdose is suspected, are there any specific antidotes? (Naloxone for opioids, atipamezole for α2 agonists, flumazenil for benzodiazepines.) See dosage charts in Appendices for more details of individual drug doses.

51.6.1 Routes of Drug Administration

51.6.1.1 Intravenous
- **Central vein > peripheral vein**.
- Follow injection with a 'flush' of 5–50 ml sterile saline (volume depends upon patient size). If a peripheral vein is used, the limb can also be raised for two minutes.

51.6.1.2 Intratracheal
Trans-mucosal absorption of drugs occurs into the broncho-oesophageal circulation that returns to both the left and right sides of the heart.

- Use **2–10 times the IV dose**, dilute in 5–10 ml sterile water or sterile saline (dogs), or 2–3 ml (cats).

- Follow instillation at the carina (via male dog or cat urinary catheter) with two good lung inflations.
- OK for epinephrine, atropine, lidocaine, methoxamine, naloxone, and vasopressin, but not bicarbonate (it is hypertonic and inactivates surfactant) or calcium salts (they precipitate in surfactant).

51.6.1.3 Intra-osseous
Useful in small animals and young animals with soft bone cortices. Intra-osseous needle power drivers are commercially available. Some people prefer this to the intratracheal route if direct intravenous access is not available.

51.6.1.4 Intracardiac
Not recommended unless open chest CPCR (allows direct visualisation of injection site).

51.6.2 Arrest Arrhythmias and Treatments

ECG essential (unless you can visualise the heart, i.e. during internal cardiac massage).

51.6.2.1 Asystole
The most common arrest arrhythmia in dogs and cats: poor prognosis. Causes include hypoxaemia, hypothermia, hypovolaemia, vagal reflexes, electrolyte abnormalities.
Treatment:

- **Atropine**, especially if high vagal tone is suspected as the cause of the arrest. Bradycardias due to hypoxaemia or hypothermia tend not to respond to anticholinergics. If hypothermia is suspected and open chest CPCR is being performed, then lavaging the open chest cavity with warmed fluids may help. Can be given every other two-minute compression cycle.
- **Epinephrine** can be given to induce ventricular fibrillation, then try electrical defibrillation (preferred to chemical defibrillation with lidocaine). High dose or low dose? High dose (0.1–0.2 mg/kg) exerts both alpha effects (peripheral vasoconstrictor effects, to 'centralise' blood volume to the vital organs, which is useful in CPCR) and beta effects (positive inotropic and chronotropic effects, which can be useful, but directly increase myocardial oxygen demand). Although high dose epinephrine may be associated with earlier ROSC, it is associated with worse myocardial (e.g. re-fibrillation) and neurological outcomes in humans. It is recommended to use 'low' dose (0.01 mg/kg) initially, and if this is unsuccessful, the subsequent doses given are then 'high'. Can be re-dosed every three to five minutes, i.e. every other two-minute compression cycle.
- **Vasopressin** is a potent vasoconstrictor (working on V1 receptors on smooth muscle), without direct positive inotropic effects on the heart; therefore, does not increase

myocardial oxygen demand directly (unlike epinephrine). It has become a first line treatment in CPCR where it can be used either instead of, or alongside, epinephrine. Whereas epinephrine, with its α and β effects, is a positive inotrope, positive chronotrope, and can cause vasodilation (especially in skeletal muscles), and/or vasoconstriction (dose- and tissue-dependent), vasopressin is a pure vasoconstrictor and the pressor response to vasopressin is not reduced by acidosis/hypoxia, whereas that of epinephrine is. It can be administered at 0.2–0.8 U/kg intravenously, although the 0.8 U/kg dose seems to be preferred. A total dose of 0.8 U/kg should not be exceeded because of the worry of splanchnic reperfusion injury post-resuscitation.

- **Electrical defibrillation is not recommended** for asystole.

51.6.2.2 Ventricular Tachycardia (VT) or Ventricular Fibrillation (VF)

Fine fibrillation can be mistaken for asystole, so, if possible, check multiple orthogonal leads of the ECG.
Treatment:

- **Electrical D.C. defibrillation** is preferred (biphasic preferred over monophasic):
  - **First shock:** 4–6 J/kg (monophasic) or 2–4 J/kg (biphasic) if external paddles, or 0.2–0.5–1.0 J/kg if internal paddles. Continue chest compressions/cardiac massage for two minutes uninterrupted, then reassess, and, if necessary, shock again. Repeat every two minutes.
  - **Successive shocks:** A 50% increase in energy may be considered if the first shock is unsuccessful (care as there is a risk of myocardial injury).
  - **Paddles** should be placed on opposite sides of the thorax at the level of the costochondral junctions.
- If no defibrillator, try **lidocaine**: Repeat boluses/infusion may be necessary. (Lidocaine does not work well if hypokalaemia or hypomagnesaemia are present.) Once lidocaine has been administered, the heart becomes refractory to electrical defibrillation. **Procainamide** may be a better choice for cats as lidocaine has profound cardiovascular side effects.
- **Amiodarone** and **magnesium sulphate** (0.15–0.3 mEq/kg slow IV over 10 minutes) are suggested for some ventricular arrhythmias that are refractory to other treatments (see Further Reading). Note that in the UK, the available injectable preparations of amiodarone tend to cause hypotensive crises/anaphylaxis, possibly due to one of the solvents, polysorbate 80.
- **Although mechanical defibrillation by precordial thump** is now discouraged in human CPCR, because it

may convert ventricular tachycardia into ventricular fibrillation or result in asystole, the situation is less clear in animals. It may therefore be considered with VF or pulseless VT, but only when electrical defibrillation is not available.

51.6.2.3 Electromechanical Dissociation (EMD)

EMD is encompassed in the term **pulseless electrical activity (PEA)**. ECG rhythm may look normal or abnormal, but no heart contractions or pulses result. Cats tend not to suffer ventricular fibrillation because their ventricular muscle mass is relatively small, however, their preferred crash rhythm is PEA. Prognosis poor. The cause is unknown, but may include acute hypovolaemia and/or hypothermia.
Treatment is often without success. Has included:

- Fluids.
- Corticosteroids.
- Naloxone (high endogenous opioids accompanying CPA may have a role in PEA).
- Electrical defibrillation is not effective.

51.6.2.4 A-V Block or Sinus Bradycardia

The causes are: hypoxaemia, vagal reflexes, hypothermia, electrolyte problems.
Treatment

- Atropine.
- β agonists (e.g. dobutamine, isoprenaline, terbutaline).
- Ephedrine (an ino-constrictor): favoured for vaso-vagal reflexes.
- Atipamezole may be indicated.
- Calcium may help to treat the effects of hyperkalaemia in the short term, but calcium is also less favoured in CPCR because it can promote cell death.

51.6.2.5 Other Drugs

The use of corticosteroids, calcium, and sodium bicarbonate are all controversial, and depend upon the individual circumstances surrounding the arrest. Calcium should be reserved for cases of acute hyperkalaemia. Current advice recommends avoidance of corticosteroids. Sodium bicarbonate should be avoided unless there was a severe pre-existing metabolic acidosis with hyperkalaemia or following prolonged CPA (dose c. 0.5–1.0 mmol/kg). Glucose should be avoided unless severe hypoglycaemia preceded the arrest as hyperglycaemia itself is detrimental to neurological outcome.

51.6.3 Fluids

Routine administration of IV fluids is not recommended (unless hypovolaemia preceded arrest), because an increase in central venous pressure can reduce coronary and cerebral perfusion. The following, however, may be considered in the case of pre-existing hypovolaemia:

- 20(−40) ml/kg 'bolus' of crystalloid for dogs; 10(−20) ml/kg for cats.
- 5(−10) ml/kg 'bolus' of colloid for dogs; 2.5(−5) ml/kg for cats.

Coronary perfusion pressure (for left ventricle) equals aortic end diastolic pressure (AEDP) minus left ventricular end diastolic pressure. Therefore, coronary perfusion pressure is about equal to diastolic arterial blood pressure minus right atrial pressure (RAP). As RAP ≡ CVP, and fluid overload increases CVP, coronary perfusion pressure is reduced by excessive intravenous fluids.

Similarly, as cerebral perfusion pressure equals mean arterial pressure minus ICP, and as increased CVP increases ICP, excessive intravenous fluids can compromise cerebral perfusion.

51.7 External or Internal Compressions/Cardiac Massage?

51.7.1 Size of Animal and Chest 'Shape'

External chest compressions, at best, can only generate around 1/3 of normal cardiac output, and in barrel-shaped dogs, external compression efforts are likely to be even less effective. Internal cardiac massage may therefore be considered earlier in the resuscitation efforts of dogs of this conformation.

51.7.2 Acute or Chronic Arrest?

Normally begin with external chest compressions for acute arrests, but be prepared to be more aggressive in the absence of an early response. For chronic arrests, it is often better to be more aggressive from the start or perhaps have 'Do not resuscitate' orders.

51.7.3 Owner Wishes?

May vary from 'do everything possible' (internal cardiac massage sooner than later), to 'do not resuscitate'.

51.7.4 Help Available?

You need facilities, drugs, and staff (**TEAM**), for the resuscitation procedure and the aftercare to be optimal.

At least three (and preferably four or five) people are needed: one to ventilate, one to perform cardiac massage (with one or two 'spare' to take turns in delivering compressions), and one (or two) to locate, draw up and administer drugs and monitor/record the animal's response. One person should be in charge. Because performing external chest compressions is rapidly tiring, it is advised to change the 'compressor' every two minutes.

51.7.5 Equipment Available?

Depending upon where (e.g. street, clinic, hospital) the arrest happens, this may be a limiting factor to the technique/s used.

In a hospital, the following are likely to be available:

- Oxygen supply
- Laryngoscope, ET tubes, suction, etc.
- Breathing systems/anaesthetic machine
- IV cannulae, etc.
- ECG
- Capnograph
- Doppler blood flow detector
- DC defibrillator
- Surgical equipment for internal cardiac massage
- Chest drains
- Syringes, needles, dog urinary catheters (useful for intratracheal O_2 administration or intratracheal deposition of drugs should IV access prove difficult), intra-osseous needles, fluids
- Drugs (see emergency dose charts)
- Selection of fluids (crystalloids, colloids, blood)

51.8 Open Chest CPCR

- Indicated immediately if:
  - Penetrating chest wounds
  - Rib fractures
  - Pleural space disease
  - Pericardial effusion
  - Owner wishes for "ALS", and especially, for barrel chested dogs >15 kg
- Potentially after two to five minutes if closed chest CPCR is not successful.

51.8.1 During Open Chest CPCR

- Cross-clamping or digital occlusion of the descending aorta is recommended to improve coronary and cerebral perfusion, but after successful resuscitation, remove the occlusion slowly and beware reperfusion injury if the descending aorta was occluded for >10 minutes.

- Squeeze the heart from apex to base, and be careful not to 'twist' it because in doing so you may twist/occlude the great vessels and reduce the potential cardiac output.

51.9 Post-resuscitation Problems

Re-arrest and arrhythmias are common, and therefore close patient monitoring is required post-arrest and ROSC. Reperfusion injury, coagulopathies, and seizures can all occur. Neurological sequelae may become apparent within hours to days. Active re-warming of patients is discouraged, and indeed permissive hypothermia may improve outcome. Seizures must be controlled in order to avoid hyperthermia, hypoxaemia, and hypoglycaemia. Tight glycaemic control is advised. Patient monitoring should include ECG, blood pressure, urine output, blood gases, and electrolytes.

It is important to have aftercare facilities and staff available to ensure adequate patient care; ideally, in an intensive care setting.

51.10 Overall

You need adequate **staff, equipment, teamwork, and regular practice** (whether real or simulated), and excellent post-resuscitation **intensive care** facilities and nursing available.

51.11 New Ideas

The 2000 International Guidelines for CPR and ECC (emergency cardiac care), later incorporated into the 2005 American Heart Association Guidelines for human cardiopulmonary resuscitation and emergency cardiovascular care, provided an evidence-based overview that ranked therapeutic interventions. This evidence classification also formed the basis of the 2012 RECOVER guidelines, the first veterinary specific CPCR guidelines for dogs and cats. RECOVER 2 has been commissioned and will provide an up-to-date resource on veterinary CPCR.

Further Reading

Small Animal

Cober, R.E., Schober, K.E., Hildebrandt, N. et al. (2009). Adverse effects of intravenous amiodarone in 5 dogs. *Journal of Veterinary Internal Medicine* 23: 657–661.

Fletcher, D.J., Boller, M., Brainard, B.M. et al. (2012). RECOVER evidence and knowledge gap analysis on veterinary CPR. Part 7: clinical guidelines. *Journal of Veterinary Emergency and Critical Care* 22 (s1): 102–131.

Hofmeister, E.H., Thompson, B.F., Brainard, B.M. et al. (2008). Survey of academic veterinarians' attitudes toward provision of cardiopulmonary cerebral resuscitation and discussion of resuscitation with clientele. *Journal of Veterinary Emergency and Critical Care* 18: 131–141.

Penson, P.E., Ford, W.R., and Broadley, K.J. (2007). Vasopressors for cardiopulmonary resuscitation. Does pharmacological evidence support clinical practice? *Pharmacology and Therapeutics* 115: 37–55.

Schmittinger, C.A., Astner, S., Astner, L. et al. (2005). Cardiopulmonary resuscitation with vasopressin in a dog. (case report). *Veterinary Anaesthesia and Analgesia* 32: 112–114.

Scroggin, R.D. and Quandt, J. (2009). The use of vasopressin for treating vasodilatory shock and cardiopulmonary arrest. *Journal of Veterinary Emergency and Critical Care* 19: 145–157.

Strachan, F. (2016). Cardiopulmonary resuscitation in small animals. *In Practice* 38: 419–438.

Horse

Corley, K.T. and Furr, M.O. (2000). Cardiopulmonary resuscitation in newborn foals. Compendium on continuing education for the practising. *Veterinarian* 22: 957–966.

Frauenfelder, C., Fessier, J.F., Latshaw, H.S. et al. (1981). External cardiovascular resuscitation of the anesthetized pony. *Journal of the American Veterinary Medical Association* 179: 673–676.

Hubbell, J.A.E., Muir, W.W., and Gaynor, J.S. (1993). Cardiovascular effects of thoracic compression in horses subjected to euthanasia. *Equine Veterinary Journal* 25: 282–284.

Jokisalo, J.M. and Corley, K.T.T. (2014). CPR in the neonatal foal- has RECOVER changed our approach? *Veterinary Clinics of North America; Equine Practice* 30: 301–316.

Ruiz, C.C. and Junot, S. (2018). Successful cardiopulmonary resuscitation in a sevoflurane anaesthetized horse that suffered cardiac arrest at recovery. *Frontiers in Veterinary Science* 5 (138): 1–5.

Self-test Section

1 Now that minimal interruption of chest compressions is advised, which of the following monitoring devices can help detect ROSC (return of spontaneous circulation) and will work despite the inevitable patient movement?
   - ECG
   - Pulse oximeter
   - Oesophageal stethoscope
   - Capnography
   - Doppler blood flow probe.

2 True or False? Vasopressin may be used as an alternative to epinephrine for its potent vasopressor effects and is efficacious in an acidic environment.

3 High dose epinephrine is no longer recommended as a first line therapy due to which concerns?

4 In a 20 kg English Bulldog, which body position would be most effective for performing chest compressions?

Appendix A

Canine Emergency Drug Doses

FOR INTRAVENOUS INJECTION, or 2–10 x dose and dilute to 5–10 ml for intratracheal deposition

DRUG	DOSE	REASON	5 kg	10 kg	25 kg	50 kg
ADRENALINE / EPINEPHRINE 1:1000 = 1 mg/ml Diluted to 1:10000 = 0.1 mg/ml	**0.01–0.1** mg/kg	CARDIAC ARREST – give IV asystole / fibrillation ANAPHYLAXIS – give IM or IV	0.05–0.5 ml	0.1–1 ml	0.25–2.5 ml	0.5–5 ml
VASOPRESSIN 20 units/ml	**(0.2 –) 0.8** U/kg	VASOPRESSOR (during CPCR)	0.2 ml	0.4 ml	1 ml	2 ml
ATROPINE 0.6 mg/ml	**0.04** mg/kg	CARDIAC ARREST, asystole Vagally-induced arrhythmias	0.33 ml	0.66 ml	1.66 ml	3.33 ml
GLYCOPYRROLATE 200 µg/ml	**(5 –) 10** µg/kg	CARDIAC ARREST, asystole Vagally-induced arrhythmias	0.25 ml	0.5 ml	1.25 ml	2.5 ml
LIDOCAINE 2% = 20 mg/ml	**1–5** mg/kg slowly can infuse at 25–50+ µg/kg/min	Ventricular arrhythmias/ Ventricular fibrillation	0.25–1.25 ml	0.5–2.5 ml	1.25–6.25 ml	2.5–12.5 ml
AMIODARONE 50 mg/ml	2–5 mg/kg slowly *Beware anaphylaxis* *with formations containing* *polysorbate 80 as preservative*	Ventricular tachyarrhythmias May be preferable to lidocaine but not always available	0.5 ml	1 ml	2.5 ml	5 ml

(*Continued*)

Veterinary Anaesthesia: Principles to Practice, Second Edition. Alexandra H. A. Dugdale, Georgina Beaumont, Carl Bradbrook, and Matthew Gurney.
© 2020 John Wiley & Sons Ltd. Published 2020 by John Wiley & Sons Ltd.
Companion website: www.wiley.com/go/dugdale/veterinary-anaesthesia

FOR INTRAVENOUS INJECTION, or 2–10 x dose and dilute to 5–10 ml for intratracheal deposition

DRUG	DOSE	REASON	5 kg	10 kg	25 kg	50 kg
ESMOLOL	0.05–0.1 mg/kg	Supraventricular tachycardias	0.025–0.05 ml	0.05–0.1 ml	0.125–0.25 ml	0.25–0.5 ml
10 mg/ml	slowly then infuse at 50–200 µg/kg/min					
ISOPRENALINE / ISOPROTERENOL	0.04–0.1 µg/kg/min	BRADYCARDIA / AV BLOCK	to effect	to effect	to effect	to effect
1 mg/ml no longer widely available	infuse to effect					
TERBUTALINE	0.01 mg/kg	BRADYCARDIA / AV BLOCK	0.1 ml	0.2 ml	0.5 ml	1.0 ml
0.5 mg/ml						
FUROSEMIDE 5%	**(1 –) 2** (– 4) mg/kg	OEDEMA / DIURETIC	0.2 ml	0.4 ml	1 ml	2 ml
50 mg/ml						
CALCIUM chloride 10%	0.1–0.2 ml/kg	HYPERKALAEMIA	0.5–1 ml	1–2 ml	2.5–5 ml	5–10 ml
100 mg/ml 1.36 mEq Ca/ml	slowly	HYPOCALCAEMIA				
CALCIUM gluconate 10%	0.5–1.5 ml/kg	HYPERKALAEMIA	2.5–7.5 ml	5–15 ml	12.5–37.5 ml	25–75 ml
100 mg/ml 0.45 mEq Ca/ml	slowly	HYPOCALCAEMIA				
ATIPAMEZOLE	5 x medetomidine dose	ANTAGONISE ALPHA 2 AGONISTS				
5 mg/ml	10 x dexmedetomidine dose slowly					
NALOXONE	10 (– 20 –) 40 µg/kg	ANTAGONISE OPIOIDS	0.125–0.5 ml	0.25–1.0 ml	0.625–2.5 ml	1.25–5 ml
0.4 mg/ml	may need repeating					
FLUMAZENIL	10 µg/kg	ANTAGONISE BENZODIAZEPINES	0.5 ml	1.5 ml	2.5 ml	5 ml
0.1 mg/ml	may need repeating					
CHLORPHENAMINE	c. 0.5 mg/kg	ALLERGIC REACTIONS	0.25 ml	0.5 ml	1.25 ml	2.5 ml
10 mg/ml	SLOWLY					
MANNITOL	0.25–**0.5 – 1** (–2) g/kg	CEREBRAL OEDEMA	12.5–25 ml	25–50 ml	62.5–125 ml	125–250 ml
20% = 200 mg/ml	slowly	Osmotic diuretic				
DIAZEPAM	**0.5** mg/kg	SEIZURES	0.5 ml	1 ml	2.5 ml	5 ml
5 mg/ml	**0.2** mg/kg	POST-OP RESTLESSNESS	0.2 ml	0.4 ml	1 ml	2 ml
DEXTROSE 5–50%	0.25–0.5 (– 1) g/kg	HYPOGLYCAEMIA				
50–500 mg/ml	slowly	not via peripheral vein if >10% soln				

Appendix B

Feline Emergency Drug Doses

FOR INTRAVENOUS INJECTION, or 2–10 × dose and dilute to 2–3 ml for intratracheal deposition

DRUG	DOSE	REASON	1 kg	2.5 kg	3.5 kg	5 kg
ADRENALINE / EPINEPHRINE	**0.01–0.1** mg/kg	CARDIAC ARREST - give IV	0.01–0.1 ml	0.02–0.25 ml	0.035–0.35 ml	0.05–0.5 ml
1 : 1000 = 1 mg/ml		asystole / fibrillation				
Diluted to 1 : 10000 = 0.1 mg/ml		ANAPHYLAXIS - give IM or IV				
VASOPRESSIN	**(0.2 –) 0.8** U/kg	VASOPRESSOR	0.04 ml	0.1 ml	0.14 ml	0.2 ml
20 units/ml		during CPCR				
ATROPINE	**0.04** mg/kg	CARDIAC ARREST, asystole	0.07 ml	0.17 ml	0.23 ml	0.33 ml
0.6 mg/ml		Vagally-induced arrhythmias				
GLYCOPYRROLATE	**(5 –) 10** µg/kg	CARDIAC ARREST, asystole	0.05 ml	0.125 ml	0.175 ml	0.25 ml
200 µg/ml		Vagally-induced arrhythmias				
LIDOCAINE	**(0.25 –) 0.5 (– 1.0)** mg/kg slowly	VENTRICULAR arrhythmias	0.025 ml	0.063 ml	0.088 ml	0.125 ml
2% = 20 mg/ml	*BEWARE TOXICITY*	Ventricular fibrillation				
AMIODARONE	2–5 mg/kg	Ventricular tachyarrhythmias	0.1 ml	0.25 ml	0.35 ml	0.5 ml
50 mg/ml	slowly	*Formulations preserved in polysorbate 80*				
		have caused anaphylaxis in dogs				
PROCAINAMIDE	1–2 mg/kg	SUPRA- / VENTRICULAR ARRHYTHMIAS	depends	upon	dilution	used
variable	slowly	may be preferable to lidocaine in cats				
	can infuse at 25–40 µg/kg/min	if amiodarone not available				

(Continued)

Veterinary Anaesthesia: Principles to Practice, Second Edition. Alexandra H. A. Dugdale, Georgina Beaumont, Carl Bradbrook, and Matthew Gurney.
© 2020 John Wiley & Sons Ltd. Published 2020 by John Wiley & Sons Ltd.
Companion website: www.wiley.com/go/dugdale/veterinary-anaesthesia

FOR INTRAVENOUS INJECTION, or 2–10 × dose and dilute to 2–3 ml for intratracheal deposition

DRUG	DOSE	REASON	1 kg	2.5 kg	3.5 kg	5 kg
ESMOLOL	0.05–0.1 mg/kg	Supraventricular tachycardias	dilute	to smaller	volume	0.025–0.05 ml
10 mg/ml	slowly then infuse at 50–200 µg/kg/min					
TERBUTALINE	0.01 mg/kg	BRADYCARDIA / AV BLOCK	0.02 ml	0.05 ml	0.07 ml	0.1 ml
0.5 mg/ml		BRONCHODILATOR during anaphylaxis/asthma				
FUROSEMIDE 5%	(1 –) **2** (– 4) mg/kg	OEDEMA / DIURETIC	0.04 ml	0.1 ml	0.14 ml	0.2 ml
50 mg/ml						
Calcium chloride 10%	0.1–0.2 ml/kg	HYPERKALAEMIA	0.1–0.2 ml	0.25–0.5 ml	0.35–0.7 ml	0.5–1 ml
100 mg/ml 1.36 mEq Ca/ml	slowly	HYPOCALCAEMIA				
Calcium gluconate 10%	0.5–1.5 ml/kg	HYPERKALAEMIA	0.5–1.5 ml	1.25–3.75 ml	1.75–5.25 ml	2.5 -7.5 ml
100 mg/ml 0.45 mEq Ca/ml	slowly	HYPOCALCAEMIA				
ATIPAMEZOLE	2.5 x medetomidine dose	ANTAGONISE ALPHA 2 AGONISTS				
5 mg/ml	5 x dexmedetomidine dose slowly					
NALOXONE	**10** (– 20) µg/kg	ANTAGONISE OPIOIDS	0.025 ml	0.06 ml	0.09 ml	0.125 ml
0.4 mg/ml	may need repeating					
FLUMAZENIL	10 µg/kg	ANTAGONISE BENZODIAZEPINES	0.1 ml	0.25 ml	0.35 ml	0.5 ml
0.1 mg/ml	may need repeating					
MANNITOL	0.25–**0.5 – 1** (–2) g/kg	CEREBRAL OEDEMA	2.5–5 ml	6.25–12.5 ml	8.75–17.5 ml	12.5–25 ml
20% = 200 mg/ml	slowly	Osmotic diuretic				
DIAZEPAM	**0.5** mg/kg	SEIZURES	0.1 ml	0.25 ml	0.35 ml	0.5 ml
5 mg/ml	**0.2** mg/kg	POST-OP RESTLESSNESS	0.04 ml	0.1 ml	0.14 ml	0.2 ml
DEXTROSE 5–50%	0.25–0.5 (– 1) g/kg	HYPOGLYCAEMIA				
50–500 mg/ml	slowly	not via peripheral vein if >10% soln				

Appendix C

Equine Emergency Drug Doses

FOR INTRAVENOUS INJECTION

DRUG	DOSE	REASON	300 kg	400 kg	500 kg	600 kg
ADRENALINE / EPINEPHRINE	**0.01**–0.1–0.2 mg/kg	CARDIAC ARREST, give IV	3+ ml	4+ ml	5+ ml	6+ ml
1 : 1000 = 1 mg/ml		asystole/fibrillation				
		ANAPHYLAXIS, give IM or IV				
ATROPINE	**0.01**–0.1 mg/kg	CARDIAC ARREST, asystole	5+ ml	6.6+ ml	8+ ml	10+ ml
0.6 mg/ml		Vagally-induced arrhythmias				
GLYCOPYRROLATE	2–10 µg/kg	CARDIAC ARREST, asystole	3+ ml	4+ ml	5+ ml	6+ ml
200 µg/ml		Vagally-induced arrhythmias				
ATIPAMEZOLE	50 (−250) µg/kg	ANTAGONISE alpha 2 agonists	3+ ml	4+ ml	5+ ml	6+ ml
5 mg/ml						
CLENBUTEROL	0.8 µg/kg	BRONCHODILATOR	8 ml	10.6 ml	13.3 ml	16 ml
30 µg/ml	SLOW i/v	pulmonary oedema, equine asthma				
	Beware sweating and tachycardia					
SALBUTAMOL	(1 -) **2** µg/kg	BRONCHODILATOR	3–6 puffs	4–8 puffs	5–10 puffs	6–12 puffs
100 µg/metered dose	aerosolised into trachea	improves V/Q matching				
NALOXONE	**10**–20 µg/kg	ANTAGONISE opioids	7.5 ml	10 ml	12.5 ml	15 ml
0.4 mg/ml						
DEXAMETHASONE	**0.1–0.2** (− 0.5) mg/kg	ALLERGIC REACTIONS/	15–30 ml	20–40 ml	25–50 ml	30–60 ml
2 mg/ml		ANAPHYLAXIS				
FUROSEMIDE	0.5–**1**–4 mg/kg	OEDEMA (diuretic)	6 ml	8 ml	10 ml	12 ml
5% = 50 mg/ml						

(Continued)

Veterinary Anaesthesia: Principles to Practice, Second Edition. Alexandra H. A. Dugdale, Georgina Beaumont, Carl Bradbrook, and Matthew Gurney.
© 2020 John Wiley & Sons Ltd. Published 2020 by John Wiley & Sons Ltd.
Companion website: www.wiley.com/go/dugdale/veterinary-anaesthesia

FOR INTRAVENOUS INJECTION

DRUG	DOSE	REASON	300 kg	400 kg	500 kg	600 kg
DIAZEPAM 5 mg/ml	0.2+ mg/kg	SEIZURES	12 ml	16 ml	20 ml	24 ml
LIDOCAINE 2% = 20 mg/ml	0.5–4 mg/kg	Ventricular arrhythmias/fibrillation	7.5–60 ml	10–80 ml	12.5–100 ml	15–120 ml

Answers to Self-test Questions

Chapter 1

1 B
2 D

Chapter 2

1 Non-technical skills are cognitive, social, and personal resource skills that complement technical skills.
2 B
3 True

Chapter 3

1 Pain is an unpleasant sensory and emotional experience associated with actual or potential tissue damage, or described in terms of such damage. Since 1996, an accompanying note has been added to this definition, which states: The inability to communicate in no way negates the possibility that an individual is experiencing pain and is in need of appropriate pain-relieving treatment. A 'working definition of animal pain', proposed by Molony and Kent (1997) following extensive work with farm species, was: 'an aversive sensory and emotional experience, representing awareness by the animal of damage to, or threat to the integrity of, its tissues … producing changes in physiology and behaviour … which help to reduce or avoid the damage, reduce the likelihood of recurrence and promote recovery'.
2 A one-off dose of analgesic/hypoalgesic given before surgery may have only a limited duration of action and may not outlast the pain and inflammation that follows surgical intervention, and therefore will not continue to pre-empt all post-operative pain. It is for this reason that analgesia should be provided before surgery and should be continued into the post-operative period for as long as the pain is likely to be present. The concept of the provision of initial pre-emptive, and then subsequent continually pre-emptive analgesia, is what is called preventive analgesia. In this case, both the establishment and the maintenance of peripheral and central sensitisation are prevented or reduced. The aim here is to provide analgesia for as long as the pet is painful.
3 Dogs with OA secondary to cruciate disease and hip dysplasia.

Chapter 4

1 D
2 C
3 A

Chapter 5

1 B
2 D
3 C
4 D

Chapter 6

Information only chapter.

Chapter 7

1 Polyethylene > Teflon > Nylon > Polyurethane
2 Careful aseptic technique
3 True

Veterinary Anaesthesia: Principles to Practice, Second Edition. Alexandra H. A. Dugdale, Georgina Beaumont, Carl Bradbrook, and Matthew Gurney.
© 2020 John Wiley & Sons Ltd. Published 2020 by John Wiley & Sons Ltd.
Companion website: www.wiley.com/go/dugdale/veterinary-anaesthesia

Chapter 8

1 MAC$_{awake}$ refers to the minimum alveolar concentration of agent at which 50% of subjects stop voluntarily responding to verbal commands (i.e. cessation of perceptive awareness) during induction of anaesthesia with that agent, or when 50% of subjects begin responding to verbal commands upon recovery from anaesthesia under that agent.
2 Desflurane > sevoflurane > isoflurane
3 B

Chapter 9

1 D
2 C

Chapter 10

1 A
2 C

Chapter 11

Information only chapter.

Chapter 12

1 B
2 Intralipid: bolus of 1.5 ml/kg over one minute, followed by a continuous infusion of 0.25–0.5 ml/kg/min (i.e. 15–30 ml/kg/h), with up to two extra 1.5 ml/kg boluses (at five minutes intervals) if required; until resolution of signs or until the maximum total dose of 12 ml/kg (for 20% lipid emulsion) has been given. Also start chest compressions and artificial ventilation as required.

Chapter 13

1 True
2 False
3 False

Chapter 14

1 B
2 C

Chapter 15

1 At least two
2 Internal abdominal oblique and transversus abdominis muscles
3 Epidural morphine, intercostal and interpleural local anaesthesia and systemic NSAID (±paracetamol), and opioid (being aware of respiratory depression); also contemplate continuous infusions of lidocaine, ketamine, and opioid, if required.

Chapter 16

1 D
2 Deep facial vein

Chapter 17

1 C
2
Various observations related to muscle activity/strength returning:

- spontaneous ventilatory efforts (curare clefts; qualitative)
- increase in compliance (quantitative)
- measurement of spontaneous tidal volume (quantitative)
- monitoring of spontaneous breath PETCO$_2$/arterial blood gases (qualitative and quantitative);
- jaw tone (qualitative)
- limb tone and reflexes (qualitative)
- ocular position and reflexes (qualitative)

Qualitative or quantitative interpretations of muscle response (usually a twitch) to electrical stimulation of a motor nerve:

- visual or tactile (qualitative) assessment of motor response (twitch) to, e.g. train-of-four or double-burst stimulation
- audible response of muscles following electrical nerve stimulation (phonomyography; can be qualitative or quantitative)
- electromyography (can be qualitative or quantitative measurement of electrical response of muscle to motor nerve stimulation)
- mechanomyography (quantitative assessment of velocity of twitch motor response to nerve stimulation)
- acceleromyography (quantitative assessment of acceleration of twitch motor response to nerve stimulation, e.g. twitch, e.g. TOF ratio)
- kinemyography (quantitative assessment of the deformation of a piezo-electric mechanosensor caused by the motor response [e.g. twitch]) to motor nerve stimulation

Chapter 18

1 Now that the pressure transducer lies 30 cm above the original site at which it was zeroed to atmospheric pressure, blood pressure will under read by the equivalent of 30 cmH$_2$O, which is (30×0.74) mmHg, i.e. 22.2 mmHg. Therefore, the MAP will now read about 48 mmHg

2
Advantages

- Non-invasive and continuous.
- Can reduce the frequency for arterial blood gas analysis.
- Real-time signal with mainstream analysers.
- Breathing rate also displayed by most modern machines.
- Many machines will also give values of inspired and expired O$_2$ tensions (called oxygraphy), which is useful when using low flow anaesthesia, medical air, or nitrous oxide, where there is always the danger of delivering a hypoxic mixture of gases to your patient.
- Some machines may also display information about the inhaled anaesthetic agent in use, e.g. its inspired concentration, its end tidal concentration, and the multiple of that agent's MAC value being administered to the patient (also warnings can be given when you are potentially delivering very high anaesthetic agent concentrations).

Disadvantages

- Sampling delay with sidestream analysers means that displayed data are slightly historical.
- Sidestream sampling can remove a significant volume of gases from the anaesthetic breathing system. These may be scavenged, but, if low flow techniques are used, it is preferable to return them to the breathing system at a site distant to the gas sampling site.
- Sidestream analysers, in particular, can be inaccurate when high sampling rates (around 200 ml/min) are used for small patients with small tidal volumes, yet high respiratory frequencies (leading to dilution of sampled gases by 'fresh gases'). Although trends are generally reliable, occasional arterial blood gas analyses may be helpful if the sampling rate cannot be reduced (e.g. to 50 ml/min).
- Occasionally, respiratory secretions may block sidestream sampling lines or obscure mainstream sampling adapter 'windows'.
- Nitrous oxide and oxygen can interfere with carbon dioxide measurement (through 'collision-broadening'), although most modern analysers are less affected.
- For sidestream analysers, sampling lines must be impermeable to CO$_2$ (e.g. Teflon).

- Water traps or special water-permeable sampling line (e.g. Nafion™ tubing) must be used with sidestream analysers.
- Machines need to be re-calibrated from time to time (e.g. every three months).
- Can be expensive. The adapters and sensors of earlier mainstream analysers tended to be prone to damage, but newer versions are more robust, reducing the need for frequent repair or replacement. Furthermore, cheaper single-use mainstream sampling adapters are now available, eliminating the costs of re-sterilisation.
- Beware addition of apparatus dead space to the anaesthetic breathing system, with both sidestream and mainstream analysers, although low dead space adapters are now available for both.
- Beware 'drag' on the anaesthetic breathing system by mainstream analysers, although modern adapters and sensors are much less bulky than earlier versions.

3 C

Chapter 19

Information only chapter.

Chapter 20

1 Radiation, convection, evaporation, conduction
2 Less than 1 °C/h; and preferably 0.25–0.5 °C/ h
3
These include:

- Cardiovascular depression, including hypotension (impaired baroreceptor reflexes), bradycardia/arrhythmias (unresponsive to anticholinergics). Overall reduced cardiac output (can lead to metabolic acidosis), and increased myocardial work (due to increased blood viscosity). Extreme hypothermia can result in ventricular fibrillation
- Hypoventilation due to impaired chemoreceptor reflexes (can lead to respiratory acidosis)
- Left shift of Hb/O$_2$ dissociation curve reduces tissue oxygen delivery (and potentially leads to lactic acidosis), but tissue oxygen demand also reduced
- Hypocoagulation
- Reduced respiratory mucociliary escalator activity, may predispose to accumulation of secretions and infection
- Reduction in anaesthetic requirements (may lead to inadvertent overdose)

- Immunodepression may enhance tumour metastasis, and at one time was thought to possibly delay would healing
- Hypothermia increases post-op shivering, which can be uncomfortable for the patient and also dramatically increases its oxygen requirement at a time when oxygen is usually not supplemented

Chapter 21

1 pH is $\log_{10}$ of the inverse of the hydrogen ion concentration (or negative $\log_{10}$ of H^+ concentration).
2 Defined as pNw, it is the pH of pure water at acid–base neutrality (which is defined as when $[H^+] = [OH^-]$, but pure water always dissociates to give equal concentrations of these ions!). Importantly, however, the degree of ionisation of water varies with temperature (it increases as temperature increases), and so pNw is near 7.0 at 25 °C, but is near 6.8 at 37 °C.

3

In order to calculate the oxygen carriage of end capillary blood, we assume it is in perfect equilibrium with the alveolar gases, and therefore we can use P_AO_2 as a substitute for $P_{c'}O2$. P_AO_2 is calculated from the alveolar gas equation, using 0.21 as F_IO_2, 760 mmHg as P_B and assuming body temperature of 37 °C, so P_{H2O} is 47 mmHg, and guessing RQ of 0.9 (middle of range, 0.8–1.0)

$P_AO_2 = F_IO_2 (P_B - P_{H2O}) - P_ACO_2/RQ$
$P_AO_2 = 0.21 (760 - 47) - 32.8/0.9 = 149.73 - 36.44$
$PAO_2 = 113.3$ mmHg; and can guess that at this oxygen tension, Hb will be 100% saturated. Can guess that (Hb) is around 11 g/dl for end-capillary blood.
$C_{c'}O2 = (1.34 \times 11 \times 1.0) + (113.3 \times 0.003) = 14.74 + 0.34 = 15.08$ ml/dl
$C_aO2 = (1.34 \times 11.2 \times 0.955) + (78.3 \times 0.003) = 14.3 + 0.23 = 14.53$ ml/dl
We assume that jugular venous blood is 'mixed venous', almost pulmonary arterial blood, so
$C_vO2 = (1.34 \times 10.8 \times 0.646) + (32.6 \times 0.003) = 9.35 + 0.10 = 9.45$ ml/dl
Shunt fraction = $(15.08 - 14.53)/(15.08 - 9.45) = 0.55/5.63 = 0.096$, which is 9.8%

Classify shunt: Just on border between normal (<10%) and mild.
Interventions: Hb saturation is >95%, so O_2 supplementation is not required at present. Ensure cat is in sternal recumbency, monitor for hypoxia and initiate O_2 supplementation if clinically indicated (F_IO_2 0.3 will correct hypoxia caused by mildly increased intrapulmonary shunt).

Chapter 22

1 Type A (inadequate tissue O_2 delivery [absolute or relative]); type B (problems with metabolism/mitochondrial oxygen utilisation [no overt tissue hypoxia]); type B1 (underlying disease); type B2 (toxins/drugs); type B3 (inborn errors of metabolism and mitochondrial dysfunction)
2 Return to [normal] within 12 hours and reduce by 50% every 1–2 hours until normal.
3 Increase by >3.3 mmol/l in the first 48 hours of hospitalisation.
4 0.5–1.2 mmol/l in the first hour and thereafter, 0.2–0.5 mmol/l/h (for at least eight hours)

Chapter 23

1 The EG plays important roles in regulation of transvascular fluid exchange, maintaining vascular homeostasis (vascular tone and permeability, and also blood clotting) and forming an important non-circulating part of the intravascular 'volume'.
2 Synthetic colloids have been associated with several problems: potential intravascular volume-overload (haemodilution and its consequences, tissue oedema, etc.), coagulopathies, acute kidney injury (various mechanisms), pruritus, tissue accumulation (with possible dysfunction/failure; especially starches), and also allergic reactions/anaphylaxis. Hyperglycaemia may occur with dextran administration.

Chapter 24

1

- Increased administration (iatrogenic)
- Reduced excretion (uro-abdomen, Addison's disease)
- Redistribution (acidosis, diabetes mellitus, hyperkalaemic periodic paralysis)
- Sample error (wrong anticoagulant)

2 Calcium if life-threatening cardiac arrhythmias. Dilution (IV fluids)/diuresis (furosemide). Glucose ± insulin. Correct acidosis (bicarbonate may be useful for some forms of metabolic acidosis). Beta 2 agonists. Mineralocorticoids have also been suggested, but require further evaluation. Haemodialysis/peritoneal dialysis. Ion-exchange resins. Treat the underlying cause.

Chapter 25

Information only chapter.

Chapter 26

1

Shock is defined as the clinical state due to inadequate cellular energy production. Main types are:

I) Hypovloaemic
II) Distributive/vasculogenic (includes anaphylactic, neurogenic, etc.)
III) Obstructive
IV) Cardiogenic
V) Metabolic/endocrine/hypoxaemic

2 Initiation, amplification, propagation
3 True

Chapter 27

Information only chapter.

Chapter 28

1 True, False, False, True
2 True, False, True, True

Chapter 29

Information only chapter.

Chapter 30

1 False; both detomidine and romifidine, but not xylazine, were shown to delay the return of swallowing.
2 True, True, True, True, True, False, False

Chapter 31

Information only chapter.

Chapter 32

1 Donkeys have a relatively large head, but disproportionately small trachea, so it can be deceiving with regard to ETT size. The angle of opening of the glottis from the pharynx is more acute than in horses; and the epiglottis is softer and easier to displace, so it may possibly retrovert more easily, obstructing passage of the tube into the trachea. Donkeys have a relatively deep pharyngeal recess, in which the tube tip may get 'stuck'. If nasopharyngeal intubation is contemplated, their ventral nasal meatus is relatively narrow, so small tubes are required.
2 True
3 False

Chapter 33

1 True, True, False, True
2 C

Chapter 34

1 20 (17.5–22) mmHg

Chapter 35

1 Pigs have a relatively narrow glottis and trachea for their size. Even proximal to the larynx, their long soft palate, excessive pharyngeal tissues, relatively large tongue, and narrow jaw-opening can make visualisation of the larynx difficult. The larynx presents a 'U' bend between the glottis and trachea, and the arytenoids are chunky with bipartite vocal folds that also may make tube passage tricky. The larynx itself contains a long, downwards-sloping thyroid cartilage and a long thyrocricoid ligament, ventrally. There is also a laryngeal recess between the base of the epiglottis and the thyroid cartilage, and a pharyngeal recess above the larynx, both of which may obstruct tube placement into the airway. They have an eparterial (tracheal) bronchus, which is easy to bypass or block (or even place a tube into) due to their short neck/trachea, and a delicate carina, so care is required if using 'sharp' intubating stylettes. Finally, their sharp teeth can damage ET tubes and their cuffs.
2 Mannitol

Chapter 36

1 Lack of familiarity/expertise, underlying disease (esp. respiratory), size (problems with IV access, prone to hypothermia; also potential problems with giving tiny drug volumes, leading to possible overdose), problems with tracheal intubation, prone to GI ileus, easy to stress and may be hard to minimise stress, pain difficult to recognise/manage.

2 Analgesia, minimal stress, minimal interruption in food/water intake; prophylactic motility enhancing drugs – ranitidine or metoclopramide.

Chapter 37

1 Closing capacity is the sum of the residual volume and the closing volume; it is the lung volume at/below which alveoli and small airways begin to close. In neonates, the closing capacity is only slightly less than the FRC (i.e. the FRC is relatively low and CC relatively high), and any factors that further reduce FRC, therefore facilitate atelectasis.

2 Pethidine is more vagolytic than other opioids and is suggested not to lower the heart rate (neonatal cardiac output is highly dependent upon heart rate). Histamine release may still occur following IM administration (it must not be given IV), and hypotension can follow; in the neonate, the baroreflex response to hypotension (i.e. tachycardia) is less well-honed, so that hypotension may be a problem. Also, pethidine stings upon IM injection and it has a short duration of action, so frequent dosing is required, which is unpleasant for the patient.

3 C

4 Hypothermia, hypoglycaemia, bradycardia, hypotension, patient size (IV access, intubation, etc.)

Chapter 38

1 True
2 True
3 Ageing patients tend to lose muscle mass, yet deposit white adipose tissue; this reduces the total body water content and can affect the various pharmacokinetic 'compartments' for drug re/distribution.

Chapter 39

1 False; progesterone reduces sensitivity to catecholamines
2 D

Chapter 40

1 True
2 BCS 9/9 is four points over the optimum 5/9; and each point represents a 10% increase in body mass; so Ideal Body Mass = 40/1.4 = 28.5 kg

Chapter 41

1 A
2 Signalment, co-morbidities, attention to pain, small size (prone to hypothermia especially with increased risk of wetting if using water-cooled drills, etc.), care with local anaesthetic doses (small size and feline) but perform blocks where possible – and consider multimodal analgesia (NSAID may be withheld until recovering from GA); beware mouth gags (avoid excessively wide jaw-opening); cuffed ET tube, or good throat protection likely required, but beware cuffed ET tubes and tracheal rupture, especially if multiple position changes during procedure/dental radiography; ensure removal of any throat packs used before recovery from anaesthesia; if likely to be anorexic post-op, consider feeding tube (especially if obese cats, which are prone to hepatic lipidosis). If air drills are used without water-cooling, beware thermal injury to tissues and also venous air emboli.

Chapter 42

1 Trigeminal (V)
2 C
3 Good analgesia, based on full mu agonist opioid. Appropriate sedation to allow calm placement of IV access and induction of anaesthesia and intubation. Topical local anaesthesia on the cornea. Gentle globe manipulation, if necessary, for positioning. NSAIDs at appropriate time and post-operatively.

Chapter 43

1

'High' opioid epidural; beware local anaesthetics at this level.

Intercostal nerve block with long-acting local anaesthetic.

Interpleural local anaesthetic – repeated post-op (or, depending on the case, may be able to be provided by continuous infusion post-op).

If no contra-indications, systemic analgesics including opioid, NSAID, lidocaine, potentially also ketamine and an α2 agonist – all of which besides the NSAID can also be given as infusions. In dogs, paracetamol can also be administered.

Slow-release formulations of bupivacaine might be infiltrated into the incision site, but are not currently widely available and require further evaluation.

2

- Flood or submerge the site with sterile saline; try to occlude the offending vessel.

- Lower the surgical site to below the heart if possible.
- Occlude both jugular veins if head/neck surgery.
- Rapid IV fluids to help increase CVP.
- Positive pressure ventilation to help increase CVP.
- Stop N_2O administration.

Chapter 44

1 C
2 B

Chapter 45

1 C
2 B

Chapter 46

1

Haemorrhage
Intra-op thyroid storm
Hypoparathyroidism (hypocalcaemia) post-op
Tracheomalacia
Post-op tissue swelling may compromise breathing/swallowing
Chronic renal failure may become apparent

2

Hyperglycaemia, hypoglycaemia probably less common because of stress response, but can happen. Hypotension.

Attention to feeding times/usual insulin dosing – try not to disrupt these.

Monitor glucose regularly throughout whole peri-anaesthetic period.

Before premedication: If pre-operative glucose <4.5 mmol/l (after food withheld): give no insulin yet; if glucose 4.5–8 mmol/l: give a quarter of the morning's insulin dose; if glucose >8–15 mmol/l, give a half of the morning's insulin dose; if glucose >15 mmol/l, give the whole morning's insulin dose.

Intra-op hypoglycaemia: if blood glucose is <4 mmol/l, a slow IV bolus (0.25–1 g/kg) of glucose may be required, followed by infusion of balanced crystalloid fluids containing 5% dextrose; if blood glucose concentration measures 4–8 mmol/l, balanced crystalloid fluids with 5% dextrose should be sufficient; if blood glucose is >8 mmol/l, balanced crystalloid fluids with 2.5% dextrose may be appropriate; if blood glucose exceeds 15 mmol/l, balanced crystalloid fluids without glucose may be most appropriate.

Intra-op hyperglycaemia: if blood glucose exceeds 15–20 mmol/l, and especially once >30 mmol/l, treatment may be warranted with soluble insulin (0.05–0.1 U/kg IM or SQ; or 0.05–0.1 U/kg IV, possibly followed by infusion 0.01–0.1 U/kg/h IV).

For hypotension, check anaesthetic depth, beware excessive PIP if artificial ventilation is employed. Good analgesia provision, including local/regional techniques where applicable, may help keep anaesthesia at relatively light level. Fluid boluses may be indicated, but beware if spiked with glucose; positive inotropes and vasopressors may be required.

3 Generalized muscle weakness may mean artificial ventilation is required to support ventilation. Tend to have expanded ECF volume (despite being PU/PD), which can alter drug pharmacokinetics; animals may be hypertensive. Prone to thrombo-embolic complications. Prone to poor wound healing and surgical site infections.

Chapter 47

1 True
2 B

Chapter 48

1 C
2 Minimise inotropic changes; maintain HR as near normal as possible; slight reduction in systemic vascular (and pulmonary vascular) resistance might be beneficial; maintain preload; keep stress to a minimum; artificial ventilation may be helpful if early pulmonary oedema present

Chapter 49

1 Upper airway obstruction due to poor conformation (stenotic nares, tortuous nasal passages [aberrant turbinates], excessive/redundant pharyngeal tissue, over-long/fleshy soft palate, macroglossia, hypoplastic trachea) leads to generation of excessive negative airway and intrathoracic pressures. These not only serve to further collapse the pharyngeal area, exacerbating the upper respiratory tract obstruction, but can also lead to laryngeal saccule eversion and laryngeal collapse, even further exacerbating the obstruction. Chronic alveolar hypoxia stimulates chronic hypoxic pulmonary vasoconstriction, which results in pulmonary hypertension and eventual cor pulmonale (right heart failure). Large negative intra-thoracic pressures

may also be to blame for a predisposition to gastric reflux/regurgitation and the development of hiatal hernias, which further predispose to gastric reflux and regurgitation. Reflux/regurgitation make patients susceptible to aspiration pneumonia, further compromising their respiratory status. Patients also struggle with the demands of exercise and hot weather as they cannot pant effectively.

2 If possible, ascertain whether the dog is already a regurgitator, and if so, put on anti-emetics or pro-motility agents and gastro-protectants for a few days before planned surgery. On the day of surgery, minimise handling stress and heat stress, but do not leave unobserved at any time. Premedication to relieve anxiety might be with opioid (also anti-tussive, possibly useful post-op) and low dose acepromazine ($\alpha2$ agonists may compromise assessment of laryngeal function, although very low doses may be considered). Further doses of gastro-protectants and anti-emetics or pro-motility drugs may be considered at this time. Try to ensure IV access gained before induction of anaesthesia. Pre-oxygenate before anaesthetic induction, if possible, to help increase time available for tracheal intubation and to allow for surgeon evaluation of upper airway. Ensure range of small cuffed ET tube sizes available, laryngoscope and bougie. Induction with injectable agents – but not always slowly to effect (i.e. depends upon how well the dog is oxygenating; if in trouble, more rapid injection may be required). Use agents that are rapidly metabolised like propofol or alfaxalone. Once trachea is safely intubated (cuffed ET tube), be vigilant for regurgitation. Chest radiographs might be prudent at this time. Vigilant eye care is also necessary. For maintenance, use agents that are not cumulative; usually inhalants. When the time comes for tracheal extubation, leave the IV catheter in until the dog is fully recovered; many brachycephalic dogs tolerate relatively late tracheal extubation. Ensure the environment is calm and not too hot. Prop into sternal recumbency and have further small ET tubes, laryngoscope, bougie, and injectable anaesthetic agent to hand, and even tracheostomy tube and surgical kit, in case of problems. (A small dose of lidocaine IV just before tracheal extubation might decrease the coughing response with tube manipulation.) Good analgesia helps reduce patient distress and attempts to pant. Consider topical nasal decongestants before tracheal extubation to improve nasal airways. Post-extubation, minor degrees of obstruction can be countered by sternal recumbency, head extended forwards, the mouth propped open and tongue pulled out. Oxygen supplementation may help, but may not always be well-tolerated. Nebulised epinephrine may also help. Corticosteroids may be considered (beware if NSAIDs already given).

Chapter 50

1 True
2 Hypoxaemia is abnormally low oxygenation of the blood (defined as $PaO_2 < 90\,mmHg$, when breathing room air or indeed when supplemental oxygen is provided); hypoxia is abnormally low tissue oxygenation.
3 Face mask, flow-by, nasal prongs (including HFOT), nasopharyngeal catheter, some sort of oxygen hood or cage/tent (E-collar-based to proper climate controlled cage); or via trachea more directly, either via ET tube or supraglottic airway device or trans-tracheal (e.g. needle tracheotomy or tracheotomy tube).

Chapter 51

1 Capnography
2 True
3 Poorer, long-term myocardial and neurological outcomes
4 Dorsal, if stable enough

Index

Note: Page numbers in *italic* refer to figures and **bold** refer to tables.

Veterinary Anaesthesia: Principles to Practice, Second Edition. Alexandra H. A. Dugdale, Georgina Beaumont, Carl Bradbrook, and Matthew Gurney.
© 2020 John Wiley & Sons Ltd. Published 2020 by John Wiley & Sons Ltd.
Companion website: www.wiley.com/go/dugdale/veterinary-anaesthesia